Cowell and Tyler's

DIAGNOSTIC CYTOLOGY AND HEMATOLOGY OF THE DOG AND CAT

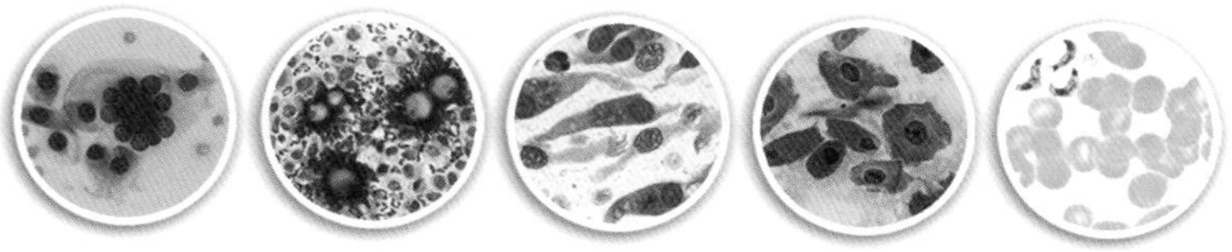

FOURTH EDITION

Cowell and Tyler's

DIAGNOSTIC CYTOLOGY AND HEMATOLOGY OF THE DOG AND CAT

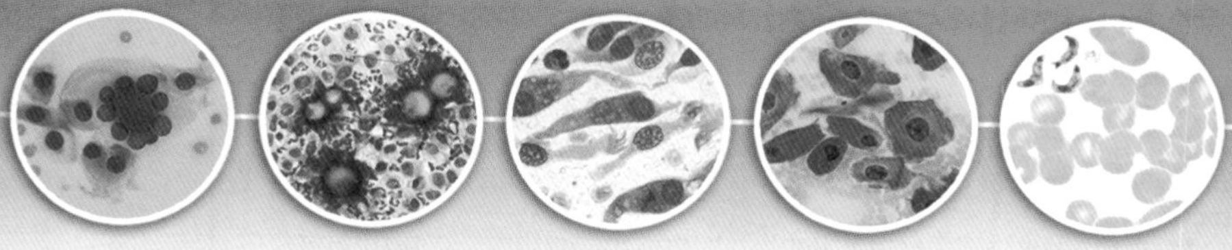

Amy C. Valenciano, DVM, MS, DACVP
Veterinary Clinical Pathologist
IDEXX Laboratories, Inc.
Dallas, Texas

Rick L. Cowell, DVM, MS, MRCVS, DACVP
Clinical Pathologist
IDEXX Laboratories, Inc.
Stillwater, Oklahoma

ELSEVIER

ELSEVIER
MOSBY

3251 Riverport Lane
St. Louis, MO 63043

COWELL AND TYLER'S DIAGNOSTIC CYTOLOGY AND HEMATOLOGY OF THE DOG AND CAT, FOURTH EDITION

ISBN: 978-0-323-08707-0

ISBN: 978-0-323-08707-0

Vice President and Publisher: Linda Duncan
Content Strategy Director: Penny Rudolph
Content Development Specialist: Brandi Graham
Publishing Services Manager: Catherine Jackson
Senior Project Manager: Sara Alsup
Designer: Jessica Williams

Printed in China

Last digit is the print number: 9 8 7 6 5 4 3 2 1

CONTRIBUTORS

Robin W. Allison, DVM, PhD, DACVP
Associate Professor
Department of Veterinary Pathobiology
Center for Veterinary Health Sciences
Oklahoma State University
Stillwater, Oklahoma
Subcutaneous Glandular Tissue: Mammary, Salivary, Thyroid, and Parathyroid
Vaginal Cytology

Tara P. Arndt, DVM, Cert LAM, DLAS (Path), DACVP
Staff Pathologist, Health & Life Sciences
Battelle Memorial Institute
Columbus, Ohio
Selected Infectious Agents
Nasal Exudates and Masses
Effusions: Abdominal, Thoracic, and Pericardial
The Liver

Anne M. Barger, DVM, MS, DACVP
Clinical Associate Professor
Department of Pathobiology
College of Veterinary Medicine University of Illinois
Urbana, Illinois
Immunocytochemistry

Deborah C. Bernreuter, DVM, MS
Veterinary Clinical Pathologist
IDEXX Laboratories, Inc.
Irvine, California
Oropharynx and Tonsils

Dori L. Borjesson, DVM, PhD, DACVP
Professor
Department of Pathology, Microbiology, and Immunology
School of Veterinary Medicine
University of California
Davis, California
The Pancreas

Seth E. Chapman, DVM, MS, DACVP
Veterinary Clinical Pathologist
IDEXX Laboratories, Inc.
Worthington, Ohio
Flow Cytometry

Jennifer R. Cook, DVM
Assistant Lecturer
Department of Veterinary Pathobiology
College of Veterinary Medicine and Biomedical Sciences
Texas A&M
University College Station, Texas
Cerebrospinal Fluid and Central Nervous System Cytology

Stephanie C. Corn, DVM, DACVP
Veterinary Clinical Pathologist
IDEXX Laboratories, Inc.
Worthington, Ohio
Flow Cytometry

Dean Cornwell, DVM, PhD
Regional Head
Department of Clinical Pathology
IDEXX Laboratories, Inc.
Dallas, Texas
Special Tests: Polymerase Chain Reaction and Lymphosarcoma

Rick L. Cowell, DVM, MS, MRCVS, DACVP
Clinical Pathologist
IDEXX Laboratories, Inc.
Stillwater, Oklahoma
Sample Collection and Preparation
Cell Types and Criteria of Malignancy
Selected Infectious Agents
Transtracheal and Bronchoalveolar Washes
The Kidneys
The Bone Marrow

Heather L. Deheer, DVM, DACVP
Clinical Pathologist
Antech Diagnostics
Newark, Delaware
Adjunct Assistant Professor
Department of Pathobiology
School of Veterinary Medicine
University of Pennsylvania
Philadelphia, Pennsylvania
The External Ear Canal

Dennis B. DeNicola, DVM, PhD, DACVP
Clinical Pathologist
Chief Veterinary Educator
IDEXX Laboratories, Inc.
Westbrook, Maine
Round Cells

Kate English, BSc, BVetMed, FRCPath, MRCVS
Lecturer, Veterinary Clinical Pathology
Department of Pathology and Pathogen Biology
Royal Veterinary College
North Mymms
Hatfield, Hertfordshire, United Kingdom
Transtracheal and Bronchoalveolar Washes

Patty J. Ewing, DVM, MS, DACVP
Director, Clinical Laboratory
Department of Pathology
Angell Animal Medical Center
Boston, Massachusetts
The Kidneys

Peter J. Fernandes, DVM, DACVP
Veterinary Clinical Pathologist
IDEXX Laboratories, Inc.
Irvine, California
Synovial Fluid Analysis

Susan E. Fielder, DVM, MS, DACVP
Clinical Pathologist
Texas A&M Veterinary Medical Diagnostic Laboratory
College Station, Texas
The Musculoskeletal System

David J. Fisher, DVM, DACVP
Veterinary Clinical Pathologist
IDEXX Laboratories, Inc.
West Sacramento, California
Cutaneous and Subcutaneous Lesions

Michael M. Fry, DVM, MS, DACVP
Associate Professor
Department of Biomedical and Diagnostic Sciences
College of Veterinary Medicine
University of Tennessee
Knoxville, Tennessee
The Lung and Intrathoracic Structures

Carolyn N. Grimes, DVM, DACVP
Professeure Adjointe
Département de Pathologie et Microbiologie
Faculté de Médecine Vétérinaire
Université de Montréal
St-Hyacinthe, Québec, Canada
The Lung and Intrathoracic Structures

Carol B. Grindem, DVM, PhD, DACVP
Professor, Clinical Pathology
Department of Population Health and Pathobiology
College of Veterinary Medicine North Carolina State University
Raleigh, North Carolina
The Bone Marrow

Jamie L. Haddad, VMD, DACVP (Anatomic and Clinical)
Veterinary Anatomic and Clinical Pathologist
Animal Medical Center
IDEXX Laboratories, Inc.
New York, New York
The Gastrointestinal Tract
The Bone Marrow

Gary J. Haldorson, DVM, PhD, DACVP
Assistant Professor
Department of Veterinary Microbiology and Pathology College of Veterinary Medicine
Washington State University
Pullman, Washington
The Adrenal Gland

Silke Hecht, DVM, DACVR, DECVDI
Associate Professor, Radiology
Department of Small Animal Clinical Sciences
College of Veterinary Medicine
University of Tennessee
Knoxville, Tennessee
The Lung and Intrathoracic Structures

Casey J. LeBlanc, DVM, PhD, DACVP
Associate Professor, Clinical Pathology
Department of Biomedical and Diagnostic Sciences
College of Veterinary Medicine
University of Tennessee
Knoxville, Tennessee
The Lung and Intrathoracic Structures

Christian M. Leutenegger, DVM, PhD, FVH
Regional Head of Molecular Diagnostics
IDEXX Laboratories, Inc.
Sacramento, California
Molecular Methods in Lymphoid Malignancies

Gwendolyn J. Levine, BS, DVM, DACVP
Clinical Assistant Professor
Department of Veterinary Pathobiology
College of Veterinary Medicine and Biomedical Sciences
Texas A&M University
College Station, Texas
Cerebrospinal Fluid and Central Nervous System Cytology

Peter S. MacWilliams, DVM, PhD, DACVP
Chief of Staff, Diagnostic Services
Professor of Clinical Pathology
Department of Pathobiological Sciences
School of Veterinary Medicine
University of Wisconsin
Madison, Wisconsin
The Spleen

Patricia M. McManus, VMD, PhD, DACVP
Veterinary Clinical Pathologist
IDEXX Laboratories, Inc.
Portland, Oregon
The Spleen

James H. Meinkoth, DVM, PhD, DACVP
Professor
Department of Veterinary Pathobiology
College of Veterinary Medicine
Oklahoma State University
Stillwater, Oklahoma
Sample Collection and Preparation
Cell Types and Criteria of Malignancy
Transtracheal and Bronchoalveolar Washes
The Kidneys

Joanne B. Messick, VMD, PhD, DACVP
Associate Professor
Department of Comparative Pathobiology
College of Veterinary Medicine
Purdue University
West Lafayette, Indiana
The Lymph Nodes

Rebecca J. Morton, BS, MS, DVM, PhD
Professor Emerita
Department of Veterinary Pathobiology
Center for Veterinary Health Sciences
Stillwater, Oklahoma
Sample Collection and Preparation

Mary B. Nabity, DVM, PhD, DACVP
Assistant Professor
Department of Veterinary Pathobiology
College of Veterinary Medicine and Biomedical Sciences
Texas A&M University
College Station, Texas
The Male Reproductive Tract: Prostrate, Testes, Penis, and Semen

Jennifer A. Neel, DVM, DACVP
Associate Professor
Department of Population Health and Pathobiology
College of Veterinary Medicine
North Carolina State University
Raleigh, North Carolina
The Gastrointestinal Tract

Reema T. Patel, DVM, DACVP
Clinical Pathologist
Department of Pathobiology
School of Veterinary Medicine
University of Pennsylvania
Philadelphia, Pennsylvania
The External Ear Canal

Emily M. Pieczarka, DVM, MS
Resident
Department of Veterinary Biosciences
The Ohio State University
Columbus, Ohio
Flow Cytometry

Brian F. Porter, DVM, DACVP
Clinical Associate Professor
Department of Veterinary Pathobiology
College of Veterinary Medicine & Biomedical Sciences
Texas A&M University
College Station, Texas
Cerebrospinal Fluid Analysis

Theresa E. Rizzi, DVM, DACVP
Clinical Associate Professor
Department of Veterinary Pathobiology
Center for Veterinary Health Sciences
Oklahoma State University
Stillwater, Oklahoma
Effusions: Abdominal, Thoracic, and Pericardial

Sonjia M. Shelly, DVM, DACVP
Clinical Pathologist
VDx; Veterinary Diagnostics
Davis, California
The Liver

Devorah A. Marks Stowe, DVM
Lecturer, Clinical Pathology
Department of Population Health and Pathobiology
College of Veterinary Medicine North Carolina State University
Raleigh, North Carolina
The Gastrointestinal Tract

Ronald D. Tyler, DVM, PhD, DACVP, DABT
Adjunct Professor
Department of Anatomy, Pathology, and Pharmacology
College of Veterinary Medicine
Oklahoma State University
Stillwater, Oklahoma
Sample Collection and Preparation
Cell Types and Criteria of Malignancy
Transtracheal and Bronchoalveolar Washes
The Kidneys
The Bone Marrow

Amy C. Valenciano, DVM, MS, DACVP
Veterinary Clinical Pathologist
IDEXX Laboratories, Inc.
Dallas, Texas
Effusions: Abdominal, Thoracic, and Pericardial

Sabrina Vobornik, DVM
Resident, Clinical Pathology
Department of Veterinary Pathobiology
College of Veterinary Medicine & Biomedical Sciences
Texas A&M University
College Station, Texas
The Male Reproductive Tract: Prostate, Testes, Penis, and Semen

Dana B. Walker, DVM, MS, PhD, DACVP
Team Lead
Global Pharmacovigilence and Epidemiology
Bristol-Myers Squibb
Wallingford, Connecticut
Peripheral Blood Smears

Koranda A. Wallace, VMD
Resident, Clinical Pathology
Department of Pathobiology
School of Veterinary Medicine
University of Pennsylvania
Philadelphia, Pennsylvania
The External Ear Canal

Heather L. Wamsley, DVM, PhD, DACVP
Assistant Professor
Department of Physiological Sciences
College of Veterinary Medicine
University of Florida
Gainesville, Florida
Examination of Urinary Sediment

Tamara B. Wills, DVM, MS, DACVP
Regional Head of Clinical Pathology
IDEXX Laboratories, Inc.
Pullman, Washington
The Adrenal Gland

Karen M. Young, VMD, PhD
Clinical Professor and Chief of Diagnostic Services
Department of Pathobiological Sciences
School of Veterinary Medicine University of Wisconsin
Madison, Wisconsin
Eyes and Associated Structures

Shanon M. Zabolotzky, DVM, DACVP
Veterinary Clinical Pathologist
IDEXX Laboratories, Inc.
West Sacramento, California
Peripheral Blood Smears

PREFACE

Cytologic evaluation of blood, fluid, and tissue specimens is an especially valuable diagnostic aid in veterinary medicine. Reliable, confident interpretation of carefully obtained, well-preserved, representative cellular samples is essential for accurate diagnosis, prognosis, and treatment. *Diagnostic Cytology and Hematology of the Dog and Cat,* fourth edition, is a comprehensive yet practical reference designed to help the reader develop and enhance the necessary clinical laboratory and interpretive skills for a wide variety of pathologic conditions seen in everyday practice, along with those less frequently encountered.

The goal of this reference text is to provide small-animal veterinary clinicians and cytology students with the knowledge and skills required to apply cytodiagnostic techniques to sample collection, preparation, microscopic assessment, and interpretation. It is intended to be a familiar and trusted bench-top reference and guide alongside the microscope. The numerous tables and flowcharts that accompany the text assist the reader in both the development of a cytologic opinion and in correlation of the cytologic findings with clinical signs and history, physical examination, diagnostic imaging, and other clinical laboratory findings to achieve the most accurate and specific diagnosis possible, while being rapid and efficient.

Written in a logical, highly visual manner, we believe we have provided a resource that will establish and maintain a secure clinical foundation for the technical as well as interpretive aspects of cytological diagnostic screening. The straightforward text is organized for quick information retrieval. Over 1000 high-resolution, full-color photomicrographs illustrate pertinent features of lesions; aid in the identification of many bacterial, fungal, and protozoal organisms and in the differentiation of normal cells from abnormal cells; and demonstrate the variability of patterns seen in certain conditions. Helpful and easy-to-follow algorithms and tables are distributed throughout the text to facilitate rapid and efficient progression through the diagnostic process. As inappropriate sample collection and poor slide preparation are often the major impediments to sample quality, we have included valuable information on collection and preparation techniques. This not only facilitates accurate on-site diagnosis but also permits the practitioner to confidently submit diagnostic-quality samples to a cytopathologist for interpretation.

The fourth edition maintains the practical diagnostic approach of its predecessors, and four new chapters—The Adrenal Gland, Immunocytochemistry, Flow Cytometry, and Molecular Methods in Lymphoid Malignancies—have been added to broaden the text's scope and to provide valuable information on important cytological diagnostic adjuncts. Many of the chapters from the previous edition have been substantially updated to include recently recognized conditions, new terminology, and new procedures. Along with numerous new photomicrographs, new to this edition, histopathology photomicrographs of both normal morphology and selected pathologic conditions have been added to enhance knowledge of tissue architecture in relation to cytology. In addition, four chapters in particular—The Spleen, The Lung and Intrathoracic Structures, The Gastrointestinal Tract, and Cerebrospinal Fluid and Central Nervous System Cytology—offer more expanded coverage and have been reorganized to integrate relevant information for better understanding.

The authors hope that you will truly find this one of the most used references in your clinical library. We also believe that, with the knowledge and skills you glean from use of this resource, you will reduce your clinical time and frustrations and, most importantly, improve the quality of care you deliver to your patients and their people.

Amy C. Valenciano
Rick L. Cowell

ACKNOWLEDGMENTS

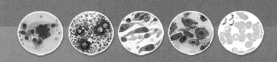

We thank our families for their support and understanding. Many other people deserve acknowledgment and sincere thanks also. These include Elsevier's excellent editors and staff and the many veterinary pathologists at IDEXX Laboratories who sent slides or pictures for use in the text, especially Drs. Dean Cornwell and Debbie Bernreuter.

It was an honor and privilege to work with each of the authors. They are exceptional veterinarians, scientists, and teachers. We thank them for sharing their time, talent, and expertise, and we thank their families for sharing them. Finally, we would like to thank IDEXX Laboratories for generously supporting veterinary education and this book in particular.

Amy C. Valenciano
Rick L. Cowell

Supported in part by IDEXX Laboratories as part of their commitment to Veterinarians, Veterinary Technicians, and Veterinary Medical Education.

IDEXX
LABORATORIES

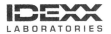

DEDICATION

To Dr. Rick Cowell, an inspiration and excellent pathologist and mentor. Thank you for sharing your projects, insights, and laughter and for entrusting to me *Diagnostic Cytology and Hematology of the Dog and Cat.* I can only hope to chase your footsteps. I dedicate my efforts to God and my family: Daniel (husband), Avery (daughter), Ty (son), Bonny (twin), and my dear parents. I thank my wonderful mentors, especially Drs. Dave Fisher, Sonjia Shelly, Carol Grindem, Jan Andrews, Mary Jo Burkhard, Gregg Dean, Christine Stanton, and Lon Rich. I also thank IDEXX Laboratories for supporting academic growth and for promoting excellence in veterinary pathology.

Amy C. Valenciano

To my parents who taught me the value of honesty and instilled in me a work ethic that has served me well through the years.

To my wife (Annette) and daughter (Anne) who have continually given support, meaning, and inspiration to my life.

To my daughter (Rebecca) who showed me the face of true courage and taught me to laugh and love even in the worst of times. While she lost her battle with cancer at the age of 11, her memories and life lessons will forever be remembered.

To the many outstanding veterinary clinical pathologists I have had the opportunity to learn from, especially Drs. Ronald D. Tyler, James Meinkoth, and Dennis DeNicola.

To the many veterinary practitioners, residents, and students who taught me much more than I could ever have hoped to teach them and have become colleagues and friends.

To IDEXX Laboratories for their continued support of veterinary education and especially to Dr. Dean Cornwell for his support and encouragement.

To Dr. Amy Valenciano for being willing to assume editorial responsibilities; I have great faith in her ability and knowledge.

Rick L. Cowell

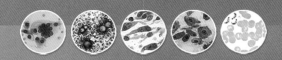

CONTENTS

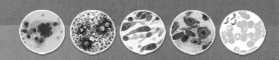

CHAPTER 1

Sample Collection and Preparation

James H. Meinkoth, Rick L. Cowell, Ronald D. Tyler and Rebecca J. Morton

Evaluation of cytologic samples has become well established as a method of obtaining a diagnosis of lesions in a wide variety of tissues. Cytology and histopathology will likely always remain complementary diagnostic procedures, reflecting a trade-off between the lower degree of invasiveness of sample collection and more rapid turnaround time with cytology and the increased amount of information available from the ability to evaluate tissue architecture with histopathology. However, the ever-increasing availability of advanced imaging techniques has resulted in an increased reliance on cytopathology to evaluate focal lesions of internal organs, which previously could not be reliably sampled. As clinicians have increased their use of this diagnostic modality and cytopathologists have become more experienced with the wider variety of lesions and tissues sampled, the spectrum of disease processes that can be identified by cytology and the reliability and precision of the diagnoses for lesions of many tissues have increased.

Other than the experience of the cytopathologist evaluating the samples, one of the major factors determining the diagnostic value of cytologic specimens is the quality of the sample. The diagnostic yield of cytology is noticeably higher in the hands of clinicians who have a great deal of experience with obtaining cytologic specimens. With histologic specimens, once the tissue sample is collected and placed in an appropriate amount of formalin, laboratory technicians handle the remainder of sample preparation. With cytology, the clinician is faced with the responsibility of not only collecting an adequately representative specimen but also preparing the slides that are to be examined and, often, staining of the slides as well. Because the cells to be examined are not grossly visible during sample collection and slide preparation, it is often difficult to tell whether an adequate specimen has been obtained at the time of the sampling procedure.

Collection and preparation of cytologic specimens is definitely a skill gained only through experience and refinement of technique based on the results obtained. Many clinicians (and owners) are understandably frustrated when a sample submitted is determined to be nondiagnostic. Fortunately, an understanding of some basic principles of sample collection and familiarity with some of the more common pitfalls related to cytologic sample preparation can increase the odds of a diagnostic result.[1-5]

METHODS OF SAMPLE COLLECTION

Several methods of collecting samples for cytologic analysis exist. The indications for each are outlined in Table 1-1.

Fine-Needle Biopsy

Fine-needle biopsy (FNB) can be performed using a standard syringe and needle with or without aspiration (as described later). This is the best overall method for sampling any cutaneous mass or proliferative lesion.[1] FNB allows collection of cells from deep within the lesion, avoiding surface contamination with inflammatory cells and organisms that often plague impression smears, swabs, or scrapings. Surface cells are often poorly preserved and may show artifacts related to cellular aging and exposure to secondary inflammation responses, especially with ulcerated masses. These changes can make evaluation of the significance of cellular atypia more difficult. A classic example of this is masses of the urinary bladder. Samples collected by traumatic catheterization often contain cells that show significant degeneration and artifact from aging and prolonged exposure to urine (Figure 1-1). Conversely, samples collected via FNB from deep within the lesion are typically well preserved and easier to evaluate (see Figure 1-1, *A*). FNB is also the only practical technique for sampling of subcutaneous or internal organs or masses.

Selection of Syringe and Needle: FNBs are collected with a 22- to 25-gauge needle and a 3- to 20-mL syringe. The softer the tissue, the smaller are the needle and syringe used. It is seldom necessary to use a needle larger than 22-gauge for aspiration, even for firm tissues. When needles larger than 22-gauge are used, tissue cores tend to be aspirated, resulting in a poor yield of free cells. Also, larger needles tend to cause greater blood contamination.

The size of syringe used is influenced by the consistency of the tissue being aspirated. Softer tissues such as lymph nodes often can be aspirated with a 3-mL syringe. Firm tissues such as fibromas and squamous-cell

TABLE 1-1

Indications for Various Methods of Sample Collection

Collection Method	Indications for Uses	Comments
Fine-needle biopsy (aspiration or non-aspiration method)	Masses (surface or internal)	Best method for cutaneous or subcutaneous masses because it avoids surface contamination
	Lymph nodes	
	Internal organs	Best method for minimally invasive sampling of internal organs or masses
	Fluid collection	
Impression smear	Exudative cutaneous lesions	Most useful for identification of infectious organisms
		May yield only surface cells and contamination (problem with ulcerated tumors)
	Preparation of cytology samples from biopsy specimens	With biopsy specimens, it is imperative to blot excess blood from sample
		Impression smears of biopsy specimens must be made before exposure of biopsy sample to formalin
Scraping	Used with flat cutaneous lesions that are not amenable to fine-needle biopsy	With dry cutaneous lesions (e.g., ringworm), it is important to scrape sufficiently to obtain some blood or serum to help cells stick to slide
	Preparation of cytology samples from poorly exfoliative biopsy specimens	
Swab		Generally used only when anatomic location not amenable to collection by other means
	Vaginal smears	
	Fistulous tracts	With fistulous tracts, most useful in classifying type of inflammatory response and identifying infectious organisms

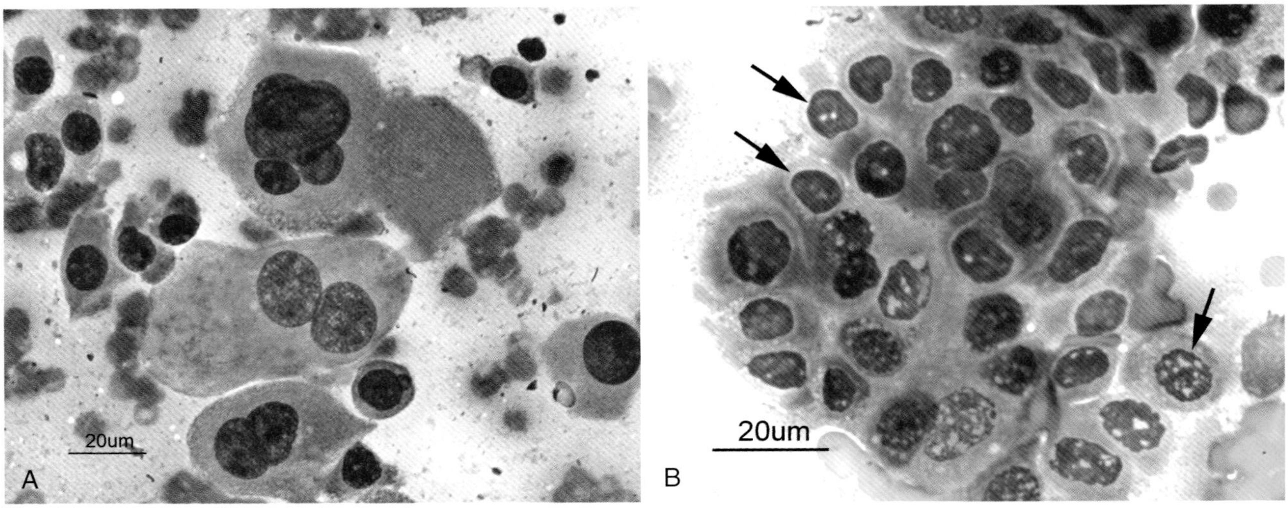

Figure 1-1 Photomicrograph of samples collected from transitional cell carcinoma. A, Sample collected by fine-needle biopsy of the mass. The cells are well preserved allowing for examination of nuclear and cytoplasmic detail. **B,** Sample collected by traumatic catheterization. These samples typically collect superficial cells that show marked changes resulting from cellular aging and exposure to urine. Nuclear degeneration is noted as a homogenous light pink-purple color as well as fragmentation with numerous clear spaces evident (*arrows*). (Courtesy Oklahoma State University Teaching Files)

carcinomas require a larger syringe to maintain adequate negative pressure (suction) for collection of a sufficient number of cells. A 12-mL syringe is a good choice if the texture of the tissue is unknown. The size of the syringe is not as critical when the samples are collected using the nonaspiration technique.

Preparation of the Site for Aspiration: If microbiologic tests are to be performed on a portion of the sample collected, or a body cavity (peritoneal and thoracic cavities, joints, etc.) is to be penetrated, the area of aspiration is surgically prepped. Otherwise, skin preparation is essentially that required for a vaccination or venipuncture. An alcohol swab can be used to clean the area. If the samples are being collected using ultrasound guidance, it is important to avoid the use of ultrasound gel, substituting alcohol as a contact agent instead. Ultrasound gel stains pink with commonly used cytology stains. Even a small amount of ultrasound gel picked up as a contaminant when the needle passes through the skin is enough to completely obscure the cells and render a slide nondiagnostic.

Aspiration Procedure: With the standard aspiration method of FNB, the mass is stabilized with one hand while the needle, with syringe attached, is introduced into the center of the mass (Figure 1-2). Strong negative pressure is applied by withdrawing the plunger to about three fourths the volume of the syringe (Figure 1-3). If the mass is sufficiently large and the patient sufficiently restrained, negative pressure can be maintained while the needle is moved back and forth repeatedly, passing through about two thirds of the diameter of the mass. With large masses, the needle can be redirected to several areas within the mass to increase the amount of tissue sampled. Alternatively, several different areas of the mass can be sampled with separate collection attempts. Care should be taken to not allow the needle to exit the mass while negative pressure is being applied because this can result in either aspiration of the sample into the barrel of the syringe (where it may not be retrievable) or contamination of the sample with tissue surrounding the mass.

The negative pressure should not be applied for more than a few seconds in any one area. Often, no material will be visible in the syringe or in the hub of the needle, even though an adequate sample has been obtained. With excessive force or prolonged application of negative pressure, disruption of blood vessels will eventually occur, and the sample will be contaminated with peripheral blood, diluting the tissue cells and rendering the sample nondiagnostic.

After several areas are sampled, the negative pressure is released, and the needle is removed from the mass and skin. The needle is removed from the syringe and air is drawn into the syringe. The needle is replaced onto the syringe and some of the tissue in the barrel and hub of the needle is expelled onto one end of a glass microscope slide by rapidly depressing the plunger. When possible, several preparations should be made, as described later in this chapter (see "Preparation of Slides").

Nonaspiration Procedure (Capillary Technique, Stab Technique): Many people prefer to collect FNB without the application of negative pressure, and this technique can yield samples of equal or better quality than those obtained with the standard aspiration technique.[4-6] The nonaspiration technique works well for most masses, especially those that are highly vascular.[1] This technique is

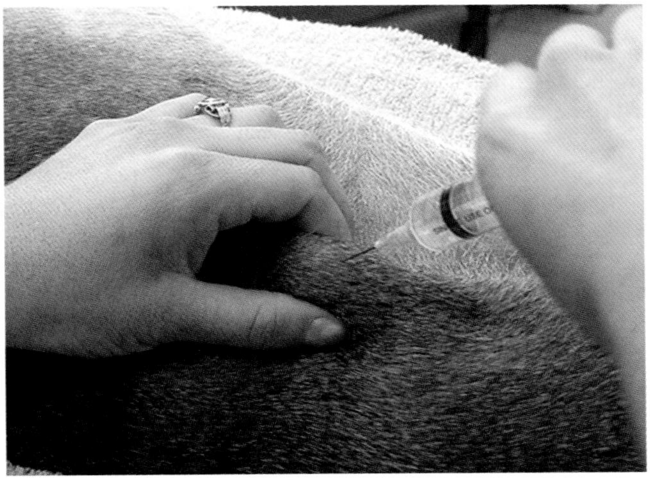

Figure 1-2 Aspiration technique of fine-needle biopsy. The mass is stabilized with one hand while the needle is introduced into the center of the mass. The hand holding the syringe is used to pull back on the plunger, creating negative pressure. (Courtesy Oklahoma State University teaching files.)

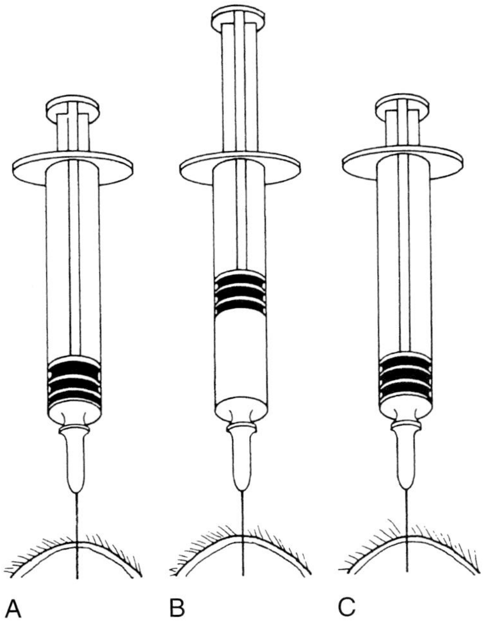

Figure 1-3 Fine-needle aspiration from a solid mass. After the needle is within the mass (*A*), negative pressure is placed on the syringe by rapidly withdrawing the plunger (*B*), usually one half to three fourths the volume of the syringe barrel. The needle is redirected several times while negative pressure is maintained, if this can be accomplished without the needle's point leaving the mass. Before the needle is removed from the mass, the plunger is released, relieving negative pressure on the syringe (*C*).

similar to the standard FNB aspiration technique, except no negative pressure is applied during collection. The procedure is performed using a small-gauge needle on a 5- to 12-mL syringe. The barrel of the syringe is filled with air prior to the collection attempt to allow rapid expulsion of material onto a glass slide. The syringe is grasped at or near the needle hub with the thumb and forefinger (much like holding a dart) to allow for maximal control (Figure 1-4). The mass to be aspirated is stabilized with a free hand, and the needle is inserted into the mass. The needle is rapidly moved back and forth in a stabbing motion in an attempt to stay along the same tract, similar to the action of a sewing machine. This allows cells to be collected by cutting and tissue pressure. Care must be taken to keep the needle tip within the mass to prevent contamination with surrounding tissue. The needle is then withdrawn and the material in the needle is rapidly expelled onto a clean glass slide, and a smear is made using one of the techniques listed later in this chapter (see "Preparation of Slides"). Having the syringe prefilled with air allows the sample to be expelled onto a slide more quickly, thereby helping to avoid desiccation (drying out) of the collected cells and coagulation of the sample.[6]

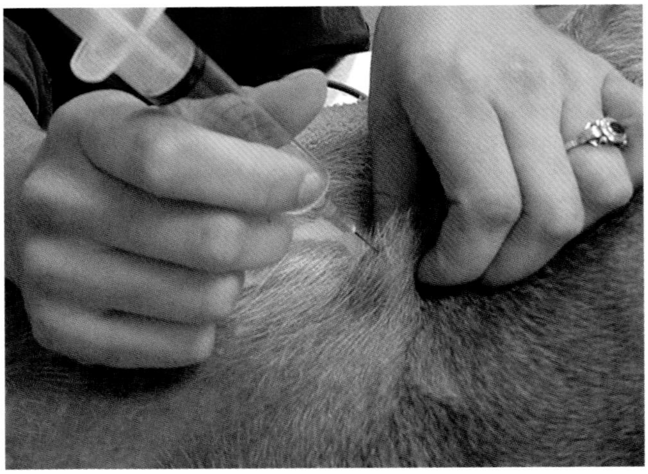

Figure 1-4 Nonaspiration technique of fine-needle biopsy. The syringe is held at or near the needle hub with the thumb and forefinger. Note that the syringe is prefilled with air. The free hand is used to stabilize the mass. This technique allows greater control over movement of the needle. (Courtesy Oklahoma State University teaching files.)

Some perform the nonaspiration technique with a needle only with no attached syringe. This may allow for even greater control of the placement and movement of the needle, although the syringe must then be attached after sample collection to expel the material from the needle. Another variation which has been recommended for ultrasound-guided collection is to have an intravenous fluid extension set placed in between the needle and the syringe.[6] This allows freedom of movement of the needle with one hand during the collection procedure. The syringe can be hung over the shoulder during collection, and then the other hand can be used to quickly expel the material onto the slide.

If possible, it is optimal to perform multiple collection attempts at various sites within the mass to increase the chance of obtaining diagnostic material and to ensure a representative sampling of the lesion.

Collection Tips

Make and Submit Multiple Slides: This is one of the most important things that can be done to increase the diagnostic yield. Small-gauge needles are used for collecting cytologic specimens, and the procedure is usually relatively painless. It takes less time to perform several collection attempts and prepare multiple slides when the animal is first presented than to repeat a procedure after finding the specimen to be nondiagnostic, often after the animal has already been discharged from the hospital. This is particularly important if sedation or anesthesia is required for collection. It is optimal to stain and briefly examine one or two slides to ensure that they are adequately cellular while the patient is still in the hospital (or before animal is recovered, if anesthesia or sedation is required). If the slides stained are not cellular, additional collection attempts can be performed immediately.

There are many possible reasons for any one slide being nondiagnostic. The slide may not have any diagnostic cells because the needle missed the lesion during collection (geographic miss) (Figure 1-5) or may have been in a nonrepresentative portion of the lesion (e.g., an area of inflammation or necrosis within a neoplasm (Figure 1-6). In

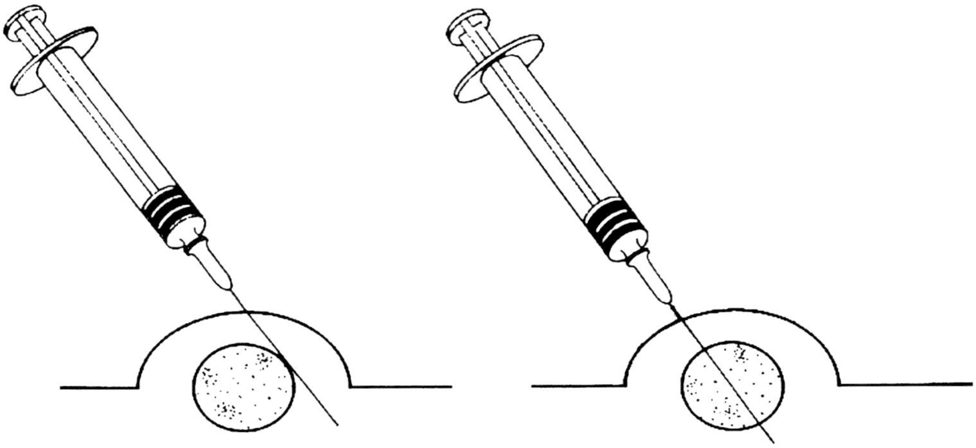

Figure 1-5 Geographic miss. Sometimes, the needle is not in the area containing representative tissue of the lesion during sample collection. This is common in obese animals where the lesion may be surrounded by abundant subcutaneous fat. (Courtesy Oklahoma State University teaching files.)

addition, some lesions simply do not exfoliate cells well. Even if adequate cells were collected, many times, the cells do not spread out well and the slides are too thick to be evaluated (especially common in the case of lymph node aspirates), or all of the cells are ruptured during smear preparation (Figure 1-7). Even in the hands of clinicians who are highly experienced in sample collection, it is not unusual to evaluate multiple slides from a single lesion and have all but one of the slides be nondiagnostic for one reason or another.

If possible, a minimum of four to five slides, representing collection attempts from several sites within the lesion, should be submitted from any lesion. If some of the samples appear to be excessively thick or if little to no material is apparent on the slides, additional slides should be made. With multiple slides, the chances of at least one of them being of diagnostic quality are increased.

If multiple masses are sampled, always a new needle and syringe should be used with each mass. If this is not done, slides from one mass may be contaminated with cells left in the needle from previous collection attempts. Each slide should be clearly labeled as to the anatomic site sampled.

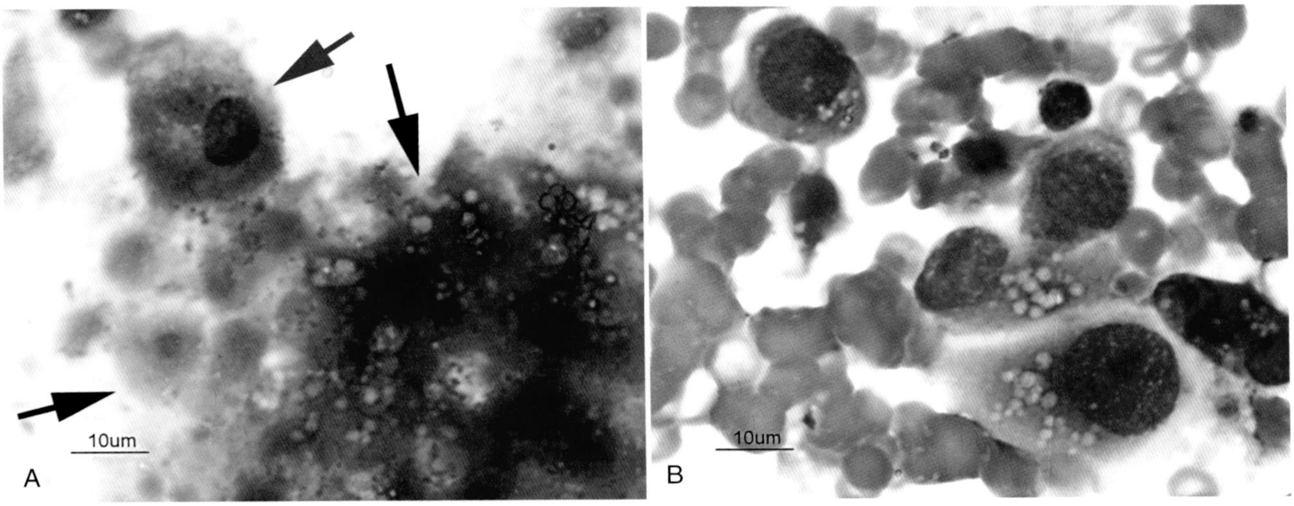

Figure 1-6 Samples collected from a prostatic carcinoma with areas of necrosis. A, Most slides were from aspirates of necrotic areas and contain predominantly necrotic cellular debris (*black arrows*). A single partially intact cell is present (*blue arrow*). These slides would be nondiagnostic. **B,** One of the aspiration attempts sampled a nonnecrotic area and the resulting slides contained numerous intact cells allowing a diagnosis to be made. This demonstrates the importance of sampling multiple sites of a mass. (Courtesy Oklahoma State University teaching files.)

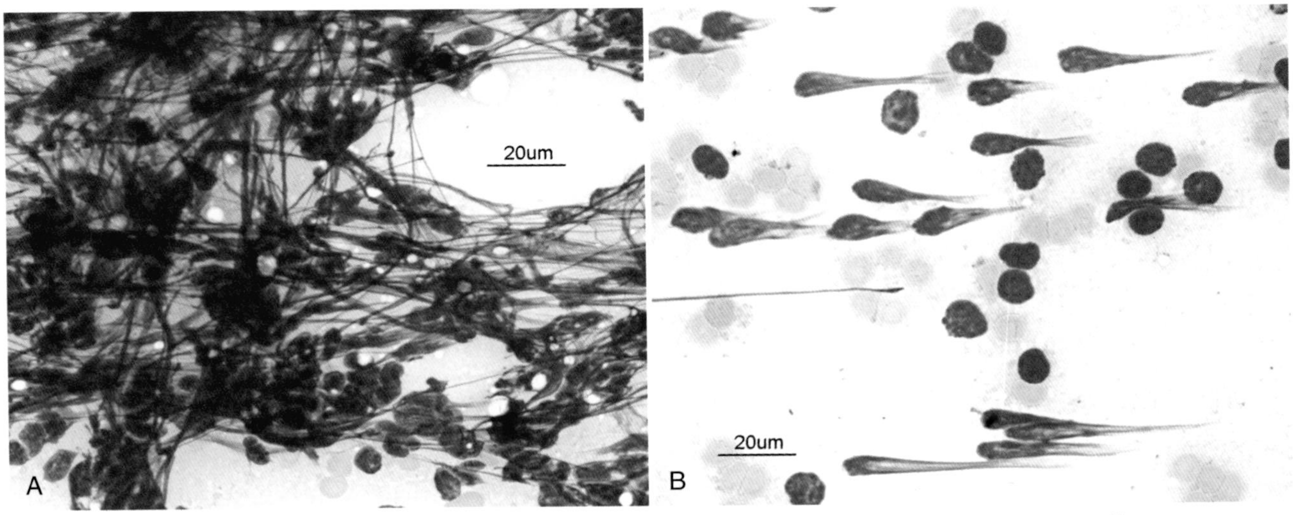

Figure 1-7 Images from an aspirate of a reactive lymph node. This sample was nondiagnostic because all of the cells have been ruptured due to excessive downward pressure being applied during sample preparation. **A,** The linear streaks of material represent nuclear chromatin of ruptured cells. **B,** Ruptured cells often appear to have "comet tails" all going the same direction. (Courtesy Oklahoma State University teaching files.)

Avoid Blood Dilution: Blood contamination (hemodilution) is another common cause of nondiagnostic slides. FNB with aspiration will collect the tissue of least resistance. If blood vessels within the lesion have been ruptured, the tissue of least resistance will be peripheral blood. Once significant blood contamination has occurred, it is difficult to salvage the sample. Additional collection attempts using a clean syringe and needle should be performed.

The two major causes of blood contamination are the use of too large a needle (<22-gauge) and prolonged aspiration. Larger-bore needles do not usually collect more cells but are more likely to rupture small blood vessels. As mentioned before, material is often not visible in the syringe during sample collection, despite adequate numbers of cells being present within the needle. Any time material is visible in the hub of the needle, the collection procedure should be stopped and slides made immediately.

Some lesions are highly vascular, making it difficult to avoid blood contamination, even with good collection technique. In these cases, use of a nonaspiration technique may result in less blood contamination and more tissue cells for evaluation.

Do Not Be Timid: Other reasons for poor cellularity of a sample are inadequate negative pressure (aspiration technique) and slow or shallow needle passages (nonaspiration technique). When using the nonaspiration technique, the clinician is relying on the cutting action of the needle going through the tissue to create a slurry of cells and tissue fluid which will enter the needle by capillary action. Needle passages should be quick and of sufficient length (although the size of the mass may limit the length of the needle pass).

Impression Smears

Impression smears can be made from ulcerated or exudative superficial lesions (Figure 1-8) or tissue samples collected at surgery or necropsy (Figure 1-9). Impression smears from superficial lesions often yield only inflammatory cells even if the inflammation is a secondary process; neoplastic cells may not exfoliate in exudates or impression smears of ulcerated masses. If possible, FNB of tissue under the ulcerated or exudative area should be collected in addition to the impression smears. Inserting the needle at a nonulcerated area will help reduce contamination during collection. Impression smears of exudates or ulcers are most beneficial for determining if bacterial or fungal organisms are present. Keep in mind that bacteria may reflect only a secondary bacterial infection.

Ulcerated areas should be imprinted before they are cleaned. The lesion should then be cleaned with a saline-moistened surgical sponge and reimprinted or scraped.

To collect impression smears from tissues collected during surgery or necropsy, the tissue should first be cut so that a fresh surface for imprinting is created (see Figure 1-9). Next, the excess blood and tissue fluid should be removed from the surface of the lesion being imprinted by blotting with a clean absorbent material (Figure 1-10). Excessive blood and tissue fluids inhibit tissue cells from adhering to the glass slide, producing a poorly cellular preparation. Also, excessive fluid inhibits cells from spreading and assuming the size and shape they usually have in air-dried smears. After excess blood and tissue fluids have been blotted from the surface of the lesion, the surface of the lesion is touched (pressed) against the middle of a clean glass microscope slide and lifted directly up (Figure 1-11). This should be repeated several times so that several tissue imprints are present on the slide. If the excess blood has been adequately removed, the tissue will stick somewhat to the slide and will appear to peel off the slide, if removed slowly. Properly made slides will have slightly opaque areas at the areas of the impressions but should not have excessively thick areas of blood (Figure 1-12).

No further smearing of the material is necessary. The tissue should not be allowed to slide around on the glass surface, as this causes cells to rupture. When possible, several slides should be imprinted so that a few can be

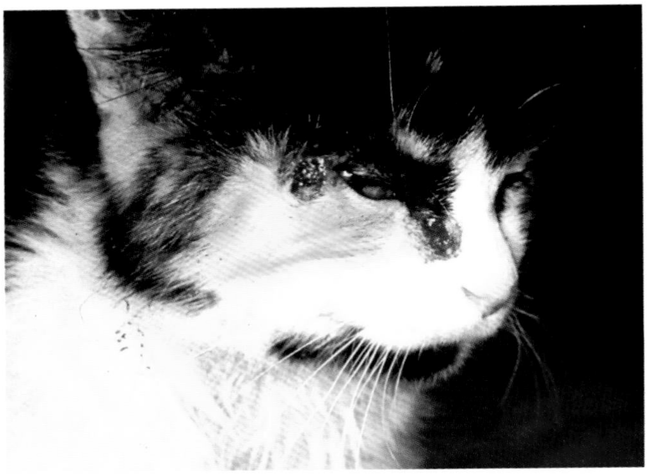

Figure 1-8 Ulcerative, exudative lesions on the face of a cat. This lesion is well suited for impression smears. Slides from these lesions revealed inflammatory cells and many Sporothrix organisms. (Courtesy Oklahoma State University teaching files.)

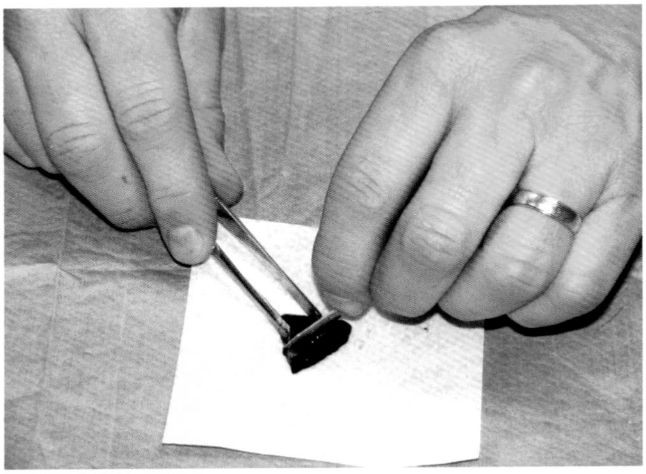

Figure 1-9 Impression smear of tissue removed at surgery. The tissue is trimmed so that a fresh surface is created for making the impression smear. If normal tissue surrounding a mass has been excised, it is important to be sure that the tissue is cut through the area of interest. (Courtesy Oklahoma State University teaching files.)

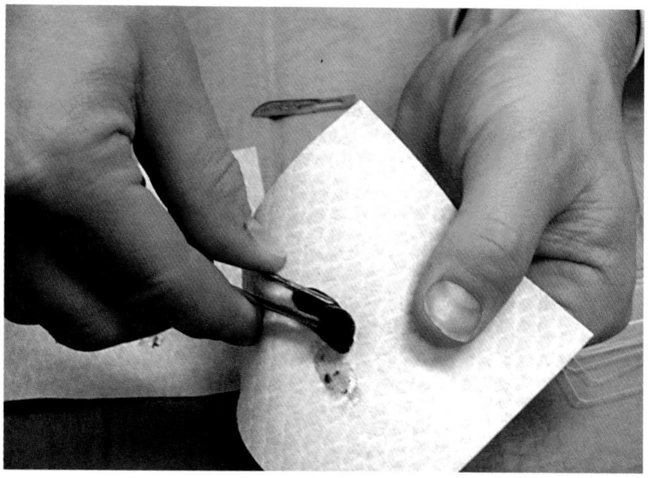

Figure 1-10 The surface of the tissue is blotted several times against an absorbent material to remove excess blood and tissue fluid. This is extremely important to avoid slides that contain only peripheral blood. (Courtesy Oklahoma State University teaching files.)

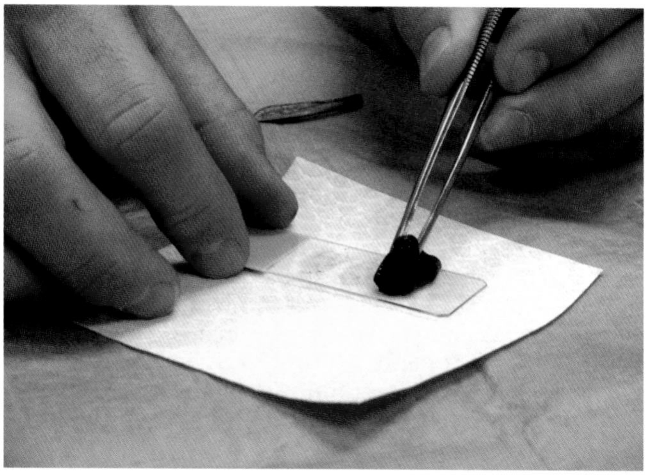

Figure 1-11 The tissue is gently pressed (not smeared) several times against the surface of a clean glass slide. (Courtesy Oklahoma State University teaching files.)

retained in case special stains are necessary. After making sufficient impression smears, the tissue used should be placed in an appropriate amount of formalin so that it may be submitted for histologic evaluation, if necessary.

Scrapings

Scrapings can be made from external lesions or tissue obtained from surgery or necropsy. Generally, scrapings will result in more cellular slides than will impression smears; however, like impression smears, scrapings may contain mostly surface contamination or inflammation if made from the surface of ulcerated cutaneous lesions. Generally, scrapings are not as valuable for diagnosing neoplasia as slides made from FNB. Scrapings are valuable in collecting samples from cutaneous lesions that are flat and dry and, thus, not amenable to FNB or impression and from samples collected at surgery or necropsy (Figure 1-13).[1] Two examples of lesions in which scrapings are beneficial are

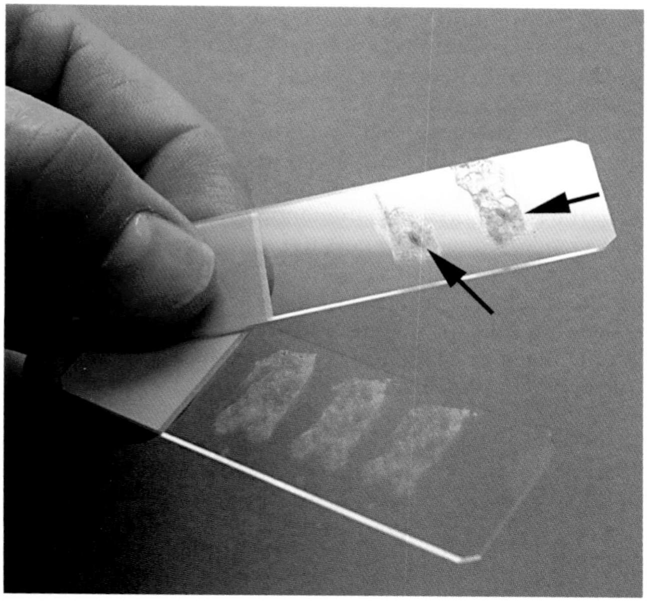

Figure 1-12 The resulting slides from an impression smear. The slide on the bottom is properly made and has several slightly opaque areas where the tissue has been touched to the slide indicating cells have probably been transferred to the slide. The slide on top has excessive peripheral blood (*arrows*), indicating that the tissue was not properly blotted against absorbent material prior to making the impression smear. This slide will likely contain only peripheral blood, or if cells are present, they may not be well spread out. (Courtesy Oklahoma State University teaching files.)

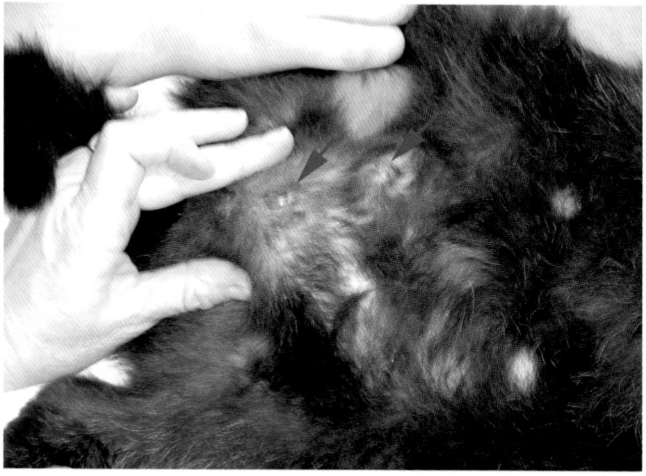

Figure 1-13 Multiple plaquelike and raised lesions on the ventrum of a cat with eosinophilic granuloma lesions. The lesions were not thick enough to obtain good aspirates but yielded diagnostic cells via scraping. The ulcerated lesions are those that have already been scraped (*arrows*). Scraping to the point of obtaining a small amount of blood or serum helps the cells adhere to the slides and also increases the chance of bypassing surface contamination and obtaining representative cells. (Courtesy Oklahoma State University teaching files.)

feline eosinophilic granuloma complex lesions and dermatophytosis.[7] Scrapings are prepared by holding a scalpel blade perpendicular to the lesion's surface and pulling the blade toward oneself several times. When scraping dry, nonulcerated lesions such as dermatophyte lesions scrapings should be sufficiently deep to cause exudation of serum or blood. This proteinaceous and fibrin-rich fluid will help the cells (and hairs when looking for dermatophytes) collected to adhere to the slide and prevent them from being washed off during staining. The material collected on the blade is transferred to the middle of a glass microscope slide and spread either by smearing gently with the scalpel blade or by one of the techniques described later for preparation of smears from aspirates of solid masses.

Swabs

Generally, swabs are used only when other collection methods are not practical, as when obtaining samples from the vagina or external ear, or within fistulous tracts. Swabs from the external ear canal and fistulous tracts are most useful for identifying infectious organisms. Swabs are collected from the site using a sterile cotton swab. If the lesion is moist, the cotton swab need not be moistened. However, if the lesion is not very moist, moistening with sterile saline is suggested. Moistening the swab helps minimize disruption of the cells that might occur during collection and sample preparation. Use of lubricant gels (such as K-Y Jelly) should be avoided when collecting swabs because they can coat the sample and interfere with staining of the cells, rendering the slide uninterpretable. Once the sample has been collected, the swab is gently rolled across the surface of a clean glass slide. It is important to not swipe the swab across the slide because this will often result in rupture of all the cells (Figure 1-14).

PREPARATION OF SLIDES: SOLID TISSUE ASPIRATES

Slide-over-Slide Smears ("Squash Preps")

When used properly, this is generally the best method for preparing slides from FNB or scrapings of solid tissue lesions. The goal is to prepare a thin film in which the cells are spread out into a single layer, without rupturing the cells. The material collected from the FNB procedure is expelled near one end (~one half inch) of a clean glass slide (sample slide). A second glass slide (spreader slide) is placed on top of and perpendicular to the slide containing the sample directly over the specimen (Figure 1-15). The specimen will usually spread out between the two slides because of the weight of the spreader slide alone. If the sample is thick or granular and does not spread out well, light momentary downward pressure may be applied to the spreader slide and then released. The spreader slide is then lightly drawn out across the length of the bottom slide, spreading the sample (Figure 1-16). Despite the name *squash prep*, it is important that no downward pressure be applied to the spreader slide while smearing the sample because this usually results in rupturing the majority of the cells.

If done properly, the smear should have a "flame shape" that does not extend to the edge of the slide. This is important because, like a blood smear, often it is only at the edges of the sample where the cells are spread out sufficiently thin to be evaluated. Smears that extend off the edge of the slides are usually too thick to evaluate. Also, many automated slide stainers do not stain the entire slide but leave an unstained area approximately one quarter to one half inch wide on either end of the slide. Cells in these areas will not be stained and, therefore, cannot be evaluated. Even when using dip-staining methods that stain the entire slide, material at the very edges of a slide may be impossible to view on some microscopes.

When done correctly, this technique does a good job of spreading out the cells, even those in clusters, so that cellular detail can be adequately evaluated. The main disadvantage of this method, particularly in inexperienced hands, is excessive cell rupturing. Lymphoid cells are particularly fragile and will often rupture if even moderate

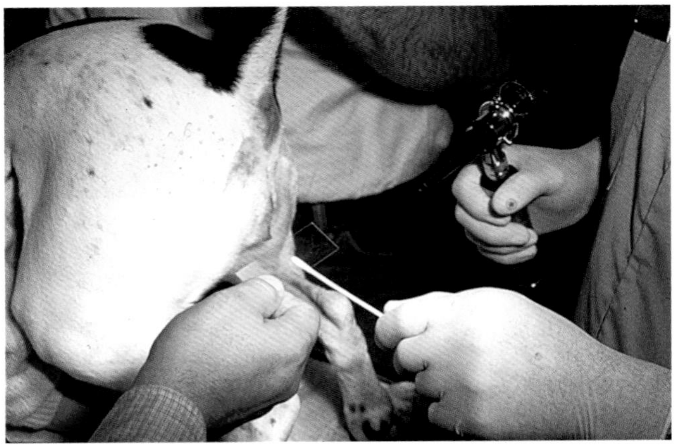

Figure 1-14 Preparation of a vaginal swab from a dog. The swab containing the sample is gently rolled along the slide. Sliding or smearing the swab across the slide will result in excessive rupturing of the cells. (Courtesy Oklahoma State University teaching files.)

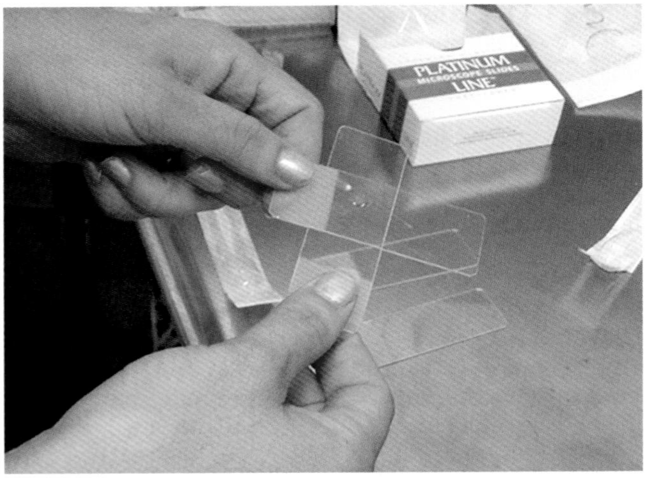

Figure 1-15 Squash preparation. Once the sample has been placed on a clean glass slide, a second slide is placed on top of the sample and will be used to spread out the sample. It is important that no downward pressure be applied with the top slide during spreading of the sample. (Courtesy Oklahoma State University teaching files.)

pressure is used when preparing slides with this technique.

Blood Smear Technique

With many samples, especially lymph node aspirates, the material expelled from the syringe onto the slide will have enough tissue fluid, blood, or both that the sample can be smeared out as if making a blood smear (Figure 1-17).[1] This technique will result in less cell rupturing, especially with fragile cell populations, and generally produces thin smears with intact cells that are well spread out.

As with the slide-over-slide technique, the sample is expelled from the syringe near one end of the sample slide. The long edge of the spreader slide is placed onto the flat surface of the sample slide in front of the sample. The spreader slide is tilted to a 45-degree angle with respect to the sample slide and pulled backward about a third of the way into the aspirated material. The spreader slide is then smoothly and rapidly slid forward, as if making a blood smear. The smear should end in a feathered edge at least 0.5 inch from the opposite end of the spreader slide. If the sample smear extends all the way to the edge of a slide, additional slides should be made, and a smaller amount of sample should be put on the slide.

"Starfish" Preps

Another technique used by some people for spreading aspirates is to drag the aspirate peripherally in several directions with the point of a syringe needle, producing a starfish shape (Figure 1-18 and Figure 1-19). This technique tends not to damage fragile cells but allows a thick layer of tissue fluid to remain around the cells. Often, the thick

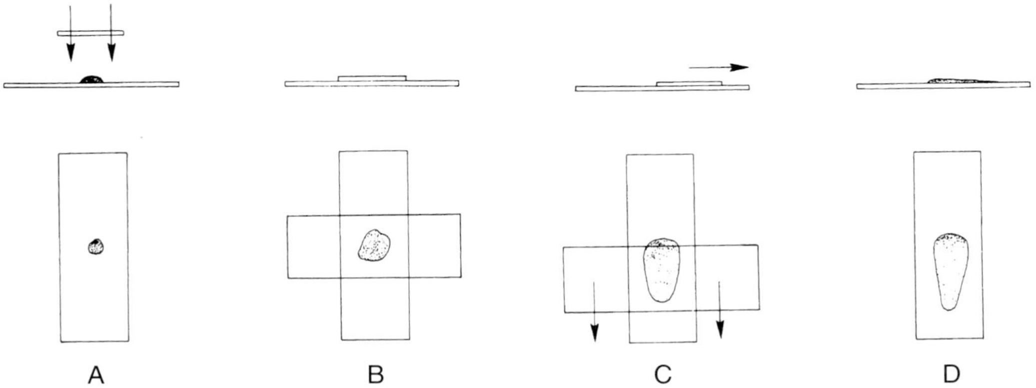

Figure 1-16 Squash preparation. A, A portion of the aspirate is expelled onto a glass microscope slide, and another slide is placed over the sample. **B,** This spreads the sample. If the sample does not spread well, gentle digital pressure can be applied to the top slide. Care must be taken not to place excessive pressure on the slide, causing the cells to rupture. **C,** The slides are smoothly slid apart. **D,** This usually produces well-spread smears but may result in excessive cell rupture.

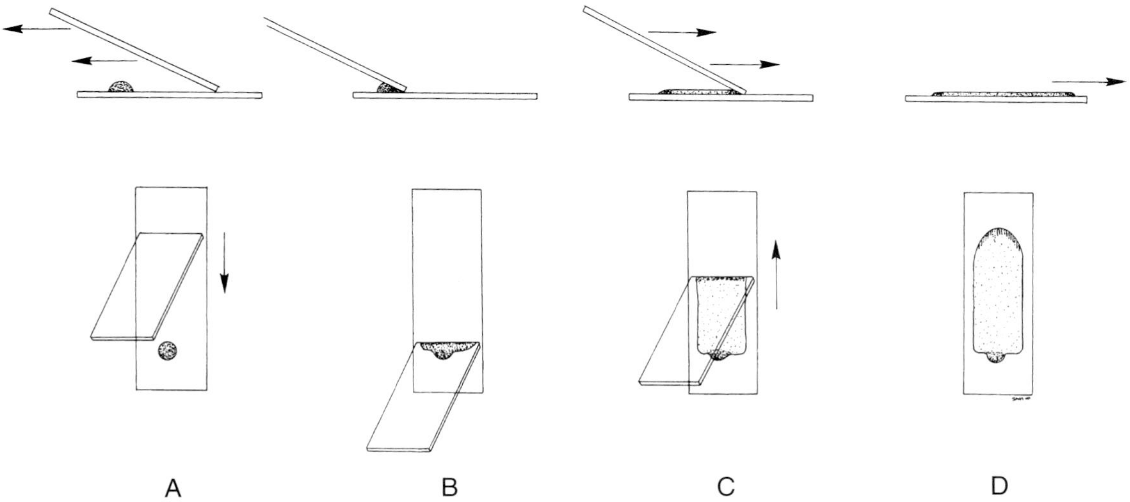

Figure 1-17 Blood smear technique. A, A drop of fluid sample is placed on a glass microscope slide close to one end, then another slide is slid backward to contact the front of the drop. **B,** When the drop is contacted, it rapidly spreads along the juncture between the two slides. **C** and **D,** The spreader slide is then smoothly and rapidly slid forward the length of the slide, producing a smear with a feathered edge.

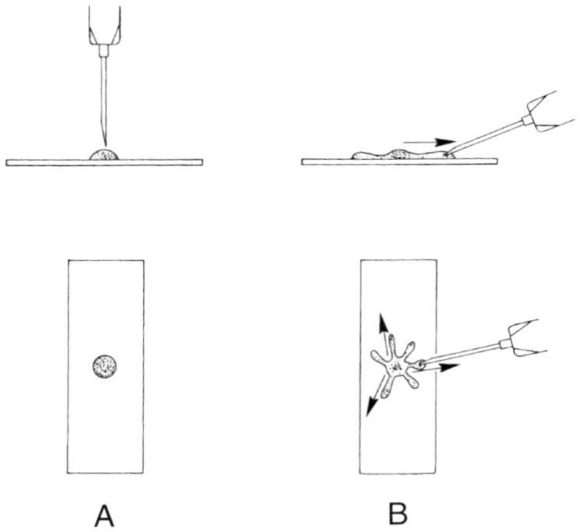

Figure 1-18 Needle spread or "starfish" preparation. A, A portion of the aspirate is expelled onto a glass microscope slide. **B,** The tip of a needle is placed in the aspirate and moved peripherally, pulling a trail of the sample with it. This procedure is repeated in several directions, resulting in a preparation with multiple projections.

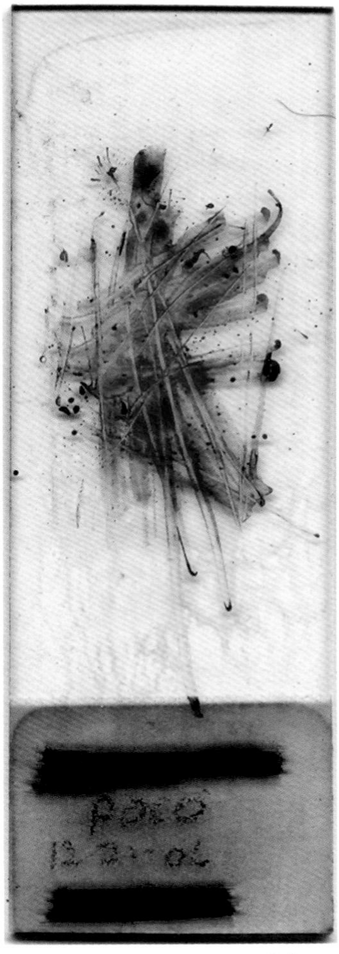

Figure 1-19 Slide prepared using starfish or needle spread technique depicted in Figure 1-18. Blue streaks indicating cellular areas are seen where the needle was dragged repeatedly across the slide and through the sample. (Courtesy Oklahoma State University teaching files.)

layer of fluid prevents the cells from spreading well and interferes with evaluation of cell detail. Typically, some acceptable areas are present; however, a well-made slide-over-slide or blood smear preparation is usually preferable.

Preparation Tips

Do Not Let the Sample Dry or Clot: If the sample clots or dries out on the slide before smears can be made, the cells may not spread out sufficiently to be evaluated. Also, the cells will often be distorted or not stain well because they are incorporated in a clot. Several clean slides should be laid out in an easily accessible area prior to the collection procedure to reduce the time between collections and final smear preparation.

One common mistake is to spray the sample from the needle onto the slide from a distance. This results in the sample being spread out in many small drops over the slide, much like a shotgun blast (Figure 1-20). The problem is that these small drops tend to dry before the operator has time to make a smear. When viewed under the microscope, small clusters of cells appear poorly spread out (Figure 1-21), and it is usually impossible to adequately visualize the morphology of the cells. When transferring the sample to the slide, the edge of the needle should be held very close to the slide, and the sample should be sprayed in one drop, if possible. The sample should then be immediately smeared using one of the techniques described previously. If sufficient sample is obtained to put on more than one slide, it is important to make all smears quickly before the sample dries. When using the non-aspiration technique, prefilling the syringe with air will shorten the time between sample collection and smear preparation and will reduce the likelihood of the sample clotting before smears can be made.

Avoid Making Too Thick a Smear: Smears that are too thick will not have cells adequately spread out, making

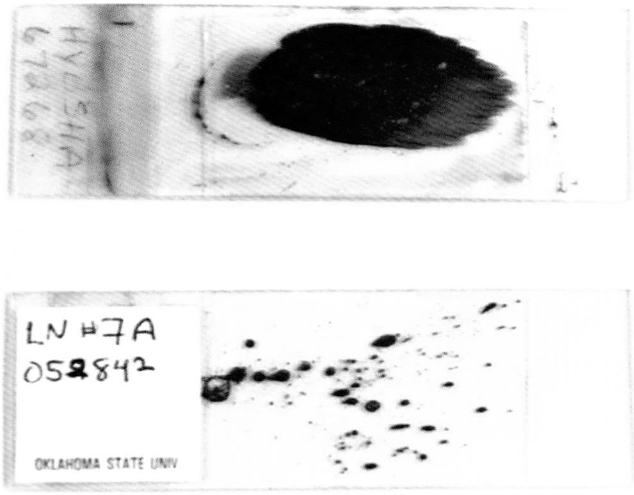

Figure 1-20 Example of a poorly smeared sample. The slide on top is well made. However, the bottom slide shows what happens when a sample is sprayed onto the slide from a distance resulting in a shotgun blast–like arrangement of small drops. These drops dry quickly and then cannot be spread out. (Courtesy Oklahoma State University teaching files.)

the cells impossible to evaluate. Samples that yield thick smears are those that are contaminated with excessive amounts of peripheral blood or samples collected from tissues that easily exfoliate large numbers of cells (e.g., lymph node aspirates). Ideally, only a small drop of sample should be applied to a slide (about the size of drop used in making a blood smear). If a large amount of sample is applied to a single smear, the smear generally ends up being too thick. If the sample extends all the way to the far end of the slide, the smear will probably be too thick.

Generally, the amount of sample being applied to the slide can be controlled when the material is expelled from the syringe. If too large a drop is applied to a slide, a thin smear can still be obtained by using the blood smear technique. The spreader slide is drawn back just to the point that it barely contacts the sample, which will begin to spread across the surface of the spreader slide by capillary action, and then is rapidly smeared forward. Alternatively, the spreader slide can be placed flat on top of the sample, as when preparing a slide-over-slide technique. Then the spreader slide is lifted up and used to transfer a portion of the sample to another clean glass slide, on which a smear can be made. This technique can be repeated more than once, if needed, and finally the remaining material on the initial sample slide is smeared out. In this way, several thin smears can be made from one large drop of sample.

PREPARATION OF SLIDES: FLUID SAMPLES

A fluid sample can be obtained when sampling body cavities (e.g., thoracocentesis, joint tap), performing washings (e.g., transtracheal wash), or when aspirating a cystic lesion (e.g., benign cyst, cystic tumor, sialocele). Proper handling of fluid samples is essential to obtaining diagnostic information. The two main considerations are preserving cell morphology during transit of the sample and preparing smears that are sufficiently cellular to allow for adequate evaluation.

Any fluid sample on which cytologic evaluation is going to be performed should be placed in an appropriate amount of ethylenediaminetetraacetic acid (EDTA). EDTA will prevent coagulation of the sample (which can alter cell counts obtained from the specimen) and help preserve cell morphology during transport to the laboratory. This is especially important if the sample will be mailed. Usually, but not always, EDTA will adequately preserve cell morphology overnight and possibly longer. Refrigeration of the sample will prolong the length of time that readable smears can be made from the sample. If culture of the fluid is anticipated, a portion of the sample should be placed separately into an appropriate transport medium or other sterile tube. It is important that a sufficient amount of sample fluid be added to the EDTA tube. EDTA has a very high refractive index, and if only a small amount of sample is added to a large EDTA tube, the total protein estimation determined by a refractometer will be artifactually elevated.

Even when fluid samples are placed in EDTA tubes and refrigerated or kept cool with ice packs, cells will undergo aging changes and eventually become too degenerate to be evaluated. Depending on the cellularity, type of cells present, and physical composition of the fluid (i.e., protein concentration), significant morphologic changes may occur within 24 hours. The best way to preserve cell morphology is to send premade, air-dried smears. Once smears are made, cell morphology will be preserved for several days, even without fixation of the slides. If possible, premade smears should always be made and sent along with the fluid sample itself. Glass slides should never be placed in the refrigerator because condensation forming on the slide can result in lysis of the cells.

Fluid samples can vary from virtually acellular (cerebrospinal fluid) to extremely cellular (septic exudate). Depending on the nature of the sample, different techniques can be used to produce slides of adequate cellularity.

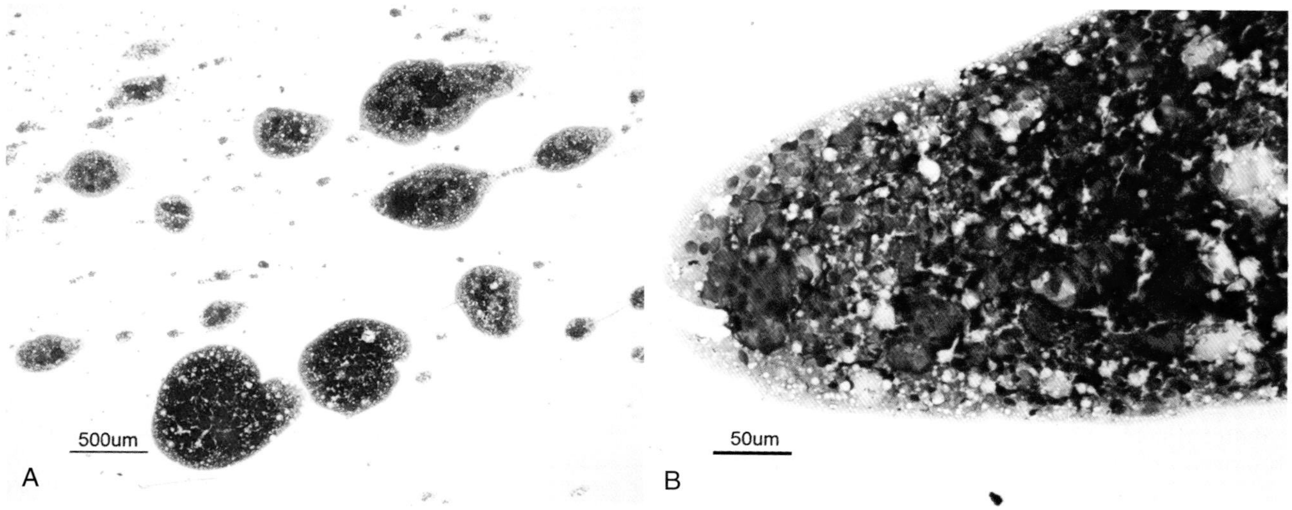

Figure 1-21 Photomicrograph of slide shown on the bottom of Figure 1-20. A, Low-magnification image shows that the cells are all present in thick drops where the sample landed and that they were not spread out before the sample dried. **B,** Higher-magnification image of one of the drops shows that the individual cells cannot be seen, resulting in a nondiagnostic sample. (Courtesy Oklahoma State University teaching files.)

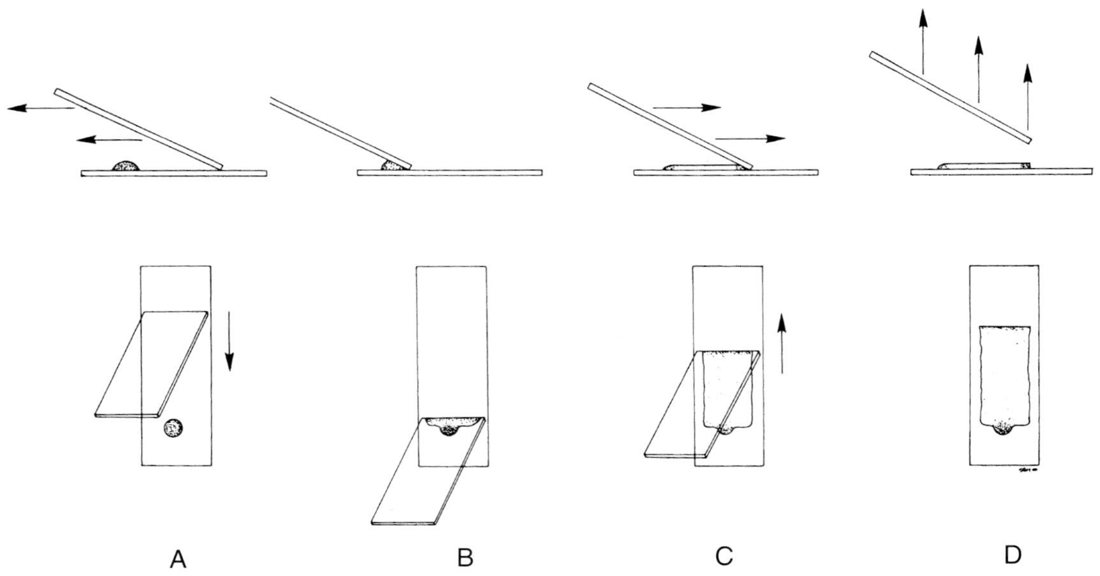

Figure 1-22 Line smear concentration technique. A, A drop of fluid sample is placed onto a glass microscope slide close to one end, and another slide is slid backward to contact the front of the drop. **B,** When the drop is contacted, it rapidly spreads along the juncture between the two slides. **C,** The spreader slide is then slid forward smoothly and rapidly. **D,** After the spreader slide has been advanced about two thirds to three fourths of the distance required to make a smear with a feathered edge, the spreader slide is raised directly upward. This produces a smear with a line of concentrated cells at its end, instead of a feathered edge.

Smears can be prepared directly from fresh, well-mixed fluid or from the sediment of a centrifuged sample using blood smear (direct smears) (see Figure 1-17), line smear (Figure 1-22 and Figure 1-23), and squash prep (see Figure 1-16) techniques. Table 1-2 outlines the samples to be prepared and submitted from fluid samples based on the characteristics of the specimen.

Blood Smear Technique (Direct Smears)

The blood smear technique (direct smear) usually produces well-spread smears of sufficient cellularity from homogenous fluids containing 5000 cells per microliter (cells/μL) but often produces smears of insufficient cellularity from fluids containing less than 5000 cells/μL. The line smear technique can be used to concentrate fluids of low cellularity but often does not sufficiently spread cells from highly cellular fluids. In general, translucent fluids are of low to moderate cellularity, whereas opaque fluids are usually highly cellular. Therefore, translucent fluids often require concentration, either by centrifugation or by the line smear technique. When possible, concentration by centrifugation is preferred. The squash prep technique often spreads viscous samples (e.g., transtracheal wash [TTW]) and samples with flecks of particulate material better than the blood smear and line smear techniques.

To prepare a smear by the blood smear technique, place a small drop of the fluid on a glass slide about one half inch from the end. Slide another slide backward at a 30- to 40-degree angle until it contacts the drop. When the fluid flows sideways along the crease between the slides, slide the second slide forward quickly and smoothly until the fluid has all drained away from the second slide. This makes a smear with a feathered edge.

Sediment Preps (Centrifugation Preps)

To concentrate fluids by centrifugation, the fluid is centrifuged for 5 minutes at 165 to 360 g (gravitational force). This is achieved by operating a centrifuge with a radial arm length of 14.6 centimeters (cm) (the arm length of most urine centrifuges) at 1000 to 1500 revolutions per minute (rpm). After centrifugation, the majority of the supernatant is separated from the sediment and analyzed for total protein concentration. The sediment is resuspended in a few drops of supernatant left in the tube by gently tapping the side of the tube. A drop of the resuspended sediment is placed on a slide, and a smear is made by the blood smear or squash prep technique (Figure 1-24). Alternatively, a plastic pipette can be placed through the supernatant and used to remove the pellet of cells from the bottom of the tube and transfer it to a glass slide and make smears using a slide-over-slide technique. An absorbent tissue may be used to wick away excess supernatant prior to smear preparation, if needed.

Sediment concentrated slides can produce highly cellular smears even from fluids of low cellularity and help identify cells present in low numbers (Figure 1-25). When possible, several smears should be made by each technique. When slides are made from the sediment of a fluid sample, it is not possible to estimate the cellularity of the sample from the slides. Therefore, it is imperative to either retain a portion of sample for cell counts or to make direct smears in addition to the sediment preps.

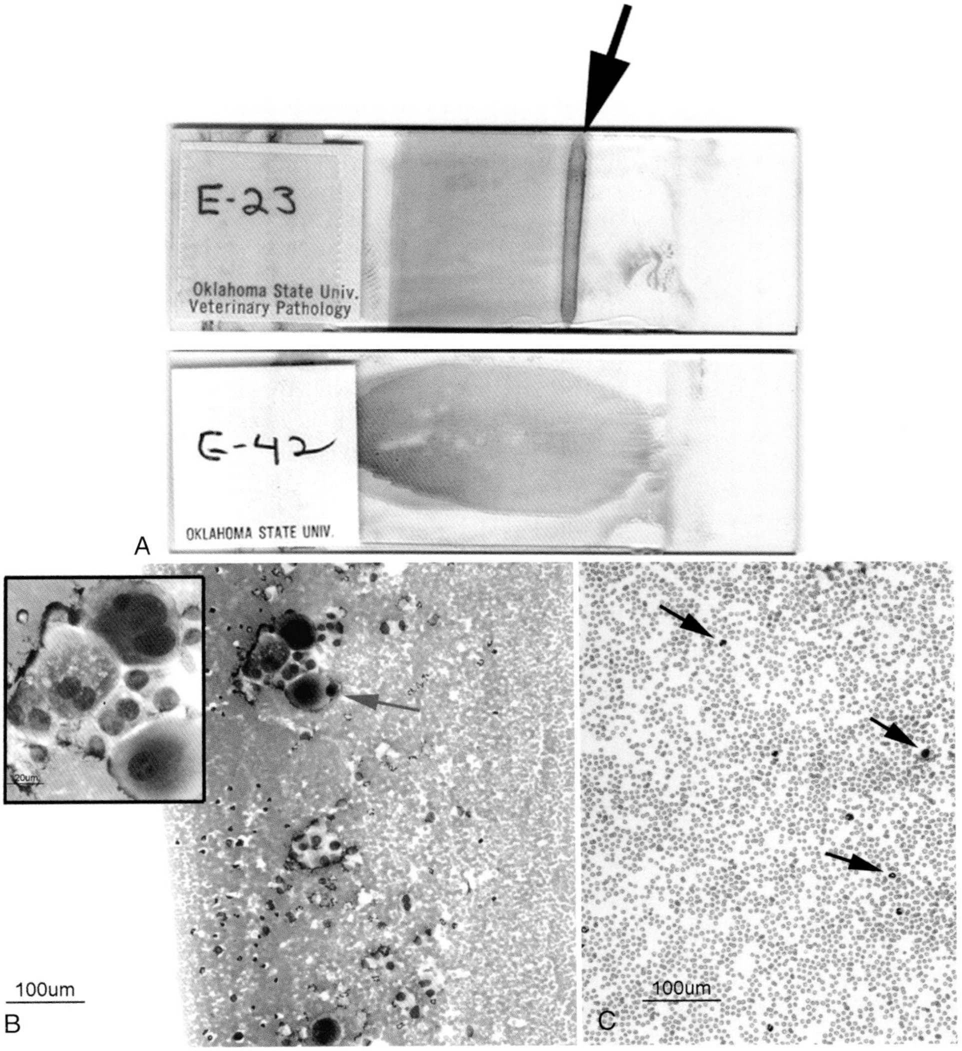

Figure 1-23 Line smear made from fluid sample. A, The slide on the bottom was made using a standard blood smear technique. Toward the right, the sample forms a typical feathered edge. The slide on the top was made using a line smear technique. Toward the right, the smear ends abruptly, forming a thick line with a higher concentration of large nucleated cells (*arrow*). **B** and **C,** Images taken from the line smear of a fluid sample. The main portion of the smear (*C*: right) is of low cellularity, consisting mostly of blood but with low numbers of nucleated cells (*black arrows*). These relatively small cells are neutrophils and macrophages. At the line edge (*B*: left), there are increased numbers of nucleated cells, especially clusters of large neoplastic epithelial cells. Inset shows higher magnification of cell cluster indicated by the red arrow. (**A,** Courtesy Oklahoma State University teaching files.)

TABLE 1-2

Methods of Preparing Cytology Slides from Fluid Samples

Types or Characteristics of Fluid	Samples to Prepare or Submit
Peripheral blood for cytology	Make several air-dried direct smears (blood smear method).
	Submit remainder in EDTA.
Clear, transparent fluids (e.g., abdominal fluid)	Make one to two direct smears (can be used to estimate cellularity) and line smears.
	Centrifuge a portion of the sample and make smears from sediment.
	Submit a portion of fluid in EDTA.
	Submit a portion of fluid in sterile container if culture is desired.
Turbid or opaque fluids	Make one to two direct smears.
	Submit a portion of the fluid in EDTA.
	Submit a portion of the fluid in sterile container if culture is desired.
Clear fluid with flecks or mucous strands (e.g., transtracheal wash fluid, bone marrow samples in EDTA)	Make several direct smears from fluid.
	Make "squash preps" (slide-over-slide preps) of particles or mucous strands removed from the fluid using either a pipette, needle, or capillary tube.
	Submit a portion of the fluid in EDTA.
	Submit a portion of the fluid in sterile container if culture is desired.

EDTA, ethylenediaminetetraacetic acid.

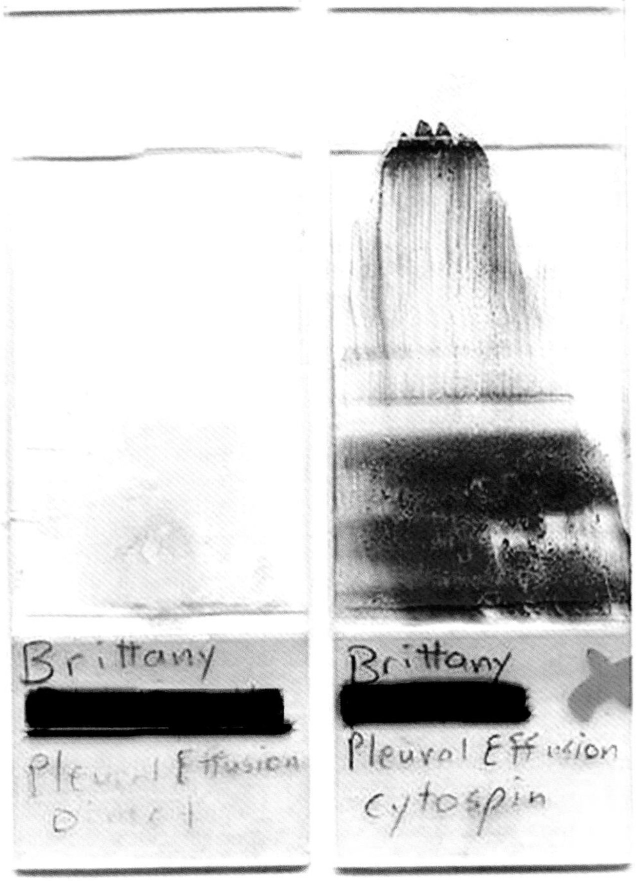

Figure 1-24 Direct smear (*left*) and concentrated smear made from sediment (*right*) of pleural effusion from a dog. The dark color on the concentrated smear is the result of markedly increased cellularity. (Courtesy Oklahoma State University teaching files.)

Line Smears

When the fluid cannot be concentrated by centrifugation or the centrifuged sample is of low cellularity, the line smear technique (see Figure 1-22) can be used to concentrate cells in the smear. A drop of fluid is placed on a clean glass slide, and the blood smear technique is used, but the spreading slide is stopped and raised directly upward about three fourths of the way through the smear. This will result in a line containing a much higher concentration of cells than the rest of the slide (see Figure 1-23). Unfortunately, the cells that are present in the line may not be well spread out, making evaluation difficult.

Sometimes fluid is obtained when sampling a mass or other proliferative lesion. When this occurs, as much fluid as possible should be drained from the lesion and handled as described previously. The lesion should then be reevaluated. If a solid tissue component still remains, that component should be sampled by FNB using either the aspiration or nonaspiration technique. Many times, cystic neoplasia will not exfoliate overtly neoplastic cells into the cystic fluid. The material obtained from direct FNB may have a completely different cell population than that present in the fluid itself.

STAINING CYTOLOGIC PREPARATIONS

To Stain or Not to Stain?

If you intend to send the slides to a laboratory for evaluation, it is not necessary to stain the slides or do any special fixation at all. Air-dried smears will hold up quite well over the length of time necessary for transport to an outside laboratory. In fact, if the slides are to be submitted for analysis, unstained slides are preferable. This will allow the cytologist to stain the smears with the type of stain he or she is used to viewing. However, it is usually advisable

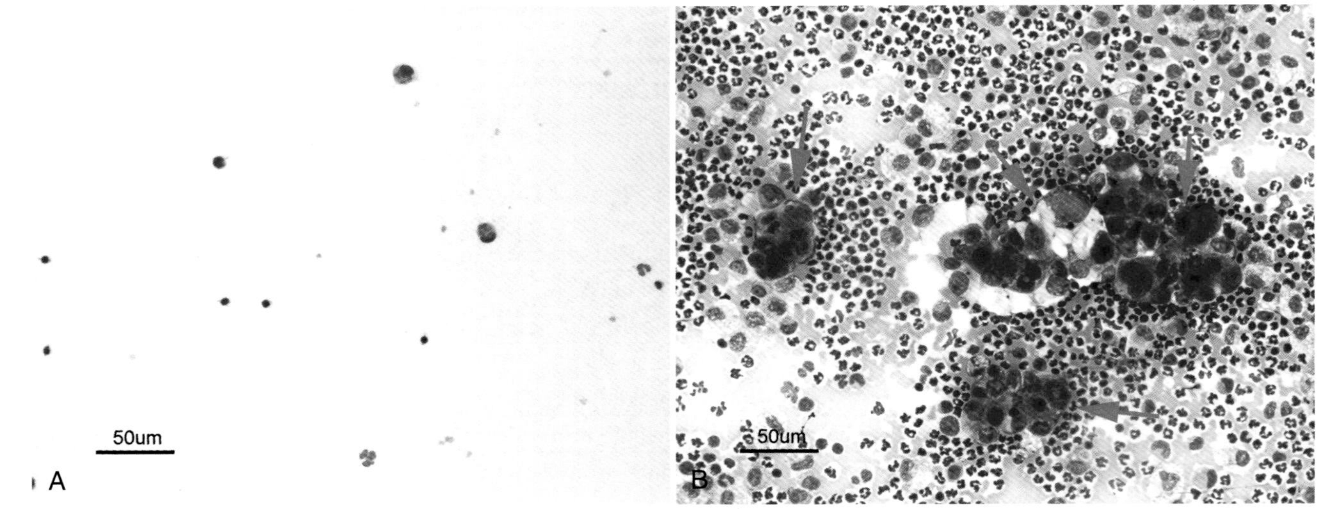

Figure 1-25 Photomicrographs taken from slides shown in Figure 1-24. A, Low-magnification image taken from direct smear of pleural fluid shows relatively sparse cellularity consisting mostly of nondegenerate neutrophils and macrophages. This image is representative of the slide. **B,** Low-magnification image taken from the concentrated sediment preparation of the same fluid sample. The slide is highly cellular. In addition to the neutrophils and macrophages seen on the direct smear, clusters of neoplastic epithelial cells (*arrows*) are easily found.

to stain at least one slide to ensure that an adequately cellular sample was obtained before paying for interpretation of the smears. All slides collected from the lesion, both stained and unstained, should be submitted for evaluation, in case not all slides were adequately cellular.

Types of Stain

Several types of stains have been used for cytologic preparations.[8] The two general types most commonly used are (1) the Romanowsky-type stains (Wright stain, Giemsa stain, Diff-Quik stain) and Papanicolaou stain and its derivatives, such as Sano's trichrome. Papanicolaou stains and their derivatives require the specimen to be wet-fixed, (i.e., the smear must be fixed before the cells have dried). Usually, this is achieved by spraying the smear with a cytologic fixative or placing it in ethanol immediately after preparation. Such procedures are not necessary and are actually undesirable if the samples are to be stained with Romanowsky-type stains. Papanicolaou-type stains give excellent nuclear detail and are routinely used in human cytopathology.[8] However, these stains require multiple staining steps, do not stain many organisms or cell cytoplasm well, and are not practical for use in most clinics. They are rarely used in veterinary cytology, even in large commercial laboratories. The remainder of this chapter (and text) deals with Romanowsky-type stains.

Romanowsky-type stains are inexpensive, readily available to the practicing veterinarian, and easy to prepare, maintain and use. They stain organisms and the cytoplasm of cells excellently. Though nuclear and nucleolar detail cannot be perceived as well with Romanowsky-type stains as with Papanicolaou-type stains, nuclear and nucleolar detail are sufficient for differentiating neoplasia and inflammation and for evaluating neoplastic cells for cytologic evidence of malignant potential (criteria of malignancy). Smears to be stained with Romanowsky-type stains are first air-dried. Air-drying partially preserves (fixes) the cells and causes them to adhere to the slide so that they do not fall off during the staining procedure.

Romanowsky stains may be either aqueous based or methanol based.[9] Wright and Giemsa stains are examples of methanol-based stains. Diff-Quik and Hema 3 are commonly used aqueous-based Romanowsky stains, but others exist. Most, if not all, Romanowsky stains are acceptable for staining cytologic preparations. Aqueous-based stains are often used in private-practice settings because of their ease of use and rapid staining times. However, the aqueous based stains may fail to stain the granules of mast cells, basophils, and large granular lymphocytes.[9] When mast cell granules do not stain, the mast cells may be misclassified as macrophages or plasma cells. This can lead to confusion in examination of some mast cell tumors. Similarly, basophils may appear as neutrophils if their granules do not stain. Although uncommonly encountered, distemper inclusions stain more prominently with aqueous-based stains than with alcohol-based stains.[9]

Each stain usually has its own recommended staining protocol. These procedures should be followed in general but adapted to the type and thickness of smear being stained and to the evaluator's preference. The thinner the smear and the lower the total protein concentration of the fluid, the less is the time needed in the stain. The thicker the smear and the greater the total protein concentration of the fluid, the more is the time needed in the stain. As a result, fluid smears with low protein and low cellularity such as some abdominal fluid samples may stain better using half or less of the recommended time. Thick smears such as smears of neoplastic lymph nodes may need to be stained twice the recommended time or longer. Each person tends to have a different technique that he or she prefers. By trying variations in the recommended time intervals for stains, the evaluator can establish which times produce the preferred staining characteristics.

Poor staining quality is a common problem for a variety of reasons. It can be confusing to the novice when trying to examine his or her own slides because the cells may appear completely unrecognizable. Most staining problems can be avoided by the following precautions:

- *Use only new, clean slides.* Attempts to reuse slides are usually doomed to failure. Even if they are cleaned and dried, the samples often do not spread out well or do not stain properly because the surface properties of the glass have been altered.
- *Use fresh, well-filtered (if periodic filtering is required) stains.* Over time, with repeated use, stains will "fatigue," form excessive precipitate, or may become contaminated with organisms or cell debris from previous slides.
- *Make sure that the slides are completely air-dried before staining.* This is particularly important when examining blood smears. Some water will remain even after slides appear grossly to have dried. Slides should be air-dried for 5 to 10 minutes or dried briefly with a hair dryer prior to staining.
- *Do not touch the surface of the slide or smear at any time.* Likewise, make sure the slide is not contaminated with ultrasound gel or other lubricant gels (e.g., K-Y Jelly).

Table 1-3 lists some problems that can occur with Romanowsky-type stains and some proposed solutions to these problems. One of the most commonly encountered problems is simply understaining the slides. Slides are often understained when they are highly cellular or stained with old stains. With well-stained smears, the nucleus of most cells should be a dark purple, and clear demarcation of the nucleus and cytoplasm should be present (see Chapter 2). When slides are understained, cells and nuclei may appear pink, it may be difficult to distinguish the boundary between the nucleus and the cytoplasm, or the cells may just appear excessively faded or "muted." It may be difficult for the beginning cytologist to recognize understaining if he or she is not familiar with what the cells should look like. However, most cytology preparations will contain some neutrophils or other peripheral blood cells whose morphology is more likely to be familiar to the observer. These cells can be used as an internal control for staining quality. If the slides appear understained, they can simply be placed in the stains for an additional period. However, restaining should optimally be done before immersion oil is placed on the slides.

SUBMISSION OF SAMPLES TO THE LABORATORY

If the clinician is not going to evaluate the slides in-house, the final step in processing of cytologic samples is ensuring that they arrive at the laboratory intact. Many well-made, potentially diagnostic slides have met their doom at the hands of various postal services. Thin cardboard slide mailers (Figure 1-26) do not offer adequate protection for slides being mailed to outside laboratories and often result in broken, unreadable slides. Rigid plastic or polystyrene foam mailers (Figure 1-27) are suitable for mailing slides and generally prevent breakage. If these are not available, slides should be wrapped in protective material (i.e., paper towel) and mailed in a small, sturdy box. Alternatively, slides can be placed in a large plastic pill bottle and then placed in a mailing envelope.

If samples of body fluids are submitted along with slides, small EDTA tubes will fit inside standard

TABLE 1-3

Some Possible Solutions to Problems Seen with Common Romanowsky-Type Stains

Problem	Solution
Excessive Blue Staining (red blood cells may be blue-green)	
Prolonged stain contact	Decrease staining time.
Inadequate wash	Wash longer.
Specimen too thick	Make thinner smears, if possible.
Stain, diluent, buffer, or wash water too alkaline	Check with pH paper and correct pH.
Exposure to formalin vapors	Store and ship cytologic preps separate from formalin containers.
Wet fixation in ethanol or formalin	Air-dry smears before fixation.
Delayed fixation	Fix smears sooner if possible.
Surface of the slide being alkaline	Use new slides.
Excessive pink staining	
Insufficient staining time	Increase staining time.
Prolonged washing	Decrease duration of wash.
Stain or diluent too acidic	Check with pH paper and correct pH; fresh methanol may be needed.
Excessive time in red stain solution	Decrease time in red solution.
Inadequate time in blue stain solution	Increase time in blue stain solution.
Mounting coverslip before preparation is dry	Allow preparation to dry completely before mounting coverslip.
Weak staining	
Insufficient contact with one or more of the stain solutions	Increase staining time.
Fatigued (old) stains	Change stains.
Another slide covered specimen during staining	Keep slides separate.
Uneven staining	
Variation of pH in different areas of slide surface (may be from slide surface being touched or slide being poorly cleaned)	Use new slides and avoid touching them before and after preparation.
Water allowed to stand on some areas of the slide after staining and washing	Tilt slides close to vertical to drain water from the surface, or dry with a fan.
Inadequate mixing of stain and buffer	Mix stain and buffer thoroughly.
Precipitate on preparation	
Inadequate stain filtration	Filter or change the stain(s).
Inadequate washing of slide after staining	Rinse slides well after staining.
Dirty slides used	Use clean new slides.
Stain solution drying during staining	Use sufficient stain, and do not leave it on slide too long.
Miscellaneous	
Overstained preparations	Destain with 95% methanol and restain; Diff-Quik–stained smears may have to be destained in the red Diff-Quik stain solution to remove the blue color; however, this damages the red stain solution.
Refractile artifact red blood cells with Diff-Quik stain (usually due to moisture in fixative)	Change the fixative.

polystyrene foam slide mailers or can be placed inside a larger cardboard box. Most overnight mailing services require that body fluids be double-sealed and placed in specially designed plastic envelopes, which they provide.

Slides mailed to an outside laboratory should be labeled with the names of the patient and the owner and the location from which the sample was collected. Microscope slides used for cytology (or hematology) should have frosted or colored edges that can be written on with a pencil. It is difficult to permanently label slides without frosted edges, and this can lead to samples being mixed up. The ink from most marking pens (even the "permanent" markers) is soluble in cytologic stains and will wash off during the staining procedure, leaving the slides unidentifiable. In contrast, pencil markings on frosted slides will not erase during staining. Many slides without frosted ends arrive at labs with patient identification written on small pieces of white bandage tapes affixed to the edge of the slide. With many types of automatic slide stainers, these labels must be removed before the slides can be stained, again leading to potential misidentification of the sample.

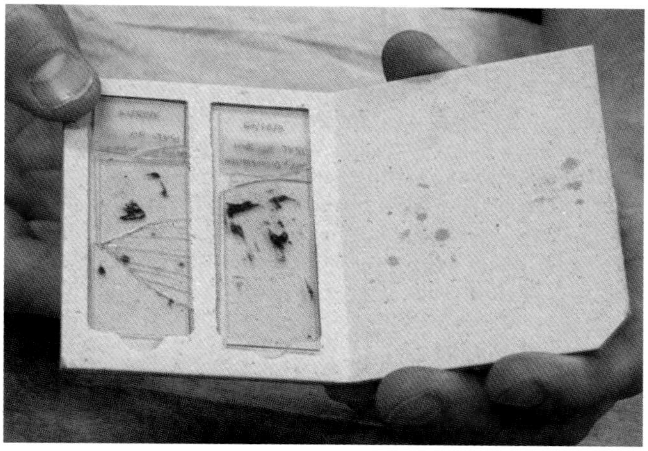

Figure 1-26 Cardboard containers do not offer sufficient protection for mailing slides. If the slides are not put in additional protective packaging, they often become broken in transit. (Courtesy Oklahoma State University teaching files.)

As a final note, unstained cytology slides should never be mailed with, or even stored near, samples in formalin. Formalin fumes will penetrate most any packaging, even biopsy samples in plastic jars with screw-top lids that are sealed in plastic zip-top bags. Formalin fumes partially fix the cells on air-dried smears and markedly interfere with subsequent staining (Figure 1-28), often making the slides totally uninterpretable.

SUBMISSION OF SAMPLES FOR CULTURE

Although this text deals primarily with cytologic evaluation of samples, with many samples (particularly fluids) submitted for cytology, culture is also indicated. Culture results are strongly influenced by sample collection, preparation, and transport. The following procedures are suggested to optimize success in culturing lesions and fluids:

- Call the laboratory before collecting the sample.
- Collect the sample as aseptically as possible.
- Submit fresh samples for culture.
- Use proper methods for collection and transport of the sample.
- Use a timely transportation service.

Call the Laboratory Before Collecting the Sample

Techniques, media, days when cultures are read or subcultures are performed, and so forth, often vary from laboratory to laboratory. By contacting the laboratory to which the sample will be submitted, such things as optimal sample type, transport medium, day of the week to submit the sample, and so on can be discussed. Also, some laboratories furnish culture supplies. Expensive supplies, quickly outdated supplies, or both, for example, blood culture tubes, may be ordered from the laboratory, as needed. Early communication with the laboratory also allows the laboratory to prepare for the sample and ensure that any special media required are available.

Collect Samples as Aseptically as Possible

All samples should be collected as aseptically as possible. Even samples collected from lesions that naturally are exposed to secondary contamination, for example,

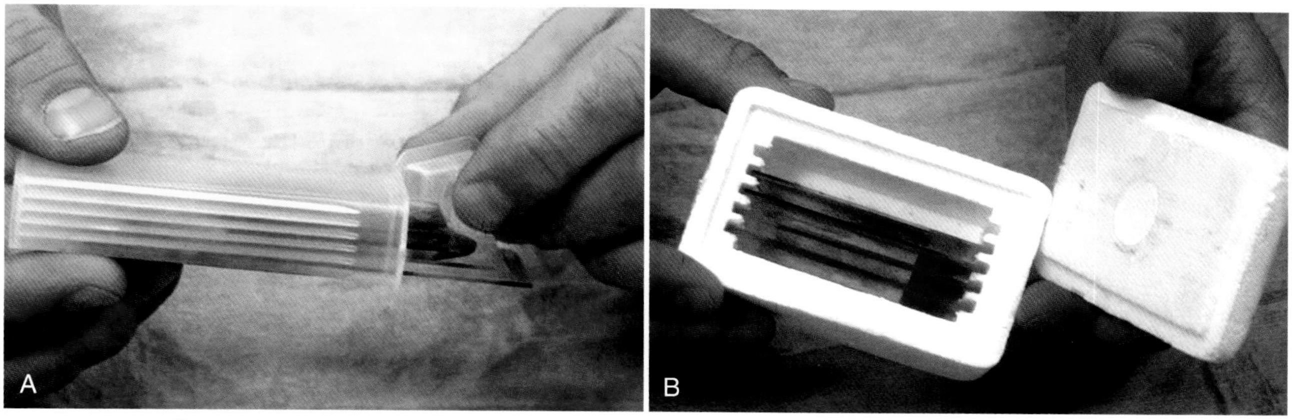

Figure 1-27 Rigid plastic (*A*) and polystyrene foam mailers (*B*), shown here, do a good job of protecting slides for mailing. Slides in these types of containers can usually be put directly in mailing envelopes with no additional protective packaging. (Courtesy Oklahoma State University teaching files.)

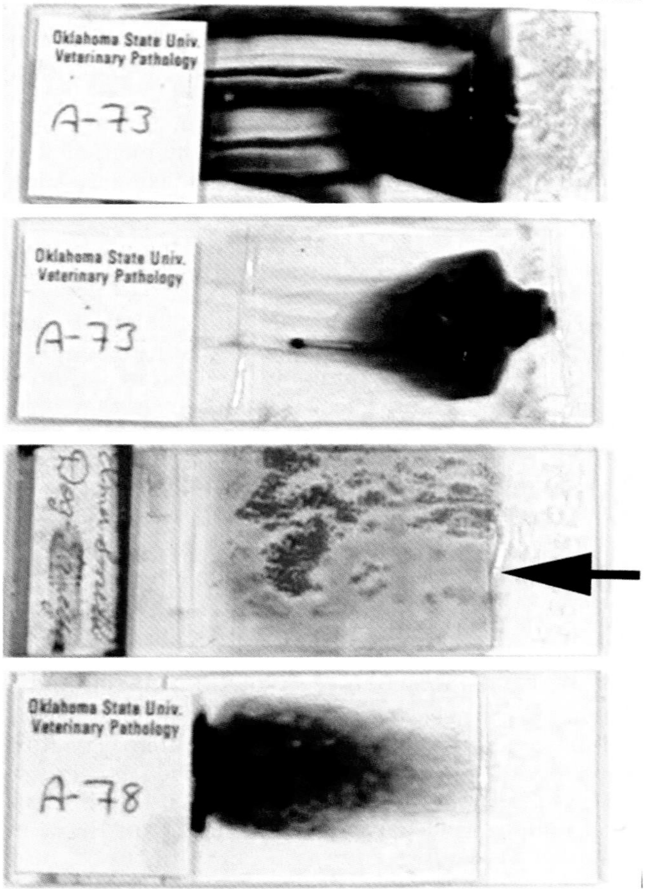

Figure 1-28 Effect of formalin fumes on unstained cytology slides. The slide second from the bottom (*arrow*) was mailed with a biopsy sample in formalin. After staining, the slide has a characteristic color that is different from the other slides that were not exposed to formalin. This partial fixation alters the staining of the cells and often makes it impossible to interpret the sample.

cutaneous ulcers, should be protected from further contamination. When samples are collected from more than one lesion, care should be taken not to cross-contaminate the samples. Finding the same organism in several different lesions is strong evidence that the organism is involved in development of the lesions. Therefore, cross-contamination of samples from different lesions can lead to misinterpretation of culture results. When fluids are collected, anticoagulant and serum tubes should not be presumed to be sterile. Serum tubes generally are identified as sterile or nonsterile on the label of the tube. Also, EDTA, because of its effect on bacterial cell walls, can be bacteriostatic or bactericidal and should therefore be avoided.

Submit Fresh Samples

Samples should be submitted as soon after collection as possible. Fluid aspiration, resection of lesions to be cultured, exploratory surgeries during which culture is anticipated, and other procedures that may produce samples to be cultured should be scheduled to allow immediate transportation of samples to the laboratory. During transport, samples should be kept cool but not frozen.

Use Proper Methods for Collection and Transport of Samples

Tissue and fluid samples usually are more rewarding than swab samples for isolation of a causative agent. Individual tissue samples submitted for culture should be about 4 cm^2 or larger. Whirl-Pak bags, which are sterile and sealable, are excellent for submitting samples for culture. If the interior of the tissue is to be cultured by the laboratory, clean and sealable plastic bags are sufficient. To avoid cross-contamination, all tissues should be packaged separately. To prevent drying during transport, small biopsies such as punch biopsies of skin lesions should be placed in a transport system with maintenance medium. Shipping biopsies in sterile saline should be avoided, as this may result in false-negative culture results.

Culture of subcutaneous or internal tissues can be collected in a minimally invasive manner by performing a fine-needle aspiration procedure into a syringe that has been prefilled with an appropriate liquid culture medium such as from blood culture bottles. Following the aspiration procedure, the culture medium in the syringe is expelled, through the needle containing the collected tissue, into a sterile tube.[10]

Fluid samples (i.e., urine, milk, joint fluid, thoracic fluid, abdominal fluid, abscess aspirates) to be cultured should be placed in containers that are sterile and leakproof such as sterile Vacutainer tubes or sterile disposable syringes.

For collection of samples for which swabs must be used (epithelial surfaces, fistulous tracts), the swabs should be placed in a maintenance medium that allows preservation with little to no replication of microbes so that the quantity and quality of the microbial flora of the swab remain as intact as possible. A variety of transport tubes containing maintenance media are commercially available for optimal transport of swabs for isolating bacteria, chlamydia, or viruses (Culturette, Transwab, Transtube, and CultureSwab). The bacterial media systems usually support a wide variety of bacteria for up to 72 hours at 20°C to 25°C. Swabs without media can dry out during transport, resulting in false-negative results, whereas swabs submitted in broth culture medium often are overgrown by contaminants. Separate swabs should be submitted if additional cultures for fungi, viruses, or both are desired.

Samples for anaerobic culturing require special handling and transport. The main objective is to limit, as much as possible, the exposure of the sample to oxygen and, thus, to air. Swabs are the least desirable means for specimen collection for anaerobes because of the difficulty of limiting the exposure of the sample to air. Fluids for anaerobic culturing should be collected in syringes, with air excluded. The needle is then plugged with a sterile rubber stopper or bent double to prevent intake of air and transported immediately to the laboratory for culture. If samples for anaerobic culturing cannot reach the laboratory within 2 hours, the sample must be placed into some type of anaerobic transport system. Several commercial systems are now available for transporting all types of specimens for anaerobic culture. Port-A-Cul systems contain a prereduced transport medium in a soft agar with reducing agents to maintain anaerobiosis and offer vials for fluid specimens, jars for small tissues and swabs, and tubes for swabs. Self-contained, gas-generating systems are also available, and these systems provide their own anaerobic atmosphere once the sample is placed in the container and the system sealed. Such systems are available for swabs (Anaerobic Culturette, Becton Dickinson Microbiology Systems) and as sealable plastic bags (Bio-Bag, Gas-Pak Pouch). The bags can be used for transporting large tissue specimens, fluids contained within syringes, and aerobic swab systems for anaerobic culturing.

In general, samples submitted for fungal culture should be collected and transported in the same manner as samples for bacterial culture, with the exception of dermatophyte cultures.

Scrapings and hair plucked from the periphery of suspected dermatophyte lesions should be submitted in clean containers that remain dry during transit. Bacterial overgrowth of dermatophyte cultures is a common problem and can be eliminated by disinfecting suspect dermatophyte lesions with alcohol prior to obtaining samples. Vacutainer tubes and similar tightly sealable containers are to be avoided because condensate tends to form within them, allowing overgrowth of contaminants. Clean paper envelopes are suitable specimen containers. For transport, the envelope should be packaged within a more durable wrapper. Swabs are the least preferred samples for fungal cultures and should never be used for dermatophyte isolation attempts.

Use a Timely Transportation Service

Care in collection of samples would be futile if the samples were not received in the laboratory in a timely manner, which generally means 48 hours or less. Most microbiology laboratories deal with various carriers on a daily basis and can advise what carrier to use. Packaging specimens to guard against breakage and leakage not only protects against specimen loss but also protects package handlers against potential infection. The clinician must be aware of special requirements to be taken when shipping biohazardous materials, including some clinical specimens. If in doubt regarding how to package specimens for transport, the microbiology laboratory to which the specimens will be sent should be contacted.

References

1. Meinkoth JH, Cowell RL: Sample collection and preparation in cytology: increasing diagnostic yield, *Vet Clin North Am* 32:1187–1207, 2002.
2. Meyer DJ, Connolly SL, Heng HG: The acquisition and management of cytology specimens. In Raskin RE, Meyer DJ, editors: *Atlas of canine and feline cytology*, ed 2, Philadelphia, 2010, Saunders, pp 1–14.
3. Lumsden JH, Baker R: Cytopathology techniques and interpretation. In Baker R, Lumsden JH, editors: *Color atlas of cytology of the dog and cat*, St. Louis, MO, 2000, Mosby, pp 7–20.
4. Menard M, Papageorges M: Fine-needle biopsies: how to increase diagnostic yield, *Comp Cont Ed Pract Vet* 19:738–740, 1997.
5. DeMay RM: *The art and science of cytopathology*, Chicago, IL, 1996, ASCP. 464–483.
6. Menard M, Papageorges M: Technique for ultrasound-guided fine needle biopsies, *Vet Rad Ult* 36:137–138, 1995.
7. Caruso K, Cowell RL, Cowell AK, et al: Skin scraping from a cat, *Vet Clin Path* 31(1):13–15, 2002.
8. Jörundsson E, Lumsden JH, Jacobs RM: Rapid staining techniques in cytopathology: a review and comparison of modified protocols for hematoxylin and eosin, Papanicolaou and Romanowsky stains, *Vet Clin Path* 28:100–108, 1999.
9. Allison RW, Velguth KE: Appearance of granulated cells in blood films stained by automated aqueous versus methanolic Romanowsky methods, *Vet Clin Path* 39:99–104, 2009.
10. Meinkoth KR, Morton RJ, Meinkoth JH: Naturally occurring tularemia in a dog, *J Am Vet Med Assoc* 225:545–547, 2004.

CHAPTER

2

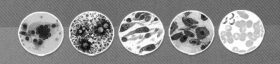

Cell Types and Criteria of Malignancy

James H. Meinkoth, Rick L. Cowell and Ronald D. Tyler

Examining cytologic preparations often presents a potentially confusing array of different cell types as well as a potentially endless variety of cell debris and contaminants. With experience, most of the common lesions are recognized quickly. In case of a lesion or sample site not previously encountered, it is helpful to keep in mind certain fundamental questions that need to be considered when evaluating a sample. Cells can usually be classified into one of a few basic categories, based on common features shared by different cells in that category.[1-4] Recognizing the common features of the different basic cell types sometimes makes it possible to classify cells that are not obvious at first.

An orderly approach to examining slides and answering certain questions in a logical order will reduce the chances of missing important information or misdiagnosing or overdiagnosing the sample.

ARE SUFFICIENT NUMBERS OF WELL-STAINED, WELL-PRESERVED, INTACT CELLS PRESENT TO BE EVALUATED?

A basic premise of cytology is that interpretations are generally based on entire populations of cells, not on low numbers of individual cells. Any one cell or few cells from a lesion may show features that are atypical or unusual. This is especially true if cells are coming from a tissue in which the cells are not well preserved or exposed to injurious stimuli. Cells coming from inflammatory reactions or areas of tissue repair often show cellular atypia that is the result of dysplasia.

In addition to atypia seen with inflammation and tissue repair, cells that undergo aging changes may be difficult to interpret. Cells present in fluid samples (e.g., thoracocentesis, abdominocentesis) may undergo morphologic changes over time if slides are not made immediately after collection. These changes can range from subtle alterations such as cellular or nuclear swelling and altered staining characteristics to overt pyknosis or lysis. Even if slides are prepared immediately after collection, cells may have undergone in vivo aging. Cells from the fluid portion of cystic lesions (such as some mammary tumors) or cells that have been in prolonged contact with urine (such as urine sediment preparations or urethral or bladder samples collected by traumatic catheterization) often have significant artifacts that must not be misinterpreted as criteria of malignancy.

Interpretations based on inadequately cellular specimens that may not contain a representative sample of the lesion could give a false impression of normalcy or, even worse, may result in a false impression of neoplasia that is not really present. Although no easily defined limit to the question, "How many cells are enough?" exists, slides should have many cells per field across a large portion of the slide. It has been said that if the question "Is the specimen adequately cellular or not?" even comes to mind when looking at the slide, it probably is not.[3] When a large lesion is being evaluated, several smears of good cellularity collected from different areas of the lesion should be evaluated to assess any variability that may be present within different parts of the lesion. Large neoplasms may have areas of inflammation or necrosis that will yield markedly different cell populations compared with adjacent areas.

The cellularity of the smear is often evident the moment the slides are stained. A slide containing high numbers of nucleated cells is visibly blue after staining. Slides that are perfectly clear after staining probably have low numbers of nucleated cells, although sufficient cells may still be present for a diagnosis. Therefore, cellularity must be confirmed by looking at the slide under the microscope. Even for practitioners who do not have the time or desire to evaluate cytology preparations themselves, it is beneficial to stain one or two smears and determine that an adequately cellular specimen is being sent off for evaluation.

When examined microscopically, the slides should first be scanned using low power (10× to 20×) to assess the cellularity of the slide and find the area(s) containing the highest number of well-stained, well-spread-out, intact cells for evaluation (Figure 2-1). Cells are often unevenly distributed across the slides, especially with impression smears or aspirates of solid tissue lesions. Even with slides made from fluid samples, large cells may all be pulled out to the feathered edge, where they can be easily overlooked if the whole slide is not scanned first (Figure 2-2).

After locating the cellular areas of the slides, it is important to determine whether the cells are sufficiently spread out for evaluation, intact and well stained. This can usually also be done on low power (10× to 20×), which

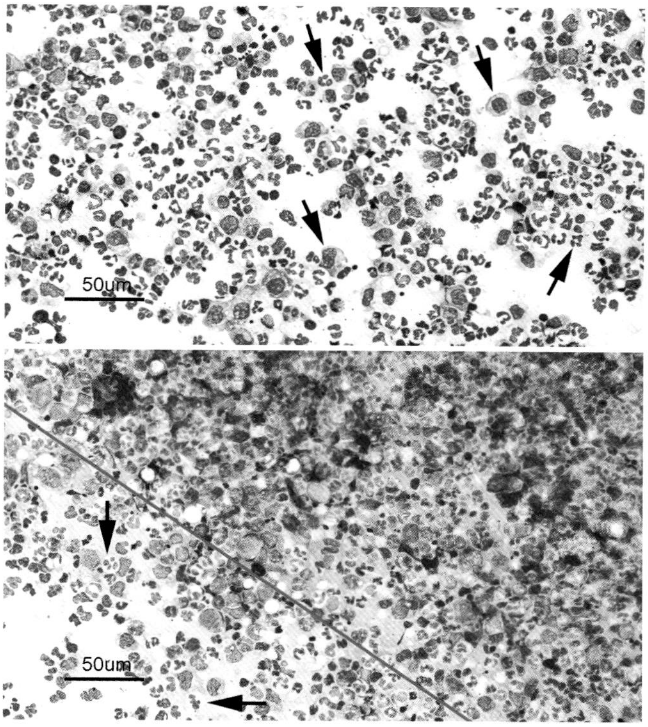

Figure 2-1 Low-power image of different areas of a slide. The top image shows an area that although highly cellular, is well spread out and the cells are well stained. Although cell detail is difficult to evaluate at this magnification, it is possible to see the characteristic nuclear shape of some well-spread-out neutrophils and to differentiate the nucleus and cytoplasm of mononuclear cells (*arrows*). The lower image shows another area from the same slide where the cells are not well spread out and thus have not stained well. Most of the area above and to the right of the red line is too thick to evaluate. A few well-spread-out cells are seen in the lower left (*arrows*).

will allow a greater portion of the slide to be evaluated in a short time. Inexperienced cytologists often frustrate themselves by spending an inordinate amount of time trying to identify cells that cannot be interpreted because they are not spread out, are poorly stained, or are ruptured. Intact, well-stained, well-spread cells should have a clearly evident demarcation between the nucleus and the cytoplasm (Figure 2-3). The nucleus may be irregularly shaped (particularly in neoplastic cells), but the nuclear outline should be smooth and distinct. A fuzzy appearance around the outline of the nucleus generally indicates that the cell has been minimally traumatized during sample collection, preparation, or both. More significant cell trauma can result in the nucleus appearing fragmented or full of holes (see Figure 2-3). Severely traumatized cells will often appear as strands of light pink nuclear chromatin (Figure 2-4). Some traumatized or ruptured cells will be present in virtually any cytologic specimen. The sample is usually still interpretable if the majority of the cells are intact; however, the traumatized cells are not evaluated. This is particularly important when determining criteria of malignancy because nuclei may appear enlarged and nucleoli may appear more prominent in traumatized cells. If the majority of the cells are traumatized or ruptured, additional samples usually need to be collected.

Cells that are not well spread out often stain diffusely dark, and it is difficult to recognize the line of demarcation and color distinction between the cytoplasm and the nucleus (Figure 2-5). Usually, the contrast between the blue cytoplasm and the purple (or pink-purple) nucleus can be seen at relatively low magnification if the cells are well spread out. Poorly spread, poorly stained cells often appear only as different shades of blue. This allows the observer to scan large areas of the slide quickly at low magnification to find areas of the slide worth examining at higher magnification.

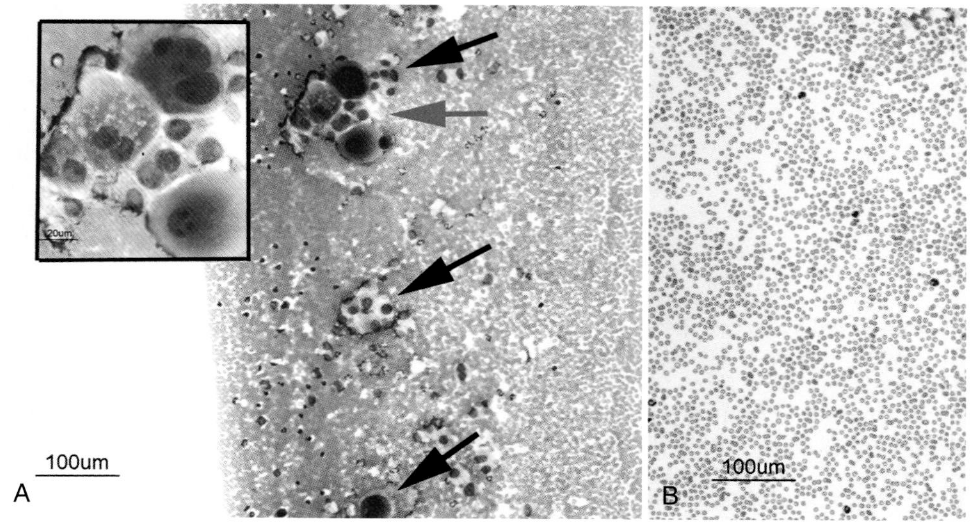

Figure 2-2 Images from a slide made from hemorrhagic pleural effusion showing uneven distribution of cells on the slide. A, Numerous large clusters of cells (*arrows*) have all been pulled out to the edge of the smear. Some of these show marked atypia allowing for a diagnosis of neoplastic effusion (carcinoma). Inset shows higher magnification of atypical cell cluster indicated by the red arrow. **B,** The majority of the smear contained predominantly erythrocytes with a few small nuclei (neutrophils and macrophages) visible. Scanning on low power quickly allowed the atypical cells to be found at the edge of the smear. These could have easily been overlooked if the observer started out at high magnification in the body of the smear.

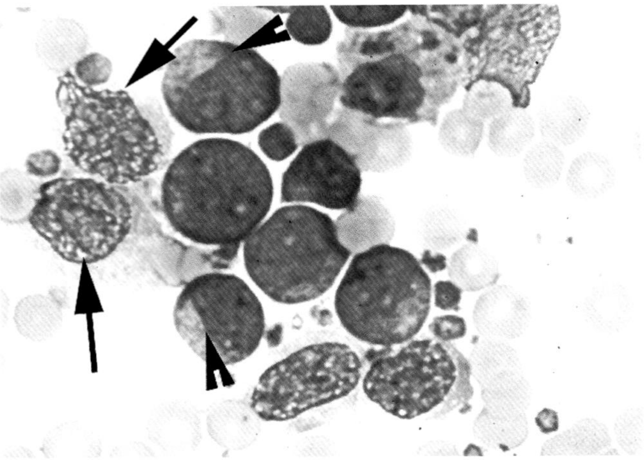

Figure 2-3 Lymph node aspirate from a dog showing well-spread-out cells. A clear distinction can be seen between the nucleus and the cytoplasm (*arrowheads*). Several traumatized cells are also present. Note that their nuclear chromatin appears excessively fragmented (*arrows*).

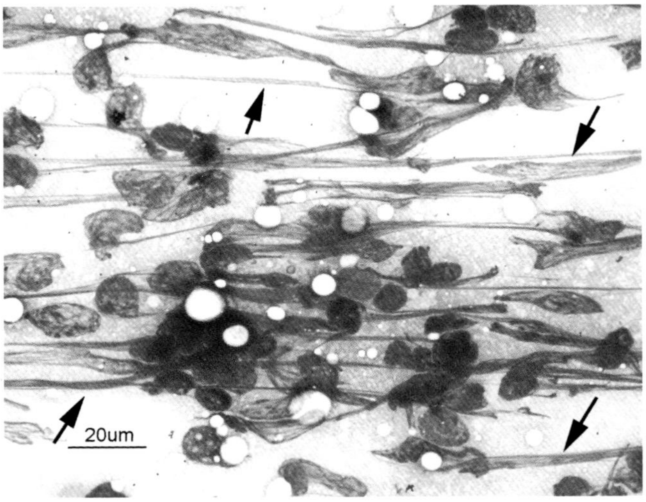

Figure 2-4 Severely traumatized cells. The streaks of material (*arrows*) represent smeared-out nuclear chromatin from ruptured cells.

Nucleoli will often be more prominent than usual in understained cells, and this can result in a false impression of malignancy if this artifact is not recognized. The nuclei of well-stained cells are usually dark purple, generally more intensely and deeply stained than the surrounding cytoplasm. Some variation will exist in the intensity and pattern of nuclear staining between cell types. In case of uncertainty as to whether light staining of nuclei is a characteristic of the cell or the result of understaining, it may be helpful to evaluate the staining of more familiar cells. Usually, some neutrophils will be present as the result of peripheral blood contamination or inflammation within the lesion and make a good reference to evaluate how well cells are stained (and spread out).

In most specimens, significant variation in cellularity, degree of cell spreading, and, hence, staining quality from area to area on the slide will exist. This is particularly true of highly cellular specimens such as lymph node aspirates, which may have areas that are of diagnostic quality even if the majority of the slide is thick and understained. Diligent scanning of the slides on low power is necessary to find these areas before attempting to evaluate the cells at higher magnification. If the entire slide is found to be understained, restaining the slide before immersion oil is added may improve the staining quality and result in a diagnostic sample.

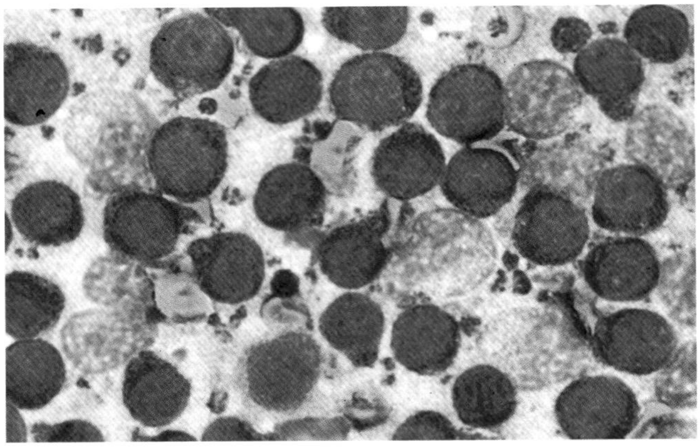

Figure 2-5 Poorly spread-out cells from a different area of the same slide shown in Figure 2-3. The cells are diffusely dark with the nuclei and cytoplasm staining different shades of blue. Compare this with the purple color of the well-spread-out nuclei in Figure 2-3. Also, it is difficult to discern the demarcation between the nucleus and the cytoplasm.

ARE ALL OF THE CELLS ON THE SMEAR INFLAMMATORY CELLS?

A good initial decision, particularly for the beginning cytologist, is to determine if the smear is composed entirely of inflammatory cells. In most general practices, inflammatory lesions are more commonly sampled compared with neoplastic lesions. Also, most clinicians initially feel more comfortable recognizing inflammatory cells because they are more familiar with the morphology of these cells, having viewed them many times in peripheral blood smears. Many clinicians choose to screen their cytology specimens, interpreting inflammatory lesions in-house and submitting those composed of tissue cells to an outside agency. Although inflammatory cells in tissues often look the same as they do in peripheral blood, some may appear different because of morphologic changes induced by their presence in a focus of inflammation or simply because they are not well spread out. It is important to remember that it may not be possible to identify every cell present on a slide, or even on any given field, and that the interpretation is based on the entire cell population present.

If a lesion is found to be composed entirely of inflammatory cells, the relative percentages of the various types of inflammatory cells should be noted because this may provide clues as to the etiology of the inflammation. Finally, a search for infectious agents should be conducted. A discussion of the various inflammatory patterns

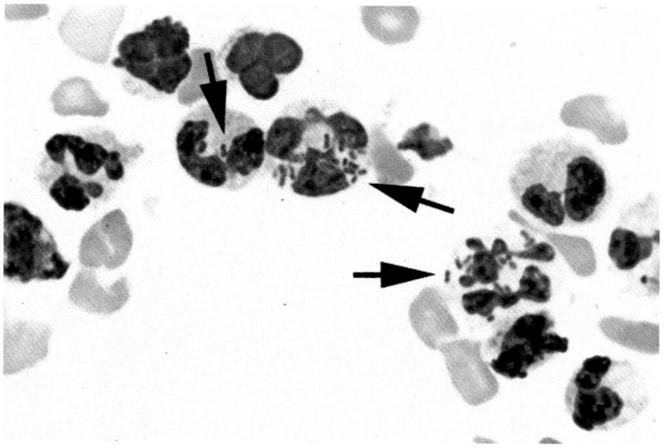

Figure 2-6 Septic neutrophilic inflammation. Many neutrophils are present, some of which contain phagocytized bacterial rods (*arrows*).

and morphology of common infectious agents will be covered more completely in Chapters 3 and 5 of this text.

Neutrophils

Neutrophils are commonly found in cytologic specimens. Their morphology is often similar to that observed in peripheral blood smears (Figure 2-6). Normal neutrophil nuclei stain dark purple and contain one to multiple distinct segments or lobes. The neutrophil cytoplasm is typically clear. Neutrophils are phagocytic cells and typically are the cells that phagocytize pathogenic bacteria, if present (see Figure 2-6). Although neutrophils contain intracytoplasmic granules, in most domestic animals, these generally do not stain prominently with cytologic stains. Sometimes, however, these granules will be discernible as elongated, faintly eosinophilic structures, and they must not be confused with bacteria or lightly staining eosinophil granules.

In thick preparations or in viscous fluids such as synovial fluid, neutrophils may not spread out well, and the segmented nature of their nucleus may be less evident. Sometimes, the nucleus will be essentially round mimicking a lymphocyte, but the cell can still be identified as a neutrophil by the lobulated outline of the nucleus. More normal neutrophil morphology can be observed in the thinner areas (often along the edges) of the smear.

Neutrophils may undergo several morphologic changes in tissues. Aging change is a commonly encountered phenomenon. The initial change seen is hypersegmentation of the nucleus (Figure 2-7). Sometimes, an elongated thin strand of nuclear material (Figure 2-8) connects the nuclear lobes of aged neutrophils. This is commonly seen in cytocentrifuged preparations from fluids. The end result of aging change is pyknosis of the nucleus. *Pyknosis* is condensation of the nuclear chromatin into one or more small discrete, densely staining spheres lacking any nuclear chromatin pattern (see Figure 2-7). Aging artifact simply represents neutrophils dying of "old age" and must not be confused with degenerative change.

Degenerative change occurs when neutrophils are present in an environment that is damaging to the cell. It is commonly seen in neutrophils from lesions in which endotoxin-producing bacteria are present. The presence of many neutrophils with marked degenerative change should prompt a diligent search for bacteria. Degenerative change is an acquired change and is distinct from the toxic changes noted in peripheral blood neutrophils. Degenerative change occurs when the neutrophil is unable to control water homeostasis and undergoes hydropic degeneration. The hallmark of degenerative change is nuclear swelling (Figure 2-9). The nucleus of the cell swells and appears thicker, stains a lighter eosinophilic color, and loses nuclear lobation. Degenerative neutrophils often resemble large band cells.

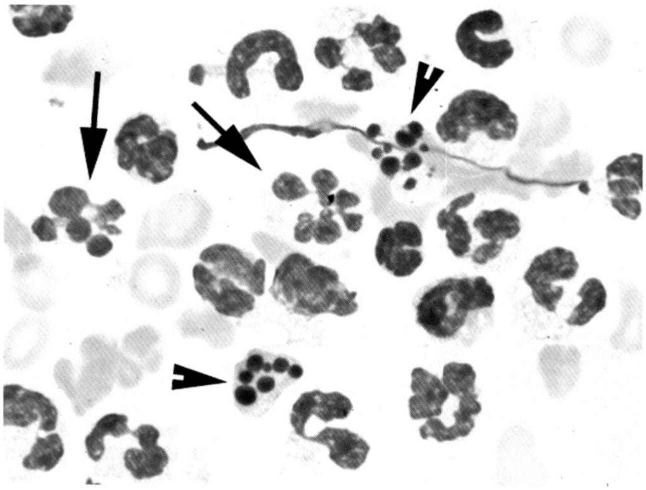

Figure 2-7 Sample from a nonseptic inflammatory lesion. Many of the neutrophils show nuclear hypersegmentation (*arrows*), an aging artifact. This will ultimately lead to pyknotic change (*arrowheads*) in which the nuclear chromatin condenses and fragments into several discrete, dense spheres.

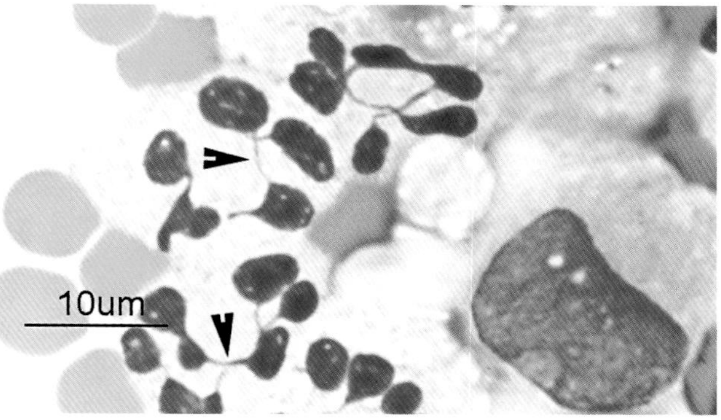

Figure 2-8 Hypersegmentation of neutrophils in which elongated thin filaments connect the nuclear lobes (*arrowheads*)**.** This is a common manifestation of aged neutrophils in fluid samples prepared by cytocentrifugation.

Macrophages

Macrophages in inflammatory lesions are derived from peripheral blood monocytes. Many tissues have low numbers of fixed tissue macrophages as normal resident cells (e.g., Kupffer cells in the liver). Macrophages may display extremely variable morphology in tissues, which can be somewhat confusing. Initially, they may resemble

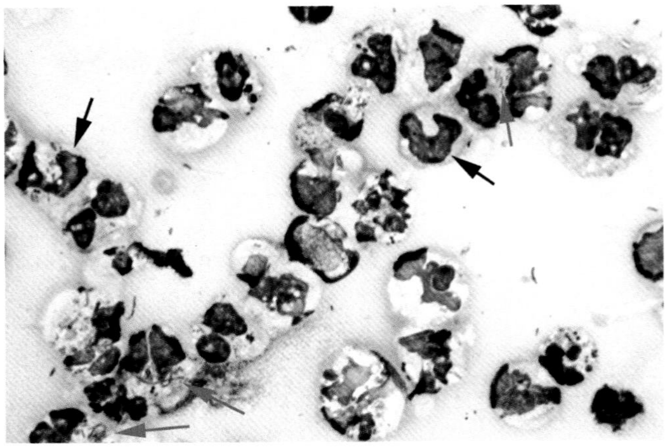

Figure 2-9 Neutrophils showing degenerative change. Degenerative change is evidenced by nuclear swelling (*black arrows*), which leads to loss of distinct segmentation. As the nucleus swells the neutrophils may appear band shaped, or in more severe change, the nucleus may appear round or overtly lytic. Degenerative change is commonly associated with the presence of endotoxin-producing-bacteria. Many bacterial rods (*red arrows*) were present on this slide.

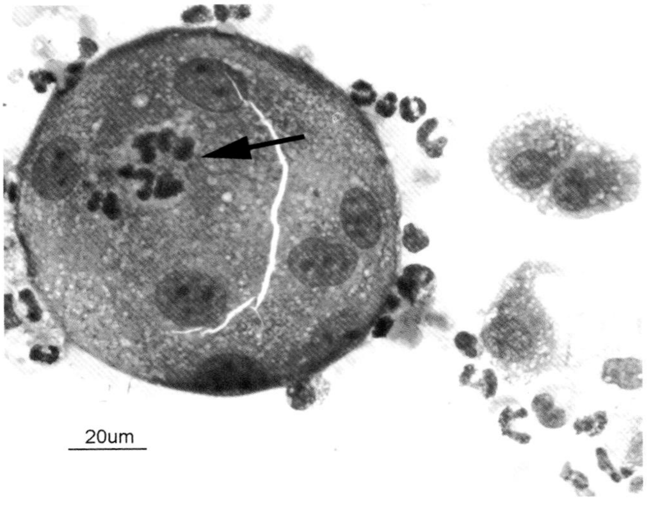

Figure 2-11 Smear from a pyogranulomatous inflammatory reaction (*Actinomyces* infection). An extremely large, multinucleated macrophage is present. The macrophage has phagocytized several neutrophils.

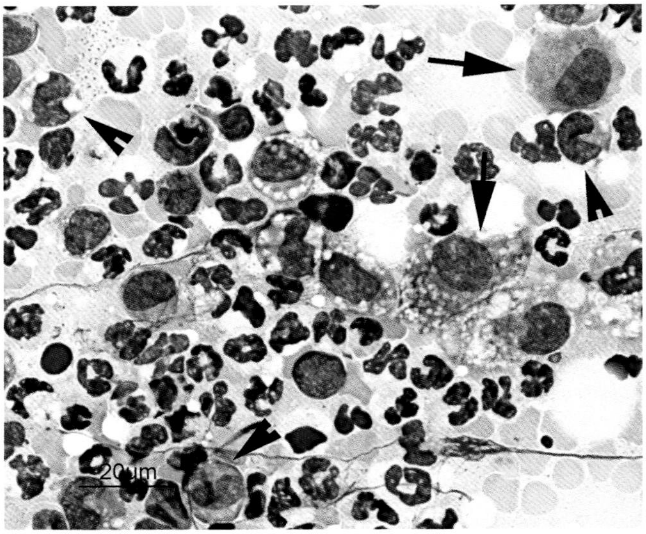

Figure 2-10 Pyogranulomatous inflammatory response demonstrating many macrophages. Some macrophages resemble peripheral blood monocytes (*arrowheads*). Other macrophages are variably increased in size resulting from increased amounts of cytoplasm that is sometimes vacuolated (*arrows*).

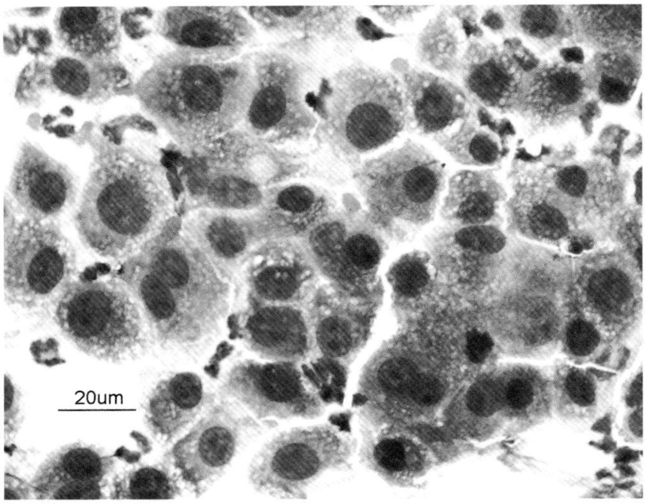

Figure 2-12 Impression smear of a nodule on pleural surface of a dog with pyothorax caused by *Actinomyces* spp. infection. Numerous large epithelioid macrophages are present. These cells have abundant basophilic cytoplasm that may be nonvacuolated to minimally vacuolated. They may also occur in large aggregates resembling epithelial cell clusters.

peripheral blood monocytes (Figure 2-10). With time, the nucleus becomes round and the cell enlarges as the cytoplasm becomes greatly expanded and, sometimes, extremely vacuolated. Macrophages are also phagocytic cells, typically phagocytizing larger structures such as fungal organisms and other cells. Many times, the cytoplasm of macrophages will contain partially phagocytized debris that cannot be identified but must not be misinterpreted as an infectious agent.

Binucleate or multinucleate macrophages are commonly encountered in longstanding inflammatory lesions (Figure 2-11). Multinucleated macrophages can get very large and are referred to as *inflammatory giant cells*. In some chronic inflammatory lesions, *epithelioid macrophages* may be encountered (Figure 2-12). This term is applied to macrophages that are enlarged with expansive cytoplasm that stains uniformly basophilic, giving the cell the look of an epithelial cell. Because these macrophages can also show variation in size and multinucleation, they could potentially be misinterpreted as neoplastic epithelial cells. Extreme caution should be exercised when diagnosing malignancy in the face of inflammation because of the potential for macrophages to display atypical criteria.

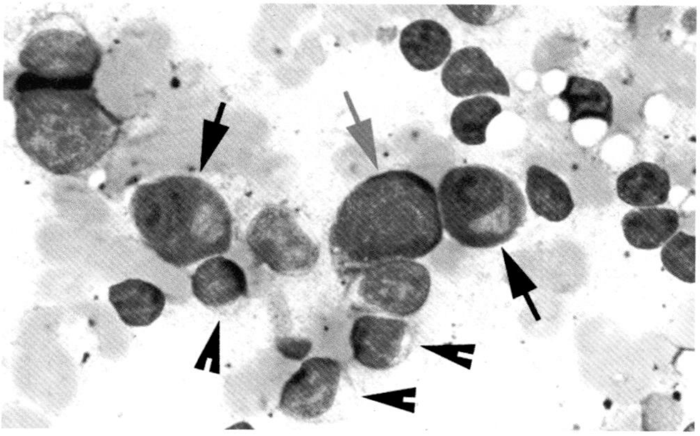

Figure 2-13 Smear made from an aspirate of a reactive lymph node. Many small lymphocytes are present (*arrowheads*). These cells have scant amounts of cytoplasm that do not appear to encircle the nucleus. Two plasma cells (*arrows*) are also present. One large, immature lymphoid cell (lymphoblast) is present (*red arrow*). Note that the lymphoblast and plasma cells are similar in size. However, the lymphoblast has a larger nucleus, whereas the nucleus of the plasma cell is similar in size to a small lymphocyte.

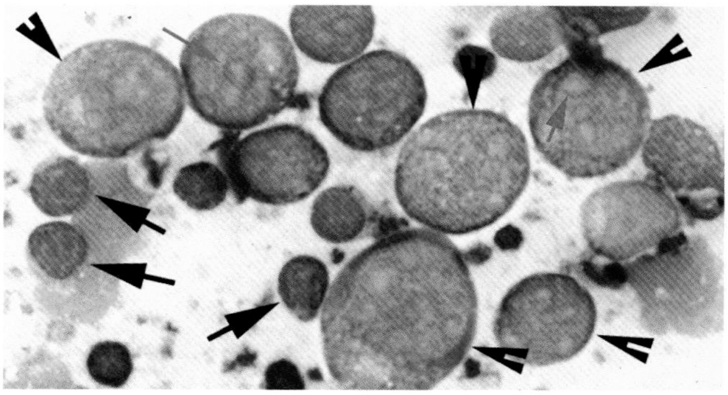

Figure 2-14 Image of a fine-needle aspirate smear of a lymph node from a dog with lymphoma containing numerous lymphoblasts (*arrowheads*) and lymphocytes (*arrows*). The lymphoblasts are larger and have more abundant cytoplasm. Nuclei are large with light staining, dispersed chromatin and often show prominent nucleoli (*red arrows*).

Lymphocytes (Small, Medium, and Large)

Small lymphocytes are smaller than neutrophils with rounded nuclei and scant basophilic cytoplasm (Figure 2-13). The nucleus is generally not perfectly round but will have a flattened or indented area on one side. The nuclear chromatin has a smudged appearance. Nucleoli are not visible; however, darker areas (heterochromatin) and lighter areas (euchromatin) are often visible. Generally, the cytoplasm is not visible completely around the circumference of the nucleus but is visible only on one side. Medium-sized lymphocytes may be present and are similar to small lymphocytes, but they have moderately increased amounts of cytoplasm and may have nucleoli visible. Large, blastic lymphocytes (lymphoblasts) (Figure 2-14), commonly encountered in aspirates of lymphoid tissue and lymphoid neoplasms, may be present in low numbers in inflammatory lesions. Lymphoblasts are large

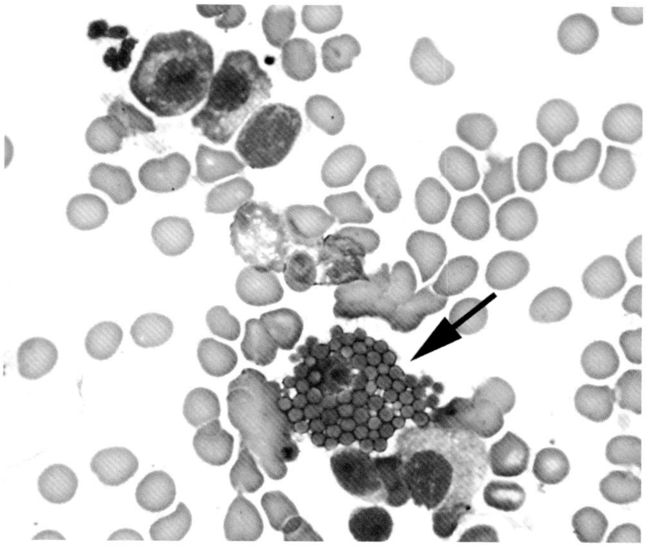

Figure 2-15 Image from a lymph node aspirate demonstrates small lymphocytes, plasma cells, and one Mott cell with numerous Russell bodies (*arrow*). The Russell bodies may range from appearing as clear vacuoles or may be somewhat basophilic as in this image. (Courtesy Dr. Robin Allison, Oklahoma State University.)

cells with enlarged nuclei and dispersed chromatin which stains a lighter pink-purple than that of mature cells (see Figure 2-14). Cytoplasm is more abundant, often visible around the complete circumference of the nucleus, and is typically deeply basophilic. Distinct nucleoli are often visible, and multiple nucleoli may be observed.

Reactive lymphocytes are those responding to antigenic stimulation. They have moderately increased amounts of basophilic cytoplasm. Plasma cells are differentiated B-lymphocytes stimulated to produce antibodies. Plasma cells have a round, eccentrically placed nucleus, moderate amounts of deeply basophilic cytoplasm, and usually a distinct clear area located next to the nucleus (see Figure 2-13). This clear area represents the Golgi apparatus and is often located between the nucleus and the greatest volume of cytoplasm. Plasma cells and lymphoblasts are both larger than small lymphocytes, but in plasma cells, most of the increase in size is caused by more abundant cytoplasm, whereas in the lymphoblast, the nucleus has enlarged (see Figure 2-13). Some plasma cells (termed *Mott cells*) have numerous large clear to basophilic vacuoles (termed *Russell bodies*) filling their cytoplasm (Figure 2-15). These vacuoles represent retained immunoglobulin.

Eosinophils

Eosinophils are slightly larger than neutrophils. Their nuclei are segmented but are commonly less lobated than those of neutrophils and often divided into only two distinct lobes (Figure 2-16). Rarely, eosinophils with perfectly round nuclei will be identified in cytologic specimens. The cytoplasm of eosinophils contains prominent orange-to-pink granules. In dogs, eosinophil granules are round and vary widely in size and number (Figure 2-17). Eosinophil granules are numerous, small, and rod shaped in cats (Figure 2-18). The delicate, densely packed granules

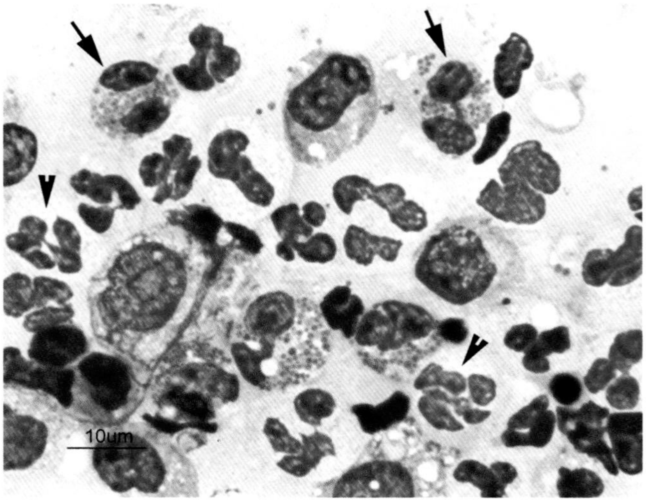

Figure 2-16 Image from an inflammatory reaction in the intestines of a dog containing a mixture of neutrophils, eosinophils, and macrophages. The nuclei of the eosinophils are typically less lobulated (*arrows*) than those of the neutrophils (*arrowheads*).

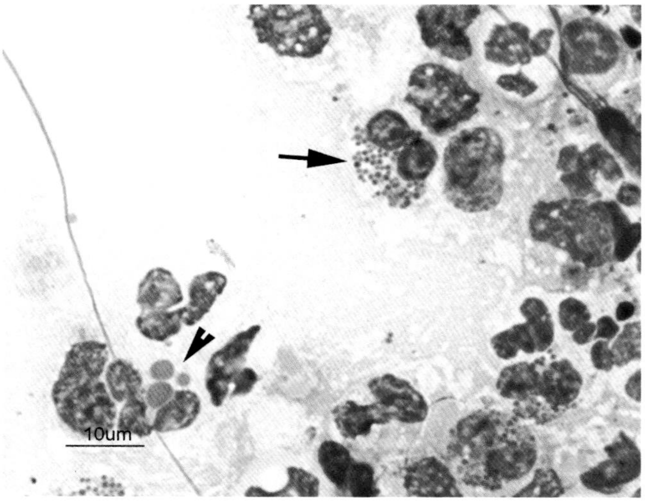

Figure 2-17 Image from the same slide as Figure 2-16. In the dog, eosinophils have numerous small granules (*arrow*) or just a few large granules (*arrowhead*).

of feline eosinophils are often less obvious than those of the dog, particularly in thick specimens such as transtracheal washes that may not stain well. Also, neutrophils in exudates will occasionally have mild eosinophilic stippling. Care must be taken not to confuse neutrophils and poorly stained eosinophils when trying to differentiate eosinophilic from neutrophilic inflammatory reactions in cats. The slightly larger and minimal nuclear lobation can help make the distinction. Often, it is easier to identify feline eosinophils that have been traumatized during slide preparation as their granules spread out and become more obvious. If many eosinophils have been ruptured during sample collection (such as with scraping of feline eosinophilic granuloma complex lesions), high numbers of eosinophil granules will be present throughout the

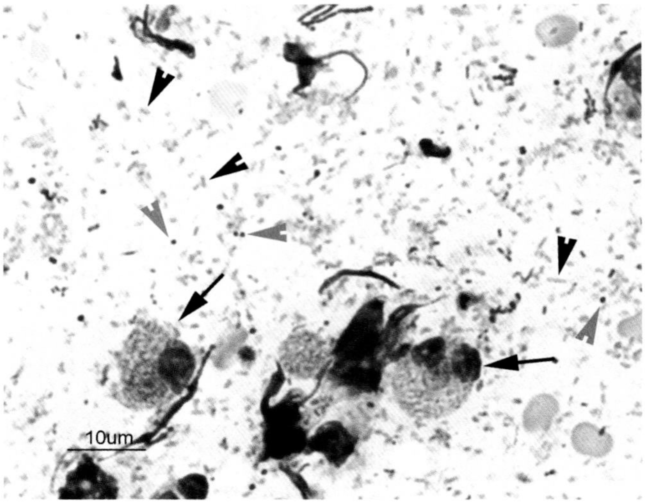

Figure 2-18 Scraping from an eosinophilic granuloma complex lesion in a cat. Cat eosinophils (*arrows*) have densely packed granules, often making it difficult to see the individual granules in intact cells. Numerous free granules (*black arrowheads*) released from ruptured cells are present and demonstrate the slender rod shape typical of feline eosinophil granules. Numerous bacteria (*red arrowheads*) are also present free in the background.

background of the smear and may be identified before intact cells are seen.

Occasionally, eosinophil granules will not stain well with Diff-Quik stain (similar to what sometimes occurs with mast cells) yet stain prominently with Wright stain or Wright-Giemsa stain.

IF A SMEAR IS COMPOSED OF TISSUE CELLS RATHER THAN INFLAMMATORY CELLS, WHAT TYPE OF CELLS ARE PRESENT?

A wide variety of specific cells may be encountered from the various normal tissues and tumors sampled cytologically. With experience, most of these cells can be easily recognized, particularly with the knowledge of what structure is being sampled. However, even if the cells are not immediately recognizable, they can generally be classified into one of three major categories on the basis of certain common cytologic features (Table 2-1):

1. Discrete cells (or round cells)
2. Epithelial cells
3. Mesenchymal cells

Categorization of cells according to the major group they belong to helps the evaluator identify the specific cell type present. Even if precise identification cannot be made, relevant information such as the presence of a cell type abnormal for the tissue sampled (e.g., epithelial cells in a lymph node aspirate) may be gained.

Discrete Cells (Round Cells)

Discrete cells are a group of cells that share certain cytologic features because they are present individually in tissues, not adhered to other cells or a connective tissue matrix. The majority of these cells are of hematogenous

TABLE 2-1

General Cytologic Characteristics of Different Tissue Cell Types

	Round Cells	Epithelial Cells	Mesenchymal Cells
Cellularity of slides	High cellularity	High cellularity	Low to high cellularity Normal mesenchymal cells and many tumors are of low cellularity because of adherence of cell in matrix Malignant tumors may yield high numbers of cells
Cell distribution	Evenly distributed across slide	Typically present in clusters Malignant cells may lose cohesion	Discretely oriented or adhered in aggregates by extracellular matrix
Cell size and shape	Small to medium sized Generally round with distinct cell borders	Small to large, depending on tissue samples Cuboidal to columnar to round depending on specific tissue Generally distinct cell borders when cells are individually oriented or at the edges of cell clusters	Often fusiform or "spindle shaped" Some cells may be plump or round (particularly cells from bone or bone tumors) Often have indistinct cytoplasmic borders
Other features suggestive of this cell type	Distinctive morphology or select individual cell types	Formation of acini or tubules Extremely large cells with abundant cytoplasm Squamous differentiation	Production of eosinophilic extracellular matrix

origin. Aspirates of normal lymphoid tissue such as the spleen and lymph nodes yield cell populations that have a discrete cell pattern. Other than normal lymphoid tissue, a discrete cell pattern usually indicates the presence of one of a group of tumors termed *discrete cell tumors* (or *round cell tumors*). Recognition of discrete cell tumors is important because these are some of the more common neoplasms encountered in small animal practice. Also, cells of most discrete cell tumors have cytologic characteristics that are sufficiently distinct to allow for a specific diagnosis.

General Cytologic Characteristics of Discrete Cell Populations: Because discrete cells are not adhered to other structures within the tissues, they generally exfoliate very readily during fine-needle biopsy (FNB). Hence, the cellularity of the resulting smears is usually very high. In addition, the individual cells are usually evenly spread throughout the smear (Figure 2-19). Cell clusters or aggregates are not present; however, the extremely high cellularity of the smears may result in cells being piled on top of each other in thicker areas of the smears and this may be misinterpreted as cell adhesion (or cell clustering). In the thinner areas of the smears, the cells can be seen to be individually oriented.

The individual cells tend to be of small to medium size and round. If the cells have not been traumatized during sample preparation, they typically have distinct cytoplasmic borders (i.e., the boundary of the cell is well defined).

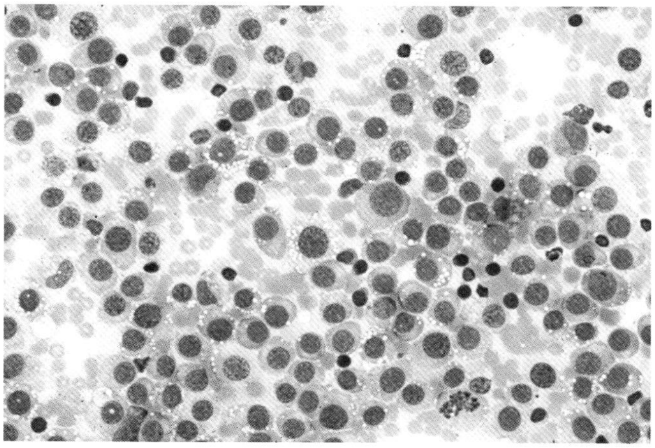

Figure 2-19 This slide, made from an aspirate of a transmissible venereal tumor, shows a typical discrete cell pattern. The slide is highly cellular and the cells are evenly spread out throughout the smear. This pattern can usually be recognized from low-power magnification.

Specific Discrete Cell Tumors: The discrete cell tumors are mast cell tumor, lymphoma (lymphosarcoma), canine cutaneous histiocytoma, histiocytocytic sarcoma, plasmacytoma, and transmissible venereal tumor. In addition, melanoma is the great imitator, yielding cell populations that may appear discrete, epithelial, or mesenchymal.

Mast Cell Tumor: Mast cell tumors are the only lesions that will yield highly cellular smears consisting entirely or predominantly of mast cells. Mast cells are recognized by their distinctive small, red-purple intracytoplasmic granules (Figure 2-20). The number of granules in mast cells varies tremendously, even within cells from the same tumor (Figure 2-21). Most mast cell tumors yield cells that contain a sufficient number of granules to be easily recognized as mast cells. Sometimes, the cells are so densely packed with granules that the cytoplasm will appear diffusely dark purple and the individual granules difficult or impossible to discern. In this situation, the granules will be evident in cells that have been ruptured. Since mast cell granules have such a high affinity for most cytologic stains, the nucleus of a heavily granulated mast cell may appear pale or even totally unstained, giving the cell the look of a photographic negative with dark cytoplasm and a pale nucleus (Figure 2-22). Some of the components of mast cell granules are chemotactic for eosinophils. The number of eosinophils present in smears from a mast cell tumor varies from very few to many. Occasionally, an aspirate from a mast cell tumor will yield predominantly eosinophils with fewer mast cells (Figure 2-23). In this case, it can be difficult to differentiate a mast cell tumor from a hypersensitivity response. Generally, if there are areas on the slides

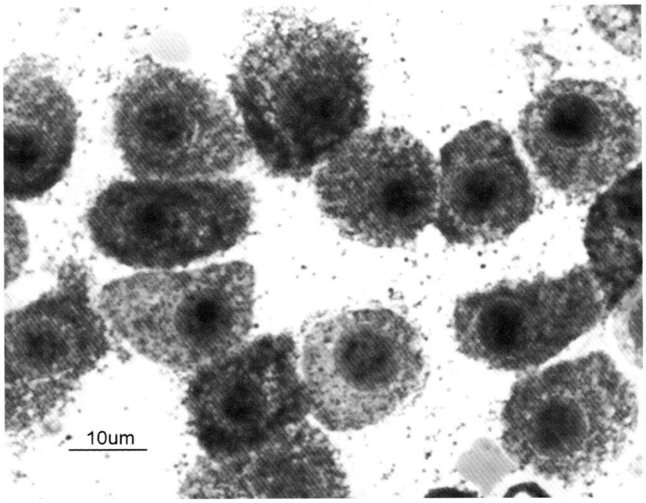

Figure 2-20 Smear made from a mast cell tumor has a pure population of heavily granulated mast cells. The nuclei of these cells are often obscured by the granulation. Numerous free granules are present in the background.

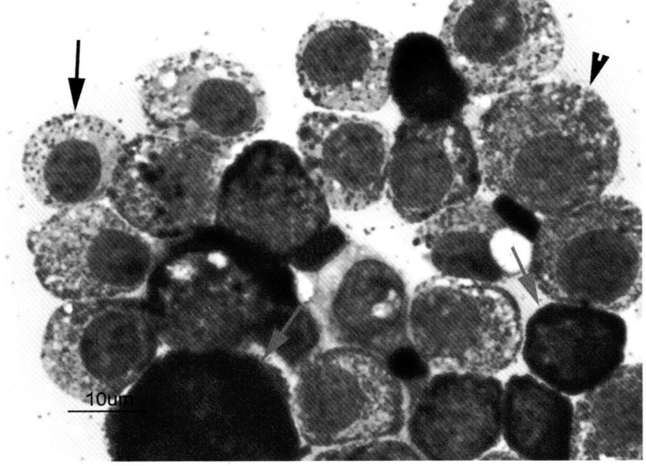

Figure 2-21 Image from a mast cell tumor. Some cells are sparsely granulated and the individual granules are easy to see (*black arrow*). In some heavily granulated cells, the cytoplasm appears diffusely pink-purple, but some individual granules can be seen and the outline of the nucleus can still be visualized (*black arrowhead*). Some cells are so densely packed with granules that neither individual granules nor the nucleus can be seen, making the cell appear as a dark purple mass (*red arrows*).

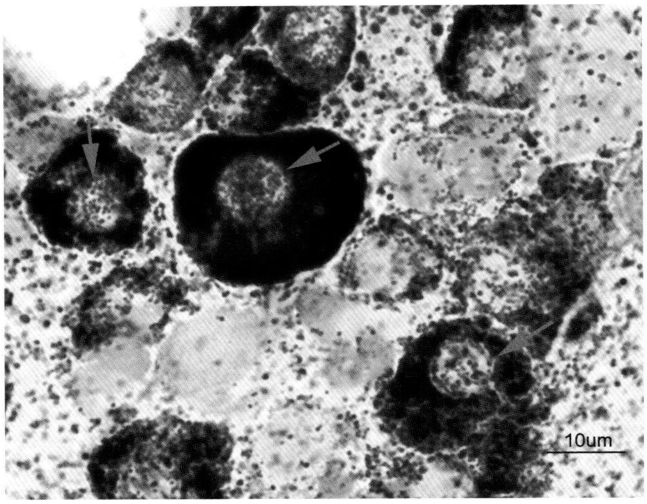

Figure 2-22 Image from a mast cell tumor. The densely packed granules in the cytoplasm have a high affinity for the stain and the nuclei of many cells are understained, giving the cells the look of a photographic negative.

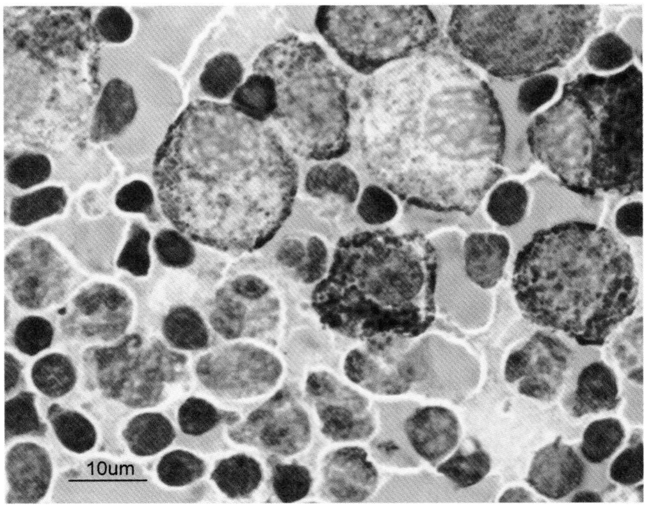

Figure 2-23 Mast cell tumor metastasis to a lymph node. Many mast cells are present, but greater numbers of eosinophils are attracted by constituents of mast cell granules. In some cases, the number of eosinophils can be greater than the number of mast cells in an aspirate from a mast cell tumor.

containing large "sheets" where mast cells are present to the exclusion of other cells, mast cell tumor is most likely.

Cells from some mast cell tumors contain relatively few granules. If a mast cell tumor had degranulated during or prior to aspiration, a percentage of the cells may have relatively few granules. Generally, some granules will still be evident in most cells, and some cells will remain heavily granulated. In addition, high numbers of free granules may be present in the background of the slides. Aspirates of degranulated mast cell tumors may be of lower than normal cellularity because of resultant tissue edema. Anaplastic (poorly differentiated) mast cell tumors may yield cells virtually devoid of granules because the cells have not differentiated sufficiently to produce them (Figure 2-24).

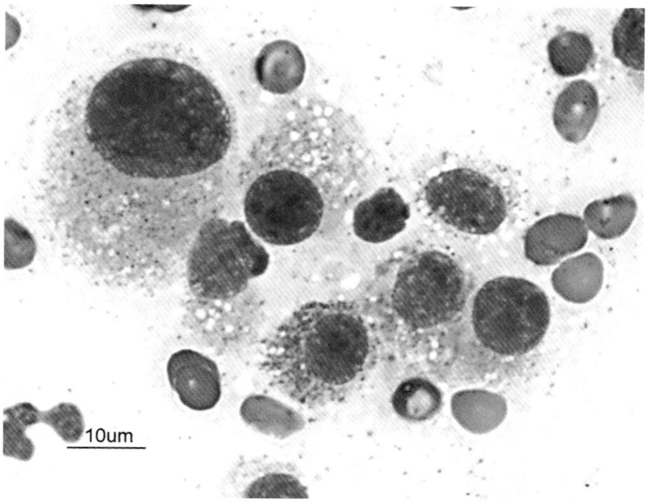

Figure 2-24 Aspirate from a poorly differentiated (grade III) mast cell tumor. The poorly differentiated cells contain relatively few granules. The individual cells show marked atypia including significant variation of cell size, nuclear size, and nuclear-to-cytoplasmic ratio.

In this case, the cells generally display marked atypia (see the section "Do the Tissue Cells Present Display Significant Criteria of Malignancy?"). Finally, the Diff-Quik stain sometimes fails to stain the granules of mast cell tumors. Slides from the same tumor stained with the Wright stain may be heavily granulated (Figure 2-25). This is an inconsistent event, occurring only in some mast cell tumors and not others. When it occurs, mast cells may resemble plasma cells or macrophages. A diligent search of the slides will usually reveal low numbers of identifiable, although poorly stained, granules in some cells. A person routinely using the Diff-Quik stain should always consider this possibility when evaluating a discrete cell population.

Cells from mast cell tumors should be evaluated for criteria of malignancy as described later in this chapter. While cytology cannot evaluate tissue invasion by neoplastic cells; a newly proposed two-tier histologic grading scheme for canine cutaneous mast cell tumors relies on nuclear atypia rather than depth of invasion.[5]

The majority of tumors composed of poorly granulated cells which display marked cytologic atypia will have an aggressive biologic behavior. A small percentage of tumors composed of heavily granulated, well-differentiated cells will be behaviorally malignant, and thus, all mast cell tumors should be removed with wide surgical excision, if possible, and submitted for histology to grade the neoplasm and evaluate completeness of excision.

Examination of peripheral blood smears or buffy coat preparations, bone marrow aspirates, and aspirates of any enlarged lymph nodes or abdominal organs (particularly liver and spleen) can be useful in detecting systemic spread of the mast cell tumor.

Lymphoma (Lymphosarcoma): Most cases of lymphoma in dogs and cats are high-grade tumors composed predominantly of large blastic lymphoid cells (Figure 2-26). If large, blastic lymphoid cells constitute greater than 50% of the cells in a highly cellular smear from lymphoid tissue containing mostly intact cells, a diagnosis of lymphoma

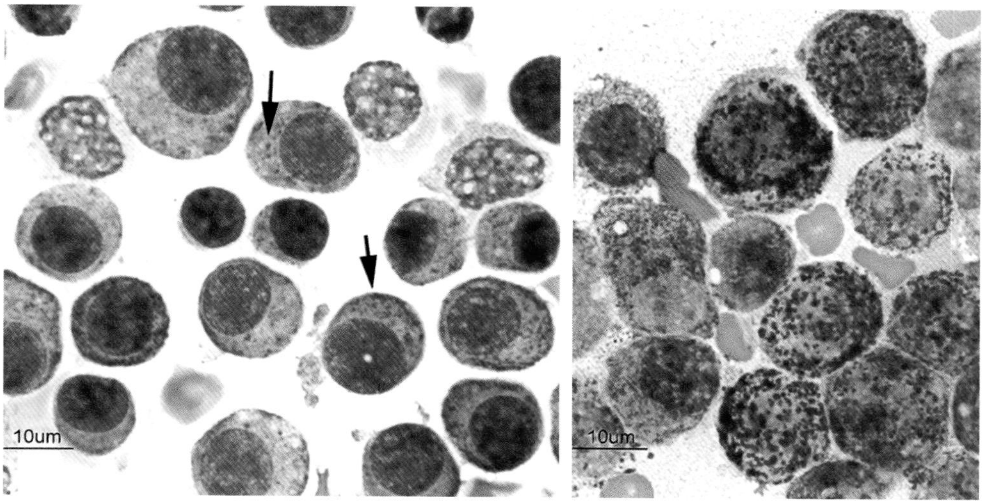

Figure 2-25 Two different slides from the same mast cell tumor were stained with either Diff-Quik (*left*) or Wright-Giemsa (*right*) stain. Although the sample stained with Wright-Giemsa stain shows that the cells are heavily granulated, Diff-Quik stain did not stain the granules of the cells well in this tumor. Some granules can be seen in the Diff-Quik–stained specimen (*arrows*).

can reliably be made. Lymphoblasts can usually be differentiated from the cells of other discrete cell tumors, on the basis of their higher nuclear-to-cytoplasmic (N:C) ratio and the intensely basophilic cytoplasm. Also, in aspirates from lymphoma, usually, numerous small, but different-sized, basophilic fragments of cytoplasm (lymphoglandular bodies) are scattered among the cells (see Figure 2-26). Lymphoid cells, particularly lymphoblasts, are fragile cells and easily ruptured during slide preparation. If an overwhelming majority of the cells on the smears are ruptured, one cannot be confident that the remaining cells accurately represent the cell population in the lymph node. In this situation, additional samples must be collected for a diagnosis. Submission of multiple slides from different lymph nodes will increased chances of a diagnostic slide.

Sometimes, lymphoma is well differentiated and composed of small- to medium-sized lymphocytes rather than large, blastic cells. Such tumors can be difficult to differentiate from normal or reactive lymphoid tissue solely on the basis of cytology, and confirmation may be required either through molecular techniques such as PARR (polymerase chain reaction for antigen receptor rearrangement) or flow cytometry (see Chapters 30 and 31) or may require histologic examination of a surgically removed lymph node which can demonstrate architectural effacement and capsular invasion.

Canine Cutaneous Histiocytoma: Canine cutaneous histiocytoma is a benign tumor of dendritic cell origin and occurs commonly in young dogs (Figure 2-27). Tumor cells are medium sized, slightly larger than neutrophils. Nuclei are generally round to oval but may be indented to irregular in shape. The nucleus has finely stippled chromatin and may have indistinct nucleoli. They have a moderate amount of light blue-gray cytoplasm. If a significant amount of protein-rich tissue fluid is present between cells, the cytoplasm of the cells may appear lighter than the background (Figure 2-28), or cell borders may be indistinct.

Histiocytomas usually regress spontaneously within a few weeks to months. Regression is associated with an infiltration of small lymphocytes into the tumor. Therefore, aspirates from these tumors will sometimes contain a mixture of tumor cells and small lymphocytes (see Figure 2-28). The presence of small lymphocytes among the larger tumor cells must not lead to misidentification of histiocytoma cells as lymphoblasts. The irregularly shaped nuclei, light color and greater volume of the cytoplasm, and the lack of lymphoglandular bodies help differentiate histiocytoma cells from lymphoid cells.

Histiocytic Sarcoma Complex: These tumors result from a proliferation of either dendritic cells or bone marrow origin macrophages.[6,7] Cytology alone may not be able to differentiate these diseases from each other or from inflammatory proliferations of macrophages (granulomatous inflammation).

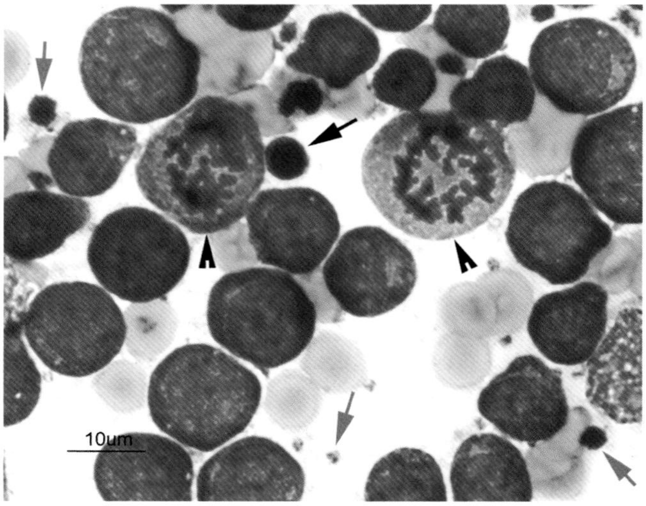

Figure 2-26 Aspirate of the lymph nodes of a dog with lymphoma. The slide consists almost entirely of large blastic lymphoid cells. One poorly spread-out small lymphocyte is present (*black arrow*). Two mitotic figures are present (*arrowheads*) and numerous cytoplasmic fragments of lymphoid cells (lymphoglandular bodies) are present in the background (*red arrows*).

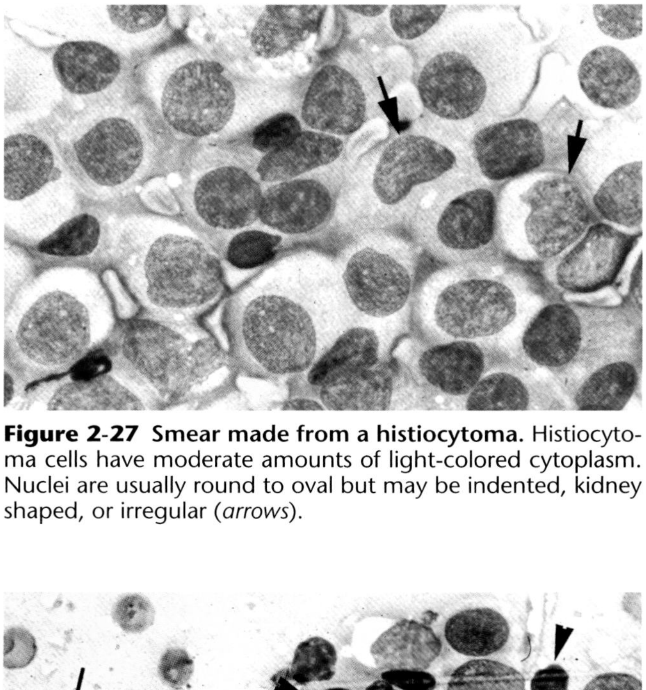

Figure 2-27 Smear made from a histiocytoma. Histiocytoma cells have moderate amounts of light-colored cytoplasm. Nuclei are usually round to oval but may be indented, kidney shaped, or irregular (*arrows*).

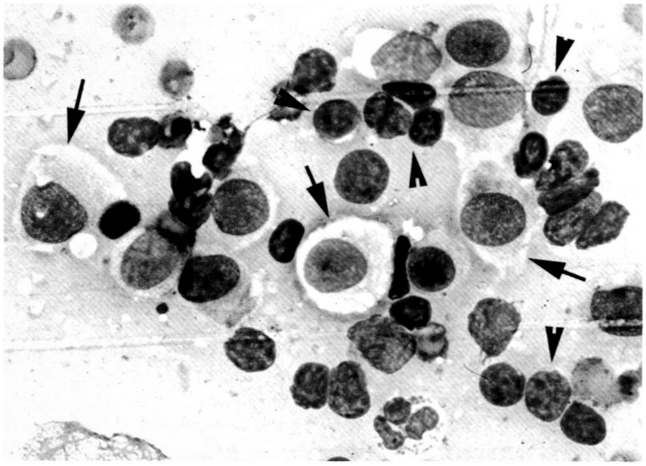

Figure 2-28 Smear made from a histiocytoma. Regression of a histiocytoma is associated with an infiltration of small lymphocytes (*arrowheads*), which may be more numerous than the histiocytoma cells (*arrows*).

Cytologic appearance of histiocytic sarcoma varies from a population of cells resembling relatively well-differentiated macrophages to histiocytic cells with marked atypia (Figure 2-29, Figure 2-30, Figure 2-31).[7] Common features include large discrete cells with abundant vacuolated cytoplasm, prominent cytophagia, and multinucleation (see Figure 2-30, *B*). With tumors of dendritic cell origin, the cytoplasmic vacuoles are often small and of uniform size and may lack the presence of phagocytic debris common in macrophages seen in inflammatory lesions (see Figure 2-29). The cells may demonstrate marked anisocytosis, anisokaryosis, and variation of N:C ratio (see Figure 2-31, *A*). Macrocytosis, karyomegaly, and the presence of large multinucleated cells are common (see Figure 2-31, *B*).

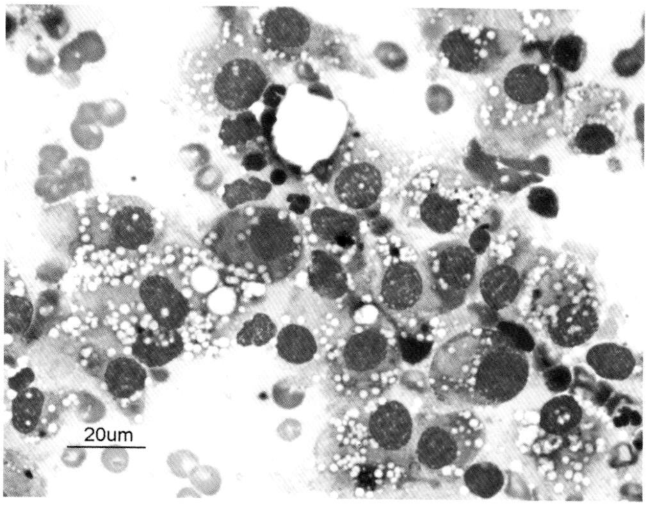

Figure 2-29 Splenic aspirate from a dog with histiocytic sarcoma. The spleen was markedly enlarged and consisted almost entirely of a population of discretely oriented, heavily vacuolated histiocytic cells. Many of the cells were fairly uniform, although other cells showed significant atypia.

When masses are composed of histiocytic cells showing marked atypia, a diagnosis of histiocytic sarcoma can be made. However, when the cells consist of macrophages that appear relatively bland, definitive diagnosis may not be possible solely on the basis of cytology. It should be noted that many of these lesions with relatively bland cytologic appearance may have an aggressive biologic behavior.

Plasmacytoma: Tumors of plasma cell origin include multiple myeloma (plasma cell myeloma), a systemic tumor arising primarily in the bone marrow, and extramedullary plasmacytomas. Extramedullary plasmacytomas are commonly cutaneous tumors but have been described from other sites, including the gastrointestinal (GI) tract. Cutaneous plasmacytomas are typically benign.[8] It has been suggested that a greater likelihood of aggressive biological behavior exists with plasmacytomas arising from the GI tract other than the oral areas.[9]

Well-differentiated plasmacytomas yield cells that resemble normal plasma cells (Figure 2-32, *A*). Distinguishing features include eccentrically placed small, round nuclei surrounded by a moderate amount of deeply basophilic cytoplasm with or without the characteristic distinct paranuclear clear zone. In some well-differentiated plasma cell tumors, the paranuclear clear zone will not be evident, even though the cells otherwise resemble well-differentiated plasma cells. Poorly differentiated plasmacytomas may yield a less distinct population of discrete cells that demonstrate significant cytologic atypia. Anisocytosis, anisokaryosis, and variation of N:C ratio can be prominent. Binucleate and multinucleate cells are common in both well-differentiated and poorly differentiated tumors (see Figure 2-32, *B*). This, together with a lack of lymphoglandular bodies, helps differentiate these tumors from lymphoma. Cytologic atypia often does not correlate with an aggressive biologic behavior. Many neoplasms effacing the bone marrow or spleen comprise uniform, well-differentiated plasma cells, whereas benign cutaneous tumors may show significant pleomorphism.

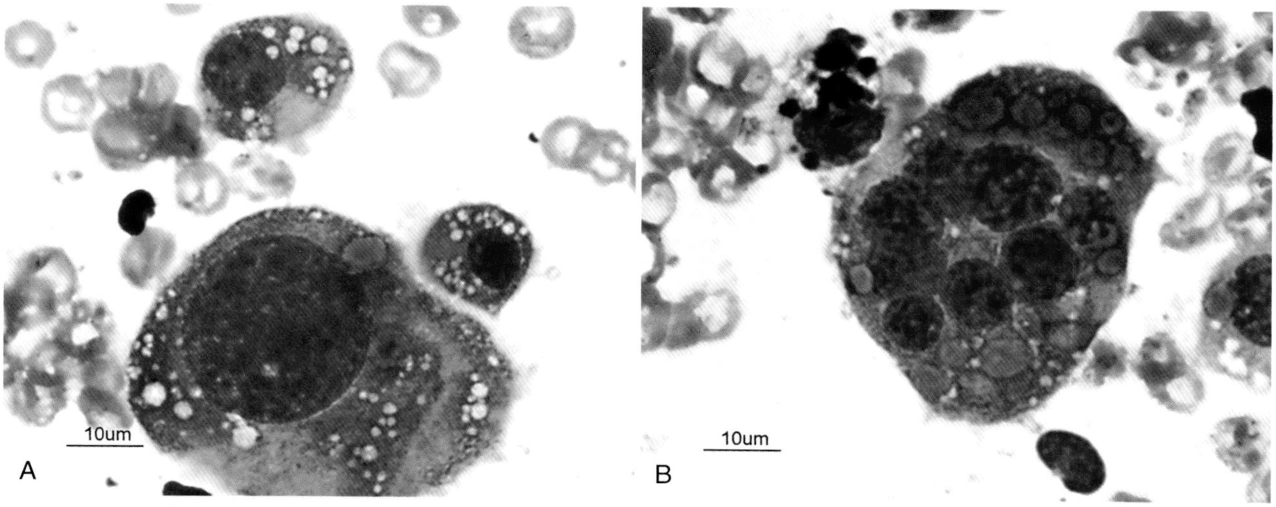

Figure 2-30 Same slide as in Figure 2-29. A, Some macrocytic, karyomegalic cells were also present. Note the phagocytosis of several red blood cells. **B,** Large multinucleated cell showing erythrophagia.

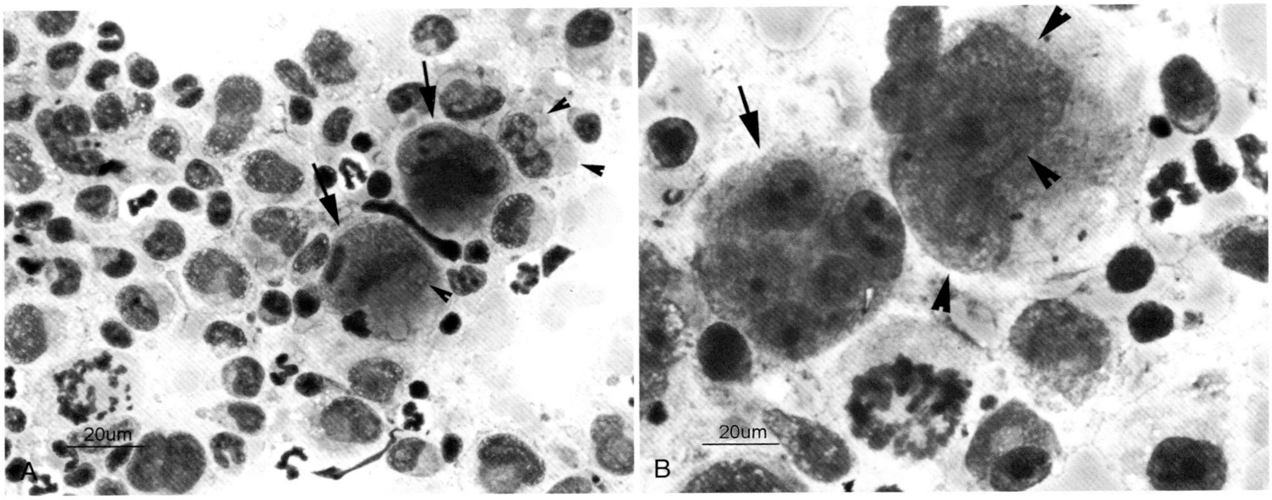

Figure 2-31 **Splenic aspirate from another dog with histiocytic sarcoma. A,** Cells from this tumor showed marked atypia including anisocytosis, anisokaryosis, and nuclear pleomorphism. Large, karyomegalic cells with large, prominent, irregularly shaped nucleoli are present (*arrows*). Many of the cells in this tumor demonstrated erythrophagia (*arrowheads*). **B,** Both large multinucleated cells and large cells with a single, pleomorphic, karyomegalic nucleus (*arrowheads*) are common in this tumor.

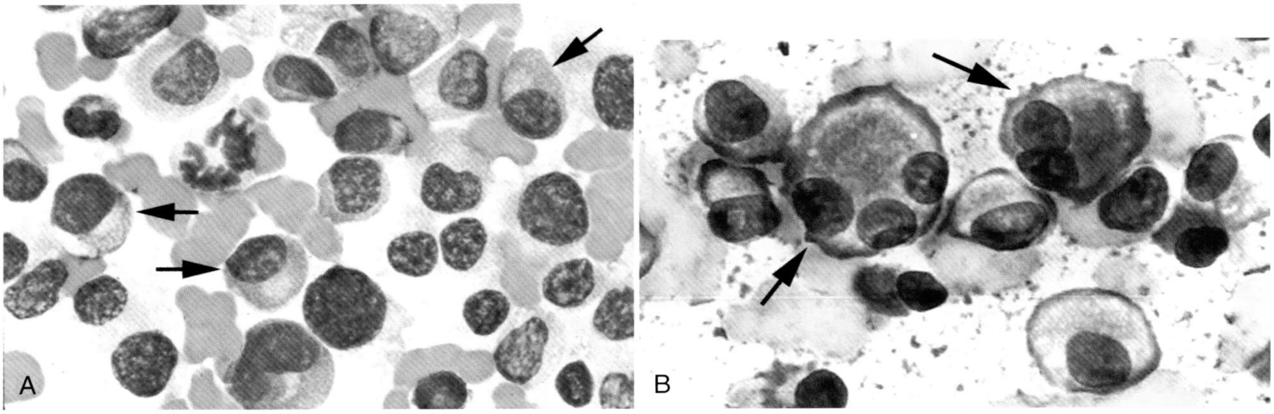

Figure 2-32 **Smears made from an extramedullary plasmacytoma. A,** Cells show a typical discrete cell pattern. Many cells resemble mature plasma cells having eccentric nuclei and distinct perinuclear clear areas (*arrows*). **B,** Binucleate and multinucleate cells (*arrows*) are common in tumors of plasma cell origin.

Some plasma cells have a distinct red color to the periphery of their cytoplasm and are referred to as *flame cells* (Figure 2-33). Rarely, an eosinophilic extracellular matrix representing amyloid (composed of immunoglobulin light chain) is seen among the neoplastic cells.

Transmissible Venereal Tumor: Except in certain geographic areas, transmissible venereal tumors (TVTs) are less commonly encountered compared with other discrete cell tumors. TVTs are often present on the external genitalia but may occur in other locations as well.

The cells from a TVT are typically more pleomorphic compared with those from most other discrete cell tumors (Figure 2-34). They have moderate amounts of smoky to light blue cytoplasm with sharply defined cytoplasmic boundaries. A prominent characteristic of TVT cells, which helps distinguish them from other discrete cell tumors, is the presence of numerous, distinctly walled, cytoplasmic vacuoles (see Figure 2-34). These vacuoles can also be found extracellularly, appearing as clear areas against a proteinaceous background of tissue fluid. Nuclei show moderate to marked anisokaryosis and have a coarse nuclear chromatin pattern. Nucleoli may be prominent and mitotic figures, often atypical, are common.

Melanoma: Tumors of melanocytic origin are the great imitators; cells may show features of discrete cells, epithelial cells or mesenchymal cells. Often, a mixture of all three of these morphologic appearances will be present within an aspirate from a single tumor. Sometimes, however, aspirates will consist entirely of discretely oriented, round cells giving the appearance of a "round cell tumor." Melanocytic tumors are usually easily recognized by their pigmentation. Individual melanin granules are rod-shaped granules that typically stain dark green to black. When these granules are densely packed within

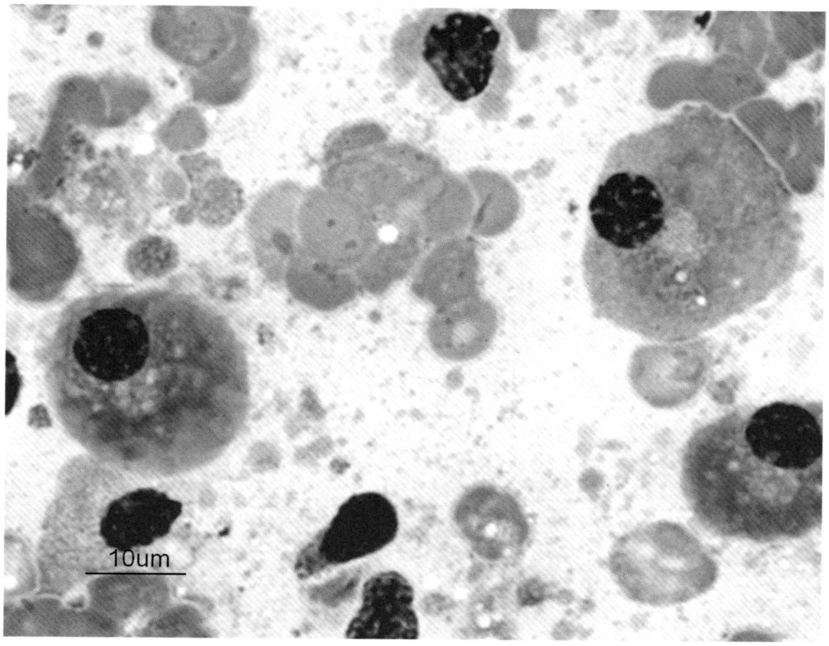

Figure 2-33 Smear made of a spleen aspirate from a dog with a plasma cell tumor. Plasma cells show a distinct red color at the periphery of their cytoplasm and are termed *flame cells*.

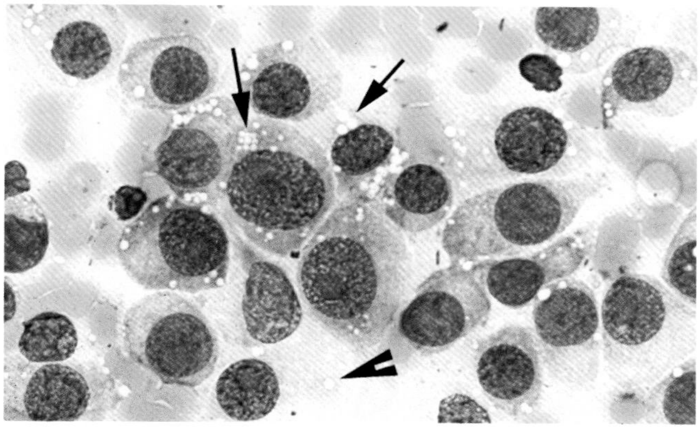

Figure 2-34 Smear made from a transmissible venereal tumor (TVT). Cells from a TVT are characterized by numerous clear vacuoles within the cytoplasm of the cells (*arrows*) and free in the background (*arrowhead*). Many of the cells have coarse nuclear chromatin and large nucleoli.

cells, they appear black. The appearance of the cells from a melanoma may range from heavily pigmented to sparsely pigmented, depending on the degree of differentiation of the tumor.

With heavily pigmented tumors, the cells often appear simply as dark black, circular to spherical objects (Figure 2-35). Visualization of cell detail is often completely obscured by the pigmentation. Nuclei may be seen in cells that are traumatized, and often, a background containing numerous free melanin granules is present (see Figure 2-35).

In poorly differentiated tumors, pigmentation may be sparse (Figure 2-36) to absent, requiring a lengthy search to find any pigment granules at all. These cells typically

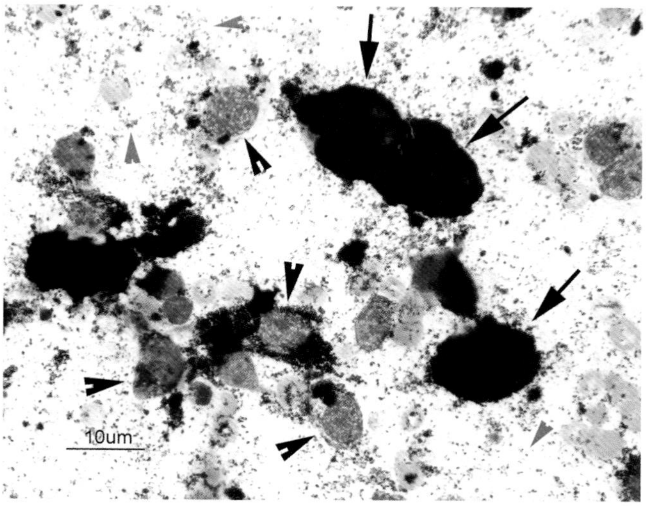

Figure 2-35 Aspirate of a heavily pigmented cutaneous melanoma from a dog. In most of the intact cells (*arrows*), the cellular detail is completely obscured by the pigmentation, preventing evaluation of these cells. Nuclei can be seen in some cells (*arrowheads*) that appear partially ruptured. Numerous free melanin granules (*red arrowheads*) are present in the background of the smear.

show marked criteria of malignancy (see subsequent section in this chapter) (see Figure 2-36).

Most poorly pigmented tumors with marked cytologic atypia have a malignant biologic behavior. It is difficult to assess the malignant potential of heavily pigmented tumors because individual cells cannot be evaluated. Although many heavily pigmented tumors are benign, some of these may also demonstrate aggressive biologic behavior. The anatomic location of the tumor greatly

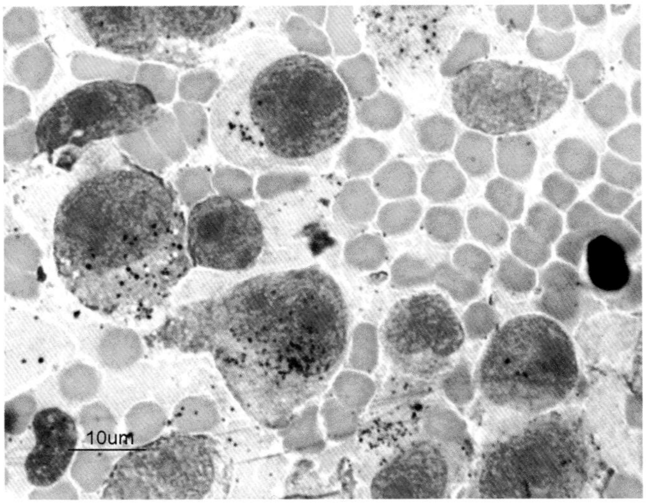

Figure 2-36 Aspirate from a poorly pigmented malignant melanoma from the oral cavity of a dog. The slide consists of large, pleomorphic cells with a high nucleus-cytoplasm ratio and large prominent nucleoli. Most cells have a few cytoplasmic melanin granules that are easily recognizable.

affects the likelihood of malignancy in dogs, with tumors of the oral cavity, mucocutaneous junctions, and nail bed carrying a greater likelihood of malignant behavior.

Epithelial Cells

Normal epithelial cells are commonly encountered in many cytologic preparations. Surface epithelium will be present in most surface scrapings or swabs (e.g., squamous cells from skin scrapings and nasal or vaginal swabs), in washings (e.g., columnar cells from transtracheal washes), and as the result of normal exfoliation (e.g., transitional cells from urine sediments). In addition, epithelial cells will be the major cellular component of smears made from FNB of many parenchymal organs (e.g., hepatocytes and bile duct epithelium from liver aspirates, renal tubular cells from kidney aspirates) and glandular aspirates (e.g., mammary, prostate).

Epithelial cells may also originate from a hyperplastic proliferation or neoplasm. Cells from benign epithelial tumors may be difficult to impossible to differentiate from their normal, or hyperplastic, counterparts solely on the basis of cytology. However, combining clinical and cytologic findings can often allow the diagnosis of a benign epithelial proliferation to be made. For example, a discrete wartlike mass on an older dog that yields numerous clusters of normal-appearing sebaceous epithelial cells suggest a sebaceous adenoma or sebaceous gland hyperplasia.

Epithelial cells that display sufficient cytologic criteria of malignancy indicate the presence of a carcinoma or adenocarcinoma. A specific diagnosis of cell type may or may not be possible solely on the basis of cytology and depends on how well differentiated and characteristic the cells are. Histopathology may be required for a more specific diagnosis of cell type. However, the ability to confirm the presence of a malignant epithelial tumor by cytology is often sufficient to guide clinical management of a case.

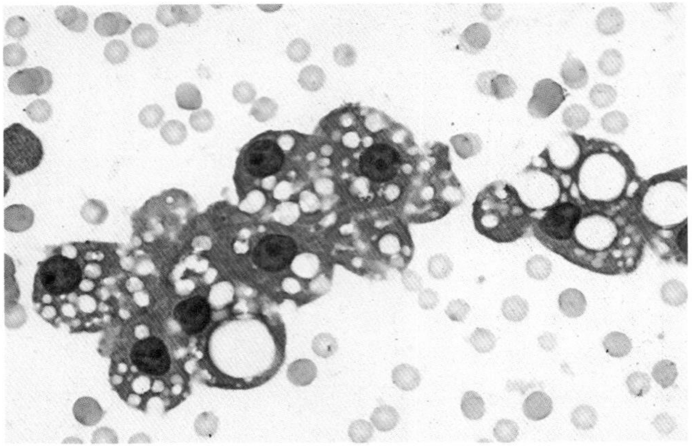

Figure 2-37 Smear made from an aspirate of a feline kidney. Numerous renal tubular epithelial cells are present. Epithelial cells tend to form cell clusters. Feline renal tubular cells may have numerous lipid vacuoles within their cytoplasm.

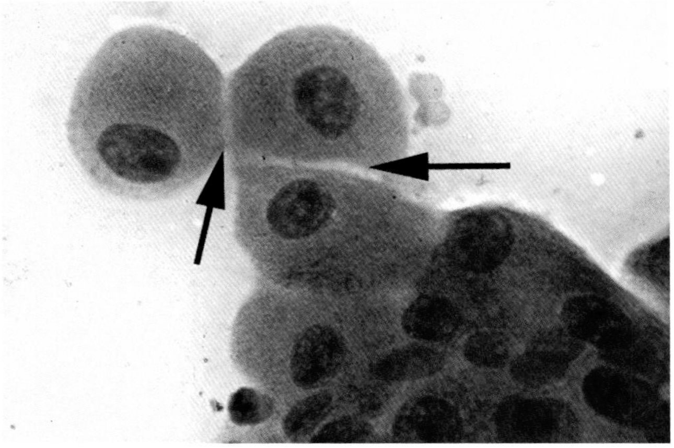

Figure 2-38 Aspirate from a perianal adenoma. The areas of cell adhesion can be seen in some cells (*arrows*).

General Cytologic Characteristics of Epithelial Cell Populations: A main feature of epithelial cells is cell-to-cell adhesion (Figure 2-37). Normal epithelial cells are typically present in different-sized sheets or clusters. Sometimes, the area of adhesion between individual cells can be seen (Figure 2-38). True cell clustering from cell-to-cell adhesion must be differentiated from crowding of cells in highly cellular aspirates of any cell type. This can usually be accomplished by looking at thinner areas of the smear. In thin areas, if the cells are still present in clusters but are separated by acellular areas, cell-to-cell adhesion is documented.

Mesenchymal cells are sometimes held together by an extracellular matrix, resulting in large aggregates of cells, which resembles cell adhesion. Often, this extracellular matrix is apparent as a brightly eosinophilic, homogeneous material between the cells and can be used to identify the type of cell present.

Normal epithelial cells vary in size from small (basal cells) to large, depending on the specific type and stage of maturation. They may be round, polygonal, columnar, or caudate in shape and typically have distinct, sharply defined cytoplasmic borders. Cytoplasmic borders within

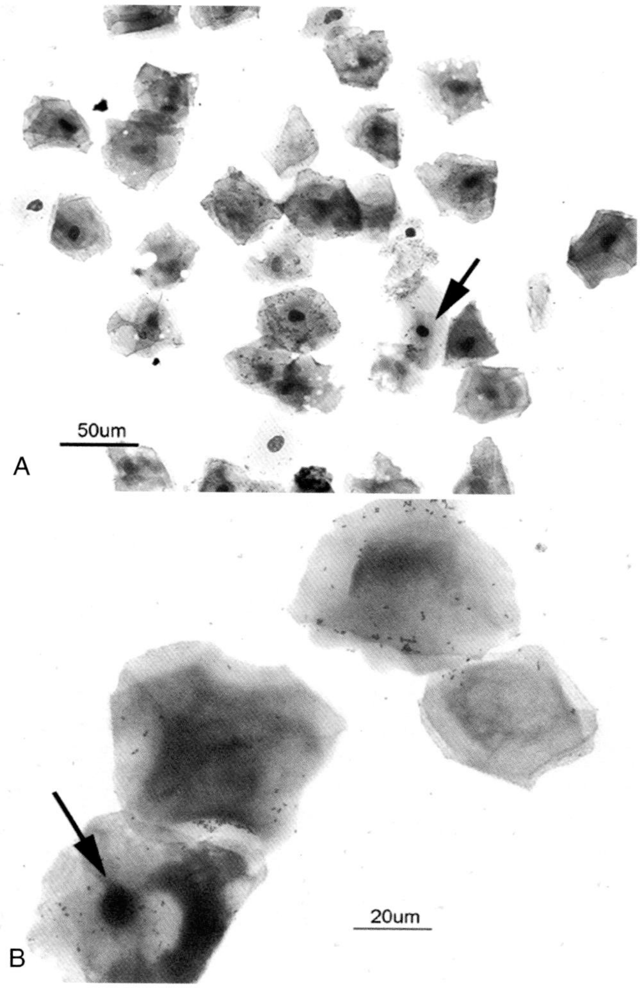

Figure 2-39 Mature, cornified cells from a canine vaginal swab. A, Low-magnification image shows that these cells tend to exfoliate individually rather than in cohesive clusters. Individual cells show angular cytoplasmic borders. Nuclei become pyknotic (*arrow*) and eventually disappear, leaving anucleate cells. **B,** High-magnification image showing three anucleate squamous cells and one mature squamous cell with a condensed pyknotic nucleus (*arrow*).

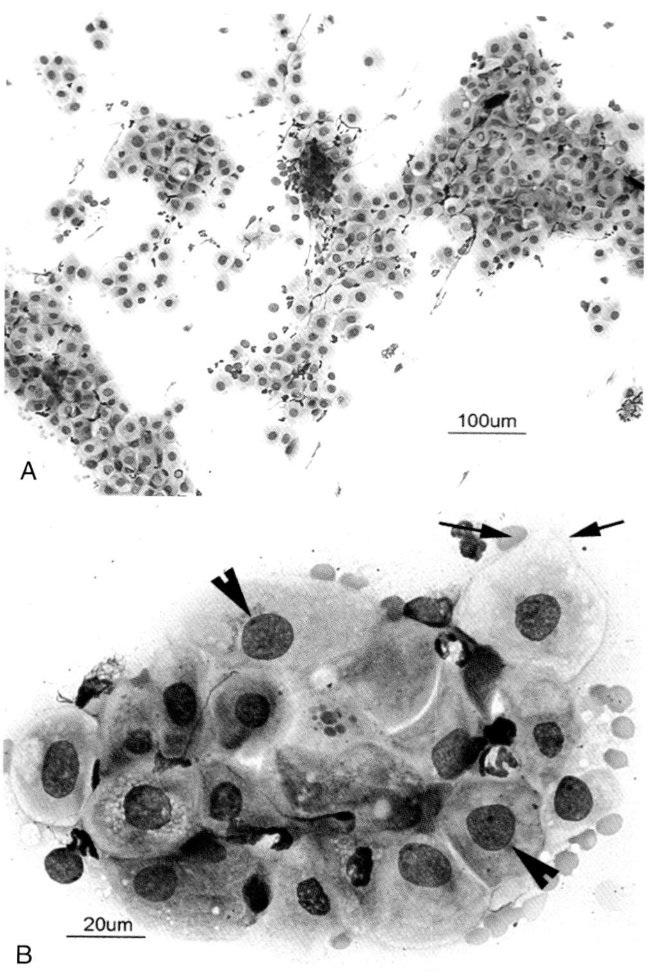

Figure 2-40 Noncornified squamous cells from a canine vaginal swab. These cells are less differentiated than those shown in Figure 2-39. These cells can be seen in surface swabs and scraping and may be intermixed with fully keratinized cells. **A,** Low-magnification image shows that these cells tend to demonstrate cell-to-cell adhesion, being present in cohesive clusters. **B,** High magnification of one cluster of noncornified squamous cells. The cells tend to be round, although some cells are beginning to develop angular borders. Amount of cytoplasm is variable, depending on stage of maturation. Cells have functional, nonpyknotic nuclei (*arrowheads*).

cell clusters may be difficult to discern; however, the outer edges of the cells in the clusters typically are clearly demarcated. Nuclei of epithelial cells are generally round to somewhat oval in shape. A single, small, round nucleolus may be visible in certain types of epithelial cells such as hepatocytes and renal tubular epithelium (see Figure 2-37).

Epithelial Criteria Specific to Certain Cell Types: Mature squamous epithelial cells are often found in samples collected from surface swabs or scrapings. These tend to be more individually oriented and may not show prominent cell clustering (Figure 2-39). Fully mature (cornified or keratinized) squamous cells have abundant cytoplasm with angular cytoplasmic borders. Their nuclei become small and pyknotic, and eventually the cell becomes anucleate (see Figure 2-39). Less differentiated squamous cells, often present in swabs or scrapings along with mature cells, are more cohesive, and have a greater tendency to be in clusters (Figure 2-40). These cells are round and have variable amounts of cytoplasm, increasing as the cell matures. Nuclei of these cells are large and round with functional (nonpyknotic) chromatin (see Figure 2-40). Because of the potential to have a mixture of cells at different stages of maturation, squamous cell populations may normally show significant variation in cell and nuclear size.

Epithelial cells from the respiratory and GI tract are distinctly columnar. Cell clusters may show long rows of cells, with nuclei lined up at the basal end of the cell (Figure 2-41). Often, cilia can be seen at the apical surface of samples from the respiratory tract (Figure 2-42). Normal epithelial cells from the GI tract are often present in large, pavemented clusters, often with clear cytoplasm, suggesting their secretory nature (Figure 2-43). The columnar nature of the cells may be evident only at the sides of the clusters, where the cells have arranged on their sides (rather than a "top down" view seen in the middle of the clusters) (Figure 2-44).

Although most tissue architecture is lost during fine-needle aspiration, some architectural arrangements may endure. Epithelial cells of glandular origin may show evidence of tubular or acinar formation (Figure 2-45 and Figure 2-46). Papillary or trabecular patterns may also be retained in some epithelial tumors.

Tumors of endocrine epithelial cells (e.g., thyroid carcinoma) and neuroendocrine cells (e.g., pheochromocytoma, chemodectoma) often yield cell populations with characteristic features (Figure 2-47). The slides are highly cellular and consist of loosely cohesive cells. In addition, these cells tend to be fragile, and smears typically contain many bare nuclei admixed with the loosely cohesive intact cells. Bare nuclei of fragile cell populations must be differentiated from bare nuclei occurring from cell rupturing caused by poor smearing technique (i.e., excessive pressure during smearing). Bare nuclei from endocrine or neuroendocrine populations often have relatively intact

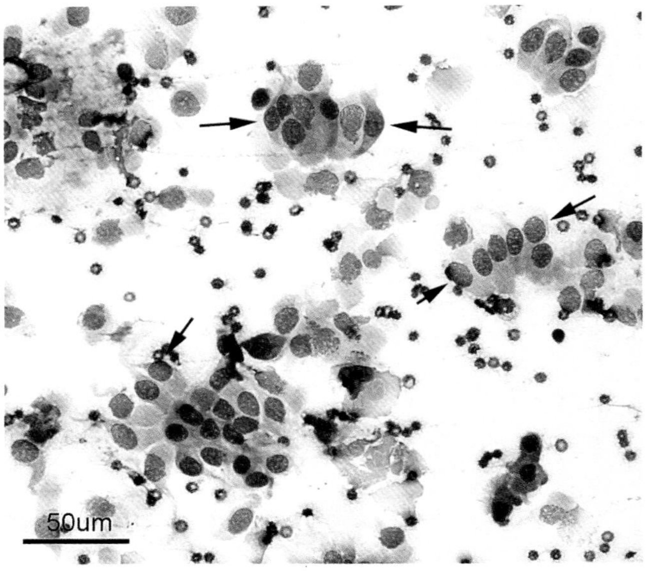

Figure 2-41 Smear of a bronchial brushing from a dog. Low-magnification image shows numerous clusters of columnar epithelial cells. In some of the well-spread-out cells, the columnar nature is evident, and the nuclei can be seen lining up on what was the basal surface of the cell.

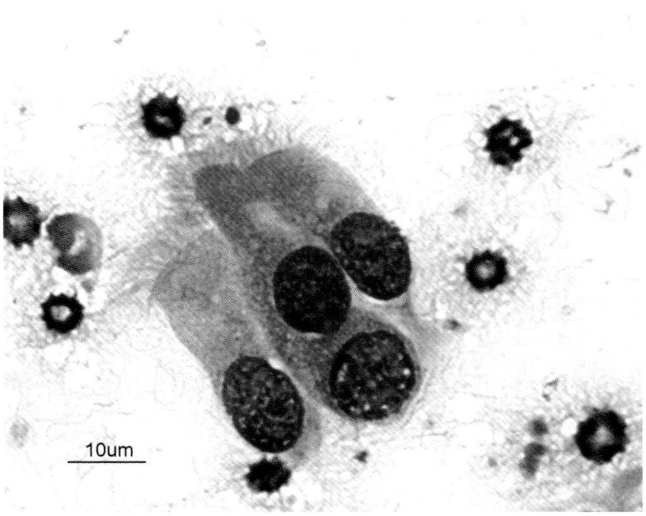

Figure 2-42 Higher magnification of slide from Figure 2-41. Cilia can be seen on the apical surface of the columnar epithelial cells.

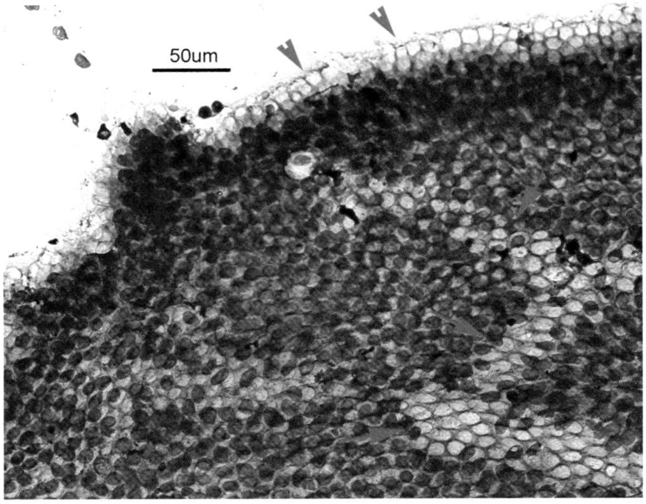

Figure 2-43 Aspirate of intestinal epithelial cells from a cat. Low magnification shows large, tightly cohesive clusters of cells in a pavemented monolayer. The secretory nature of the cells is evident by the clear nature of the cytoplasm of many of the cells (*red arrows*). The columnar nature of the cells is evident only at the edges of the cluster (*red arrowheads*).

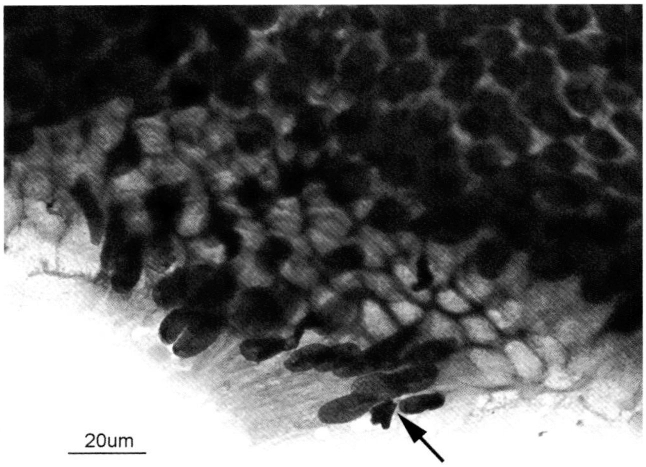

Figure 2-44 Higher magnification of intestinal epithelial cells shown in Figure 2-43. The columnar nature of the cells and palisading nuclear arrangement can be seen on the edge of the cluster (*arrow*). Again, many of the cells have clear, distended cytoplasm typical of secretory cells.

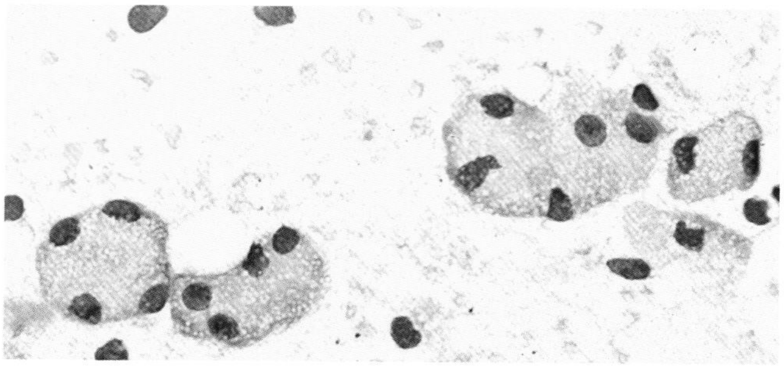

Figure 2-45 Smear from an aspirate of a normal salivary gland (accidentally aspirated instead of the submandibular lymph node). The cells are arranged in an acinar pattern with nuclei at the periphery of the acinus. Individual cells are relatively small with small, round nuclei showing mature chromatin and abundant cytoplasm yielding a low nucleus-to-cytoplasm ratio.

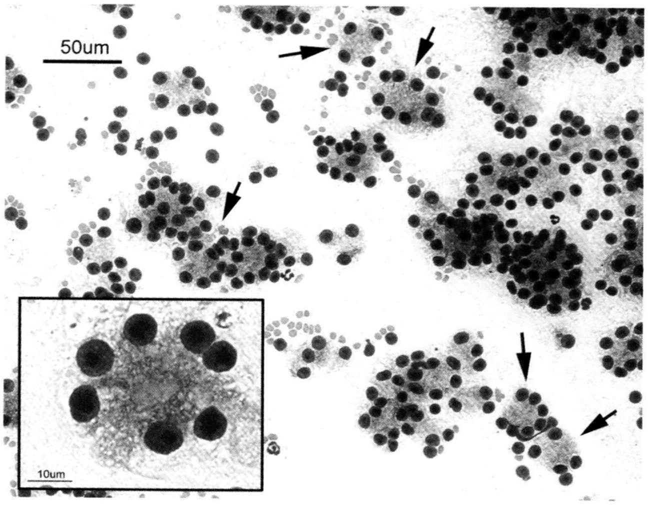

Figure 2-46 Smear of a pancreatic aspirate from a cat. Uniform epithelial cells are in clusters and show acinus formation (*arrows*) indicating a glandular origin. Inset, Higher magnification of a single acinus with evidence of secretory material (*slightly pink*) in the center of the acinus.

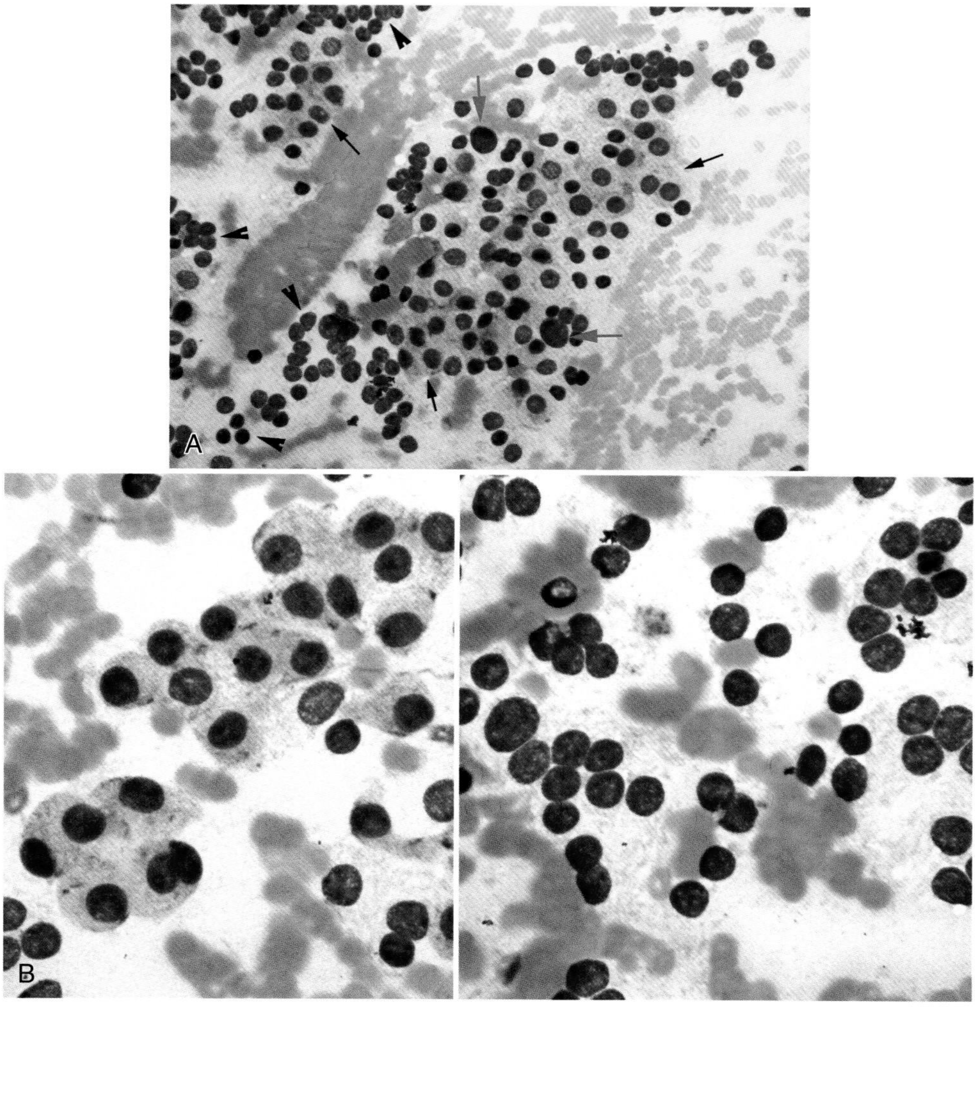

Figure 2-47 A, Low-magnification image of a neuroendocrine (heartbase) tumor from a dog. The slide is highly cellular and consists of a mixture of loosely cohesive intact cells (*black arrows*) and bare nuclei of ruptured cells (*black arrowheads*). The cells are fairly uniform, although some karyomegalic cells are seen (*red arrows*). **B,** Higher magnification of same slide as *A*. On the left, the intact cells appear fairly uniform and have small nuclei with mature, condensed chromatin and moderate amounts of lightly basophilic cytoplasm. On the right, a different field shows many bare nuclei suggesting the fragile nature of the cells. Note that although the cells are ruptured, the bare nuclei appear intact rather than the nuclear streaming often seen when cells are ruptured from excessive pressure during slide preparation.

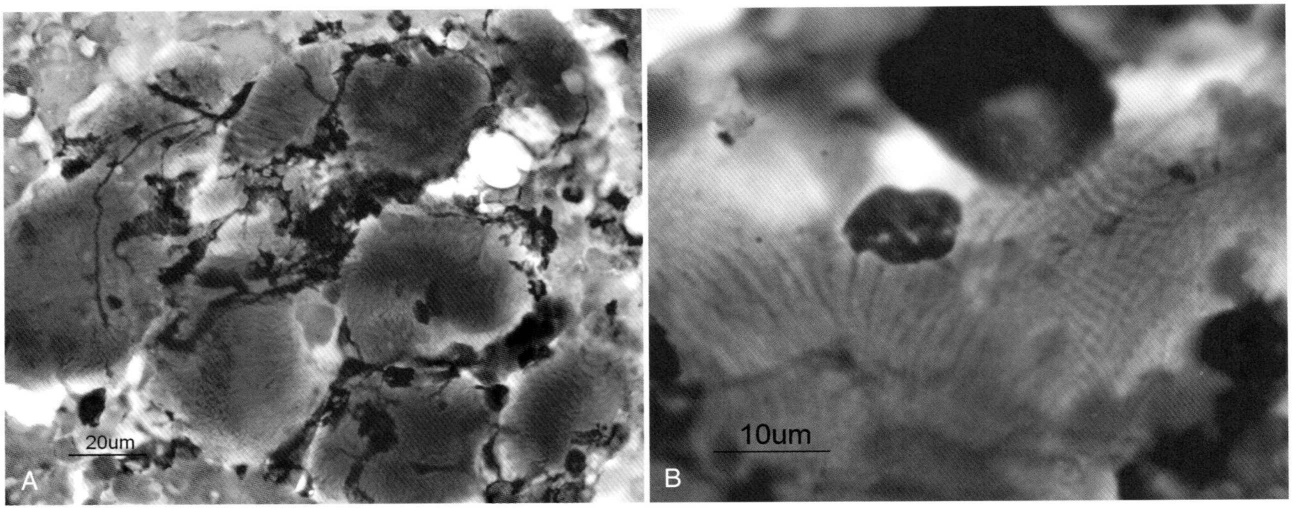

Figure 2-48 Aspirate of a perianal gland tumor from a dog. A, Numerous circular to oval, basophilic structures represent fragments of normal striated muscle. **B,** Higher magnification of another area from the same slide shows distinct striations within the cytoplasm.

nuclear outlines, as opposed to the traumatized, irregular appearance often seen with poor smearing technique.

Mesenchymal Cells

Origin of Mesenchymal Cells in Cytologic Samples: Mesenchymal cells are cells that form connective tissue, blood vessels, and lymphatics. Because blood is considered a connective tissue, hematopoietic cells (including many of the cells described in the section about discrete cells) are typically classified as mesenchymal cells. However, because these hematopoietic cells have a cytologic appearance that is highly distinct from the other connective tissues, they are typically considered a separate classification. Most often, the discussion of mesenchymal cells in cytology texts implies stromal connective tissue cells.

Most normal connective tissues exfoliate very few, if any, cells when sampled by FNB. Sometimes, small fragments of mature muscle will be seen in samples as inadvertent sampling of muscle surrounding a lesion (Figure 2-48). Muscle fragments appear as basophilic, irregularly shaped structures from low magnification. At high magnification, regularly spaced, ovoid nuclei may be noted, and striations may be seen in the cytoplasm by focusing up and down on the tissue fragment. Fibroblasts and fibrocytes are the one nonneoplastic mesenchymal cell type that is commonly encountered in cytologic specimens. Clusters of normal stromal cells can be seen in aspirates of internal organs, particularly the spleen. Scattered individual fibroblasts may be seen in aspirates from virtually any tissue. Reactive fibroblasts may be present in significant numbers in aspirates from areas of inflammation or tissue repair (e.g., surgical scars). Reactive fibroblasts (fibroplasia) may show many of the cytologic criteria of malignancy, so caution should be exercised in evaluating mesenchymal cells when a significant inflammatory response is present. Reactive fibroblasts should be suspected when scattered mesenchymal cells are present along with a population of inflammatory cells (Figure 2-49).

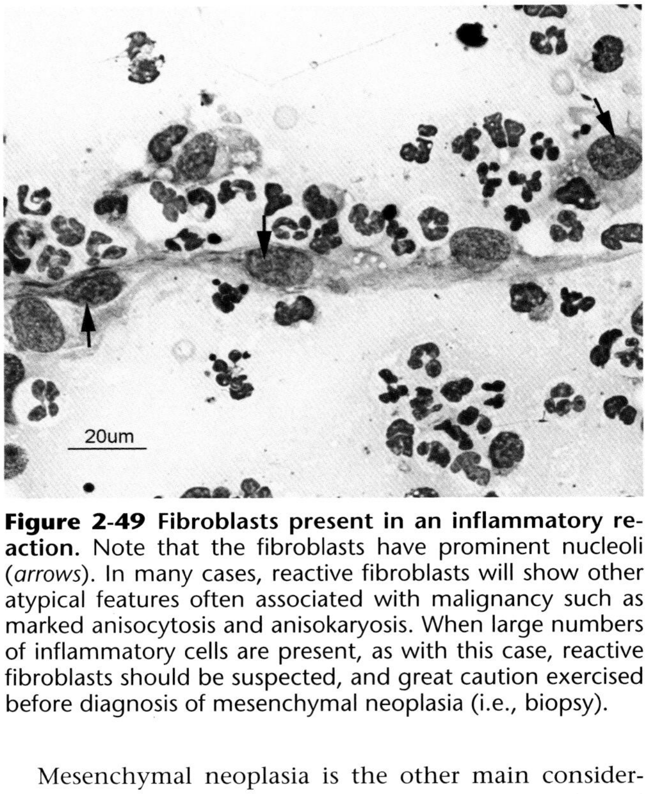

Figure 2-49 Fibroblasts present in an inflammatory reaction. Note that the fibroblasts have prominent nucleoli (*arrows*). In many cases, reactive fibroblasts will show other atypical features often associated with malignancy such as marked anisocytosis and anisokaryosis. When large numbers of inflammatory cells are present, as with this case, reactive fibroblasts should be suspected, and great caution exercised before diagnosis of mesenchymal neoplasia (i.e., biopsy).

Mesenchymal neoplasia is the other main consideration for a cytologic specimen containing mesenchymal cells. Highly cellular smears containing a pure population of mesenchymal cells that show cytologic atypia are likely to indicate mesenchymal neoplasia. Malignant tumors of mesenchymal origin are by definition sarcomas, although the names of some tumors do not follow the standard nomenclature (e.g., malignant fibrous histiocytoma, hemangiopericytoma).

General Cytologic Characteristics of Mesenchymal Cell Populations: As previously mentioned, aspirates of normal mesenchymal tissue are usually sparsely

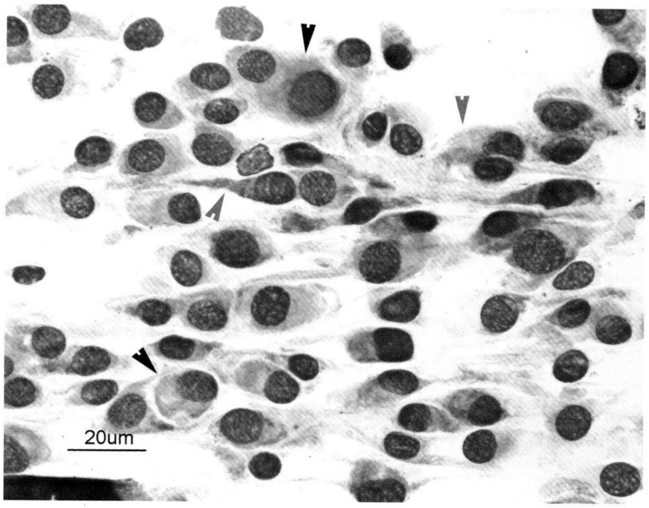

Figure 2-50 Aspirate from a tumor of mesenchymal origin. The slide is highly cellular and the population of mesenchymal cells has a mixture of tapered cells (*red arrowheads*) to cells that are essentially round (*black arrowheads*), demonstrating the need to evaluate the entire cell population to determine the cell type present. Contrast this with the appearance of the cells in Figure 2-51.

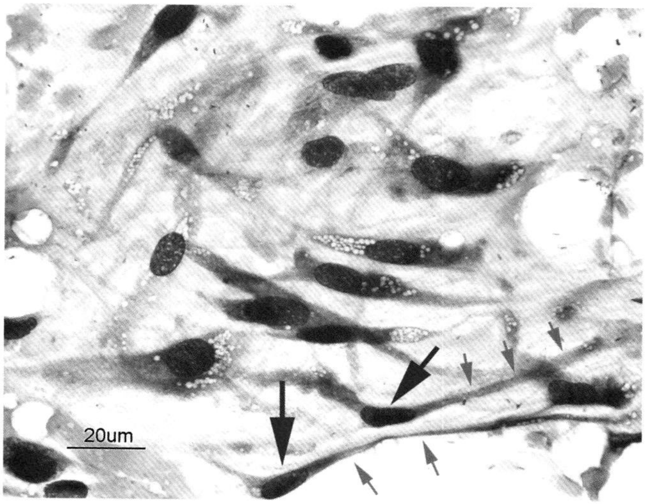

Figure 2-52 Cells from a malignant mesenchymal tumor (fibrosarcoma). Note that most cells are extremely elongated with thin, tapered cytoplasm (*red arrows*). The majority of the nuclei are also fusiform (*blue arrows*).

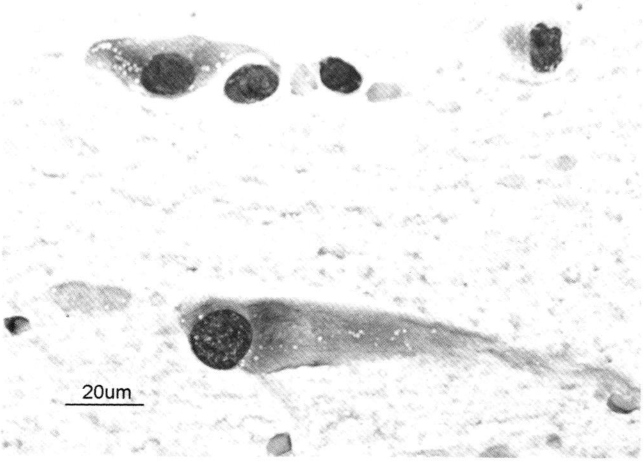

Figure 2-51 Spindle cells from a malignant tumor of mesenchymal origin (myxosarcoma). Note the elongated appearance of the cells with cytoplasm that tapers in one or more directions.

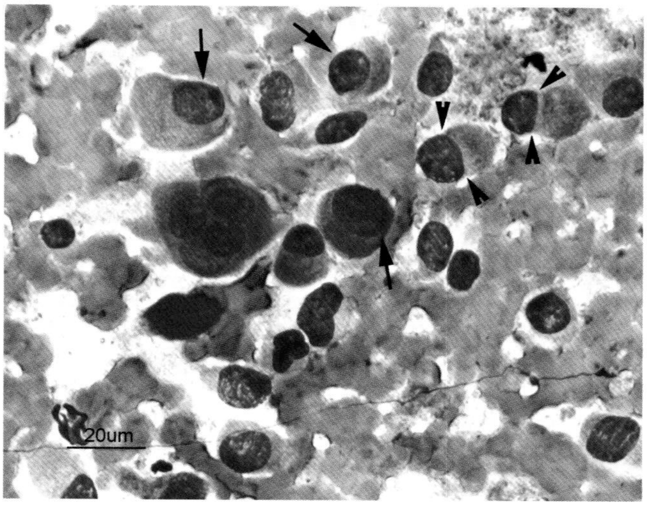

Figure 2-53 Cells from a canine osteosarcoma. The osteoblasts show little to no spindling and have distinct cytoplasmic borders. Note that most of the cells have eccentrically placed nuclei (*arrows*). Often, the nuclei appear to be partially outside the cytoplasmic borders (*arrowheads*). The mesenchymal nature of these cells is suggested by the presence of an extracellular matrix.

cellular because of the tightly cohesive nature of connective tissue. Benign mesenchymal tumors tend to exfoliate very few cells, and samples of diagnostic quality may be difficult to obtain. In contrast, malignant mesenchymal tumors may yield highly cellular aspirates (Figure 2-50). The cells are usually individually oriented, although large aggregates may be present, particularly if held together by an extracellular matrix (see below).

Mesenchymal cells are often fusiform cells with cytoplasm that tapers in one or more directions (Figure 2-51). These are commonly referred to as spindle cells. Mesenchymal cells may range from extremely elongated, fusiform cells with thin, rod-shaped nuclei (Figure 2-52) to cells that are plump and minimally tapered and have round nuclei (Figure 2-53). Aspirates from malignant mesenchymal tumors often show a mixture of cells of various shapes, so the entire population must be examined to determine the cell type (see Figure 2-50). Depending on the histologic subtype, cells from primary bone tumors (e.g., osteosarcoma, chondrosarcoma) may show virtually no spindling and may have well-defined cytoplasmic borders mimicking discrete cells or epithelial cells (see Figure 2-53). Usually, these are identified as being mesenchymal in nature on the basis of clinical suspicion (i.e., lytic bone lesion), the presence of extracellular matrix, the presence of osteoclasts (Figure 2-54), and the characteristic appearance of the cells (see Figure 2-53).

In contrast to other cell types (discrete and epithelial), the cytoplasmic borders of mesenchymal cells are often very indistinct (Figure 2-55). The cytoplasm may blend imperceptibly with the background, making it nearly impossible to distinguish the limits of the cell membrane. Ruptured cells may also have indistinct cytoplasmic borders. In these traumatized cells, the nuclear membrane is usually also disrupted, whereas the nuclear outline of intact mesenchymal cells is well defined. Another characteristic of mesenchymal cells is production of an extracellular matrix (Figure 2-56). This is seen as a variably eosinophilic material present between cells, often holding them in large aggregates.

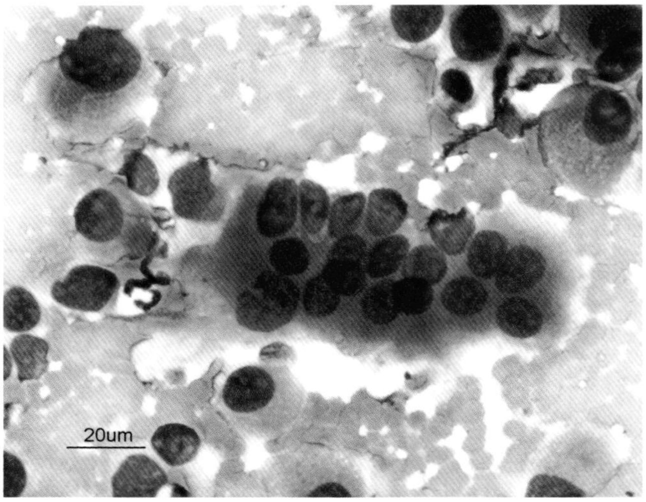

Figure 2-54 High magnification of slide from Figure 2-53. A large osteoclast is present in the center surrounded by osteoblasts. Osteoclasts often have 10 to 20 nuclei or more.

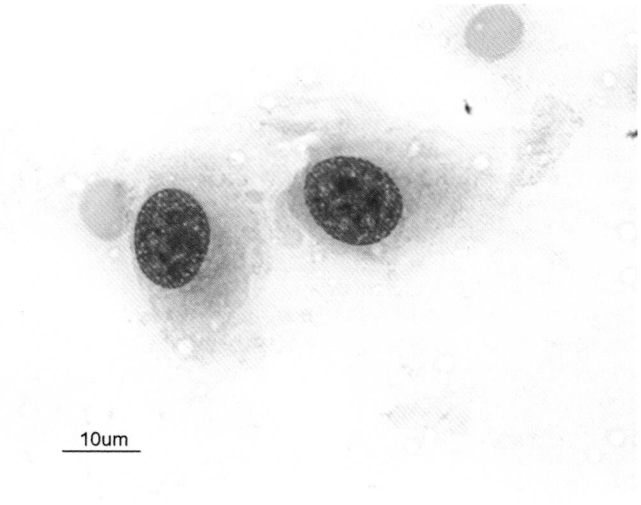

Figure 2-55 Cells from a tumor of mesenchymal origin. The cytoplasmic boundary of these cells is extremely indistinct; the cytoplasm seems to fade gradually into the background. This is another common feature of cells of mesenchymal origin.

These descriptions outline general characteristics. The entire cell population present should be carefully evaluated because no single criterion will definitively identify a cell population. Sometimes, particularly with poorly differentiated malignant tumors, the cells will show criteria of more than one category. In these cases, it may be impossible to accurately classify the type of cell present. If cell type cannot be categorized, the cells should be evaluated for criteria of malignancy because identification of a malignant tumor may be sufficient information to direct management of the case. Surgical biopsy and histopathology may be able to provide a more specific diagnosis as to tissue of origin, if needed.

DO THE TISSUE CELLS PRESENT DISPLAY SIGNIFICANT CRITERIA OF MALIGNANCY?

Tissue cells should be evaluated for cytologic atypia (criteria of malignancy). If sufficient criteria are present, a diagnosis of malignant neoplasia can be made. Cells from normal tissue, hyperplastic tissue, and benign neoplasia generally do not contain significant criteria of malignancy.

Cytologic Criteria of Malignancy

Although some assessment of the arrangement of cells within cell clusters can be made, cytologic samples often lack the architectural information that is available on histologic sections. Therefore, factors such as disruption of normal architecture and invasion of suspect cells into adjacent normal tissue or lymphatics usually cannot be made. Evaluation of malignant potential in cytology specimens involves evaluating cell populations for lack of differentiation and cellular atypia. In general, benign lesions yield morphologically uniform populations of

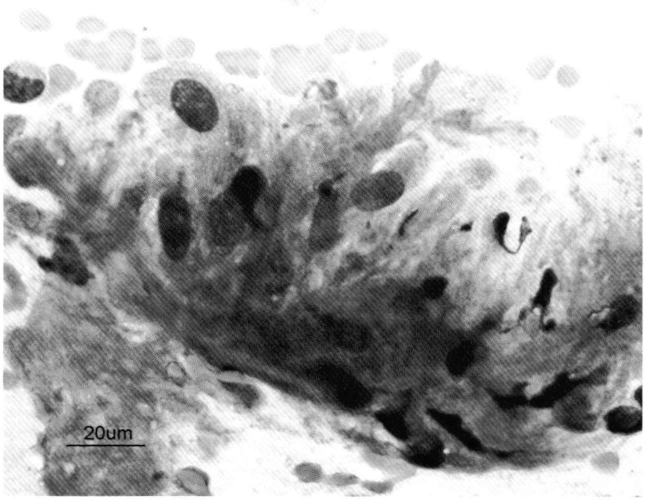

Figure 2-56 Aspirate from a mesenchymal tumor showing extracellular matrix production. Numerous mesenchymal cells are present, which appear to be embedded in a brightly eosinophilic extracellular matrix.

well-differentiated cells, whereas malignant tumors are characterized by variability of cell features. Cytologic criteria are divided into general criteria of malignancy and nuclear criteria of malignancy (Table 2-2). Nuclear criteria of malignancy are more reliable because they are less likely to be induced by nonneoplastic processes such as inflammation-induced dysplasia. No single criterion indicates the presence of malignancy, and any of the features described below may be seen in certain cells or cell populations.

TABLE 2-2

Easily Recognized General and Nuclear Criteria Of Malignancy

Criteria	Description	Schematic Representation
General Criteria		
Anisocytosis and macrocytosis	Variation in cell size, with some cells ≥2 times larger than normal	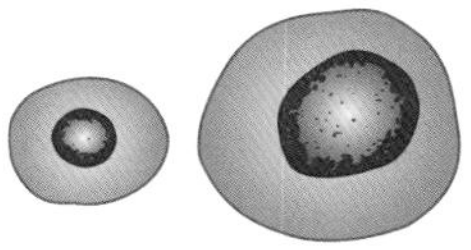
Hypercellularity	Increased cell exfoliation caused by decreased cell adherence	Not depicted
Pleomorphism (except in lymphoid tissue)	Variable size and shape in cell of the same type	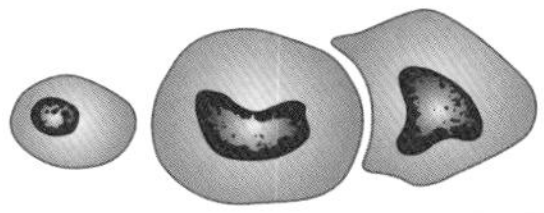
Nuclear Criteria		
Macrokaryosis	Increased nuclear size; cell with nuclei larger than 20 micrometers (μm) in diameter suggest malignancy	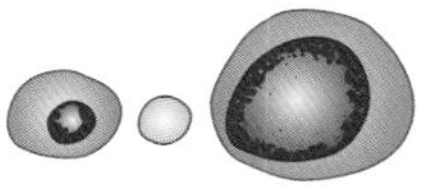 RBC
Increased nucleus-to-cytoplasm ratio (N:C)	Normal nonlymphoid cells usually have a N:C of 1:3 to 1:8, depending on the tissue; increased ratio (1:2,1:1, etc.) suggests malignancy	See "macrokaryosis"
Anisokaryosis	Variation in nuclear size; especially important if the nuclei of multinucleate cells vary in size.	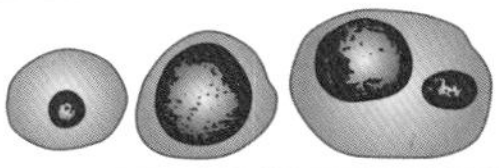
Multinucleation	Multiple nuclei in a cell; especially important if the nuclei vary in size	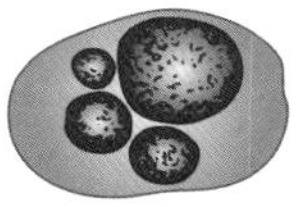
Increased mitotic figures	Mitosis is rare in normal tissue	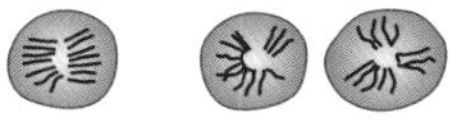 normal abnormal
Abnormal mitosis	Improper alignment of chromosomes	See "increased mitotic figures"
Coarse chromatin pattern	The chromatin pattern is coarser than normal; may appear ropy or cordlike	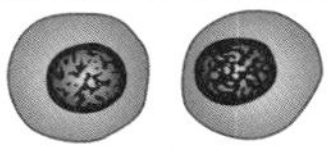
Nuclear molding	Deformation of nuclei by other nuclei within the same cell or adjacent cells	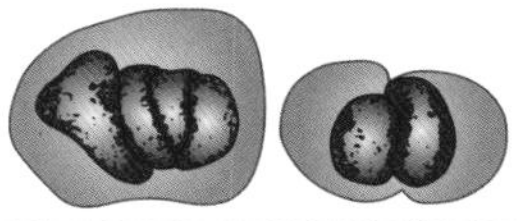
Macronucleoli	Nucleoli are increased in size; nucleoli ≥5 μm strongly suggest malignancy. For reference, RBCs are 5-6 μm in the cat and 7-8 μm in the dog.	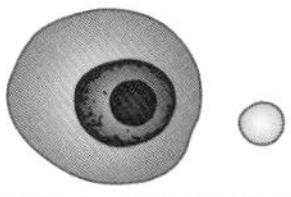 RBC
Angular nucleoli	Nucleoli are fusiform or have other angular shapes instead of their normal round to slightly oval shape	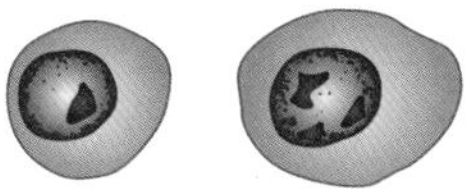
Anisonucleoliosis	Variation in nucleolar shape or size (especially important if the variation is within the same nucleus)	See "angular nucleoli"

RBC, red blood cell.

General Criteria of Malignancy

Anisocytosis and Macrocytosis: *Anisocytosis* (Figure 2-57) refers to variation in cell size, whereas *macrocytosis* (Figure 2-58) refers to exceptionally large cells. Macrocytic cells are most commonly observed in tumors of epithelial origin. Both are atypical findings in most cell populations, although exceptions do exist. In samples of normal or reactive lymphoid tissue, variation in cell size is an expected finding because of the variety of different cell types present (i.e., mature lymphocytes, lymphoblasts, plasma cells). In contrast, lymphoid malignancy yields a uniform, monomorphic population of lymphoblasts. In scrapings from skin surfaces and some vaginal swabs, moderate to marked anisocytosis of the squamous epithelial cells may exist. This relates to the fact that such samples can collect squamous cells of varying degrees of maturation, ranging from small, immature basal or parabasal cells to mature, fully keratinized, superficial squamous cells. Transitional epithelial cells also show moderate anisocytosis as a normal feature of that cell type. Finally, macrophages in inflammatory reactions can show marked variation in size (see Figure 2-10 and Figure 2-11) as well as many other atypical features.

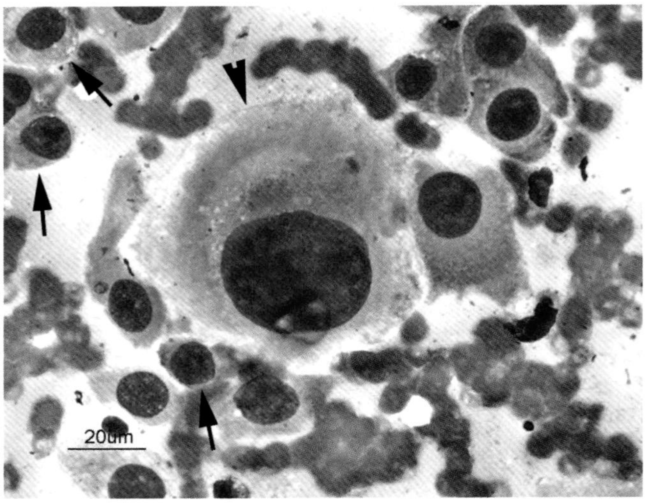

Figure 2-57 Aspirate from a transitional cell carcinoma. The cells show significant anisocytosis and anisokaryosis. Some cells (*arrowhead*) are several times larger than other cells in the population (*arrows*).

Some degree of anisocytosis is normal in any cell population. The tendency of many beginning cytologists is to overinterpret normal variability in cell size rather than to ignore significant variation when it is present; therefore, caution is warranted in evaluating subjective parameters. Significant variation in cell size is when one cell is multiple times the size of other cells from the same population. No easily defined objective criteria of macrocytosis exist, although this usually indicates cells that are decidedly larger than what is normal for the cell population. Obviously, this requires having sufficient experience to recognize the limits of normal. If normal cells from the tissue in question are present along with neoplastic cells, this can give a valuable reference point from which to judge the degree of variability (Figure 2-59).

Hypercellularity: Malignant tumors tend to exfoliate high numbers of cells, even when arising from tissues that would not normally exfoliate any cells. A classic example of this is primary bone tumors such as osteosarcoma and chondrosarcoma. Normal bone will obviously exfoliate very few, if any, cells. However, aspirates from primary bone tumors are often highly cellular (Figure 2-60). Cells in malignant tumors are often anaplastic and have not differentiated to the point where they develop cell receptors or produce the extracellular matrix that makes them adhesive to other tissues in the body. Therefore, these cells will exfoliate very well by FNB. Similarly, these cells will often demonstrate a loss of cohesion.

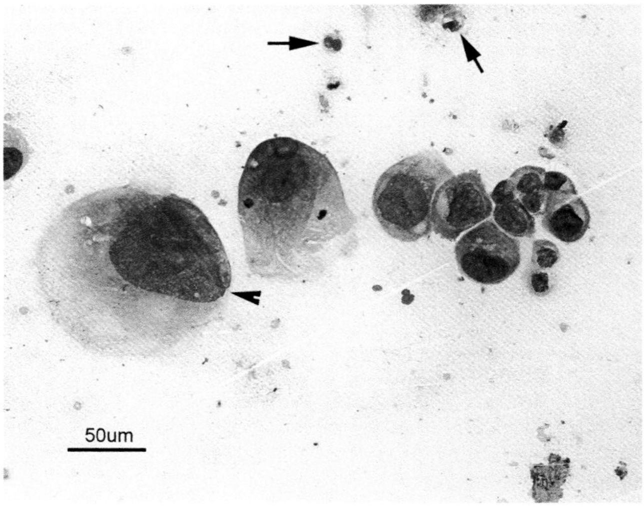

Figure 2-58 Low-power photomicrograph of smears made from thoracic fluid of a cat with a metastatic carcinoma. Atypically macrocytic cells almost 100 micrometers (μm) in diameter with macronuclei (karyomegaly) greater than 50 μm are present. Macrophages (*arrows*) are present for size comparison.

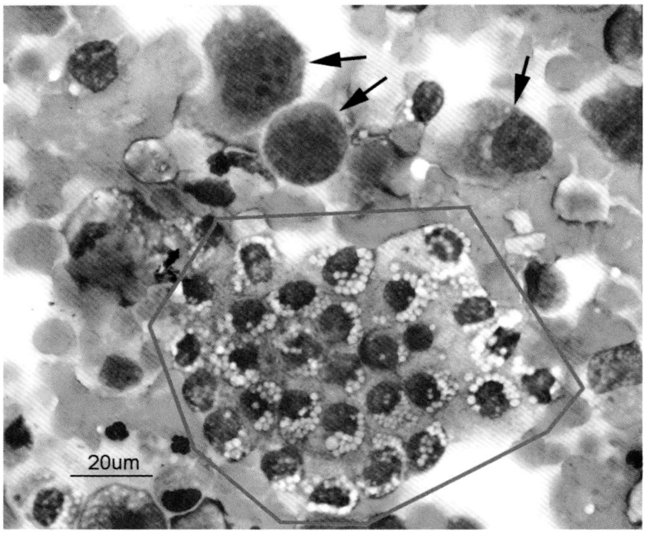

Figure 2-59 Aspirate of a carcinoma from the prostate of a dog. In this case, the presence of relatively normal, uniform prostatic cells in the middle (*surrounded by the red boundary*) allows for easier recognition of the surrounding abnormal larger cells with larger nuclei and prominent nucleoli.

Highly malignant epithelial tumors may yield cells that distribute in more of a discrete cell pattern, with fewer cell clusters (Figure 2-61).

Obviously, hypercellularity as a criterion of malignancy must be viewed in terms of the tissue sampled. Inflammatory lesions (see Figure 2-1), lymphoid tissue, and some other tissues normally yield high numbers of cells. In these instances, hypercellularity cannot be considered a criterion of malignancy. However, highly cellular slides containing a single population of mesenchymal cells is not a normal finding (see Figure 2-50). Hypercellularity is also important because the sample is more likely to be representative of the lesion than if relatively few cells are present. A definitive diagnosis of malignancy should be made with extreme caution if the sample is of low cellularity.

Pleomorphism: *Pleomorphism*, which refers to variability in the shape of cells, may be normal if more than one cell type is present on a smear. Also, pleomorphism among cells of a single cell type is seen in some normal tissue such as transitional cells from the urinary tract and samples containing squamous cells of varying degrees of maturation (skin scrapings and vaginal smears).

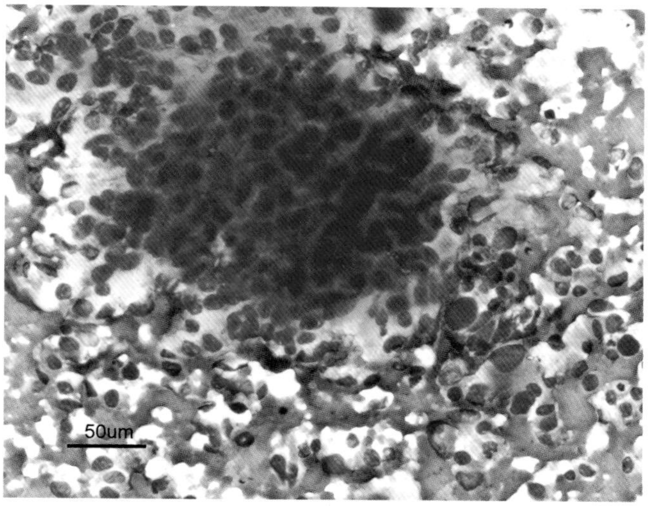

Figure 2-60 Aspirate from a canine osteosarcoma demonstrating the hypercellularity that may be seen with malignant tumors. Normal bone would exfoliate no cells, whereas an osteosarcoma often yields highly cellular slides.

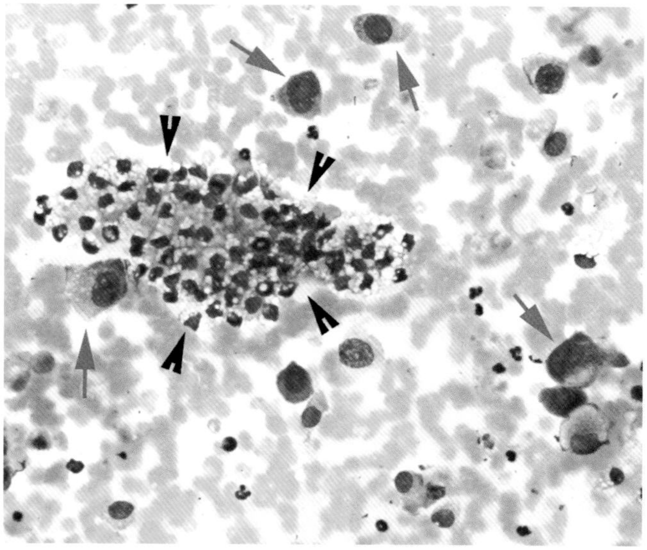

Figure 2-61 Aspirate from a carcinoma in the prostate of a dog. Note that the smaller, uniform cells representing normal prostatic epithelium (*black arrowheads*) are in a tightly cohesive cluster, whereas the larger, neoplastic cells are largely individually oriented because of loss of cellular cohesion (*red arrows*).

Nuclear Criteria of Malignancy

Anisokaryosis and Macrokaryosis (Karyomegaly): *Anisokaryosis* and *macrokaryosis* are terms that refer to variation in nuclear size (see Figure 2-57) and excessively large nuclei (see Figure 2-58), respectively. Nuclei that are multiple times the size of those in other cells within the same population represent significant anisokaryosis. In some malignant tumors, particularly carcinomas, macronuclei, which may be larger than some entire cells of the same population, may be present.

Anisokaryosis is a normal finding in samples containing squamous epithelial cells. As squamous cells mature, the nucleus becomes small and pyknotic, eventually disappearing from the cell.

Multinucleation: Cells with multiple nuclei may be seen in malignant tumors of any cell type. Multinucleation is particularly important when anisokaryosis is present among nuclei within a single cell (Figure 2-62). Multinucleation in neoplastic cells results from nuclear division without cell division. Usually, in multinucleate cells, even numbers of nuclei are present. Odd numbers of nuclei indicate atypical nuclear division and are an important finding (Figure 2-63).

Multinucleation can also be seen in nonneoplastic lesions. Inflammatory lesions may have macrophages that are multinucleate (multinucleate inflammatory giant cells) (see Figure 2-11). Osteoclasts are also normally

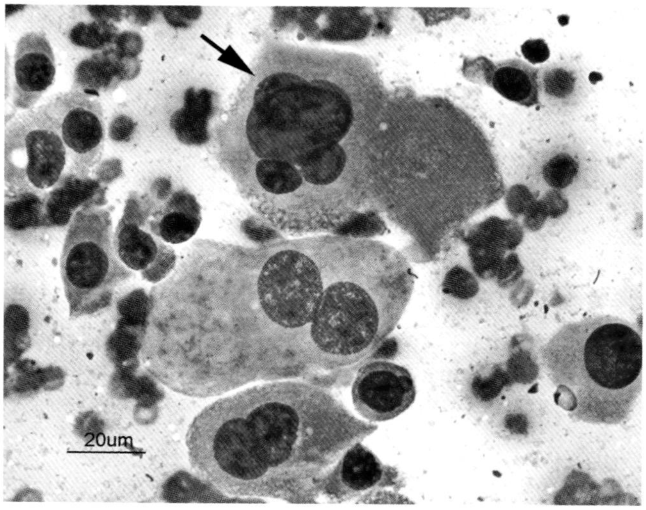

Figure 2-62 Aspirate of a transitional cell carcinoma from a dog. Two binucleate cells are present with equally sized nuclei. However, one multinucleated cell (*arrow*) shows significant variation in nuclear size.

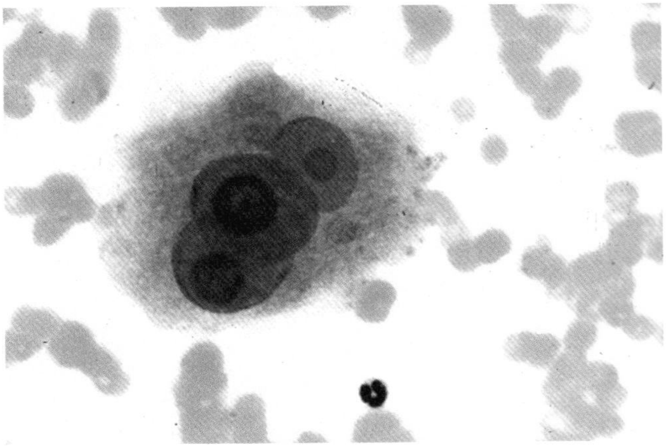

Figure 2-63 A multinucleated cell with an odd number of nuclei. Prominent, large nucleoli of varying size are also present. The erythrocytes and neutrophil can be used for size comparison.

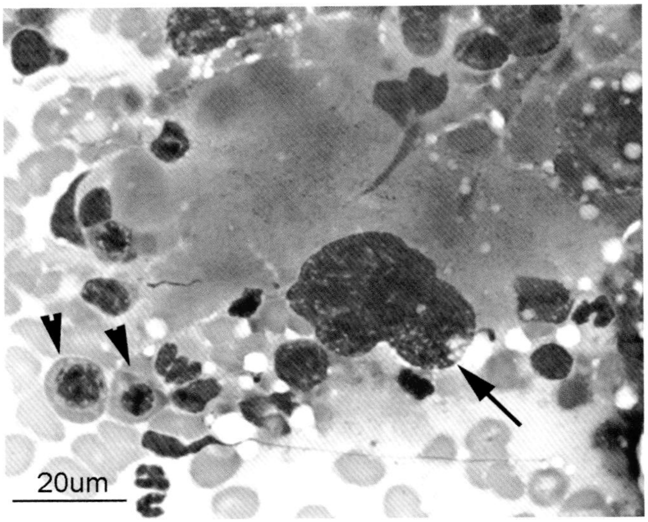

Figure 2-64 Splenic aspirate from a dog with extramedullary hematopoiesis. A single megakaryocyte is present. This large cell has expansive cytoplasm and a single, multilobulated nucleus and can resemble a multinucleate cell.

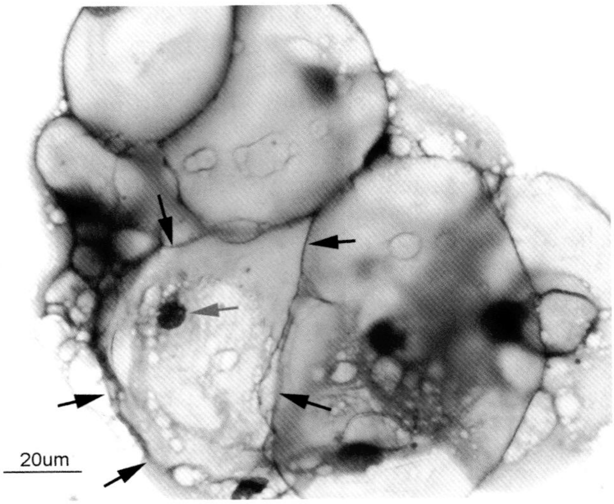

Figure 2-65 Aspirate of mature adipose tissue (lipoma) demonstrates a low nuclear-to-cytoplasmic ratio. The cells are extremely large (*black arrows* outline the cytoplasmic boundaries of a single adipocyte) yet have very small nuclei (*red arrow*).

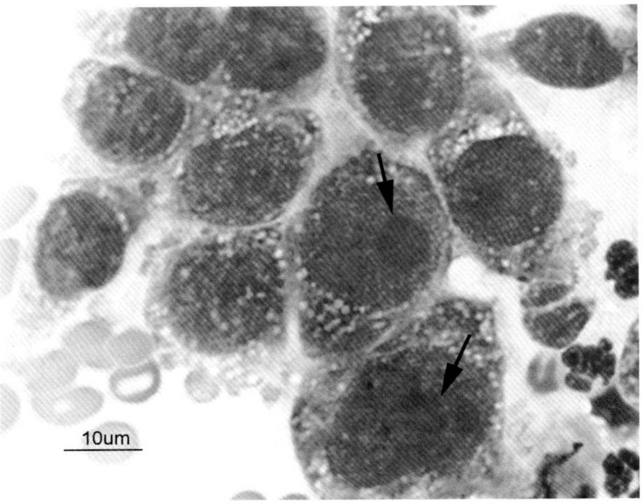

Figure 2-66 Carcinoma from a sample of canine pleural fluid. The neoplastic cells demonstrate a high nuclear-to-cytoplasmic (N:C) ratio. Note that the nucleus takes up well over half of the volume of the entire cell. Some cells have only scant amounts of visible cytoplasm. A high N:C ratio is normal in some cells such as lymphocytes and basal epithelial cells, but in large cells such as this, it generally indicates undifferentiated cells. Also, note the large nucleoli (*arrows*).

multinucleate (see Figure 2-54). Megakaryocytes, which are commonly present in the spleen as a reflection of extramedullary hematopoiesis, may have multiple nuclear lobes (Figure 2-64) and may appear to be multinucleate. Binucleate cells are commonly found in aspirates of epithelial tissue undergoing hyperplasia or regeneration (e.g., hepatic nodular hyperplasia). Also, some benign tumors, such as cutaneous plasmacytomas, may have many binucleate and multinucleate cells (see Figure 2-33).

Abnormal Nuclear-to-Cytoplasmic Ratio: *N:C ratio* refers to the relative areas occupied by the nucleus and cytoplasm of the cell. A low N:C ratio indicates a cell with a relatively small nucleus and vast amounts of cytoplasm (Figure 2-65). In contrast, cells with only scant amounts of cytoplasm have a high N:C ratio (Figure 2-66). Epithelial and mesenchymal cells having a high N:C ratio are suggestive of malignancy. A high N:C ratio is a particularly important finding in very large cells because some small cells (e.g., mature lymphocytes, basal epithelial cells) normally have a high N:C ratio. A high N:C ratio in a large cell generally indicates a poorly differentiated cell.

Marked variation in the N:C ratio of cells within a single population is also an abnormal finding (Figure 2-67). Again, exceptions exist. Slides of normal lymphoid tissue and scrapings containing normal squamous cells of varying stages of maturation will demonstrate variation in N:C ratio.

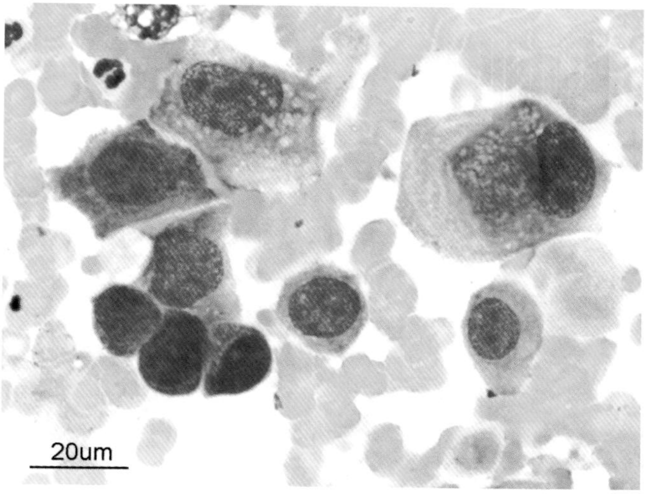

Figure 2-67 Aspirate from a carcinoma. Note the variation in nuclear-to-cytoplasmic ratio.

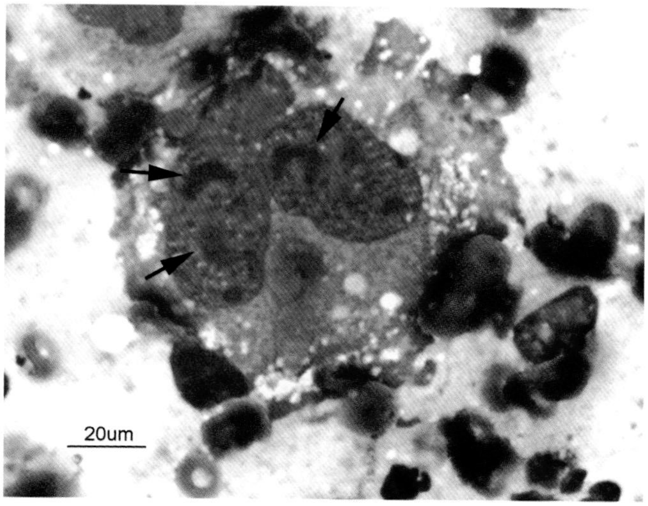

Figure 2-68 Cell from a carcinoma. Note the large, irregularly shaped nucleoli (*arrows*).

Abnormal Nucleoli: Nucleoli are areas within the nucleus that are responsible for production of ribosomal ribonucleic acid (RNA). All cells have nucleoli, but they are usually small and often not readily visible. Nucleoli that are abnormally large (macronucleoli) that are atypically shaped (angular) or that vary in size are strong indicators of malignancy. Nucleoli in normal cells are small, approximately 1 to 2 micrometers (μm) in diameter. Nucleoli greater than 5 μm in diameter are suggestive of malignancy (see Figure 2-66). Erythrocytes can be used as a reference for evaluating the size of nucleoli. Canine erythrocytes are 7 to 8 μm, whereas feline erythrocytes are approximately 5 to 6 μm in diameter, if well spread out.

Normal cells have round nucleoli. Fusiform, pleomorphic, or angular nucleoli are indicative of malignancy (Figure 2-68). Diff-Quik stain often stains nucleoli more prominently than do other cytologic stains, so this must be considered when evaluating cells for malignant potential. Also, nucleoli may be more prominent than normal in cells that are either ruptured or understained.

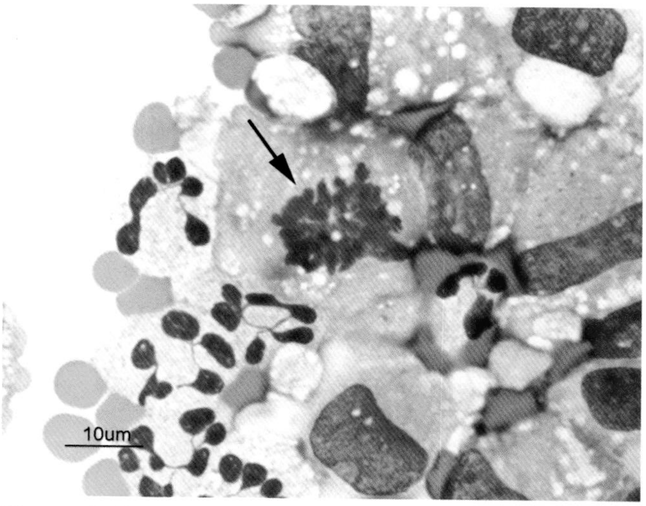

Figure 2-69 Transtracheal wash fluid from a cat. Several neutrophils and macrophages are shown. One macrophage is undergoing mitosis (*arrow*).

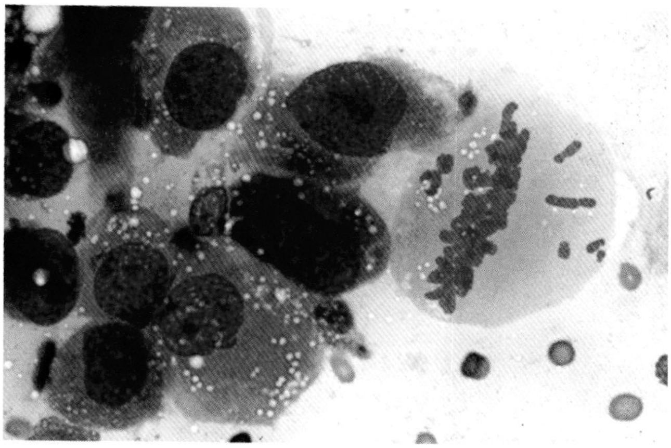

Figure 2-70 Smear from a malignant tumor in the lung of a cat. One abnormal mitotic figure is present, which demonstrates some lagging chromosomes.

Abnormal Mitosis: Mitotic figures are rare in samples from most normal tissue cell populations. Exceptions are lymphoid tissue and bone marrow, where mitoses may be common. Also, macrophages can divide in tissues and so mitotic figures are frequently seen in inflammatory responses with numerous macrophages (Figure 2-69). Increased numbers of mitoses in other tissues or mitotic figures showing abnormal alignment of chromosomes are suggestive of malignancy (Figure 2-70, Figure 2-71, and Figure 2-72).

Coarse or Immature Nuclear Chromatin: Nuclear chromatin patterns are not as distinctive and evident in cells stained with Romanowsky-type stains as they are when cells are wet fixed and stained with Papanicolaou-type stains. Still, an abnormally coarse nuclear chromatin pattern is often visible in malignant cells. Also, mature cells tend to have nuclear chromatin that is condensed and, thus, stains a dark purple. Immature cells may have light staining chromatin lacking aggregates of

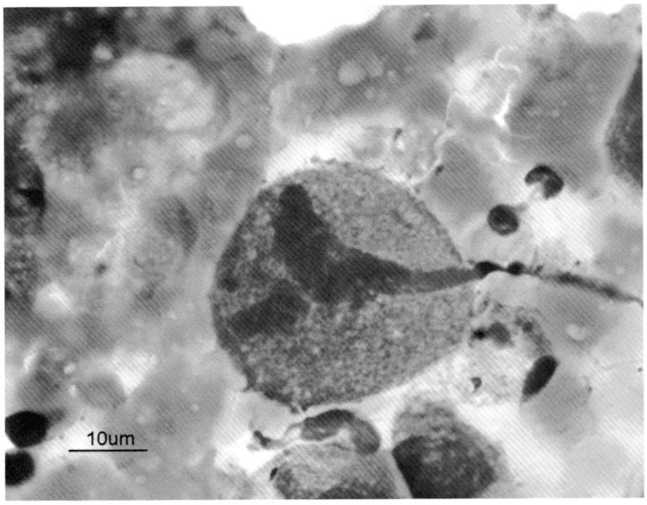

Figure 2-71 Abnormal mitotic figure in a sample of a malignant tumor from a dog. The nuclear material has formed a "Y" shape rather than forming a straight line.

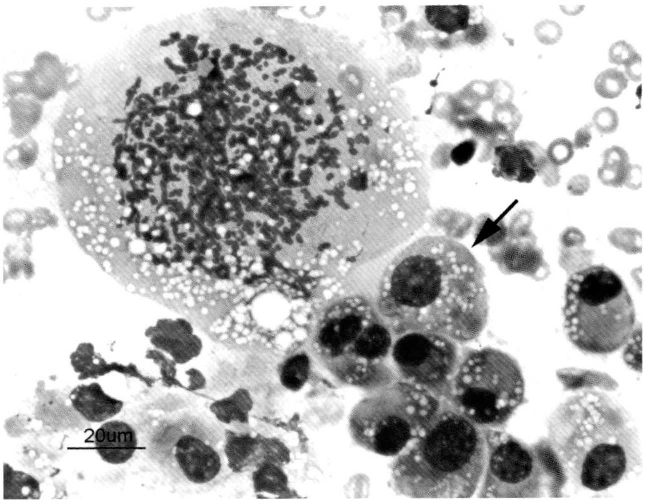

Figure 2-72 Extremely large, bizarre mitotic figure from a spleen aspirate of a dog with histiocytic sarcoma. Several other histiocytic cells are present, one of which shows erythrophagocytosis (*arrow*).

heterochromatin often described as "dispersed" or "open" (see Figure 2-14).

Abnormal Nuclear Arrangement: Although the majority of tissue architecture is lost when performing fine-needle aspiration, some cellular structure is still evident in cell clusters. Normal cell clusters tend to have a very uniform arrangement of the nuclei, giving them a honeycomb appearance (Figure 2-73). Because mature cells typically have a lower N:C ratio, the nuclei often appear evenly spaced and not touching each other (see Figure 2-73). In contrast, clusters of neoplastic cells often show irregular arrangement (Figure 2-74). Lack of normal contact inhibition can result in nuclei that are crowded together and piled on top of each other (see Figure 2-74).

Sometimes, the nucleus of one cell can be seen to deform around the nucleus of another cell (or another nucleus within a multinucleated cell). This is referred to as nuclear molding and indicates rapid growth and loss of contact inhibition (Figure 2-75).

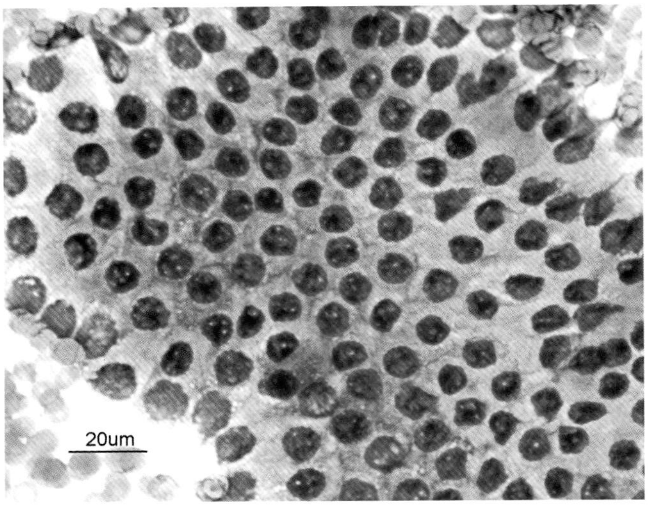

Figure 2-73 Prostatic aspirate from a dog with benign prostatic hyperplasia. The slide consists of mature, well-differentiated prostatic epithelial cells. Note the uniform and even spacing of the nuclei in the center of this cell cluster. The nuclei are round and have densely stained, mature chromatin. Around the edges of the cell cluster, some of the cells have been traumatized, resulting in lighter staining nuclei with irregular outlines.

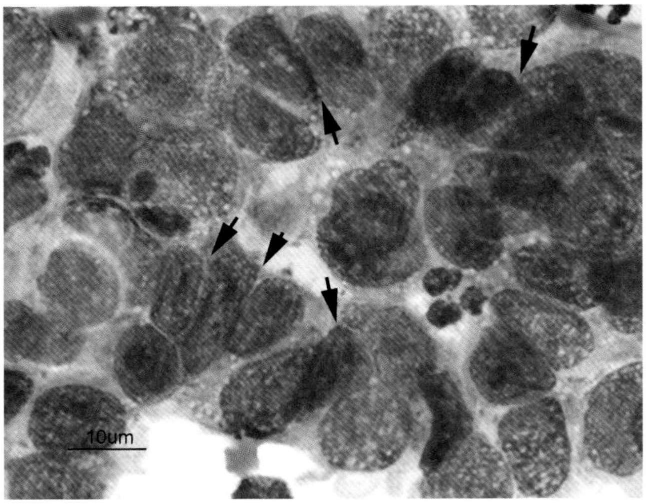

Figure 2-74 Aspirate of a carcinoma from a dog. The cells lack the regular arrangement of benign well-differentiated cells. Nuclei are crowded together and pile on top of each other. The cells have a high nucleus-to-cytoplasm ratio and many have prominent nucleoli.

General Cautions Regarding Evaluating Cytologic Criteria of Malignancy

No single cellular feature reliably distinguishes malignant from benign cells. A reliable diagnosis of malignancy can usually be made if three or more nuclear criteria of malignancy are present in a majority of the cells present in the smear. If cytologic features of malignancy are not unambiguous, the diagnosis should be confirmed with a biopsy

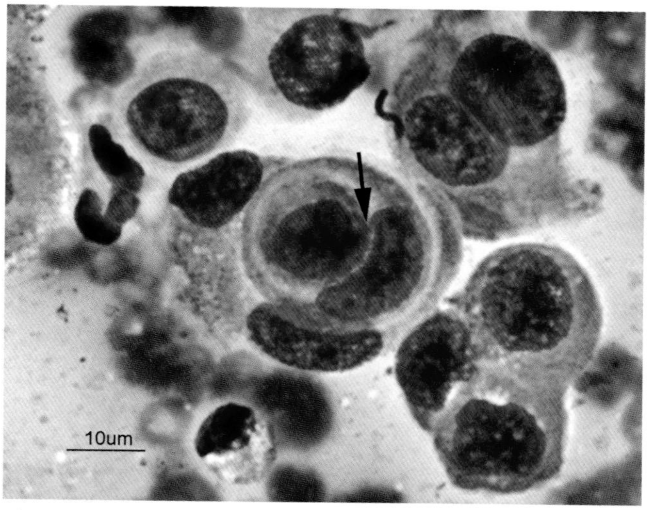

Figure 2-75 Cells from a transitional cell carcinoma from a dog. Nuclear molding is seen in the center, where the nucleus of one cell is wrapping around that of another.

and histologic evaluation. It is imperative that a representative sample (highly cellular) is available and that only intact (nontraumatized), well-spread-out, well-stained cells are evaluated. Nucleoli are often more distinct in understained cells present in thick areas of the smears. When cells are partially ruptured, the nuclear chromatin spreads out and uncoils. This results in the nucleus appearing larger than it really is and also makes nucleoli, normally obscured by the condensed chromatin, more visible.

Also, caution should be exercised in diagnosing neoplasia in the face of inflammation. Inflammation can induce dysplastic changes in tissue cells that can mimic neoplasia. Inflammatory lesions may also contain large, epithelioid macrophages and proliferating fibroblasts, both of which may have some features that are similar to malignant cells.

Conversely, not every malignant tumor shows marked cellular atypia and variability. Some tumors may yield relatively uniform populations of cells, yet exhibit aggressive biologic behavior. This finding is frequently encountered in endocrine tumors. The majority of thyroid tumors in dogs are malignant, yet samples from some thyroid carcinomas contain relatively uniform cells without marked criteria of malignancy. The same situation is described in other tumors of endocrine and neuroendocrine origin. Many other well-differentiated carcinomas (e.g., perianal gland tumors) are difficult to distinguish from a benign proliferation solely on the basis of cytologic examination. In some cases, this differentiation is also difficult to make on histologic examination. Thus, although an understanding of general features of cellular atypia is helpful, experience with the peculiarities of each individual tumor type is needed for correct interpretation of many samples.

References

1. Meinkoth JH, Cowell RL: Recognition of basic cell types and criteria of malignancy, *Vet Clin North Am* 32:1209–1235, 2002.
2. Raskin R: General categories of cytologic interpretation. In Raskin RE, Meyer DJ, editors: *Atlas of canine and feline cytology*, ed 2, Philadelphia, PA, 2010, Saunders, pp 15–25.
3. McKinley ET: General cytologic principles. In Atkinson BF, editor: *Atlas of diagnostic cytopathology*, ed 2, Philadelphia, PA, 2004, Saunders, pp 1–30.
4. Kocjan G: *Fine needle aspiration cytology: diagnostic principles and dilemmas*, New York, 2006, Springer. 35–58.
5. Kiupel M, Webster JD, Bailey KL, et al: Proposal of a 2-tier histologic grading system for canine cutaneous mast cell tumor to more accurately predict biological behavior, *Vet Pathol* 48:147–155, 2011.
6. Affolter VK, Moore PF: Localized and disseminated histiocytic sarcoma of dendritic cell origin in dogs, *Vet Pathol* 39:74–83, 2002.
7. Moore PF, Affolter VK, Vernau W: Canine hemophagocytic histiocytic sarcoma: a proliferative disorder of CD11d+ macrophages, *Vet Pathol* 43:632–645, 2006.
8. Clark GN, Berg J, Engler SJ, et al: Extramedullary plasmacytomas in dogs: results of surgical excision in 131 cases, *J Am Anim Hosp Assoc* 28:105–111, 1992.
9. Vail DM: Plasma cell neoplasms. In Withrow SJ, Vail DM, editors: *Small animal clinical oncology*, ed 4, St. Louis, MO, 2007, Saunders, pp 769–794.

CHAPTER 3

Selected Infectious Agents

Rick L. Cowell and Tara P. Arndt

Evaluating cytologic samples often results in the observance of microorganisms, some of which may be primary etiologic agents, opportunistic secondary overgrowths, or part of the normal flora of the location sampled. In some cases, the challenge is not only the identification of the organisms but also the recognition of the significance or insignificance of the organism in the overall pathologic process. This chapter is intended to aid in recognizing selected organisms found during the cytologic evaluation of samples from dogs and cats. It is beyond the scope of this book and chapter to discuss all of the organisms noted in cats and dogs; however, this chapter is intended to serve as a reference for the more commonly encountered infectious agents in canine and feline cytopathology. Discussions of the pathologic changes and conditions that these organisms produce are found in the following relevant chapters. Sample collection, staining and submission of samples for culture were previously covered in Chapter 1.

IDENTIFICATION OF ORGANISMS

Size, shape, and staining characteristics are important in the cytologic identification of organisms. The remainder of this chapter contains brief descriptions of organisms, including routine staining characteristics, which can be identified by cytologic analysis, and one or more photomicrographs of each organism to aid in its identification. The staining characteristics indicated in this chapter are for commonly available, routine hematologic stains such as Wright, modified Wright, Wright-Giemsa, Diff-Quik, or Dip-Stat stains, unless otherwise stated.

BACTERIA

Staining Characteristics

With the routine hematologic stains described previously, all bacteria, whether gram positive or gram negative, stain blue to purple, with a few exceptions such as *Mycobacterium*. The lipid cell wall of *Mycobacterium* spp. prevents uptake of hematologic stains, causing the organisms to appear as nonstaining "negative" rods.

Gram stains can be used, but it is much more difficult to find bacteria with Gram stains than with hematologic stains and Gram stains often do not give reproducible, accurate results for bacteria in exudates. Cells, exudative proteins, and bacteria (whether gram positive or gram negative) tend to stain red in cytologic smears made from exudates.

Primary and Opportunistic Secondary Infection versus Normal Microflora

Intracellular bacteria indicate an active bacterial infection (primary or secondary), whereas extracellular bacteria are nonspecific and may represent an active bacterial infection, normal microflora, or contamination. Concomitant intracellular and extracellular bacteria are indicative of true bacterial infection, whereas normal microflora and contamination yield only extracellular bacteria. Also, a monomorphic bacterial population (only one bacterial type present) suggests infection, whereas a pleomorphic population (mixture of rods and cocci or different-sized rods) may be seen with contamination, normal microflora, or a mixed bacterial infection. Mixed bacterial populations may occur with infectious conditions such as gastrointestinal (GI) infections, bite wounds, and foreign bodies.

Bacterial Cocci

Pathogenic bacterial cocci are usually gram positive and of the genera *Staphylococcus*, *Streptococcus*, *Peptostreptococcus*, or *Peptococcus* (Figure 3-1). Staphylococci usually occur in clusters of 4 to 12 bacteria; however, *Streptococcus*, *Peptostreptococcus*, and *Peptococcus* spp. tend to occur in short or long chains of organisms. *Staphylococcus* and *Streptococcus* spp. are aerobic, and *Peptostreptococcus* and *Peptococcus* spp. are anaerobic. When cocci are identified in cytologic preparations, aerobic and anaerobic cultures and sensitivity testing should be performed to identify the organism and to guide optimal antibiotic therapy. As most cocci are gram positive, antibiotic therapy effective against gram-positive organisms should be used when it is deemed necessary to start therapy before culture and sensitivity results are received.

Dermatophilus congolensis replicates by transverse and longitudinal division, producing long chains of coccoid bacterial doublets that resemble small, blue railroad tracks (Figure 3-2). It infects the superficial epidermis,

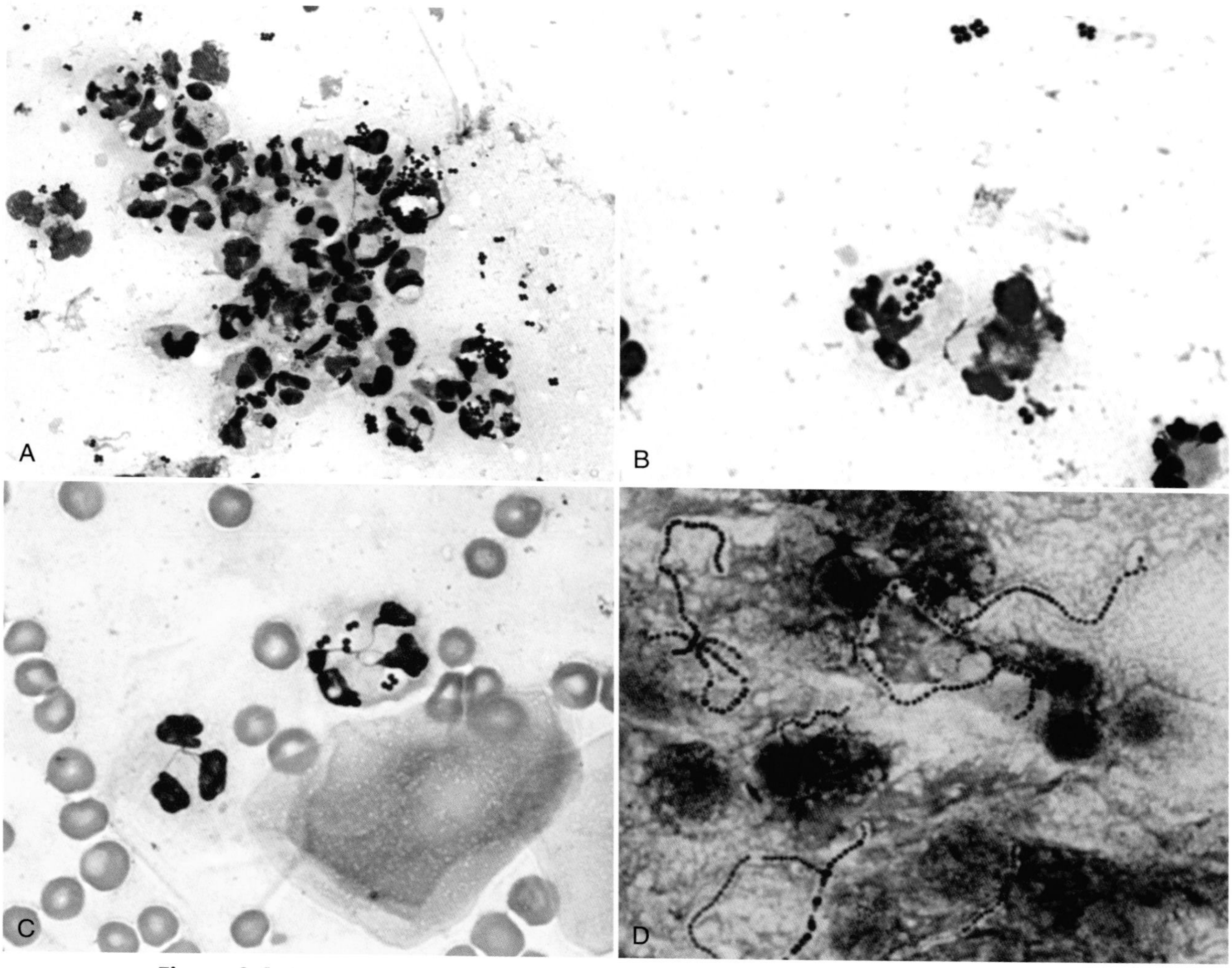

Figure 3-1 **A,** Neutrophilic inflammation with moderate numbers of bacterial cocci present both intracellularly and extracellularly. (Wright stain.) **B,** Higher magnification showing a neutrophil containing phagocytized bacterial cocci. (Wright stain.) **C,** Scattered red blood cells, two neutrophils, and a superficial squamous epithelial cell are shown. One of the neutrophils contains phagocytized bacterial cocci. (Wright stain.) **D,** Bacteria cocci chains. (Wright stain).

causing crusty lesions. Cytologic preparations from the undersurface of scabs from these crusty lesions are most rewarding in demonstrating organisms. The preparations usually contain mature epithelial cells, keratin bars, debris, and organisms. A few neutrophils may also be found.

Small Bacterial Rods

Most small bacterial rods are gram negative and some can be recognized as bipolar rods (Figure 3-3). It is safe to assume that all pathogenic, bipolar bacterial rods are gram negative. Common small bacterial rods include *Escherichia coli* and *Pasteurella* spp. Infections with bacterial rods are usually associated with a marked neutrophilic inflammatory response. When small bacterial rods are recognized in cytologic preparations, the lesion should be cultured to identify the organism, and sensitivity tests should be performed to determine the optimal antibiotic therapy. If it is necessary to institute antibiotic therapy before the culture and sensitivity results are received, the therapy employed should be effective against gram-negative organisms as most pathogenic small rods are gram negative.

Filamentous Rods

Pathogenic filamentous rods that cause cutaneous or subcutaneous lesions are typically *Nocardia* or *Actinomyces* spp. Other anaerobes such as *Fusobacterium* and *Mycobacterium* spp. may also be filamentous but are rarely so. *Nocardia* and *Actinomyces* spp. generally have a distinctive morphology in cytologic preparations stained with routine hematologic stains. They are characterized by long, slender (filamentous) strands that stain pale blue and have intermittent small pink or purple areas giving a "beaded" appearance to the organism (Figure 3-4). This morphology is characteristic of both *Nocardia* and *Actinomyces* spp. and the filamentous form of *Fusobacterium* spp. When these features are recognized cytologically, cultures should be performed specifically for *Nocardia* and *Actinomyces* spp. as well as for other anaerobes.

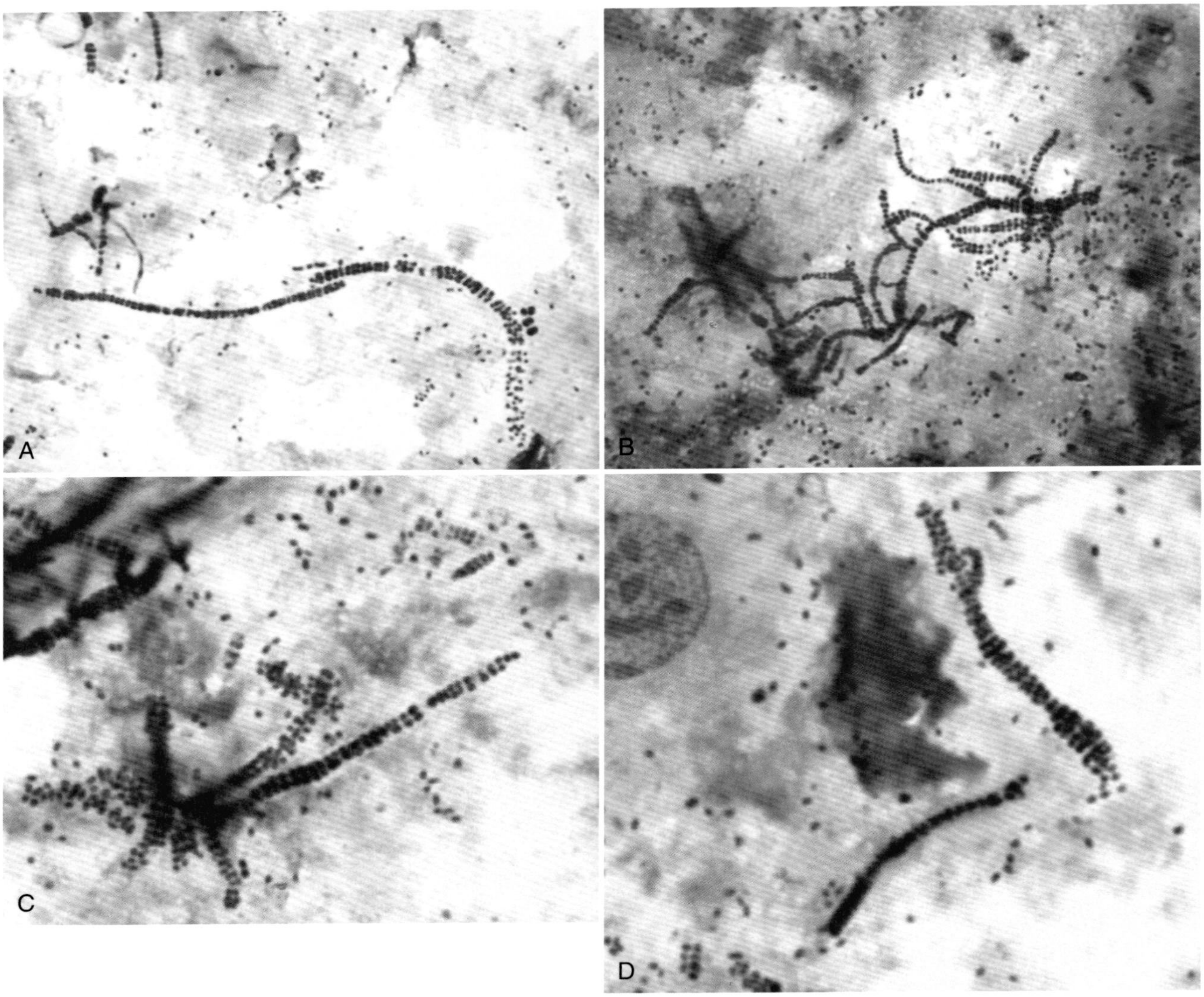

Figure 3-2 A-D, Impression smear from skin lesions showing bacterial cocci replicating by transverse and longitudinal division, producing long chains of coccoid bacterial doublets that resemble small, blue railroad tracks. This pattern of bacterial cocci is typical of *Dermatophilus congolensis*. (Wright stain.).

Mycobacterium spp. does not stain with routine hematologic stains. As a result, negative staining rods (Figure 3-5) may be observed in the cytoplasm of macrophages, inflammatory giant cells, or both. When epithelioid macrophages, inflammatory giant cells, or both are encountered in cytologic preparations that do not contain any obvious organisms, a careful search for negative images of *Mycobacterium* spp. should be made. *Mycobacterium* spp. stain with acid-fast stains; therefore, when the character of the lesion suggests that *Mycobacterium* spp. be considered, and negative images are not identified, an acid-fast stain can be performed to aid in organism identification (see Figure 3-5, *C*). Cultures, and/or polymerase chain reaction (PCR) testing of tissue samples for *Mycobacterium* spp. may be helpful. Specific breeds of cats and dogs, including Siamese cats, Bassett dogs, and Miniature Schnauzer dogs, appear to be predisposed to *Mycobacterium* infections.

Because these organisms are often refractory to common antibiotic therapy and reliable culture has special requirements, cytology is very useful in indicating to the practitioner that special cultures are needed. Multiple species of mycobacteria cause disease in dogs and cats and many of these species are zoonotic, which raises possible public health concerns. (See Mycobacterial infections. In: Greene CE, editor: *Infectious diseases of the dog and cat*, ed 4, St. Louis, MO, 2012, Saunders.)

Large Bacterial Rods

Large bacterial rods that are pathogenic and sometimes infect the cutaneous and subcutaneous tissues include *Clostridia* spp., and infrequently, *Bacillus* spp. When large bacterial rods are thought to be pathogenic, both aerobic and anaerobic cultures should be performed. Also,

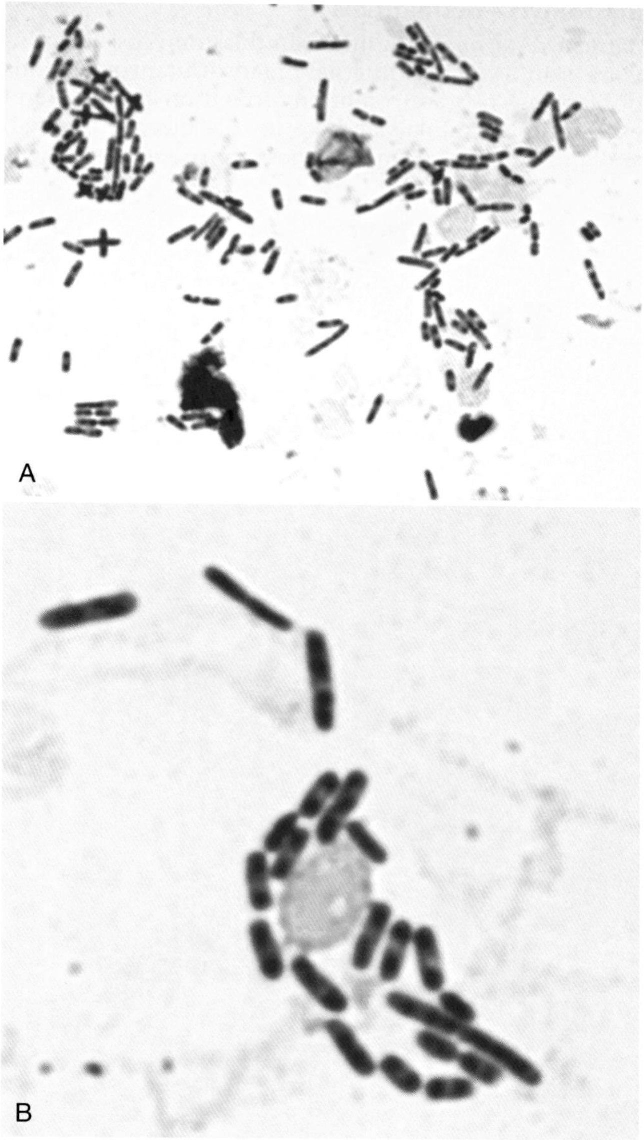

Figure 3-3 **A,** Bipolar rods in cat (Wright stain). **B,** Higher magnification of bipolar rods (Wright stain).

the smears should be inspected for large rods containing spores (Figure 3-6), as this may indicate *Clostridium* spp. infection.

Occasionally, the large nonpathogenic bacterial rods of *Simonsiella* spp. are observed in cytologic specimens (e.g., contaminated tracheal washes). *Simonsiella* spp. are part of the normal oral flora of many domestic species and divide lengthwise, yielding parallel rows of bacteria that give the impression of a single, large bacterium with the characteristic "footprint" (Figure 3-7). Finding these organisms in cytologic samples from various locations indicates oral contamination; for example, if found in nasal flush samples, it may indicate a nasal–oral fistula, or if found in a lesion on a limb, it indicates licking and potentially could complicate the interpretation of an atypical mesenchymal population as neoplastic versus reactive.

YEAST, DERMATOPHYTES, HYPHATING FUNGI, AND ALGAE

Mycotic agents produce lesions that tend to be more granulomatous; that is, the inflammatory reaction has more macrophages compared with bacterial lesions. However, neutrophils may still be the predominant cell type, and eosinophils may be plentiful with certain hyphating fungi. Mycotic lesions often contain low numbers of lymphocytes, plasma cells, and fibroblasts, and smaller organisms that tend to be phagocytized by macrophages, but can be found phagocytized by granulocytic cells as well. Many factors, including the infectious agent, the animal demographics, the location of the lesion, the chronicity of the lesion, and the immune status of the animal, will influence the nature of the lesion in these infections. A comparison of the common fungi that form yeasts in tissues is presented in Table 3-1.

Sporothrix schenckii

In many species, *Sporothrix schenckii* infection (sporotrichosis) can cause raised proliferative skin lesions that are often ulcerated. In cats, lesions tend to have many organisms, and cytologic evaluation readily leads to a diagnosis. In dogs, however, organisms are scant, and cytologic preparations must be carefully screened, as often only the inflammatory reaction is recognized. If no cause for a robust inflammatory reaction is identified, the lesion should be cultured, or a biopsy of the lesion should be submitted for histopathologic evaluation.

In cytologic preparations stained with hematologic stains, *S. schenckii* (Figure 3-8) are round to oval shaped or fusiform (cigar shaped), 3 to 9 micrometers (μm) long and 1 to 3 μm wide and stain pale to medium blue with a slightly eccentric pink or purple nucleus. Caution in interpreting is warranted, as occasionally these organisms can be confused with *Histoplasma capsulatum* if only a few yeasts are found and if they are not classically fusiform.

S. schencki is naturally found in soil, hay, sphagnum moss, and plants and has been termed "rose gardener's disease." Caution is warranted with handling feline cases, as zoonotic potential exists, particularly for humans with impaired or compromised immune systems.

Histoplasma capsulatum

Histoplasma capsulatum primarily affects the lungs; however, symptoms can vary greatly. In cases of systemic histoplasmosis, infections can involve other internal organs, including skin. Cutaneous histoplasmosis lesions are typically raised and proliferative and may ulcerate, rarely producing draining tracts. These lesions usually yield copious organisms that can be found extracellularly and phagocytized more commonly by macrophages and rarely by neutrophils. In routinely stained cytologic preparations, *Histoplasma* organisms (Figure 3-9) are round to slightly oval in shape; however, they are not fusiform as *Sporothrix* spp. classically are. *Histoplasma* spp. range in diameter from 2 to 4 μm, have a thin clear halo, stain pale to medium blue, and have an eccentric crescent-shaped eosinophilic to metachromatic nucleus.

H. capsulatum is found throughout the world and is endemic in certain areas of the United States, particularly in states bordering the Ohio River valley and the lower Mississippi River. It is also common in caves in southern and eastern Africa. *H. capsulatum* grows in soil and material contaminated with bird or bat droppings (guano).

Blastomyces dermatitidis

Blastomyces dermatitidis infection (blastomycosis) can involve skin, eyes, and internal organs. Cutaneous lesions of blastomycosis are commonly found on the nose and extremities of animals and are usually ulcerated, raised, and proliferative. Cutaneous lesions should be sought

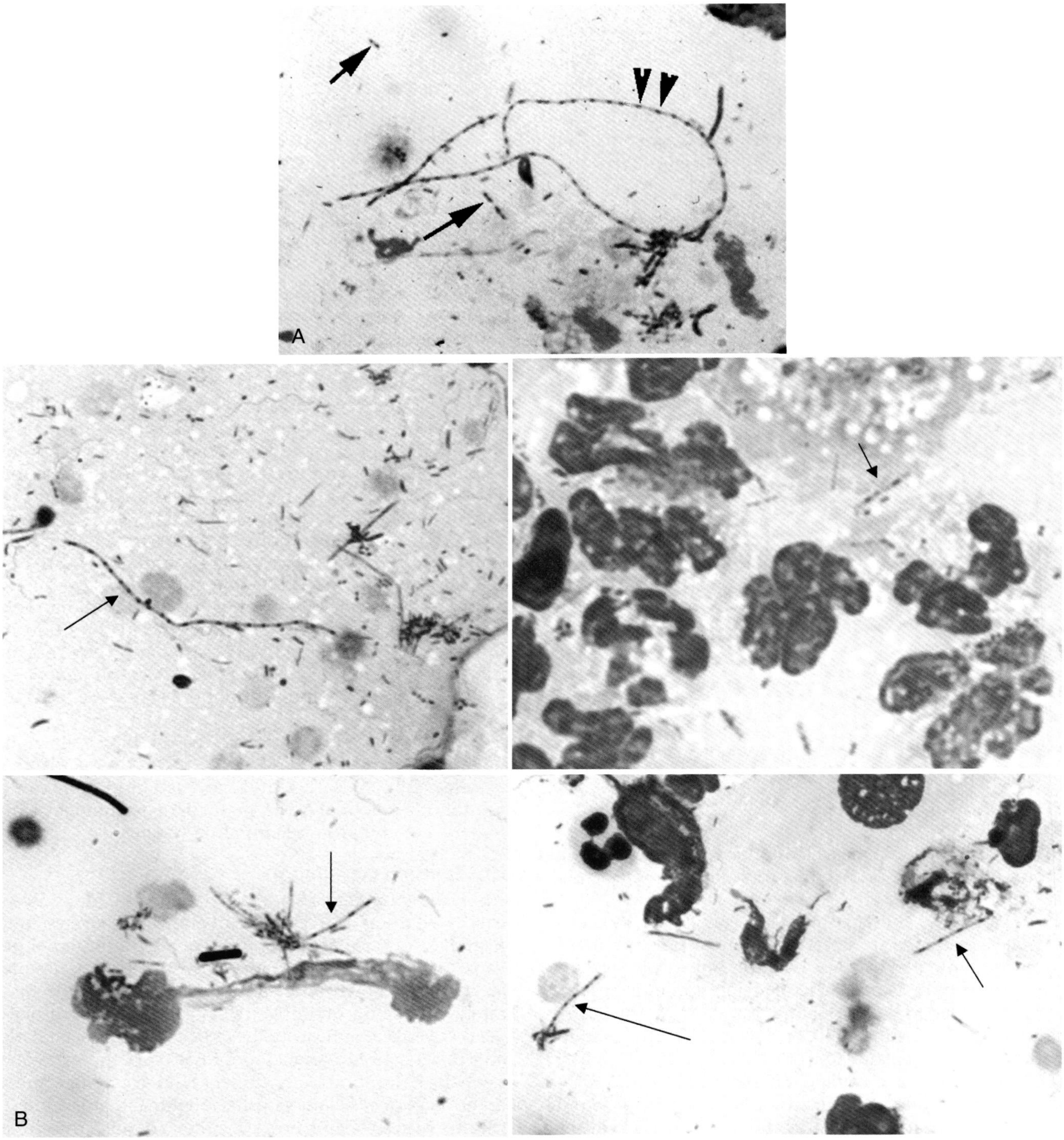

Figure 3-4 **A,** A long filamentous rod staining pale blue with intermittent small pink or purple dots (*arrowheads*) and smaller filamentous rods (*arrows*) are shown (Wright stain). **B,** Composite picture showing filamentous rods (*arrows*) typical of *Actinomyces* or *Nocardia* spp. (Wright stain.)

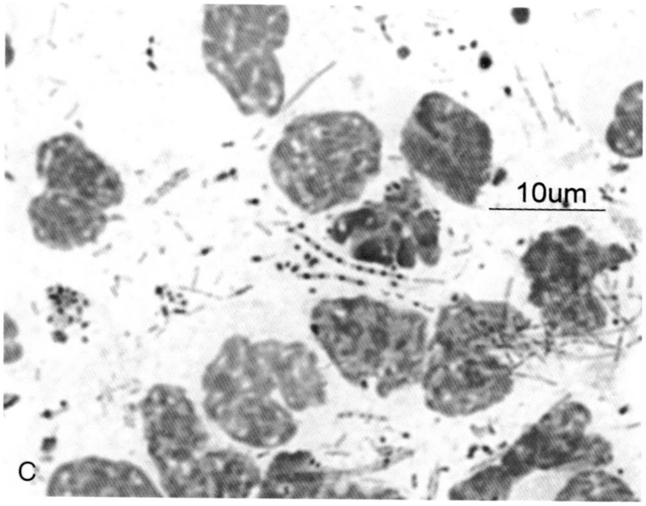

Figure 3-4 cont'd, **C,** Multiple filamentous rods and ruptured cells are shown. (Wright stain.)

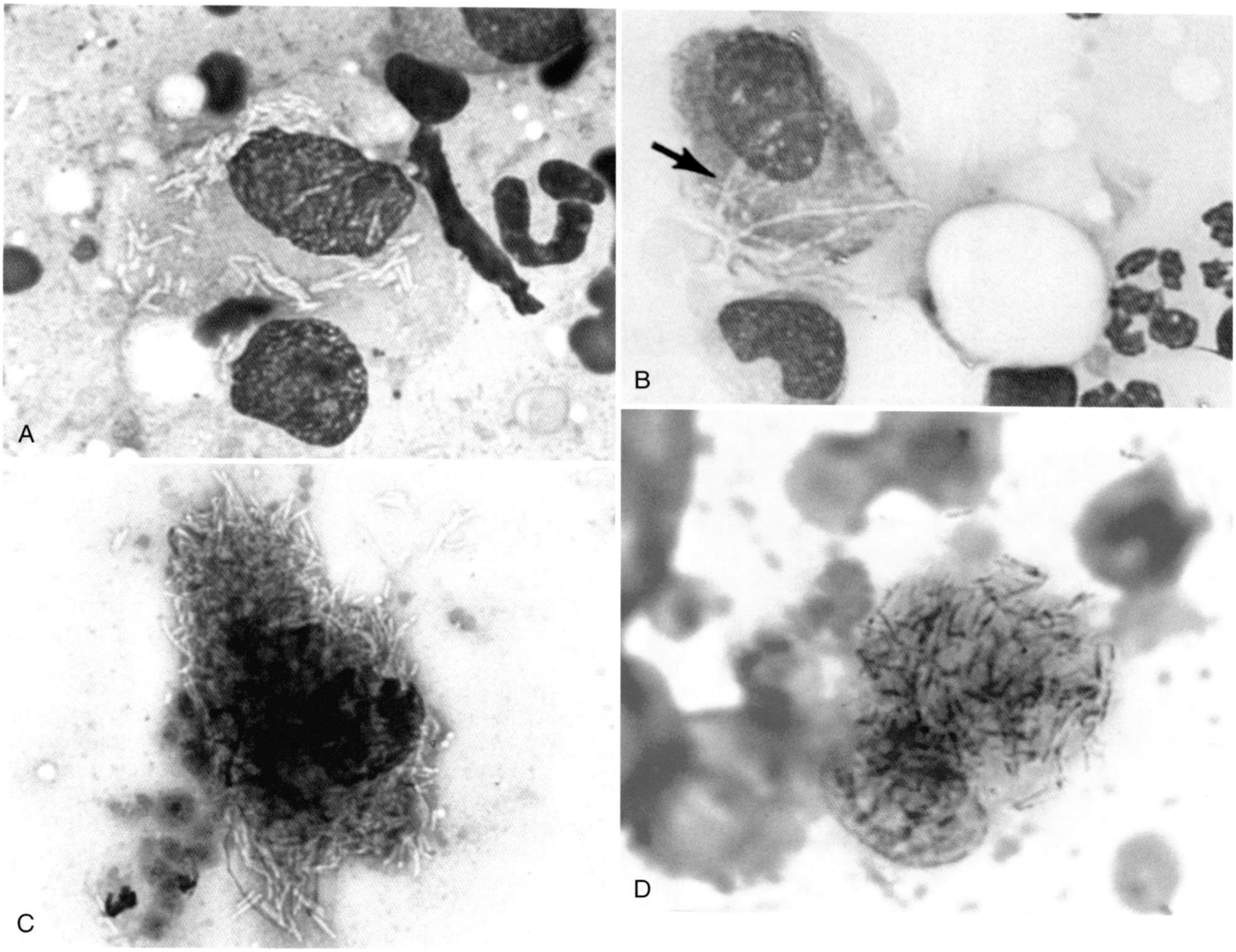

Figure 3-5 **A,** Negative images of *Mycobacterium* organisms in macrophage from cat liver aspirate (Wright stain). **B,** Fine-needle aspirate of a consolidated pulmonary mass. An alveolar macrophage, which contains nonstaining bacterial rods identified as clear streaks through the cell (*arrow*), is indicative of a *Mycobacterium* infection. (Wright stain.) **C,** Cat liver *Mycobacterium* (Wright stain). **D,** Cat liver *Mycobacterium*. (Acid-fast stain.)

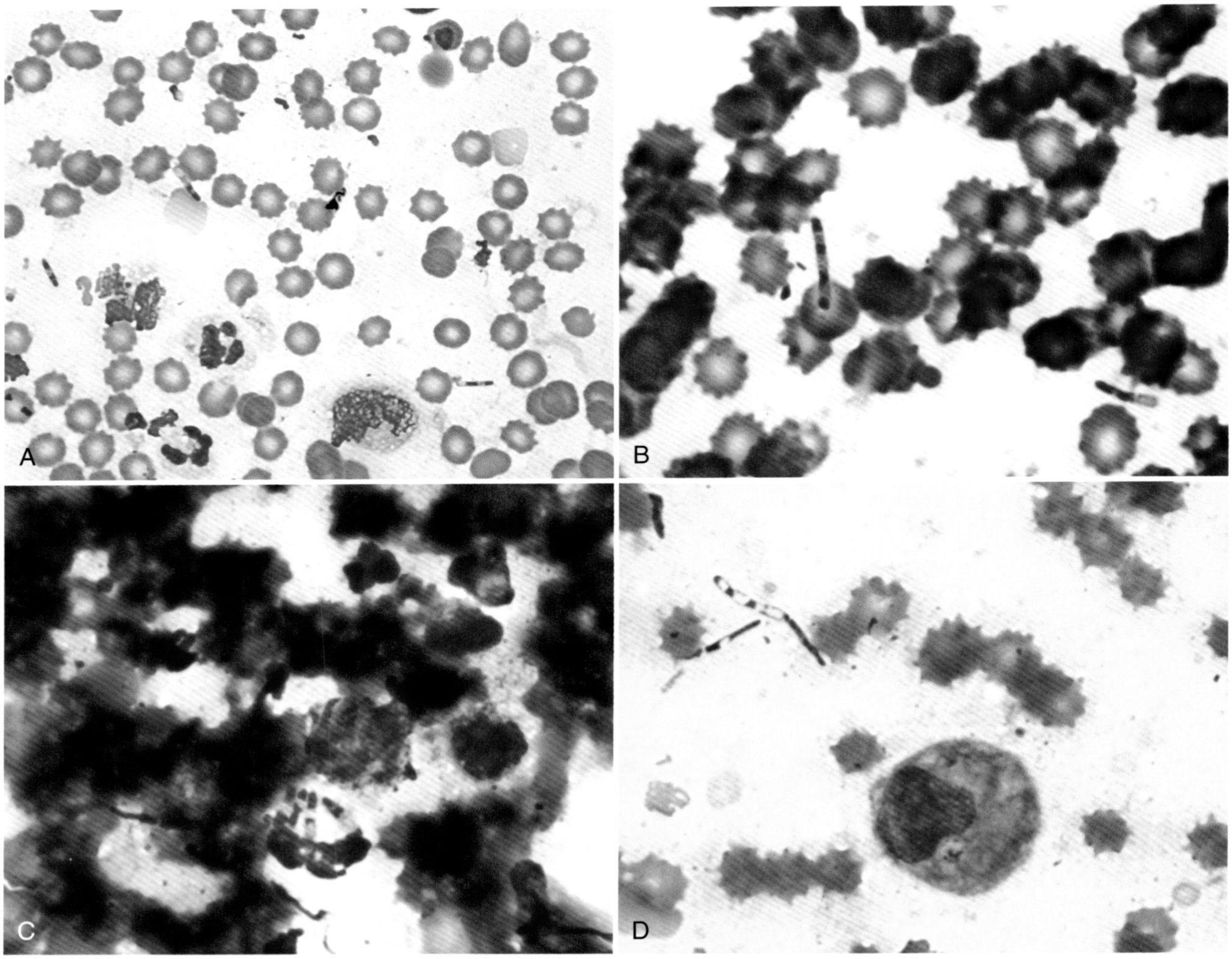

Figure 3-6 **A,** Scattered inflammatory cells, red blood cells (RBCs), and large spore-forming bacterial rods typical of *Clostridium* spp. (Wright stain.) **B,** Higher-power view from same case as in *A.* Scattered RBCs and two large extracellular spore-forming bacterial rods are shown. (Wright stain.) **C,** Same case as in *A.* Multiple phagocytized spore-forming bacterial rods are shown. (Wright stain.) **D,** *Clostridium* organisms from mass on dog (Wright stain).

when any form of blastomycosis is suspected. Aspirates or impression smears taken from these lesions often are composed of degenerate neutrophils, macrophages, lymphocytes, and few multinucleate giant cells. Organisms will range in number from a rare single organism to many, and with routine hematologic staining, the organisms (Figure 3-10) are found to be deeply basophilic, spherical, 8 to 20 μm in diameter, and thick walled. Most organisms are found to be single, but occasionally, organisms showing broad-based budding are found, and few may be phagocytized by macrophages. Blastomyces are distinctly larger than *S. schenckii* or *H. capsulatum* and are differentiated from *Cryptococcus neoformans* by their tinctorial staining qualities, absence of a negative staining capsule, and broad-based budding. They are distinguished by their smaller size and lack of endospores compared with *Coccidioides immitis*. Blastomyces is found primarily in the midwestern and northern United States and Canada and is endemic to the Mississippi and Ohio river valleys and the vicinity of the Great Lakes.

Cryptococcus neoformans

Cryptococcus neoformans infection (cryptococcosis) can involve the subcutaneous tissues causing crusting nodular lesions of the nose; however, commonly, it involves the upper respiratory and central nervous systems as well. Cryptococcosis generally elicits a granulomatous response, including epithelioid macrophages with few multinucleate giant cells and lower numbers of lymphocytes and rare granulocytes. Particularly in immune-suppressed or immune-compromised animals, a minimal inflammatory response may be seen, and *Cryptococcus* organisms may outnumber inflammatory cells and tissue cells. The organism (Figure 3-11) can be pleomorphic, ranging from spherical shape to fusiform but typically is easily recognized because of its thick nonstaining mucoid capsule. Occasionally, small, nonencapsulated, or rough forms are found. The organism ranges from 4 to 15 μm in diameter without its capsule and about 8 to 40 μm in diameter with its capsule. In cytologic preparations stained with routine hematologic stains, the organism appears eosinophilic to

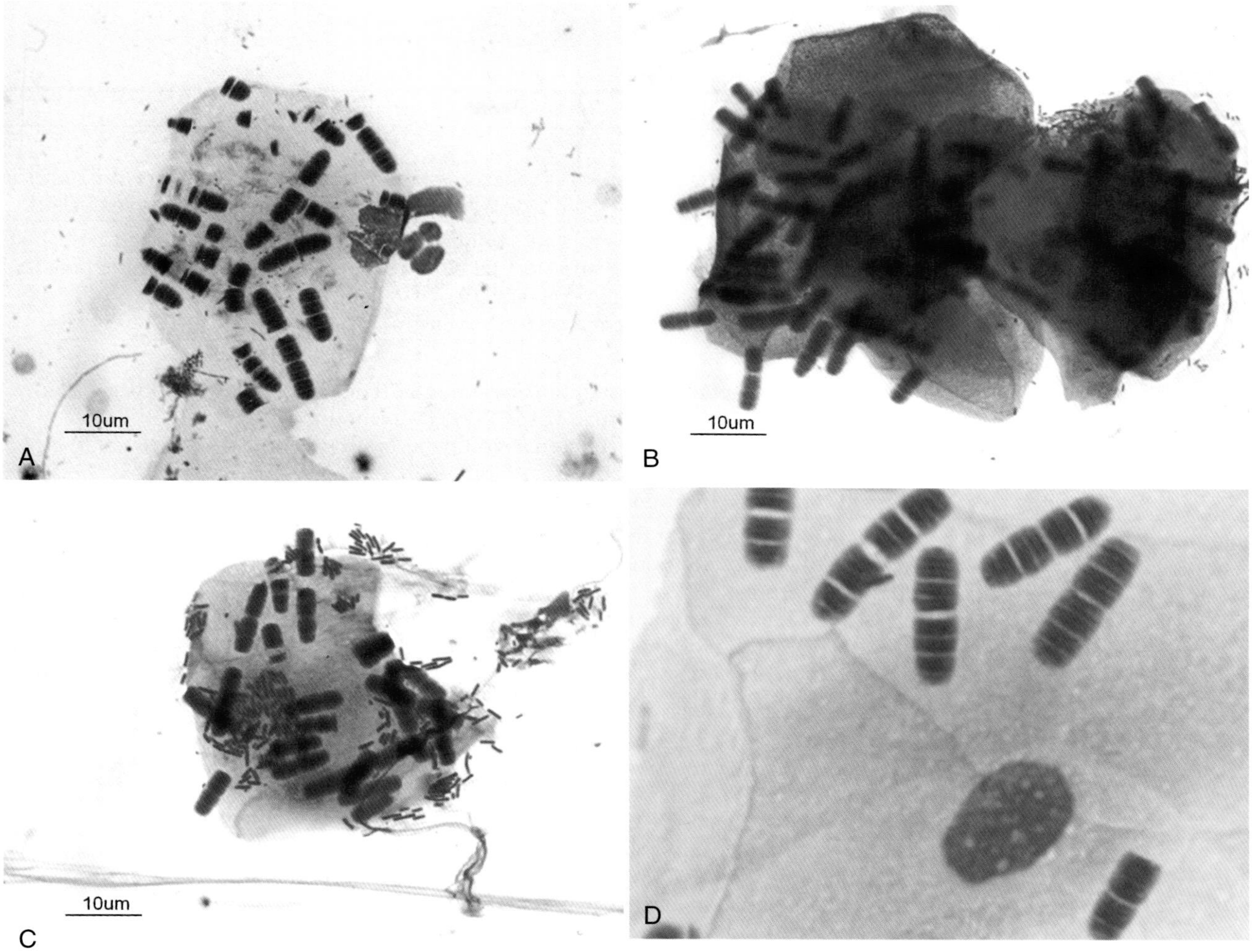

Figure 3-7 **A,** Superficial squamous epithelial cell with adherent bacteria. *Simonsiella* organisms are large striated rodlike organisms. Other bacteria are present, adhered to the squamous cell and free in the background of the smear. (Wright stain.) **B,** Two superficial squamous epithelial cells with many *Simonsiella* organisms. (Wright stain.) **C,** One superficial squamous epithelial cell with many *Simonsiella* organisms and bacterial rods. (Wright stain.) **D,** Higher magnification, *Simonsiella* organisms (Wright stain).

metachromatic and may be slightly granular. The capsule is commonly clear and homogenous; however, in some cases, it may appear to have a pale eosinophilc staining quality. Unlike *Blastomyces* spp., *Cryptococcus* spp. demonstrate narrow-based budding, referred to as "wasp-waist budding." Although India ink is often proposed as an aid in identifying *C. neoformans*, air bubbles and fat globules can be mistaken for organisms, particularly in low-yielding samples with a paucity of material to examine, and therefore routine staining is recommended. More than 37 recognized species of *Cryptococcus* spp. exist in many different geographic regions of the world and have been reported to be found in pigeon droppings. Many are not harmful to animals or humans; however, some do have zoonotic potential. *Cryptococcus gattii* was once restricted to tropical and subtropical regions of the world such as Australia, South America, and Southeast Asia and has recently emerged in North America (particularly the Pacific northwest and Vancouver Island), and this has prompted its reevaluation as a significant pathogen in animals with great zoonotic potential.

Coccidioides immitis

Coccidioides immitis infections generally involve the lungs and bones of dogs. In some cases, however, masslike cutaneous lesions and draining tracts extend from bony lesions. Cytologic preparations usually have a cell composition characteristic of pyogranulomatous or granulomatous inflammation. *Coccidioides* organisms (Figure 3-12) are infrequent in lesions; therefore, systematic and exhaustive examinations are often required to identify organisms from suspected coccidioidomycosis lesions. In cytologic preparations stained with routine hematologic stains, spherules are large, measuring 10 to 200 μm in diameter, double-contoured, blue or clear spheres with finely granular protoplasm and may appear folded or crumpled because of the large size. Multiple round endospores 2 to 5 μm in diameter may be seen in some of the larger

TABLE 3-1

Common Fungi That Form Yeasts in Tissue

Yeast	Distinguishing Characteristics
Small Yeasts	
Sporothrix spp.	Round to oval to fusiform (cigar-shaped) organisms that are about 3-9 micrometers (μm) long and 1-3 μm wide, and stain pale to medium blue with a slightly eccentric pink or purple nucleus.
Histoplasma spp.	• Round to oval but not fusiform; yeasts are about 2-4 μm in diameter (one fourth to one half the size of a red blood cell [RBC]), and stain pale to medium blue with an eccentric pink-to-purple staining nucleus that is often crescent shaped. • Usually, a thin, clear halo is present around the yeast.
Medium-Sized Yeasts	
Blastomyces spp.	• Organisms are blue, spherical yeasts that are about 8-20 μm in diameter and thick walled. • Occasional organisms showing broad-based budding are found. • Blastomyces organisms are differentiated from *Cryptococcus neoformans* by their color, lack of a clear-staining capsule, and broad-based budding. • They are distinguished from *Coccidioides immitis* by their smaller size and lack of endospores.
Cryptococcus spp.	• Extremely pleomorphic yeast that ranges from spherical to fusiform shape, has a smooth (encapsulated) and rough (nonencapsulated) form, and is about 4-15 μm in diameter (not including the capsule). • The yeast stains pink to blue-purple and may be slightly granular. *Cryptococcus* spp. demonstrate narrow-based budding. • The smooth form usually is easily recognized because of its thick mucoid capsule, which usually is clear and homogeneous.
Large Yeasts	
Coccidioides spp.	• These organisms are scarce in many cytology specimens; therefore, cytologic preparations from suspected coccidioidomycosis lesions should be examined carefully. • When present, the organisms are large (10-100 μm in diameter), double-contoured, blue or clear spheres with finely granular protoplasm, and will often appear folded or crumpled. • Round endospores from 2-5 μm in diameter may be seen in some of the larger organisms. • The tremendous variation in the size and presence of endospores differentiates *Coccidioides immitis* from nonbudding *Blastomyces dermatitidis.*

organisms and occur extracellularly in cases of ruptured spherules. The tremendous variation in the size and presence of endospores differentiates *C. immitis* from the small broad-based budding of *B. dermatitidis*. Coccidiodes can be found in the soil in certain parts of the southwestern United States, northern Mexico, and a few other areas in the Western Hemisphere—commonly desert regions—and causes valley fever in humans. Although *Coccidioides* spp. can be grown in culture from patient samples, this is not recommended, as it can take weeks to grow and poses a public health risk, thus necessitating special precautions to be taken by the laboratory. It has been declared a select agent ("…. has the potential to pose a severe threat to public health and safety") by both the U.S. Department of Health and Human Services and the U.S. Department of Agriculture and is considered a "biosafety level 3" pathogen. Caution is warranted in cases of, or suspected cases of, *C. immitis*.

Malassezia spp

Malassezia canis, also called *Malassezia pachydermatis*, is a small, broad-based, budding, gram-positive, nonmycelioid yeast, typically peanut shaped but may be globose or ellipsoidal in shape as well (Figure 3-13). It is a common skin commensal and opportunistic pathogen and contributing factor in otitis externa and *Malassezia*-associated dermatitis, which is commonly diagnosed in dogs, particularly small white dogs (commonly as yeast-associated pododermatitis).

Dermatophytes

Microsporum and *Trichophyton* spp. commonly cause dermatophytosis or ringworm in dogs and cats. The lesions are often crusty, focal, scaly, and occur with alopecia on the head, feet, and tail of dogs and cats. Dermatophytosis is also zoonotic, and similar lesions can be noted in humans who come in close contact with the affected animals. Scrapings from the edge of active lesions are the best cytologic samples for visualizing dermatophytes. They can be identified in cytologic preparations using the standard 10% potassium hydroxide stain for hair, in wet-mount preparations stained with new methylene blue, or air-dried preparations stained with routine hematologic stains. Cytologically, fungal mycelia and arthrospores are found adhered to the surface of epithelial cells and free in the background of the smear, as well as within hair shafts (*Trichophyton* spp.) or on the hair shaft surface (*Microsporum* spp.). With hematologic stains, the mycelia and spores stain medium to dark blue with a thin, clear halo (Figure 3-14).

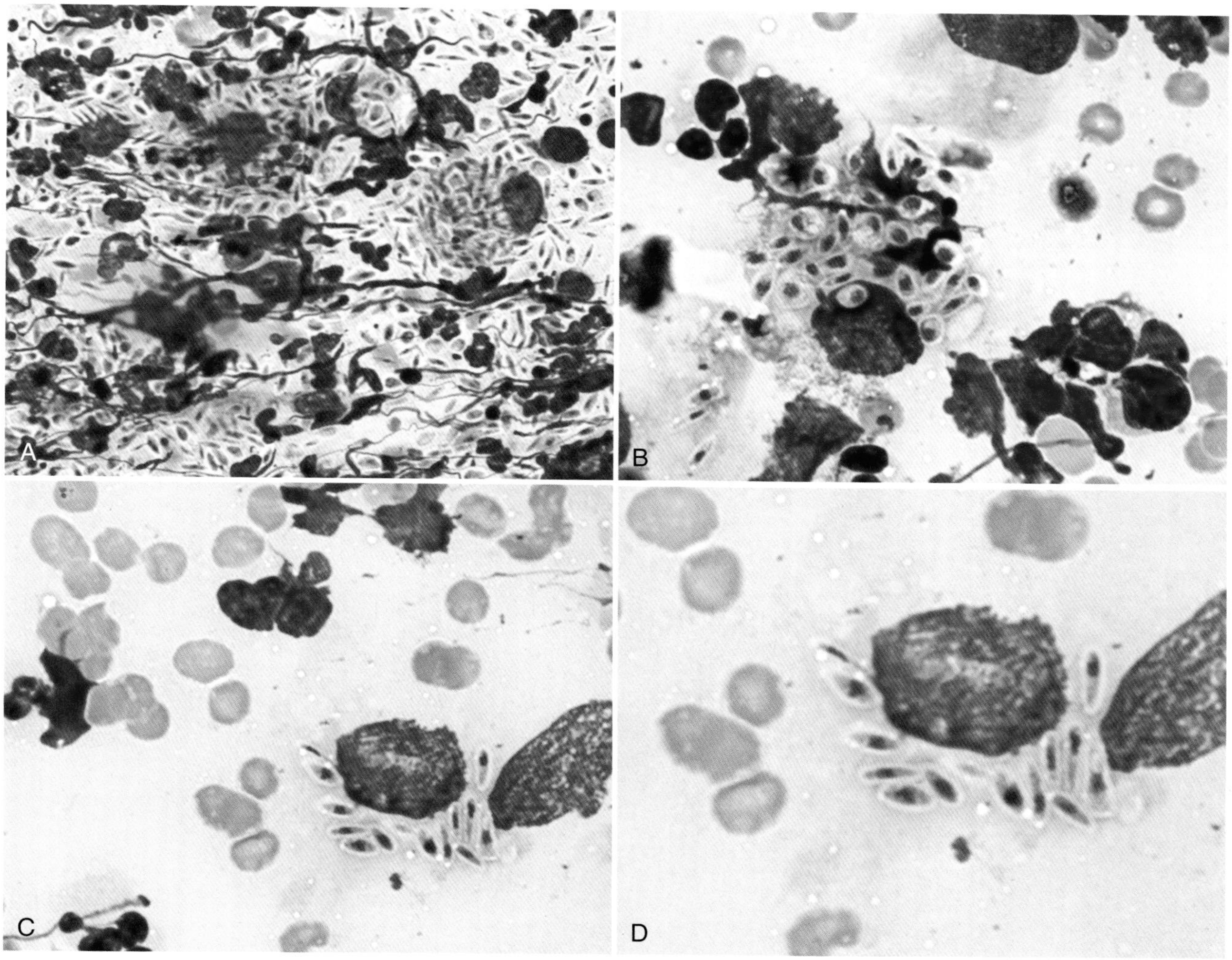

Figure 3-8 **A,** Scraping from a skin lesion in a cat. Pyogranulomatous inflammation and high numbers of sporotrichosis organisms are present in the smear. (Wright stain.) **B,** Macrophage containing round, oval, and fusiform sporotrichosis organisms. (Wright stain.) **C,** A ruptured macrophage containing many fusiform sporotrichosis organisms. (Wright stain.) **D,** Higher magnification, *Sporothrix* organisms in cat. (Wright stain).

The inflammatory reaction is often an admixture of neutrophils, macrophages, lymphocytes, and plasma cells and may be seen in cytologic preparations from skin scrapings. Silver staining (e.g., Gomori methenamine silver [GMS]) or periodic acid-Schiff (PAS) staining highlights the arthrospores. Fungal culture is often needed for definitive identification.

Rhinosporidium seeberi

Rhinosporidium seeberi is a eukaryotic pathogen responsible for rhinosporidiosis, which affects many species, including humans, dogs, cats, horses, and cattle, and is found in tropical regions of the world. Rhinosporidiosis in dogs is characterized by polypoid nasal growths with a granular surface that can resemble neoplastic lesions. It is diagnosed by finding round to oval spores, approximately 7 µm in diameter, in nasal exudates or tissue imprints. Spores stain bright pink, have internal eosinophilic globules, and are surrounded by thin bilamellar cell walls (Figure 3-15). Finding large sporangia containing numerous endospores supports the diagnosis; however, these structures are infrequently seen. Additional information can be found in the Chapter 7 in this book.

Pneumocystis spp

Pneumocystis is considered an endemic, opportunistic fungal pulmonary pathogen, which may be observed in either cystic (5 to 10 µm diameter that may contain up to eight intracystic bodies) or trophic form (1 to 2 µm). Several species that affect animals and humans, with little crossover, have been identified. Routine stained samples will have distinctive intact cysts with the notable intracystic bodies (Figure 3-16); however, the smaller, free trophic form may be difficult to differentiate from background debris. Cytologically, *Pneumocystis* organisms may appear morphologically similar to protozoal organisms; however, *Pneumocystis* is classified as a fungus and has recently undertaken an expansion of speciation in domestic animals and humans.

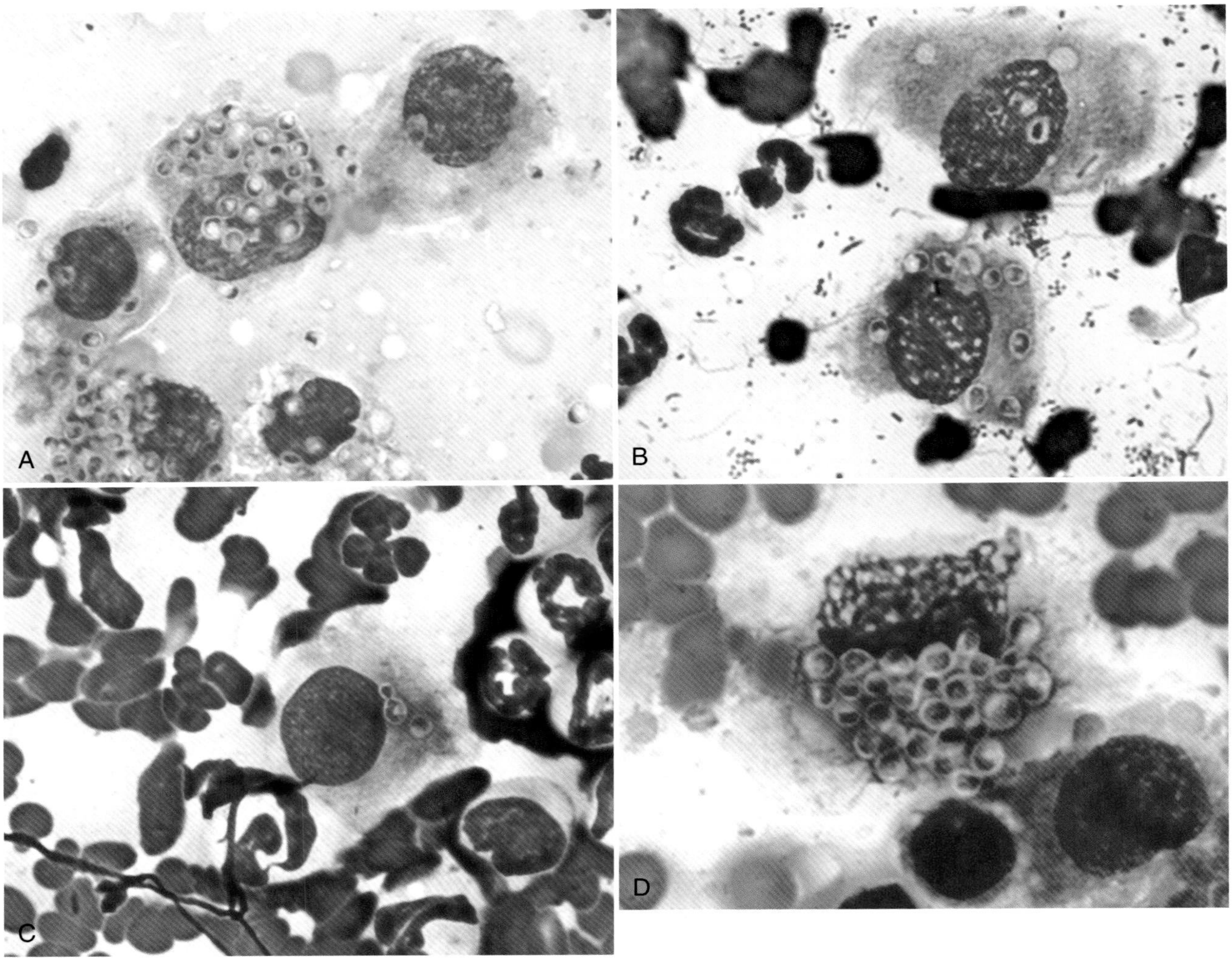

Figure 3-9 **A,** Lung aspirate showing macrophages containing high numbers of *Histoplasma* organisms. (Wright stain.) **B,** Scraping from an ulcerated mass in the mouth of a cat. High numbers of mixed bacteria, blood, pyogranulomatous inflammation, and many *Histoplasma* organisms are shown. (Wright stain.) **C,** Pyogranulomatous inflammation and a macrophage containing a budding *Histoplasma* organism and a round nonbudding *Histoplasma* organism. (Wright stain.) **D,** Histoplasma organisms from intraabdominal aspirate (Wright stain).

Fungi That Form Hyphae in Tissues

Many different fungi can infect the cutaneous and subcutaneous tissues or internal organs and form hyphae (Figure 3-17). With cutaneous lesions, these fungi usually cause small-to-large, raised, proliferative lesions that often ulcerate. They often induce a granulomatous, inflammatory response, which is characterized by epithelioid macrophages and inflammatory giant cells. The number of neutrophils, lymphocytes, plasma cells, and eosinophils varies. Some hyphating fungi do not stain well with hematologic-type stains and are recognized as negative images (Figure 3-18). The organisms that cause phycomycosis typically do not stain with hematologic stains and induce an eosinophilic, granulomatous response in the affected tissue. A fungal culture or histopathology with special immunohistochemical stains may be needed to definitively classify the organism involved.

Algae: *Prototheca* spp. (*P. zopfii* and *P. wickerhami*) are colorless algae, which are ubiquitous in the southern regions of America but only rarely cause systemic protothecosis. In dogs, the disease is often disseminated, frequently with ocular manifestations; however, only cutaneous protothecosis has been reported in cats. Cytologic preparations reveal an inflammatory response characteristic of pyogranulomatous or granulomatous inflammation and organisms ranging from very few to many. The organisms (Figure 3-19) are round to oval in shape and are 1 to 14 μm wide and 1 to 16 μm long. When stained with routine stains, they are seen to have granular basophilic cytoplasm and a clear cell wall roughly 0.5 μm thick. Mature organisms contain a small nucleus that stains pink to deep purple. A single alga may consist of two to four or more endospores. Most organisms are extracellular, but small forms may be found phagocytized in macrophages and neutrophils.

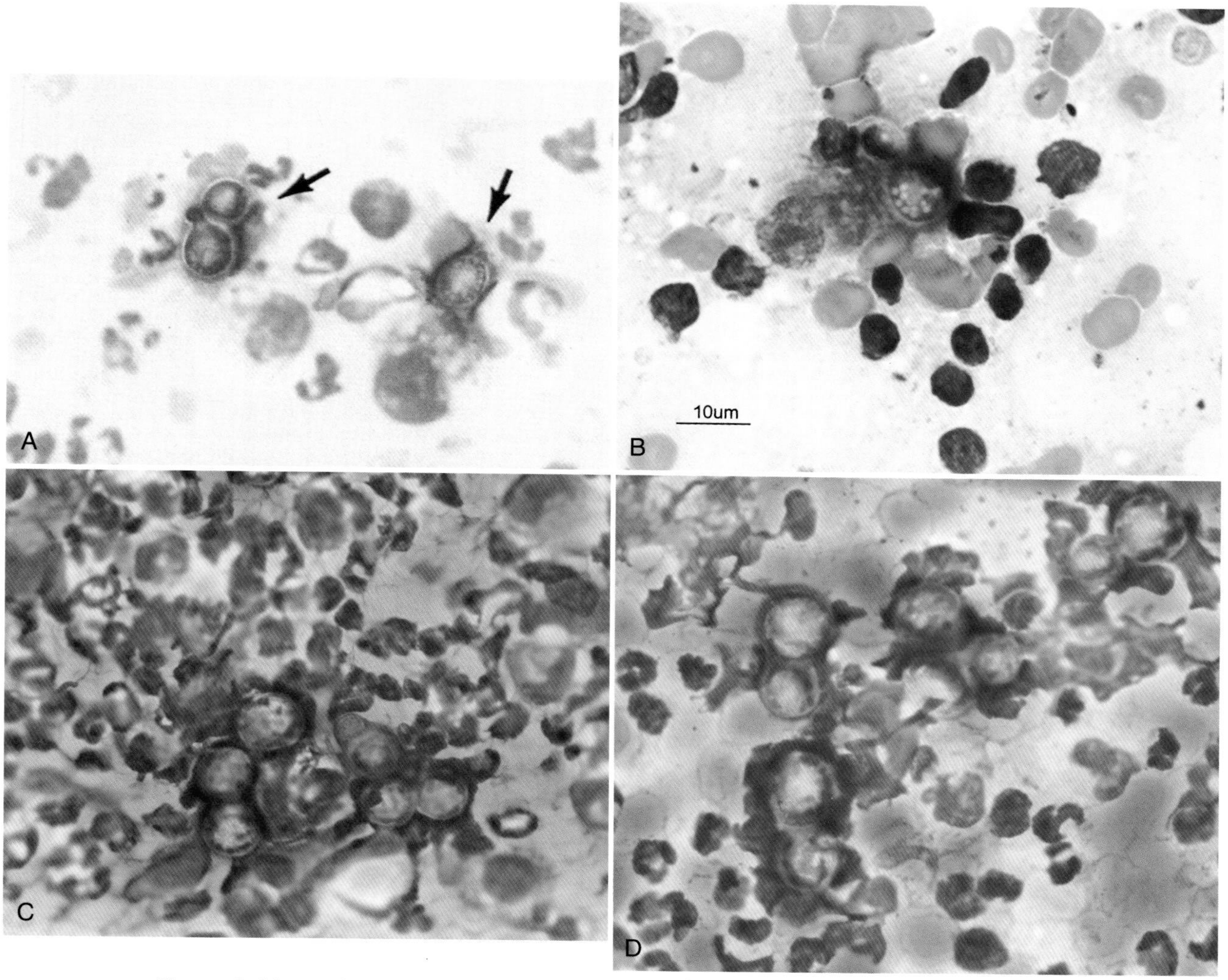

Figure 3-10 A, *Blastomyces dermatitidis* is a bluish, spherical, thick-walled, yeastlike organism in Romanowsky-stained smears (*arrows.*) The organisms are about 8 to 20 micrometers (μm) in diameter. Occasionally, a single broad-based bud may be present. (Wright stain.) **B,** A budding *Blastomyces* organism in a lymph node aspirate is shown. (Wright stain.) **C,** *Blastomyces* organisms in lung aspirate from a dog (Wright stain). **D,** *Blastomyces* organisms in lung aspirate from a dog (Wright stain).

PROTOZOA

Leishmania spp.

Until recently, leishmaniasis was an endemic disease occurring in the Mediterranean region. However, natural cases of leishmaniasis have begun appearing in dogs in North America since 2000, and *Leishmania*-positive foxhounds have been reported in 22 states and two provinces of Canada since 2008. *Leishmania* spp. of the *Leishmania donovani* complex can infect the skin and subcutaneous tissues of dogs, producing different-sized, thickened, ulcerative dermatitis lesions. Imprints, scrapings, and aspirates yield numerous cells, which are an admixture of predominantly neutrophils and macrophages, with fewer lymphocytes and plasma cells. Frequently, numerous organisms are found phagocytized within macrophages and free in the background of sample preparations. *Leishmania* organisms are oval shaped and small, approximately 2 to 4 μm (Figure 3-20). They have an oval, light-purple nucleus and a characteristic small, dark-purple, rod-shaped kinetoplast. The position of the kinetoplast with respect to the nucleus is variable; however, the kinetoplast tends to be located between the nucleus and the greatest volume of cytoplasm. The presence of a kinetoplast distinguishes this organism from *Toxoplasma* spp. and small fungal yeasts such as *Histoplasma* spp.

Toxoplasma gondii

Toxoplasma gondii is a coccidial organism, which is found in contaminated water, soil, and other substances. It causes toxoplasmosis, which can affect most warm-blooded animals, birds and mammals alike, but most often affects feline fetuses and cats with compromised immune systems. Although it is uncommon for animal infections to lead to serious clinical disease, toxoplasmosis can result

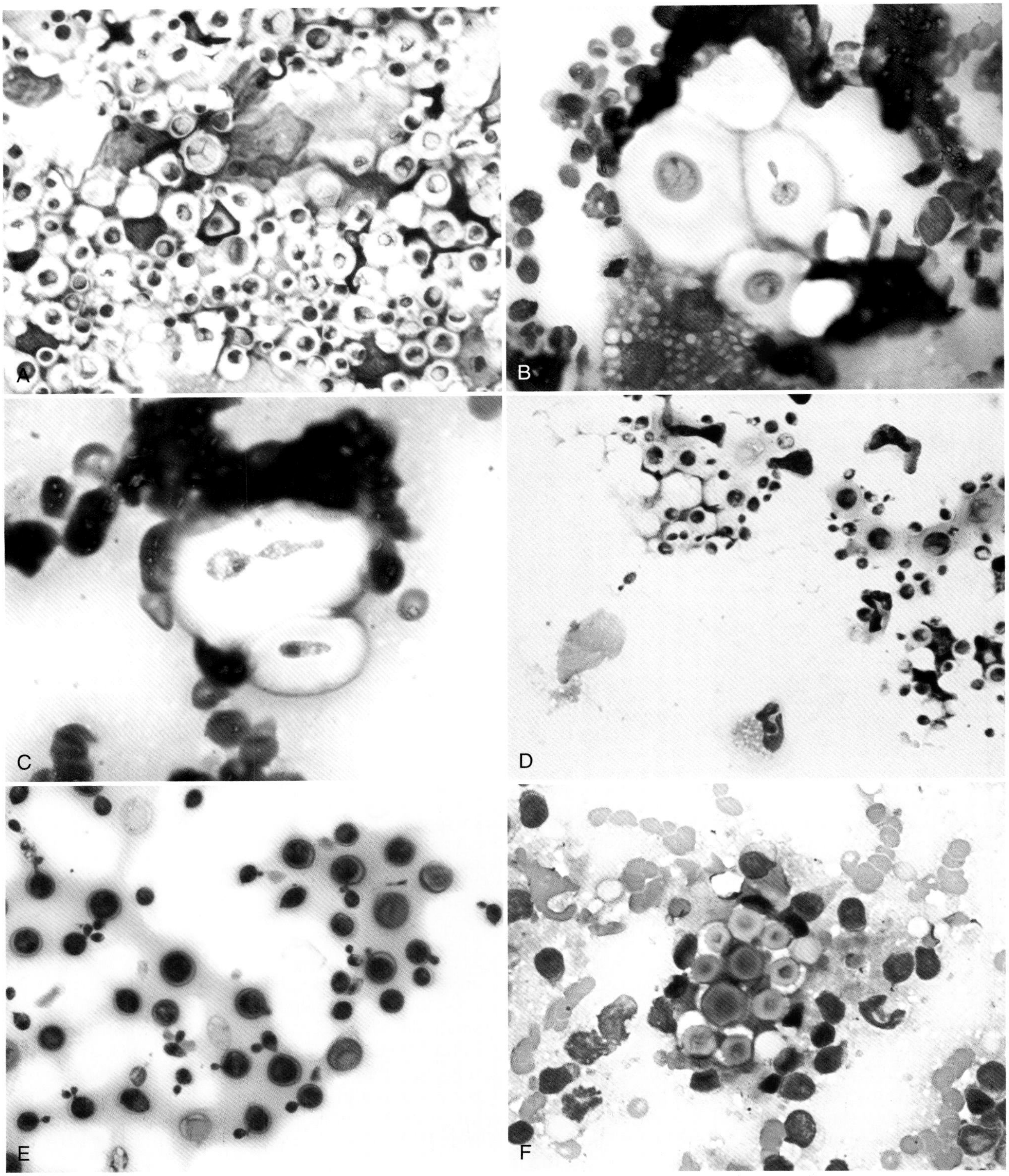

Figure 3-11 **A,** Low-power view of high numbers of *Cryptococcus* organisms characterized by medium-sized yeasts with clear capsules. Note the lack of an inflammatory response. (Wright stain.) **B,** *Cryptococcus* organisms with large clear capsules and narrow-based budding. (Wright stain.) **C,** Two *Cryptococcus* organisms showing narrow-based budding. (Wright stain.) **D,** *Cryptococcus* organisms found in cerebrospinal fluid. (Wright stain.) **E,** Higher-power magnification from same case as shown in *D*. (Wright stain.) **F,** Lymph node aspirate showing a group of *Cryptococcus* organisms, scattered lymphocytes, a single neutrophil, and scattered red blood cells. (Wright stain.)

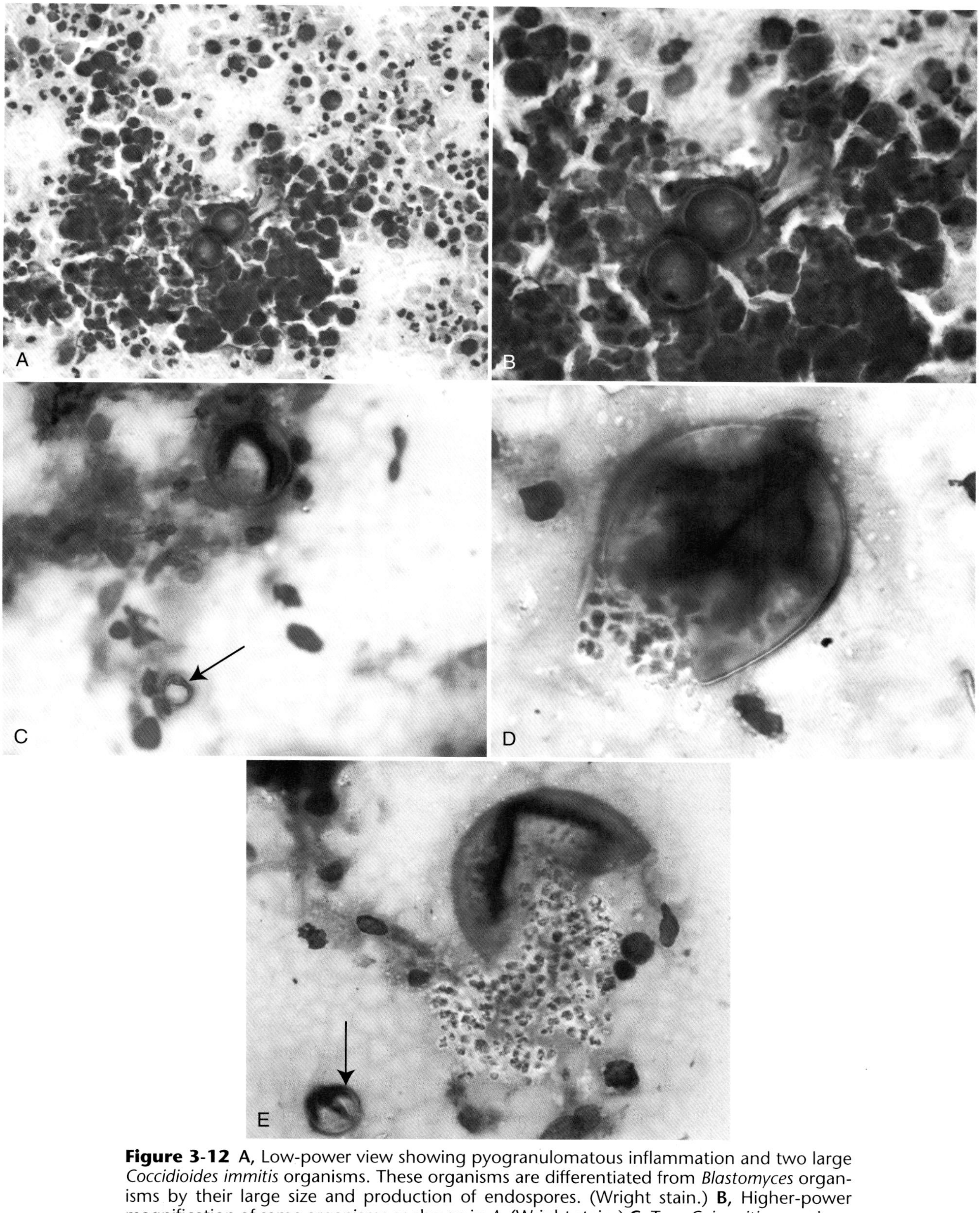

Figure 3-12 **A,** Low-power view showing pyogranulomatous inflammation and two large *Coccidioides immitis* organisms. These organisms are differentiated from *Blastomyces* organisms by their large size and production of endospores. (Wright stain.) **B,** Higher-power magnification of same organisms as shown in *A.* (Wright stain.) **C,** Two *C. immitis* organisms (*arrows*) showing the marked variation in size that can occur with the organisms. (Wright stain.) **D,** Large *C. immitis* organism with endospores. (Wright stain.) **E,** Large *C. immitis* organism, which has ruptured and released the endospores. Also, a small *C. immitis* organism (*arrow*) is present. (Wright stain.)

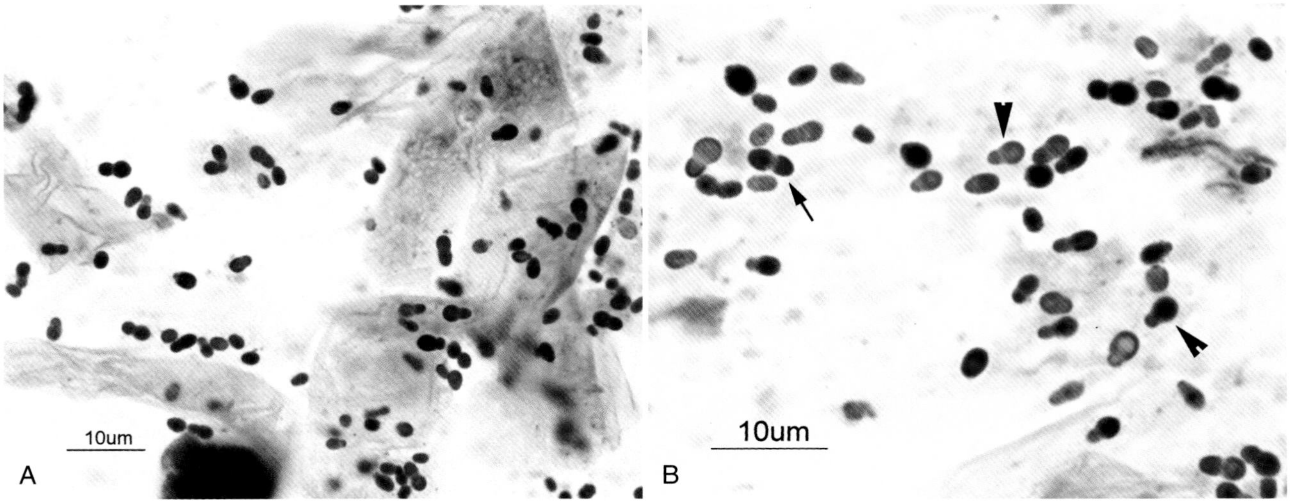

Figure 3-13 **A,** Canine ear swab showing numerous *Malassezia canis* organisms (*Malassezia* overgrowth) adhered to cornified epithelial cells and free in the background. **B,** Individual *Malassezia* organisms are spherical, but broad-based budding produces figure-of-8 (*arrow*) and snowman (*arrowheads*) shapes.

in ophthalmic damage. In addition, in severe cases, it can cause GI, respiratory, and neurologic disorders that may be fatal. In cats, *T. gondii* infection is common, although clinical disease caused by *T. gondii* is uncommon. Roughly 50% of all cats are believed to have been infected with this organism at some point in their lives, and most show no outward clinical signs.

T. gondii may be found in tissue or fluid samples from animals with toxoplasmosis. Tachyzoites are spindle shaped to crescent shaped, 2 to 4 μm in length, with light-blue cytoplasm and red-purple nuclei (Figure 3-21). Tachyzoites of *T. gondii* and *Neosporum caninum* cannot be distinguished cytologically from one another, and polymerase chain reaction (PCR) is the most reliable method for definitively identifying these organisms.

Neospora spp. (*Neosporum caninum*)

Neosporum caninum is a coccidial parasite, very similar to *T. gondii*. Infection, in the dog, is usually congenital and often lethal. Tissues targeted and clinical signs are variable and include brain, skeletal muscle, and ocular diseases (e.g., chorioretinitis, uveitis, dermatitis, encephalitis, and myositis). Tachyzoites of *N. caninum* can be found in tissue or fluid samples of infected animals and have the same cytologic appearance as *T. gondii* tachyzoites, making PCR the most reliable method for definitively differentiating these organisms.

Cytauxzoon felis

Cytauxzoonosis is an often fatal disease in cats caused by the protozoan parasite *Cytauxzoon felis*. It is transmitted to domestic cats by ticks, and its natural reservoir host is the bobcat. In tissues, developing merozoites may be seen in macrophages. These macrophages are typically large with visible nucleoli and contain either small, dark-staining bodies or larger irregularly defined clusters of developing merozoites of *Cytauxzoon* (Figure 3-22). The macrophages may contain other cellular and phagocytic debris also. It is important not to confuse these macrophages with neoplastic cells. Red blood cells in the background of the smear may contain *Cytauxzoon* organisms appearing as signet-rings. *C. felis* was originally recognized in Missouri in 1976 and was believed to be limited to south central and southeastern United States; though it is now recognized in the mid-Atlantic and northeastern parts of the United States as well.

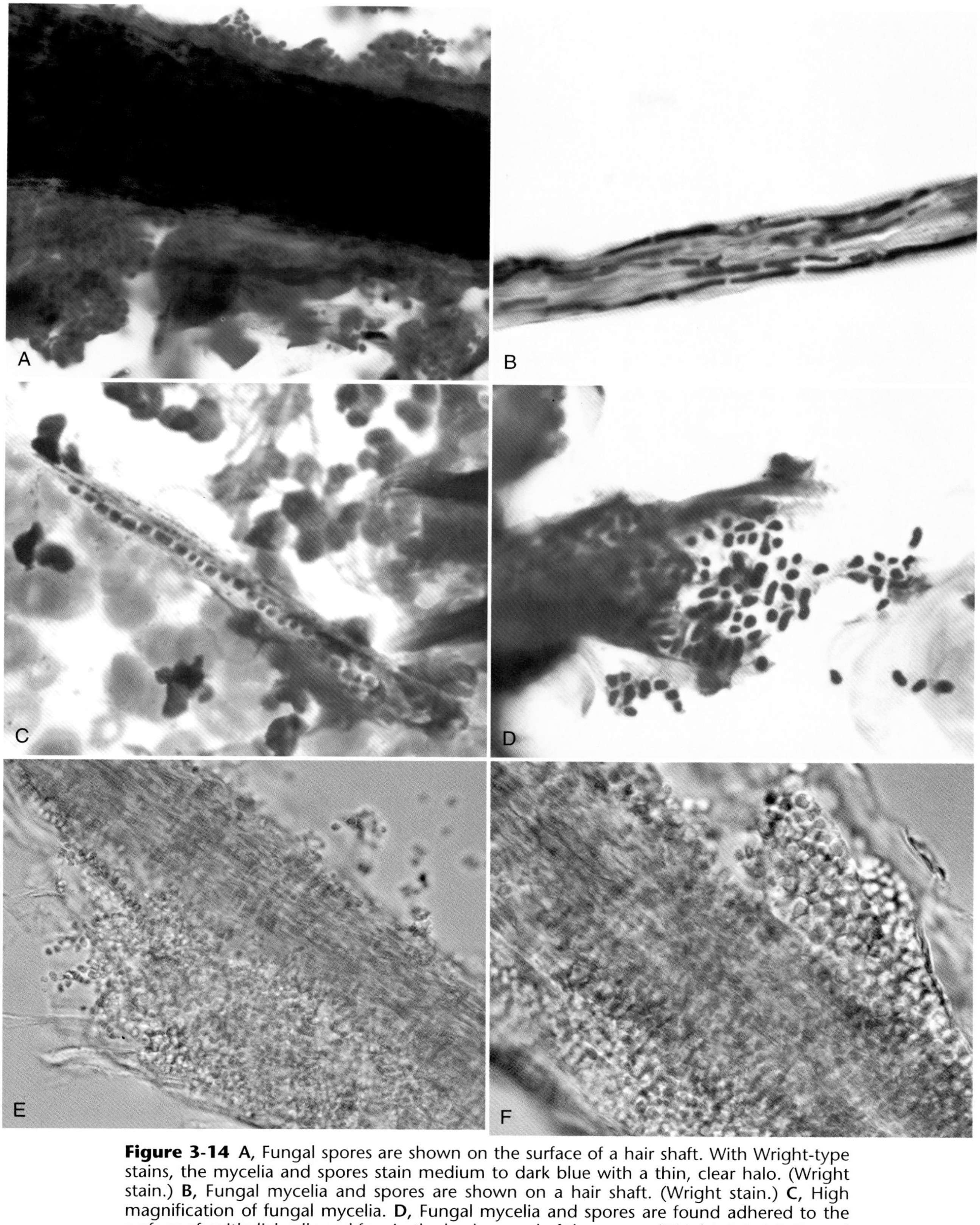

Figure 3-14 A, Fungal spores are shown on the surface of a hair shaft. With Wright-type stains, the mycelia and spores stain medium to dark blue with a thin, clear halo. (Wright stain.) **B,** Fungal mycelia and spores are shown on a hair shaft. (Wright stain.) **C,** High magnification of fungal mycelia. **D,** Fungal mycelia and spores are found adhered to the surface of epithelial cells and free in the background of the smear. (Wright stain.) **E,** Fungal (ringworm) mycelia and spores on unstained smears. **F,** Higher magnification from same case as E. (Unstained).

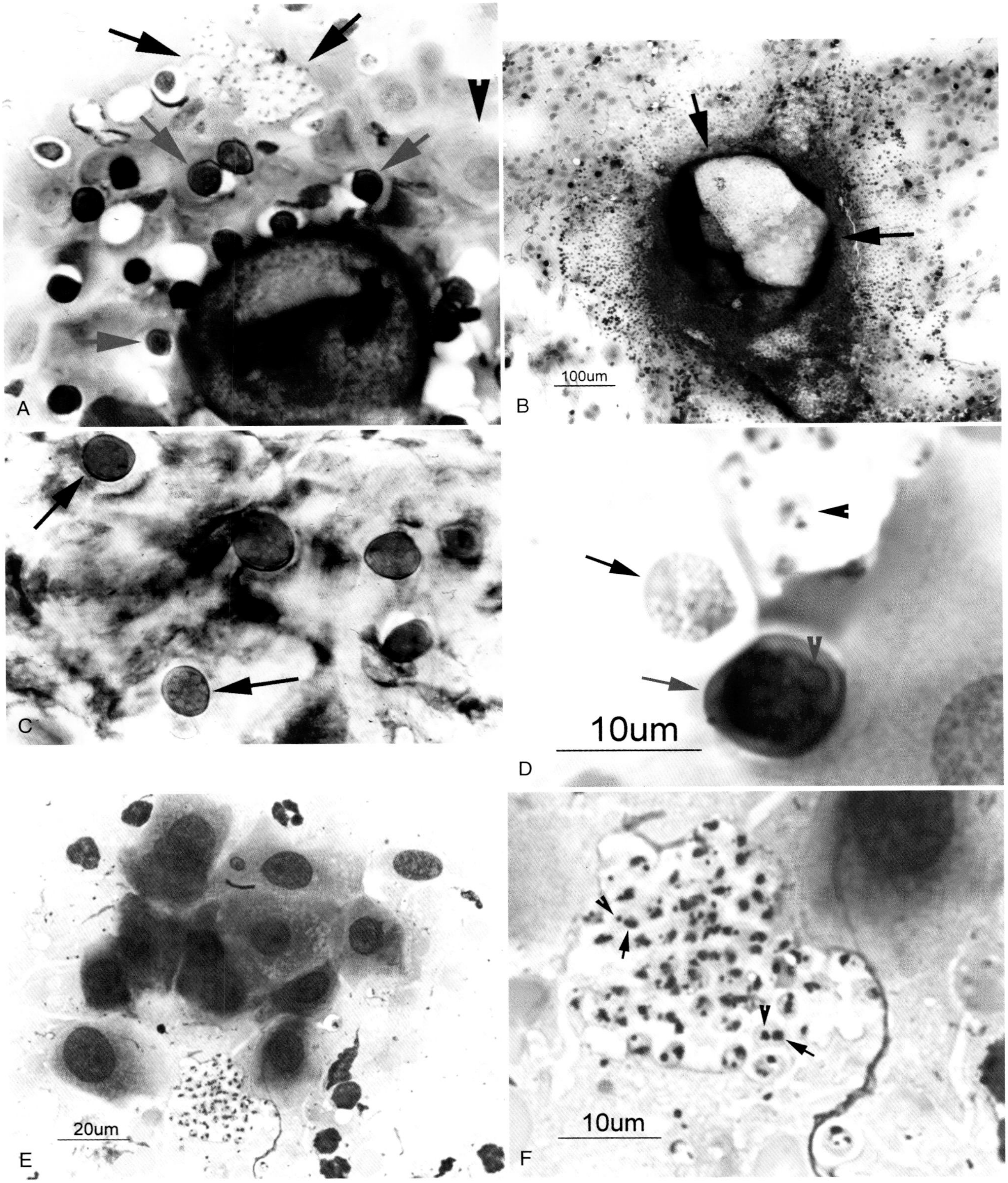

Figure 3-15 **A,** Impression smear of a nasal biopsy from a dog with rhinosporidiosis. Three distinct forms of the organism can be seen along with nasal epithelial cells (*black arrowhead*). The large circular structure at the bottom is a relatively small sporangium. Surrounding this are numerous spores or endospores (*blue arrows*), which stain dark when not well spread out but pink to pink-purple when well spread out. Also present are small immature spores or endospores (*black arrows*). (Wright stain.) **B,** Low-magnification image showing a large, ruptured sporangium surrounded by hundreds of developing spores or endospores (*arrows*). (Wright stain.) **C,** Canine rhinosporidiosis. Numerous well-spread-out spores or endospores are present among cellular debris (*arrows*). (Wright stain.) **D,** Higher magnification of a mature spore or endospore (*blue arrow*) demonstrating thick cell wall and eosinophilic globular bodies (*blue arrowhead*). Also present are immature spores or endospores (*black arrowhead*) as well as an intermediate form (*black arrow*). (Wright stain.) **E,** Immature spores or endospores of *Rhinosporidium seeberi*. Low-magnification image showing numerous epithelial cells with a cluster of immature spores or endospores near the bottom of the image. (Wright stain.) **F,** Higher magnification from same field as shown in *E* shows details of the immature spores or endospores. They are spherical, lightly basophilic structures, which contain purple areas thought to be nuclear material (*arrows*) and one or more darker blue spherical structures (*arrowheads*). (Wright stain.)

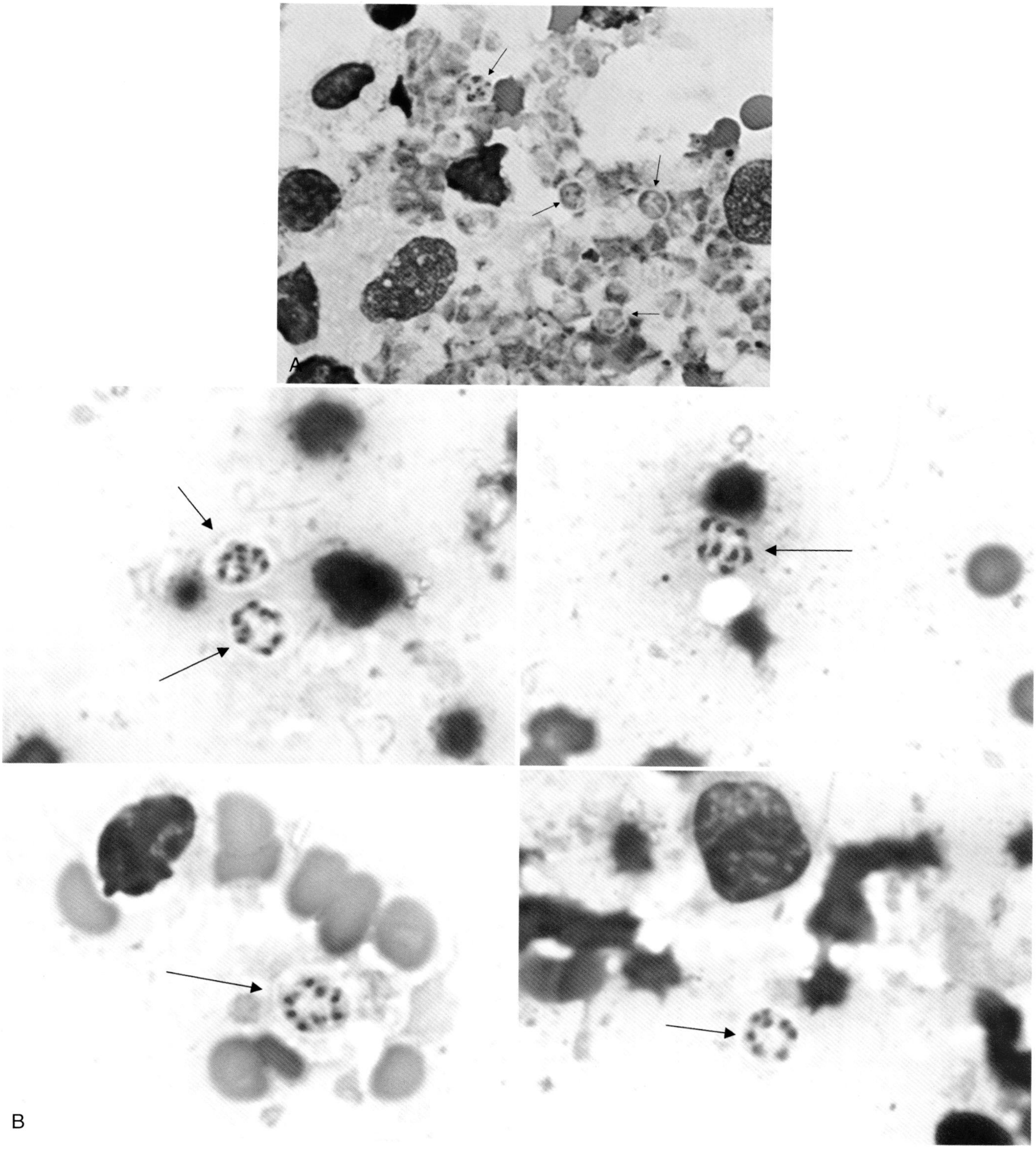

B

Figure 3-16 **A,** Transtracheal wash from a dog with pneumocystosis. High numbers of *Pneumocystis carinii* cysts (*arrows*) are present. *P. carinii* cysts are 5 to 10 micrometers (μm) in diameter and usually contain four to eight intracystic bodies that are 1 to 2 μm in diameter. (Wright stain.) **B,** Composite showing *P. carinii* cysts (*arrows*). (Wright stain.)

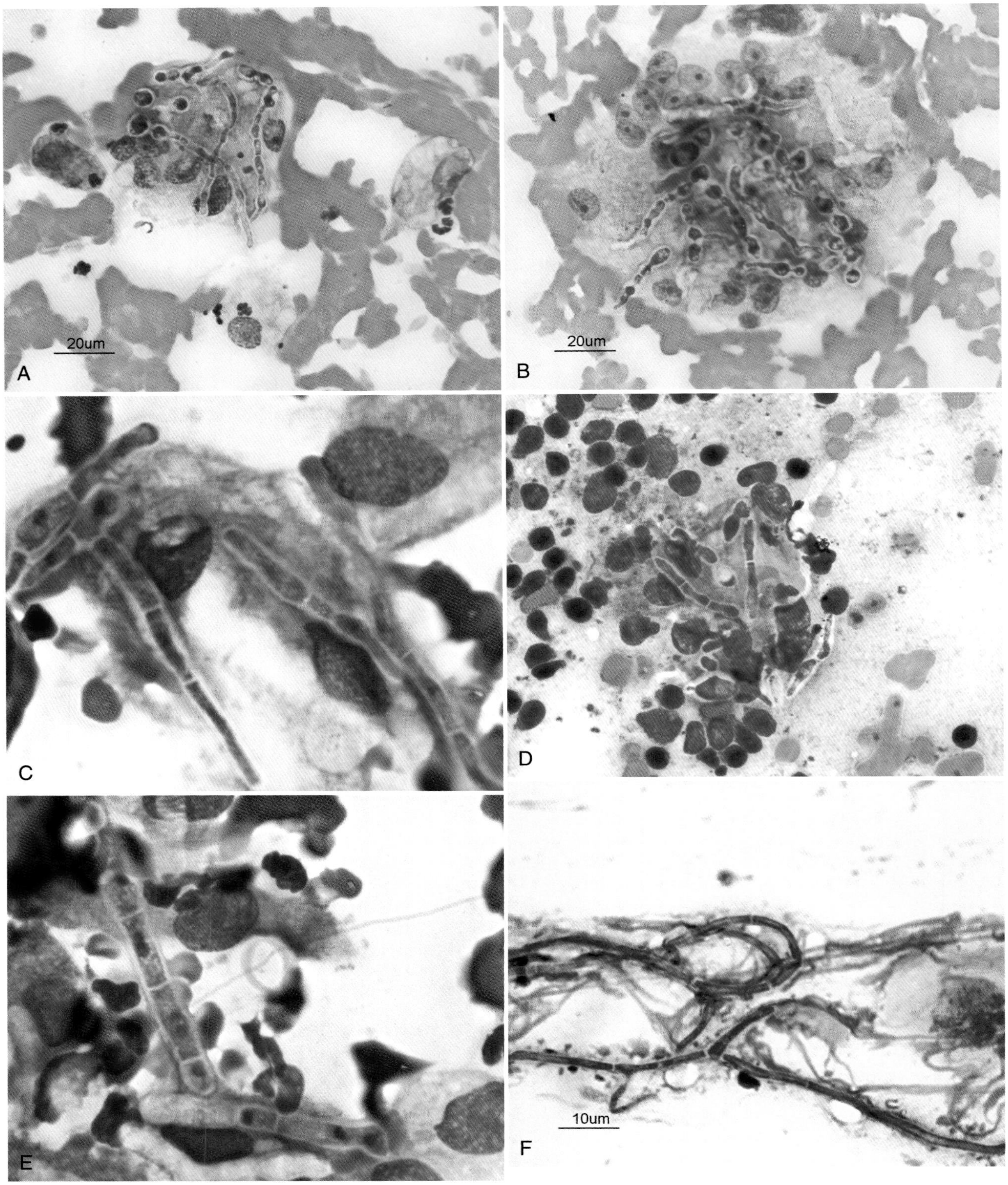

Figure 3-17 **A**, Granulomatous inflammation, red blood cells, and a giant cell (macrophage) containing several fungal hyphae are shown. (Wright stain.) **B**, Multinucleated inflammatory giant cell containing several fungal hyphae. (Wright stain.) **C**, Fungal hyphae in nose of cat (Wright stain). **D**, Lymph node aspirate. High numbers of lymphocytes and a group of macrophages containing several fungal hyphae are shown. (Wright stain.) **E**, Fungal hyphae in nose of cat (Wright stain). **F**, Nasal swab, diagnostic of fungal infection even with excessive cell rupturing. (Wright stain).

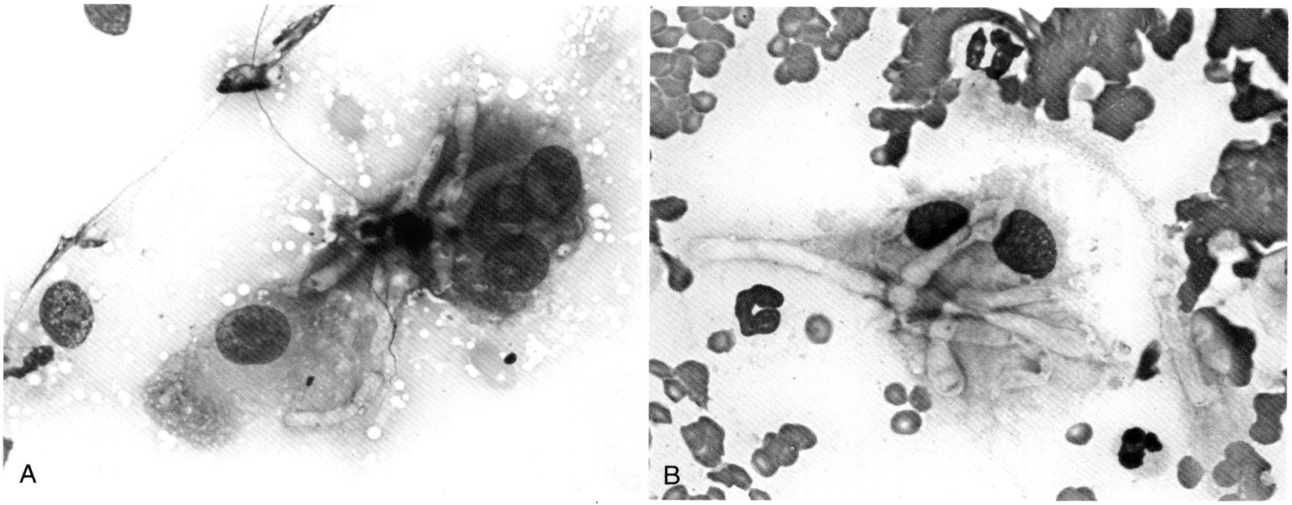

Figure 3-18 **A,** Fine-needle aspirate from a lytic bone lesion on a dog showing granulomatous inflammation and negative images of fungal hyphae. (Wright stain.) **B,** Fine-needle aspirate from a mass in the nose of a cat showing negative images of fungal hyphae within macrophages and free in the background of the smear. (Wright stain.)

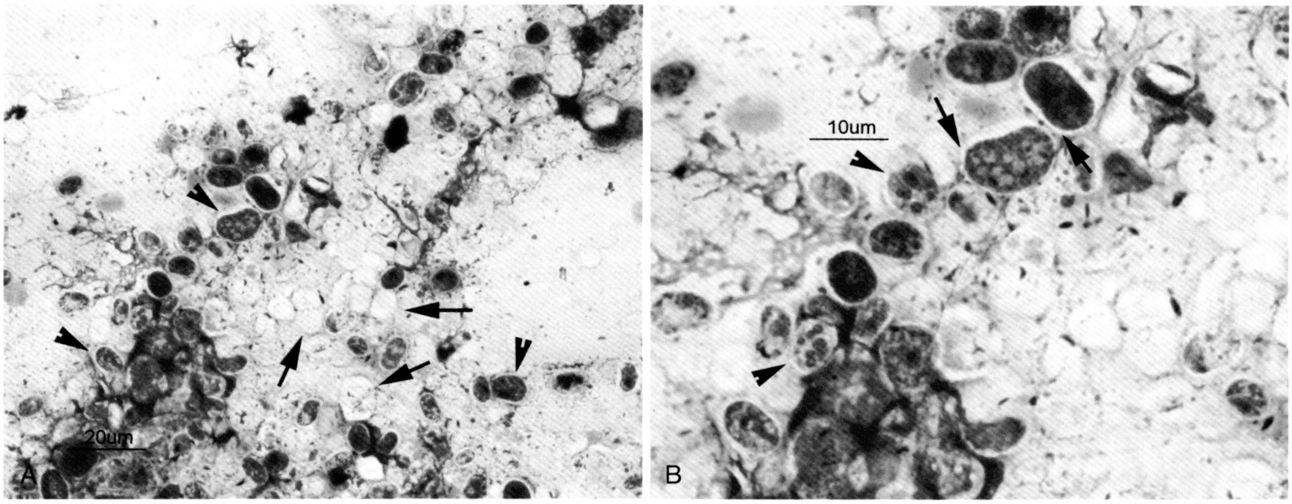

Figure 3-19 **A,** Ocular (fluid from areas of retinal separation) aspirate from a dog with protothecosis. Numerous round to oval organisms are present (*arrowheads*), as well as clear, negatively staining areas representing empty casings of ruptured organisms (*arrows*). (Wright stain.) **B,** Higher magnification of same slide as *A*, shows numerous round to oval organisms, many of which contain endospores (*arrowheads*). A thin, clear cell wall can be seen surrounding most organisms (*arrows*). (Wright stain.)

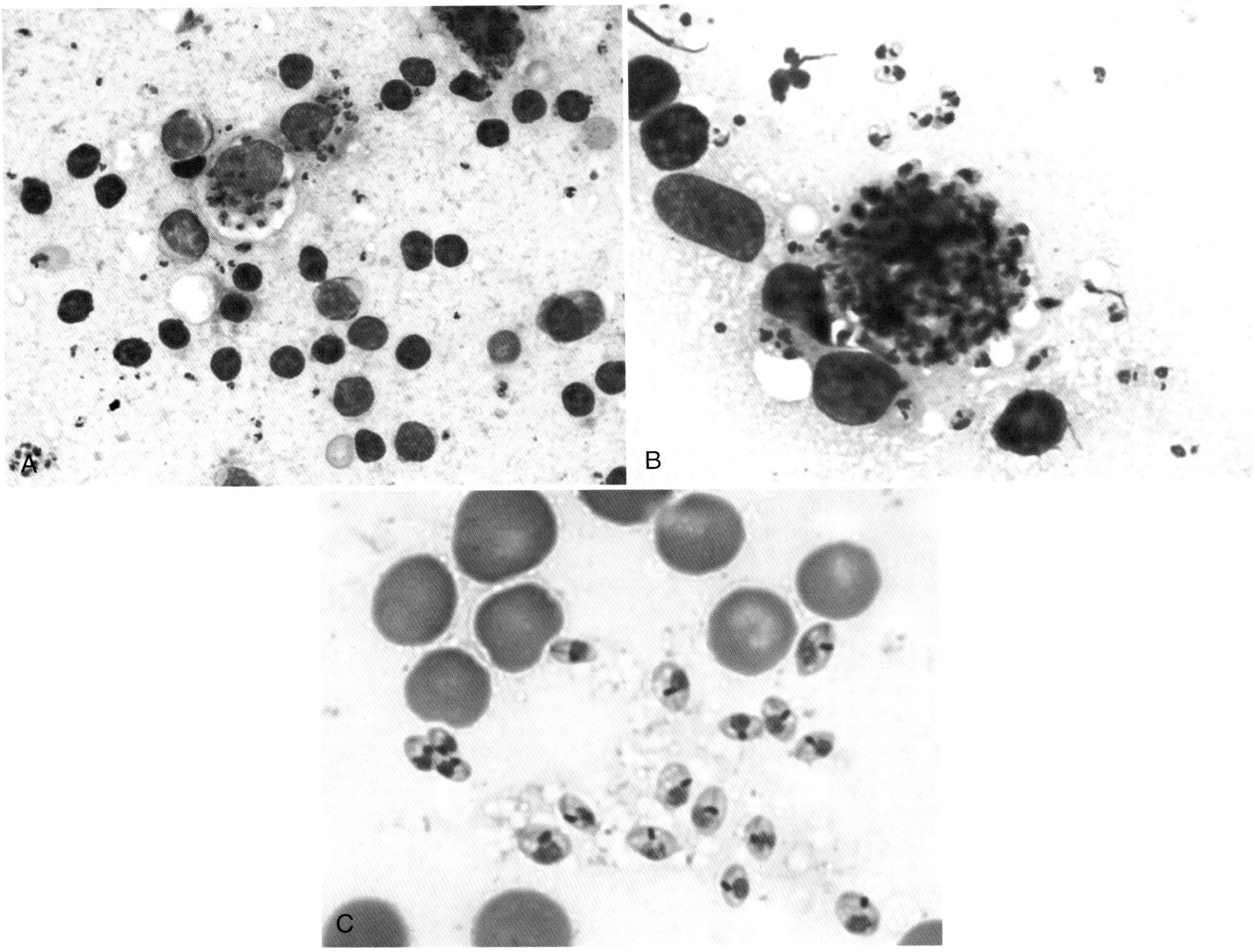

Figure 3-20 **A,** Lymph node aspirate from a dog showing many lymphocytes, a few red blood cells, and macrophages. *Leishmania* organisms are present within the macrophages and in the background of the smear. (Wright stain.) **B,** Higher magnification showing *Leishmania* organisms in a macrophage and free in the background of the smear. (Wright stain.) **C,** *Leishmania* organisms (Wright stain).

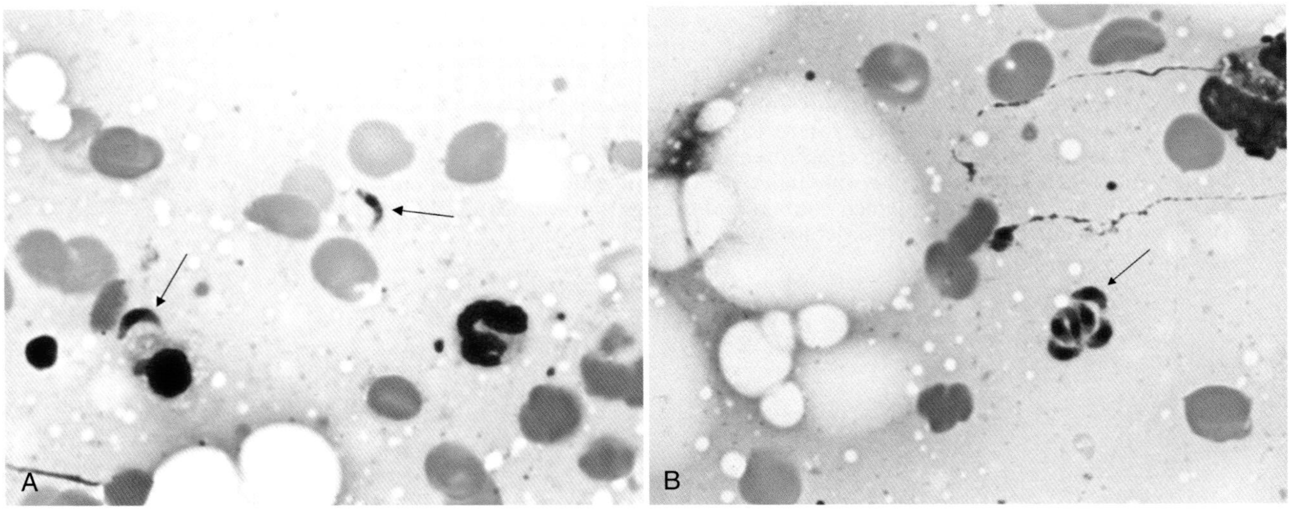

Figure 3-21 **A,** Bronchoalveolar lavage (BAL) from a cat showing two small crescent-shaped bodies with light-blue cytoplasm and dark-staining pericentral nucleus typical of *Toxoplasma* tachyzoites (*arrows*). (Wright stain.) **B,** A group of *Toxoplasma* tachyzoites (*arrow*) in a BAL. (Wright stain.)

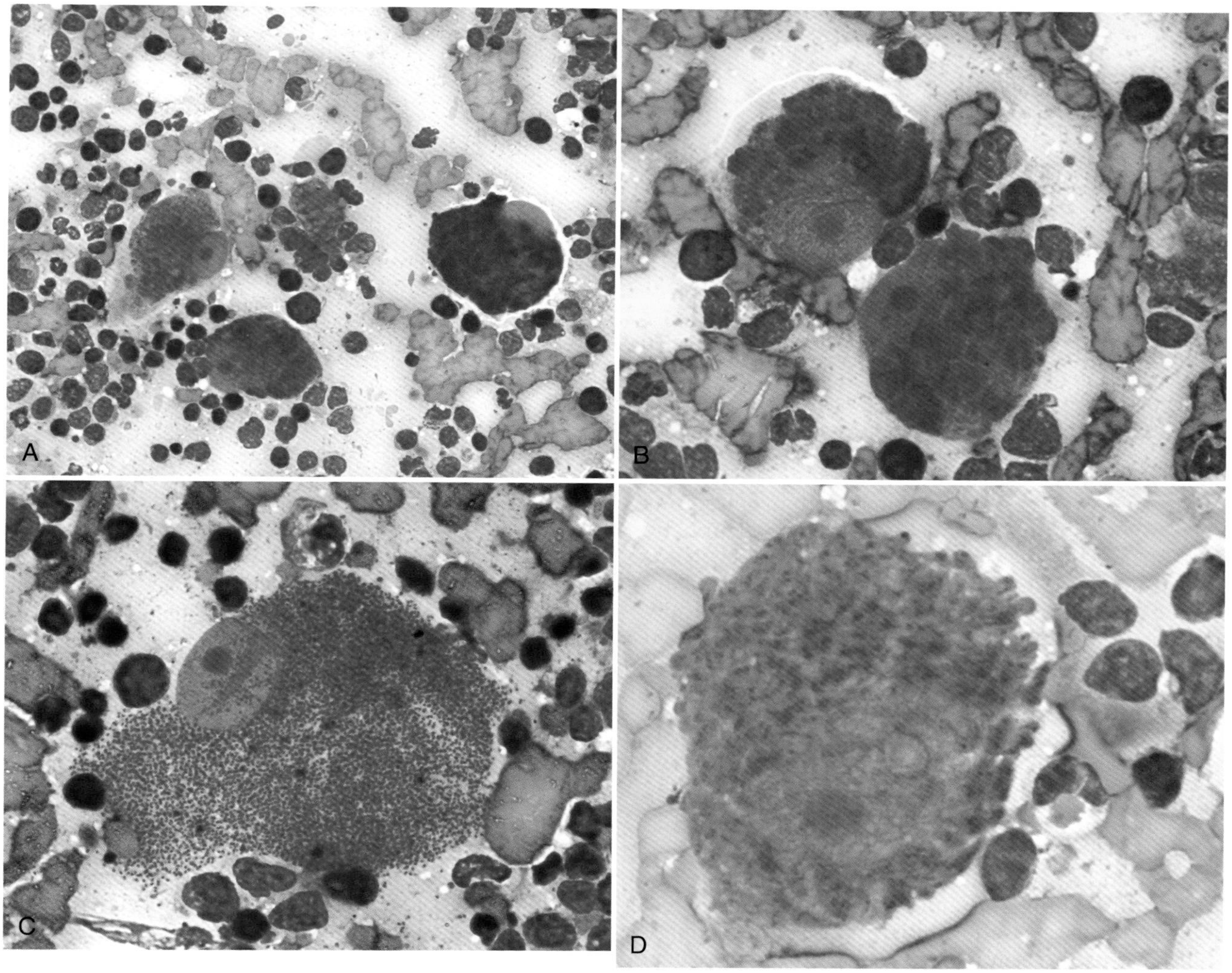

Figure 3-22 **A,** Lymph node aspirate from a cat with cytauxzoonosis. Many lymphocytes, red blood cells, scattered neutrophils, and three macrophages containing developing merozoites of *Cytauxzoon* are shown. (Wright stain.) **B,** Same case as *A*. Two macrophages with large prominent nucleoli are shown. Both macrophages contain intracytoplasmic irregularly defined clusters of developing *Cytauxzoon* organisms. (Wright stain.) **C,** Same case as *A*. A single macrophage containing high numbers of small, dark-staining bodies of *Cytauxzoon* merozoites. (Wright stain.) **D,** *Cytauxzoon* in cat splenic aspirate. (Wright stain.)

References

1. Bottles K, Miller TR, Cohen MB, et al: Fine needle aspiration biopsy: has its time come? *Am J Med* 81:525–531, 1986.
2. Caruso KJ, et al: Skin scraping from a cat, *Vet Clin Pathol* 31(1):13–15, 2002.
3. Duprey ZH, Steurer FJ, Rooney JA, et al: Canine visceral leishmaniasis, United States and Canada, 2000-2003, *Emerg Infect Dis* 12(3):440–446, 2006.
4. Greene CE, editor: *Infectious diseases of the dog and cat*, ed 4, Philadelphia, PA, 2011, Saunders.
5. Lester SJ, et al: Cryptococcosis: update and emergence of *Cryptococcus gattii*, *Vet Clin Path* 40(1):4–17, 2011.
6. Nelson RW, Couto G, editors: *Small animal internal medicine*, ed 4, Philadelphia, PA, 2009, Mosby, 2009.
7. Raskin RE, Meyer DJ, editors: *Canine and feline cytology, a color atlas and interpretation guide*, ed 2, Philadelphia, PA, 2010, Elsevier, 2010.
8. Rebar AH: Diagnostic cytology in veterinary practice. Proceedings of the 54th Annual Meeting of the AAHA, 1987 [pp. 498-504]. In Kirk RW, editor: *Current veterinary therapy, vol. VII*, Philadelphia, PA, 1980, Saunders, pp 16–27.
9. Sukura A, Saari S, Järvinen AK, et al: *Pneumocystis Carinii* pneumonia in dogs—a diagnostic challenge, *J Vet Diagn Invest* 8:130–133, 1996.
10. Seybold I, Goldston RT, Wikes RD: Exfoliative cytology, *Vet Med Small Anim Clin* 77:1029–1033, 1982.
11. Cowell RL, editor: Cytology Part I, *Vet Clin North Am Small Animal Pract* 32(6), 2002.
12. Cowell RL, editor: Cytology Part II, *Vet Clin North Am Small Animal Pract* 2003. 32(6), 2003.

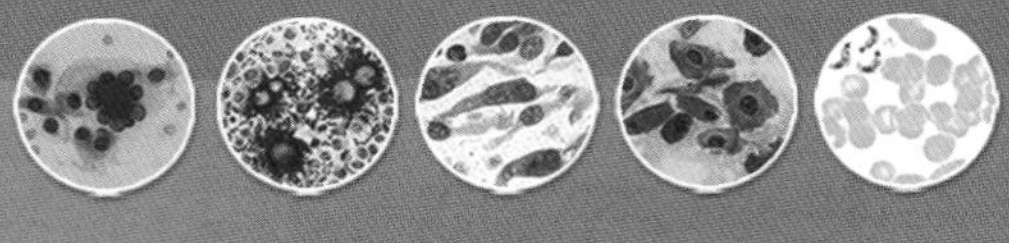

CHAPTER 4

Round Cells

Dennis B. DeNicola

The category of discrete round cell neoplasms is composed primarily of cells of the hemolymphatic system. The title of these types of neoplastic conditions is highly descriptive of the cytomorphologic presentation. Neoplastic cells in this category are typically discrete in nature and round in shape. However, the round shape of these cells is not always definitive for a round cell neoplasm, as in many other neoplastic processes the neoplastic cells also are predominantly round in shape. For example, many epithelial neoplasms and some poorly differentiated mesenchymal neoplasms are composed of neoplastic cells that are round to ovoid in shape. Even a few well-differentiated mesenchymal neoplasms such as osteoblastic osteosarcoma and chondrosarcoma are composed of round to ovoid neoplastic cells.

The distinguishing morphologic feature of the discrete round cell neoplasms is the discrete nature of the neoplastic cells. Because no cellular junctions connect individual neoplastic cells, as with epithelial neoplasms, this becomes a highly distinguishing feature. Mesenchymal neoplasms composed of round to oval cells often also have extracellular matrix material produced by the neoplastic cells which sometimes causes loose groupings of cells resembling cohesion between cells. This apparent grouping is not typically seen with discrete round cell neoplasms.

General comments on the cytomorphologic features, tissue distribution, and biologic behavior of discrete round cell neoplasms are outlined next:

- *Cell shape:* As was noted above, these cells are typically round to oval in shape; however, an amoeboid or irregular shape may be seen particularly with cells of histiocytic lineage.
- *Nuclear shape:* Cell nuclei of discrete round cell neoplasms are generally round to slightly oval; however, irregularly shaped nuclei are often present within the histiocytic group of discrete round cell neoplasms.
- *Cytoplasmic characteristics:* The cytoplasmic features of the various discrete round cell neoplasms are among the most important morphologic features used to differentiate one from the other. The presence or absence of cytoplasmic vacuoles, the presence or absence of cytoplasmic granules, and the color and distribution of cytoplasmic granules prove extremely helpful in making a definitive diagnosis.
- *Tissue distribution:* Discrete round cell neoplasms can be found essentially in any anatomic location, including both cutaneous and visceral tissue distributions. Some have relatively consistent locations of origin, which will be discussed later with each neoplasm type, and other chapters will highlight various visceral locations for discrete round cell neoplasms.
- *Biologic behavior:* Discrete round cell neoplasms have dramatically variable biologic behaviors. In many instances, although cytomorphologic atypia may be seen, these morphologic features often do not prove helpful in predicting potential biologic behavior.

The list of processes included in the discrete round cell neoplasm varies in the literature because of either including or excluding melanocytic neoplasms from the group. Since many of the cutaneous melanocytic neoplasms have a prominent round cytologic presentation, these are often included. A brief comment on the clinical and cytologic presentation of melanoma is included in this chapter. The entire group of discrete round cell neoplasms is as follows:[1-6]

- Transmissible venereal tumor
- Mast cell tumor
- Histiocytic tumors
- Lymphoproliferative disease
- Melanocytic tumors

TRANSMISSIBLE VENEREAL TUMORS

Presentation and Biologic Behavior

Transmissible venereal tumors (TVT) were the first described transplantable neoplastic process. They are more commonly seen in more tropic urban areas, where large numbers of free-roaming dogs are present. Young sexually active dogs are most commonly affected because of direct contact and transplantation of neoplastic cells; external genitalia are most commonly affected. The typical social behavior of dogs licking and sniffing results in transplantation in other locations, including the oral and nasal cavities. The TVT is considered mostly to be a benign neoplastic process, which, with the aid of a competent immune system, will often spontaneously regress; however, metastatic disease, particularly to the intraocular space, may rarely occur.[7,8]

Cytologic Presentation

Aspirates and touch preparations of a TVT generally yield a large number of neoplastic cells. The typical TVT cell is the epitome of the discrete round cell neoplasm group. The distinctive discrete round cells have eccentric round nuclei with uniform granular chromatin patterns and, often, a single round prominent nucleolus. Mitotic figures are common and abnormal mitotic figures may be present, but these abnormal figures are not useful in predicting biologic behavior. Neoplastic cells range from 12 to 24 micrometers (μm) in diameter, and they have moderate amounts of granular and moderately blue-staining cytoplasm. Distinguishing cytoplasmic granules are not present; however, low-to-moderate numbers of TVT cells have distinguishing, clear, distinct, punched-out cytoplasmic vacuoles. These vacuoles are commonly similar in size and arranged in a linear array along the inner surface of the cell membrane (Figure 4-1).[5,9]

In addition to the neoplastic cells, normal-appearing small lymphocytes, few well-differentiated plasma cells, and rarely seen histiocytes or macrophages are commonly present.[5] These cells tend to increase in relative numbers during spontaneous regression of the neoplastic process secondary to a localized immune response.

MAST CELL TUMORS

Presentation and Biologic Behavior

Mast cell tumors are among the most common cutaneous neoplasms of dogs and cats; however, they may occur at any anatomic location both as primary and secondary neoplastic disease.[8] They are most commonly seen in middle-aged dogs and cats, but an animal of any age is susceptible. In the dog, mast cell tumors are considered malignant, with the potential for widespread dissemination. A histologic grading scheme has been used to help predict biologic behavior; however, even well-differentiated grade I mast cell tumors have the potential for dissemination. Cytologic identification of metastatic or disseminated mast cell tumor, regardless of degree of differentiation, is of great value. MCT can also be found in the subcutaneous tissue and may be less aggressive than the cutaneous form. Histologic grading schemes for cutaneous mast cell tumors cannot be applied to assess the behavior of subcutaneous mast cell tumors.

Determination of prognostic behavior of canine mast cell tumors is primarily based on histological grading. However, also of importance are several clinical factors such as: clinical signs related to mast cell disease, location and size of the MCT, clinical stage, completeness of surgical excision, and determination of the rate of tumor growth. Further prognostication can be achieved by immunohistochemical and histochemical staining of MCT for markers of cellular proliferation such as: AgNOR, Ki67, and PCNA. Additionally, immunohistochemical staining for the presence and quantification of, and cellular location of c-KIT (a protooncogene) can be performed on tumor tissue and used as indicators of proliferative activity. Identification of c-KIT mutations by polymerase chain reaction (PCR) may be used as an indicator of potential aggressive biological behavior of canine mast cell tumors.

The general features of the histologic grading system with canine cutaneous mast cell tumors are outlined next:[5,7]

Grade I: well-differentiated, generally well-defined, superficial, low mitotic index

Grade II: moderately differentiated, moderate to poorly circumscribed, mild to moderate infiltration into deeper dermal tissues, moderate mitotic index, potential slight cytomorphologic atypia

Grade III: potentially poorly differentiated, poorly circumscribed, deep infiltration into subcutis, potential high mitotic index, potential moderate cytomorphologic atypia

Feline mast cell tumor has multiple presentations. Isolated cutaneous mast cell tumor is generally considered a benign lesion in the cat, and complete excision typically proves curative; however, dissemination may even be seen in cases with suspected isolated cutaneous mast

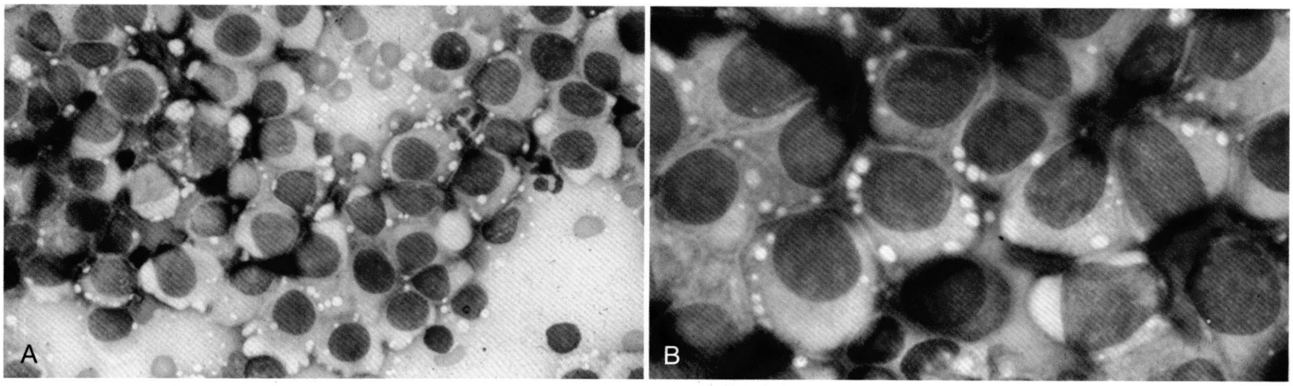

Figure 4-1 Transmissible venereal tumor. Aspirates of a transmissible venereal tumor on the prepuce of a dog. A, Highly cellular specimen containing a monotonous population of discrete round mononuclear cells mixed with small amounts of peripheral blood. (Wright stain.) **B,** Higher magnification of a similar field of view demonstrating the discrete round nature of the cells, the eccentric round to slightly oval nuclei, the uniform chromatin patterns and the moderate amounts of pale blue cytoplasm with multiple, discrete, clear vacuoles at the periphery of the cell. (Wright stain.)

cell tumor.[10-12] A guarded prognosis with short median survival times is reported in cats with multiple cutaneous mast cell tumors, recurring mast cell tumors and primary splenic mast cell neoplasia. Degree of differentiation is commonly considered a poor prognostic finding; however, the literature is contradictive with regard to the more poorly differentiated mast cell tumor in the cat. One study found no correlation between degree of cell differentiation and prognosis.[1,13]

Cytologic Presentation

The diagnosis of mast cell tumor in dogs and cats is relatively straightforward in most cases. Cytologic specimens are commonly very cellular and peripheral blood contamination is common. In addition to the distinctive discrete round cell characteristics, mast cell tumors have distinguishing fine-to-coarse purple granules when stained with a Romanowsky-type stain (Figure 4-2).[1] These granules allow a definitive diagnosis in most cases; however, it is reported that one of the most commonly used stains in practice, Diff-Quik, often fails in staining these granules, making accurate identification of mast cell tumor from other discrete round cell tumors difficult or impossible. Anecdotal reports suggest that approximately 15% of canine mast cell tumors will not stain with Diff-Quik (Figure 4-3). In reality, if one examines the specimen very carefully, although staining may be significantly less with Diff-Quik, identifiable purple granules are able to be visualized. Additional anecdotal reports suggest that prolonged fixation of mast cell tumors in the first solution of the Diff-Quik stain improves staining of mast cell granules.

Although canine mast cell tumor grading is based on histologic evaluation, where comments on degree of tissue invasion becomes an important criterion, degree of differentiation of mast cell tumor cells is possible cytologically, and correlation to histologic grading is good. The less differentiated cells are less granulated and have greater variability of cell size, nuclear size, and nucleus-to-cytoplasm (N:C) ratios. Prognosis should be considered guarded for the less differentiated canine neoplasms; however, it should be noted that well-differentiated mast cell tumors may also disseminate. Identification of metastasis to regional lymph nodes or parenchymal organs proves most useful in characterizing the biologic behavior of mast cell tumors in dogs and cats (Figure 4-4). With feline mast cell tumors, the distribution of neoplasms (isolated, multiple or disseminated) and the degree of circumscription of the neoplasm are potentially more predictive of biologic behavior compared with degree of differentiation (Figure 4-5).

Mast cell tumor cell nuclei are generally round to slightly oval and paracentral in location. If discernible, nuclear chromatin patterns are finely stippled and uniform; however, irregularly clumped chromatin patterns may be seen in less-differentiated mast cell tumors. Nuclei are often obscured from view with heavily granulated mast cells, or they stain extremely pale because of the high affinity of the cytoplasmic granules for the stain. Eosinophils may be present in the background, and these are more commonly seen in canine mast cell tumors than in feline mast cell tumors (Figure 4-6). They are not predictive of biologic behavior. Low numbers of normal-appearing small lymphocytes may be seen in feline cutaneous mast cell tumors.

In addition to the mast cell tumor cells and the potential of eosinophils, many cutaneous mast cell tumor cytologic preparations also have significant numbers of hyperplastic fibroblasts. Collagenolysis and reactive fibroplasia are common histologic findings. Fibroblasts are identified as nongranulated, large, plump, spindle-to-polygonal mononuclear cells, with large oval central nuclei, uniform chromatin patterns, potentially prominent nucleoli, and moderate-to-abundant amounts of deeply blue–staining granular cytoplasm (Figure 4-7). These cells are often embedded in densely packed groups of mast cell tumor cells and may be incorrectly identified as a component of the mast cell tumor population or a potential

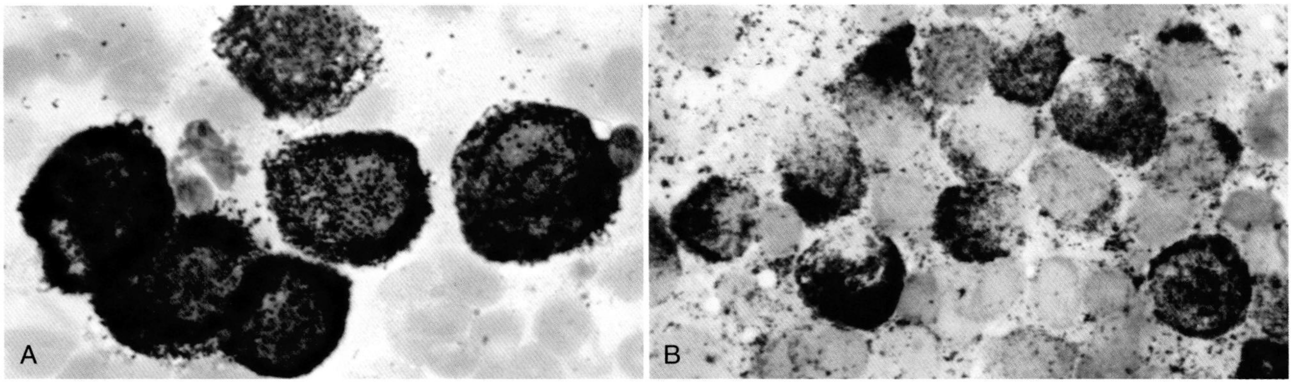

Figure 4-2 Mast cell tumor. Aspirates of two well-differentiated mast cell tumors on the skin of two different dogs. A, Moderately cellular specimen with significant peripheral blood contamination, which is common with mast cell tumor aspirates. The neoplastic cells are uniform and well differentiated. Nuclei are almost obscured from view because of the many coarse purple granules. Note the one eosinophil in the center left of the field of view. (Wright stain.) **B,** Highly cellular preparation with densely packed sheets of mast cells, where neoplastic cell nuclei are stained very pale blue because of the heavy degree of granulation and lack of stain penetration to the nucleus. (Wright stain.)

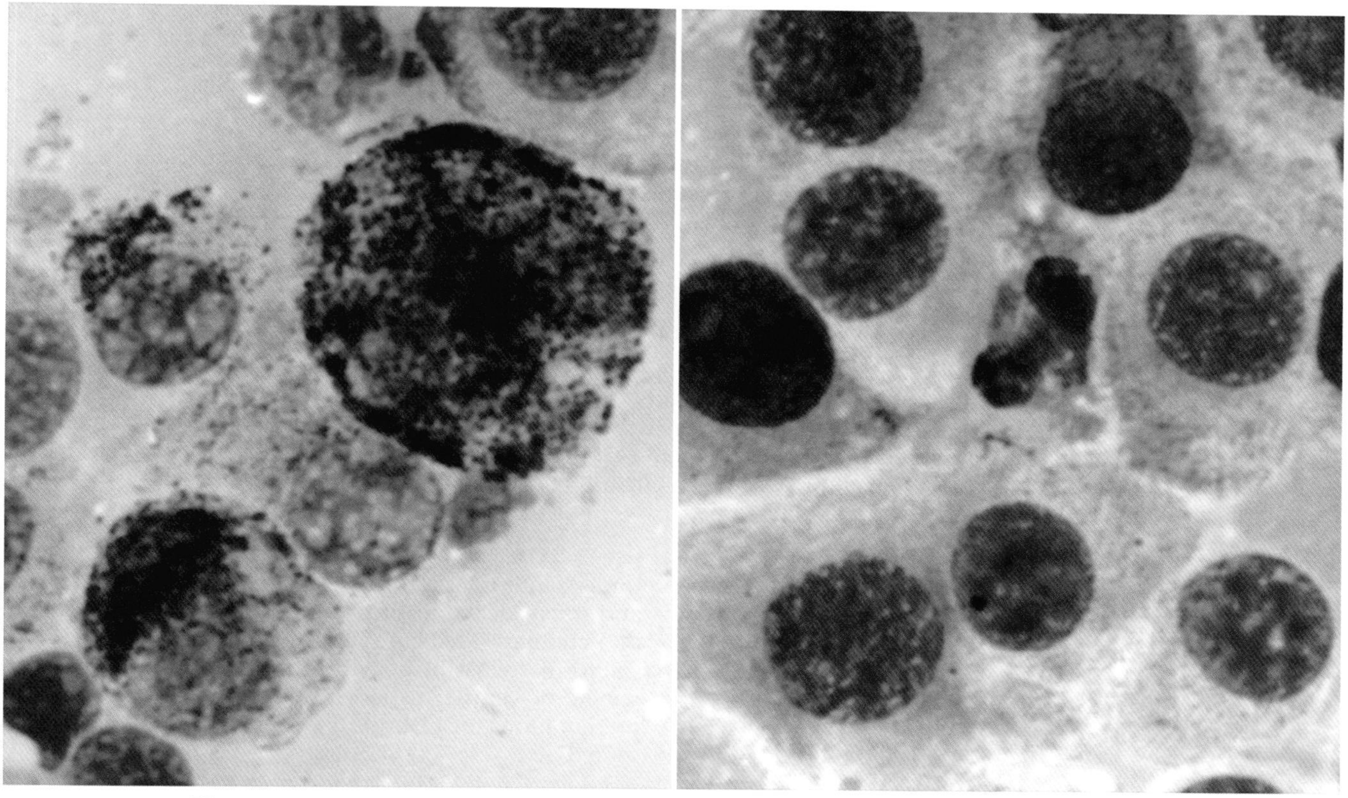

Figure 4-3 Aspirates of a cutaneous mast cell tumor on a dog. The image on the left is from a Wright-stained preparation, and the image on the right is from a Diff-Quik–stained preparation from the same aspirate. On the basis of the Wright-stained preparation (*left*), the tumor is characterized as moderately well differentiated with neoplastic cells containing variable numbers of fine to coarse, purple to pink granules. On the Diff-Quik–stained preparation (*right*), only extremely few cytoplasmic granules are distinguishable. The eosinophil in the center of the field of view gives a possible clue to an underlying poorly differentiated mast cell tumor, or one of those mast cell tumors that do not stain well with Diff-Quik stain.

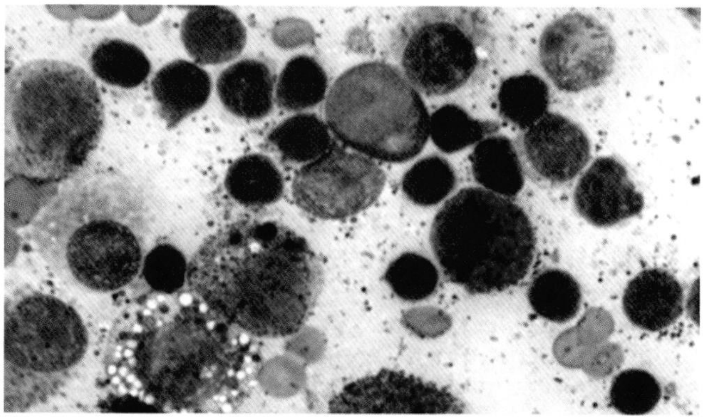

Figure 4-4 Aspirate of a popliteal lymph node from a cat with multiple cutaneous mast cell tumors. Note the mixture of moderately well-differentiated mast cells mixed with many normal-appearing small lymphocytes, which represent a population of residual normal lymphoid elements in the lymph node. A single eosinophil is noted in the top right region of the field of view; eosinophils are not as commonly seen in feline mast cell tumor as in the canine counterpart. (Wright stain.)

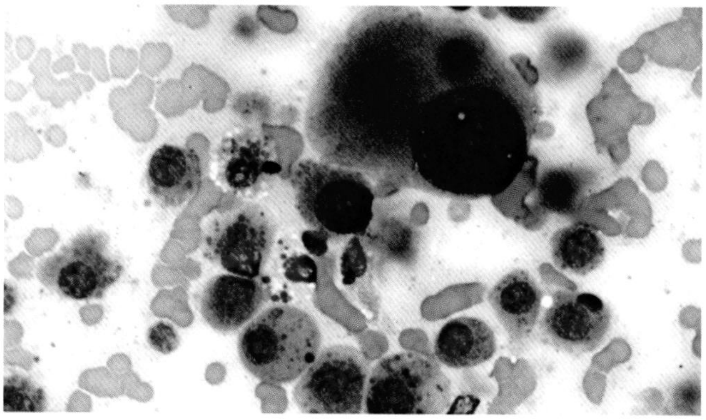

Figure 4-5 Aspirate of an isolated and well-defined cutaneous mast cell tumor in the skin of a cat. Intermixed with moderate amounts of peripheral blood, many poorly granulated mast cells are present. Marked cytomorphologic atypia is seen; however, on complete surgical excision, this animal was disease free with no recurrence of neoplastic disease. (Wright stain.)

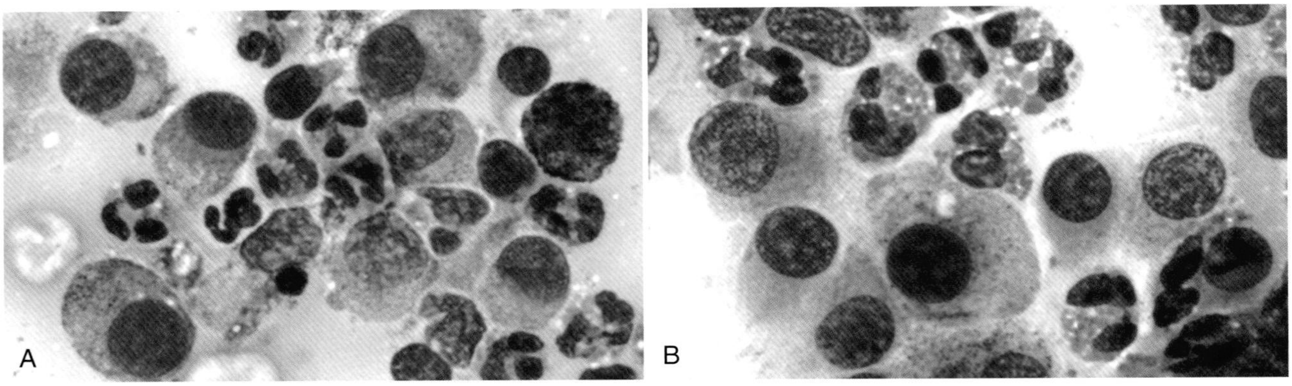

Figure 4-6 Aspirates from cutaneous mast cell tumors on two different dogs. **A,** Wright-stained specimen. **B,** Diff-Quik–stained specimen. The samples are highly cellular, containing a mixture of poorly granulated mast cells and numerous eosinophils. The high number of eosinophils may suggest that the underlying discrete cell neoplastic process is a poorly differentiated mast cell tumor.

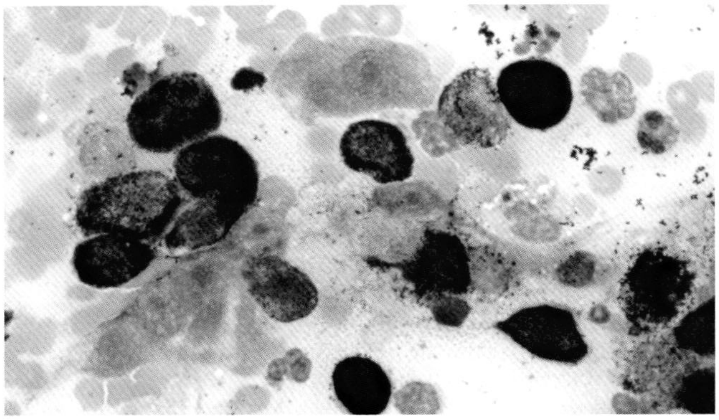

Figure 4-7 Aspirate from a cutaneous well-differentiated mast cell tumor on a dog. Many well-granulated mast cells mixed with peripheral blood, low numbers of eosinophils, and plump spindle to irregularly shaped hyperplastic fibroblasts are seen. Fibroplasia is commonly seen in mast cell tumors of the skin and should not be interpreted as a second neoplastic process. (Wright stain.)

second neoplastic process. If an area of fibroplasia is aspirated and high numbers of the hyperplastic fibroblasts and fewer well-differentiated mast cells are present, a diagnosis of a primary mesenchymal neoplasm with mast cell infiltration is also possible. Specimen collection ensuring sampling from different areas of the primary mass can help minimize this possibility.

HISTIOCYTIC TUMORS

Presentation and Biologic Behavior

Histiocytic neoplastic disease is extremely complex, particularly in the dog. The wide range of clinical presentations and biologic behaviors are dependent on the cell of lineage. In many cases, cytomorphologic features of the neoplastic histiocytes are highly predictive of biologic potential; however, tissue distribution of two of the benign histiocytic proliferative diseases cannot be predicted on the basis of cytomorphologic features alone. In recent years, tremendous advances have been made in the understanding of canine histiocytic neoplastic processes, and the reader is directed to the laboratory at the School of Veterinary Medicine, University of California, Davis, California (www.histiocytosis.ucdavis.edu) for a detailed review of canine histiocytic disease.[14-17] The four basic presentations for histiocytic neoplasia in the dog are presented next.

Canine Cutaneous Histiocytoma: Canine cutaneous histiocytoma is typically a benign solitary cutaneous lesion in young dogs; however, it may be seen in dogs of any age. Most commonly, it is seen in dogs younger than 1.5 to 3 years of age. Complete excision is typically curative, and spontaneous regression is reported. These neoplasms may be found anywhere on the body, but extremities and ears are common locations.

Cutaneous Histiocytosis: Cutaneous histiocytosis is considered a benign process, even though multiple lesions are common.[17] Lesions are present in cutaneous and subcutaneous tissues, and distribution of lesions is relatively widespread on the body. The lesions may wax and wane, and spontaneous regression is reported. These lesions most likely represent a reactive histiocytosis of dendritic cells rather than a true neoplastic process.[14] Local and systemic immune modulation prove helpful in lesion management in many cases.

Systemic Histiocytosis: In the past, systemic histiocytosis was considered a separate entity from cutaneous histiocytosis because in addition to the possible multiple cutaneous lesions, peripheral lymph nodes and occasionally visceral organs may be affected. Recent studies suggest that systemic histiocytosis and cutaneous histiocytosis are variants of the same reactive histiocytic proliferative process.[14,18] Because of the apparent disseminated nature of this disease process, euthanasia was commonly suggested in the past. Clinical management is more difficult than with cutaneous histiocytosis; immunosuppression therapy directed toward inhibition of T-cell activation is recommended more for patients with systemic histiocytosis than with cutaneous histiocytosis.

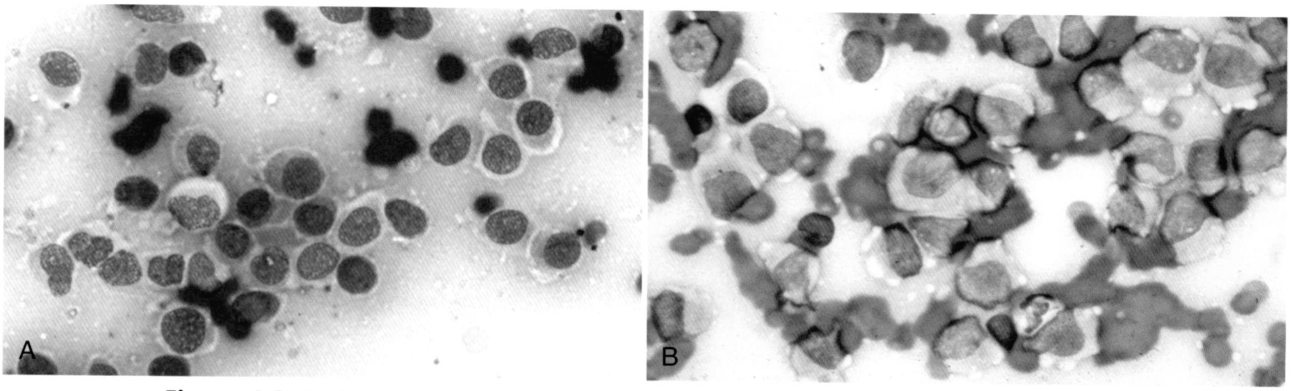

Figure 4-8 Aspirates of two canine histiocytomas from the skin of two different dogs. **A,** Aspirates are from an early-developing canine histiocytoma containing many relatively uniform discrete round mononuclear cells with eccentric round to oval to slightly indented nuclei with finely stippled and uniform chromatin patterns. The cytoplasm is moderate in amount, pale blue, and granular. Erythrocytes are found in the background. **B,** Aspirates are from a late-stage resolving canine histiocytoma containing slightly larger discrete round mononuclear cells compared with cells from *A*. Nuclei are more irregularly shaped, and the nuclear chromatin pattern resembles chromatin patterns of peripheral blood monocytes.

Histiocytic Sarcoma Complex: Histiocytic sarcoma complex is a group of neoplastic processes in the dog, which encompasses histiocytic sarcoma, which is typically a solitary lesion, and malignant histiocytosis or disseminated histiocytic sarcoma, which occurs when the disease process extends beyond regional lymph nodes and involves various visceral tissues.[19] This disease complex is best described in the Bernese mountain dog but has been seen in many breeds of dogs.[19,20] This disease complex presents with cytomorphologically distinguishing features of cellular atypia and, in many cases, multinucleate giant pleomorphic neoplastic cells.

Feline histiocytic disorders are less common and much less understood than are the canine counterparts. A benign cutaneous histiocytoma, as seen in the dog, does not exist in the cat. Histiocytic disease in the cat appears progressive in nature both with a morphologically benign appearing neoplastic cell population and a population of histiocytes with significant cytomorphologic atypia. Lesions often present as solitary cutaneous nodules with either gradual progression and possible eventual multiple cutaneous lesions or potential progression to involve regional lymph nodes and, terminally, visceral organs. A cytomorphologically malignant-appearing histiocytic neoplastic process, histiocytic sarcoma, resembles the canine counterpart. These tumors are typically locally invasive, and metastatic disease primarily to regional lymph nodes is possible.

Cytologic Presentation

Although significant variations exist in clinical presentation for histiocytic proliferative disease in the dog and in the cat, cytomorphologic variations are relatively few, which makes it difficult sometimes to make a definitive diagnosis on cytologic presentation alone. All of the different variants of histiocytic proliferative disease typically present with moderate-to-high cellularity, with varying amounts of peripheral blood contamination.

Canine Cutaneous Histiocytoma, Cutaneous Histiocytosis, and Systemic Histiocytosis: The proliferative histiocytes in canine cutaneous histiocytoma, cutaneous histiocytosis, and systemic histiocytosis in the dog have similar morphologic features.[19,21,22] These discrete cells are relatively round and range from 12 to 30 μm in diameter. They may present with an irregular or amoeboid cell shape; this is seen more in later stages of resolution, particularly in the cutaneous histiocytoma in young dogs. Nuclei are mostly round to oval and eccentric in location, but blunt indentations of the nucleus or irregular shapes may also be seen. Nuclear chromatin patterns are finely stippled and uniform and, in many cases, resemble the nuclear chromatin patterns of normal-appearing peripheral blood monocytes. The cytoplasm is variable in amount but generally moderate to abundant. Cytoplasm stains pale blue and is granular, with no distinguishing granules or vacuoles (Figure 4-8 and Figure 4-9).

Low numbers of normal-appearing small lymphocytes and rarely seen macrophages and well-differentiated plasma cells may be distributed among the histiocytic cells. These nonhistiocytic cells may increase in number during phases of resolution.

Histiocytic Sarcoma Complex: Neoplastic cells within the histiocytic sarcoma complex of neoplasms are distinctively different from the more benign-appearing counterparts noted previously. Anisocytosis, anisokaryosis, variation in N:C ratios, and overall pleomorphism are common. In addition, multinucleate giant cell formation is often seen. Nuclear chromatin patterns can be irregularly clumped and prominent; multiple or irregularly shaped nucleoli may be seen. Cytoplasm is typically moderate to abundant in mount, pale blue staining, granular, and sometimes vacuolated (Figure 4-10 and Figure 4-11). Phagocytosis of erythrocytes, leukocytes, and other neoplastic cells may be seen and is particularly common in a variant of the histiocytic sarcoma complex called *hemophagocytic histiocytic sarcoma*.

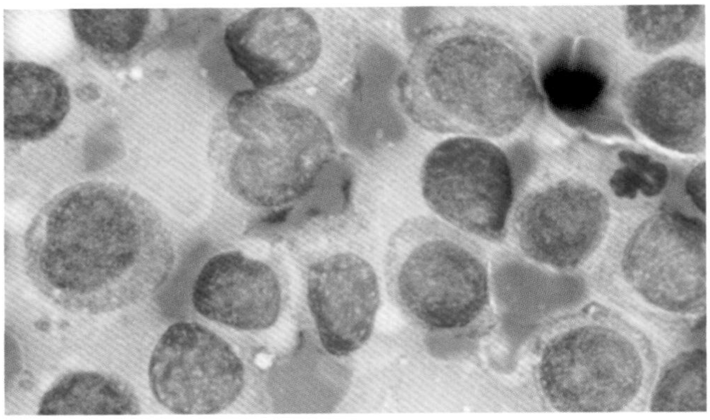

Figure 4-9 Aspirate of one of multiple cutaneous masses on a dog. Morphologic features of the primary neoplastic cell population are similar to those of the typical cutaneous histiocytoma commonly found in young dogs. Erythrocytes are present in the background. This aspirate is from a case of cutaneous histiocytosis. (Wright stain.)

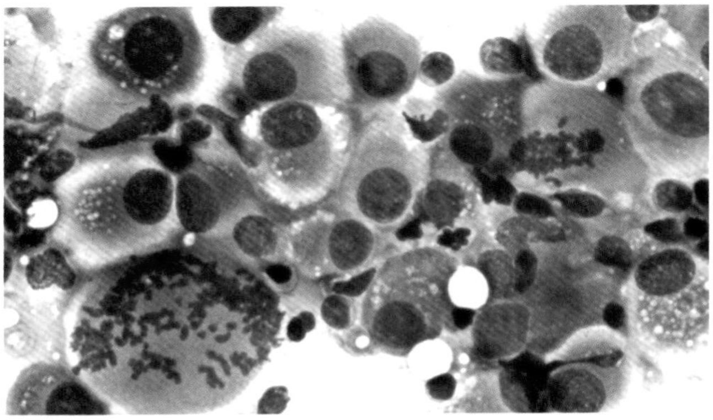

Figure 4-10 Aspirate of an enlarged prescapular lymph node on a dog with multiple skin and internal organ space-occupying lesions. The sample is highly cellular, containing a population of discrete round and mostly mononuclear cells with moderate anisocytosis, anisokaryosis, and variation in nucleus-to-cytoplasm ratios. Two abnormal mitotic figures are present. This aspirate is from a case of histiocytic sarcoma complex.

A hemophagocytic syndrome with observed anemia and possible other peripheral cytopenias may occur.

LYMPHOPROLIFERATIVE DISEASE

Presentation and Biologic Behavior

Detailed discussion of lymphoproliferative disease is found in Chapter 11; however, some general comments related to the discrete round cell nature of this group of neoplastic diseases is warranted because anatomic locations for lymphoproliferative disease overlap locations of origin for other discrete round cell neoplasms. Morphologic distinction between the different types of tumors is important because biologic behavior is potentially dramatically different from one tumor to the next. Malignant lymphoma or lymphosarcoma presenting with classic localized or generalized lymphadenomegaly itself has a variety of potential biologic behavior patterns. Different forms of malignant lymphoma range from the low-grade, smoldering type to the high-grade and rapidly progressive type. Cutaneous and other nonlymphoid tissue originating lymphoproliferative disease is generally considered malignant, and progressive disease with eventual dissemination.[7]

A variant of lymphoproliferative disease, *plasma cell neoplasia*, commonly presents differently from malignant lymphoma. Cutaneous and other extramedullary plasmacytomas are most commonly considered benign lymphoproliferative disease, and complete excision typically proves curative.[23] This is in significant contrast to the predominating pattern for multiple myeloma, a plasma cell tumor originating in the bone marrow. These latter neoplastic processes may present with isolated lesions but more commonly present with multiple lesions within the marrow, resulting in multiple lytic lesions that can be identified radiographically. Even though most cutaneous or isolated extramedullary plasmacytomas are considered benign, the potential for disseminated disease exists regardless of cytomorphologic presentation (atypia or no atypia), so investigation into possible systemic disease is always warranted.

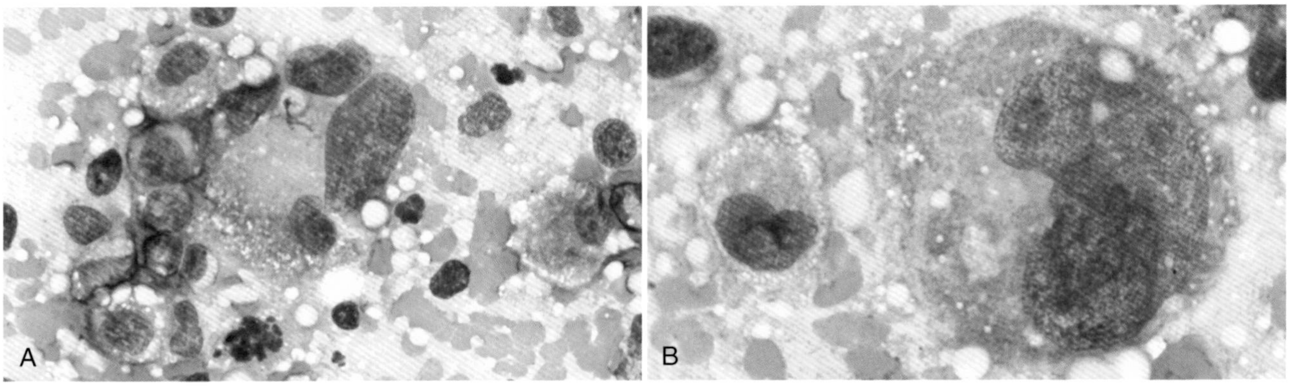

Figure 4-11 Aspirates from a mediastinal mass from a dog with histiocytic sarcoma complex. A, The specimen is highly cellular and has much peripheral blood contamination mixed with the neoplastic cell population. Significant cytomorphologic atypia is consistent with this malignant variant of histiocytic disease in the dog. A single mitotic figure is noted in the bottom center region of the field of view. (Wright stain.) **B,** Higher-magnification field of view of a different area of the same lesion as presented in *A*. Cytomorphologic atypia is characterized by the presence of a giant cell with a giant nucleus. Nuclear chromatin patterns are open with irregular clumping of chromatin. (Wright stain.)

Cytologic Presentation

The key cytologic feature of malignant lymphoma other than the discrete round nature of the neoplastic cells is that these tumors are generally composed of a homogeneous population of lymphocytes at one state of differentiation. Cytologic specimens are typically highly cellular, even when presented with aspirates of plaquelike lesions in the skin of a dog. Inflammatory lesions with high numbers of infiltrating lymphocytes are also highly cellular, but these specimens typically contain a highly heterogeneous population of lymphocytes. Normal small lymphocytes typically predominate, and many prominent reactive lymphocytes, plasmacytoid lymphocytes, well-differentiated plasma cells, and very few large and immature appearing lymphocytes are present.

The neoplastic lymphocytes are commonly very similar to the primary tissue's normal-appearing cellular elements. A small cell malignant lymphoma is composed mostly of relatively normal-appearing small lymphocytes with potentially slightly greater than normal amounts of pale blue–staining cytoplasm or clefted nuclei. The N:C ratios are high, and the nuclear chromatin patterns are somewhat smudged and dense in contrast to the cells of a TVT or canine cutaneous histiocytoma (Figure 4-12). Intermediate-sized to large-cell-type malignant lymphomas are composed of a vastly predominating population of morphologically normal-appearing medium-to-large lymphocytes commonly seen in reactive lymphoid tissues or in very low numbers in normal lymphoid tissue. Even these lymphocytes have distinctively high N:C ratios, which helps distinguish them from other discrete round cell tumors (Figure 4-13). In some cases of malignant lymphoma, the potential for significant variation in cell size and shape, as well as significant cellular atypia, exists; however, many malignant lymphoma cases have no significant cytomorphologic criteria of malignancy beyond the lack of heterogeneity typically found in normal or reactive lymphocytic tissue. The mitotic activity (mitotic index) is better classified with histopathologic evaluation of fixed tissue specimens; however, both normal and abnormal mitotic figures may be easily seen in cases of malignant lymphoma with a histologically identified high mitotic index.

A special morphologic variant of lymphoproliferative disease is the plasma cell tumor. Cutaneous plasmacytoma, noncutaneous extramedullary plasmacytoma, and multiple myeloma present with a similar cytologic picture.[1,24,25] Neoplastic cells have morphologic features of differentiated plasma cells. These cells are round to oval mononuclear cells mixed with potentially low numbers of binucleate cell forms. The cells mostly range from 15 to 30 μm in diameter. Nuclei are commonly round with uniform and sometimes coarse but regular chromatin patterns. Nuclei are peripherally located and unlike other lymphoid tumor cells, plasmacytoma cells typically have moderate amounts of cytoplasm giving the cells a moderate rather than a high N:C ratio. Cytoplasm is commonly deeply blue staining because of the density of cytoplasmic ribonucleic acid (RNA). A prominent perinuclear clear zone representing the Golgi apparatus of cytoplasmic organelles is commonly seen (Figure 4-14). Extramedullary plasmacytomas and multiple myelomas may present with a monotonous population of very uniform well-differentiated plasma cells or with neoplastic cells with some plasmacytoid differentiation and moderate cellular atypia or a combination of these presentations. Morphologic features are not predictive of biologic behavior, but the more atypia present, the greater the concern for disseminated disease; and investigation into possible other anatomic locations of disease is strongly warranted.

MELANOCYTIC TUMORS

Presentation and Biologic Behavior

Benign and malignant melanoma can originate from any pigmented location; however, the haired skin and oral cavity are among the most common locations of occurrence.[8]

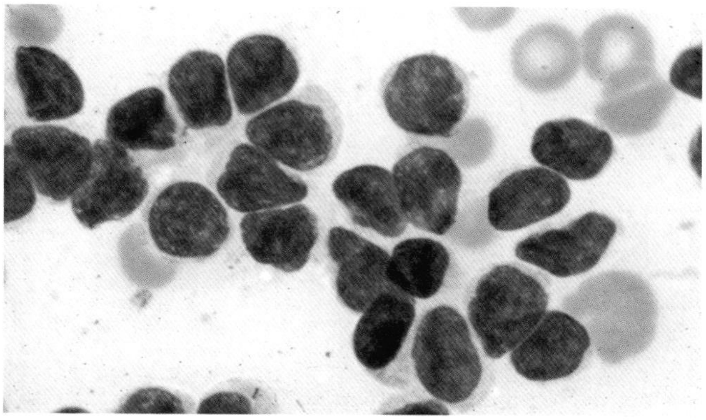

Figure 4-12 Aspirate from a case of cutaneous malignant lymphoma in a dog. Aspirates of multiple cutaneous lesions yielded highly cellular specimens containing primarily a single population of normal-appearing small lymphocytes mixed with peripheral blood. The lack of heterogeneity within the lymphoid cell population provides strong support for the existence of a lymphoproliferative process because most reactive lymphoid reactions result in the finding of many lymphocytes in different stages of reactivity and maturation. (Wright stain.)

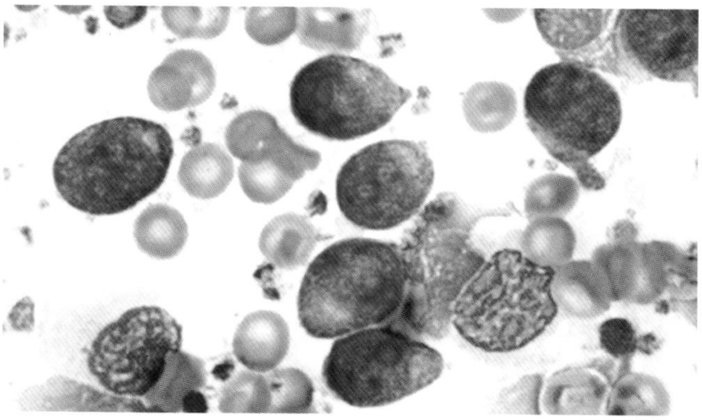

Figure 4-13 Aspirate of an intraabdominal mass in a dog. This specimen is highly cellular containing a primarily monotonous population of intermediate-sized to large and immature-appearing lymphocytes, often with eccentric round nuclei with single and sometimes multiple prominent nucleoli. The cytoplasm is moderate in amount, deeply blue, and granular with no distinguishing granules or vacuoles. The relatively high nucleus-to-cytoplasm ratios are supportive of lymphoid lineage. Many erythrocytes and lymphoglandular bodies are present in the background. (Wright stain.)

Biologic behavior is dramatically variable, and in many cases, cytomorphologic criteria of malignancy are helpful indicators of biologic behavior; the more cytomorphologic atypia, the greater is the metastatic potential. However, there are exceptions.

In the dog, anatomic location or origin plays a significant role in predicting biologic behavior. Melanocytic neoplasms originating from the digit and lip and oral melanomas have a worse prognosis than cutaneous tumors elsewhere. However, location alone is not always predictive of prognosis. Evidence of distant metastasis, regardless of the primary tumor's site of origin, is associated with a poor prognosis. In some studies, histologic assessment of mitotic index and nuclear atypia may be helpful in prognostication of canine melanocytic tumors. Immunohistochemical staining for Ki67 can also be performed on tumor tissue, which is an index of the growth fraction of neoplastic cells, and used as a prognostic indicator.

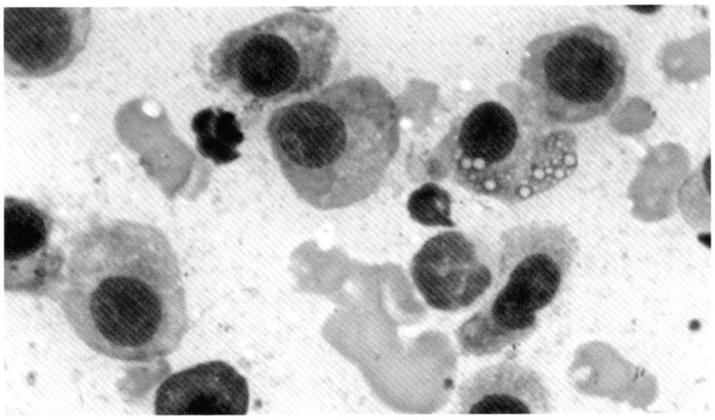

Figure 4-14 Aspirate of a solitary, well-defined, cutaneous, extramedullary plasmacytoma on a dog. The sample is highly cellular, containing a primary population of well-differentiated plasma cells with eccentric round dense nuclei and moderate to abundant amounts of deeply blue cytoplasm, often with poorly defined perinuclear clear zones. The monotony of the plasma cell population with no other significant inflammatory process is highly supportive of a diagnosis of extramedullary plasmacytoma.

Cytologic Presentation

As mentioned earlier, melanocytic tumors actually belong to a distinct class of neoplastic tissue—neuroendocrine tumors. However, they often have a presentation that can be confusing to even the expert cytologist. Melanoma cell morphology ranges from round to polygonal to plump spindle or even stellate; however, if the more round-shaped cells are predominant, a poorly differentiated melanoma can resemble other round cell tumors. It is important to examine the entire specimen because in most cases, a mixture of cellular morphologic presentations will be observed when looking at many of the neoplastic cells. Typically, these neoplasms exfoliate well, so many cells are available for evaluation. Cell sizes can be quite variable, ranging from as small as 12 to 20 μm in greatest dimension and as large as 20 to 30 μm or more in dimension. Nuclei are commonly paracentral in location and round to oval in shape. Nuclear chromatin patterns in the benign neoplasms are uniform and finely stippled; however, in the malignant variants, chromatin patterns are often coarsely and irregularly clumped. Nucleoli can be multiple, prominent, and irregularly shaped. Good nuclear criteria of malignancy are easily documented in many of the malignant melanomas. A moderate to high number of mitotic figures may be seen with the more malignant variants of melanoma, and rarely seen abnormal mitotic figures may be present.

The cytoplasm is typically moderate to abundant in amount, giving the cells a moderate to low N:C ratio. It is granular and lightly to moderately blue staining. One of the distinguishing features of this class of neoplasms is the presence of variable numbers of melanin pigment granules. In contrast to normal melanin granules, these are often rounded and variably sized and sometimes clumped to varying degrees. The granules stain black to green-black with commonly used Romanowsky stains in contrast to the purple staining granules of mast cell tumors (Figure 4-15). Histologically, a class of melanocytic

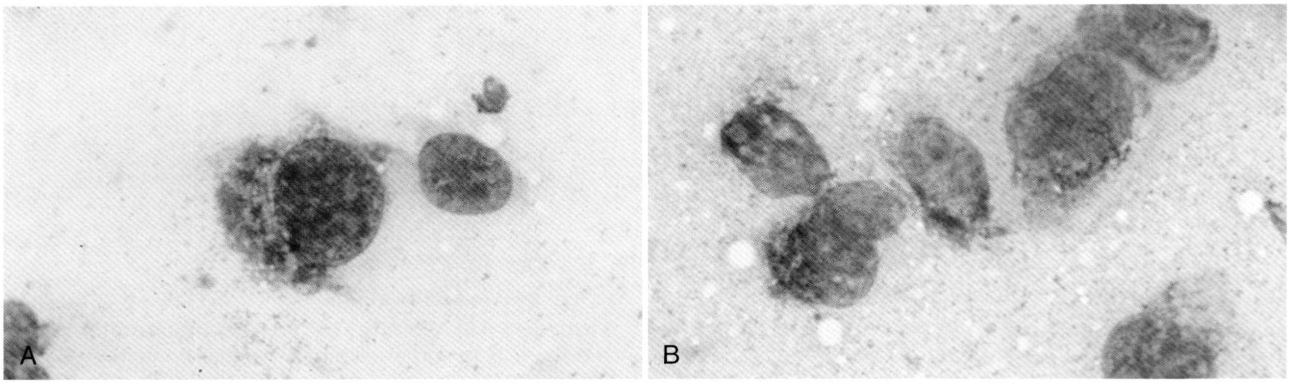

Figure 4-15 Aspirates of a lip mass on a dog. A, One intact round to polygonal mononuclear cell is adjacent to a broken mononuclear cell. The intact cell has an eccentric round to oval nucleus with slightly irregularly clumped chromatin. The cytoplasm is moderate in amount and filled with fine, black melanin granules. (Wright stain.) **B,** A different field of view from the same aspirate as *A*. Slightly greater amounts of cellular pleomorphism are noted. (Wright stain.)

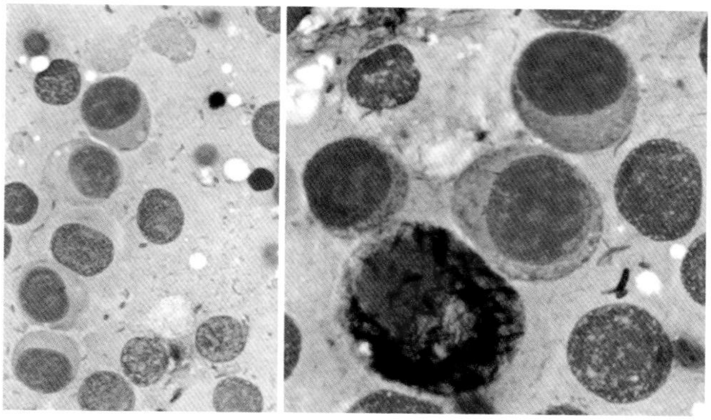

Figure 4-16 Aspirate of an amelanotic melanoma on the lip of a dog. Low-magnification view (*left*) of the specimen reveals a primary population of apparent discrete round mononuclear cells with no obvious melanin pigment. (Wright stain.) On evaluation of the complete specimen at high-magnification field of view (*right*), isolated neoplastic cells have obvious delicate needlelike melanin granules in the cytoplasm and few other cells have only a minimal dusting of the cytoplasm with melanin granules. (Wright stain.)

tumors are identified as amelanotic melanomas because of the apparent absence of melanin pigment granules with standard histologic staining procedures. Cytologically, even in the least pigmented melanomas, few melanin granules can be identified with deliberate microscopic review of the specimen (Figure 4-16). It should be noted that simple identification of melanin granules does not allow the making of a diagnosis of melanoma. The novice cytologist commonly misidentifies a pigmented basal cell tumor as melanoma; normal melanocytes pass melanin to epithelial cells of the epidermis. Additionally, some may confuse the presence of hemosiderin granules in a macrophage as melanin granules in a melanocyte; hemosiderin typically stains more brown to brown-black with commonly used Romanowsky stains.[5]

References

1. Baker R, Lumsden JH: The skin. In Baker R, Lumsden JH, editors: *Color atlas of cytology of the dog and cat*, St. Louis, MO, 2000, Mosby, pp 39–50.
2. Barton C: Cytologic diagnosis of cutaneous neoplasia: an algorithmic approach, *Comp Cont Ed* 9:20–33, 1987.
3. Duncan JS, Prasse KW: Cytologic examination of the skin and subcutis, *Vet Clin North Am* 6:637–645, 1976.
4. Duncan JS, Prasse KW: Cytology of canine cutaneous round cell tumors, *Vet Pathol* 16:673–679, 1979.
5. Raskin RE: Skin and subcutaneous tissues. In Raskin RE, Meyer DJ, editors: *Atlas of canine and feline cytology*, Philadelphia, PA, 2001, Saunders.
6. Rebar A: *Handbook of veterinary cytology*, St. Louis, MO, 1979, Ralston Purina Co.
7. Goldschmidt H: Tumors of the skin and soft tissues. In Meuten D, editor: *Tumors in domestic animals*, ed 4, Ames, IO, 2002, Blackwell Publishing Company.
8. Yager JA, Wilcock BP: Tumours of the skin and associated tissues. In Yager JA, Wilcock BP, editors: *Color atlas and text of surgical pathology of the dog and cat*, St. Louis, MO, 1994, Mosby.
9. Richardson RC: Canine transmissible venereal tumor, *Compend Cont Ed Pract* 3:951–956, 1981.
10. Buerger RG, Scott DW: Cutaneous mast cell neoplasia in cats: 14 cases:1975-1985, *J Am Vet Med Assoc* 190:1440–1444, 1987.
11. Miller MA, et al: Cutaneous neoplasia in 340 cats, *Vet Pathol* 28:389–395, 1991.
12. Wilcock BP, Yager JA, Zink MC: The morphology and behaviour of feline cutaneous mastocytomas, *Vet Pathol* 23:320–324, 1986.
13. Molander-McCrary H, et al: Cutaneous mast cell tumors in cats: 32 cases—1991-1994, *J Am Anim Hosp Assoc* 34:281–284, 1998.
14. Affolter VK, Moore PF: Canine cutaneous and systemic histiocytosis: reactive histiocytosis of dermal dendritic cells, *Am J Dermatopathol* 22:40–48, 2000.
15. Moore PF, Rosin A: Malignant histiocytosis of Bernese mountain dogs, *Vet Pathol* 23:1–10, 1986.
16. Moore A, et al: Canine cutaneous histiocytoma is an epidermotropic Langerhans cell histiocytosis that expresses CD1 and specific beta 2-integrin molecules, *Am J Pathol* 148:1699–1708, 1996.
17. Moore PF: Canine histiocytic diseases: proliferation of dendritic cells is key. Proceedings of the 55th Annual Meeting of the American College of Veterinary Pathologists, Amelia Island, FL, December 2000.
18. Moore PF: Systemic histiocytosis of Bernese mountain dogs, *Vet Pathol* 21:554–563, 1984.
19. Affolter VK, Moore PF: Histiocytosis. In: Proceedings of the 14th Annual Congress ESVD-ECVD, Pisa, Italy, September 5–7, 1997.
20. Hayden DW, et al: Disseminated malignant histiocytosis in a Golden Retriever: Clinicopathologic, ultrastructural, and immunohistochemical findings, *Vet Pathol* 30:256–264, 1993.
21. Bender WM, Muller GH: Multiple resolving cutaneous histiocytoma in a dog, *J Am Vet Med Assoc* 194:535–537, 1989.
22. Paterson S, Boydell P, Pike R: Systemic histiocytosis in the Bernese mountain dog, *J Small Anim Pract* 36:233–236, 1995.
23. Rowland PH, et al: Cutaneous plasmacytomas with amyloid in six dogs, *Vet Pathol* 28:125–130, 1991.
24. Rakich PM, et al: Mucocutaneous plasmacytomas in dogs: 75 cases: 1980-1987, *J Am Vet Med Assoc* 194:803–810, 1989.
25. Rogers KS: Diagnostic dilemma of extramedullary plasmacytomas, *Vet Cancer Soc Newslett* 15:12–14, 1991.

CHAPTER 5

Cutaneous and Subcutaneous Lesions

David J. Fisher

Cutaneous and subcutaneous lesions are commonly sampled sites for cytologic evaluation. Several reasons for this are possible, but perhaps some of the primary reasons are that these lesions are easily seen by the owners of the animals and thus cause concern and their sites are easily sampled by veterinarians. For the most part, sampling from skin lesions does not require imaging aid, nor does it necessarily require sedation or anesthesia. Just as important, many lesions are highly exfoliative, and skin or subcutaneous cytologic samples tend to have a high diagnostic yield. In one study comparing cytologic and histopathologic test results of cutaneous and subcutaneous lesions in 243 specimens, diagnosis was in agreement in 90.9% of the cases.[1]

Despite the potential usefulness of cytologic sampling, it is important to recognize that dermatologic disease encompasses a broad range of inflammatory, noninflammatory, and neoplastic lesions. Not all of these lesions exfoliate well, and many of the diagnoses are dependent on tissue distribution of cells, not just cytomorphologic appearance. Cytology interpretation is only based on cells, organisms, and background material, but since these have no architectural arrangement, as can be evaluated in biopsy samples, the results often are less specific compared with histologic interpretation (Figure 5-1). Finally, all cytology samples have some degree of artifact such as smudging of round cells that makes them appear spindloid, thick background material resulting in cells shrinking and appearing more round, or artifactual aggregates of cells resembling cohesive clusters; this artifact may make it difficult to be certain about cell types in some cases.

For these reasons, histopathology is often necessary for definitive diagnosis of dermatologic diseases. When taking cytologic samples from skin or subcutaneous lesions, it is useful to explain to the owner that the sampling process, in the best case scenario, will yield a clear-cut diagnosis, failing which, it would be a preliminary step to aid in determining what needs to be done next (Table 5-1).

Although cytologic evaluation is often straightforward, a better interpretation of cytologic findings can often be made when all relevant clinical information is integrated. This should include signalment, history, duration, location, and distribution, as well as other laboratory findings. If samples are to be forwarded to a clinical pathologist for review, it is important to provide this information along with the sample to allow for the best interpretation of the cytologic findings. Instead of describing a lesion as a "skin" mass, it would be more helpful to describe it more completely, for example, "solitary 1 × 1 cm, round, raised, red, hairless mass confined to skin, duration 3 weeks on left pinna, in a 2-year-old Cocker spaniel dog." A clinical pathologist is likely to interpret the cytologic findings for this case differently from those made in a 10-year-old dog with multiple similar-appearing lesions that had been present for several months with progressive growth.

COLLECTION TECHNIQUES

Multiple methods are used for collecting samples for cytologic evaluation. These include needle aspiration, skin swabs, scrapings, and impression smears. Each method has advantages and disadvantages. For mass lesions, the most useful technique is needle aspiration as this allows sampling from a variety of areas in the lesion, including cells found in deeper tissues that are not accessible by other cytologic methods. Many lesions in skin and subcutaneous tissues are highly exfoliative when aspirated, and often a good cell yield is available for interpretation. Fine-needle sampling may be done by aspiration or nonaspiration techniques, depending on the expected degree of exfoliation and the likelihood of blood contamination. If a syringe is used to create negative pressure while the needle is embedded in the lesion of interest, then care must be taken to make sure the pressure is released prior to removing the needle from the mass, as otherwise, the cells may easily be lost into the syringe, or surrounding normal fatty tissue may contaminate the sample. Material collected from solid masses should be carefully expelled onto a slide. A second slide or cover slip should be used to gently spread the material on the first slide into a thin layer. The sample should be allowed to air-dry before being stained with a Romanowsky-type stain. If the lesion is fluid filled, preparation of both direct and sediment smears of the fluid may be useful, but typically, a complete fluid analysis (i.e., protein

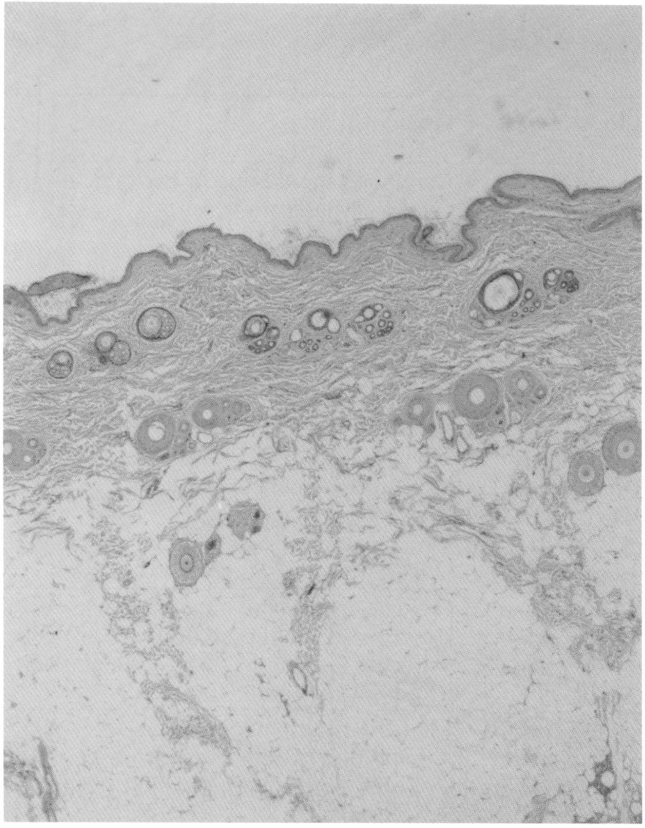

Figure 5-1 Biopsy sample from normal skin. Skin is divided into three general areas: epidermis, dermis, and hypodermis. Adnexal structures found in skin include sebaceous glands, sweat glands, and hair follicles. The dermis contains the adnexal structures as well as smooth muscle, blood vessels, lymphatic vessels, collagen, and elastic fibers. This histologic section shows adnexal structures in cross-section rather than longitudinally, which is related to tissue processing. The hypodermis (or subcutis) contains adipose tissue and collagen bundles. Histologic diagnoses incorporate specifically what areas of the skin are being affected by inflammatory, degenerative, or neoplastic processes. This is not possible with cytologic methods. (H&E, 2× objective.)

concentration, cell count, differential in addition to cytology) is not necessary for evaluation, and cytology alone generally will indicate whether an inflammatory, noninflammatory, or neoplastic process is present. If a solid mass is associated with a fluid-filled lesion, then the solid areas as well as the fluid areas of the mass should be sampled.

If the lesion is not amenable to aspiration (e.g., superficial, fistulous), then other sampling techniques such as scrapings, impression smears, or swabs should be considered. Scrapings are collected by rubbing the edge of a scalpel or spatula across the lesion and then spreading the accumulated material onto a slide. Impression smears are made by pressing the surface of a slide against the lesion with several imprints made on separate areas of the slides. If excess fluid or blood is on the surface of the lesion, then the lesion should be blotted dry before sampling. Swab samples are most commonly collected from a mucosal surface such as the vaginal cavity. Using a sterile cotton swab, material is collected from the site of interest. After sample collection, the swab is gently rolled (not rubbed) along the surface of a slide.

Samples collected by these latter methods may only demonstrate surface abnormalities and not underlying pathology. If a lesion is ulcerated, a swab or impression smear likely will reveal neutrophils, blood, protein, and debris, as well as possibly some microorganisms, but these are all nonspecific findings that should be expected from an ulcerated surface. Nevertheless, with superficial or exudative lesions, these types of samples may be useful for demonstrating microorganisms, including mites, bacteria, yeast, and fungal and protozoal organisms.

GROSS APPEARANCE

Knowledge of the gross appearance of skin and subcutaneous masses is helpful in interpreting cytologic findings. Descriptions of gross appearance should include location, distribution, size, shape, color, haired versus nonhaired, sessile versus pedunculated, intact epithelium versus ulceration, mobility, and firmness, as well as duration and growth characteristics, when known. The gross appearance of the mass often aids in limiting the types of lesions that need to be considered cytologically.

GENERAL CYTOLOGIC EVALUATION

The approach to cytologic evaluation of skin and subcutaneous lesions is similar to other tissues. Multiple slides should be prepared for review by using standard smear preparation techniques. For the most part, cytology smears need only be stained with a Romanowsky-type stain (Wright, Wright-Giemsa, and quick stains such as Diff-Quik). In some instances, additional stains may be desirable, particularly if it is thought that rare or difficult-to-see microorganisms may be present, in which case, other stains such as acid-fast stains for *Mycobacterium* or *Nocardia* and Gomori methenamine silver (GMS) or periodic-acid-Schiff (PAS) stains for fungal organisms may help find these organisms. For this reason, it may be useful to leave some slides unstained in case additional staining is needed. It is possible, however, to destain slides, then restain them with a variety of different special stains and achieve adequate staining quality for interpretation.[2]

Slides should first be reviewed at low power (4 to 10× objective) to assess the adequacy of the smear. Degree of cellularity, adequate separation of cells, thickness of smear, and good staining quality are some of the factors that should be evaluated. The entire smear area should be reviewed on low power to review for the presence of any large structures such as infrequent cell clusters or large fungal organisms (e.g., *Coccidioides spherules*) that could be missed with a higher-power lens. The low-power scan should also help identify areas where the cytologist would want to go to a higher-power review. Most cytologic abnormalities may be seen with a good 50× oil immersion objective lens. This lens is preferable to a 40× high-dry lens, although this latter lens is an

TABLE 5-1

CYTOLOGIC FINDINGS AND FOLLOW-UP STEPS

Primary Finding	Cell Types/ Additional Findings	Other Findings/Conclusions	Follow-Up Steps
Low-nucleate cellularity	Acellular	Lipid droplets before staining; lipid may wash off slide during staining; possible lipoma	Continued monitoring or excision, as clinically indicated
		No lipid droplets prior to staining – possible cyst. Epithelial cysts usually benign May be poorly exfoliative fibrous lesion	Diagnosis will require histopathology; however, since cystic and fibrous lesions are often benign, monitoring may be considered
	Blood	Platelets present; no erythrophagia, hemosiderin or hematoidin	Likely blood contamination of poorly exfoliative or vascular lesion; diagnosis likely will require biopsy
		No platelets present; erythrophagia, hemosiderin, hematoidin, or all found	Likely true hemorrhage; rule out coagulopathy or trauma May be vascular tumor, in which case diagnosis will require biopsy
Lysed cells	Only disrupted cells	Lysed cells cannot be cytologically interpreted	Evaluate smear preparation technique Consider reaspiration If necrosis suspected, reaspirate at the edge of lesion rather than center
Inflammatory cells	Neutrophils	Neutrophilic inflammation may occur secondary to bacterial infection as well as noninfectious causes (foreign body, keratin, immune-mediated disease)	May respond to medical therapy If lesion is persistent and nonresponsive, surgical exploration +/– biopsy may be necessary
	Lymphocytes	Lymphocytic inflammation suggests immunologic reactivity Well-differentiated lymphoproliferative disorder should be considered	May spontaneously improve or regress If persistent, then biopsy should be considered
	Eosinophils	Eosinophilic inflammation suggests a hypersensitivity reaction possibly due to arthropod bite or sting Can be seen secondary to chronic infectious agents and some tumors (particularly mast cell tumor)	May spontaneously resolve or regress Some lesions may be corticosteroid responsive but the possibility of fungal or protozoal infection or tumor such as mast cell or lymphoma should be considered
	Mixed	Mixed (pyogranulomatous, granulomatous) inflammation may be caused by chronic infectious agents but also can be secondary to foreign bodies, keratinizing cysts, immune-mediated disease	If an etiologic agent cannot be identified, surgical exploration and biopsy (for both histopathology and culture) may be necessary
Tissue cells	Minimal pleomorphism	Uniform cells, minimal pleomorphism, low mitotic rate suggest hyperplastic or benign lesion	Lack of malignant criteria does not completely exclude the possibility of malignancy, but monitoring for progression and invasiveness should be considered Mass excision should be considered, as appropriate
	Marked pleomorphism	Marked anisocytosis and anisokaryosis, open chromatin, prominent nucleoli, numerous mitotic figures, nuclear molding are features of malignancy	If large numbers of pleomorphic cells are present, malignancy should be suspected Evaluation for metastatic disease (staging) should be considered prior to any surgical approach

TABLE 5-1—cont'd

CYTOLOGIC FINDINGS AND FOLLOW-UP STEPS

Primary Finding	Cell Types/ Additional Findings	Other Findings/Conclusions	Follow-Up Steps
Mixed inflammatory and tissue cells	Both inflammatory cells and tissue cells are prominent	Inflammation may often cause changes in epithelial and mesenchymal cells that resemble neoplastic cells Alternatively, some tumors may cause inflammatory reactions (e.g. squamous cell carcinoma)	When prominent inflammation exists, it is difficult to ascertain the significance of tissue cells based on cytomorphology alone Surgical exploration and biopsy should be considered for further evaluation

adequate alternative. The 100× oil lens is needed only to confirm small structures such as bacteria, intercellular granules or inclusions, and small fungal spores or protozoa.

Once the adequacy of the smear has been assessed, a determination may then be made about the pathologic process. On initial review, a definitive diagnosis may be made based purely on the cells, any organisms present, or both. Many times, however, a clear-cut definitive answer is not based on cytology findings alone. In these cases, a systematic approach should be taken to narrow down differentials and, just as importantly, make a decision about what the next diagnostic or therapeutic step needs to be (see Table 5-1). A consistent approach includes a thorough review of all areas of the sample and then systematically classifying the type of pathologic process and likely etiologies. In general, if a mass lesion is aspirated and only tissue cells are collected, then the lesion is caused by either hyperplasia or neoplasia. If only inflammatory cells are present, then the underlying cause may be infectious or noninfectious, keeping in mind that some tumors may elicit an inflammatory response. Mixtures of inflammatory and tissue cells may be difficult to interpret for this reason, in addition to the fact that inflammation may induce morphologic changes in tissue cells.

INFLAMMATORY CELLS

Sampling from inflammatory lesions tends to yield large numbers of cells often with no obvious tissue cells. Inflammatory lesions may result from infectious and noninfectious causes. Noninfectious inflammatory diseases may ultimately require histopathology to further investigate underlying causes such as immune-mediated skin disease. The types of inflammatory cells that are present, however, may aid in determining the underlying process.

Samples with primarily neutrophils are often referred to as displaying neutrophilic, suppurative, or purulent inflammation (Figure 5-2). The neutrophils should be characterized as "well preserved" or "showing some signs of degeneration." Degenerative changes in neutrophils include nuclear swelling with paler staining chromatin (karyolysis). Severely degenerate neutrophils may have round

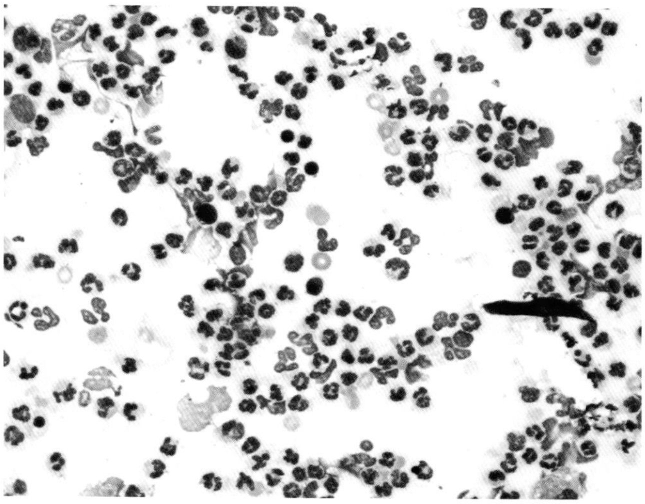

Figure 5-2 Neutrophilic inflammation is characterized by the predominance of neutrophils. (Wright stain.)

nuclei, and the cell type may be virtually unrecognizable. Degenerative changes are not pathognomonic for infection but should raise the clinical suspicion of infection. Neutrophilic inflammation is often caused by bacterial infection but may also be seen with fungal or yeast infection as well as noninfectious problems.

Samples with mostly small lymphocytes are characterized as lymphocytic inflammation, reactivity, or both. Increased numbers of mature lymphocytes suggest immunologic reactivity or chronic inflammation. This pattern is often seen with vaccine reactions or arthropod bites or stings. Sometimes, increased numbers of eosinophils are also noted. When lymphocytic infiltrates are more chronic, then a chronic lymphoproliferative disorder needs to be considered, but a biopsy of these infiltrates will be required for diagnosis.

Eosinophilic inflammation (Figure 5-3) in skin has similar considerations as in other tissues. In skin, it is often related to a hypersensitivity response to the bite or sting of an arthropod (e.g., flea, bee, spider, or tick). Other parasites, including mites and nematodes, may also cause eosinophilic inflammation. It is sometimes noted as a component of inflammation secondary to

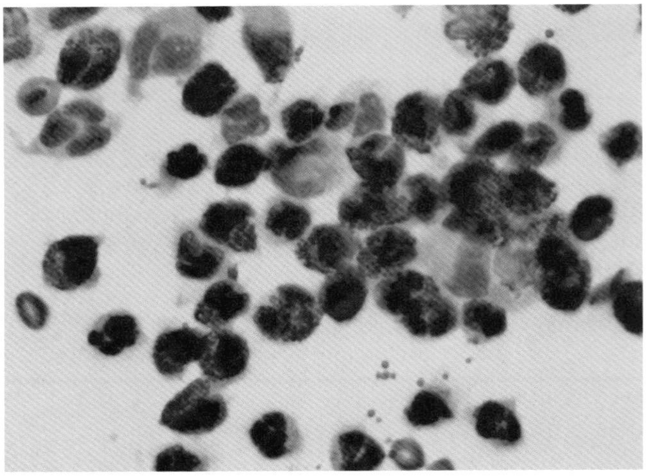

Figure 5-3 Fine-needle aspirate from subcutaneous swelling in a dog. Mixed inflammatory cells are present, however, the majority are eosinophils. Fewer macrophages and neutrophils are also noted. (Wright-Giemsa, 100× objective.)

infection, possibly more commonly with fungal infection, and may also be seen as a component of some vaccine reactions. Solid masses or linear plaques with large numbers of eosinophils may be an eosinophilic granuloma, but care must be taken to rule out infectious agents or neoplasia, as an eosinophilic infiltrate may also be seen as a paraneoplastic response to some tumors, most notably mast cell neoplasia as well as others such as lymphoma.

Granulomatous inflammation and *pyogranulomatous inflammation* are terms that should be reserved for histopathologic diagnosis, as these are associated with a specific type of inflammatory cell arrangement in tissues. Nevertheless, these terms are used by some cytologists as well. Others will use *chronic inflammation, macrophagic inflammation*, or *mixed cell inflammation*. These terms imply that macrophages are present, with some mixture of lymphocytes and possibly other cells, including sheets of epithelioid macrophages and multinucleate cells (Figure 5-4). This type of inflammation typically is associated with chronic inflammatory disorders, and these often involve chronic infectious agents such as higher bacteria (*Actinomyces, Nocardia, Mycobacterium*

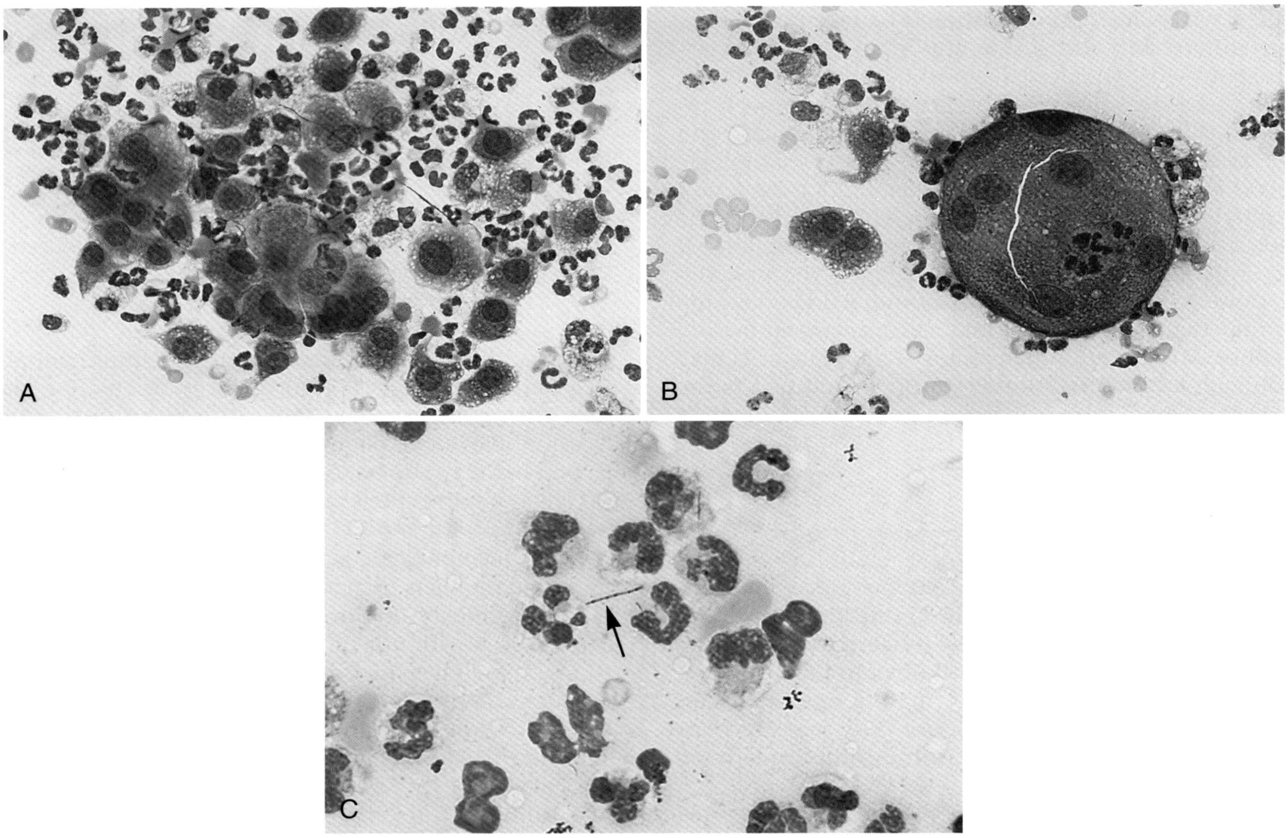

Figure 5-4 Impression smears of a pyogranulomatous nodule in a dog. A, Pyogranulomatous inflammation includes a mixture of neutrophils and macrophages with the macrophages often noted in sheets. (Diff-Quik, original magnification 160×.) **B,** Multinucleate inflammatory giant cell with scattered neutrophils and macrophages from the same lesion shown in *A*. (Diff-Quik, original magnification 132×). **C,** Long, slender, filamentous bacterial rod (*arrow*) present among inflammatory cells. (Diff-Quik, original magnification 400×).

spp.), fungal or protozoal organisms, or noninfectious agents such as foreign bodies. If nothing else, this type of inflammation indicates the lesion may be unresponsive to routine antibiotic therapy alone.

INFECTIOUS AGENTS

Many types of infectious agents, including mites, fungi, protozoa, and bacteria, may be seen with cutaneous and subcutaneous lesions. All of these organisms may be seen either through Romanowsky staining or as a nonstaining outline. Nonstaining organisms sometimes may be highlighted with other stains.

Bacteria

Superficial or deep pyoderma and bacterial abscesses: bacterial infection of the skin may present as surface or superficial disease or deep pyoderma. Infection may be caused by primary skin disease but may also occur secondary to bite or puncture wounds. In addition, cystic lesions and tumors may become secondarily infected, particularly if ulcerated. When stained with Romanowsky-type stain, most bacteria will stain blue to purple, similar to chromatin. Bacterial organisms tend to be uniform in size and shape, which is helpful in distinguishing them from particulate debris, which tends to be irregular. Further characterization of bacterial organisms may be done with a Gram stain, but definitive identification requires culture. Both aerobic and anaerobic culture should be considered for subcutaneous infections.

Surface or superficial pyoderma presents with skin surface abnormalities, including pustules, papules, crusts, and erythema. Bacteria may be identified with impression smears or scrapings, but these techniques potentially could miss other underlying disease. Deeper pyoderma results from infection extending deeper into follicular tissue, resulting in nodules and abscesses. The most common bacterial pathogen for superficial and deep pyoderma is *Staphylococcus intermedius* (Figure 5-5, *A*); however, other secondary invaders may also exist, and in chronic cases, bacterial culture and sensitivity may be advisable.[3] Bacterial infection may also occur as a consequence of a bite or other penetrating wound. These often result in a mixed infection with both aerobic and anaerobic organisms (see Figure 5-5, *B*).

Mycobacterium *Spp:* Mycobacterial infection manifests in several different forms, including slow-growing tuberculous; lepromatous, cutaneous nodular; slow-growing, nontuberculous, cutaneous; and fast-growing, cutaneous and subcutaneous. All of these forms may result in cutaneous lesions. Disseminated infection may also occur particularly with tuberculous disease. Cutaneous lesions include draining nodules, ulceration, and nodules.[3] Definitive identification of organisms requires specialized culture for both rapid growers and slow growers. In some cases, polymerase chain reaction (PCR) testing of tissue samples may be helpful.

In cytologic samples, *Mycobacterium* spp. on rare occasions may be seen as filamentous organisms but are more commonly found as short rods. Mycobacterial organisms do not stain with Romanowsky stains because of their thick lipid walls. They still may be readily identifiable on Romanowsky-stained slides as nonstaining short rods, often noted in macrophages (Figure 5-6). These organisms will stain positive with an acid-fast stain.

Actinomyces *Spp. and* Nocardia *Spp:* These organisms are often associated with chronic draining or nodular lesions. Infection is typically secondary to a bite wound or penetrating foreign body. These filamentous bacteria are often branching and may be found in thick mats on

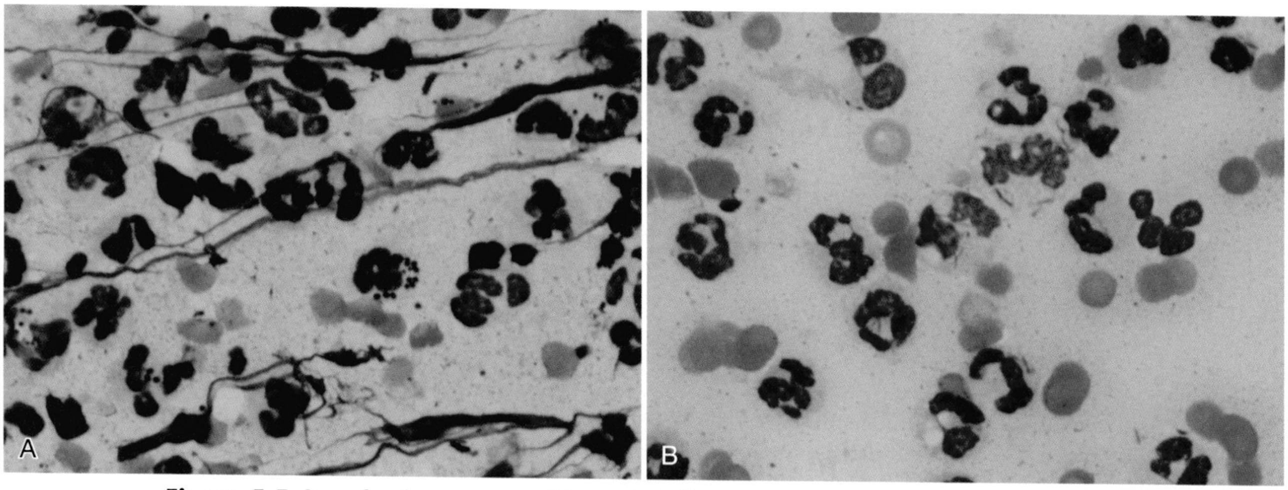

Figure 5-5 Samples from areas with septic inflammation. A, Most cells are degenerating neutrophils. Some contain phagocytized bacterial cocci. Streaming nuclear material is also present in addition to scattered erythrocytes. (Wright-Giemsa stain, 100× objective.) **B,** This sample also contains many degenerating neutrophils as well as erythrocytes. Many of the neutrophils contain thin rods in the cytoplasm. Some bacteria appear to be free in the background. The organisms suggest the infection is secondary to a bite wound, foreign body, or other penetrating wound. (Wright-Giemsa, 100× objective.)

smear preparations. *Actinomyces* and *Nocardia* spp. sometimes stain poorly with Romanowsky stains and may only be noted as a faint outline, often best visualized in the cytoplasm of epithelioid macrophages (Figure 5-7, *A*). When stained, they are light blue in color with an intermittent pink beading appearance. *Nocardia* spp. also may be partially acid-fast positive, which may help distinguish them from *Actinomyces* spp. (see Figure 5-7, *B*). Culture is required to definitively identify these organisms.

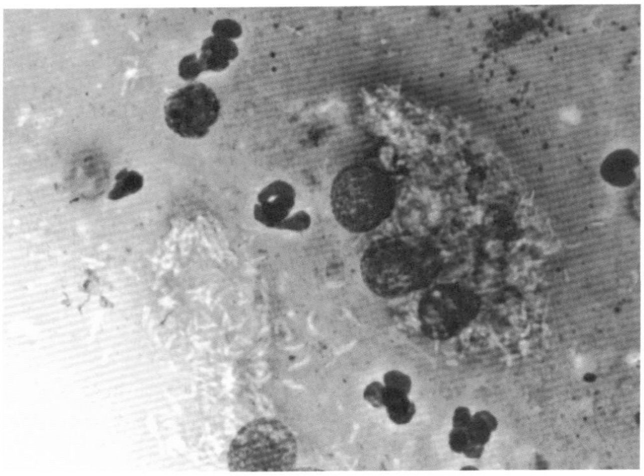

Figure 5-6 Aspirate from a canine leproid granuloma. Large numbers of nonstaining short bacterial rods (mycobacteria) are seen within a multinucleate cell. Numerous rods are also free in the background, as well as scattered neutrophils and free nuclear material. The nonstaining rods must be distinguished from artifact or other debris and can be confirmed as bacterial organisms with an acid-fast stain (*not shown*). (Wright-Giemsa, 100× objective.)

Yeast, Fungi, and Algae

Malassezia pachydermatitis: Overgrowth of these organisms typically occurs on the skin surface and usually is not associated with a significant exudative process. These yeast are small (3-8 micrometers [μm] diameter) and typically shaped like a "footprint" (Figure 5-8). They are considered normal flora of skin, so just finding a few does not necessarily indicate abnormality. Greater than two organisms per 100× field has been suggested as indicative of overgrowth.[3] It is not unusual to find large numbers of organisms as well as large numbers of anucleate squames but minimal to no evidence for inflammation. Overgrowth of these organisms is usually thought to be secondary to other diseases such as skin allergies, seborrhea, bacterial pyoderma, and skin conformation problems or secondary to antibiotic use.

Dermatophytes: Dermatophyte infections may manifest in varying ways. In dogs, infection typically manifests as expanding annular areas of alopecia, scales, and crusts. Infection may be localized but may also occasionally be seen with extensive skin involvement. On occasion, infection may result in a solid, raised, nodular lesion, referred to as a *kerion*. In cats, infection usually causes one or more areas of annular to irregular alopecia with or without scales. Skin impressions or scrapings from the edge of annular lesions typically will demonstrate cellular debris and mixed inflammation, including neutrophils, macrophages, lymphocytes, and eosinophils. Accumulations of hair follicle structures and, particularly around these areas, small fungal spores may be found, sometimes in dense aggregates (Figure 5-9). On rare occasions, septate hyphae may be found. Similar findings may be noted with aspiration of kerion lesions. The causative agents for dermatophytosis are most commonly *Microsporum canis*, *M. gyseum*, and

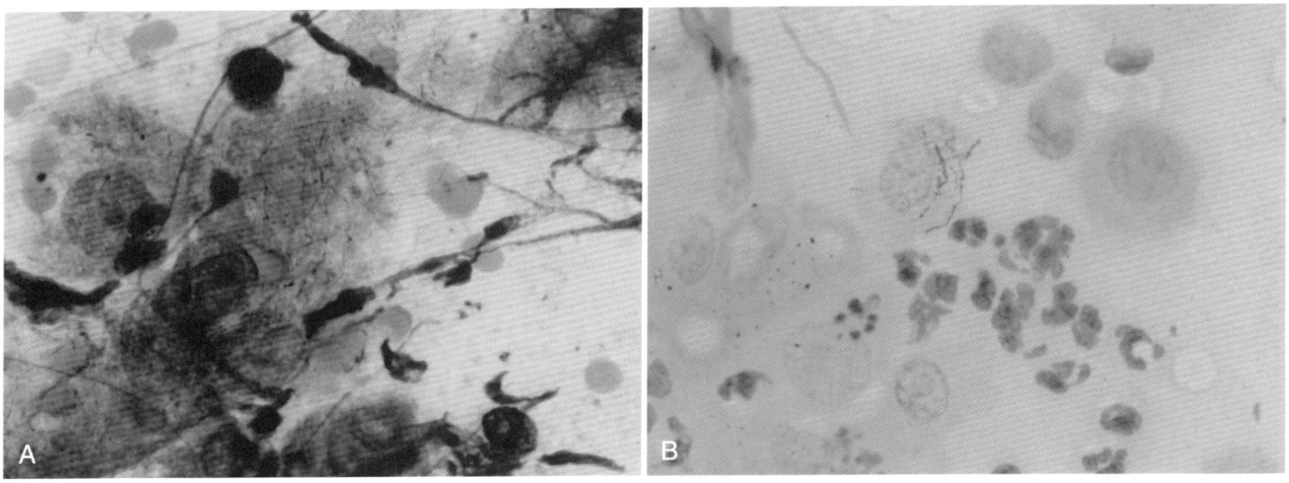

Figure 5-7 Fine-needle aspirate from a draining nodule in a cat. A, Large epithelioid macrophages or spindle cells mixed with degenerating cells and nuclear debris. Thin, beaded, branching bacterial rods are present and particularly evident in the cytoplasm of the central cell. (Wright-Giemsa, 100× objective.) **B,** Slide stained with acid-fast stain. Note pink staining thin branching organisms in cell cytoplasm supporting the diagnosis of *Nocardia* spp. infection. Mycobacterial organisms more typically are short rods but, on rare occasions, may be filamentous, and definitive identification as *Nocardia* requires culture. *Actinomyces* spp. may appear morphologically similar as in *A* but do not stain with acid-fast stain. (100× objective).

Trichophyton mentagrophytes. Fungal culture is required to definitively identify the organism.

Histoplasma capsulatum: Infection with this organism typically causes systemic disease, and animals may present with a variety of clinical signs, including fever, weight loss, anorexia, coughing, and gastrointestinal signs. Infection may also cause cutaneous lesions that are characterized by papules, nodules, ulcers, and draining tracts. Impression smears from oozing tracts or fine-needle aspirate of nodular lesions reveal mixed inflammation with variable numbers of small (2-4 μm diameter) round yeast, with a thin nonstaining capsule and a basophilic nucleus that often is crescent shaped (Figure 5-10). These organisms may be noted free in the background and may be phagocytized by macrophages as well as neutrophils.

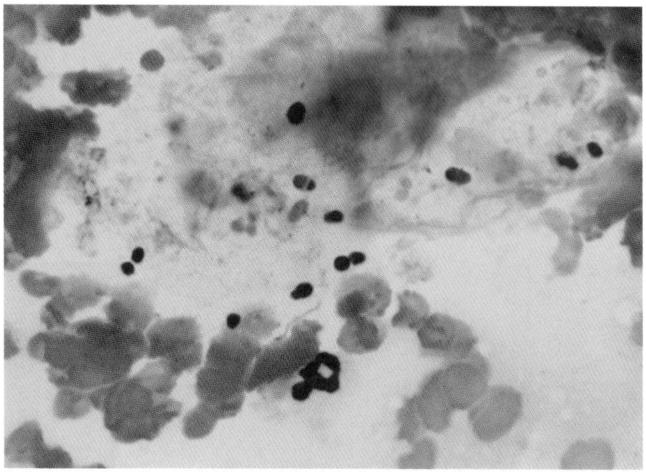

Figure 5-8 Malassezia pachydermatitis from a skin lesion on a dog. Numerous small oval to "footprint" shaped organisms are noted associated with squamous debris. Large numbers of erythrocytes are also present, as well as a single neutrophil in the lower center region. (Wright-Giemsa, 100× objective.)

Sporothrix schenckii: Infection with this agent may cause cutaneous, cutaneolymphatic, or disseminated lesions. In dogs, cutaneous lesions often occur on the head or trunk and typically present as nodules. These may ulcerate with purulent discharge and crusts. In cats, draining tracts are typically noted on distal limbs, head, or tail base. Samples from these sites typically reveal neutrophilic to pyogranulomatous inflammation, with variable numbers of yeast organisms noted in the macrophages, in the neutrophils, and in the background. In particular, cats often will have large numbers of organisms in discharge material, and for this reason, cats with this infection need to be handled with caution to prevent zoonotic spread. The yeast organisms are pleomorphic in shape, varying from round to oval to cigar shape, 2 to 10 μm in length, and 1 to 3 μm wide (Figure 5-11). Although similar in size to *Histoplasma*, *Sporothrix* may be distinguished by its variety of shapes.

Blastomyces dermatitidis: Clinical signs associated with blastomycosis include anorexia, weight loss, cough, ocular disease, lameness, and skin lesions. Skin lesions may be found in up to 40% of cases.[3] These lesions include firm papules, nodules, plaques, ulcers, draining tracts, and abscesses. Material for cytologic evaluation may be collected from draining tracts or aspirated from nodules or abscesses. These samples reveal neutrophilic to pyogranulomatous inflammation with variable numbers of organisms. These are dimorphic fungus, which are typically found in the yeast phase in infected animals, although on rare occasion may form hyphae in tissues.[4] The yeast organisms are variably sized (5-20 μm in diameter), with a thick, blue wall and a thin, nonstaining capsule (Figure 5-12). Occasionally, broad-based budding will be seen, which is useful in distinguishing from *Cryptococcus*. Blastomyces

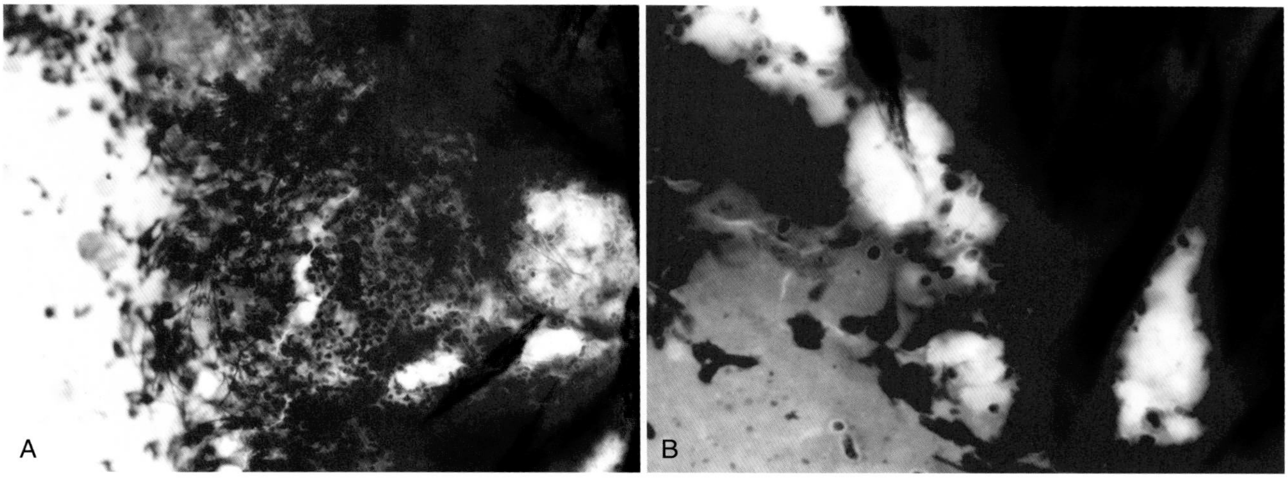

Figure 5-9 Aspirate from a dermatophytic kerion in a dog. A, Large numbers of small round to slightly oval fungal spores are in the center of the figure. The spores have a small nonstaining capsule and are surrounded by a large amount of nuclear material primarily from degenerating neutrophils. Small fragments of hair are noted at the right. (Wright-Giemsa, 50× objective.) **B,** Same lesion with 100× objective. Note the mild variation in spore shape, as well as the diffuse stippled internal appearance. (Wright-Giemsa.)

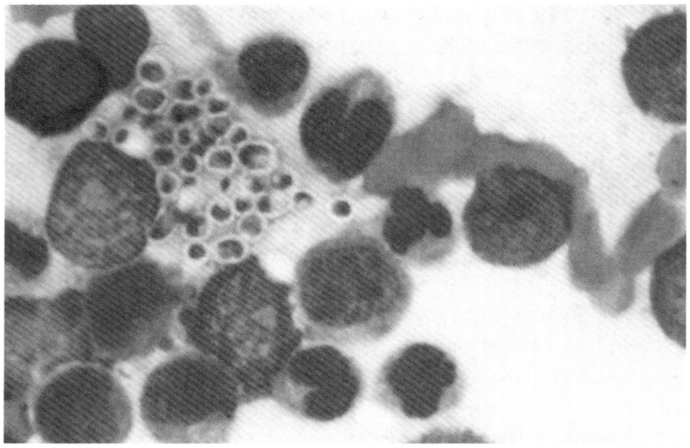

Figure 5-10 A large macrophage containing numerous *Histoplasma capsulatum* organisms is shown. (Wright stain.)

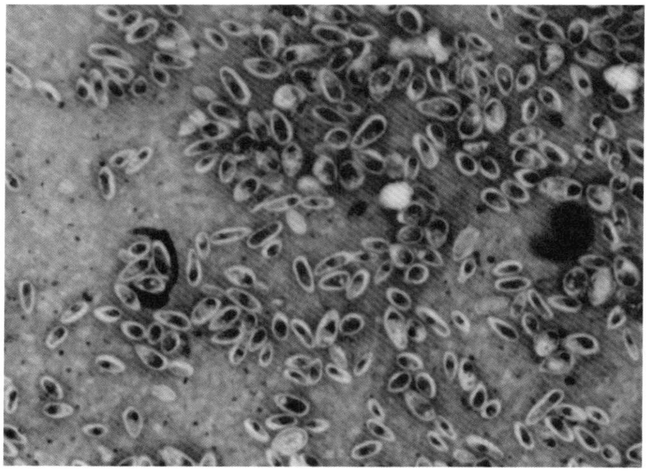

Figure 5-11 Impression smear from a draining lesion in a cat with *Sporothrix schenckii* infection. Large numbers of small pleomorphic yeast are present. The yeast vary from round to cigar shaped with a thin, nonstaining capsule. A small lymphocyte is seen to the right. (Wright-Giemsa, 100× objective.)

are larger than *Histoplasma* and *Sporothrix*, but typically smaller than *Coccidiodes* spherules.

Cryptococcus *Spp:* Cryptococcosis is most commonly associated with nasal signs (sneezing, snuffling, nasal discharge) in cats and central nervous system or ocular signs in dogs. Both species may also have skin lesions, which, however, are more common in cats. The skin lesions may occur as solitary lesions or as part of disseminated disease. Lesions include papules, nodules, ulcers, abscesses, and draining tracts. Sampling from these lesions often reveals large numbers of organisms. These are yeast organisms that are round in shape (occasionally fusiform) and variably sized (2-20 µm in diameter). The organisms stain pale pink to purple and often have a granular appearance. They typically have a large nonstaining capsule, which may be up to 40 µm in diameter (Figure 5-13). Sometimes, only smaller yeast organisms with thinner capsules are found, and thus, the lack of a thick capsule should not be used to

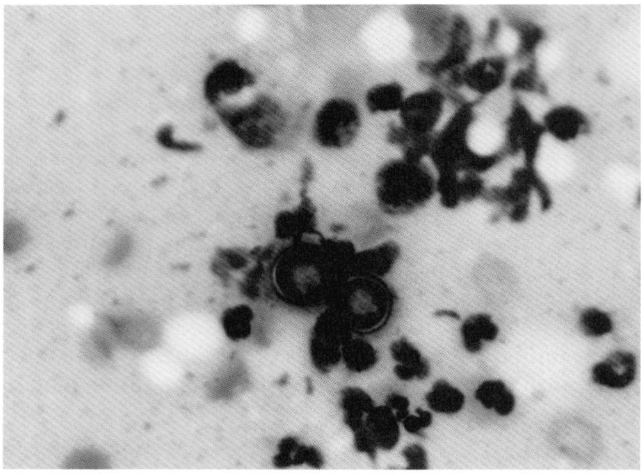

Figure 5-12 Two *Blastomyces dermatitidis* **yeast.** The yeast are adjacent to one another. When budding is present (*not shown*), it is thick and broad based. The organisms tend to be uniform in size, stain deep stippled blue, and have a thin nonstaining capsule. Scattered degenerating neutrophils, lymphocytes, macrophages, and nuclear debris are also present. (Wright-Giemsa, 100× objective.)

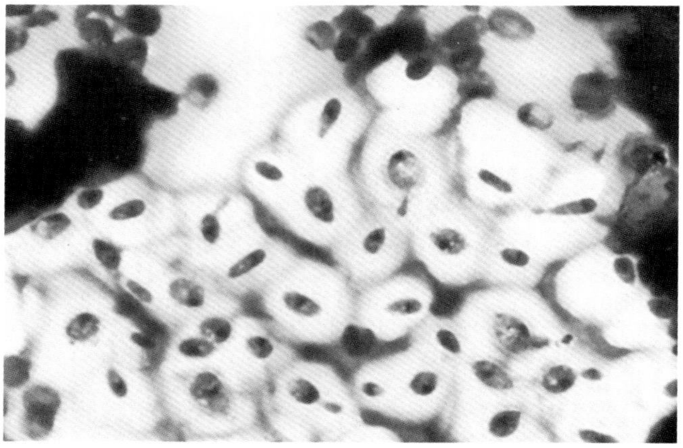

Figure 5-13 *Cryptococcus* spp. are spherical yeast that frequently have a thick, nonstaining mucoid capsule. Organism size may vary, and the thick capsule is not always present. Narrow-based budding is a characteristic feature. This figure has numerous budding and nonbudding organisms with prominent thick capsules. (Wright stain.)

rule out *Cryptococcus* spp. infection. On occasion, narrow-based budding, which is a useful diagnostic feature, may be seen. Minimal associated inflammation may be present, in which case, it is typically granulomatous. The etiologic agent is typically *Cryptococcus neoformans*; however, *Cryptococcus gattii* has emerged as another pathogen occurring in the tropical and subtropical regions of Australia, South America, Southeast Asia, and Africa and also in the North American Pacific Northwest.[5] Morphologic features do not distinguish these two species.

Coccidioides immitis: Infection with this organism usually causes lung disease but may disseminate systemically and cause skin involvement. Skin lesions may occur as subcutaneous nodules or draining tracts. Cytologic preparations

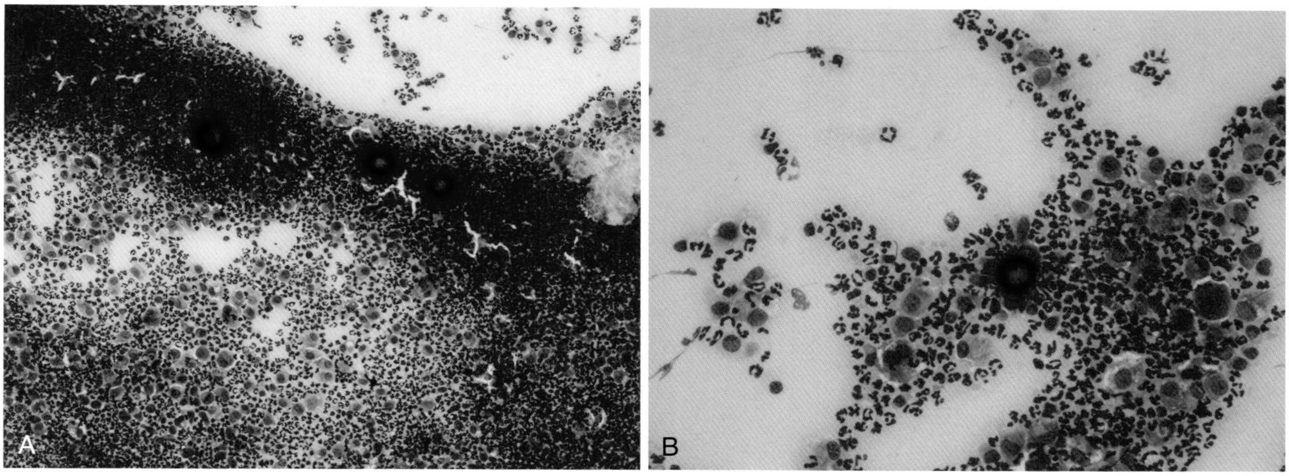

Figure 5-14 *Coccidiodes immitis* **spherules, which are large, spherical structures with a thick wall and stippled blue internal appearance. A,** Low-power magnification from draining cutaneous lesion in a cat. Three large dark-blue spherules are found with marked pyogranulomatous inflammation. The spherules are thick walled and usually keep a three-dimensional shape on cytology smears. Because of this, it is usually not possible to see the spherules sharply in focus in the same plane of focus as the inflammatory cells. Focusing up and down can aid in showing the thick spherule wall as well as the stippled internal appearance. (Wright-Giemsa, 10× objective.) **B,** Same lesion as *A* under higher magnification. (Wright-Giemsa, 20× objective.)

from these lesions typically contain large numbers of inflammatory cells, including neutrophils and macrophages. The organisms are often scarce and not finding an organism does not rule out infection. When present, the organisms are usually found as spherules, which are variable in size but may be large (10-100 μm in diameter) (Figure 5-14). Because of the large size and low numbers of spherules in a sample, these are often easiest to find at low-power (4 to 10×) scans and may be missed if microscopic examination is only done at high power. The spherules have a thick, blue wall with a finely granular internal appearance (endospores). It is often necessary to focus up and down to see the internal detail because of the thickness of the spherules relative to the accompanying cells. On rare occasions, small (2-5 μm) endospores may be seen free in the background or phagocytized by cells. The smaller-sized spherules may be mistaken for *Blastomyces*, but *Coccidiodes* spherules do not show budding.

Opportunistic Fungi: Many different fungal organisms may infect animals and cause either localized or disseminated skin disease as well as systemic disease. The terminology applied to these infections is complex and beyond the scope of what is possible to diagnose via cytology alone. Fungal skin infections typically present with chronic draining lesions or nodules. Animals with these infections frequently are immunocompromised or have a history of immunosuppressive therapy. Cytologic samples from these lesions will typically reveal pyogranulomatous to granulomatous inflammation. Some cases will also have increased numbers of eosinophils. When organisms are present, usually they occur as hyphal segments (Figure 5-15), although on occasion conidial structures may be found. Categories of opportunistic fungal infection include phaeohyphomycosis (pigmented septate hyphae), hyalohyphomycosis (non-pigmented septate hyphae), mycetoma (localized nodular infections) and zygomycosis (broad, poorly septate hyphae). The structure of the hyphae (septate versus nonseptate; pigmented versus nonpigmented; hyphal width) may be helpful in suggesting a particular species of fungus, but as a rule, fungal culture is necessary to definitively identify the organism.

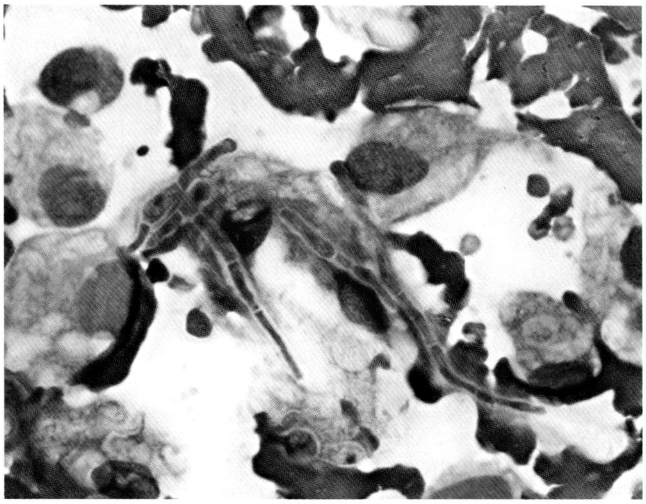

Figure 5-15 Fungal hyphae and granulomatous inflammation are shown. (Wright stain.)

Pythium insidiosum: *Pythium* spp. are not true fungi but are water molds that infect dogs more commonly than cats. Infection results in gastrointestinal signs but may also cause cutaneous lesions. Infection usually is thought to occur from standing in or drinking infected water. Cutaneous lesions often involve the extremities and typically

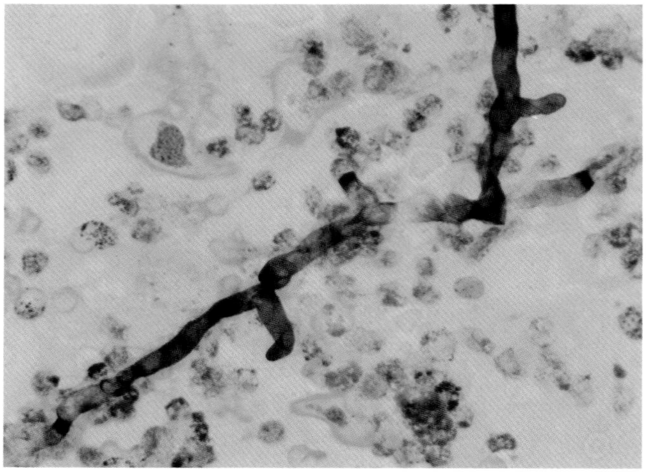

Figure 5-16 Pythium hyphal element. These organisms have poorly septated, branching hyphae with relatively parallel walls ranging in diameter from 2 to 7 micrometers. The hyphae stain poorly or not at all with Romanowsky stain and are easy to miss with routine cytologic staining. If infection is suspected, then Gomori methenamine silver (GMS) staining should be performed. Periodic acid-Schiff (PAS) does not stain this organism. (GMS, 50× objective.)

are ulcerated nodules with draining tracts. Cytologic samples from these lesions reveal pyogranulomatous inflammation, usually with an eosinophilic component. When organisms are present, they are found as poorly staining, broad, poorly septate hyphae ranging from 2 to 7 μm in diameter. The hyphae do not stain well with Romanowsky stains but are easily visualized with GMS stain (Figure 5-16). A related organism that also may cause skin infections, *Lagenidium* sp., has hyphae with broader (diameter ranging from 25 to 40 μm) and more irregular or bulbous hyphae than *Pythium*. Definitive identification of these organisms may require a combination of fungal culture, serology testing, and biopsy with immunohistochemical testing, other molecular diagnostics, or both.[3]

Prototheca Spp

Prototheca spp., which are colorless algae that are ubiquitous in the southern regions of the United States, only rarely cause disease. In dogs, infection is often disseminated, but only cutaneous protothecosis has been reported in cats.[3] Cutaneous protothecosis is caused by *Prototheca wickerhamii* in both dogs and cats, whereas disseminated infections in dogs is almost always caused by *Prototheca zopfii*. Dermatologic lesions include multiple papules and nodules, often over pressure points, or nodules and ulcers involving the mucocutaneous junctions (especially nostrils), scrotum, and footpads. Samples from these lesions reveal pyogranulomatous to granulomatous inflammation, with few to numerous organisms. The organisms are found as spherules or cells (Figure 5-17), which are round to oval and 2 to 30 μm in diameter. The organisms reproduce by endosporulation, and most commonly, two to four (occasionally up to 20) endospores are visible inside the spherule. Most organisms are extracellular, but smaller organisms may be phagocytized by macrophages or neutrophils.

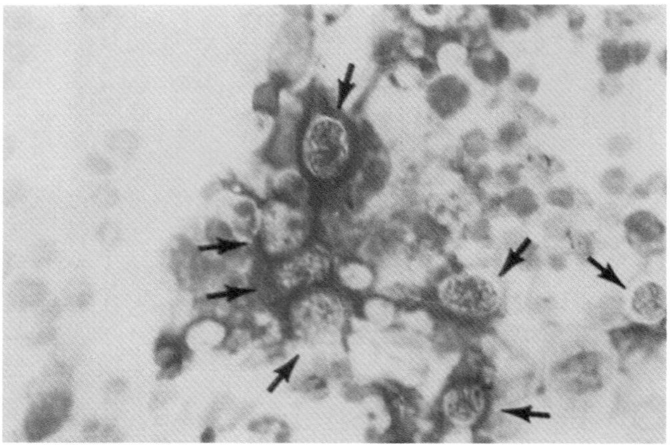

Figure 5-17 Prototheca organisms (*arrows*) are round to oval and have a granular basophilic cytoplasm and a clear cell wall. (Wright stain.)

OTHER INFECTIOUS AGENTS

Leishmania Spp

Leishmaniasis is a disease caused by protozoal infection. It is caused by a variety of *Leishmania* species. *Leishmania* spp. infection is most commonly seen in the Mediterranean region but has also been reported elsewhere, including in the United States. Infection with this organism occurs more commonly in dogs than in cats. Skin lesions occur commonly in animals infected with *Leishmania* spp. This is typically an exfoliative dermatitis which may be generalized. Other dermatologic lesions may also be seen. Other clinical findings include weight loss, muscle wasting, cachexia, intermittent fever, lameness, and lymphadenopathy, among other signs. Diagnosis may be aided by identifying the amastigotes in cytologic samples. Unless nodular skin lesions are present, it may be difficult to find organisms in cytology samples from skin. Often, diagnosis is made by finding organisms in draining lymph nodes or internal organs. Amastigotes are ovoid to round 2.5 to 5 × 1.5 to 2.0 μm in size and may be found in macrophages as well as free in the background (Figure 5-18). They have a small nucleus, with a characteristic small, rod-shaped structure adjacent to the nucleus (kinetoplast). Although unusual, other protozoal organisms may cause cutaneous lesions also.[6] The kinetoplast aids in distinguishing this organism from other protozoal organisms or small yeast such as *Histoplasma* spp.

Parasites

Ectoparasites are a common cause of skin disease in both dogs and cats. Ectoparasites include fleas and mites. The diagnosis is based on history of pruritus, direct observation of the organisms (fleas), or observation via microscopic examination of skin scraping material (mites). The details of mite identification are beyond the scope of a cytology textbook, and readers are referred to any veterinary parasitology text for specifics of mite identification. *Demodex* spp. are sometimes noted in superficial skin samples, including impression smears or superficial scrapings, and it is important to note that on occasion the outline of these organisms may be seen and should not be ignored as just nonstaining debris (Figure 5-19).

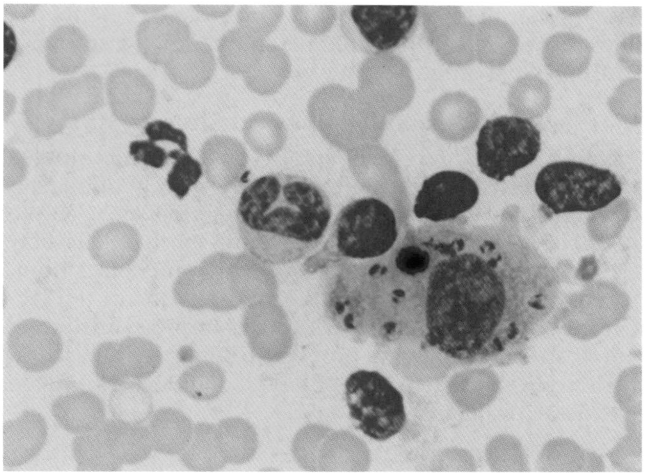

Figure 5-18 Moderate numbers of *Leishmania* spp. organisms within a macrophage. Note the small, bar-shaped kinetoplast next to the organism nucleus. Two lymphocytes, one neutrophil, one monocyte, and several bare nuclei are also present. (Wright-Giemsa, 100× objective.)

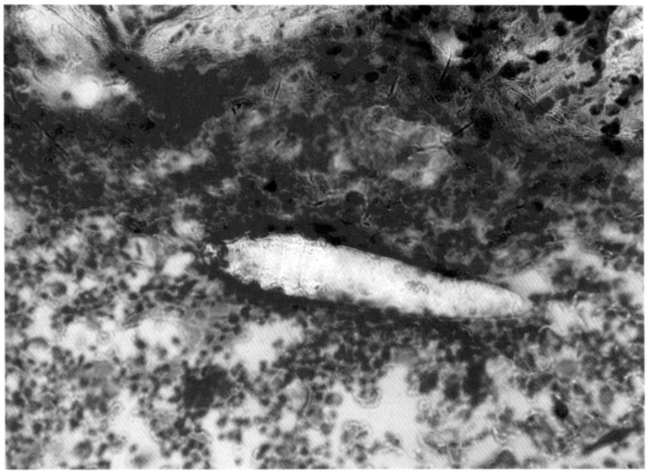

Figure 5-19 Skin scraping from dog with chronic skin disease, including alopecia, crusts, and scaling. An adult *Demodex* spp. mite is in the center of the figure (nonstained). It is surrounded by large numbers of degenerating neutrophils and abundant cellular debris, as well as erythrocytes. The cellular elements are out of focus, as the large mite is not in the same focal plane. (Wright-Giemsa, 20× objective, condenser down.)

In addition to ectoparasites, other types of parasites, including different types of helminths, may also cause skin disease. Types of skin disease caused by helminths include hookworm dermatitis, *Pelodera* spp. dermatitis, *Strongyloides stercoralis*–like infection, cutaneous larval migrans, schistosomiasis, and dracunculiasis, as well as filarial infections (*Dirofilaria immitis, D. repens*). Diagnosis of these conditions is often dependent on history, lesion distribution, environmental exposure, and biopsy, but on occasion, cytologic methods such as skin scraping (*Pelodera* spp. larvae) or fine-needle aspiration (filarial organisms) may yield a diagnosis.[7,8]

NONINFECTIOUS INFLAMMATORY LESIONS

Inflammation in skin may occur for reasons other than infection. Inflammation may occur secondary to foreign bodies, penetrating wounds, arthropod bite or sting, trauma, allergy, immune-mediated disease, and cystic lesions, as well as inflammation secondary to neoplastic lesions related to necrosis or a paraneoplastic effect. Noninfectious inflammatory lesions may be well-encapsulated, discrete subcutaneous lesions that are not responsive to antibiotic therapy or drainage alone. Neutrophilic, pyogranulomatous, eosinophilic, and granulomatous types of lesions are seen. Definitively diagnosing these lesions often is dependent on ruling out other underlying or systemic diseases and surgical exploration to identify a foreign body and to collect tissue for both histopathology and culture purposes.

Noninfectious inflammatory lesions may also present with nonnodular or masslike lesions. These lesions may present as macules, papules, pustules, wheals, scales, crusts, pigmentary abnormalities, plaques, excoriations or ulcerations, fissures, and draining tracts, among others. These nonnodular lesions are the type in which cytologic methods may only offer limited, if any, diagnostic information. In many instances, the distribution of the inflammatory cells in the tissue (e.g., follicular, perifollicular, vascular, epidermis–dermis interface) as well as other findings such as edema, fibrosis, and clefting, are all important findings that help characterize disease processes, all of which are not identifiable by cytologic methods.

Injection Site and Foreign Body Reactions

Inflammatory reactions at the site of injections, most typically vaccinations, are not uncommon. Even with an unclear history of injection, these may be suspected if a nodular lesion develops in an area associated with vaccination or injection (e.g., intrascapular, hindlimb muscles). These may occur within days to several weeks after injection. Aspiration from these lesions typically is moderately cellular, with a thin proteinaceous background. Usually, a mixed inflammatory process, including lymphocytes, macrophages, and variable numbers of eosinophils and neutrophils, is present. Low numbers of moderate- to large-sized spindle cells are also usually present. Most characteristically, aspiration often will reveal abundant pink to purple, globular to amorphous material, which may be noted as being free in the background as well as in macrophages (Figure 5-20). On occasion, the globular-to-amorphous material may be blue in color, rather than pink or purple. In cats, it may be difficult to cytologically distinguish vaccine reactions from vaccine-associated sarcomas; if a mass persists (>3 months) in the area of vaccination, then these should be biopsied for histopathologic evaluation.

Sterile Panniculitis

Panniculitis refers to inflammation of subcutaneous fat, which results in deep cutaneous and subcutaneous nodules that may become cystic and ulcerated. The etiology is multifactorial, and this inflammation may occur in both dogs and cats. It may occur secondary to infectious agents but also from noninfectious processes and thus may be sterile. Noninfectious causes include trauma, foreign body, pancreatic disease, vitamin E deficiency, immune-mediated disorders, adverse drug reactions, and idiopathic disease. Aspirates from these lesions often will have large amounts of nuclear and cellular debris admixed with free lipid and a proteinaceous background. Sometimes, this material is noted in dense aggregates, and it may be difficult to discern intact cells. When inflammatory cells are found, they include variable numbers of neutrophils, macrophages, multinucleate inflammatory cells, and a few small lymphocytes (Figure 5-21). A few spindle cells may also be present. Because of the large amount of cellular debris that is often present, it may be difficult to rule out whether bacteria or other organisms are present, and culture should be considered before therapy with immunosuppressive drugs.

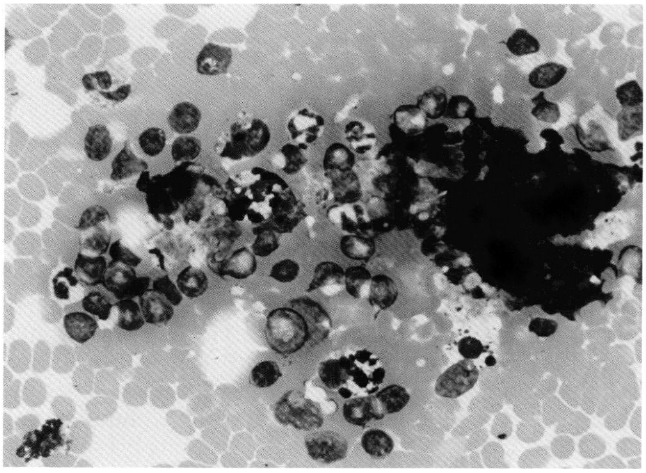

Figure 5-20 Fine-needle aspirate from subcutaneous interscapular swelling in a dog with recent history of vaccination at the site. Mixed inflammatory cells are present including small lymphocytes, macrophages, fewer neutrophils, and rare eosinophils. Aggregates of globular purple material are noted extracellularly as well as irregular globular purple material in macrophages. (Wright-Giemsa, 50× objective.)

Allergic Reactions and Arthropod Bites or Stings

Aspirates from these lesions are typically predominated by eosinophils with lesser numbers of small lymphocytes as well as a few neutrophils and macrophages. A few to moderate numbers of mast cells and spindle cells may also be present. In some cases, in which moderate numbers of mast cells are present, it may be difficult to cytologically distinguish mast cell tumor from an arthropod bite or sting. If moderate numbers of mast cells exist and the lesion is persistent, then biopsy should be considered for further evaluation.

Eosinophilic Granuloma

Eosinophilic granulomas are most common in cats but may also occur in dogs. In cats, these occur in different forms, including indolent ulcer (mucocutaneous and oral mucosal ulcerative lesion), eosinophilic plaque (plaque lesions on ventral abdomen and medial thigh) and eosinophilic granuloma (linear raised lesions on caudal thigh, face, or oral cavity). Diagnosis is typically based on the gross appearance. Samples from these lesions are predominated by eosinophils, but other mixed inflammatory cells as well as a few spindle cells may be present.

Reactive Histiocytosis

This is an uncommon disorder that occurs in dogs and is characterized by proliferation of dermal dendritic cells (histiocytes).[9] Two general forms occur: (1) cutaneous and (2) systemic. Both forms primarily result in cutaneous and subcutaneous lesions. The systemic form also has lesions in other tissues. The lesions are characterized by multiple, nonpruritic, haired to partially alopecic, cutaneous nodules and plaques. These are sometimes noted in linear rows. Aspirates from the nodules contain histiocytes, small

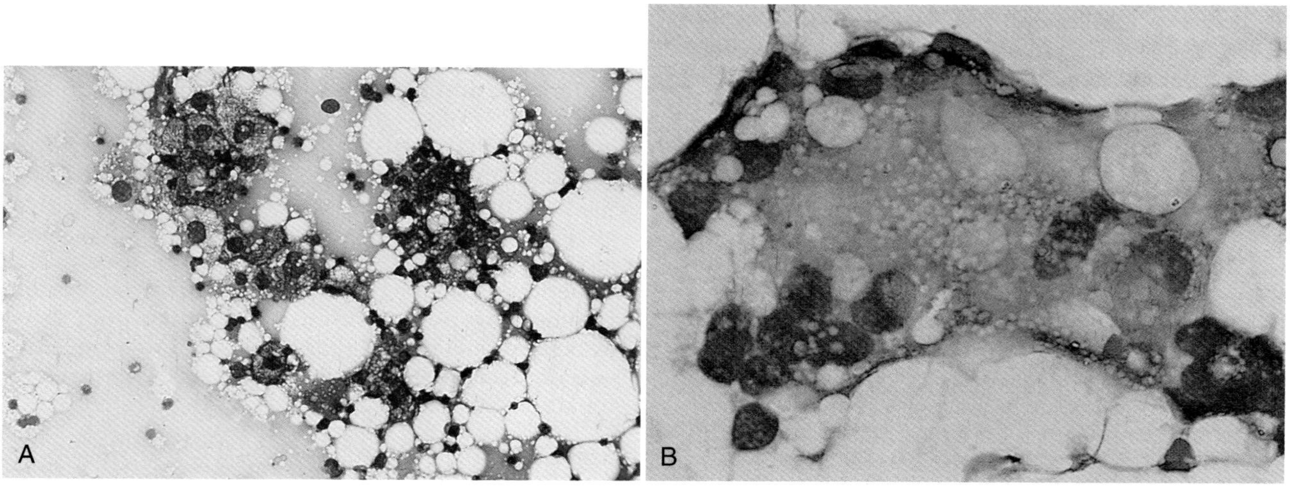

Figure 5-21 Aspirates of a cutaneous nodule from a dog with panniculitis. A, Many macrophages, which have foamy appearances from phagocytizing lipids, are scattered among lipid droplets. (Wright stain, original magnification 100×.) **B,** Higher magnification of epithelioid macrophages or multinucleate inflammatory cells with small to large vacuoles in their cytoplasm. Cell borders are indistinct. (Wright stain, original magnification 250×.) (Courtesy of University of Georgia, College of Veterinary Medicine.)

lymphocytes, and neutrophils. Small lymphocytes may account for up to 50% of the cells and neutrophils may be found in increased numbers secondary to necrosis. Because of the mixture of cells, definitive diagnosis of this disorder based on cytology alone is not possible.

Immune-Mediated Skin Lesions

Many immune-mediated skin disorders occur in dogs and cats. Examples include the pemphigus complex, lupus disorders, and drug reactions. In general, no specific cytologic findings for these disorders are made, and diagnosis is based on signalment, clinical presentation, and histopathology. Acantholytic cells are a diagnostic finding in cases of pemphigus. However, these types of cells may be seen with other causes of inflammation, and these cells are not pathognomonic for pemphigus (Figure 5-22).

NONINFLAMMATORY (TISSUE) LESIONS

The skin is a common site for neoplasia in dogs and cats. Skin tumors account for approximately 30% of all dog neoplasms and about 20% of all cat neoplasms.[7] The three most common skin tumors in dogs include lipoma, benign adenoma, and mast cell tumor, accounting for more than 50% of all skin tumors.[10] When tissue cells are the predominant finding in cytology smears that implies that the lesion is noninflammatory in nature. That, by itself, does not mean the lesion is neoplastic, as hyperplastic lesions may also form nodules or masses. Cells from hyperplastic lesions may appear similar to those from benign tumors. In addition, some benign tumors display some degree of cytologic atypia. Finally, some malignant tumors may have relatively unremarkable cells and the lack of cytologic criteria of malignancy does not always rule out malignancy. Nevertheless, using cytomorphology assessing for cytologic features of malignancy may aid in determining tumor type and further steps necessary for diagnostics and therapy. Cytologic features of malignancy include variable anisocytosis and anisokaryosis, open or stippled chromatin, prominent large or irregular nucleoli, nuclear molding, and mitotic figures. Prominent features of malignancy in numerous cells with no inflammatory cells suggest the lesion is a malignant neoplasm. In many cases, biopsy will be necessary to definitively characterize a lesion as benign or malignant or determine the cell of origin. Some features that would be looked for on biopsy samples (histopathology) that cannot be evaluated by cytologic methods include invasion into the deeper subcutis, irregular tissue borders, growth pattern, and vascular or lymphatic invasion.

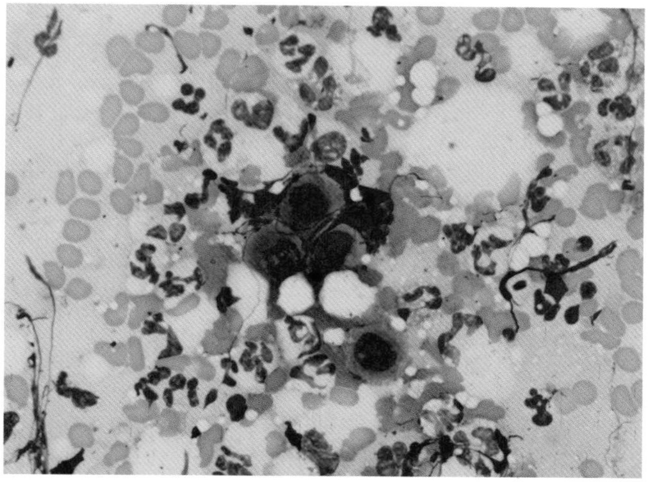

Figure 5-22 Acantholytic cells from a dog with chronic skin disease. Four acantholytic epithelial cells are in the center of the figure. These cells are round with a large round nucleus and dark-blue cytoplasm. They are surrounded by numerous relatively well-preserved neutrophils with rare eosinophils and lymphocytes, as well as nuclear debris. The acantholytic cells should not be confused with neoplastic epithelial cells and can be found in many cases with chronic inflammatory skin disease, not just pemiphigus lesions. (Wright-Giemsa, 50× objective).

When a neoplastic process is suspected on the basis of clinical presentation and the predominance of tissue cells on a cytology sample, typically the next step is to try to characterize the cells as either round cells, epithelial cells, or spindle (mesenchymal) cells. This categorization helps limit the possible differentials. However, some tumors display mixed cytomorphology. In some cases, it may be difficult to even make the limited distinction of round versus epithelial versus spindle cell neoplasia, particularly with anaplastic tumors. It may only be possible to characterize a tumor as round cell, epithelial, or spindle cell tumor and not as any specific tumor type. It is also important to note that the tumors discussed in the following sections are not a comprehensive list of all tumors that may occur in the skin or subcutaneous tissues but only those that have characteristic cytomorphology that aids in diagnosis (Table 5-2).

In general, round cell tumors have discrete noncohesive round cells as a characteristic finding. Epithelial tumors typically have clusters of cohesive cells, although cells may also be noted individually. Cell shape varies from round to cuboidal to stellate or angular. Cytoplasmic borders are often distinct. Finally, spindle cell tumors often have cells found individually, although they are also noted in loose aggregates. The cells will typically have an irregular to wispy or spindloid shape. When found in aggregates, the cells often are enmeshed in a fibrillar background material that is usually extracellular matrix.

Round (Discrete) Cell Tumors

Round cell tumors are sometimes referred to as *discrete cell tumors* because the cells are found individually and not in cohesive clusters. They are typically highly exfoliative, and their characteristic cytologic features often lead to a specific diagnosis. Round cell tumors include mast cell tumors, histiocytoma, histiocytic sarcoma, plasmacytoma, lymphoma, and transmissible venereal tumor. In some cases, epithelial or spindle cell tumors may have individual cells which may appear round.

Lymphoma: Cutaneous lymphoma is divided into two general types: (1) epitheliotropic and (2) nonepitheliotropic. Distinguishing these requires a biopsy sample to assess the tissue distribution of lymphocytes in relation to the epidermis which cannot be done with cytologic samples.

TABLE 5-2

CYTOLOGIC FEATURES OF CUTANEOUS OR SUBCUTANEOUS TUMORS AND DIFFERENTIAL DIAGNOSES

Cell Shape	Characteristic Cytologic Features	Cytologic Interpretation	Differential Diagnoses or Other Comments
Discrete round cells	Pale cytoplasm with no granules or vacuoles; relative uniform nuclear and cell size	Histiocytoma	Lymphoma, amelanotic melanoma, agranular mast cell tumor, plasmacytoma, transmissible venereal tumor (TVT)
	Pale cytoplasm, moderate to marked pleomorphism, variable vacuolization, multinucleated cells	Histiocytic sarcoma	Anaplastic sarcoma, fibrosarcoma, amelanotic melanoma, lymphoma
	Large cells with a high nucleus-to-cytoplasm (N:C) ratio, open chromatin, prominent nucleoli	Lymphoma	Histiocytoma, plasmacytoma
	Blue cytoplasm with pale perinuclear zone and a few binucleate or multinucleate cells.	Plasmacytoma	Histiocytoma, osteosarcoma (rare to occur in skin)
	Fine to coarse purple cytoplasmic granules	Mast cell tumor	Lymphoma of granular lymphocytes (rare in skin), agranular mast cell tumor may resemble histiocytic or other anaplastic tumor
	Pale cytoplasm, small numbers of punctate cytoplasmic vacuoles	TVT	Histiocytoma
Round, stellate, polygonal, columnar cells found individually and in sheets or clusters (epithelial)	Accumulations of sky blue material with angular edges and debris; anucleate squames; cholesterol crystals; +/− cell clusters and inflammation	Follicular cyst or cystic follicular tumor	Numerous epithelial tumors may have cyst formation with keratin debris accumulation
	Densely packed cells with a high N:C ratio; palisades or fronds of cells	Benign basaloid tumors (trichoblastoma, others)	Definitive diagnosis of tumor type requires histopathology
	Angular to polygonal cells; sky blue cytoplasm; N:C asynchrony	Squamous cell carcinoma	Many epithelial tumors may have areas of squamous differentiation.
	Clusters of highly vacuolated, minimally pleomorphic cells	Sebaceous adenoma	Sebaceous epithelial cells should be distinguished from highly vacuolated macrophages
	Pale granular cytoplasm, round to indistinct cell borders, cells found individually and in sheets	Sweat gland tumor	Liposarcoma, spindle cell tumor, plasmacytoma, amelanotic melanoma
	Pink granular cytoplasm with minimal pleomorphism	Perianal gland adenoma	Perianal gland adenocarcinoma
	Sheets of variably pleomorphic cells with pale cytoplasm, indistinct cytoplasmic borders	Apocrine gland tumor of anal sac origin	Neuroendocrine tumor (rare in skin)
Irregular, wispy or spindle-shaped cells found individually, in loose aggregates (spindle cell), or both	Low N:C ratio, clear cytoplasm	Lipoma	Cannot cytologically be distinguished from normal fat
	Variable N:C, pale vacuolated cytoplasm, round to irregular cells, free lipid in background	Liposarcoma	Granulomatous steatitis, sweat gland tumor, plasmacytoma, amelanotic melanoma

TABLE 5-2—cont'd

CYTOLOGIC FEATURES OF CUTANEOUS OR SUBCUTANEOUS TUMORS AND DIFFERENTIAL DIAGNOSES

Cell Shape	Characteristic Cytologic Features	Cytologic Interpretation	Differential Diagnoses or Other Comments
	Elongated cells with wispy to diaphanous cytoplasmic borders	Spindle cell tumor	Reactive fibroplasia
	Round to spindle-shaped, pleomorphic cells, giant multinucleated cells	Anaplastic sarcoma	Granulomatous inflammation, plasmacytoma
	Round to spindle-shaped cells found individually and in sheets, fine to dusty dark (black) pigment	Melanocytic tumors	Some epithelial tumors are pigmented
	Bloody sample with pleomorphic spindle cells found individually and in sheets	Hemangiosarcoma	Hematoma with secondary fibroplasia

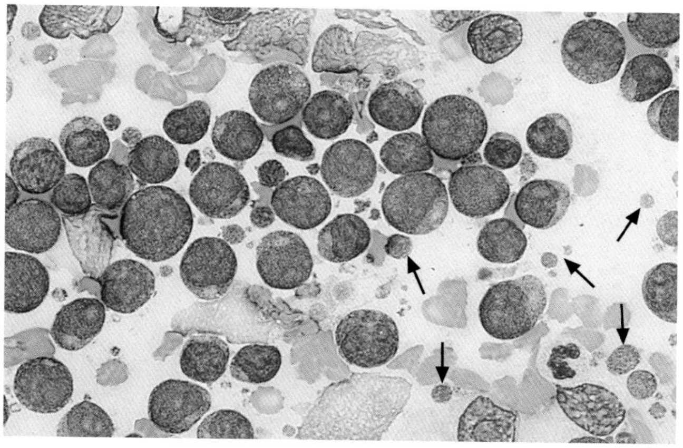

Figure 5-23 Smear consisting primarily of large lymphoblasts from a dog with lymphoma. Scattered lymphoglandular bodies (*arrows*), which are cytoplasmic fragments, are present in the background of the smear. (Wright stain.)

Nonepitheliotropic lymphoma typically presents with nodules, which may be dermal or subcutaneous, may be alopecic, and may be red to purple in color. Usually, evidence exists for systemic involvement with this form of lymphoma. Aspirates from the nodules reveal a monomorphic population of lymphocytes, but the cells may be small to large in size and may have clumped to open chromatin. Aspirates containing a monomorphic population of cells that are large and lymphoblastic in appearance are consistent with an intermediate to high grade lymphoma (Figure 5-23), but those containing only small cells or a mixed cell population need biopsy to rule out the possibility of small cell or mixed cell lymphoma.

Epitheliotropic lymphoma may present variably. These may include generalized pruritus, erythema, and scaling; depigmentation and ulceration; and solitary or multiple cutaneous plaques or nodules. Sampling from these lesions may be difficult if not in the nodular form. The lymphocytes are often described as large or histiocytic in appearance, and associated inflammation may be present (Figure 5-24).

Mast Cell Tumor: Mast cell tumors may be one of the easier types of tumors to diagnose by using cytologic methods. Because mast cell granules typically stain well with Romanowsky-type stains, diagnosing these tumors in some ways is easier by cytology than on hematoxylin and eosin (H&E)–stained biopsy samples (Figure 5-25). The key cytologic feature is variable to large numbers of discrete, fine to coarse, purple cytoplasmic granules in a cell with a round nucleus and abundant pale cytoplasm. Sometimes, the cells are so densely granulated that it may be difficult to discern individual granules. Mast cell tumors occur in the skin of both dogs and cats but also may occur elsewhere, including liver, spleen, and intestine. These tumors have a variable gross appearance but typically are erythematous, alopecic, edematous masses or plaques. Larger tumors may be ulcerated. Aspirates may be hemodiluted and have a variable degree of associated inflammation. Mast cells have moderate-sized round nuclei with a moderate amount of cytoplasm. Nuclear and cytoplasmic details are often obscured by large numbers of small, round, purple granules, which are characteristic of these cells. In some cases, the cells may be poorly granulated, which is thought to be one feature of more poorly differentiated tumors (Figure 5-26 and Figure 5-27). It is important to note that some quick stains used in-clinic may not stain mast cell granules well.

Individual mast cells may be found as part of an inflammatory reaction, so just finding a few mast cells scattered throughout a field of inflammatory cells is of questionable significance. Finding large numbers of mast cells individually but also in aggregates is more diagnostic for neoplasia. These tumors often will have a paraneoplastic infiltrate of eosinophils and may also elicit a stromal reaction with prominent spindle cells and pink fibrillar material between cells. Grading schemes for these tumors require assessment of features that are not all evident with cytology (e.g., subcutaneous infiltration). However, cytomorphologic changes such as poor granulation, anisocytosis or anisokaryosis, and prominent nucleoli suggest a higher-grade tumor.

Histiocytoma: These tumors most commonly occur in dogs under 2 years of age but may also be seen in older dogs.[7]

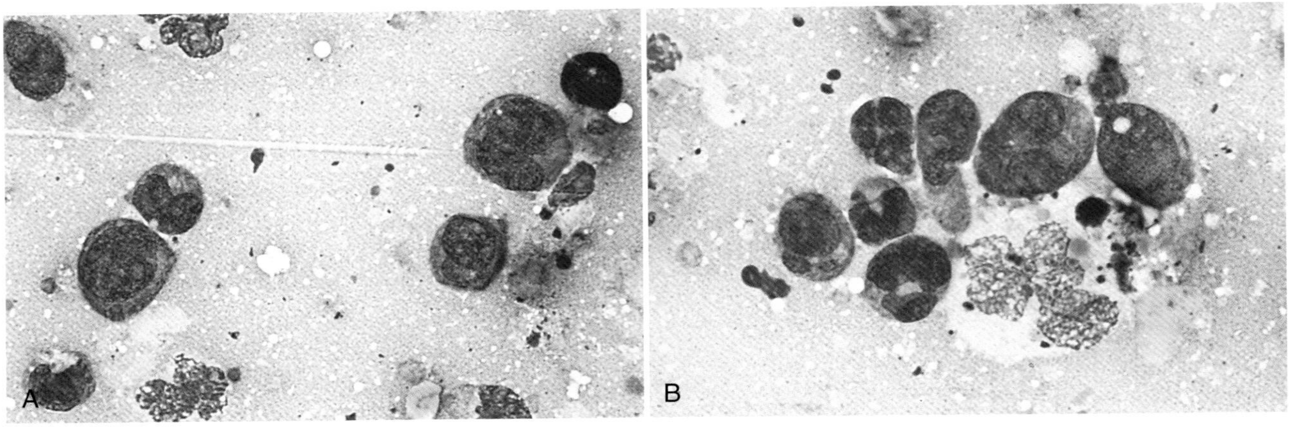

Figure 5-24 Aspirates from a dog with epitheliotropic lymphoma. Cells from this form of lymphoma sometimes have a histiocytic appearance. **A** and **B,** Blasts with irregularly-shaped, monocytoid nuclei and more typical lymphoblasts. (Wright stain, original magnification 250×.)

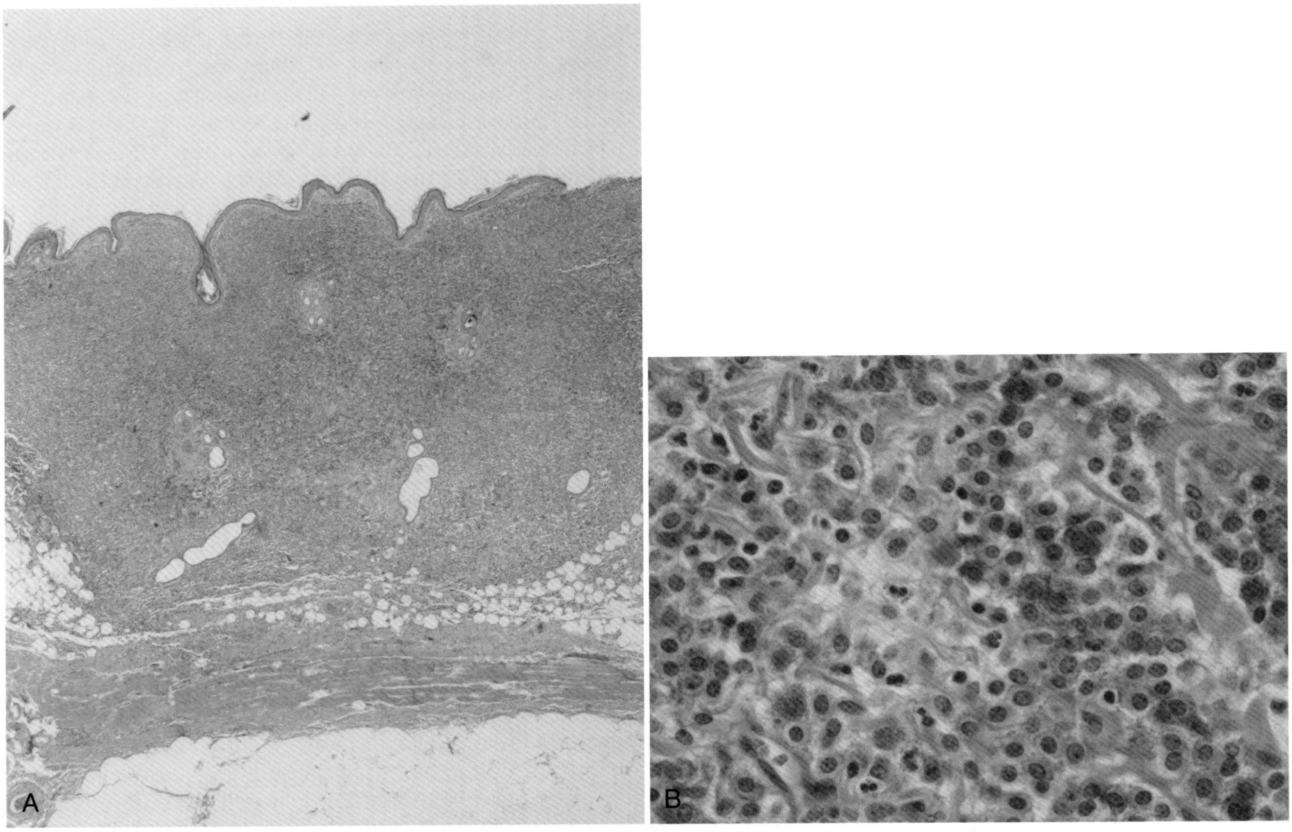

Figure 5-25 Biopsy sample from canine mast cell tumor. A, Low-power view (2× objective) showing intact epithelium with neoplastic round cell infiltrate just under epidermis and extending down into deeper dermis region. (H&E.) **B,** Higher-power view (40× objective) of neoplastic round cells admixed with eosinophils. Note purple granules are not apparent with H&E stain. Additional stains (toluidine blue or Giemsa) must be used to visualize the granules (*not shown*). (Case material provided courtesy of Dr. Shane Stiver, IDEXX laboratories.)

Only rare anecdotal reports of this tumor in cats have been published. The tumors comprise Langerhans cells, which are intraepithelial, dendritic, antigen-presenting cells of skin. These usually occur as solitary tumors, although, on rare occasions, they may be multiple or involve regional lymph nodes. They are typically firm, dome or button-shaped, and dermal in location. They often become ulcerated and may be secondarily infected. The majority of these tumors regress spontaneously, and increased numbers of small lymphocytes may be seen in samples

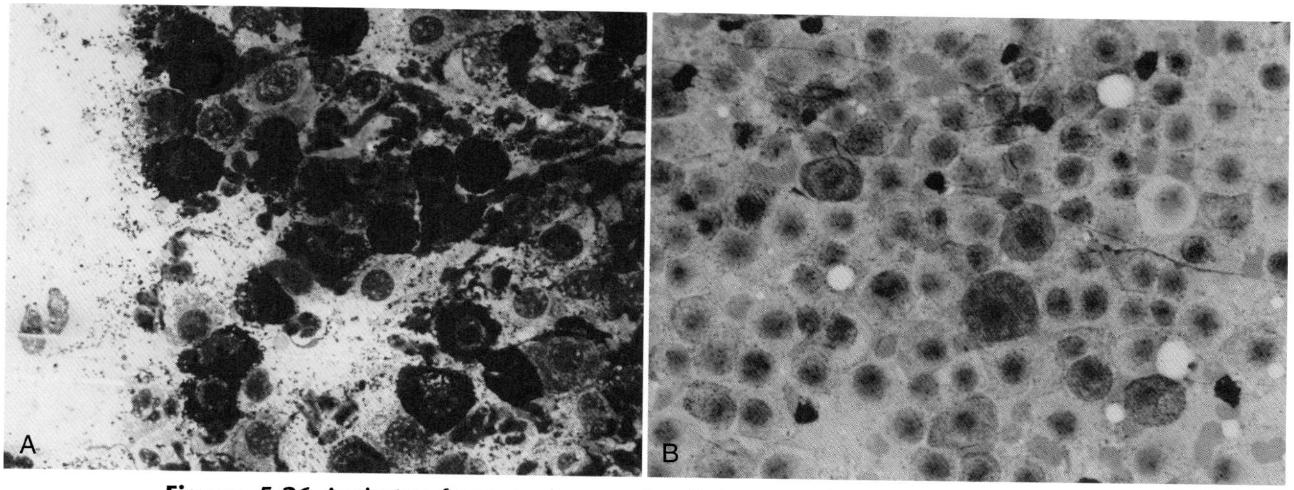

Figure 5-26 Aspirates from canine mast cell tumors. **A,** Large numbers of well-granulated mast cells are present. The large numbers of granules obscure the nuclear detail. Many free granules are also present in addition to neutrophils, eosinophils, and spindle cells. (Wright-Giemsa, 50× objective.) **B,** Large numbers of poorly granulated mast cells are present, suggesting a poorly differentiated mast cell tumor. Nuclear detail is more evident than in *A*. The use of some quick stains may also result in poor granule staining. (Wright-Giemsa, 50× objective.)

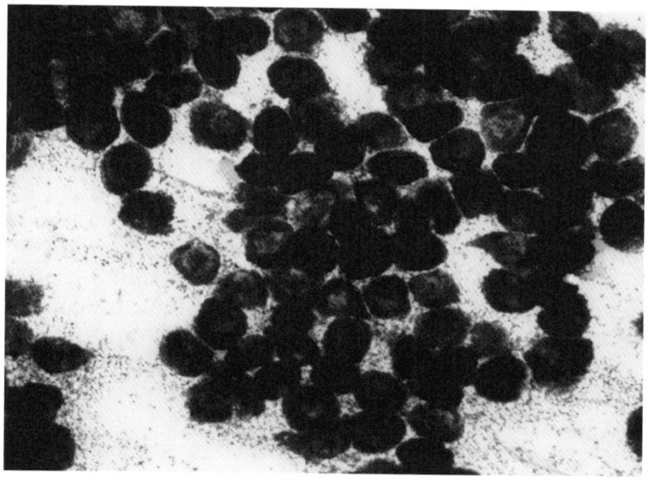

Figure 5-27 Aspirate from feline cutaneous mast cell tumor. Large numbers of well-granulated mast cells often found in dense aggregates. Free mast cell granules are noted in the background. (Wright-Giemsa, 50× objective.)

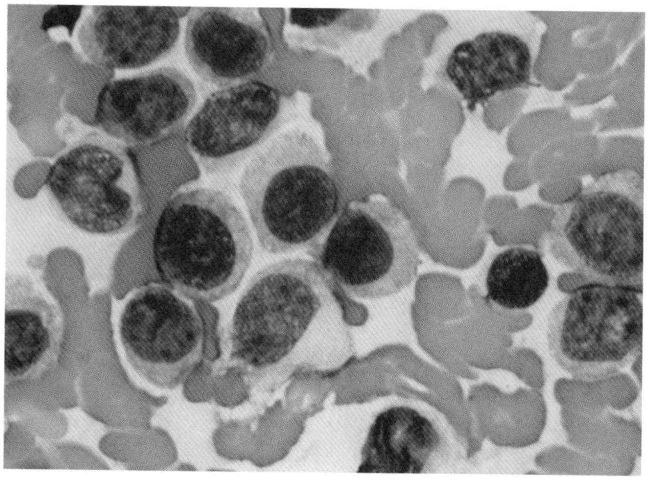

Figure 5-28 Aspirate from a cutaneous histiocytoma. Large discrete round cells are found. They have a large round to slightly indented nucleus with a moderate amount of pale cytoplasm and stippled chromatin. Aspirates from these tumors often will have increased numbers of small lymphocytes as the tumor begins to regress or have neutrophils if the lesion is ulcerated (*not shown*). (Wright-Giemsa, 100× objective.)

from these tumors, presumably related to immunologic reactivity associated with the regression. Aspirates from this tumor typically are moderately to highly cellular. Cells are found individually and have a discrete round shape. The cells may be noted in aggregates, but they are not cohesive. The cells usually have a moderate-sized, round to slightly indented nucleus with finely reticulated to stippled chromatin and a moderate amount of pale, slightly granular cytoplasm (Figure 5-28). It is not unusual to find low numbers of mitotic figures. The background is often proteinaceous in appearance.

Histiocytic Sarcoma (Malignant Histiocytosis): These tumors can occur as localized masses as well as disseminated disease. The disseminated form is also referred to as *malignant histiocytosis*. Histiocytic sarcoma occurs more commonly in the dog than in the cat. Localized histiocytic sarcoma often originates in subcutaneous tissue but can occur as localized disease in internal organs also. The tumors are firm and often large and typically are infiltrative into surrounding tissue. Aspiration from these lesions may be moderately to highly exfoliative. Cells are often noted individually but can also be found in small loose aggregates. The cells are large and round to spindloid in shape (Figure 5-29). They have large round nuclei with abundant pale cytoplasm. The cytoplasm is often vacuolated, and the cells may demonstrate cytophagia. These nominally

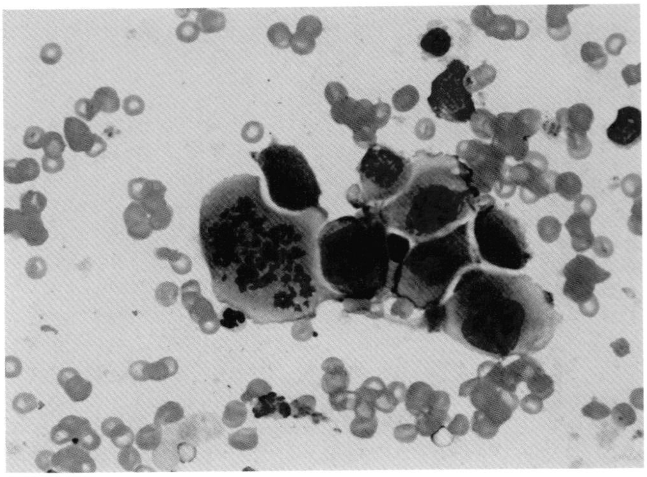

Figure 5-29 Aspirate from dog with histiocytic sarcoma. Neoplastic cells are large (note size relative to red blood cells) with a variable nucleus-to-cytoplasm ratio but generally abundant blue cytoplasm. The cells may or may not be vacuolated, and erythophagia and cytophagia are sometimes found (*not shown*). Mitotic figures (*cell on left*) are usually present and may be aberrant in appearance. The cells cannot be distinguished from other anaplastic tumor types, and definitive identification of histiocytic lineage usually requires immunophenotyping by cytologic or histologic methods. (Wright-Giemsa, 50× objective.)

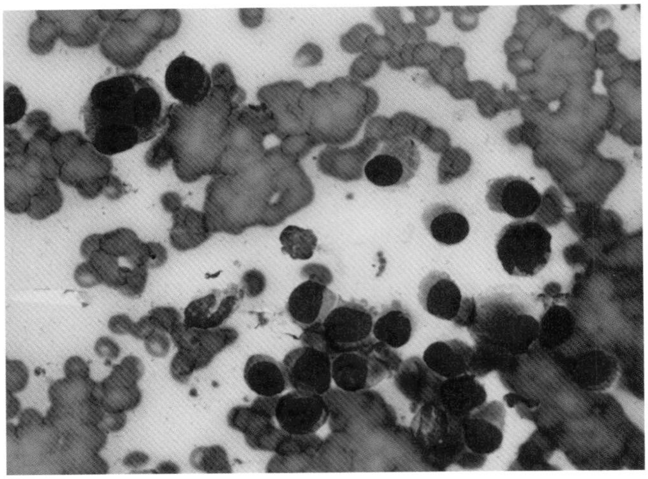

Figure 5-30 Aspirate from cutaneous plasmacytoma in a dog. The cells from plasmacytoma often have a plasmacytoid appearance (eccentric nucleus, pale perinuclear area) but are larger and more pleomorphic than typical plasma cells. Multinucleate cells are a relatively common finding. (Wright-Giemsa, 50× objective.)

resemble macrophages but display more prominent anisocytosis and anisokaryosis. Mitotic figures are usually apparent and multinucleate cells can sometimes be seen.

Feline Progressive Dendritic Cell Histiocytosis: This is thought to be a rare disorder in cats, as only a few cases have been reported. Cats with this disorder typically present with a solitary skin nodule on the head, neck, or extremities. Over time, multiple nodules develop that may be limited to one extremity or noted in more widespread locations. Nodules may wax and wane in size but do not completely regress. Clinical behavior in late disease may be similar to histiocytic sarcoma.[9] Aspirates from the lesions can contain mixed cell types, including predominantly histiocytes, some of which may be multinucleate. The cytomorphology may resemble lymphoid or plasmacytoid cells. Inflamed lesions may also contain variable numbers of neutrophils and lymphocytes. Definitive diagnosis of the disorder requires a good clinical history as well as histopathology and immunohistochemistry.

Plasmacytoma: Cutaneous plasmacytomas are common in dogs but are thought to be rare in cats. In dogs, cutaneous plasmacytomas usually are not associated with systemic multiple myeloma and often are benign. The clinical behavior in cats is less well known.

These tumors are typically found in older dogs and usually are solitary, although multiple plasmacytomas can be seen. The tumors are well circumscribed, raised, smooth, and often pink to red in color. Aspirates tend to be moderately to highly cellular and contain discrete round cells (Figure 5-30). Aggregates of the cells may be noted, but cell-to-cell cohesion is not present. The cells have a large, round nucleus, which is typically eccentric in placement. The chromatin is coarsely reticulated to stippled, and some cells may have indistinct nucleoli. Usually, abundant blue cytoplasm is present, and many cells have a lighter staining perinuclear area (i.e., Golgi zone). Cutaneous plasmacytomas often display moderate anisocytosis and anisokaryosis. In addition, binucleate and multinucleate cells are typically found. Despite the moderate atypia these tumors may display, they usually are benign in dogs. In a small percentage of tumors, extracellular pink fibrillar material may exist, and it is often speculated to be amyloid. On rare occasions, rod-shaped to spiculated granules may be noted in the tumor cells.

Transmissible Venereal Tumor: These tumors occur in sexually active dogs and are most commonly found on the external genitalia, although they may also be found in skin. Tumors can be single or multiple and vary from nodular to pedunculated to cauliflower-like forms. They usually are firm and friable and often ulcerated. Aspirates from these lesions usually are cellular and predominated by large discrete round cells with moderate-sized, round nuclei, stippled chromatin, small nucleoli, and a moderate amount of pale cytoplasm (Figure 5-31). Many of the cells have a few small distinct cytoplasmic vacuoles, which is a helpful distinguishing finding from histiocytoma.

Epithelial Tumors

Many types of epithelial tumors can occur in skin. In general, epithelial cells tend to be cohesive, and cell clusters are often apparent when these tumors are aspirated. The cell shapes can vary from round to cuboidal, columnar, or stellate and can have a variable amount of cytoplasm. Epithelial cells tend to display cellular atypia in response to inflammation, and interpreting cytomorphology should be done carefully when inflammation is present. In many cases, histopathology is necessary to specifically identify the exact type of tumor.

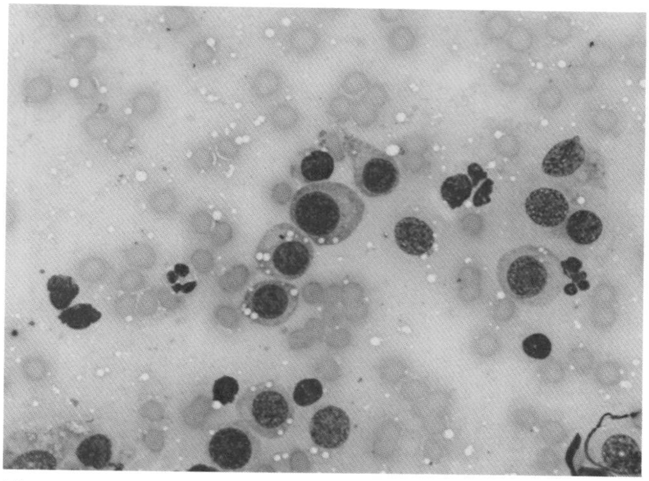

Figure 5-31 Aspirate from a transmissible venereal tumor. Tumor cells are round and similar in appearance to histiocytes. A distinguishing feature is the presence of discrete cytoplasmic vacuoles. Several neutrophils and free nuclei are also seen in this figure. (Wright-Giemsa, 50× objective.)

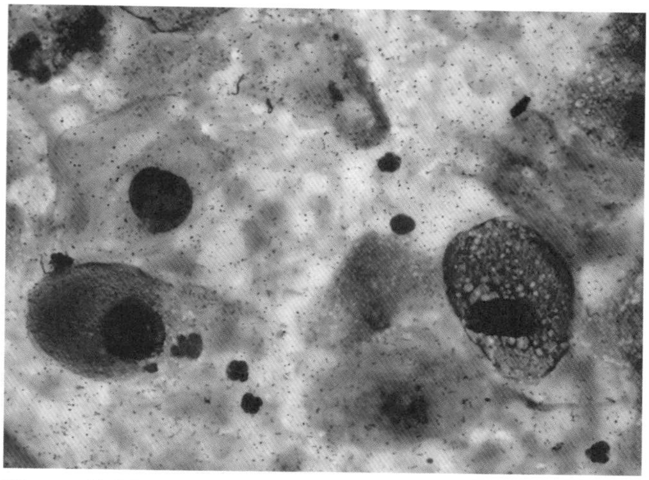

Figure 5-32 Aspirate from a squamous papilloma. Large ovoid nucleated squamous cells are present, as well as anucleate cells, neutrophils, bare nuclei, bacteria, and precipitate debris. Despite the large nucleus, these tumors are benign and, if viral induced, may regress on their own. The cytoplasm may have a stippled purple appearance as the cell in the lower left or may appear vacuolated as the cell in the lower mid-right (koilocyte). (Wright-Giemsa, 50× objective.)

Some epithelial tumors that have a fairly unique cytomorphologic appearance include circumanal (hepatoid or perianal) gland adenoma, basal cell tumors (usually trichoblastoma), apocrine gland tumor of anal sac origin, squamous papilloma, squamous cell carcinoma, sebaceous adenoma or epithelioma, and sweat gland tumor. Keratin-producing cystic lesions are common, and aspiration from these often yields abundant keratin debris. These lesions include cysts but also cystic neoplasms. Cystic epithelial lesions are usually benign; however, histopathology is necessary to specifically identify them.

Papilloma: A variety of types of papillomas exist. They are common in dogs but are rare in cats. These tumors can have a variable gross appearance, but classically, exophytic papillomas occur as single or multiple, sessile to pedunculated, or papillated masses. They often have a waxy appearance to the surface because of hyperkeratosis. These occur most commonly on the head and extremities. Aspiration from these lesions typically is moderately cellular. The cells often are found individually. In many cases, they may only resemble relatively normal squamous epithelial cells. Some epithelial cells may be large and ovoid to fusiform with a large, eccentrically placed nucleus, coarsely reticulated chromatin, and a small nucleolus (Figure 5-32). The cytoplasm may have a stippled pink to purple appearance. Other cells may appear vacuolated. Mitotic figures are uncommon. The larger ovoid to fusiform cells with vacuolated or stippled cytoplasm are thought to be hypertrophied keratinocytes (also called *koilocytes*), and these are a common feature of papillomavirus infection.[11] Not all papillomas are related to papillomavirus infection.

Follicular Cysts and Cystic Follicular Tumors: Several masslike lesions, when aspirated, yield large amounts of keratin debris that is often in thick accumulations separated by a thinner proteinaceous background. The keratin material is sky blue in color and may be admixed with variable numbers of anucleate cornifying squamous epithelial cells (Figure 5-33, *A* and *B*). In addition, cholesterol crystals are often noted as well as fragments of hair (see Figure 5-33, *C*). Sometimes, sheets and clusters of relatively uniform epithelial cells may also be noted. Because keratin may be irritative to surrounding tissues, if these lesions rupture, they may incite moderate to marked neutrophilic to pyogranulomatous inflammation.

Lesions that may have these types of findings include follicular cyst, dilated pore, warty dyskeratoma, trichofolliculoma, trichoepithelioma, acanthoma, and pilomatricoma. Distinguishing these by cytology alone is generally not possible; however, these all are usually benign lesions (malignant forms of pilomatricoma and trichoepithelioma also exist), although excision of the cyst wall or tumor may be necessary for definitive characterization of the lesion, for resolution, and to prevent recurrent inflammation and ulceration.

Trichoblastoma (Basal Cell Tumor): These tumors are what previously have been referred to as *basal cell tumors* in dogs and cats. These are neoplasms that are derived from primitive hair germ and, thus, are thought to actually be of follicular origin.[9] Basal cell carcinoma and other epitheliomas may have a similar cytologic appearance and definitive characterization of these tumors require histopathology. *Basal cell tumor* continues to be a general diagnostic term to encompass these tumors for cytologic diagnosis, although the majority of "basal cell tumors" are trichoblastomas. These are common in both cats and dogs. The tumors are usually solitary, firm, alopecic nodules, which are dome shaped to polypoid. Larger masses may be ulcerated. The appearance in cats is similar, although the tumors also are often pigmented and may have areas of central necrosis and cyst formation. Aspirates from these

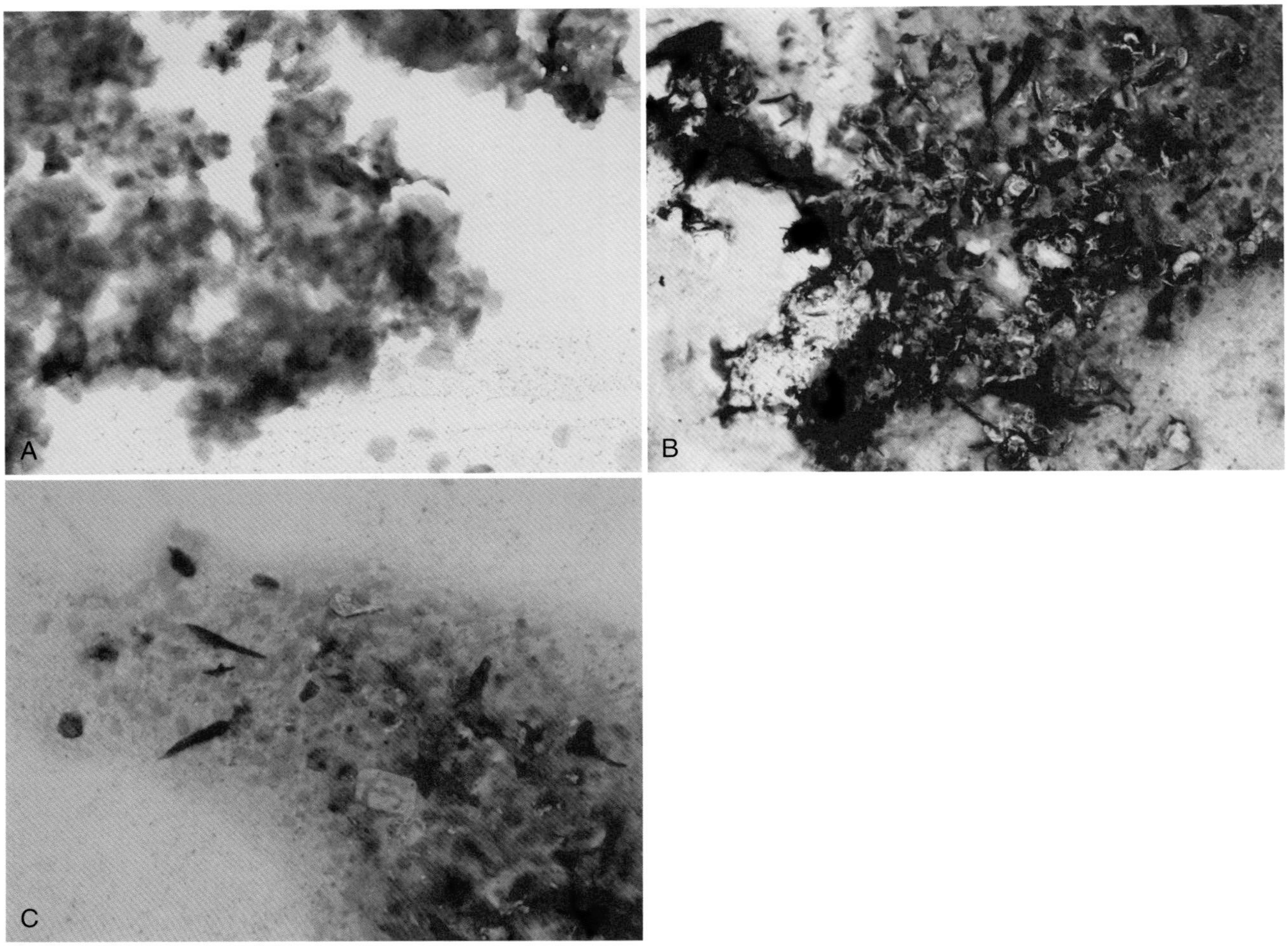

Figure 5-33 Aspirates from follicular cysts or hair follicle tumors. Aspirates from these lesions often cannot be distinguished from each other as they are predominated by keratin and squamous material. **A,** Thick accumulations of keratin and anucleate squames separated by a thin blue background material. (Wright-Giemsa, 10× objective.) **B,** Individualized variably cornifying squames separated by a proteinaceous background and cellular debris. (Wright-Giemsa, 10× objective.) **C,** Blood, protein, and cell debris from a cystic lesion. A cholesterol crystal is noted in the center. (Wright-Giemsa, 20× objective.)

lesions tend to be moderately to highly cellular. They may have a thin background separating sheets and clusters of cells, particularly if accompanied by cyst formation (Figure 5-34, *A*). The clusters often form palisades, fronds, or ribbons (see Figure 5-34, *B*). The cells have small- to moderate-sized, round nuclei with a small amount of blue cytoplasm. They are often densely packed together. Sometimes, a small amount of fibrillar pink material may be seen along the edge of clusters, which may be basement membrane. Scattered individualized cells may be noted along with a few thin spindle cells. Mitotic figures are usually not apparent.

Squamous Cell Carcinoma: These tumors are common in both cats and dogs. They may occur anywhere in skin, but they occur most frequently in areas where sun damage can occur and, thus, have a higher incidence in white-furred cats and short-coated dogs. They are most common on the pinnae, nasal planum, and eyelids in cats; in dogs, tumors occur more frequently on the ventral abdomen and flank and on medial stifles. These tumors present as plaquelike, papillary, and fungiform masses, which can vary from small to large in size. They may be alopecic, erythemic, and ulcerated, and crusts are often present. Sampling from these lesions may be complicated by the lack of discrete mass lesions and ulceration. In addition, the keratin that is produced by these tumors often induces a moderate to marked inflammatory reaction, which can make interpreting the epithelial changes difficult. The tumor may be highly exfoliative if a discrete mass region is available to aspirate. If not, a scraping sample from the edge of a plaque or ulcer may be diagnostically helpful. The epithelial cells are typically found in sheets, in clusters, and individually. When found individually, the cells vary from round to large and angular (Figure 5-35). The cells have variably sized nuclei with reticulated to open chromatin and indistinct nucleoli. Moderate to marked anisocytosis and anisokaryosis are often noted. The cytoplasm will vary from deep blue to more sky blue in appearance. In some cases, mild to moderate perinuclear

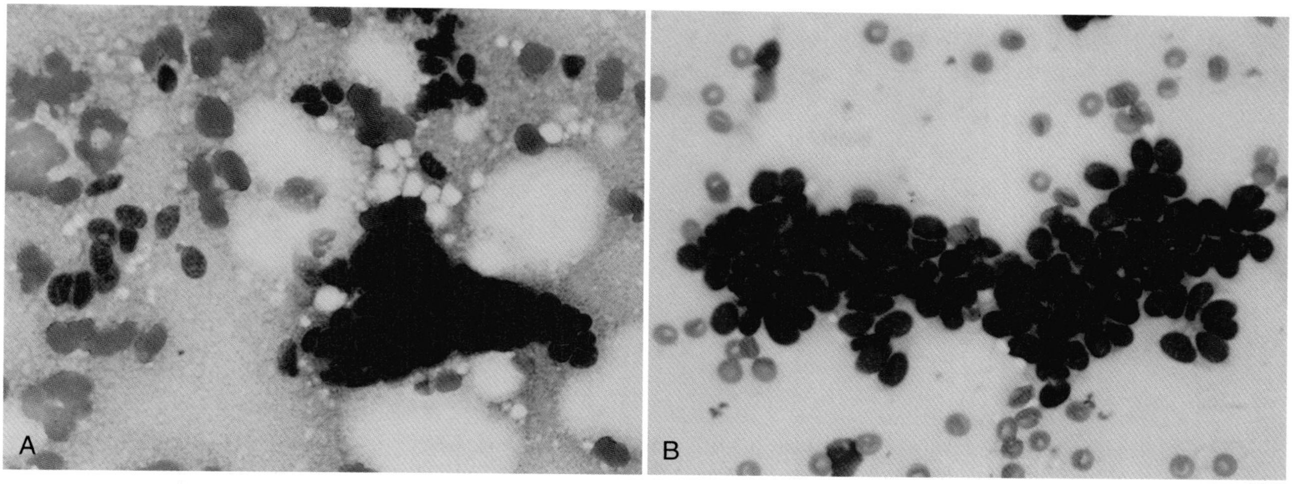

Figure 5-34 Aspirate from trichoblastoma (basal cell tumor). A, A dense, tightly packed cluster of cohesive cells is noted in the lower right. The cells have round to oval nuclei with a small amount of blue cytoplasm. Cells are also noted in rows (*mid-left*) and sometimes found individually. Cystic lesions such as this one may have a stippled proteinaceous background. (Wright-Giemsa, 50× objective.) **B,** Higher-power view of elongated frond of "basaloid" cells. (Wright-Giemsa, 100× objective.)

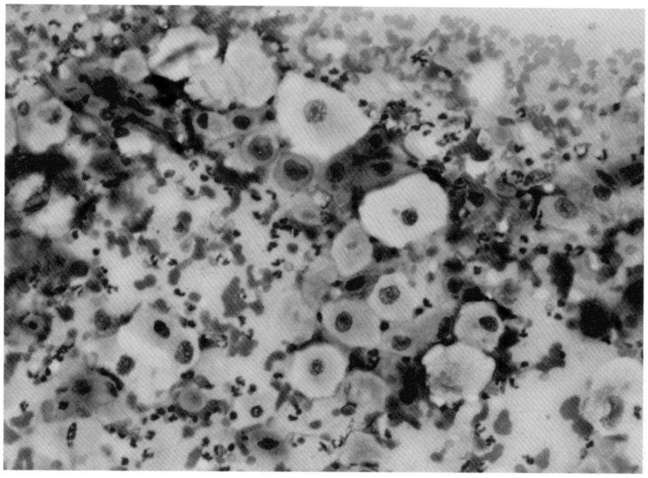

Figure 5-35 Well differentiated squamous cell carcinoma. The epithelial cells are noted individually in this figure but also may occur in sheets and clusters. The cells display anisocytosis and mild anisokaryosis with variably cornifying cytoplasm. Some cells with abundant cornified cytoplasm have relatively large nuclei (nuclear, cytoplasmic asynchrony) with open chromatin and nucleoli. Numerous neutrophils are present, as well as blood in the background. The presence of inflammation often makes it difficult to discern neoplastic from hyperplastic or dysplastic cells. (Wright-Giemsa, 20× objective.)

vacuolization may be present. Some of the large angular cells will have large nuclei and prominent nucleoli. Large cells with abundant sky blue cytoplasm (i.e., mature cytoplasmic features) with a large nucleus with open chromatin (i.e., immature nuclear features) are present. These cells demonstrate asynchronous maturation of the nucleus and cytoplasm and are referred to as *dyskeratotic*. Sometimes, dense clusters of pleomorphic cells may be found, and often, a large amount of squamous and keratin debris is noted. The lack of marked atypia does not exclude malignancy, and some of these tumors may only have well differentiated cells. Mitotic figures are sometimes seen.

Sebaceous Adenoma and Epithelioma: These tumors are common in dogs and uncommon in cats. They occur most commonly on the limbs, trunk, and eyelids in dogs and on the head, neck, and trunk in cats. The lesions are usually solitary, well circumscribed, raised, smooth to lobular, or wartlike. Aspiration from these tumors is usually at least moderately cellular, with numerous variably sized clusters of highly vacuolated, minimally pleomorphic cells (Figure 5-36). These vacuolated cells have a low nucleus-to-cytoplasm (N:C) ratio, and mitotic figures are usually not evident. The cells from sebaceous adenomas are well differentiated and cannot be distinguished from hyperplastic cells. Sebaceous epithelioma has a similar cytologic appearance to sebaceous adenoma, but admixed with the clusters of vacuolated cells are sheets of densely packed basophilic cells, which are smaller in size and have a higher N:C ratio.

Sweat Gland Tumor: Sweat gland tumors are uncommon in both the dog and the cat. They can occur in benign and malignant forms and have numerous histopathologic classifications, including cystadenoma, glandular adenoma, ductular adenoma, and a variety of carcinoma subtypes (solitary, papillary, tubular, glandular, ductular, clear cell, and signet ring). The definitive characterization of these tumors requires histopathology, although a general diagnosis of sweat gland tumor is usually possible on the basis of cytomorphology. Grossly, these tumors are most common on the head, dorsal neck, and limbs. These tend to be solitary, well circumscribed, firm, raised tumors that often are ulcerated. On occasion, the tumors may be poorly circumscribed, infiltrative, and plaquelike.

Aspiration from these lesions tends to be moderately to highly exfoliative. Cells are noted individually as well

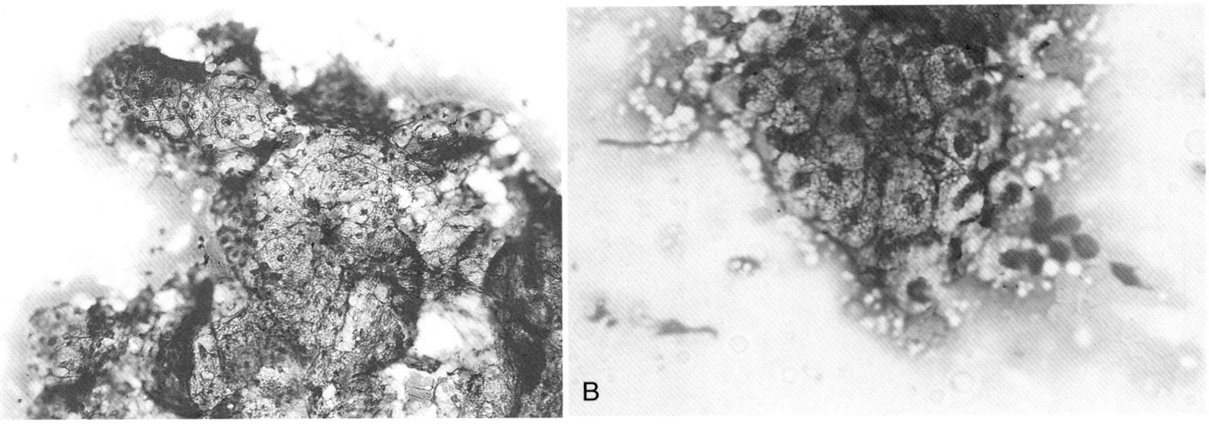

Figure 5-36 Aspirate from a sebaceous adenoma in a dog. A, A large cluster of cohesive sebaceous epithelial cells is present. (Wright stain, original magnification 80×.) **B,** Higher magnification of cells in *A*. The cells resemble normal sebaceous cells. Nuclei are uniform, and the nucleus-to-cytoplasm ratio is low. Note the vacuolation of the cytoplasm. (Wright stain, original magnification 160×.)

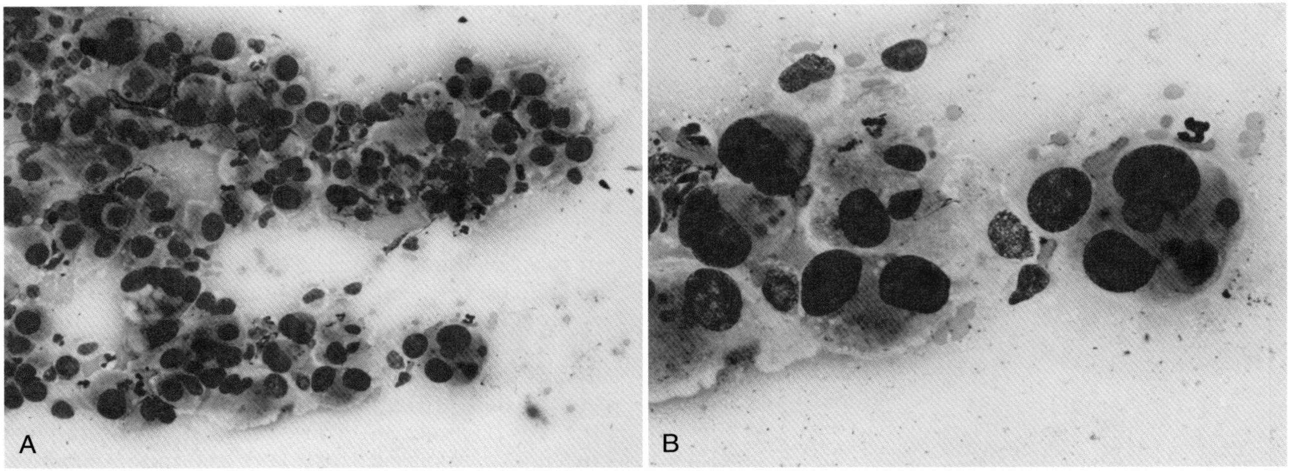

Figure 5-37 Aspirate from a sweat gland carcinoma in the neck of a dog. A, Cells are noted in aggregates, although it is difficult to discern whether the cells are cohesive. Many appear to be individualized and round to ovoid. Marked anisocytosis and anisokaryosis are evident, aiding in a diagnosis of malignancy in this case, although not all sweat gland tumors display this much atypia. (Wright-Giemsa, 20× objective.) **B,** Higher power view of *A*. Note the open chromatin pattern with prominent multiple nucleoli. Low numbers of surrounding red blood cells and a single neutrophil are present and aid in emphasizing the large size of the cells. Several cells appear to be binucleate or multinucleate. (Wright-Giemsa, 50× objective.)

as within cohesive sheets (Figure 5-37). The cells usually have moderate-sized round nuclei, with eccentric placement and a variable amount of pale granular cytoplasm. When found individually, the cells are round to slightly angular in shape, but when found in sheets, the cytoplasmic borders may be indistinct. The cells often may be smudged and may take on a spindloid appearance, and thus, aspiration from these tumors may resemble soft tissue spindle cell tumors such as liposarcoma. Other tumors with similar cells include amelanotic melanoma and plasmacytoma.

Circumanal Gland Tumor (Perianal or Hepatoid Gland Tumor): Circumanal gland tumors (also called *hepatoid gland* or *perianal gland tumors*) are common particularly in older intact male dogs; however, they may also occur in younger, neutered, or female dogs. They typically are found in the perianal region but also may be found on the tail, perineum, prepuce, thigh, and dorsal lumbosacral area. They may be solitary or multiple. Smaller lesions tend to be spherical to ovoid, but as they grow, these can become multinodular and ulcerated. Aspirates from these lesions tend to be highly exfoliative, characterized by sheets and clusters of large ovoid to cuboidal cells with round eccentrically placed nuclei and abundant pink granular cytoplasm (Figure 5-38). Typically, minimal pleomorphism is present, although some admixed smaller reserve cells may also be present. These latter cells

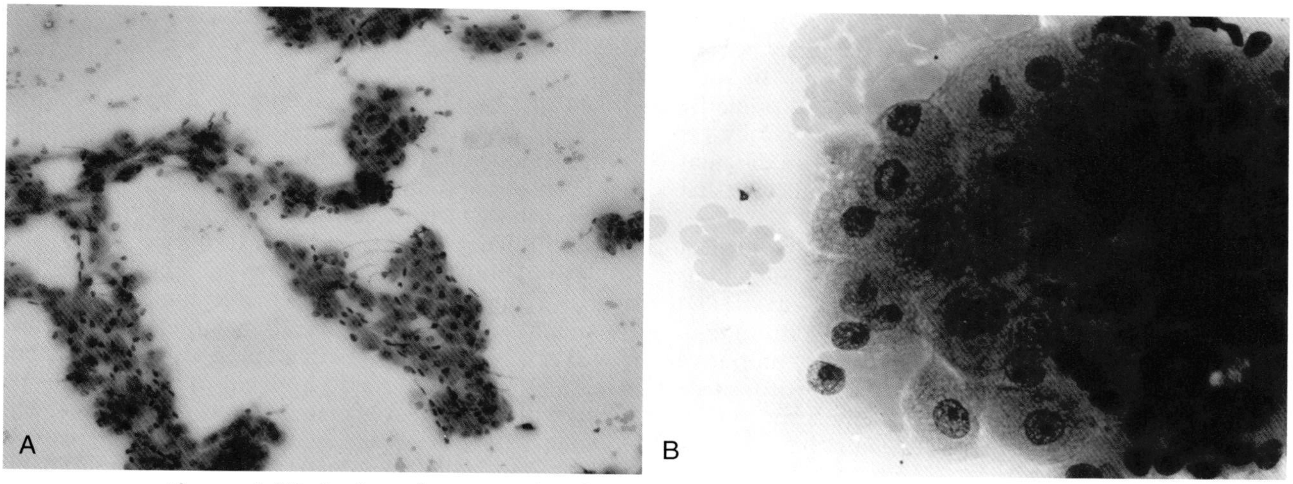

Figure 5-38 Aspirate from a perianal gland tumor in a dog. A, Sheets of cohesive epithelial cells are present. The cells are round to low cuboidal in shape but can have a slightly irregular or spindloid shape because of preparation technique (Wright-Giemsa, 10× objective.) **B,** On high-power view, the cells have pink granular cytoplasm; hence, these are also referred to as *hepatoid tumors*. Nucleoli are present, but not necessarily indicative of malignancy. The majority of hepatoid tumors are benign (e.g., adenomas), but histopathology is necessary to definitively characterize malignant potential. (Wright-Giemsa, 50× objective.)

are more densely packed together with basophilic cytoplasm and a high N:C ratio. These lesions can become secondarily inflamed or have areas of necrosis and cyst formation. This type of tumor is typically benign; however, the cytomorphology does not correlate well with clinical behavior, requiring histopathology for definitive characterization.

Apocrine Gland Tumor of Anal Sac Origin: This type of tumor also is found in the perianal area but occurs in the anal sac region (ventrolateral to anus). These mostly occur in older dogs and are rare in cats. These tumors often are adenocarcinomas. They occur as an intradermal or subcutaneous mass and often invade deep into perirectal tissue along the pelvic canal. This tumor is sometimes associated with hypercalcemia of malignancy. Although usually adenocarcinomas, the cells typically do not display prominent pleomorphism. The cells are usually found in variably sized sheets, although individualized cells and free nuclei may be seen (Figure 5-39). The cells have moderate-sized, round nuclei, with moderate to abundant pale cytoplasm. When found in sheets, the cytoplasmic borders may be indistinct, but when found individually, the cells tend to have a round shape. This morphology resembles what some cytologists will call a "neuroendocrine appearance." The chromatin is usually stippled, and small indistinct nucleoli may be present.

Other Epithelial Tumors: Many other epithelial tumors, for the most part, cannot be distinguished by cytomorphology alone. It is important to note that not all tumors that occur in skin or subcutaneous tissue are primary skin tumors but may, in fact, be metastatic tumors. As an example, feline lung tumors have a predisposition to metastasize to the nailbed and may be found elsewhere in skin.

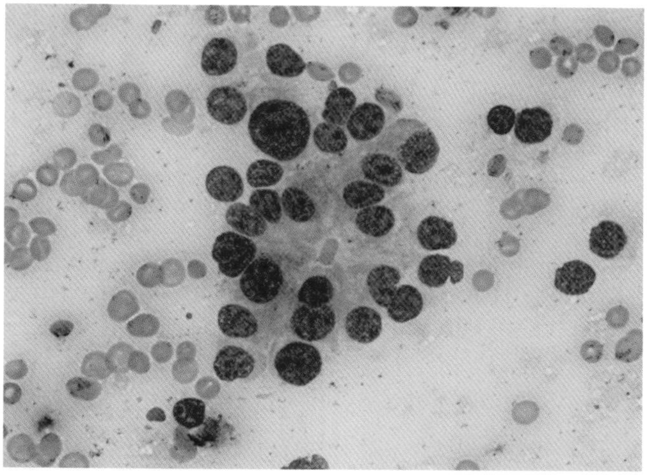

Figure 5-39 Aspirate from apocrine adenocarcinoma of anal sac gland origin. Aspirates from these lesions can be highly cellular and often contain sheets of cells with indistinct cytoplasmic borders. The cells have round nuclei, with a moderate amount of pale blue cytoplasm. In this case, moderate anisokaryosis is present, but these tumors often have minimal anisocytosis or anisokaryosis despite being malignant. (Wright-Giemsa, 50× objective.)

Subcutaneous Glandular Tissues: Tumors and other lesions of salivary, mammary, and thyroid glandular tissue are discussed in Chapter 6.

Mesenchymal (Spindle Cell) Tumors

Mesenchymal tumors (sometimes referred to as *spindle cell tumors*) are characterized by cells that have irregular to wispy to indistinct cell borders, particularly when of soft tissue origin. Although these tumors are often said to be poorly exfoliative, some may be moderately to highly exfoliative. These tumors are diverse, and, for the most part, are difficult to definitively identify by cytomorphology alone. In some cases, immunocytochemical staining may be beneficial in further identifying histogenic origin.[12] In addition, although most "spindle cell tumors" are primarily mesenchymal tumors, some tumors morphologically get lumped into this category. However, they have a different histogenesis (e.g., melanocytic tumors—melanocytes that are neuroectodermal in derivation).

Of all the masses that occur in skin, probably the most care needs to be taken when evaluating spindle cells from mass lesions, as reactive spindle cells associated with fibroplasia cannot be easily distinguished from neoplastic cells. A history of progressive growth, infiltrative behavior, and irregular mass borders, along with a lack of inflammatory cells, should increase the suspicion for a neoplastic process. Mesenchymal tumors have benign (e.g., fibroma) and malignant (e.g., fibrosarcoma) forms, but unless marked cytologic atypia exists, making this distinction requires histopathology. Definitively characterizing a lesion as a mesenchymal neoplasm almost always requires histopathology. This is particularly true if any admixed inflammation is present.

Lipoma: Lipomas are common subcutaneous tumors in dogs and less common in cats. They may be single or multiple in site and occur over the thorax, abdomen, thighs, and proximal limbs. They seldom ulcerate. Aspirates yield variable numbers of adipocytes noted individually and in variably sized clusters (Figure 5-40). These are often admixed with a few thin spindle cells and bare nuclei. Typically, free lipid is also present. Slides with fat on them do not dry and have an oily appearance. Because most Romanowsky-type stains use alcohol as a fixative, the fat sometimes is washed off the slide during the staining process, and after staining, the slide may be essentially acellular. Adipocytes from a lipoma cannot be distinguished from normal subcutaneous fat cells, so care must always be taken when collecting samples from subcutaneous masses to avoid contamination with surrounding normal tissue.

Liposarcoma: These are rare tumors in both the dog and the cat. They are usually solitary in occurrence and are most frequently found on the ventral abdomen, thorax, and proximal limbs. These tumors tend to be poorly circumscribed, firm to fleshy, and subcutaneous. They behave similarly to other soft tissue sarcomas.

Aspiration from these tumors may be moderately to highly cellular. Typically, a variable amount of free lipid material is also present. Cells are noted individually as well as in sheets and are often found around the lipid material. The cells are round to ovoid to spindloid in shape and typically have moderate to large, round nuclei with a variable amount of pale cytoplasm. A few punctate cytoplasmic vacuoles are sometimes noted. The chromatin is stippled to lacy, and some cells may have small multiple nucleoli. Mitotic figures may be observed. The morphology of the cells can be similar to sweat gland tumor or amelanotic melanoma, and the free lipid can be a useful distinguishing finding (Figure 5-41).

Soft Tissue Spindle Cell Tumor: These tumors encompass several different types of sarcomas that are named on the basis of their presumptive progenitor cell. A few minor cytologic differences exist between these tumors, but otherwise, even with histopathology, it is not always clear what the actual origin of the neoplastic cells is. Thus, from a cytologic perspective, it is probably best just to lump these tumors into the category of soft tissue spindle cell tumor, at least in the dog. These include fibrosarcoma, myxosarcoma, hemangiopericytoma, and peripheral nerve sheath tumor. As a generalization, these tumors tend to behave similarly regardless of cell origin.

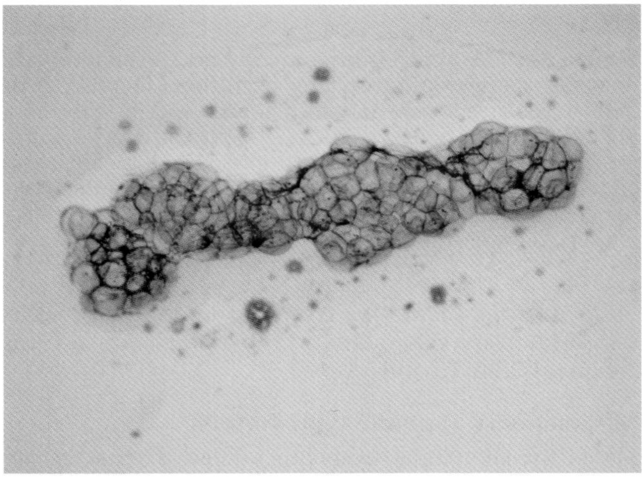

Figure 5-40 Aspirate from a lipoma. A single large cluster of well differentiated adipocytes is present surrounded by small droplets of blood. Adipocytes from a lipoma cannot be distinguished from normal subcutaneous fat. (Wright-Giemsa, 4× objective.)

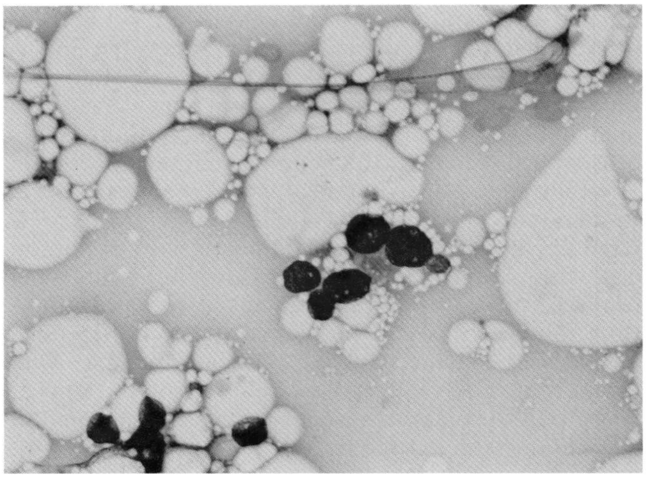

Figure 5-41 Aspirate from liposarcoma in a dog. Aspirates from these lesions typically have a large amount of free lipid, and this sometimes results in lysis of the cells during smear preparation. The cells are often noted among the lipid material, and sometimes, it may appear as if only free nuclei are present. The cytoplasm tends to be pale and can blend into the background. When cell borders are distinct, the cells may appear round to ovoid in shape rather than spindloid. (Wright-Giemsa, 50× objective.)

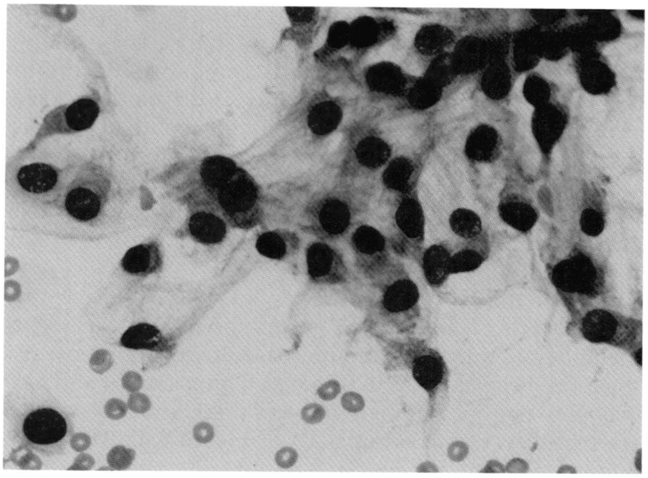

Figure 5-42 Aspirate from spindle cell tumor in a dog. Large numbers of irregularly shaped spindle cells are found in loose aggregates. The cells have moderate- to large-sized nuclei with abundant pale blue cytoplasm and wispy cytoplasmic borders. Red blood cells are noted, but inflammatory cells are not apparent. On biopsy, this lesion was diagnosed as hemangiopericytoma. (Wright-Giemsa stain, 50× objective.)

They usually are low to moderate grade malignancies with local invasiveness and a propensity to recur after excision. In the cat, soft tissue sarcomas often are fibrosarcomas, which may have a slightly higher metastatic potential when vaccine associated.

Most of these tumors arise in subcutaneous tissue and may occur in various anatomic sites. Aspiration from spindle cell tumors vary in the degree of cellularity, but these may be moderately to highly exfoliative lesions. Cells are found both individually as well as within loosely arranged aggregates. The cells are usually elongated with irregular to wispy borders (Figure 5-42). The nuclei are moderate to large in size and often centrally located with cytoplasm extending from each pole of the nucleus. The chromatin is reticulated to stippled, and small distinct nucleoli may be present. Some of these tumors (e.g., myxosarcoma) may have abundant pink-stippled to fibrillar background material, with prominent windrowing of the cells (Figure 5-43). Others may have denser accumulations of pink fibrillar material noted between cells (e.g., fibrosarcoma). A variant of fibrosarcoma that has been reported in dogs is keloidal fibrosarcoma.[13] This may occur in a benign form also (e.g., fibroma). These have a characteristic appearance with striking accumulations of

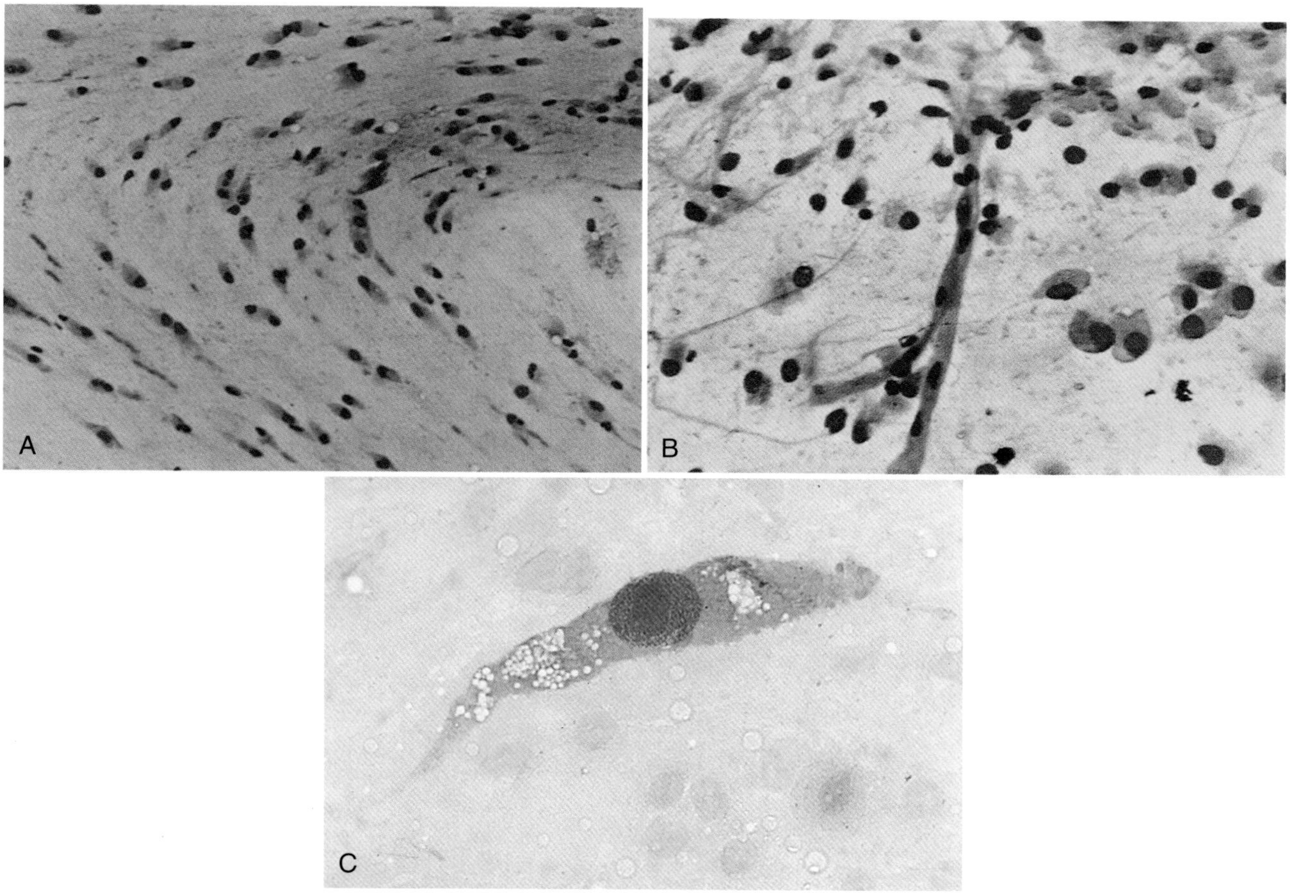

Figure 5-43 Aspirate from a myxosarcoma in a dog. A, Low magnification shows many rows of cells embedded in a pink substance. (Wright stain, original magnification 50×.) **B,** A higher magnification shows many cells with a plasmacytoid appearance and a background of pink material. A few cells are spindle shaped. (Wright stain, original magnification 100×.) **C,** Cell from a myxosarcoma, showing a large, prominent nucleolus. (Wright stain, original magnification 250×.)

bright pink to blue, hyalinized collagen in addition to the spindle cells (Figure 5-44).

Anaplastic Sarcoma with Giant Cells (Malignant Fibrous Histiocytoma, Giant Cell Tumor of Soft Parts): This tumor type has a fairly distinctive cytologic appearance. It has previously been called *malignant fibrous histiocytoma,* but this is considered controversial nomenclature. More recent studies have suggested this tumor is not a distinct morphologic entity and likely represents a group of poorly differentiated sarcomas with morphologic similarities, including fibrosarcoma, leiomyosarcoma, rhabdomyosarcoma, liposarcoma, synovial sarcoma, and histiocytic sarcoma.[9,14] These tumors appear similar to other soft tissue sarcomas and often present as large, solitary, firm, poorly circumscribed, subcutaneous and dermal masses. With aspiration, these tumors may be moderately to highly exfoliative. Cells are typically found individually but may be in loose aggregates. Most of the cells are large and round to slightly spindloid in shape. They usually have a large nucleus, with open chromatin and prominent nucleoli. The cytoplasm is usually abundant, pale, and granular and may be variably vacuolated. The distinctive feature is the presence of variable numbers of giant multinucleate cells (Figure 5-45). The cells may have up to 30 nuclei and usually have abundant pale granular cytoplasm. Mitotic figures are commonly noted in the round cell population.

Melanocytic Tumors: The terminology for classifying melanocytic tumors is complex, but in general, most use the term *melanocytoma* to denote a benign tumor and *melanoma* to denote a malignant tumor. Melanocytic tumors are relatively common in both dogs and cats. When involving just skin, the majority in dogs are benign. Tumors involving the nailbed or oral cavity often have a more

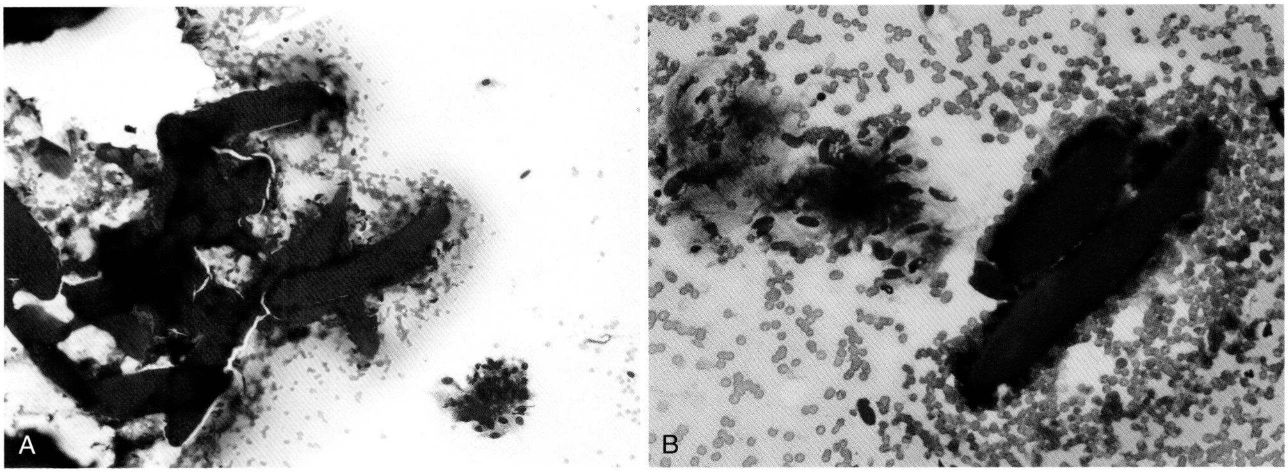

Figure 5-44 Aspirate from keloidal fibrosarcoma. A, Thick rectangular accumulations of pink to blue hyalinized collagen characterizes this lesion. Note small aggregates of irregular spindle cells in lower right mixed with more typical pink fibrillar matrix found with soft tissue spindle cell tumors. (Wright-Giemsa, 10× objective.) **B,** Higher-power view of hyalinized collagen next to spindle cells. (Wright-Giemsa, 20× objective.) (Slide courtesy of Dr. J. Johnsrude, IDEXX Laboratories.)

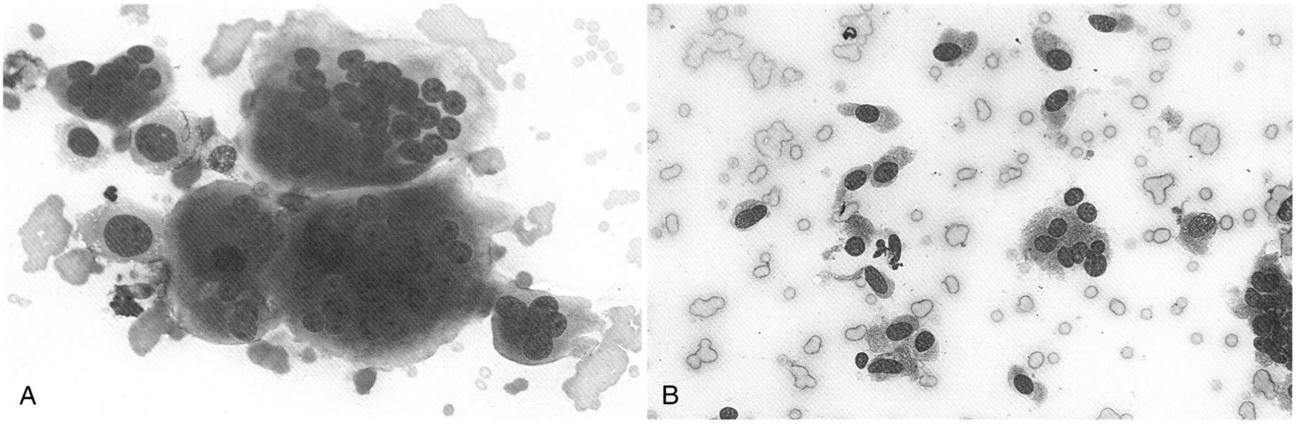

Figure 5-45 A, Aspirate from anaplastic sarcoma with giant cells from a cat. These tumors contain a mixture of large, multinucleated cells mixed with pleomorphic round to spindle-shaped cells. (Diff-Quik, original magnification 132×.) **B,** Mesenchymal cells (Wright stain, original magnification 160×.)

aggressive clinical course. In cats, benign and malignant tumors occur with about equal frequency.[7]

These tumors typically occur in older animals. They are usually solitary and mostly occur on the head, neck, trunk, and paws. The lesions are usually well circumscribed, firm to fleshy, darkly colored, and alopecic and vary from dome shaped to pedunculated or papillomatous in appearance.

Aspirates from these lesions are typically moderately to highly cellular with some degree of blood contamination. Cells are found individually as well as in aggregates or sheets. When found individually, the cells vary from round to stellate to spindloid in shape (Figure 5-46). They may be densely pigmented with fine to moderately coarse dark-brown to black melanin granules. The pigment may be so abundant that all other cytologic detail is obscured. In other cases, the cells are variably or less well pigmented, and nuclear detail may be evident. The presence of more prominent nuclear atypia such as anisokaryosis, pleomorphism, open chromatin, and prominent nucleoli are suggestive of a malignant process. Mitotic figures may be common in malignant tumors. Often, free pigment will also be noted in the background, as well as macrophages with phagocytized pigment. These latter cells are referred to as *melanophages*, and these may be seen in nonneoplastic lesions as well as in lymph nodes draining pigmented skin. It is also important to note that some epithelial tumors (e.g., basal cell tumors) often have large numbers of admixed melanocytes, with the epithelial cells having readily visible melanin granules, and these should not be interpreted as melanocytic tumors.

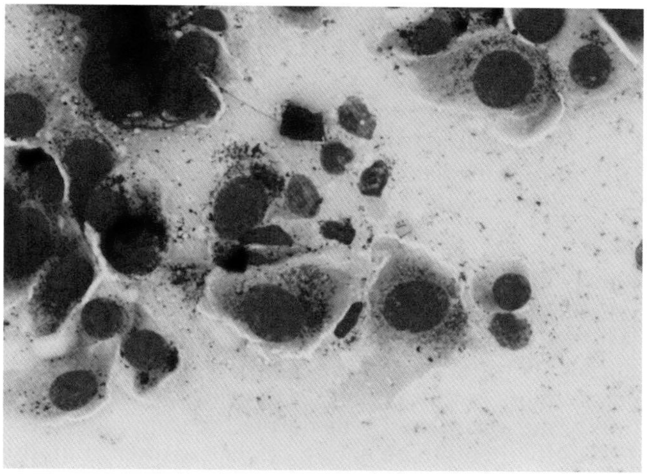

Figure 5-46 Aspirate from melanoma. Cells are mostly noted individually in this figure but also can be found in sheets. The cell shape varies and often is irregular. The cytoplasm contains fine, dark pigment, indicating that these are melanocytes. The cellular and nuclear atypia (anisocytosis, anisokaryosis, open chromatin, and small nucleoli) suggest this is a malignant neoplasm. (Wright-Giemsa, 50× objective.)

Hemangiosarcoma: This tumor is a difficult cytologic diagnosis, as *hemangiosarcoma* comprises vascular tissue and may be cavernous. Aspiration often is very bloody and not very cellular, although some forms of these tumors may be densely cellular with higher cell exfoliation. The tumor cells may be found individually and in sheets. They typically have a pleomorphic appearance but usually are irregular to spindloid in shape (Figure 5-47). As with other spindle cells, interpreting their significance on the basis of cytomorphology alone is difficult, as reactive spindle cells found in an organizing hematoma may also appear somewhat pleomorphic. Accompanying cytologic findings may include erythrophagic macrophages as well as extramedullary hematopoiesis.

FLUID-FILLED LESIONS

Fluid-filled lesions in skin or subcutaneous lesions may be caused by infection (abscess); trauma; cystic or necrotic or infarcted areas of glands; or neoplasia. When lesions are confined to skin, they may reflect true cysts developing from apocrine tissue. In almost all of these cases, aspiration of the fluid may aid in defining whether an inflammatory process exists or not as well as aid in finding infectious

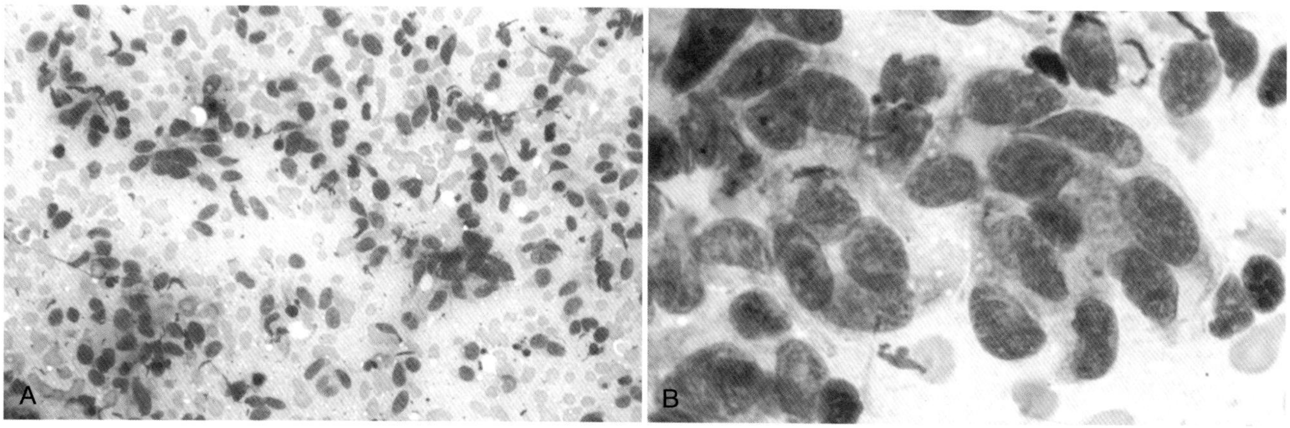

Figure 5-47 A, Scraping from a hemangiosarcoma. Scattered red blood cells, spindle cells, and bare nuclei are shown. **B,** Higher magnification of spindle cells shown in *A*. (Wright stain.) (Slide courtesy of Dr. D. DeNicola, IDEXX Laboratories.)

agents, if present. However, usually, tissue cells surrounding the fluid cavity do not exfoliate well into the fluid, and thus, evaluation of the fluid by itself may not entirely reflect the pathologic process. Examples of fluid-filled lesions with typically low to moderate numbers of nucleate cells include seroma, hematoma, hygroma, sialocele, synovial cyst, and apocrine cyst.

Seroma, Hygroma, and Synovial and Apocrine Cysts

Aspirates from these lesions are generally poorly cellular and consist of primarily macrophages or reactive mononuclear cells but no tissue cells. The fluid typically appears clear to pale yellow and may be thin or viscous. The location of the swelling aids in distinguishing these lesions: Apocrine cysts are typically superficially located in the skin; synovial cysts occur around joints; hygromas are noted over bony prominences or areas of chronic trauma; and seromas are found in areas of prior trauma such as surgery sites.

Hematoma

The fluid from hematomas is cloudy and red to red-brown. The total protein concentration of the supernatant approaches that of peripheral blood. Smears contain primarily red blood cells (RBCs) with low numbers of leukocytes, which are primarily the same as those noted in peripheral blood. In addition, if the hematoma has been present for more than 12 to 24 hours, some macrophages should be present, including some that are more highly vacuolated and display phagocytosis of RBCs (erythrophagocytosis) as well as hemoglobin breakdown material such as hematoidin (Figure 5-48). Platelets are generally absent unless hemorrhage into the site has occurred within a few hours of sample collection (or if blood contamination has occurred). Some vascular tumors (hemangioma, hemangiosarcoma) may have large cavitated areas filled with blood, and aspiration from these areas will not necessarily contain neoplastic cells; thus, the lack of overtly neoplastic cells in these samples does not exclude the possibility of neoplasia.

Sialocele

Sialoceles have characteristic findings. Aspiration from these lesions (which are found under the mandible or intermandibular space) yields a viscous fluid that is often blood tinged. Smears are bloody with low to moderate numbers of macrophages and neutrophils. Usually, scattered thick accumulations of amorphous blue material that is consistent with mucus is present (Figure 5-49).

MISCELLANEOUS

Calcinosis Circumscripta

These lesions are characterized by tumorlike nodules in subcutaneous tissue. They are mostly seen in young, large-breed dogs and are rare in cats. They consist of focal deposition of mineral salts forming well-circumscribed subcutaneous nodules, often over areas of chronic focal trauma. Aspirates from these lesions typically "feel" gritty. Often, a large amount of pasty material is present, but when stained, the cellularity is actually low. The stained surface of the slide often will have a characteristic blue chalklike appearance. On microscopic examination, usually a large amount of poorly staining irregular crystalline material with few intact cells, including macrophages and spindle cells, is seen (Figure 5-50).

Poorly Cellular Samples

When a solid skin or subcutaneous mass is aspirated and very few cells are subsequently found on the slides, it suggests that the lesion may be poorly exfoliative. Other possibilities exist for poorly cellular slides, such as aspiration of fat with loss of cells during the staining process. Tissues that tend to be poorly exfoliative often comprise dense fibrous tissue. In many cases, these turn out to be benign lesions such as fibromas, collagenous hamartomas, or related lesions. However, definitive identification almost always requires histopathology, and thus, if the lesion is growing, feels infiltrative, becomes ulcerated, or otherwise is bothering the patient, then biopsy will be necessary for diagnosis.

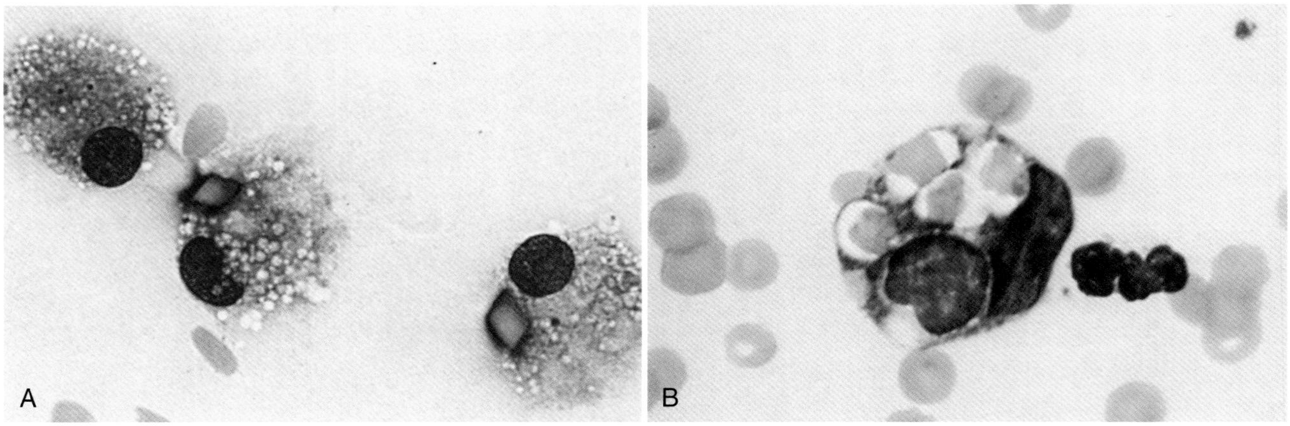

Figure 5-48 **A,** Large, vacuolated macrophages with intracytoplasmic golden hematoidin crystals. Hematoidin is a product of red blood cell breakdown and is sometimes referred to as *tissue bilirubin*. (Wright stain.) **B,** A macrophage with erythrophagocytosis. (Wright stain.)

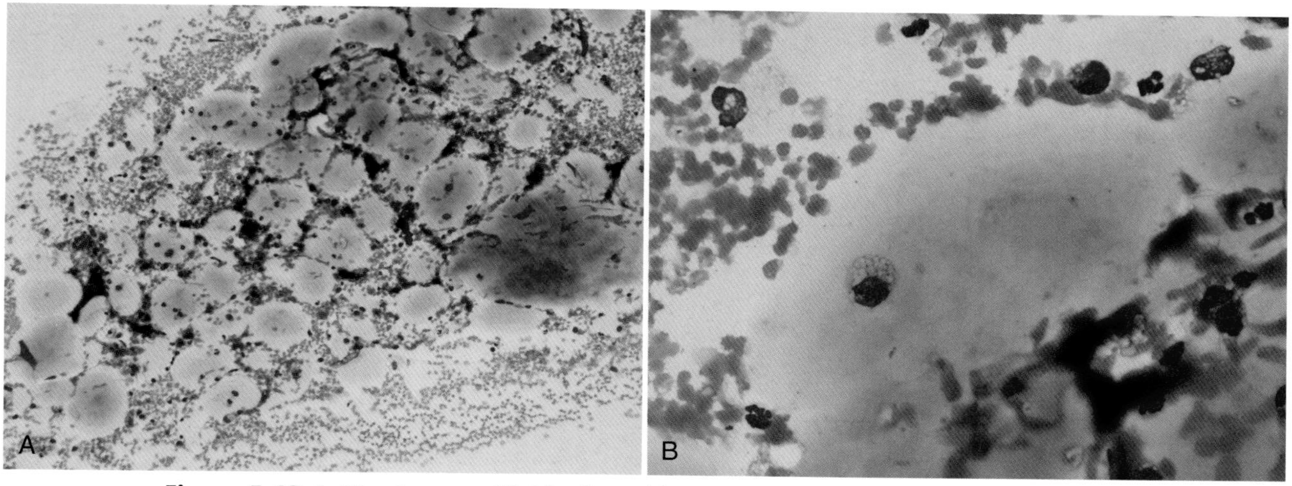

Figure 5-49 A, Direct smear of fluid collected from a sialocele. Large numbers of red blood cells surround different-sized thick accumulations of blue-staining mucus. The color of the mucus resembles what is seen with cornifying squames or keratin debris, and care must be taken not to interpret the material as squamous in origin. The mucous accumulations have rounded edges, unlike maturing squames. The dark structures in the mucus are cells. (Wright-Giemsa, 10× objective.) **B,** Higher power view of *A*. Note smooth rounded margins of mucus surrounded by red blood cells and low numbers of macrophages, neutrophils, and bare nuclei. A large vacuolated macrophage is embedded mucus. (Wright-Giemsa, 50× objective.)

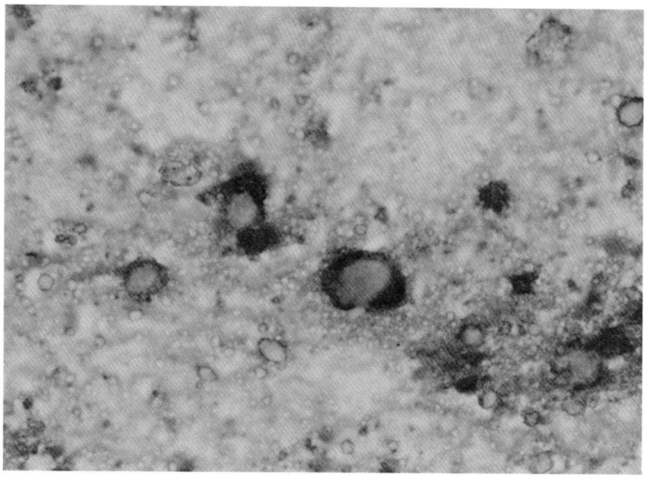

Figure 5-50 Calcinosis circumscripta in a dog. After staining, slides from these lesions often have a dark-blue, gross appearance to the sample area, but under microscopic examination, the samples are typically poorly cellular with a large amount of irregular, poorly staining calcified material. (Wright-Giemsa, 50× objective.)

References

1. Ghisleni G, Roccabianca P, Ceruti R, et al: Correlation between fine-needle aspiration cytology and histopathology in the evaluation of cutaneous and subcutaneous masses from dogs and cats, *Vet Clin Pathol* 35(1):24–30, 2006.
2. Marcos R, Santos M, Santos N, et al: Use of destained cytology slides for the application of routine special stains, *Vet Clin Pathol* 38(1):94–102, 2009.
3. Greene C: *Infectious diseases of the dog and cat*, ed 3, Philadelphia, 2006, Saunders.
4. Bulla C, Thomas JS: What is your diagnosis? Subcutaneous mass fluid from a febrile dog, *Vet Clin Pathol* 38(3):403–405, 2009.
5. Lester SL, Malik R, Bartlett KH, et al: Cryptococcosis: update and emergence of *Cryptococcus gattii*, *Vet Clin Pathol* 40(1):4–17, 2011.
6. Gupta A, Stroup S, Dedeaux A, et al: What is your diagnosis? Fine-needle aspirate of ulcerative skin lesions in a dog, *Vet Clin Pathol* 40(3):401–402, 2011.
7. Scott DW, Miller Jr WH: *Griffin CE: Muller & Kirk's small animal dermatology*, ed 6, Philadelphia, 2001, Saunders.
8. Giori L, Garbagnoli V, Venco L, et al: What is your diagnosis? Fine-needle aspirate from a subcutaneous mass in a dog, *Vet Clin Pathol* 39(2):255–256, 2010.
9. Gross TL, Ihrke PJ, Walder EJ, et al: *Skin diseases of the dog and cat: clinical and histopathologic diagnosis*, ed 2, Oxford, U.K, 2005, Blackwell Science.
10. Villamil JA, Henry CJ, Bryan JN, et al: Identification of the most common cutaneous neoplasms in dogs and evaluation of breed and age distributions for selected neoplasms, *J Am Vet Med Assoc* 239(7):960–965, 2011.
11. Sprague W, Thrall MA: Recurrent skin mass from the digit of a dog, *Vet Clin Pathol* 30(4):189–192, 2001.
12. Höinghaus R, Hewicker-Trautwein M, Mischke R: Immunocytochemical differentiation of canine mesenchymal tumors in cytologic imprint preparations, *Vet Clin Pathol* 37(1):104–111, 2008.
13. Little LK, Goldschmidt M: Cytologic appearance of a keloidal fibrosarcoma in a dog, *Vet Clin Pathol* 36(4):364–367, 2007.
14. Fulmer AK, Mauldin GE: Canine histiocytic neoplasia: an overview, *Can Vet J* 48(10):1041–1050, 2007.

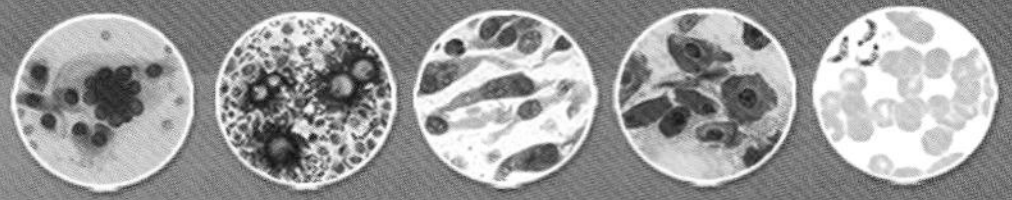

CHAPTER 6

Subcutaneous Glandular Tissue: Mammary, Salivary, Thyroid, and Parathyroid

Robin W. Allison

Mammary, salivary, thyroid, and parathyroid glands are located in the subcutaneous fat layer. Knowledge of the normal microanatomy of these glands and of other structures in proximity is important for accurate cytologic interpretation. Except for the thyroid and parathyroid glands, regional locations of these glands differ considerably. Cytologically, normal exocrine glands (mammary and salivary) may appear similar, but they differ from normal endocrine glands (thyroid and parathyroid). Lymphoid and adipose tissues may be found near any of these glands; salivary tissue may be inadvertently aspirated when attempting to aspirate submandibular lymph nodes. Thymic tissue may be near the thyroid and parathyroid, especially in young animals or when any of these tissues exist in ectopic locations.

Cytologic evaluation of subcutaneous glandular tissue is a valuable extension of clinical examination. Collection of samples by fine-needle aspiration (FNA) is simple, quick, and avoids the trauma and anesthetic risk of surgical biopsy. Most lesions are readily palpable and, therefore, easily aspirated. Although aspiration is the usual means of obtaining specimens, cytologic evaluation of mammary glands may also be performed on imprints of excised tissue, scrapings of ulcerated surface lesions, and secretions.

A primary goal of aspiration cytology is to distinguish inflammatory lesions from neoplastic lesions and to differentiate, when possible, benign neoplasms from malignant neoplasms. However, endocrine tumors (e.g., thyroid and parathyroid) frequently exhibit few cellular criteria of malignancy, appearing cytologically benign even when malignant. These tumors require histopathologic evaluation of invasion and other features to determine their malignant potential.

Mammary gland lesions present special challenges because of the diversity of cell types that may be involved and the often-overlapping cell populations within hyperplastic, dysplastic, benign, and malignant lesions. Reported diagnostic accuracy for cytologic differentiation of benign neoplasms from malignant mammary neoplasms in dogs varies from 33% to 93%.[1-5] Best agreement with the histologic diagnosis was achieved when multiple aspirates from each lesion were evaluated collaboratively by two experienced cytologists.[1] A cytologic grading system for differentiation of benign from malignant mammary tumors in dogs based on 10 important criteria of malignancy has been proposed.[2] In that study, the predictive value of a positive result was higher (90% to 100%) than that of a negative result (59% to 75%), suggesting that cytologic evaluation tends to underdiagnose mammary gland malignancies. Wet fixation and a Papanicolaou-type stain were used in that study, which are less frequently used by most cytologists, and were thought to allow better appreciation of some criteria of malignancy.

A high rate of false-negatives in cases of malignancies may result from several factors. Sampling errors occur if the needle is not directed into a representative area of the tumor. This problem is proportional to tumor size, and sampling of multiple sites in large tumors may increase the likelihood of aspirating neoplastic cells.[1] Multiple mammary tumors in an animal may be of different types, thus requiring examination of all lesions. Tumors containing an abundance of connective tissue may exfoliate poorly, leading to nondiagnostic samples. Mammary gland malignancies may be diagnosed based on histopathologic evidence of tissue invasion regardless of cellular atypia.[6] It is no surprise that cytologic samples from such tumors may be misleading. Conversely, some encapsulated tumors containing areas with significant cell pleomorphism may be considered benign based on absence of tissue invasion. Cytologic samples from these tumors may falsely suggest a malignant process. Accuracy of evaluation will also depend on the experience of the cytologist. Samples yielding equivocal results, for example, cystic fluid, nonseptic inflammatory changes, or those cytologically suggestive of benign neoplasia, should be evaluated histologically. Presence of marked criteria of malignancy makes malignant neoplasia most likely, but histopathology should still be employed to confirm the diagnosis. Samples yielding definitive nonneoplastic diagnoses may not need to be evaluated histologically.

MAMMARY GLANDS

Normal Cytologic Appearance

Mammary tissue of dogs and cats consists of five pairs of modified sweat glands that extend along the ventral body wall from the cranial thorax to the inguinal region. Glands consist of secretory acini and a series of excretory ducts. Myoepithelial cells lie between glandular epithelial cells and the basement membrane. During lactation the glands undergo marked hypertrophy to produce colostrum and then milk (Figure 6-1). Normal mammary secretions contain large amounts of protein and lipid droplets and are of low cellularity. The predominant cell type in milk is the foam cell—a large, vacuolated epithelial cell that resembles an active macrophage (Figure 6-2). These cells usually occur singly. Small numbers of lymphocytes and neutrophils may also be present.

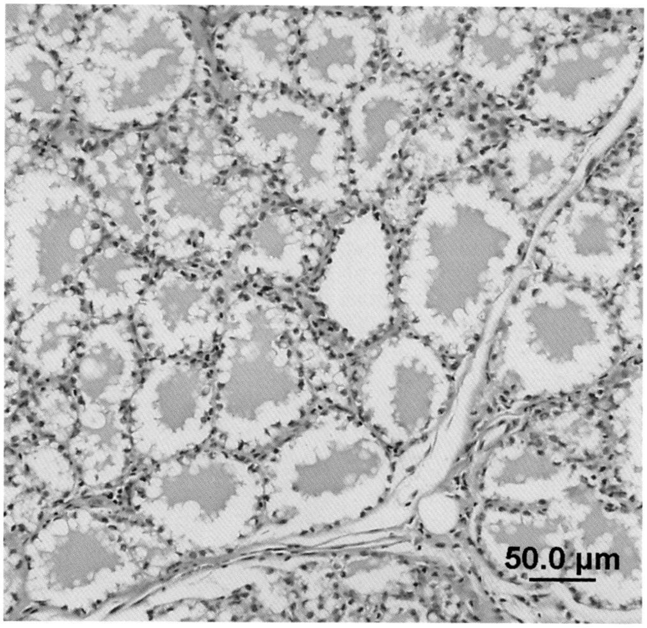

Figure 6-1 Biopsy of mammary tissue from lactating cat. Glandular acini are hyperplastic and distended with eosinophilic secretory product. (H&E, 200×.)

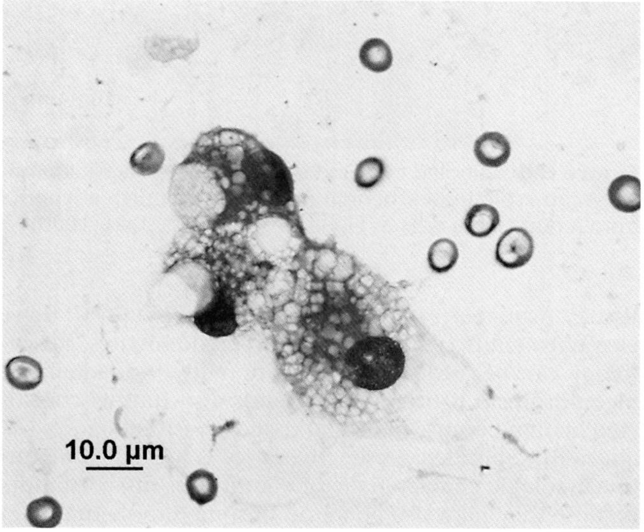

Figure 6-2 Several vacuolated foam cells from a mammary gland aspirate contain eccentric oval nuclei and abundant vacuolated cytoplasm with a variable amount of basophilic secretory product. (Wright stain, 1000×.)

Aspirates of normal mammary tissue are frequently acellular or contain only blood. When mammary tissue is present, secretory cells are arranged in an acinar pattern. Individual cells have moderate amounts of basophilic cytoplasm and round, dark nuclei of uniform size. Duct epithelial cells have basal, ovoid nuclei and scanty cytoplasm and are arranged in small sheets or fragments of ductules. Myoepithelial cells appear as dark-staining, naked, oval nuclei or as spindle-shaped cells. Adipocytes and lipid droplets may be present.

Benign Lesions

Mastitis: Mastitis, or inflammation of the mammary glands, may occur either as a diffuse form involving two or more mammae or as a focal lesion. Mastitis is usually associated with postpartum lactation or pseudopregnancy and may result from ascending or hematogenous infections.[7] Mammary secretions are usually adequate for diagnosis in cases of diffuse inflammation, whereas aspirates may be required for diagnosis of focal lesions. Smears are very cellular and contain large amounts of debris. Inflammatory cells may include neutrophils, lymphocytes, and macrophages in variable numbers, depending on the causative agent (Figure 6-3). Bacteria may be seen within phagocytes. Offending agents are usually coliforms, *Streptococcus* or *Staphylococcus* spp., although other bacteria and fungi may occasionally be isolated.[8] Nonseptic mastitis, usually affecting the most caudal pair of glands, may occur secondary to milk stasis. Inflammatory cells will be present in variable numbers without accompanying bacteria.[8] Focal, nonseptic inflammatory nodules may occur secondary to lobular hyperplasia. These are characterized by epithelial metaplasia, pigment-laden macrophages, nondegenerate neutrophils, lymphocytes, and plasma cells.[7]

Cysts: Mammary cysts result from a dysplastic process in which dilated ducts expand to form large cavitations.[6] Cyst linings may consist of single layers of flattened epithelium or may have papillary projections. Cysts may be

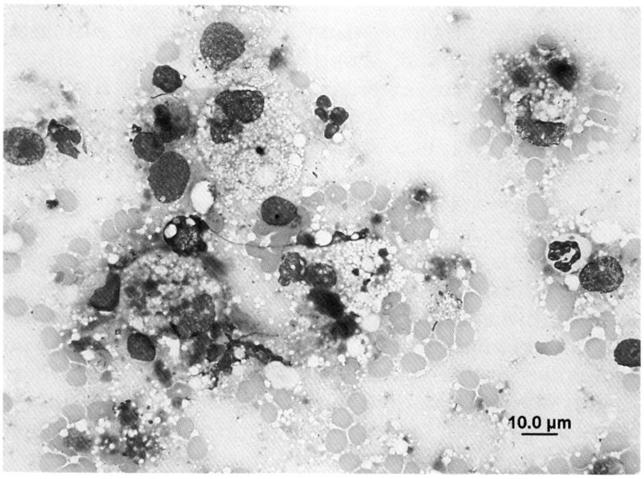

Figure 6-3 Aspirate from an inflamed mammary gland contains macrophages, foam cells, and neutrophils with amorphous basophilic secretory material in the background. (Wright stain, 1000×.)

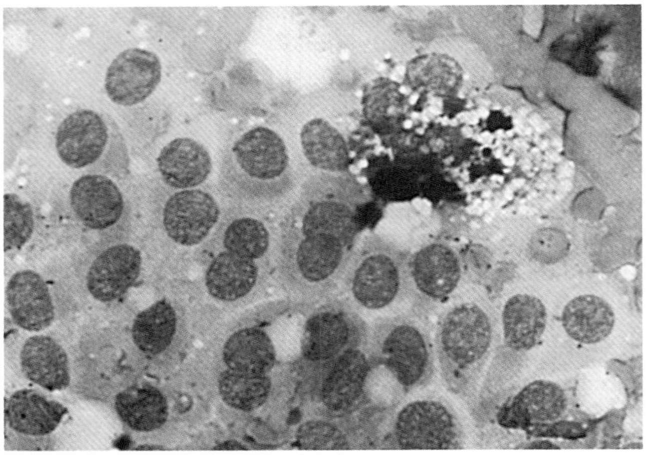

Figure 6-4 Sheet of glandular cells exhibiting little nuclear or cytoplasmic pleomorphism and a fine granular chromatin pattern characteristic of a mammary adenoma. A large, pigment-laden macrophage is present. (Wright stain, 1250×.)

present as single nodules or multinodular masses that grow slowly and have a bluish surface. Cysts are common in middle-aged and older female dogs, but may occasionally appear in young dogs. Fluid aspirated is usually yellow, brown, green, or blood-tinged and of low cellularity unless concurrent inflammation is present. Cells are primarily vacuolated or pigment-laden macrophages. Epithelial cells aspirated from cysts lined by papillary projections may occur in dense clusters and exhibit a minor degree of nuclear pleomorphism.[7] Because mammary cysts may be present along with benign or malignant neoplasia, sampling of solid tissue in addition to cystic fluid is recommended.

Solid Masses: Dysplastic lesions and benign epithelial neoplasms of mammary tissue include lobular hyperplasia, adenosis, adenomas, and papillomas, all of which contain similar cell populations.[7,9] Smears made from aspirates contain many epithelial cells occurring singly or arranged in sheets and clusters. These cells generally exhibit little pleomorphism, having evenly dispersed chromatin and small, round nucleoli. However, dilated ducts can contain exfoliated epithelial cells that may have more criteria of malignancy than the rest of the mass.[10] Sampling those cells for cytologic evaluation may result in a false impression of malignancy. Pigment-laden macrophages may be present (Figure 6-4). Some of these processes can also involve myoepithelial cells and connective tissue, further complicating the cytologic picture.[9] Benign tumors involving stromal and epithelial elements, for example, complex adenomas (Figure 6-5), fibroadenomas, and benign mixed tumors, are common in dogs and sometimes seen in cats.[7,9] Smears of aspirates from these lesions contain spindle-shaped cells of myoepithelial or connective tissue origin, in addition to clusters of epithelial cells similar to those described previously (Figure 6-6). These lesions can be difficult to differentiate even with histopathology because of the spectrum of cell types involved. Benign mixed tumors may produce cartilage, bone, or fat, in addition to fibrous tissue and epithelial tissue.[9] Aspirates from these lesions may contain all these elements, but if a single population predominates, the cytology can be misleading.[11] Additionally, individual cell pleomorphism is occasionally marked in tumors considered benign because of lack of tissue invasion (Figures 6-7 and 6-8).[5] Spindled mesenchymal cells are not a definitive cytologic characteristic of complex or mixed tumors because they may also be found in some simple tumors.[2]

A specific form of mammary hyperplasia, termed *fibroepithelial hyperplasia* or fibroadenomatous change, has been recognized in cats. This condition may affect young female cats that are pregnant or actively cycling or cats of

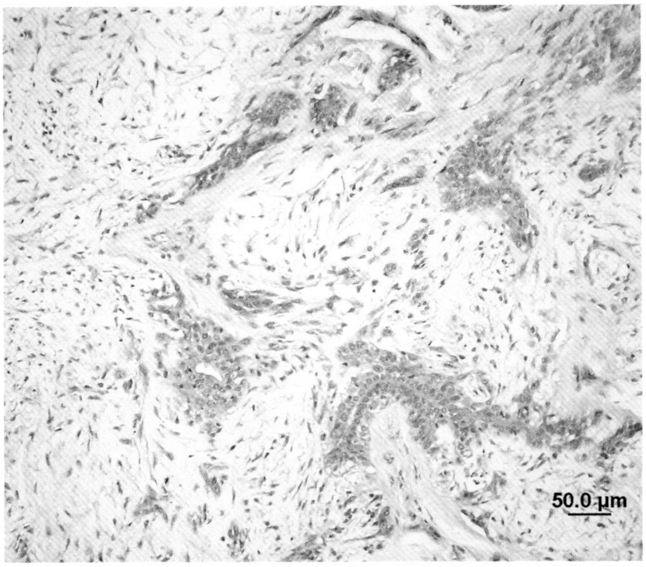

Figure 6-5 Biopsy of a benign mammary complex adenoma from a dog contains mixed mesenchymal and epithelial components. Aspirates from this mass are shown in Figures 6-6, 6-7, and 6-8. (H&E, 200×.)

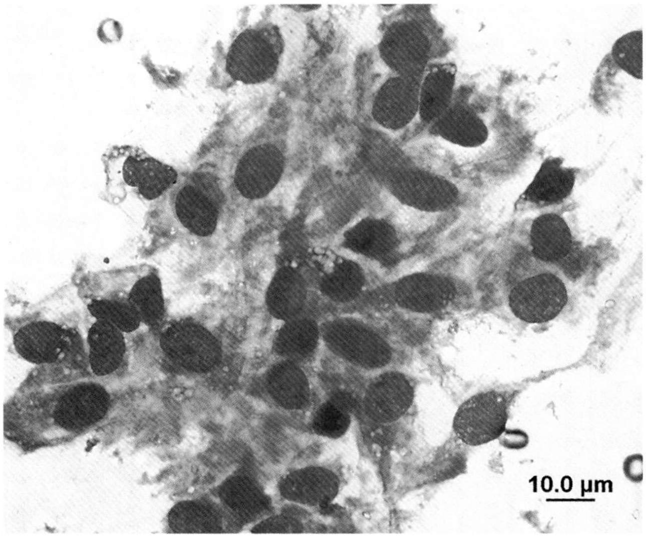

Figure 6-6 Spindled cells and eosinophilic extracellular matrix in an aspirate of a benign mammary complex adenoma from a dog, same case as Figure 6-5. (Wright stain, 1000×.)

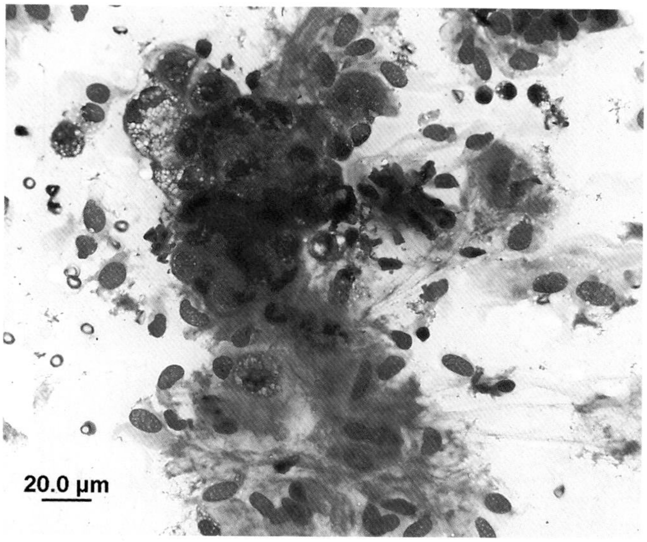

Figure 6-7 Canine mammary complex adenoma, same aspirate as Figure 6-6. Abundant eosinophilic matrix material and spindled mesenchymal cells near a cluster of vacuolated mammary epithelial cells. Epithelial cells exhibit moderate criteria of malignancy. (Wright stain, 500×.)

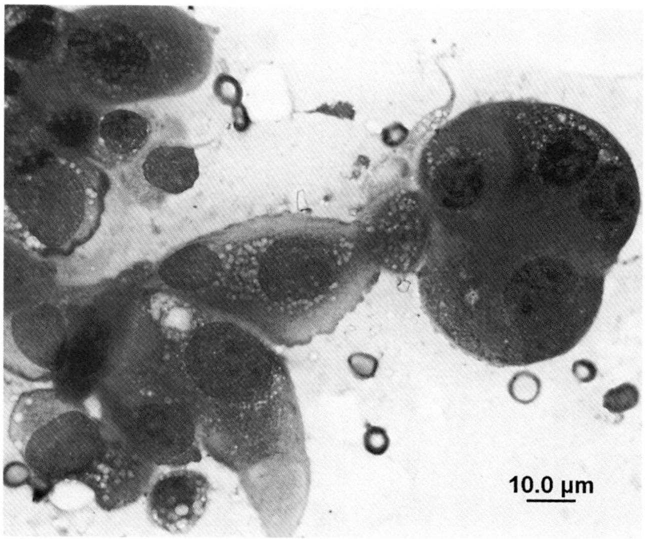

Figure 6-8 Canine mammary complex adenoma, same aspirate as Figure 6-6. These epithelial cells exhibit moderate to marked criteria of malignancy including anisocytosis, anisokaryosis, and multiple prominent nucleoli. Histopathology revealed this tumor to be well-encapsulated and benign, despite individual cell pleomorphism. (Wright stain, 1000×.)

either gender that have received progesterone-containing compounds.[12,13] Typically, rapid enlargement of multiple glands occurs. Aspirates from affected mammary glands contain both uniform epithelial cells and spindled mesenchymal cells, usually associated with abundant pink extracellular matrix material.[14] The epithelial cells are of ductal origin and have a relatively high nucleus-to-cytoplasm (N:C) ratio with dense, round nuclei and a small amount of basophilic cytoplasm. The mesenchymal cells may exhibit moderate anisocytosis and anisokaryosis.[14] Ovariohysterectomy or removal of the progesterone-containing compound is generally curative. Drug therapy with a progesterone antagonist has also been an effective treatment.[15]

Malignant Neoplasms

Mammary gland tumors are common in both dogs and cats; however, the biologic behavior of the tumors varies greatly between these species. Mammary tumors comprise up to 50% of neoplasms in the canine female, and 40% to 50% of those tumors are malignant, with adenocarcinomas the most common histologic type.[7,16] Mammary tumors are the third most common neoplasm in cats and account for about 17% of all neoplasms in queens.[9] In contrast to dogs, up to 80% of feline mammary gland tumors are malignant. Similar to dogs, adenocarcinomas are diagnosed most frequently.[17,18] Mammary tumors are rare in males of both species.[7,19]

A new histologic classification and grading scheme was proposed for canine mammary tumors in 2011.[6] Significant criteria recognized for the diagnosis of malignant canine mammary tumors include tumor type, degree of pleomorphism, mitotic index, presence of necrosis, peritumoral or lymphatic invasion, and regional lymph node metastasis.[6] Multiple morphologic types of carcinoma are recognized histologically on the basis of the pattern of cell arrangement and degree of cell differentiation.[6,9] Carcinomas are also graded on the basis of histologic features such as tubule formation, mitotic rate, and cell pleomorphism. Many different types of carcinomas may contain collagenous stroma, sometimes in large amounts. Both histologic type and grade, as well as degree of invasion, have been shown to have prognostic significance in dogs.[6,20] Dogs frequently have multiple tumors, which are often of different histologic types.[16] A study by Sorenmo et al. provided evidence that canine mammary tumors may progress from benign to malignant over time and showed a strong association between tumor size and malignancy.[21] In cats with mammary carcinomas, tumor size has been shown to be the single most important prognostic factor.[18,22]

Cytologic criteria that best correlate with malignancy include variable nuclear size, nuclear giant forms, high N:C ratio, variable numbers of nucleoli, abnormal nucleolar shape, and the presence of macronucleoli (Figures 6-9 and 6-10).[2] However, as previously discussed, mammary malignancies may be well differentiated and show little cellular pleomorphism, and moderate criteria of malignancy may be present in tumors considered benign because of lack of tissue invasion.[6] Smears of aspirates from adenocarcinomas generally contain epithelial cells occurring singly and in clusters of variable size. Adenocarcinoma cells are usually round, with round to oval, eccentrically placed nuclei and variable quantities of basophilic cytoplasm that occasionally contains vacuoles that may be filled with secretory product (Figure 6-11). Cell borders are usually distinct, and cells may be arranged in acinar or tubular patterns. Binucleate or multinucleate cells may be seen. Mesenchymal cells may be present in variable numbers. Necrosis, readily identifiable in histologic sections, may also be observed in cytologic samples from

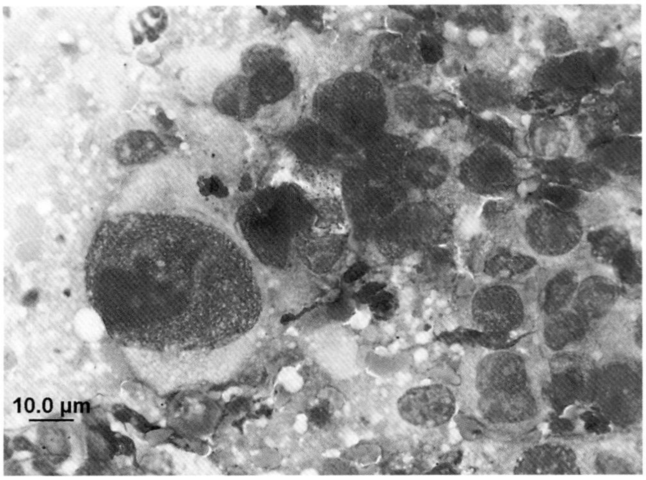

Figure 6-9 Epithelial cells from a feline mammary carcinoma have marked variation in cell and nuclear morphology. One large nucleus contains an abnormally shaped macronucleolus. (Wright stain, 1000×.)

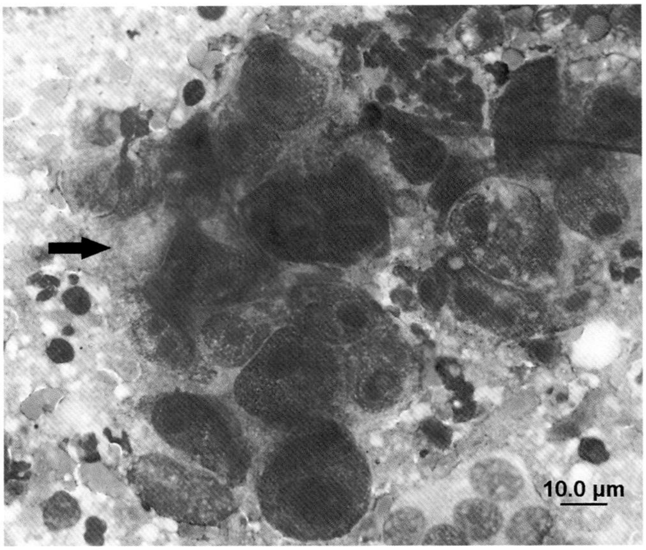

Figure 6-11 Aspirate from a feline mammary carcinoma. Eosinophilic secretory product is visible within the cytoplasm of one cell (*arrow*). (Wright stain, 1000×.)

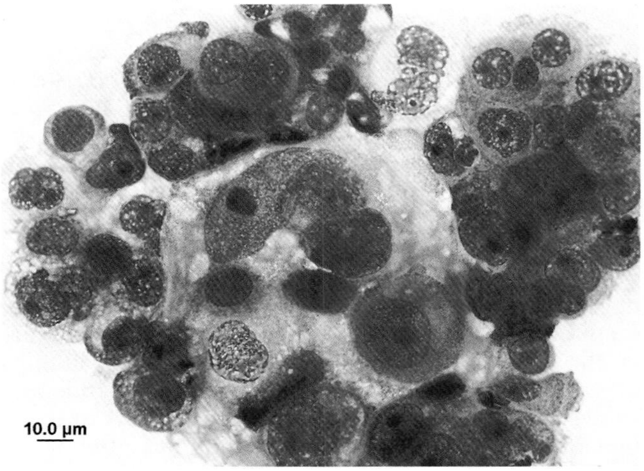

Figure 6-10 Pleural fluid from the same cat as Figure 6-9 contains tightly cohesive clusters of epithelial cells with marked criteria of malignancy, confirming presence of intrathoracic metastatic disease. (Wright stain, 1000×.)

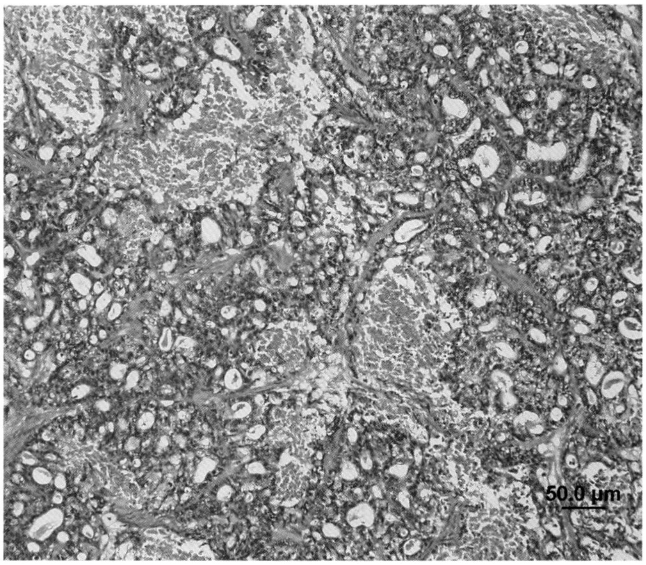

Figure 6-12 Biopsy of a ductular adenocarcinoma from a cat. Pale pink areas represent necrosis randomly distributed between neoplastic epithelial cells. Aspirates of this mass are shown in Figure 6-13. (H&E, 200×.)

malignant tumors, appearing as amorphous smudged basophilic material (Figures 6-12 and 6-13).

Anaplastic carcinomas are diffusely infiltrative tumors composed of large, pleomorphic epithelial cells with bizarre nuclear and nucleolar forms (Figure 6-14).[6,9] These cells occur singly and in variably sized clusters and have a high N:C ratio (Figure 6-15). Multinucleate cells and mitotic figures are common (Figures 6-16 and 6-17). These tumors may contain abundant collagenous stroma infiltrated by inflammatory cells.[6,9] Anaplastic carcinomas are considered highly malignant, frequently metastasize, and have a poor prognosis.

Inflammatory carcinomas have distinctive clinical and histologic features and are aggressive tumors associated with a poor prognosis.[23,24] These tumors may be clinically misdiagnosed as mastitis because of the marked local tissue swelling and edema with signs of systemic disease; however, inflammatory cells are not a prominent histologic feature. Inflammatory carcinomas have been reported in dogs and cats, with a variety of histologic types represented.[23-26] In one report, cytology of mammary gland aspirates revealed malignant epithelial cells in 15 of 33 dogs and contributed to the diagnosis; the other 18 cytologic samples had low cellularity.[25] The hallmark of inflammatory carcinoma is the histologic finding of dermal lymphatic involvement.[6,25]

Nonglandular carcinomas may be simple, with only epithelial proliferation, or complex, with cells of epithelial and myoepithelial origin. Accordingly, cytology

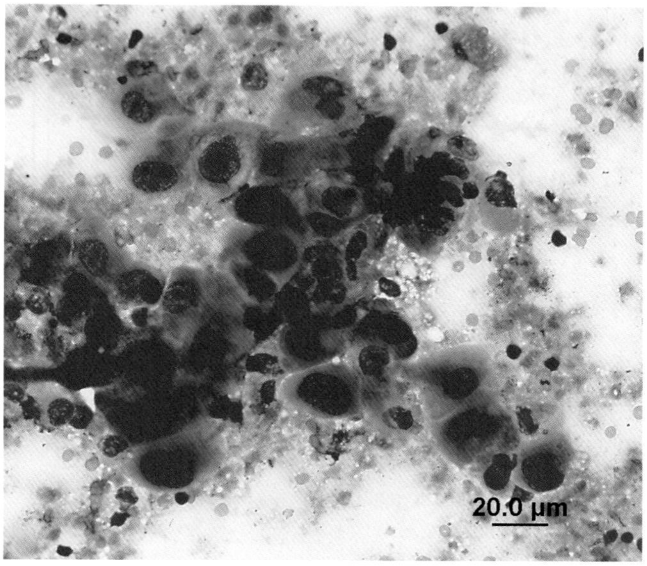

Figure 6-13 Aspirate of a ductular adenocarcinoma from a cat, same case as Figure 6-12. Pleomorphic cohesive malignant epithelial cells are present in an amorphous basophilic background of necrotic material. (Aqueous Romanowsky stain, 500×.)

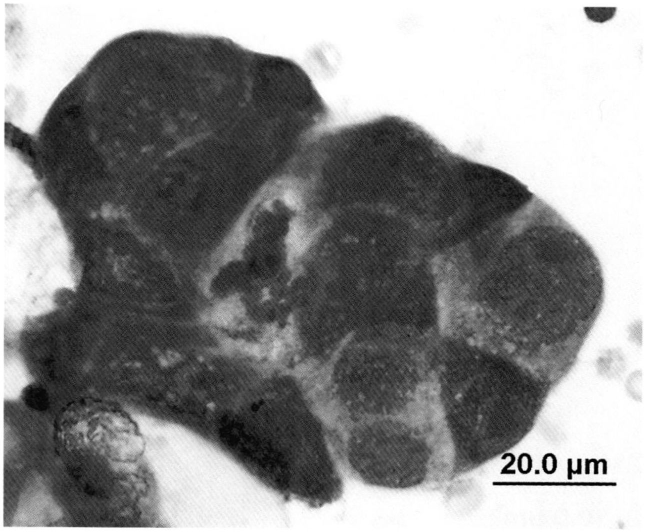

Figure 6-15 Aspirate of an anaplastic mammary carcinoma from a dog, same case as Figure 6-14. Cohesive cluster of malignant mammary epithelial cells with a high nucleus to cytoplasm ratio and multiple prominent nucleoli. A mitotic figure is visible in the center of the cluster. (Wright stain, 1000×.)

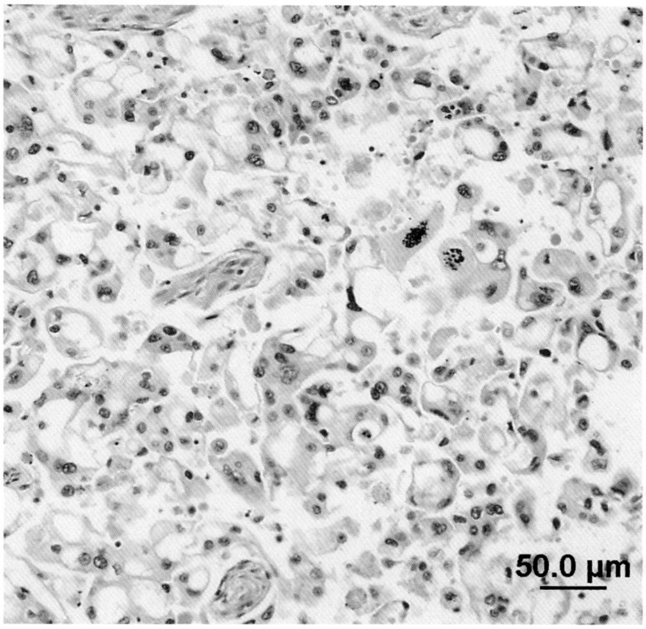

Figure 6-14 Biopsy of an anaplastic mammary carcinoma from a dog. These cells are markedly pleomorphic and variably cohesive. Aspirates from this mass are shown in Figures 6-15, 6-16, and 6-17. (H&E, 200×.)

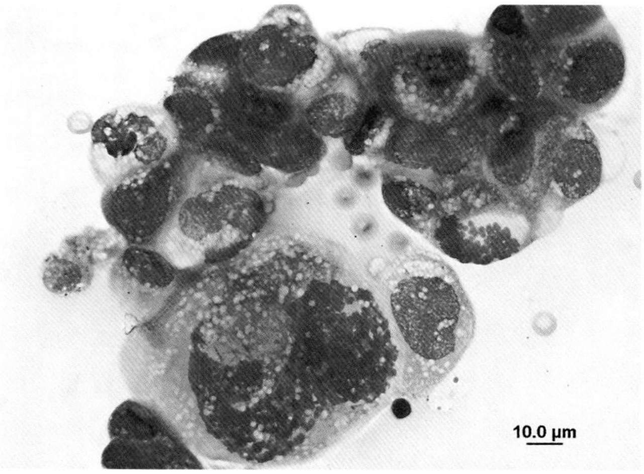

Figure 6-16 Anaplastic mammary carcinoma, same aspirate as Figure 6-15. Malignant epithelial cells have cytoplasmic vacuoles in this cluster, and two mitotic figures are present. (Wright stain, 1000×.)

samples may contain predominantly epithelial cells or a mixture of cell types. In contrast to adenocarcinomas, epithelial cells from nonglandular carcinomas may not contain intracytoplasmic vacuoles (Figure 6-18). Squamous cell carcinomas in mammary glands appear cytologically similar to those in other body regions. Tumor cells occur singly or in small sheets and may be keratinized or nonkeratinized. Nuclei are variable in size, from small and pyknotic to large with immature chromatin and prominent nucleoli. Cytoplasm is variably abundant and basophilic, appearing glassy and blue-green with keratinization (see Chapter 5 for further discussion of the features of squamous cell carcinoma). These tumors frequently adhere to the overlying dermis and may be ulcerated, leading to the presence of many inflammatory cells and bacteria in samples taken from ulcerated areas. It is important to realize that squamous metaplasia may occur in other tumor types; thus, finding squamous cells on a cytologic sample is not specific for squamous cell carcinoma (Figure 6-19).[6,9,10]

Mammary sarcomas are less common than carcinomas. They are usually large, firm tumors that have an un-

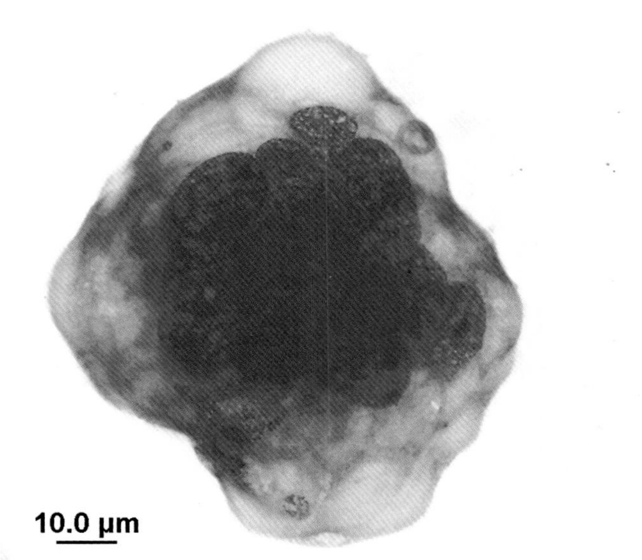

Figure 6-17 A large multinucleated epithelial cell from the same anaplastic mammary carcinoma as Figure 6-15. Note the nuclear fragments visible in the cytoplasm. (Wright stain, 1000×.)

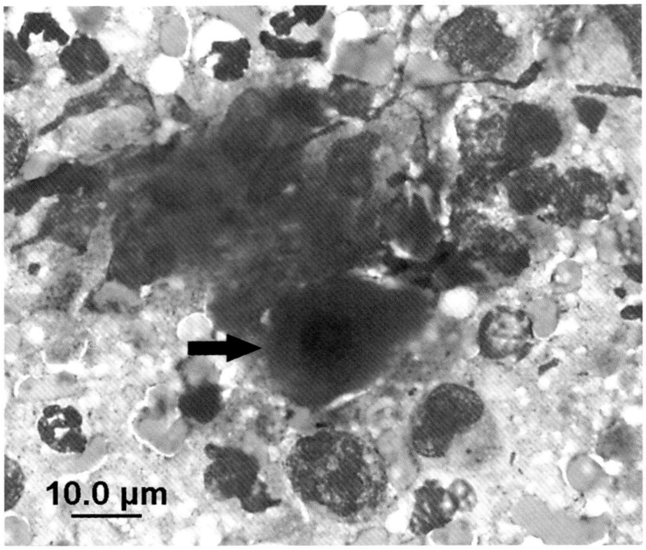

Figure 6-19 Aspirate from a feline mammary carcinoma. A single cell contains glassy dark-blue cytoplasm and angular cytoplasm (*arrow*), consistent with squamous differentiation. (Wright stain, 1000×.)

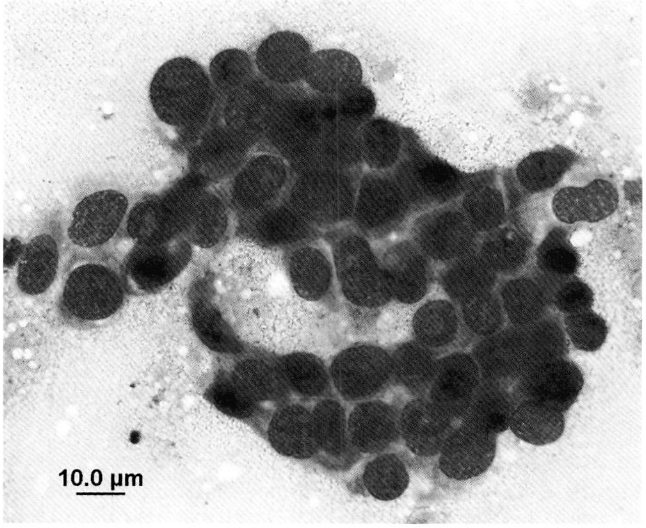

Figure 6-18 These cohesive epithelial cells from an aspirate of a canine papillary mammary carcinoma have no cytoplasmic vacuoles and minimal cellular atypia, emphasizing the need for histopathologic confirmation when neoplasia is suspected. (Wright stain, 1000×.)

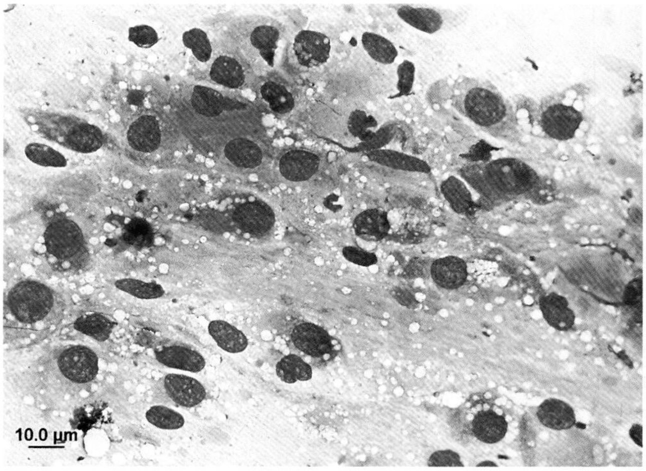

Figure 6-20 Spindled cells and extracellular matrix in an aspirate of a malignant mixed mammary gland tumor in a dog. (Wright stain, 1000×.) (Glass slide courtesy of Boone et al., Texas A&M University, presented at the 2000 ASVCP case review session.)

favorable prognosis because of local recurrence and metastasis.[9] Osteosarcoma is the most frequent type in the dog.[6] Cells from sarcomas are often irregular or spindle shaped, occur singly or in small aggregates, and have indistinct cell borders. Pink matrix material may be associated with cell aggregates. The degree of pleomorphism and mitotic activity is variable and indicative of tumor malignancy. In general, cytologic criteria of malignancy described for carcinomas apply to sarcomas. Because mesenchymal cells, collagenous stroma, cartilage, and even bone formation may also be found in benign mixed tumors, mixed-type carcinomas and carcinosarcomas, cytologic interpretation of these cell populations may be confusing (Figures 6-20 and 6-21).[6,11] Histologically (and presumably cytologically), fibrosarcoma may be confused with other spindle cell neoplasms (spindle cell carcinoma, malignant myoepithelioma). Immunohistochemistry is required for differentiation.[6] Carcinosarcomas (malignant mixed mammary tumors) are uncommon tumors of mixed origin, containing both malignant epithelial and malignant mesenchymal populations.[6,9]

Table 6-1 presents a summary of the most common cytologic findings in aspirates from mammary lesions.

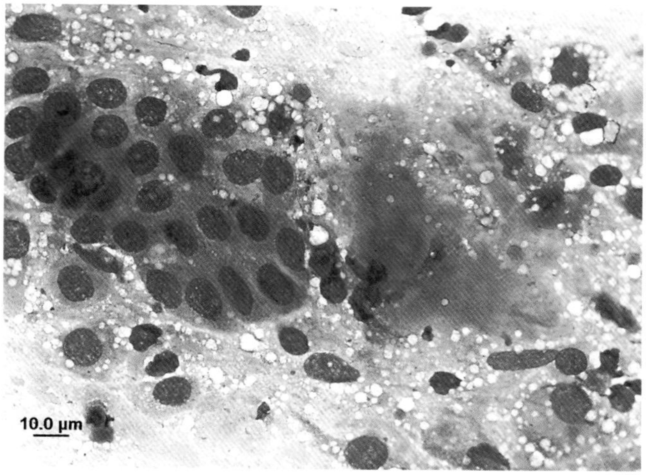

Figure 6-21 Malignant mixed mammary gland tumor, same aspirate as Figure 6-20. A few clusters of well-differentiated epithelial cells and an abundance of spindled cells and extracellular matrix. Despite the lack of cellular pleomorphism, neoplastic epithelial cells within lymphatics and evidence of metastases to lung and lymph node confirmed malignancy in this case. (Wright stain, 1000×.)

SALIVARY GLANDS

Normal Cytologic Appearance

The major salivary glands in dogs and cats are the parotid, mandibular, sublingual, and zygomatic glands. Minor, or buccal, salivary glands are spread over the oral mucosa. Salivary glands are composed of secretory cells arranged in acini and an extensive ductular network. A layer of myoepithelial cells lies between the glandular cells and basement membrane. Aspirated samples from normal salivary glands reveal secretory epithelial cells with small, round nuclei and abundant cytoplasm distended with clear vacuoles. Acinar cells usually occur in clusters (Figure 6-22). When seen individually, these cells are difficult to differentiate from foamy macrophages. Ductal epithelial cells are seen less frequently and have a higher N:C ratio (Figure 6-23). Basophilic mucin may be present in the background. Samples may also include occasional spindle-shaped myoepithelial cells, adipocytes, and lipid droplets. Hemorrhage is frequent upon aspiration of salivary glands. Erythrocytes in smears assume a characteristic linear pattern (windrowing) caused by the mucin content of the sample.

TABLE 6-1

COMMON CYTOLOGIC FINDINGS IN MAMMARY GLAND ASPIRATES

Cell Types	Key Features	Differential Diagnoses	Comments
Foam cells Inflammatory cells: Neutrophils, lymphocytes, plasma cells, macrophages Epithelial cell clusters	Predominance of inflammatory cells Proteinaceous debris ± Bacteria Epithelial cells may be reactive	Mastitis	Mild atypia in epithelial cells expected with inflammation
Vacuolated macrophages ± Epithelial cell clusters	Low-cellularity fluid aspirated Minimal atypia in epithelial cells	Cyst	Cysts may occur along or with benign or malignant neoplasia Sample solid tissue as well as cystic fluid
Epithelial cell clusters Spindled mesenchymal cells Extracellular matrix	Uniform epithelial cells, high nucleus-to-cytoplasm ratio Mildly pleomorphic mesenchymal cells with abundant matrix	Fibroepithelial hyperplasia	Typically affects young intact female cats, or cats previously treated with progesterone drugs Affects multiple glands Rapid growth Cytologic appearance similar to many benign tumors
Variable numbers of epithelial cells and mesenchymal cells ± Extracellular matrix, cartilage, or bone (osteoblasts) ± Inflammatory cells	Variable depending on specific process Usually mild pleomorphism, but may be moderate to marked	Benign neoplasia (adenoma/complex adenoma, benign mixed tumors, etc.) Lobular hyperplasia	Multiple possible cell types result in confusing cytology Inflammatory nodules may occur with lobular hyperplasia Tumors exfoliating numerous atypical cells may suggest malignancy despite lack of tissue invasion Histopathologic confirmation required.
Variable numbers of epithelial cells and mesenchymal cells ± Extracellular matrix, cartilage, or bone (osteoblasts) ± Inflammatory cells	Variable depending on specific process Cellular pleomorphism can be minimal or marked	Malignant neoplasia (adenocarcinoma, various carcinomas, inflammatory carcinoma, fibrosarcoma, osteosarcoma, etc.)	Canine: ~50% are malignant Feline: ~80% are malignant Multiple possible cell types result in confusing cytology Marked pleomorphism increases likelihood of malignancy Tumors with minimal atypia may be malignant based on tissue invasion Histopathologic confirmation required

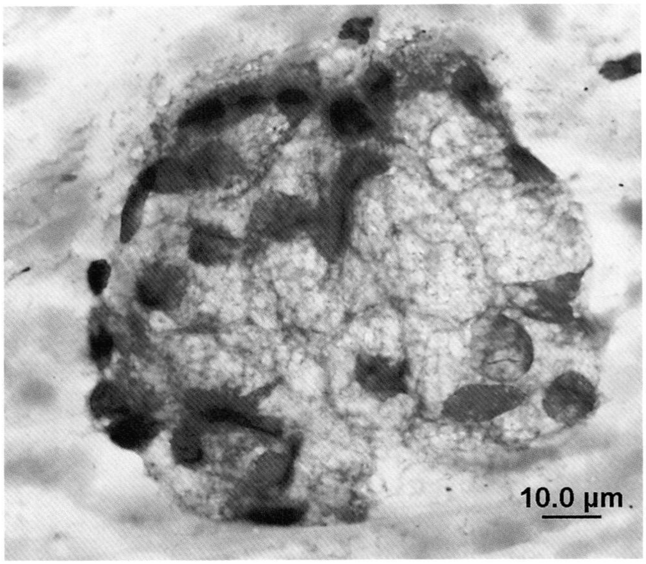

Figure 6-22 Cohesive cluster of vacuolated secretory cells from a normal salivary gland. (Wright stain, 1000×.)

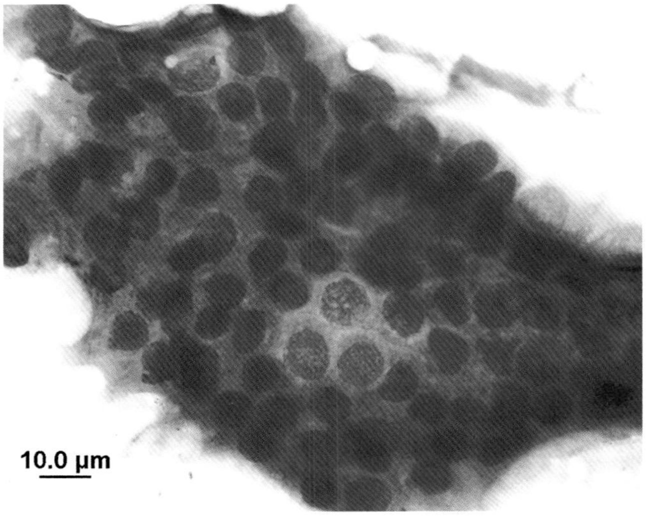

Figure 6-23 Sheet of nonsecretory epithelial cells with a high nucleus to cytoplasm ratio from a normal salivary gland most likely represent ductal epithelium. (Wright stain, 1000×.)

Nonneoplastic Lesions

Sialoceles: The most common salivary gland disorder in dogs is the sialocele.[27] These are nonepithelial-lined cavities filled with salivary secretions. Leakage of salivary secretions into fascial tissues usually follows blunt trauma but may occasionally be secondary to calculi or duct obstruction by bite wounds, abscesses, and ear canal surgery. Swellings occur most commonly on the floor of the mouth (ranulae) or the cranial cervical area and less frequently in pharyngeal or retrobulbar areas. Aspirated fluid is viscous, clear, or blood tinged and contains low to moderate numbers of nucleated cells.

Cytologic evaluation of sialocele aspirates usually reveals diffuse or irregular clumps of homogeneous eosinophilic to basophilic mucin. Large phagocytic cells with small, round nuclei and abundant foamy cytoplasm may be found individually or in small clusters (Figure 6-24). Salivary gland epithelial cells may be present but are not easily distinguished from macrophages cytologically. Erythrocytes often occur in linear patterns (windrows) because of the mucin content. Nondegenerate neutrophils are present in variable numbers, depending on the extent of the inflammatory response. Neutrophil nuclear segmentation may be difficult to appreciate because the cells often do not spread out well in the viscous fluid. Lymphocytes may increase in number with extended duration of the lesion. Macrophages containing phagocytized erythrocytes or debris may also be present. Golden, rhomboidal hematoidin crystals seen extracellularly or within the cytoplasm of macrophages result from erythrocyte degradation secondary to intracyst hemorrhage and suggest chronicity (Figure 6-25).

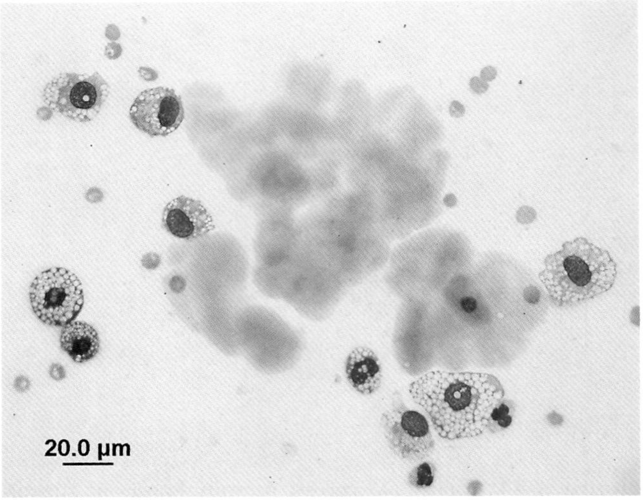

Figure 6-24 Foamy macrophages, vacuolated epithelial cells, or both, and a few erythrocytes from a salivary sialocele. Note the extracellular clumps of amorphous basophilic material, consistent with mucin. (Wright stain, 500×.)

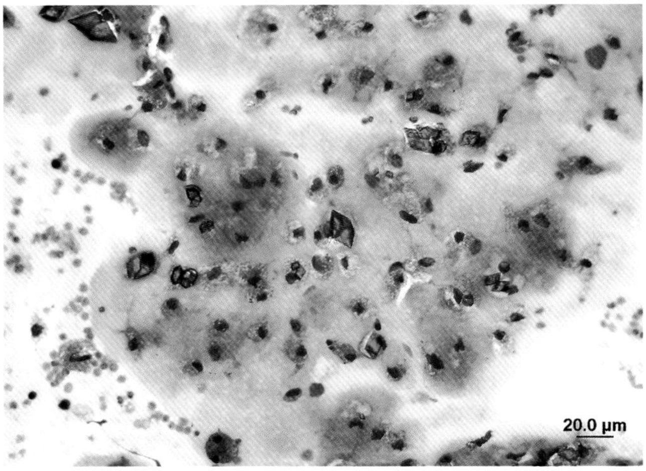

Figure 6-25 Numerous vacuolated cells and large, golden, rhomboidal hematoidin crystals indicating previous hemorrhage in an aspirate from a sialocele. Erythrocytes and basophilic mucin are present in the background. (Wright stain, 500×.)

Sialadenosis: Idiopathic bilateral enlargement of the mandibular salivary glands (sialadenosis) has been reported in both dogs and cats as a cause of excessive salivation.[28-31] Aspirates from affected glands have shown normal salivary epithelium, and histopathologic evaluation has revealed either normal or hypertrophied salivary tissue. Some of these animals have responded to oral phenobarbital therapy, suggesting a neurogenic cause.

Sialadenitis: Inflammatory lesions of the salivary gland are uncommon.[32] Inflammation may be primary or secondary, extending into the gland from surrounding tissues. Primary inflammation is often associated with a sialocele, as described previously, or rarely with infarction. In both situations, mixed inflammatory cells (neutrophils, lymphocytes, and macrophages) may be present.[32] Sialadenitis may occur with systemic viral infections (canine distemper virus, rabies virus, paramyxovirus).[33] Viral lesions may contain significant numbers of lymphoid cells. Secondary inflammation may occur from trauma or bacterial infections in surrounding tissues. The inflammatory cell infiltrate will vary, depending on the primary process. In bacterial infections, degenerate neutrophils with phagocytized bacteria may be observed. Depending on the extent of the infection, salivary epithelial cells may not be evident in cytologic samples.

Neoplastic Lesions

Salivary gland neoplasia is uncommon in dogs and cats. It occurs most frequently in animals older than 10 years, and some evidence suggests that poodles, spaniel breeds, and Siamese cats may be predisposed.[34] Both the parotid and mandibular salivary glands are frequent sites for salivary neoplasia.[32,34] Carcinomas occur most often, and a wide variety of tumor types can be recognized histologically, including acinic cell carcinomas, adenocarcinomas, squamous cell carcinomas, mucoepidermoid tumors, basal cell carcinomas, sebaceous carcinomas, and undifferentiated carcinomas.[35-37] Acinic cell carcinomas and adenocarcinomas represent the most common malignant neoplasms of the salivary glands in dogs and cats (Figure 6-26).[34,35,38]

Cytology samples from salivary carcinomas contain cohesive epithelial cells with round to oval nuclei and basophilic cytoplasm with a relatively high N:C ratio. These cells may show little differentiation toward normal vacuolated salivary epithelium (Figures 6-27 and 6-28).[39] Criteria of malignancy may be mild, consisting only of mild anisocytosis and anisokaryosis, or may be more pronounced with the presence of prominent nucleoli and mitotic figures in addition to marked pleomorphism.[40,41] Eosinophilic secretory product may be seen extracellularly or within the cytoplasm of the neoplastic cells in varying amounts (Figures 6-29 to 6-31).

Squamous epithelial cells can be a component not only of salivary squamous cell carcinomas but also of mucoepidermoid carcinomas and necrotizing sialometaplasia. Salivary squamous cell carcinomas have a similar cytologic appearance to squamous cell carcinomas in other locations (see Chapter 5 for further discussion of the features of squamous cell carcinoma). Mucoepidermoid carcinomas contain both squamous and mucus-producing cell types. The cytologic appearance of necrotizing sialometaplasia has been described, consisting of mixed salivary glandular cells, pleomorphic spindled cells, and rafts of mononuclear epithelioid cells with increased numbers of neutrophils.[42] In that case, the cytologic diagnosis was sialadenitis and possible mesenchymal neoplasia, but histopathology revealed necrosis and ductal squamous metaplasia leading to the final diagnosis. Thus, accurate cytologic interpretation may be limited when multiple cell types are present.

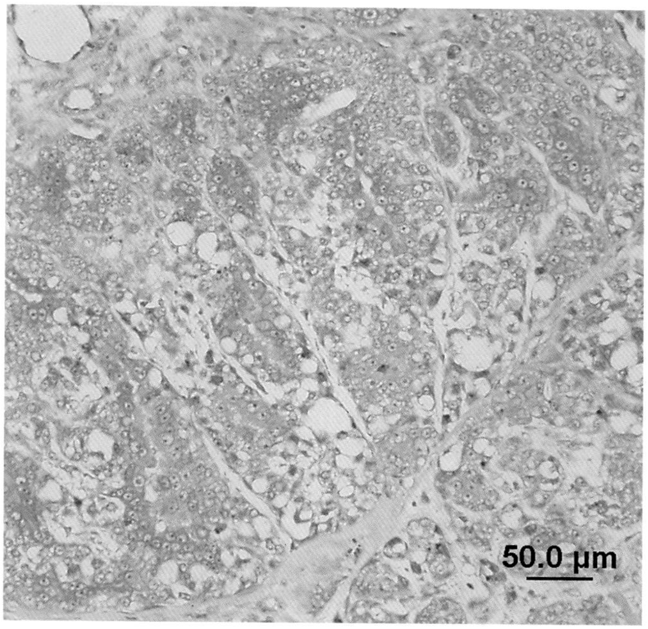

Figure 6-26 Biopsy of a salivary adenocarcinoma from a dog. Aspirates from this mass are shown in Figures 6-29, 6-30, and 6-31. (H&E, 200×.)

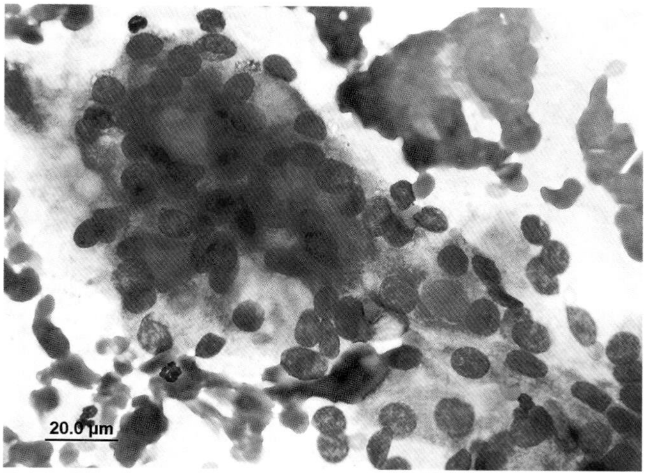

Figure 6-27 Aspirate of a salivary adenocarcinoma from a cat. Cluster of nonvacuolated epithelial cells that have a disorganized appearance and indistinct cell borders. A small amount of eosinophilic secretory product is visible. (Wright stain, 1000×.)

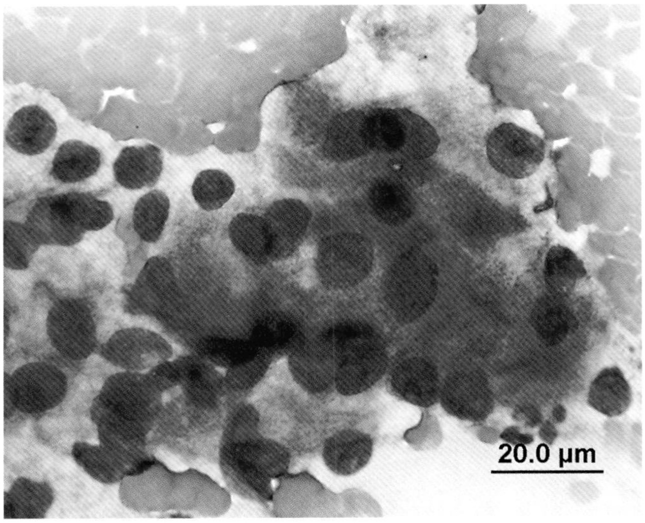

Figure 6-28 **Salivary adenocarcinoma, same aspirate as Figure 6-27.** Granular, eosinophilic, intracytoplasmic secretory material is present within epithelial cells. (Wright stain, 1000×.)

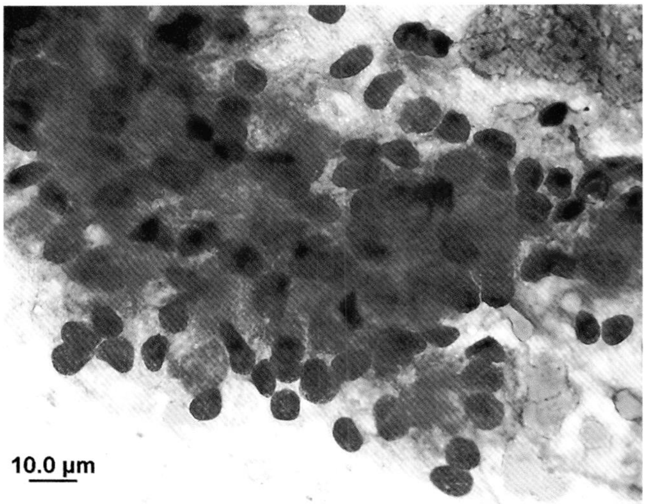

Figure 6-29 Aspirate of a salivary adenocarcinoma from a dog, same case as Figure 6-26, contains abundant extracellular secretory material and monomorphic epithelial cells. (Wright stain, 1000×.)

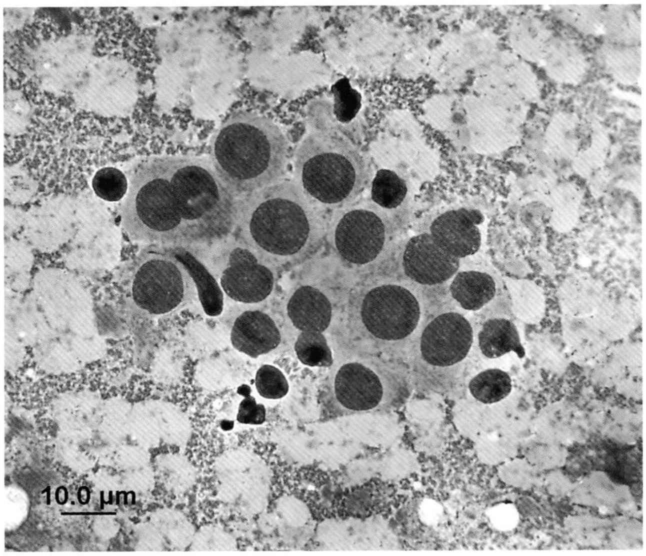

Figure 6-30 **Salivary adenocarcinoma, same aspirate as Figure 6-29.** Individual epithelial cells with round nuclei and lightly basophilic cytoplasm are present in a thick eosinophilic background of secretory material. Cellular pleomorphism is minimal. (Wright stain, 1000×.)

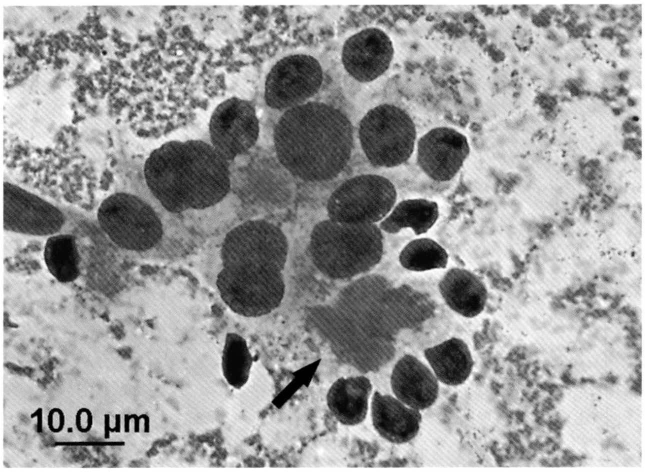

Figure 6-31 **Salivary adenocarcinoma, same aspirate as Figure 6-29.** The arrow indicates a rare acinar structure containing eosinophilic secretory material. (Wright stain, 1000×.)

Malignant mixed tumors of salivary glands are rare, but have been described in both dogs and cats.[35,43,44] These tumors may be the result of carcinoma arising in a previously benign pleomorphic adenoma. Rarely, true carcinosarcomas have been reported, containing both sarcoma and carcinoma elements. Cytology would be expected to reveal a mixture of epithelial and mesenchymal cell types with criteria of malignancy.

Benign salivary tumors are rare in dogs and cats. Pleomorphic adenomas contain epithelial, myoepithelial, and stromal elements and may include areas of cartilage or bone. Sebaceous adenomas and cystadenomas have also been reported.[35]

Table 6-2 presents a summary of the most common cytologic findings in aspirates from salivary gland lesions.

THYROID GLANDS

Normal Cytologic Appearance

The thyroid glands of dogs and cats are paired endocrine glands in the ventral cervical region. Their exact location may vary from the laryngeal region to the thoracic inlet. Ectopic thyroid tissue may also occur in the cranial mediastinum near the heart base. The normal thyroid gland is not readily palpated and is, therefore, not usually aspirated for cytologic examination. Palpable abnormalities may occur unilaterally or bilaterally as diffuse swelling, multinodular swelling, or solitary nodular masses. Aspiration cytology may help differentiate benign lesions from malignant lesions and help rule out other causes of

TABLE 6-2

COMMON CYTOLOGIC FINDINGS IN SALIVARY GLAND ASPIRATES

Cell Types	Key Features	Differential Diagnoses	Comments
Secretory epithelium Background red blood cells (RBCs)	Clusters and individual cells Low nucleus-to-cytoplasm ratio Abundant cytoplasmic vacuoles	Normal salivary tissue Sialadenosis	± Clusters of ductal epithelium (high nucleus-to-cytoplasm ratio, no vacuoles) RBCs often line up (windrowing)
Secretory epithelium and vacuolated macrophages Background RBCs ± Neutrophils, lymphocytes	Viscous sample Abundant amorphous basophilic mucin background	Sialocele	Sialocele may have associated inflammation Hematoidin crystals from previous hemorrhage indicate chronicity
Mostly inflammatory cells (neutrophils, lymphocytes) ± Secretory epithelium ± Bacteria	Cell types vary with cause Degenerate neutrophils suggest bacterial infection	Sialadenitis	May see bacteria phagocytized by neutrophils Epithelial cells may be lacking
Epithelial cell clusters Background RBCs ± Eosinophilic secretory material (intracellular or extracellular)	Clusters of cells with high nuclear-to-cytoplasmic ratio Cells may not be vacuolated Pleomorphism variable	Salivary carcinoma	Carcinomas more common than benign tumors Malignant cells may have few criteria of malignancy, but often do not resemble normal salivary epithelium Histopathologic confirmation desirable

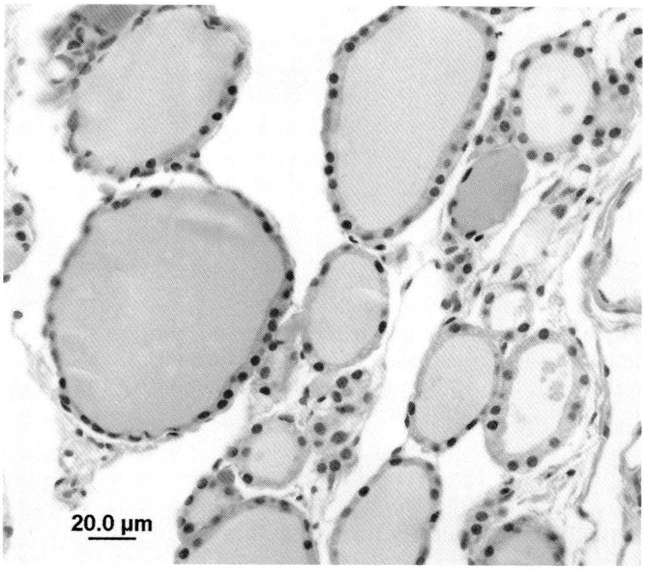

Figure 6-32 Histologic appearance of normal canine thyroid tissue. Follicles are lined by cuboidal epithelium and are filled with eosinophilic colloid. (H&E, 500×.)

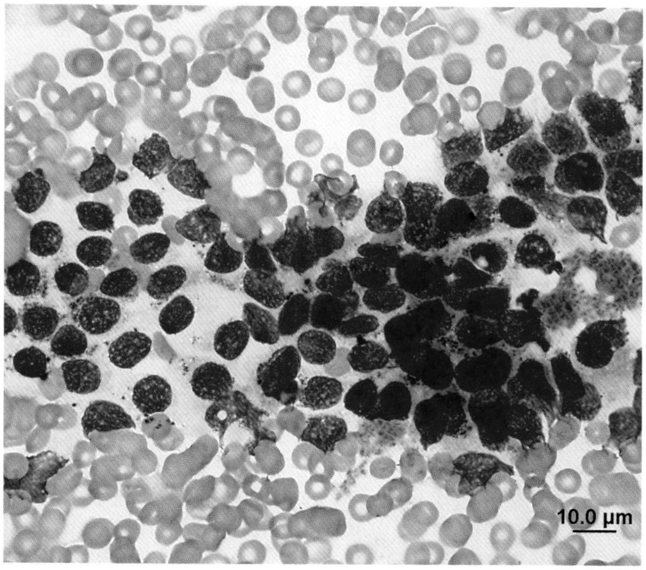

Figure 6-33 Sheet of normal canine thyroid gland epithelial cells. Cells are slightly disrupted but have central nuclei with clumped chromatin and a small amount of basophilic cytoplasm that sometimes contains blue granular pigment. (Aqueous Romanowsky stain, 1000×.)

cervical masses, including abscesses, lymphadenopathy, sialoceles, and nonthyroid neoplasms.

Thyroid tissue consists of numerous follicles lined by cuboidal to polygonal epithelial cells and filled with colloid (Figure 6-32). Each gland is enclosed in a connective tissue capsule and has a rich vascular supply. Scrapings or imprints of normal thyroid tissue contain clusters of typical follicular epithelial cells (Figure 6-33). Nuclei are of uniform size with finely stippled chromatin and are located centrally in a moderate amount of lightly basophilic, granular cytoplasm. Cytoplasmic borders are indistinct, and many naked nuclei from broken cells are often present. Blue-black granular pigment, thought to represent tyrosine accumulation or thyroglobulin, may be seen within the cytoplasm.[39,45] Large macrophages containing variable amounts of pigment believed to be digested colloid are occasionally seen. Amorphous colloid may be present extracellularly, usually appearing pink but occasionally grayish-blue.

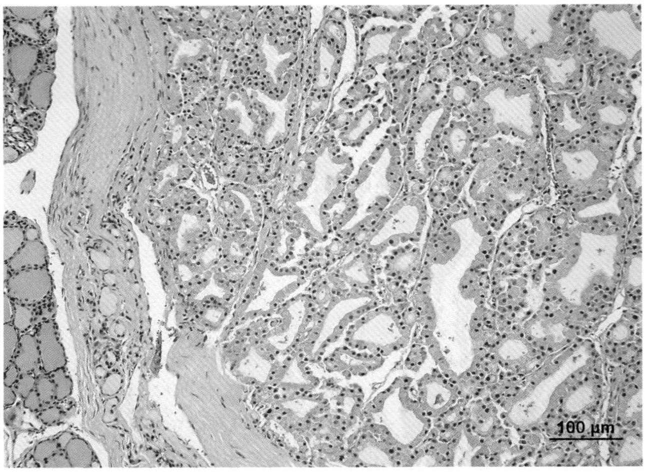

Figure 6-34 Biopsy of a thyroid adenoma from a cat. The benign neoplasm is encapsulated and compressing normal thyroid tissue, visible on the far left. (H&E, 200×.)

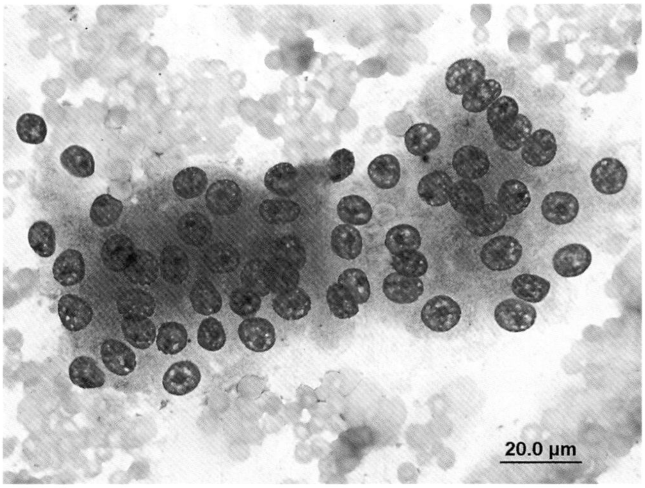

Figure 6-35 Cluster of cells from a feline thyroid adenoma. Cells have monomorphic nuclei and abundant granular cytoplasm. Cells at the edge of the cluster have lysed. (Wright stain, 1000×.)

Benign Lesions

Inflammation: Chronic lymphocytic thyroiditis is an immune-mediated lesion that is a rare cause of thyroid gland enlargement in dogs.[46,47] Dogs with this syndrome usually have no signs of disease in early stages when the thyroid gland is most likely to be enlarged. When clinical signs of hypothyroidism appear, the thyroid gland has usually atrophied, is not palpable, and, therefore, is not aspirated. Affected thyroid glands contain numerous lymphocytes, plasma cells, and macrophages in addition to normal and degenerating follicular cells.

Hyperplasia and Adenoma: Functional multinodular (adenomatous) hyperplasia and functional thyroid adenoma are the most common causes of clinical hyperthyroidism in older cats.[48,49] Distinguishing between the two processes requires histopathologic examination to evaluate compression of adjacent thyroid tissue and presence of a capsule, and it is likely that considerable overlap has occurred in these histologic diagnoses (Figure 6-34). In contrast to these typically functional masses in cats, thyroid adenomas in dogs are less common and generally nonfunctional.[48,50] In dogs, the majority of thyroid adenomas are incidental findings at necropsy. Cytologic specimens have variable cellularity with clusters of follicular cells and scattered naked nuclei as the predominant finding. Aspirates are often bloody because of extensive vascularity. Follicular cells are uniform in appearance, with small round nuclei placed centrally in a moderate amount of basophilic cytoplasm (Figure 6-35). The presence of blue-black intracytoplasmic granules is variable (Figure 6-36). Follicular cells may form acinar arrangements, sometimes surrounding central colloid (Figure 6-37).

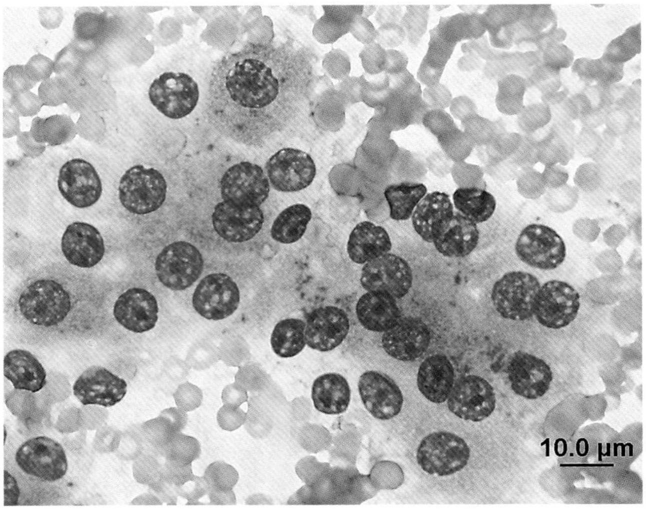

Figure 6-36 Feline thyroid adenoma. Blue intracytoplasmic pigment is present within some of these follicular cells. (Wright stain, 1000×.)

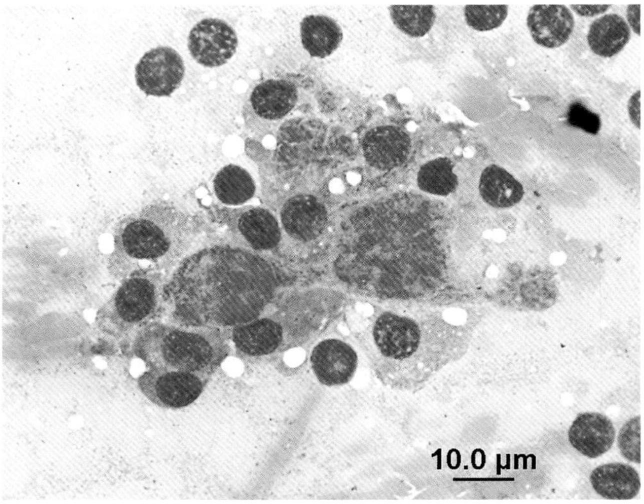

Figure 6-37 An acinar structure surrounding eosinophilic colloid in an aspirate of a thyroid adenoma. Note the naked nuclei and lightly basophilic background from ruptured cells. (Wright stain, 1000×.)

Uncommon causes of thyroid hyperplasia in animals include iodine deficiency, iodine excess, and errors of

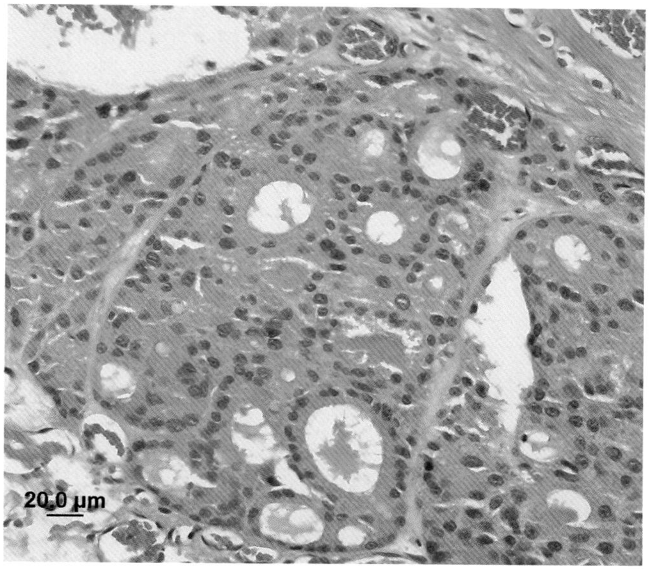

Figure 6-38 Biopsy of a functional follicular thyroid carcinoma from a dog, showing solid areas and a few follicular structures. Aspirates from this mass are shown in Figures 6-39, 6-40, and 6-41. (H&E, 400×.)

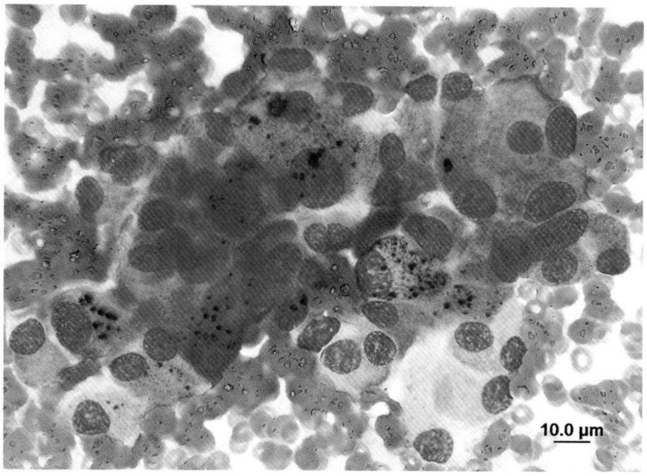

Figure 6-39 Aspirate of a functional follicular thyroid carcinoma from a dog, same case as Figure 6-38. Neoplastic thyroid epithelial cells are present in a cohesive cluster along with abundant erythrocytes. Some of these cells contain blue-black cytoplasmic pigment. These cells exhibit more criteria of malignancy than are typical for most thyroid carcinomas. (Wright stain, 1000×.)

thyroid hormone synthesis (dyshormonogenesis).[48,51,52] Thyroid follicular cells may appear hyperplastic, and the amount of colloid present is variable.[48]

Malignant Neoplasms

The vast majority of clinically evident thyroid tumors in dogs are carcinomas (80% to 90%), in contrast to only 5% in cats.[50] Thyroid carcinomas usually occur in older dogs, with no sex predilection. A breed predisposition has been shown for Boxers, Beagles, and Golden Retrievers.[48] Malignant tumors are poorly encapsulated and usually tightly adherent to underlying tissues because of extensive local invasion. Pulmonary metastases are frequent because of early invasion into thyroid veins.[48] Larger tumors may have a greater potential for metastasis.[53] Areas of mineralization and bone formation may be present within the tumor. Most thyroid carcinomas are nonfunctional in both dogs and cats.

A good correlation between results of aspiration cytology and histopathologic examination has been found with thyroid carcinomas.[54] The problem of excessive blood contamination in many specimens may require repeated aspirations. In the absence of excessive blood contamination, smears tend to be highly cellular and may or may not contain colloid. Follicular thyroid carcinomas yield cells that occur both singly and in dense clusters, sometimes forming acinar structures (Figures 6-38, 6-39 and 6-40). Typical blue-black cytoplasmic granules may be seen, and fine needle–shaped cytoplasmic inclusions

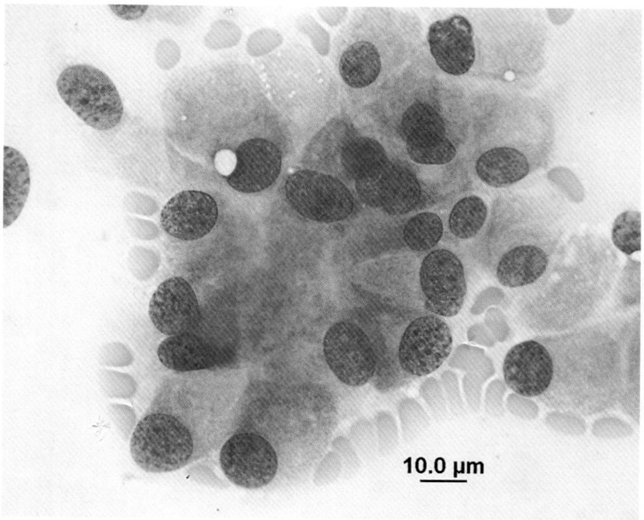

Figure 6-40 Thyroid carcinoma, same aspirate as Figure 6-39. An acinar structure without colloid is present. (Wright stain, 1000×.)

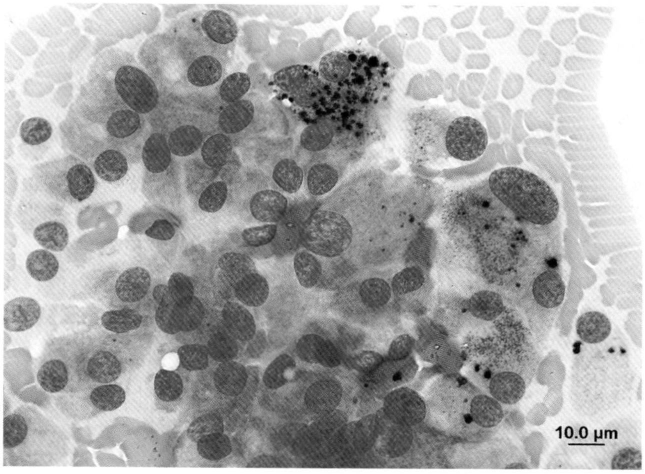

Figure 6-41 Thyroid carcinoma, same aspirate as Figure 6-39. Some cells contain blue-black cytoplasmic pigment, while others do not. (Wright stain, 1000×.)

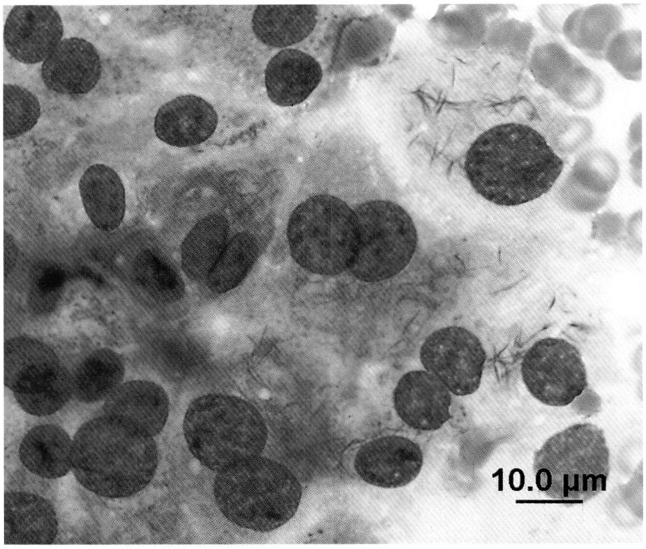

Figure 6-42 Aspirate of a nonfunctional follicular thyroid carcinoma from a dog demonstrating needle-shaped intracytoplasmic inclusions in many cells. The significance of these inclusions is not known. (Wright stain, 1000×.)

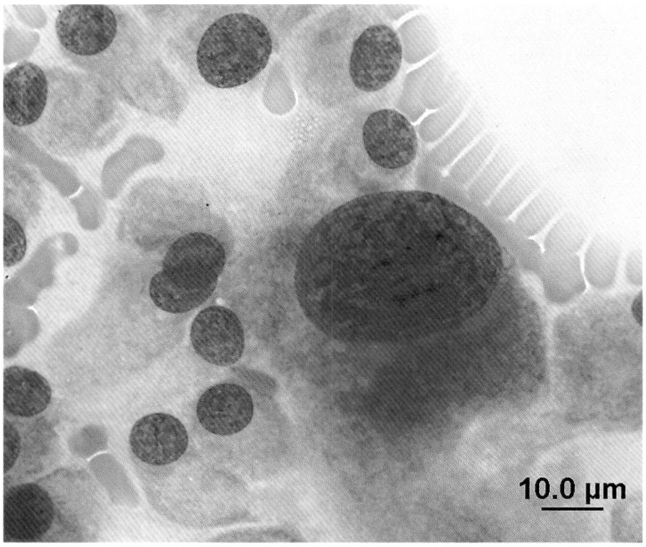

Figure 6-43 Marked anisocytosis and anisokaryosis are present in this aspirate of a follicular thyroid carcinoma from a dog. (Wright stain, 1000×.)

have also been observed (Figures 6-41 and 6-42). Anisocytosis and anisokaryosis are variable. Cytologic criteria of malignancy are subtle or completely lacking in many carcinomas. Nuclei may be mildly enlarged and have indistinct nucleoli; mitotic figures are uncommon. When marked anisocytosis and anisokaryosis are present, a diagnosis of carcinoma can be made with confidence (Figure 6-43). Otherwise, histopathologic evaluation of tumor encapsulation and invasion is required to distinguish adenoma from carcinoma.

Although most carcinomas arise from follicular thyroid epithelium, medullary parafollicular C-cell tumors have also been described in dogs. Previously thought to

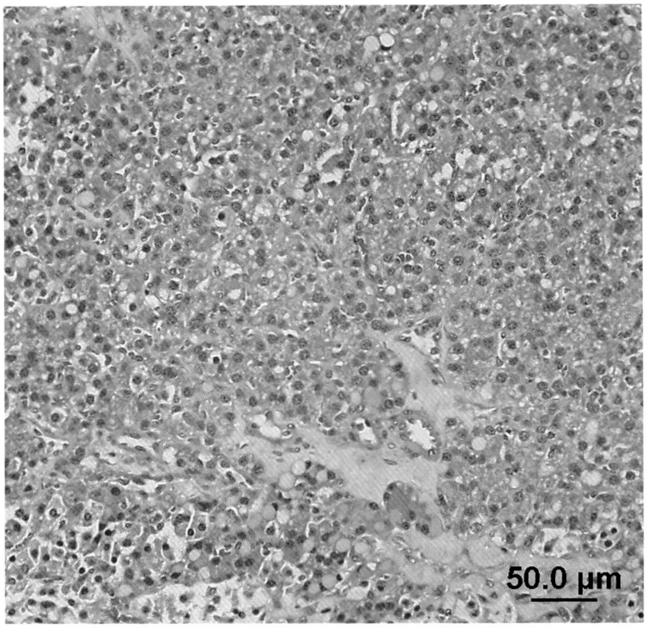

Figure 6-44 Biopsy of a follicular thyroid carcinoma from a dog. Neoplastic cells are present in solid sheets with only rare follicular structures. (H&E, 200×.)

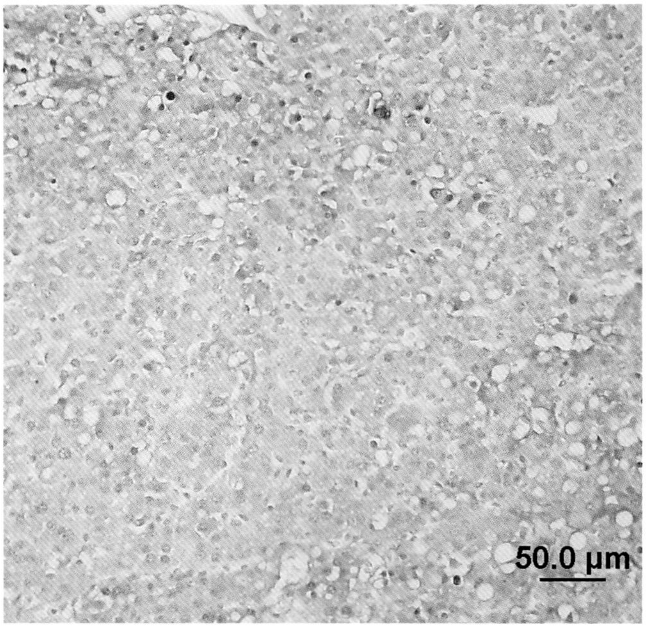

Figure 6-45 Follicular thyroid carcinoma from a dog, same case as Figure 6-44. Neoplastic cells have variable expression of thyroglobulin (brown stain) confirming follicular origin. (Immunohistochemical stain for thyroglobulin, DAB chromagen, hematoxylin counterstain, 200×.)

be uncommon, evidence suggests that medullary carcinomas may be recognized more frequently with increasing use of immunohistochemical stains (thyroglobulin, chromogranin A, and calcitonin).[53,55,56] Follicular tumors are expected to express thyroglobulin (Figures 6-44 and 6-45), and medullary tumors are expected to express calcitonin (Figures 6-46 and 6-47). Because medullary C-cell tumors

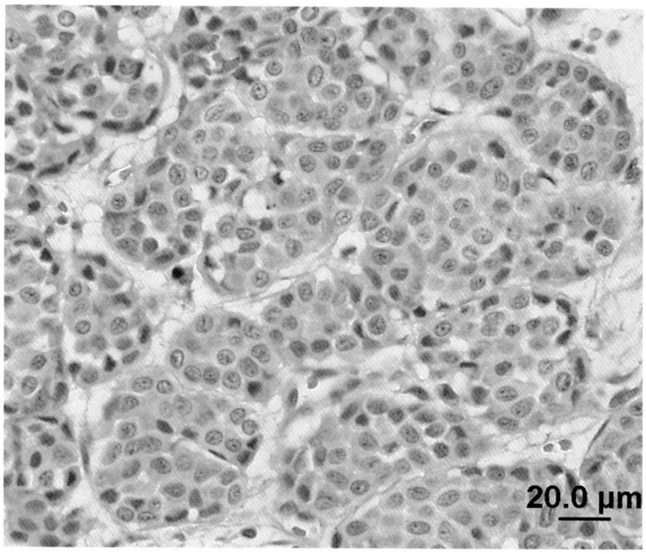

Figure 6-46 Biopsy of a medullary thyroid carcinoma from a dog. Aspirates of this mass are shown in Figures 6-48 and 6-49. (H&E, 400×.)

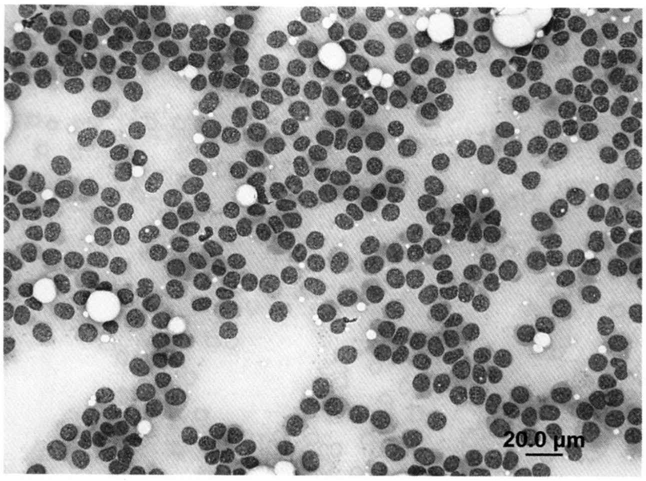

Figure 6-48 Aspirate of a medullary thyroid carcinoma from a dog, same case as Figure 6-46. Neoplastic cells are relatively uniform and present in loose clusters with rare acinar structures. (Aqueous Romanowsky stain, 400×.)

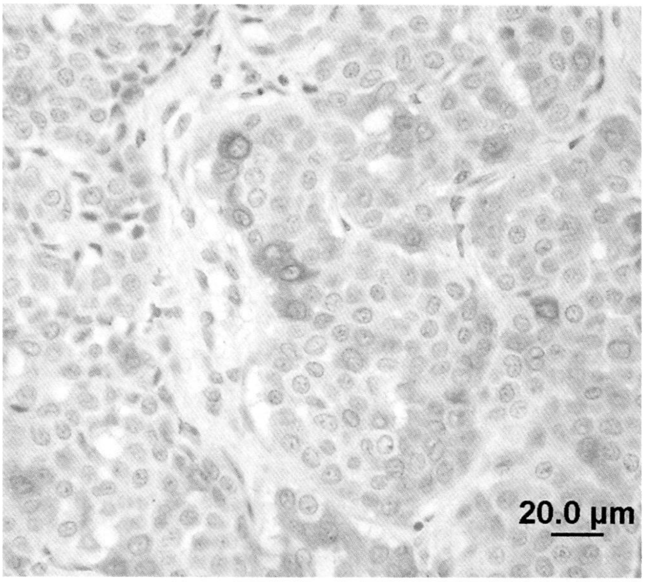

Figure 6-47 Medullary thyroid carcinoma from a dog, same case as Figure 6-46. Neoplastic cells have variable expression of calcitonin (brown stain) confirming C-cell origin. (Immunohistochemical stain for calcitonin, DAB chromagen, hematoxylin counterstain, 400×.)

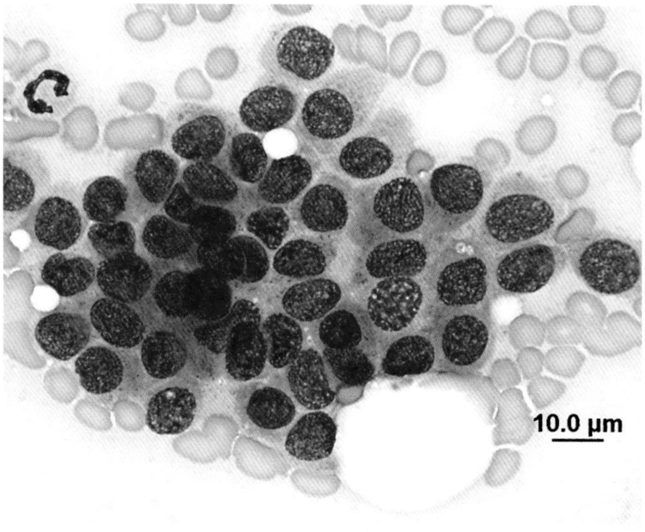

Figure 6-49 Medullary thyroid carcinoma, same aspirate as Figure 6-48. Faint cytoplasmic granulation is visible within this cluster of cells. (Aqueous Romanowsky stain, 1000×.)

tend to be well encapsulated and less likely to metastasize, differentiating them from follicular carcinomas may have prognostic implications.[55] The cytologic features of medullary carcinomas are virtually identical to follicular carcinomas, with epithelial cells occurring in clusters and acinar patterns (Figure 6-48 and 6-49).[57] Pink amorphous material consistent with colloid was observed in one case, but blue-black intracytoplasmic pigment was not.[57]

Undifferentiated carcinomas of the thyroid are rare in dogs and cats.[58] These tumors may contain spindle-shaped cells, suggestive of a sarcoma. Malignant mixed thyroid tumors are also rare, being composed of epithelial and mesenchymal elements (Figures 6-50 and 6-51).[48]

Cystic Lesions

Cystic lesions have been reported in association with both thyroid adenomas and carcinomas in dogs and cats.[48,59-61] Aspirated fluid may appear serous but is more commonly brown and turbid because of previous hemorrhage and necrosis. Foamy, pigment-laden macrophages, lymphocytes, erythrocytes, and occasionally cholesterol crystals are seen along with clusters of follicular cells (Figures 6-52 and 6-53). Thyroid hormone levels in the cystic fluid can be measured to confirm thyroid origin.[60]

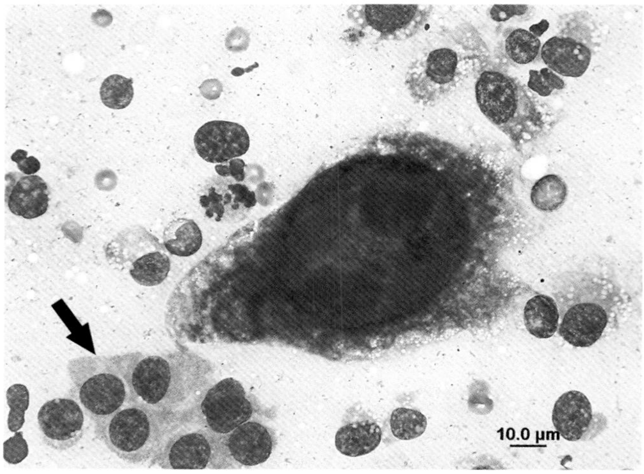

Figure 6-50 A cluster of epithelial cells (*arrow*) and several pleomorphic mesenchymal cells in a malignant mixed thyroid tumor from a dog. (Wright-Giemsa stain, 1000×.) The central mesenchymal cell contains a macronucleus with two macronucleoli. (Glass slide courtesy of Juopperi et al., North Carolina State University, presented at the 2002 ASVCP case review session.)

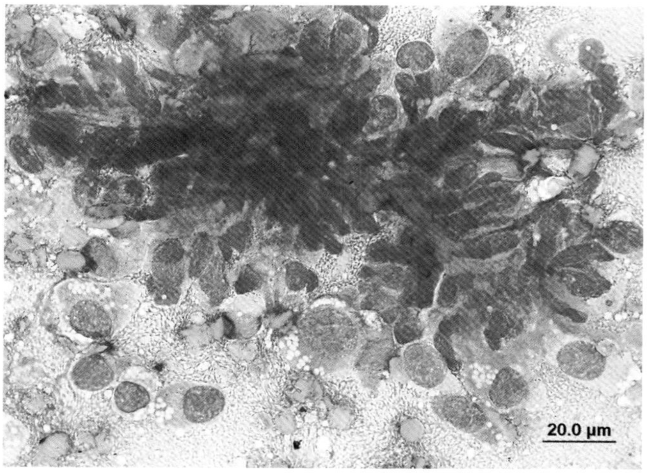

Figure 6-51 This aspirate of a malignant mixed thyroid tumor from a dog contains only pleomorphic mesenchymal cells and abundant extracellular eosinophilic matrix, suggesting a diagnosis of sarcoma. Histopathology revealed neoplastic epithelial cells as well. (Wright stain, 1000×.)

THE PARATHYROID GLANDS

The parathyroid glands are located adjacent to the thyroid glands. Tumors involving the parathyroid chief cells are uncommon but have been reported in both dogs and cats (Figure 6-54).[62-64] Parathyroid tumors in dogs are not usually palpable because of their small size and location but are more often identified with ultrasound during a search for causes of hypercalcemia in animals showing clinical signs of primary hyperparathyroidism.[65] Cats may be more likely to have a palpable parathyroid nodule.[64,66] Adenomas are diagnosed more frequently than carcinomas in both dogs and cats, and either may be

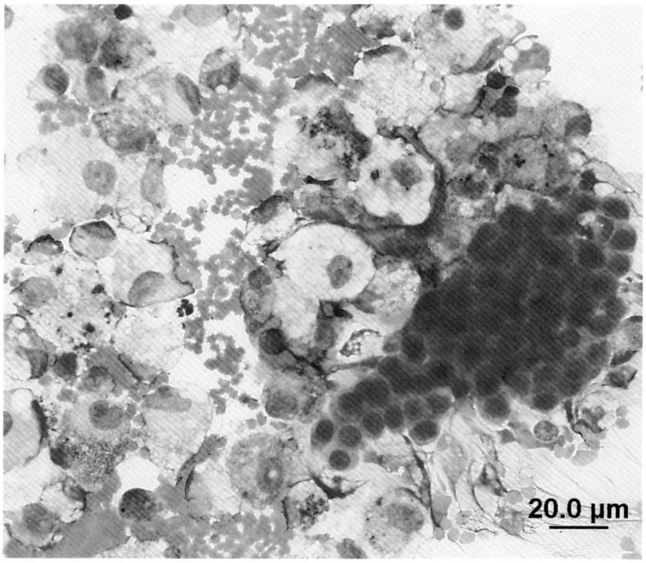

Figure 6-52 Aspirate of a cystic thyroid mass from a cat with hyperthyroidism. A cohesive cluster of thyroid epithelial cells is present along with numerous vacuolated macrophages and erythrocytes. (Wright stain, 1000×.) (Glass slide courtesy of Theresa Rizzi, Oklahoma State University.)

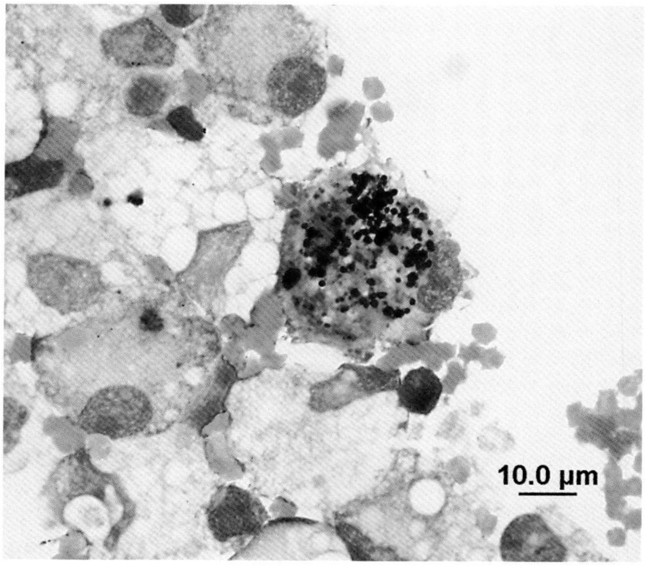

Figure 6-53 Cystic thyroid mass, same aspirate as Figure 6-52. Many macrophages contain blue-black phagocytized pigment, likely representing thyroglobulin. (Wright stain, 1000×.)

functional, producing excess parathormone. Adenomas are usually encapsulated and compress adjacent normal parathyroid and thyroid tissues. Carcinomas are generally larger than adenomas and are fixed to underlying tissues because of local infiltration.[67] Because both tumors are composed of well-differentiated chief cells, differentiating adenoma from carcinoma relies on a combination of gross appearance and microscopic evidence of invasion, although cells from carcinomas may exhibit greater pleomorphism.[67]

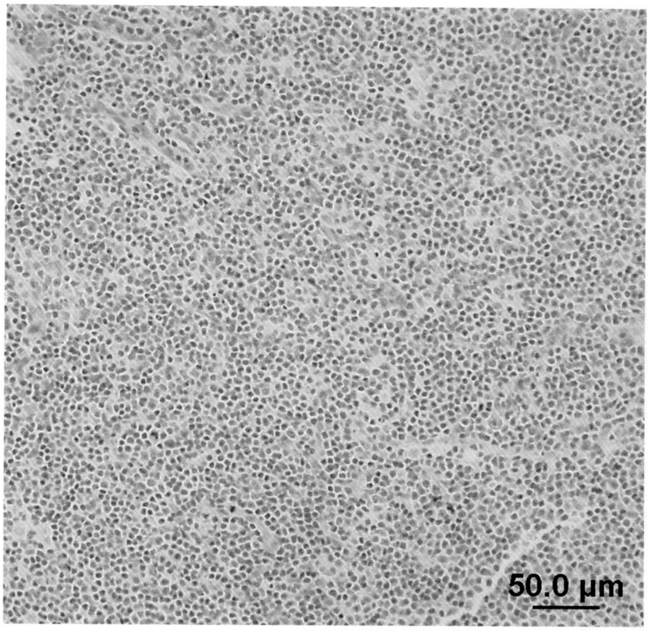

Figure 6-54 Biopsy of a functional parathyroid carcinoma from a dog. Neoplastic cells form cords and trabeculae. Aspirates from this mass are shown in Figures 6-55 and 6-56. (H&E, 200×.)

Cells from both adenomas and carcinomas have a similar cytologic appearance. Many naked nuclei are seen in a background of lightly basophilic cytoplasmic material (Figure 6-55). Nuclei are round to oval and generally uniform in size; mild anisokaryosis may be noted in carcinomas (Figure 6-56). When present in clusters these cells have indistinct cytoplasmic borders, and may form acinar structures. Eosinophilic needle-like structures were noted within the cytoplasm in one report of a canine parathyroid carcinoma.[68] The significance of these inclusions is not known, but they have also been seen in aspirates of follicular thyroid neoplasia (see Figure 6-42).

Table 6-3 presents a summary of the most common cytologic findings in aspirates from thyroid and parathyroid gland lesions.

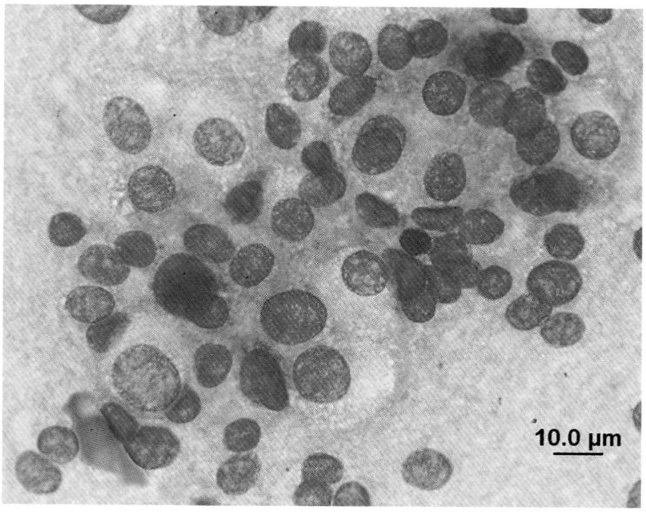

Figure 6-55 Aspirate of a functional parathyroid carcinoma from a dog, same case as Figure 6-54. Sheets and small clusters of cells with round nuclei, stippled chromatin, and lightly basophilic cytoplasm. Many cells are ruptured, and basophilic cytoplasm fills the background. (Wright stain, 1000×.)

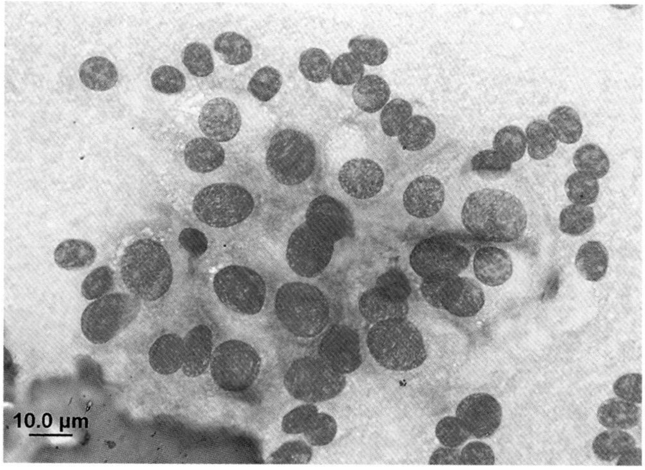

Figure 6-56 Parathyroid carcinoma, same aspirate as Figure 6-55. Moderate anisocytosis and anisokaryosis are seen in the intact cells. (Wright stain, 1000×.)

TABLE 6-3

COMMON CYTOLOGIC FINDINGS IN THYROID OR PARATHYROID ASPIRATES

Cell Types	Key Features	Differential Diagnoses	Comments
*Follicular epithelium Abundant red blood cells (RBCs) ± Colloid	Naked nuclei in background Intact cells in clusters or singly ± Acinar structures ± Blue-black cytoplasmic granules ± Needle-shaped cytoplasmic inclusions ± Colloid (eosinophilic or basophilic)	Thyroid follicular hyperplasia Thyroid follicular tumor	Hyperplasia, adenoma, and many carcinomas appear identical with cytology Carcinomas often exhibit little or no atypia, but can show marked pleomorphism Feline: most are functional and benign Canine: most are nonfunctional and malignant Histopathologic confirmation desirable
*Parafollicular epithelium (C cells) Abundant RBCs	Naked nuclei in background Intact cells in clusters or singly ± Acinar structures	Thyroid medullary tumor	Less common than follicular tumors Animal may be hypocalcemic Colloid may be present Histopathologic confirmation desirable Special stains assist identification
*Epithelial cells (Chief cells)	Naked nuclei in background Intact cells in clusters or singly ± Acinar structures ± Needle-shaped cytoplasmic inclusions May have fewer RBCs than thyroid tumors	Parathyroid tumor	Less common than thyroid tumors Adenomas or carcinomas may be functional Animal may be hypercalcemic Carcinomas may exhibit little or no atypia Histopathologic confirmation desirable

*Cytologically identical

References

1. Simon D, Schoenrock D, Nolte I, et al: Cytologic examination of fine-needle aspirates from mammary gland tumors in the dog: diagnostic accuracy with comparison to histopathology and association with postoperative outcome, *Vet Clin Pathol/Am Soc Vet Clin Pathol* 38(4):521–528, 2009.
2. Allen SW, Prasse KW, Mahaffey EA: Cytologic differentiation of benign from malignant canine mammary tumors, *Vet Pathol* 23(6):649–655, 1986.
3. Griffiths GL, Lumsden JH, Valli VE: Fine needle aspiration cytology and histologic correlation in canine tumors, *Vet Clinical Pathol/Am Soc Vet Clin Pathol* 13(1):13–17, 1984.
4. Hellmen E, Lindgren A: The accuracy of cytology in diagnosis and DNA analysis of canine mammary tumours, *J Comparat Pathol* 101(4):443–450, 1989.
5. Cassali GD, et al: Evaluation of accuracy of fine needle aspiration cytology for diagnosis of canine mammary tumours: comparative features with human tumours, *Cytopathology* 18(3):191–196, 2007.
6. Goldschmidt M, et al: Classification and grading of canine mammary tumors, *Vet Pathol* 48(1):117–131, 2011.
7. Brodey RS, Goldschmidt MH, Roszel JR: Canine mammary gland neoplasms, *J Am Anim Hosp Assoc* 19:61–81, 1983.
8. Feldman EC, Nelson RW: Preparturient diseases: *Canine and feline endocrinology and reproduction*, ed 3, St. Louis, MO, 2004, Saunderspp, pp 831–832.
9. Misdorp W: Tumors of the mammary glands. In Meuten DJ, editor: *Tumors of domestic animals*, ed 4, Ames, IA, 2002, Iowa State Press, pp 575–606.
10. Klaassen JK: Cytology of subcutaneous glandular tissues, *Vet Clin North Am* 32(6):1237–1266, 2002. v-vi.
11. Fernandes PJ, Guyer C, Modiano JF: Mammary mass aspirate from a Yorkshire terrier, *Vet Clinical Pathol / Am Soc Vet Clin Pathol* 27(3):79, 1998.
12. Hayden DW, Barnes DM, Johnson KH: Morphologic changes in the mammary gland of megestrol acetate-treated and untreated cats: a retrospective study, *Vet Pathol* 26(2):104–113, 1989.
13. MacDougall LD: Mammary fibroadenomatous hyperplasia in a young cat attributed to treatment with megestrol acetate, *Can Vet J* 44(3):227–229, 2003.
14. Mesher CI: What is your diagnosis? Subcutaneous nodule from a 14-month-old cat, *Vet Clinical Pathol / Am Soc Vet Clin Pathol* 26(1):4, 1997.
15. Wehrend A, Hospes R, Gruber AD: Treatment of feline mammary fibroadenomatous hyperplasia with a progesterone-antagonist, *Vet Rec* 148(11):346–347, 2001.
16. Sorenmo K: Canine mammary gland tumors, *Vet Clin North Am* 33(3):573–596, 2003.
17. Hayes HM Jr, Milne KL, Mandell CP: Epidemiological features of feline mammary carcinoma, *Vet Rec* 108(22):476–479, 1981.

18. MacEwen EG, Hayes AA, Harvey HJ, et al: Prognostic factors for feline mammary tumors, *J Am Vet Med Assoc* 185(2):201–204, 1984.
19. Skorupski KA, Overley B, Shofer FS, et al: Clinical characteristics of mammary carcinoma in male cats, *J Vet Intern Med / Am Coll Vet Intern Med* 19(1):52–55, 2005.
20. Karayannopoulou M, et al: Histological grading and prognosis in dogs with mammary carcinomas: application of a human grading method, *J Comparat Pathol* 133(4):246–252, 2005.
21. Sorenmo KU, Kristiansen VM, Cofone MA, et al: Canine mammary gland tumours: a histological continuum from benign to malignant: clinical and histopathological evidence, *Vet Comp Oncol* 7(3):162–172, 2009.
22. Viste JR, et al: Feline mammary adenocarcinoma: tumor size as a prognostic indicator, *Can Vet J* 43(1):33–37, 2002.
23. de M Souza CH, Toledo-Piza E, Amorin R, et al: Inflammatory mammary carcinoma in 12 dogs: clinical features, cyclooxygenase-2 expression, and response to piroxicam treatment, *Can Vet J* 50(5):506–510, 2009.
24. Pena L, Perez-Alenza MD, Rodriguez-Bertos A, Nieto A: Canine inflammatory mammary carcinoma: histopathology, immunohistochemistry and clinical implications of 21 cases, *Breast Cancer Res Treat* 78(2):141–148, 2003.
25. Perez Alenza MD, Tabanera E, Pena L: Inflammatory mammary carcinoma in dogs: 33 cases (1995-1999), *J Am Vet Med Assoc* 219(8):1110–1114, 2001.
26. Perez-Alenza MD, et al: First description of feline inflammatory mammary carcinoma: clinicopathological and immunohistochemical characteristics of three cases, *Breast Cancer Res* 6(4):R300–R307, 2004.
27. Smith MM: Oral and salivary gland disorders. In Ettinger SJ, Feldman EC, editors: ed 6, *Textbook of veterinary internal medicine*, vol 2, St. Louis, MO, 2005, Elsevier, Inc, pp 1290–1297.
28. Boydell P, Pike R, Crossley D: Presumptive sialadenosis in a cat, *J Small Anim Pract* 41(12):573–574, 2000.
29. Boydell P, et al: Sialadenosis in dogs, *J Am Vet Med Assoc* 216(6):872–874, 2000.
30. Sozmen M, Brown PJ, Whitbread TJ: Idiopathic salivary gland enlargement (sialadenosis) in dogs: a microscopic study, *J Small Anim Pract* 41(6):243–247, 2000.
31. Stonehewer J, Mackin AJ, Tasker S, et al: Idiopathic phenobarbital-responsive hypersialosis in the dog: an unusual form of limbic epilepsy? *J Small Anim Pract* 41(9):416–421, 2000.
32. Spangler WL, Culbertson MR: Salivary gland disease in dogs and cats: 245 cases (1985-1988), *J Am Vet Med Assoc* 198(3):465–469, 1991.
33. Brown NO: Salivary gland diseases. Diagnosis, treatment, and associated problems, *Prob Vet Med* 1(2):281–294, 1989.
34. Hammer A, Getzy D, Ogilvie G, et al: Salivary gland neoplasia in the dog and cat: survival times and prognostic factors, *J Am Anim Hosp Assoc* 37(5):478–482, 2001.
35. Head KW, Else RW: Tumors of the salivary glands. In Meuten DJ, editor: *Tumors of domestic animals*, ed 4, Ames, IA, 2002, Iowa State Press, pp 410–416.
36. Sozmen M, Brown PJ, Eveson JW: Sebaceous carcinoma of the salivary gland in a cat, *J Vet Med* 49(8):425–427, 2002.
37. Sozmen M, Brown PJ, Eveson JW: Salivary gland basal cell adenocarcinoma: a report of cases in a cat and two dogs, *J Vet Med* 50(8):399–401, 2003.
38. Carberry CA, et al: Salivary gland tumors in dogs and cats: a literature and case review, *J Am Anim Hosp Assoc* 24:561–567, 1988.
39. Baker R, Lumsden JH: The head and neck. In Baker R, Lumsden JH, editors: *Color atlas of cytology of the dog and cat*, St. Louis, MO, 2000, Mosby, pp 119–127.
40. Mazzullo G, Sfacteria A, Ianelli N, et al: Carcinoma of the submandibular salivary glands with multiple metastases in a cat, *Vet Clin Pathol / Am Soc Vet Clin Pathol* 34(1):61–64, 2005.
41. Militerno G, Bazzo R, Marcato PS: Cytological diagnosis of mandibular salivary gland adenocarcinoma in a dog, *J Vet Med* 52(10):514–516, 2005.
42. Duncan RB, Feldman BF, Saunders GK, et al: Mandibular salivary gland aspirate from a dog, *Vet Clin Pathol / Am Soc Vet Clin Pathol* 28(3):97–99, 1999.
43. Perez-Martinez C, Garcia Fernandez RA, Reyes Avila LE, et al: Malignant fibrous histiocytoma (giant cell type) associated with a malignant mixed tumor in the salivary gland of a dog, *Vet Pathol* 37(4):350–353, 2000.
44. Smrkovski OA, LeBlanc AK, Smith SH, et al: Carcinoma ex pleomorphic adenoma with sebaceous differentiation in the mandibular salivary gland of a dog, *Vet Pathol* 43(3):374–377, 2006.
45. Perman V, Alsaker RD, Riis RC: *Cytology of the dog and cat*, South Bend, IN, 1979, American Animal Hospital Association.
46. Gosselin SJ, et al: Autoimmune lymphocytic thyroiditis in dogs, *Vet Immunol Immunopathol* 3(1-2):185–201, 1982.
47. Graham PA, et al: Lymphocytic thyroiditis, *Vet Clin North Am* 31(5):915–933, 2001. vi-vii.
48. Capen CC: Tumors, hyperplasia, and cysts of thyroid follicular cells. In Meuten DJ, editor: *Tumors in domestic animals*, ed 4, Ames, IA, 2002, Iowa State Press, pp 634–654.
49. Feldman EC, Nelson RW: *Feline hyperthyroidism (thyrotoxicosis). In: Canine and feline endocrinology and reproduction*ed 3, St. Louis, MO, 2004, Saunderspp. 152–215.
50. Feldman EC, Nelson RW: *Canine thyroid tumors and hyperthyroidism. In: Canine and feline endocrinology and reproduction*ed 3, St. Louis, MO, 2004, Saunders. 219–248.
51. Chastain CB, et al: Congenital hypothyroidism in a dog due to an iodide organification defect, *Am J Vet Res* 44(7):1257–1265, 1983.
52. Fyfe JC, Kampschmidt K, Dang V, et al: Congenital hypothyroidism with goiter in toy fox terriers, *J Vet Intern Med / Am Coll Vet Intern Med* 17(1):50–57, 2003.
53. Leav I, Schiller AL, Rijnberk A, et al: Adenomas and carcinomas of the canine and feline thyroid, *Am J Pathol* 83(1): 61–122, 1976.
54. Thompson EJ, et al: Fine needle aspiration cytology in the diagnosis of canine thyroid carcinoma, *Can Vet J* 21(6): 186–188, 1980.
55. Carver JR, Kapatkin A, Patnaik AK: A comparison of medullary thyroid carcinoma and thyroid adenocarcinoma in dogs: a retrospective study of 38 cases, *Vet Surg* 24(4):315–319, 1995.
56. Patnaik AK, Lieberman PH: Gross, histologic, cytochemical, and immunocytochemical study of medullary thyroid carcinoma in sixteen dogs, *Vet Pathol* 28(3):223–233, 1991.
57. Bertazzolo W, et al: Paratracheal cervical mass in a dog, *Vet Clin Pathol / Am Soc Vet Clin Pathol* 32(4):209–212, 2003.
58. Anderson PG, Capen CC: Undifferentiated spindle cell carcinoma of the thyroid in a dog, *Vet Pathol* 23(2):203–204, 1986.
59. Hofmeister E, Kippenes H, Mealey KL, et al: Functional cystic thyroid adenoma in a cat, *J Am Vet Med Assoc* 219(2):190–193, 2001.
60. Phillips DE, et al: Cystic thyroid and parathyroid lesions in cats, *J Am Anim Hosp Assoc* 39(4):349–354, 2003.
61. Wisner ER, Nyland TG: Ultrasonography of the thyroid and parathyroid glands, *Vet Clin North Am* 28(4):973–991, 1998.
62. Berger B, Feldman EC: Primary hyperparathyroidism in dogs: 21 cases (1976-1986), *J Am Vet Med Assoc* 191(3): 350–356, 1987.

63. den Hertog E, et al: Primary hyperparathyroidism in two cats, *Vet Q* 19(2):81–84, 1997.
64. Kallet AJ, et al: Primary hyperparathyroidism in cats: seven cases (1984-1989), *J Am Vet Med Assoc* 199(12):1767–1771, 1991.
65. Feldman EC, et al: Pretreatment clinical and laboratory findings in dogs with primary hyperparathyroidism: 210 cases (1987-2004), *J Am Vet Med Assoc* 227(5):756–761, 2005.
66. Feldman EC, Nelson RW: Primary hyperparathyroidism in cats. *Canine and feline endocrinology and reproduction*, St. Louis, MO, 2004, Saunders, pp 711–713.
67. Capen CC: Tumors and nonneoplastic cysts of the parathyroid gland. In Meuten DJ, editor: *Tumors in domestic animals*, ed 4, Ames, IA, 2002, Iowa State Press, pp 665–669.
68. Ramaiah SK, et al: A mass in the ventral neck of a hypercalcemic dog, *Vet Clin Pathol / Am Soc Vet Clin Pathol* 30(4):177–179, 2001.

CHAPTER 7

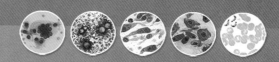

Nasal Exudates and Masses

Tara P. Arndt

INDICATIONS

Pathologic conditions in the nasal cavity of cats and dogs are often characterized by sneezing, nasal discharge, epistaxis, ocular discharge, pawing at the nose, or facial deformity. Epistaxis may also result from primary coagulopathies, secondary coagulopathies (e.g., canine ehrlichiosis), and hyperviscosity syndromes. Cytologic findings are interpreted in light of historical, physical, rhinoscopic, radiographic, and clinical laboratory findings to arrive at a diagnosis. Rhinoscopy and cytologic evaluation are simple noninvasive procedures that may yield a definitive diagnosis. Cytologic evaluation is a method of screening the nasal cavity for the underlying etiology; however, negative or nonspecific findings do not exclude a fungal infection, neoplasm, or foreign body if only superficial inflammatory cells are obtained. The limiting factor for nasal cytology is obtaining a representative sample. In some cases, surgical exploration of the nasal cavity with cytology and/or biopsy assessments may be necessary for definitive diagnosis.

Detailed examination of the nasal cavity and most sample collections are optimally performed while the animal is under general anesthesia, with an endotracheal tube in place and the cuff inflated. Radiographs and rhinoscopy should be performed before biopsy or flushing techniques so that radiographic detail and visualization are not altered by potential trauma and hemorrhage caused by manipulation of the nasal tissues.[1] The major landmarks and communication of the airways and food passages are schematically indicated in Figure 7-1.

The nasal cavity may be examined with equipment that varies from simple to sophisticated. In some animals, an otoscope may be used to examine the rostral nares; however, a flexible 4-mm fiberoptic endoscope should be used to view the ventral nasal meatus or nasopharynx.[2] The oronasal cavity can be examined by retracting the soft palate with forceps and using a dental mirror or flexible endoscope. These procedures can aid visualization of abnormal tissues although copious exudates or hemorrhage may preclude adequate examination.

SAMPLING TECHNIQUES

Cytologic specimens from the nasal cavity may be obtained by flushing or aspiration techniques. These methods are safe if care is taken not to penetrate the cribriform plate with the instruments used for obtaining samples and if precautions are taken to prevent inhalation of blood and fluids by the animal during sampling. Some hemorrhage may occur during manipulation of the nasal cavity, however this should not be a complicating factor unless a coagulopathy is present.

For the nasal flushing technique, the depth of the nasal cavity is estimated, and a soft rubber catheter is passed caudad through the external nares or in a retrograde direction from caudal to the nasopharynx. A syringe containing approximately 10 milliliters (mL) of nonbacteriostatic sterile saline is attached to the catheter, and multiple flushes are performed using intermittent positive and negative pressure.[1,2] Dislodged particulate matter can be caught in a gauze sponge placed caudal to the soft palate or rostral to the nares, depending on the direction of the flushing procedure. Aqueous cytologic material can be collected within the syringe barrel by aspiration.

Aspiration, the second means of obtaining samples from the nasal cavity, is useful when a mass is localized radiographically or visually. This technique involves use of a large-gauge polypropylene urinary catheter, a Sovereign plastic needle guard (Monoject, Sherwood Medical, St. Louis, MO), or a tomcat catheter cut at a 45-degree angle to form a sharp cutting edge.[3] Proper catheter length is determined by measuring the distance from the external nares to the medial canthus of the eye. Catheter length is important to prevent penetration of the cribriform plate during the procedure. The catheter is attached to a syringe and advanced into the nasal cavity until moderate resistance is felt. Suction is applied while several advances are made into the mass. Gentle negative pressure is maintained as the catheter is removed from the mass and nasal cavity to retain solid tissue fragments.

Alternatively, a biopsy needle (Tru-Cut, Baxter Healthcare Corp., Deerfield, IL) may be passed through the nares to the mass and a biopsy obtained. Samples may also be obtained with a biopsy forceps attachment during endoscopic examination. Needle and endoscopic biopsies are large enough for cytologic touch imprint preparations and, if necessary, histopathologic examination.

Nasal swabs often do not yield satisfactory diagnostic material because they cannot be inserted far enough into the nasal cavity and are not abrasive enough to obtain representative samples of deep mucosal lesions. A diagnosis may be obtained using nasal swabs if a causative agent such as *Cryptococcus neoformans* is present in the nasal exudate or rostral nares.

Cytologic preparations are made from touch imprints or squash preparations of tissue fragments, smears of flush samples and swabs, and smears of centrifuged nasal flush sediments. These preparations are air-dried, stained, and examined by routine methods. (See Chapter 1 for further discussion concerning specimen preparation and staining.) A portion of the samples can be reserved for microbiologic culture and sensitivity testing if an infectious agent is suspected or found on stained cytologic preparations. If samples are used for microbiologic testing, a sterile swab or sterile tube should be submitted that does not contain an anticoagulant such as ethylenediaminetetraacetic acid (EDTA) as EDTA can be bacteriostatic. If the fluid is submitted for cytologic examination, EDTA is useful for preservation of cell morphology. After imprinting for cytologic evaluation, tissue fragments can be preserved in 10% neutral buffered formalin for histopathologic evaluation.

Flow charts are provided to aid in the evaluation of nasal cytologic smears containing primarily inflammatory cells (Figure 7-2) and those containing primarily epithelial cells, mesenchymal cells, or both (Figure 7-3).

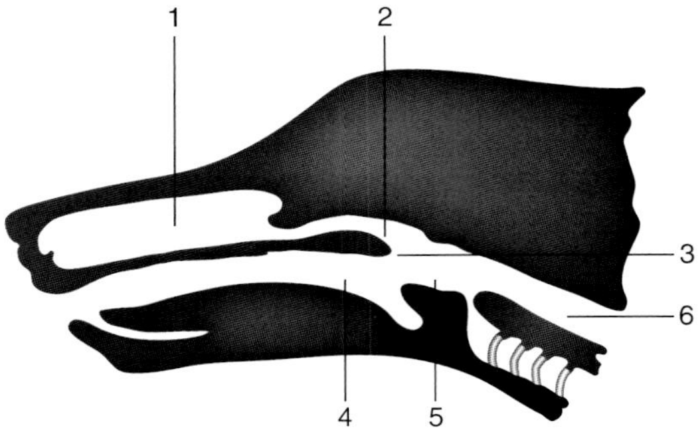

Figure 7-1 Schematic diagram indicating major landmarks and communication of the airways and food passages. 1, Nasal cavity. **2,** Nasopharynx. **3,** Palate. **4,** Oropharynx. **5,** Epiglottis. **6,** Esophagus. The nasal cavity (*1*) may be sampled rostrad through the nares or caudad through the nasopharynx (*2*) as the soft palate (*3*) is retracted.

NORMAL CYTOLOGIC FINDINGS

It is important to distinguish normal from pathologic cells and bacterial populations in cytologic preparations. In nasal flush specimens, oropharyngeal organisms of variable morphology and epithelial cells may be obtained from healthy animals. *Simonsiella* spp. are large, stacked, rod-shaped bacteria that are inhabitants of the oral cavity of dogs and cats and are seen commonly in smears contaminated by oral secretions (Figure 7-4).[4] Epithelial cell morphology varies with the site and depth of the specimen. Nonkeratinized squamous epithelial cells, often with adherent bacteria, are obtained from the external nares and oropharynx. Ciliated pseudostratified columnar epithelial cells and associated mucus originate from the nasal turbinates (Figure 7-5 and Figure 7-6). Basal epithelial cells are smaller and rounded and have darker blue cytoplasm. Hemorrhage during sampling results in the presence of red blood cells (RBCs) and white blood cells (WBCs) in similar proportions to peripheral blood (approximately 1 WBC for every 500 to 1000 RBC).

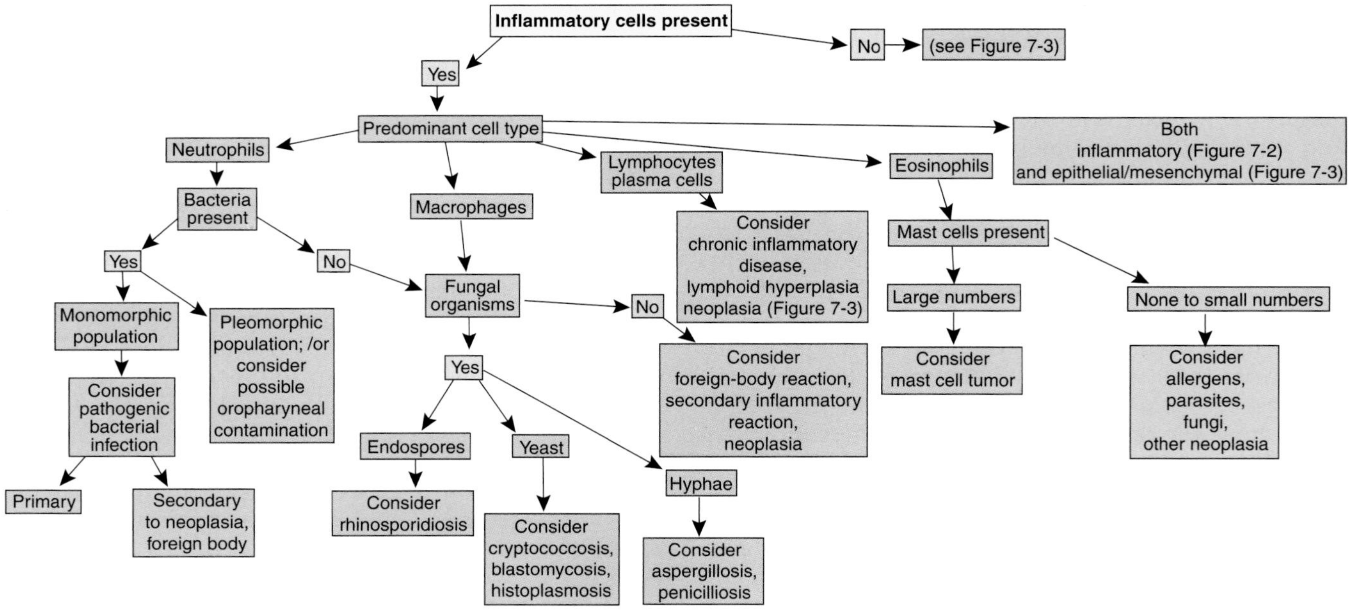

Figure 7-2 Flow chart of nasal cytologic evaluation with inflammatory cells.

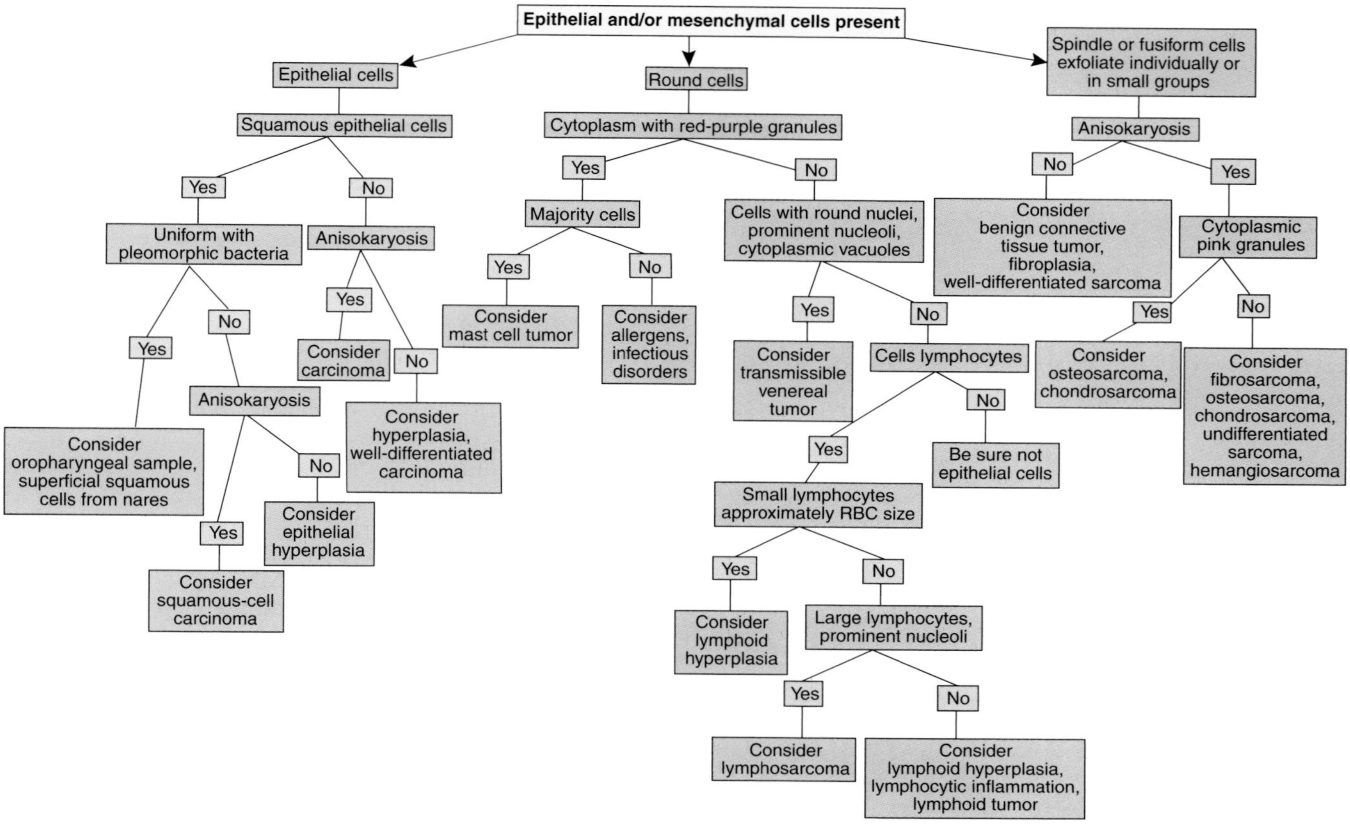

Figure 7-3 Flow chart of nasal cytologic evaluation with epithelial cells, mesenchymal cells, or both.

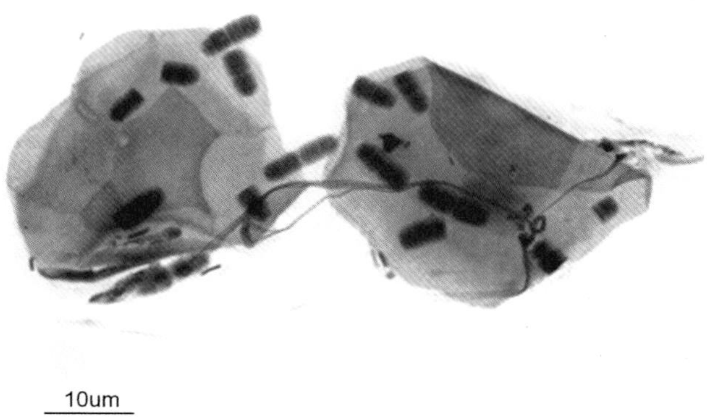

Figure 7-4 Two superficial squamous epithelial cells with many *Simonsiella* organisms and scattered bacterial rods. *Simonsiella* organisms appear as a single large bacterium but are actually several bacterial rods lying side by side, giving the striated appearance. *Simonsiella* organisms are inhabitants of the oral cavity of dogs and cats and are seen commonly in smears contaminated by oral secretions. (Wright stain.) (Courtesy of Dr. R. L. Cowell.)

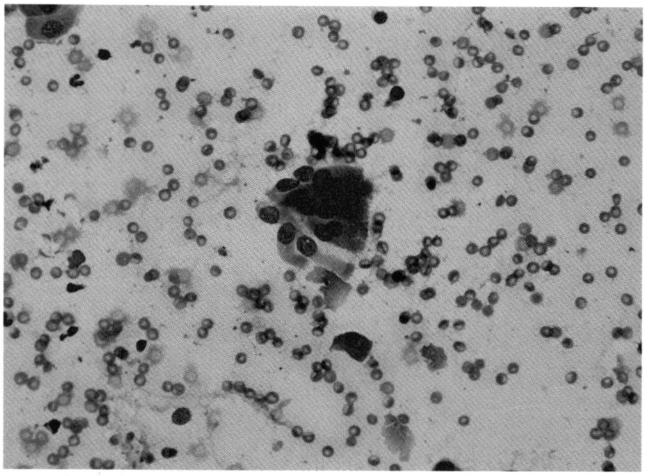

Figure 7-5 A cluster of normal ciliated columnar respiratory epithelial cells. (Wright stain)

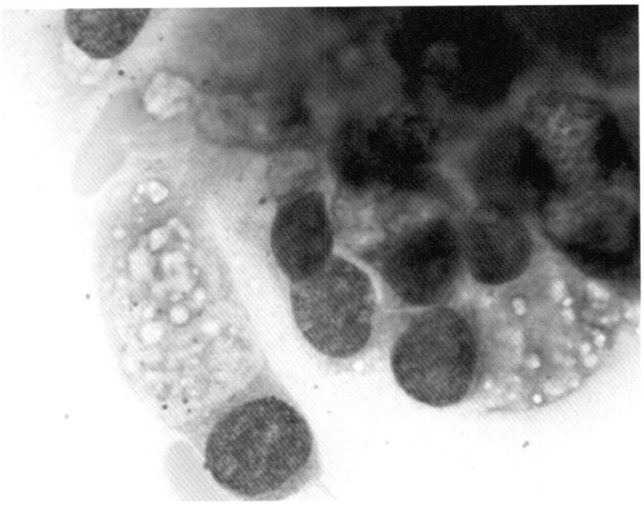

Figure 7-6 Mucin secreting tall columnar respiratory epithelial cells. (Wright stain, 100×.)

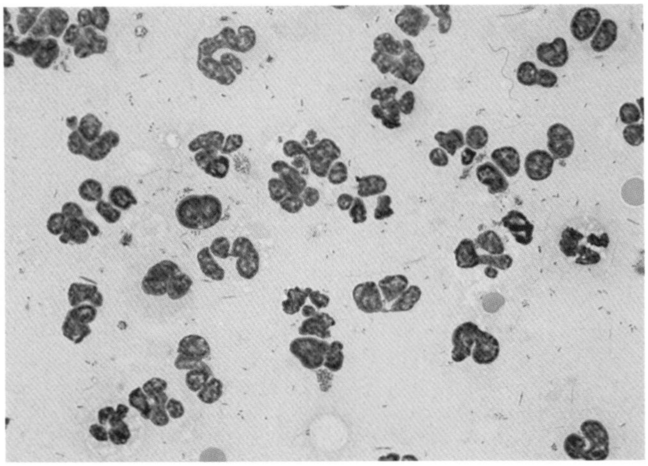

Figure 7-7 Septic purulent exudate with a mixed population of intracellular and extracellular bacteria that suggests septic inflammation associated with oronasal fistula. (Wright stain.)

INFECTIOUS AGENTS

Neutrophils usually predominate in exudates associated with bacterial, viral, and some fungal infections (Figure 7-7). In addition to neutrophils, variable numbers of macrophages, lymphocytes, and plasma cells may be present with any inflammatory condition. Pathogenic bacterial infection should be suspected when bacterial organisms are seen within neutrophils compared with normal bacterial flora that colonize squamous epithelial cells in the absence of neutrophils. As bacteria from the oral cavity are generally a pleomorphic population, a monomorphic bacterial population suggests overgrowth or infection.[5]

Identification of bacteria only on the basis of a Gram-stained exudate is often unreliable. With routine hematologic stains, homogeneous populations of cocci usually represent gram-positive organisms, such as *Staphylococcus* or *Streptococcus* spp., whereas homogeneous populations of rods often indicate gram-negative organisms. Prior treatment with antibiotics may preclude identification of bacteria from cytologic preparations. Samples should therefore be submitted for microbiologic culture, identification, and sensitivity testing prior to initiating antibiotic therapy.

Bacterial infections are usually secondary to mucosal injury from trauma or foreign bodies but also may be associated with viral infection, fungal infection, and neoplasia. Oronasal fistulas can result in chronic bacterial rhinitis. These fistulas most commonly involve canine, premolar, and/or molar teeth.[6]

Viral inclusions are infrequently seen in nasal cytology specimens. Herpesvirus infection in cats may produce intranuclear inclusions within epithelial cells.[7] As viral inclusions are rarely found in Wright-stained cytologic preparations, definitive diagnosis of such inclusions is best accomplished by fluorescent antibody examination or viral isolation.

Fungal infections, foreign bodies, and neoplasia of the nasal cavity should be suspected when sinusitis is unresponsive to antibacterial therapy. In the case of mycotic rhinitis, fungal hyphae frequently are present within dense accumulations of cells and debris (Figure 7-8). Hyphae may be difficult to discern because they may not stain well with Romanowsky stain and new methylene blue

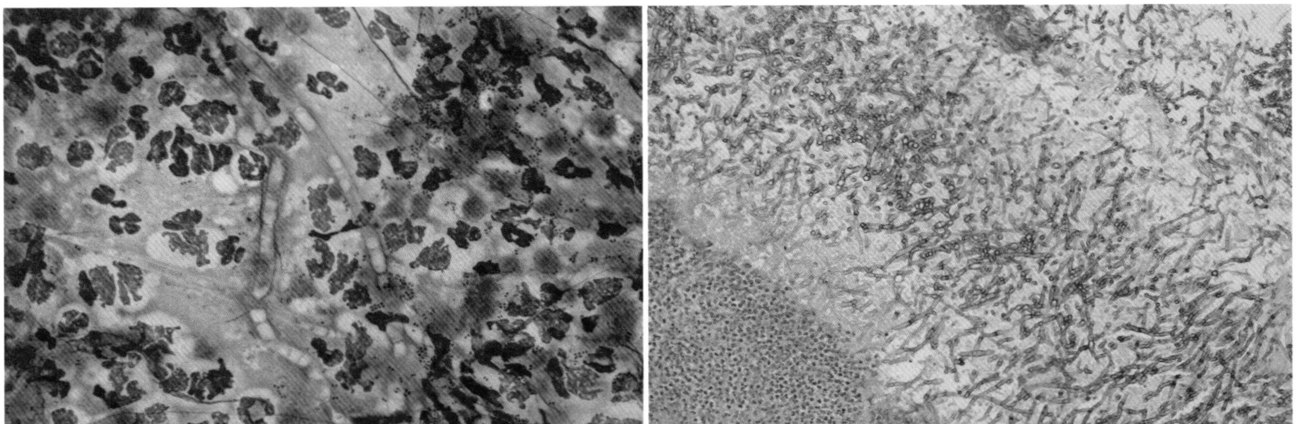

Figure 7-8 **A,** Numerous fungal hyphae and pyogranulomatous inflammation. (Wright stain, 250×.) **B,** Mat of fungal hyphae with subjacent accumulation of neutrophils. (H&E stain.)

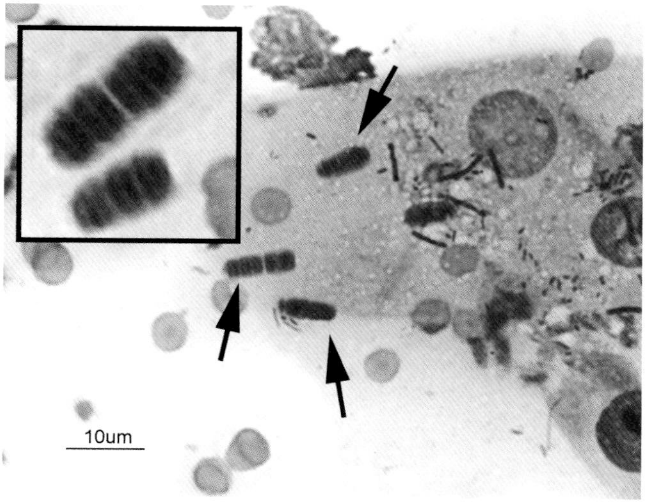

Figure 8-4 Mature squamous cells with *Simonsiella* spp. bacteria (arrows). *Simonsiella* spp. is a normal inhabitant of the oropharynx and must not be mistaken for a pathogen. What appears to be one very large organism is actually numerous slender bacterial rods lined up side to side. *Inset*, Higher magnification of *Simonsiella* organisms in which the individual organisms can be seen.

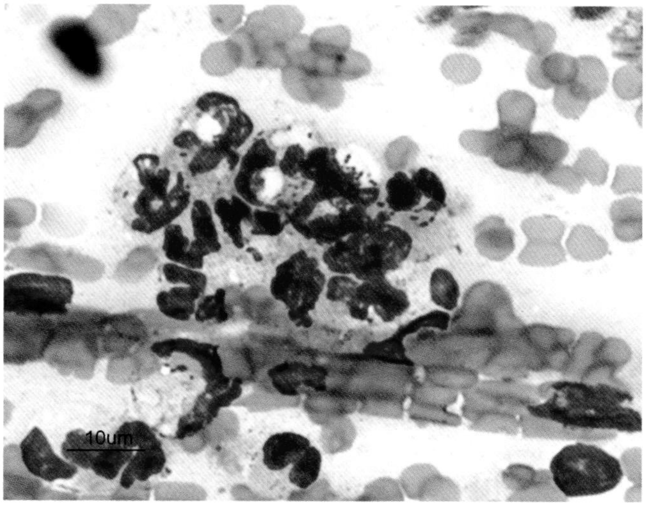

Figure 8-5 Septic, purulent inflammation. Scraping of a lesion in the oral cavity of a cat shows many neutrophils with phagocytized bacteria. Bacteria that are associated with an inflammatory reaction and are phagocytized by neutrophils likely represent pathogens (primary or secondary).

Reactive hyperplasia of the tonsils is characterized by a population of lymphoid cells that are predominantly small mature lymphocytes, with variably increased numbers of plasma cells (Figure 8-8). Lymphoblast numbers remain low. Variable numbers of neutrophils and macrophages may be present, depending on the degree of concurrent inflammation. Bacterial or fungal organisms can be present. Because tonsils have no afferent lymphatics, malignancies and inflammation in the oropharynx drain into the submandibular and pharyngeal lymph nodes rather than into the tonsils.

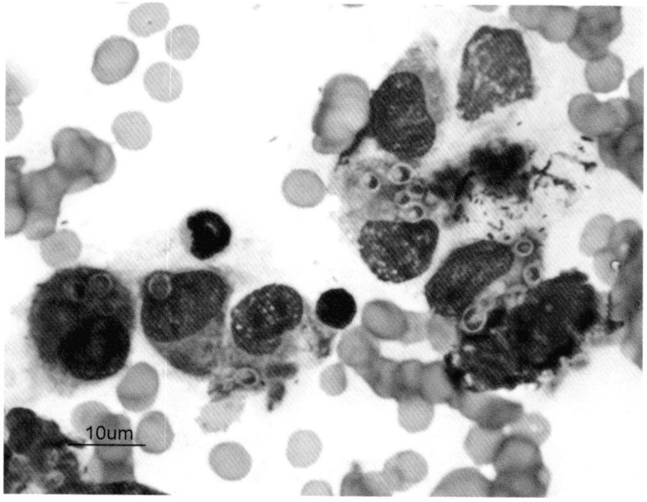

Figure 8-6 Scraping of an oral lesion of a cat with histoplasmosis. The lesion was pyogranulomatous, yielding a mixture of neutrophils and macrophages. In this image, many macrophages are present and contain phagocytized *Histoplasma* organisms.

Eosinophilic Granuloma Complex: Eosinophilic ulcers, granulomas, and plaques are common within the oropharynx. Cytologically, they are identified by a predominance of eosinophils (Figure 8-9). Macrophages, fibroblasts, lymphocytes, and plasma cells can also be observed in variable numbers because they are all normal components of eosinophilic granuloma lesions. As with other oropharyngeal lesions, secondary opportunistic bacterial inflammation can be observed if the sample is superficial. Eosinophils can also be the dominant cell type in some mycotic lesions and foreign-body reactions, so these possibilities must be differentiated from eosinophilic granuloma complex by the gross appearance of the lesion, fungal culture, fungal serology, or excisional biopsy.

Neoplastic Lesions

Tumors in this region can be classified cytologically as being of epithelial origin, of mesenchymal origin, or as discrete round cell tumors. They can be evaluated for malignant criteria and for any secondary inflammation caused by tissue necrosis from an expanding tumor or by opportunistic bacterial infection. Malignant tumors in the oropharynx usually have a poor prognosis unless they are detected early and completely excised before any microscopic metastasis has occurred.

Tumors of Epithelial Origin: Epithelial tumors of the oropharynx include papillomas, epulides, squamous cell carcinomas, epithelial odontogenic tumors, and adenocarcinomas. Cytologically, an epithelial origin of a tumor is suggested by cells that display adhesion (i.e., cell clustering, although this may be variable, depending on the specific tumor and degree of differentiation), round nuclei with stippled chromatin, and sparse to abundant amounts of cytoplasm with generally distinct cell margins.

Canine oral papillomas are caused by a transmissible papovavirus and usually occur in animals younger than

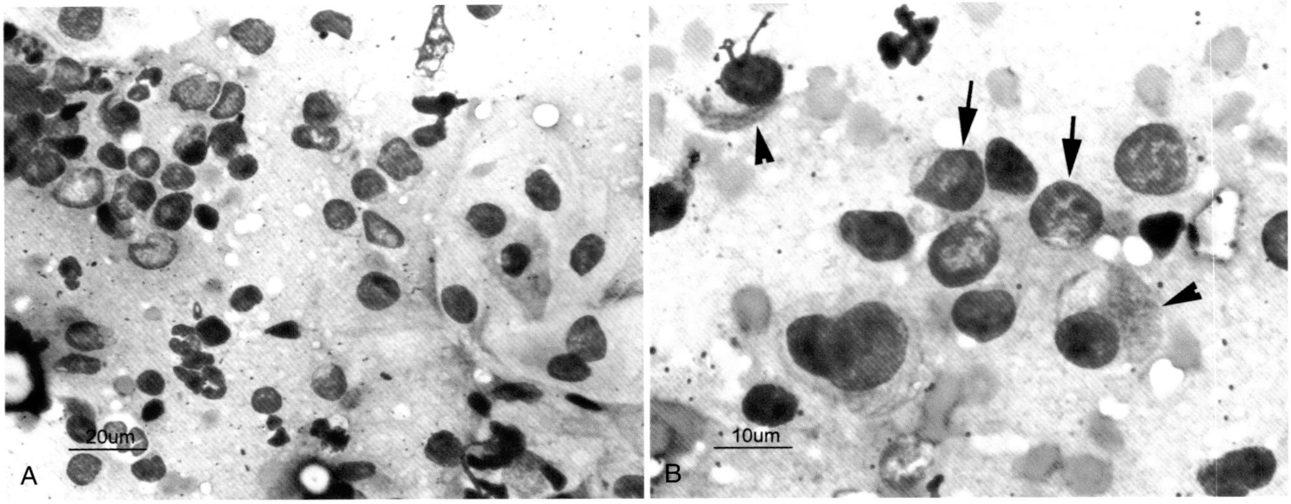

Figure 8-7 **Scrapings of a cat with lymphocytic-plasmacytic gingivitis. A,** Low-magnification image shows normal squamous cells (*right*) and a dense infiltrate of inflammatory cells. **B,** Higher-magnification image of inflammatory cells shows a predominance of small lymphocytes (*arrows*) as well as increased numbers of mature plasma cells (*arrowheads*).

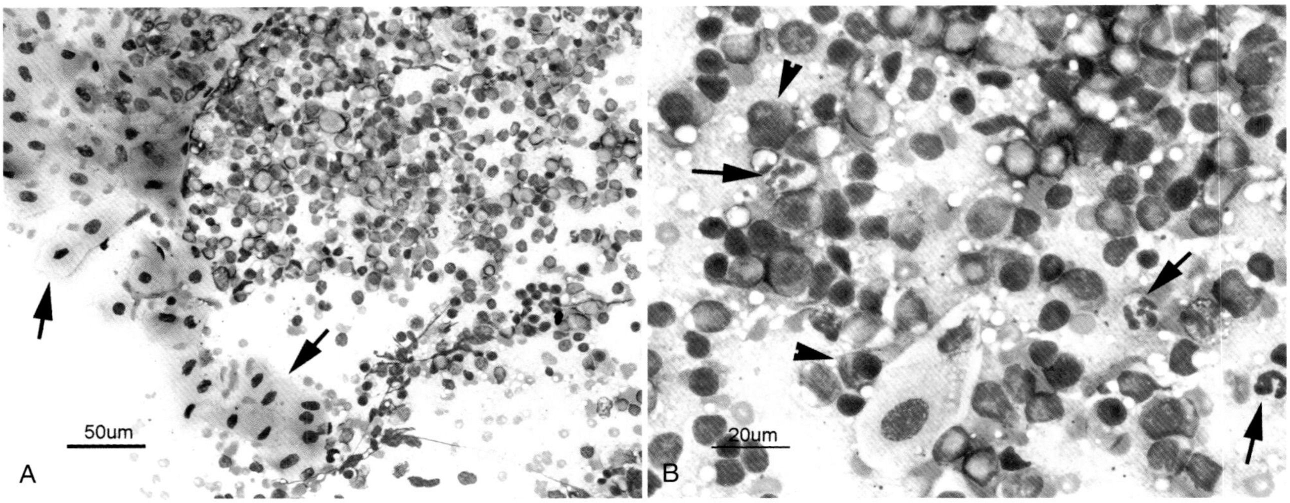

Figure 8-8 **Impression smears of a biopsy of an enlarged tonsil from a dog with a hyperplastic, inflamed tonsil. A,** Low-magnification image shows normal surrounding squamous epithelium (*arrows*) and a lymphoid population from the tonsil itself. **B,** Higher-magnification image shows the lymphoid population to be a predominance of small lymphocytes. Increased numbers of neutrophils (*arrows*) and plasma cells (*arrowheads*) are present.

1 year. They are usually identified by their gross appearance. When aspirated, they yield variable numbers of squamous cells that appear intermediate to mature, with keratinization of the superficial cells.

Epulides are a group of common benign tumors, or tumorlike masses, that are located on the gingiva. They are identified and differentiated from each other only by histopathologic examination of the tissue architecture, not by cytology. Because epulides are composed of squamous epithelium and fibrous tissue, aspirates of these tumors are composed of variable numbers of mature squamous cells and occasional small spindle cells. The fibrous portion of the epulis is nonexfoliative or minimally exfoliative, which causes many aspirates to be almost acellular and nondiagnostic. The more cellular samples are usually composed almost entirely of intermediate and mature squamous cells. Ossifying epulides can exhibit some eosinophilic, amorphous, extracellular material representing osteoid. Excisional biopsy is the treatment of choice for epulides so that they can be classified correctly on the basis of the tissue architecture of an adequate number of representative cells. This can lead to complete resolution, although some can recur at the same site and some can invade alveolar bone. Biopsy will also differentiate an epulis from a well-differentiated squamous cell carcinoma and from epithelial odontogenic neoplasms.

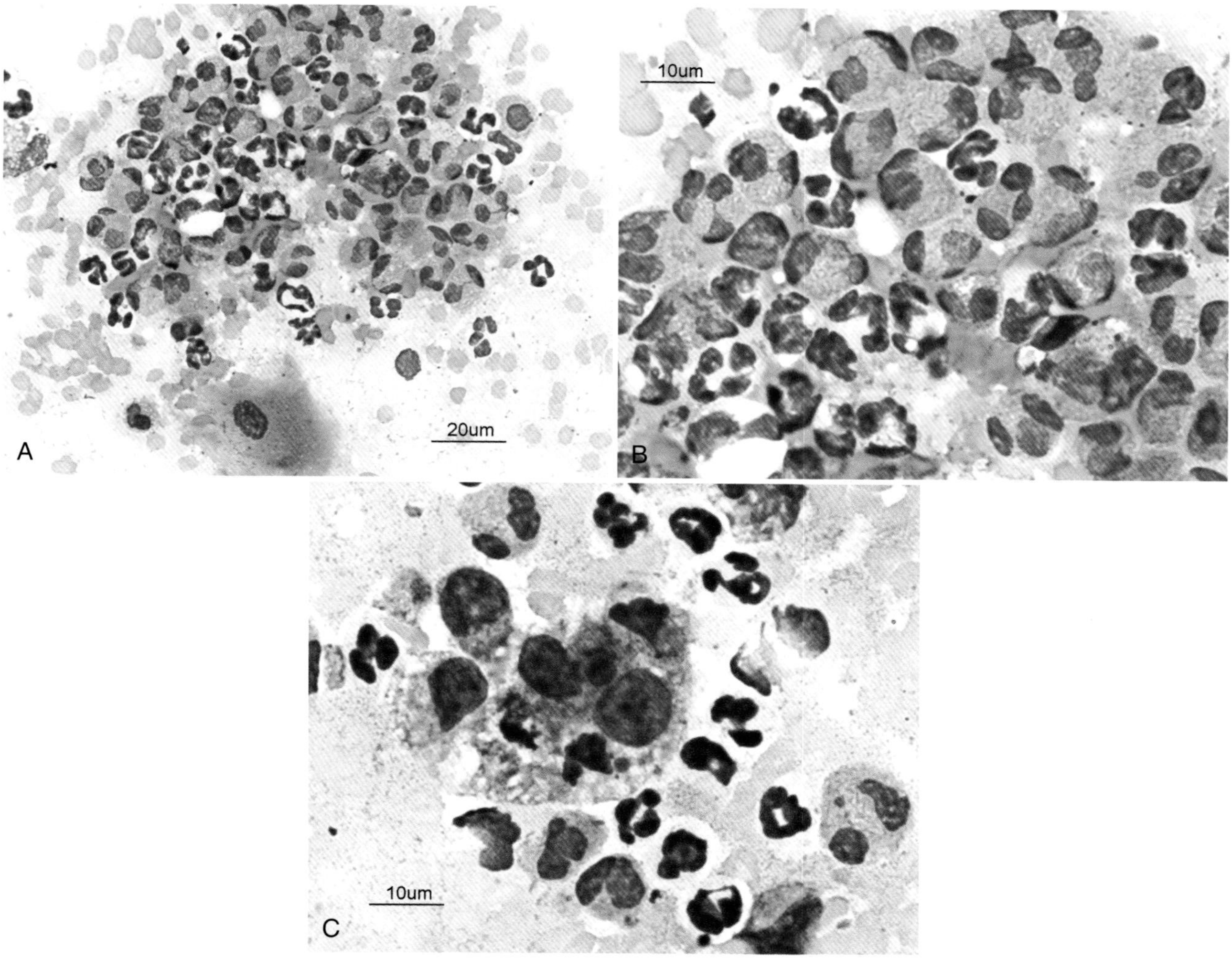

Figure 8-9 Scrapings of an oral lesion from a cat with an eosinophilic granuloma complex lesion ("rodent ulcer"). A, Low-magnification image shows one mature squamous cell and many inflammatory cells. **B,** Higher-magnification image of the inflammatory cells shows a predominance of eosinophils and some neutrophils. The eosinophils can be easily differentiated from the neutrophils by the orange color of their cytoplasm imparted by the granules. In contrast, the cytoplasm of the neutrophils is clear. The eosinophil granules are so densely packed in the cell that individual granules are often difficult to see. **C,** Another field from the same slide. Although eosinophils predominate in these lesions, variable numbers of macrophages are also present.

Epithelial odontogenic neoplasms are a group of neoplasms that can occur in young or old animals. They usually occur near teeth. All are characterized by epithelial cells that can exhibit many criteria of malignancy or can appear rather well differentiated. Examination of the tissue architecture is necessary for accurate classification of these neoplasms and for accurate prognosis. Thus, surgical biopsy and histopathology is needed for these lesions.

Squamous cell carcinomas are common oropharyngeal malignant neoplasms. They can occur in any squamous epithelial tissue, including the squamous covering of the tonsils. The individual appearance of malignant squamous cells varies widely, depending on the degree of differentiation of the tumor. Some squamous carcinoma cells (e.g., from poorly differentiated tumors) are round and exhibit sparse to moderate amounts of moderately to deeply basophilic, finely granular cytoplasm with elevated nucleus-to-cytoplasm (N:C) ratio and prominent large nucleoli (Figure 8-10). In addition, perinuclear, punctate hyaline vacuoles are frequently observed in squamous cell carcinomas (Figure 8-11). Mitotic figures and abnormal nuclear and cellular division can be observed. Other more well-differentiated but malignant carcinomas yield cells that have a more mature squamous appearance with fewer malignant criteria (see Figure 8-11). These can exhibit lighter basophilia and more abundant cytoplasm; however, moderate anisocytosis, anisokaryosis, and variability of the N:C ratio remain. With well-differentiated tumors, diligent searching can reveal low numbers of cells with marked criteria of malignancy admixed among more well-differentiated cells (see Figure 8-11, *B*). Because such cells can be rare to nonexistent, biopsy should be

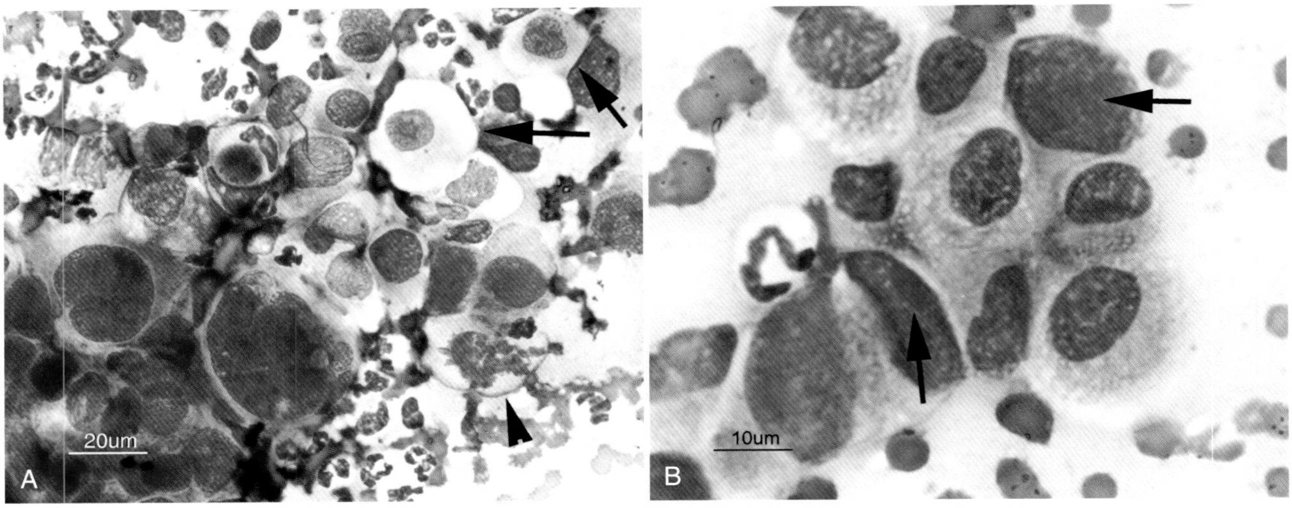

Figure 8-10 Aspirates from a poorly differentiated squamous cell carcinoma in the oral cavity of a cat. A pleomorphic population of epithelial cells is present. Two large, karyomegalic cells are present. Only rare cells show evidence of squamous differentiation having more abundant, lightly colored cytoplasm that is beginning to show angular borders (*arrows*). A mitotic figure is present (*arrowhead*).

performed on any oropharyngeal squamous cell neoplasm before it is classified as benign. When inflammation is present, epithelial cells can exhibit some criteria that are common to epithelial hyperplasia, dysplasia, and malignancy. Then biopsy can be necessary to differentiate primary malignancy with secondary inflammation from a site of primary inflammation with secondary epithelial dysplasia.

Adenocarcinomas are rarely observed in the oral cavity, although tumors of salivary epithelium are possible. Refer to Chapter 6 for characteristics of benign and malignant salivary epithelial cells.

Tumors of Mesenchymal Origin: Fibrosarcomas are common mesenchymal tumors in cats and dogs, even in young dogs (Figure 8-12). Since they are fibrous, they can be poorly exfoliative. If inadequate numbers of cells are obtained by fine-needle aspiration, a scraping can yield more numerous cells. However, care must be taken to spread the scraped cells into a monolayer for evaluation. Malignant fibroblasts are large spindle cells that exhibit oval nuclei, reticular chromatin, and one or more prominent, large nucleoli. Sometimes, the nucleoli can be larger than erythrocytes. Mitotic figures and abnormal nuclear and cytoplasmic division can be observed. Anisocytosis and anisokaryosis can be moderate to marked. Occasional multinucleate cells can be observed. More primitive fibrosarcoma cells can appear almost round; however, cytoplasmic tails can eventually be found on careful examination. More well-differentiated fibrosarcomas yield cells with fewer malignant criteria. If inflammation is present concurrently, biopsy can be necessary to differentiate a primary, well-differentiated fibrosarcoma with secondary inflammation from primary inflammation with secondary reactive fibroplasia.

Other soft tissue sarcomas, including liposarcomas and hemangiosarcomas, can rarely occur in the oral cavity. Most soft tissue sarcomas have a similar cytologic appearance, consisting of poorly exfoliative spindle cells. Histopathologic examination of the tissue architecture is necessary for correct classification and prognosis. Hemangiosarcomas are typically nonexfoliative, and aspirates usually consist entirely of peripheral blood.

The bones and joints around the oropharynx can be the source of osteosarcomas and chondrosarcomas. Their appearance is identical to those described in Chapter 13. Oral squamous cell carcinomas can also metastasize to bone.

Benign fibromas can occur in the oropharynx. They are composed of poorly exfoliative, elongated spindle cells that do not exhibit criteria of malignancy. Because they are very fibrous, they usually require biopsy so that an adequate number of representative cells can be evaluated.

Melanomas are traditionally discussed with tumors of mesenchymal origin, although they are actually of neural crest origin, and many exhibit cytologic morphology that is more epithelioid than spindle shaped. Greater than 90% of oral melanomas are malignant. If detected early, they can be completely excised. However, when detected, they have frequently metastasized to the submandibular lymph nodes and then to the thorax. In fact, the ultimate cause of death from malignant melanoma is thoracic metastasis. For this reason, if a melanoma is identified in the oropharynx, evaluation of the submandibular lymph nodes and thoracic radiographs should be included in the workup. If the submandibular lymph nodes are enlarged, cytology or biopsy can be performed to check for metastasis. Individual cellular morphology of malignant melanomas can vary from round to spindle-shaped large cells. They exhibit reticular chromatin, frequently with prominent large nucleoli (Figure 8-13). The N:C ratio is high. The cytoplasm is usually light blue and finely granular, with variable numbers of punctate, round black melanin granules. The nuclear shape varies from round to oval. Some malignant melanomas

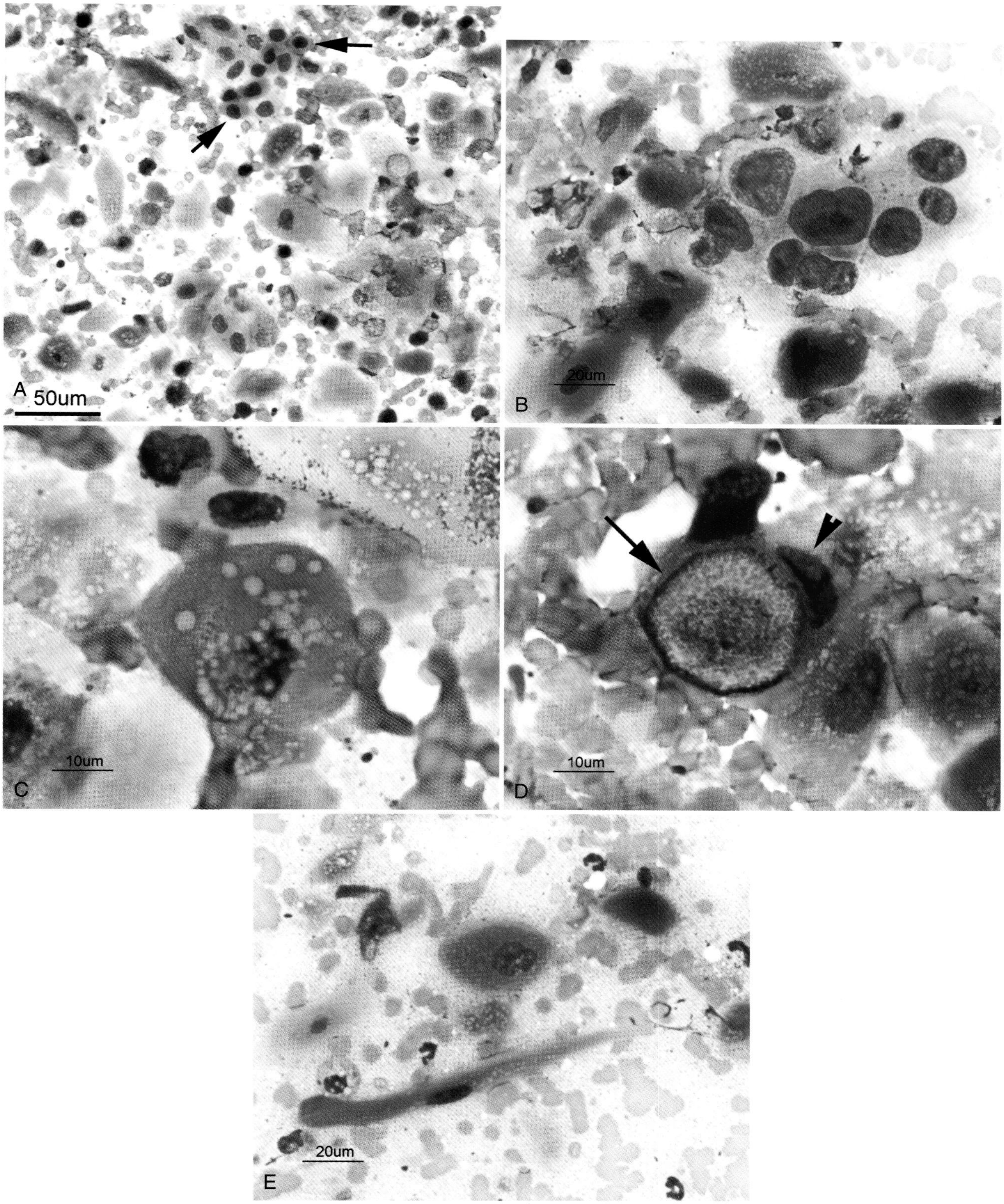

Figure 8-11 Images from an aspirate of a well-differentiated squamous cell carcinoma. A, Low-magnification image shows a dense population of squamous cells. The majority of the cells are fully cornified superficial cells, either with pyknotic nuclei or anucleate. A cluster of relatively uniform noncornified cells is present (*arrows*). Overall, the majority of the cells do not show marked criteria of malignancy. **B,** Another image of the same tumor shows some cells with significant atypia, including marked anisocytosis, nuclear pleomorphism, and large prominent nucleoli. Although these cells were present, they were in low numbers and required diligent searching to find. **C,** Squamous cell showing perinuclear vacuolization. Note the pink-purple color of the cytoplasm, which is seen in some cells undergoing keratinization. **D,** Large eosinophilic cytoplasmic inclusion. This is a common finding in aspirates from a squamous cell carcinoma. **E,** An elongated cornified epithelial cell. This morphologic presentation is seen in some squamous cell carcinomas.

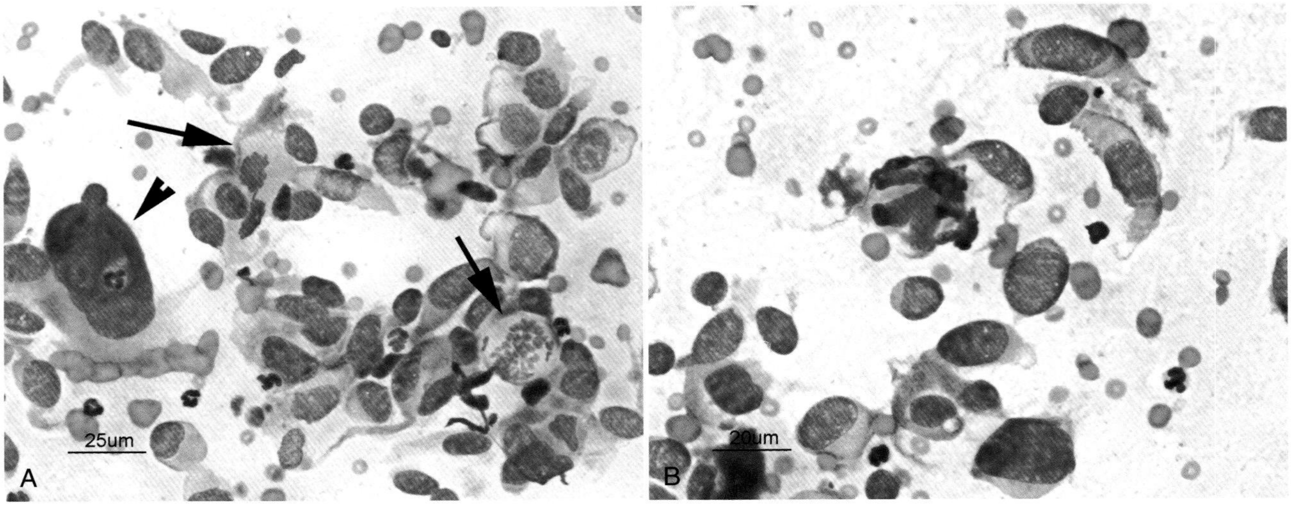

Figure 8-12 Fibrosarcoma from the oral cavity of a cat. A, Dense population of mesenchymal cells. A large, karyomegalic cell (*arrowhead*) and two mitotic figures (*arrows*) are present. **B,** Another image from same aspirate shows cellular pleomorphism, moderate anisokaryosis, and variation of nucleus-to-cytoplasm ratio.

are very poorly melanotic or completely amelanotic, which can make definitive identification almost totally dependent on histopathologic examination. However, such tumors are readily identified as malignant on cytology, and the possibility of an amelanotic melanoma should be considered if cytology demonstrates malignant tumor cells that have variable characteristics, including some cells that are epithelioid and some slightly more spindle shaped. Wide excisional biopsy would be warranted. The highly variable cytologic and histologic appearance of melanomas can make their identification and prognosis problematic by both methods. Ancillary diagnostic techniques such as immunohistochemical stains and monoclonal antibodies to melanocytes can be helpful to identify some melanomas. Currently, no single diagnostic technique is capable of differentiating benign melanocytic neoplasms from malignant ones or predicting survival time.

Malignant Lymphoma: Malignant lymphoma can be found in any lymphoid tissue, and it is the most common tumor of the tonsils. In high-grade lymphoma, greater than 50%, and usually greater than 90%, of the lymphoid cells are large lymphoblasts that exhibit one or more large, prominent nucleoli. The cytoplasm is sparse and deeply basophilic. In some lymphomas, punctate lipid vacuoles are observed in the cytoplasm. The remaining cells are small- and intermediate-sized lymphocytes that appear mature. Small-cell and intermediate-cell lymphomas are less than 10% of canine lymphomas but are more frequent in cats. These are characterized by a predominance of small lymphocytes or intermediate lymphocytes (approximately the size of a neutrophil), and for this reason, they cannot be identified by cytology alone. By definition, they are identified by abnormalities in the tissue architecture while individual cell morphology remains relatively normal. If small-cell or intermediate-cell lymphoma is suspected in the oropharynx, biopsy will be necessary for accurate diagnosis and for differentiation from lymphoid hyperplasia caused by nonspecific immune stimulation.

Discrete Round Cell Tumors: Histiocytomas can occur in dogs of any age, although most occur in young dogs. Mastocytomas occur in the mouth; many are poorly granulated. Some are almost agranular, although careful examination will usually lead to the identification of a few granules that are necessary to differentiate mastocytomas from other discrete round cell tumors. When an oral mastocytoma is identified, the submandibular lymph nodes should be checked for any evidence of metastasis. Consultation with an oncologist for possible treatment options would also be warranted because of the difficulty of obtaining adequate margins when excising a mastocytoma from the oropharynx. Transmissible venereal tumors are occasionally observed in the oropharynx. All discrete round cell tumors in the mouth are cytologically identical to those in the subcutaneous tissues. Refer to the cytologic description of these tumors in Chapter 4.

ALGORITHMIC INTERPRETATION OF SAMPLES

A logical approach to the evaluation of cytology samples is necessary to minimize evaluation time and especially to ensure that the evaluation is thorough and the interpretation is logical. One example of a logical algorithm is presented in this chapter (Figure 8-14). Ultimately, if cytology determines that a tumor is possible or likely, biopsy (excisional if possible) will be warranted, in addition to evaluation of regional lymph nodes and thoracic radiographs. If inflammation is present, bacterial culture, fungal culture or both could be warranted. If appropriate treatment does not lead to complete resolution, biopsy should be performed for further evaluation.

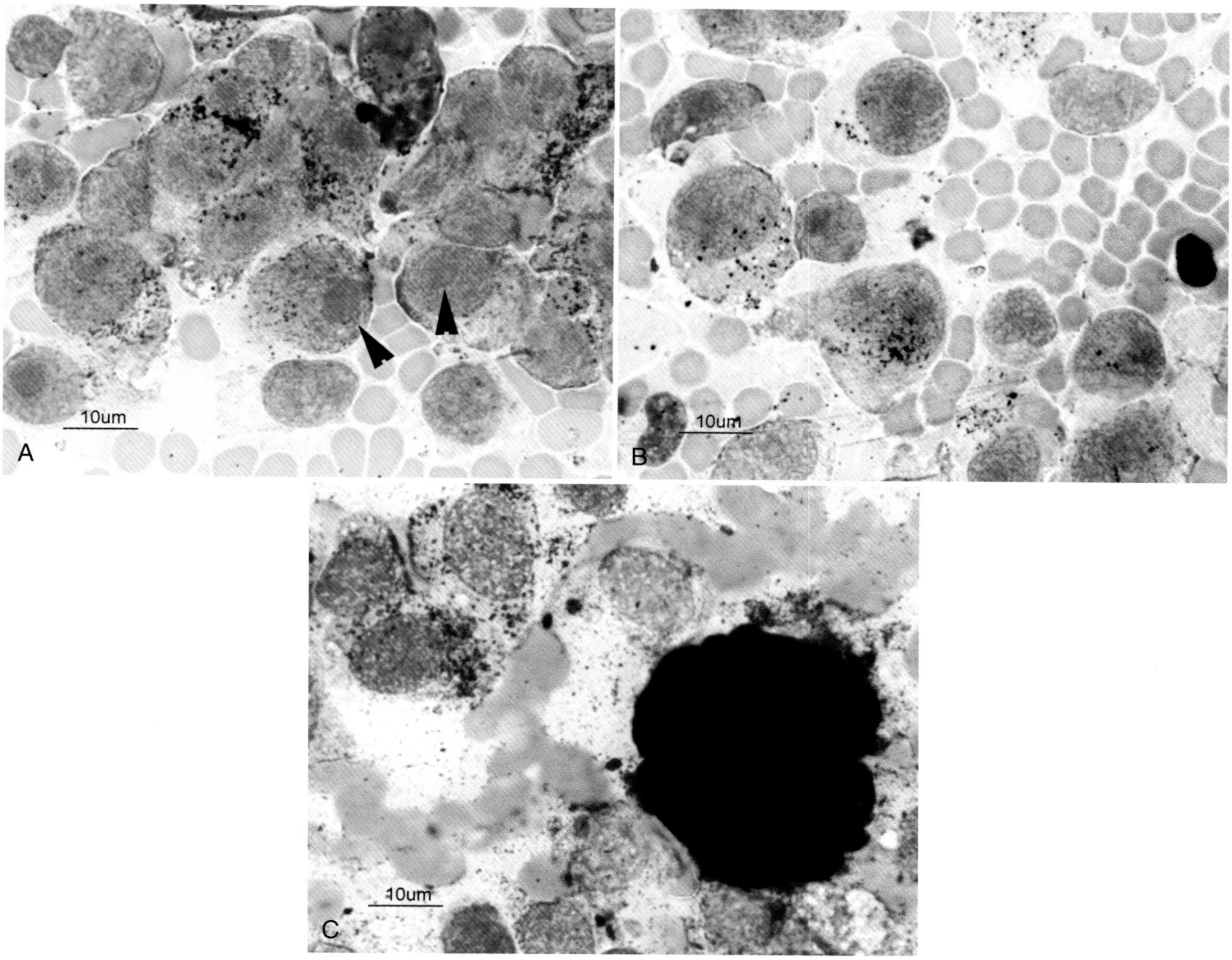

Figure 8-13 Aspirates from a melanoma in the oral cavity of a dog. A, A population of melanocytes showing the marked atypia common with oral melanoma. The cells appear poorly differentiated, being large cells with a high nucleus-to-cytoplasm ratio, noncondensed chromatin, and large prominent nucleoli (*arrowheads*). Although the tumor is poorly pigmented, melanin granules are present in most cells. **B,** Another image from the same slide as in *A*. In this image, the cells appear to have a discrete cell appearance and are individually oriented. Cells from a melanoma may have features of mesenchymal cells, epithelial cells, or discrete cells. Sometimes, cells with each of these morphologies will be present in the same tumor. **C,** Image from another oral melanoma. In addition to the poorly pigmented cells, rare cells are so densely pigmented that the cellular detail is completely obscured and the cell appears simply as a large black sphere.

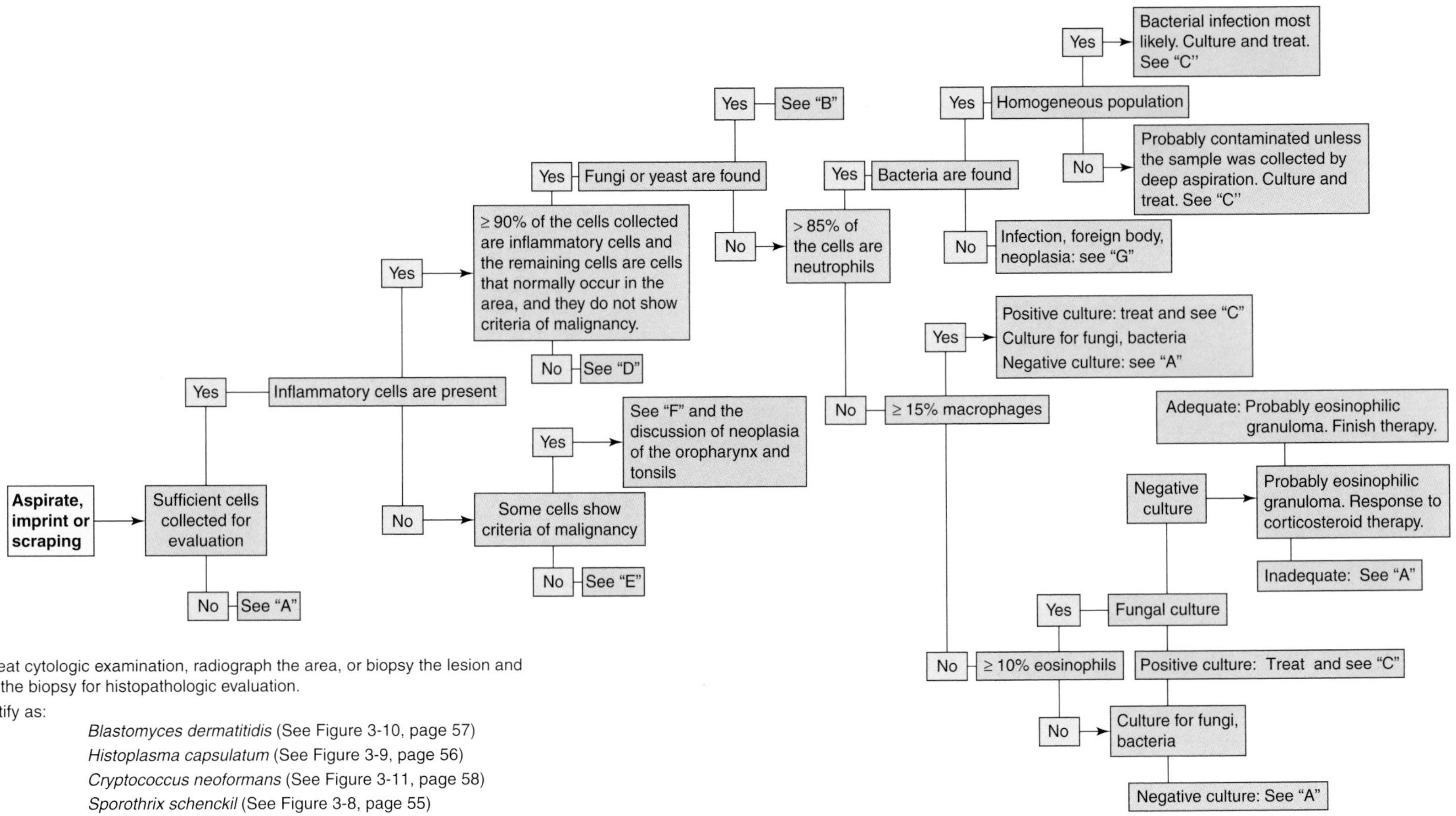

A. Repeat cytologic examination, radiograph the area, or biopsy the lesion and submit the biopsy for histopathologic evaluation.

B. Identify as:

Blastomyces dermatitidis (See Figure 3-10, page 57)
Histoplasma capsulatum (See Figure 3-9, page 56)
Cryptococcus neoformans (See Figure 3-11, page 58)
Sporothrix schenckil (See Figure 3-8, page 55)
Coccidioldes immitis (See Figure 3-12, page 59)

Culture, or refer the slide if unsure of the organism or if specific identification of a hyphating fungus is needed.

C. If there is no response to therapy, the patient should be re-evaluated. Occasionally, tumors become infected and yield cytologic samples containing inflammatory cells and bacteria, but not cells from the tumor. In these cases, antibiotic therapy often eliminates the infection, and subsequent cytologic samples contain sufficient tumor cells to diagnose neoplasia.

D. When there is an admixture of inflammatory cells and noninflammatory cells, the lesion should be evaluated for causes of inflammation and for indications of neoplasia. The more the shift of the admixture is an one direction, the more likely that process is occuring, *ie*, if 85% of the cells are inflammatory cells, then inflammation is very likely and neoplasia is less likely. On the other hand, if 15% of the cells are inflammatory and 85% are noninflammatory cells, neoplasia with secondary inflammation is more likely.

Also, the greater the proportion of inflammatory cells, the stronger the criteria of malignancy must be in cells suspected to be neoplastic for neoplasia to be diagnosed.

Re-evaluation by cytologic, radiographic and/or histopathologic examination after treatment of the inflammatory condition may be necessary.

E. If no inflammatory cells are present and no cells show criteria of malignancy, the lesion is probably due to hyperplasia, benign neoplasia, cyst formation (such as salivary cysts) or collection from normal tissue surrounding the lesion, but malignant neoplasia cannot be ruled out. Re-evaluation by cytologic, radiographic and/or histopathologic examination may be necessary.

F. If no inflammatory cells are present and some of the cells show criteria of malignancy, neoplasia is likely. The morphology of the cells collected should be evaluated to determine, if possible, the tumor cell type and the level of criteria of malignancy. Depending on the tumor cell type and level of criteria of malignancy present, a prediction of the malignant potential of the tumor may be possible. However, histopathologic examination may be necessary for definitive diagnosis.

G. Infection (mycotic or bacterial), neoplasia or foreign body are all possible. At this time, the cytologic preparation may be referred for interpretation, another sample may be collected, the lesion may be cultured and treated accordingly, or radiographic examination or biopsy with histopathologic examination may be performed. If the patient is treated, a cytologic sample collected 1-2 weeks after therapy is begun may reveal the true nature of the lesion.

Figure 8-14 An algorithm for cytologic evaluation of oropharyngeal lesions.

References

1. Raskin RE, Meyer DJ: *Atlas of canine and feline cytology*, St. Louis, MO, 2001, Saunders.
2. Baker R, Lumsden JH: *Color atlas of cytology of the dog and cat*, St. Louis, MO, 2000, Mosby.
3. Bernreuter DC: Cytology of the skin and subcutaneous tissues. In Ettinger SJ, Feldman EC, editors: *Textbook of veterinary internal medicine*, ed 6, St. Louis, MO, 2005, Elsevier, pp 305–307.
4. Smith SH, Goldschmidt MH, McManus PM: A comparative review of melanocytic neoplasms, *Vet Pathol* 39:6651–6678, 2002.

CHAPTER 9

Eyes and Associated Structures

Karen M. Young

Cytologic evaluation of specimens collected from diseased ocular structures may be a valuable aid in both the diagnosis and management of ocular diseases. Although cytologic analysis alone may provide a diagnosis, it is often used in conjunction with other tests such as culture, immunofluorescent staining, polymerase chain reaction (PCR) assays, and biopsy. Proper collection (including appropriate cautions when sampling damaged tissue), sample processing (including concentration techniques), slide preparation, and staining are prerequisites to obtaining accurate and useful information from the microscopic evaluation, as is familiarity with the normal cytologic appearance of the sampled site. If possible, several slides containing adequate sample volume should be prepared to permit the use of special stains, if indicated. When slides are sent to a cytopathologist, it is essential to identify the source of the specimen (e.g., cornea or conjunctiva). The first slide prepared often contains the best material for evaluation and should be included even if it has been stained. In this chapter, cytologic findings are reviewed by anatomic location following some general considerations. Certain lesions, particularly of the eyelids and orbit, are common to other body systems, and illustrations may appear elsewhere in the text.

GENERAL CONSIDERATIONS

Stains

Romanowsky stains are standard and, in general, are excellent for observing the morphologic characteristics of cells, organisms, and other structures. The major artifact is stain precipitate, which can mimic clusters of bacterial cocci. Quick stains (such as Diff-Quik) are often adequate but do not stain cytoplasmic features as well as do parent stains, especially methanolic stains. In some instances, for example, mast cell granules do not stain with quick stains, and the presence of these cells may go undetected if other stains are not used. Also, quick stains must be maintained well, or the stains themselves may contain organisms such as *Malassezia* from previously stained specimens or from contamination. Other stains that may be used as adjuncts include stains for fungal organisms, such as periodic acid-Schiff (PAS) and Gomori methenamine silver stain (GMS). Gram stain may be used to determine if bacteria are Gram-positive or Gram-negative. Gram-stained slides can be tricky to read and require experience to avoid misinterpretation. Indirect fluorescent antibody (IFA) staining requires special reagents and a fluorescence microscope.

Microscopic Evaluation

Ocular specimens are often small in volume, and therefore examination of the entire sample is easy. The observer should be familiar with the normal cytologic and histologic characteristics of the tissue sampled and recognize cellular patterns, other structures, and background material.[1,2] Identification of specific types of inflammatory cells permits classification of inflammation as neutrophilic (synonyms include suppurative and purulent); eosinophilic (often accompanied by mast cells); lymphocytic–plasmacytic; mixed, including pyogranulomatous; and granulomatous. If neoplasia is suspected on the basis of the presence of a mass and a homogenous population of noninflammatory cells, the observer should be able to identify the cell type (epithelial, mesenchymal or connective tissue, and discrete round cells) and the cytologic features of benign and malignant tumors. It is important to recognize that neoplasms can induce an inflammatory response. Finally, the observer should be familiar with the cytologic characteristics of cysts, acute and chronic hemorrhage, and degenerative diseases.

When identifying cell types, it is essential to examine cells in an area where they can be evaluated individually. However, thick collections of material—often consisting of clustered epithelial cells, aggregates of mesenchymal cells, or necrotic material—tend to be understained, and cells with granules that stain more readily than other components (mast cell and eosinophil granules), naturally pigmented elements (melanin), bacteria, and fungal hyphae may be visualized within or on top of the thick tissue (Figure 9-1). Inclusions found in epithelial or inflammatory cells may be normal elements, artifacts of treatment, or evidence of the pathologic process or etiology (Table 9-1). Normal tissue also may be present.

Once a category is identified, a more specific diagnosis may be possible. For example, search for an etiologic agent is indicated if inflammation is present. At the very least, the category can guide additional testing or therapy.

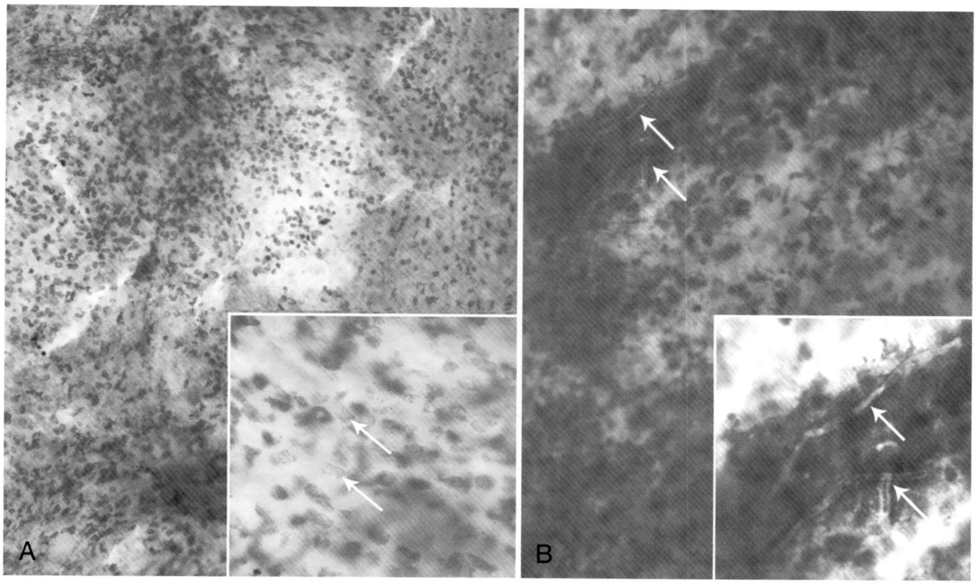

Figure 9-1 Thick understained tissue from two corneal scrapes in which significant structures or cells may be visualized. A, Eosinophils and eosinophil granules (*arrows*). **B,** Fungal hyphae (*arrows*). (Wright stain, original magnification 200×; insets 600×.)

TABLE 9-1

Inclusions in or on Cells from Ocular Tissue

Inclusions	Significance
Inclusions in or on Epithelial Cells	
Melanin granules	Normal in pigmented tissue Small granules may be confused with *Mycoplasma* organisms
Mucin or mucin granules	Normal goblet cells
Surface mixed bacteria	Contaminants
Drug inclusions	Artifact of treatment with topical ophthalmic ointments
Mycoplasma spp.	Pathogen
Chlamydophila spp.	Pathogen
Neutrophils	Intact neutrophils within squamous cells: no known significance
Inclusions in Neutrophils	
Bacteria	Pathogen
Small fungal organisms (e.g., *Histoplasma* spp.)	Pathogen
Pyknotic nuclei	Aging-related change or accelerated apoptosis
Inclusions in Macrophages	
Red blood cells (erythrophagia)	Hemorrhage
White blood cells (leukophagia): whole or degraded	Longstanding inflammation
Iron pigment (macrophages are termed *hemosiderophages*)	Chronic or previous hemorrhage
Melanin (macrophages are termed *melanophages*)	Pigmented tissue with release of melanin from ruptured or degraded epithelial cells
Certain bacteria (e.g., *Mycobacterium* spp.)	Pathogen
Some fungal organisms (e.g., *Histoplasma* spp.)	Pathogen
Protozoal organisms (e.g., *Leishmania* spp.)	Pathogen

TABLE 9-2

Special Cytologic Features and Their Significance

Cytologic Feature	Significance
Neutrophils	
Nondegenerate: well-lobulated condensed nuclei, intact nuclear and plasma membranes	Neutrophilic or purulent inflammation: septic or nonseptic
Degenerate: swollen hypolobulated nuclei, fragmented nuclear or cytoplasmic membrane	Septic inflammation likely
Pyknotic: shrunken, condensed, rounded, and disconnected nuclear lobes	Aging-related change or accelerated apoptosis
Intracytoplasmic bacteria	Usually pathogen(s)
Epithelial Cells	
Dysplastic change: nucleus-to-cytoplasm (N:C) asynchrony	Secondary to inflammation; differentiate from epithelial neoplasia with secondary inflammation
Cornification or keratinization; keratin does not stain with Romanowsky stains; its presence is inferred when squamous cells are angular or folded	Abnormal for corneal epithelial cells; occurs in keratitis
Extracellular Material	
Bacteria	Possible contaminants, but may be significant, especially if found in corneal samples or if many bacteria of a single morphology are noted
Fungal organisms: yeast forms of *Blastomyces*, *Cryptococcus*, *Coccidioides*, *Histoplasma*; hyphae of *Aspergillus* and other fungi	Pathogens
Parasites: larvae rarely seen cytologically	Pathogens
Free eosinophil, mast cell, or melanin granules	Indicate presence of ruptured eosinophils, mast cells, or epithelial cells; granules may be mistaken for bacteria
Cell fragments, especially stringy nuclear chromatin	Artifact of slide preparation; may resemble fungal hyphae when surrounded by mucus
Cholesterol crystals	Epithelial degeneration
Stain precipitate	Artifact; may be mistaken for bacterial cocci
Mucus	Normal in areas where goblet cells are located; may be increased with some pathologic processes

Special cytologic features of neutrophils, epithelial cells, and extracellular material (Table 9-2) often provide additional information about the pathologic process; misinterpretation of these features (e.g., mistaking free mast cell granules for bacterial cocci) could lead to erroneous conclusions.

EYELIDS

The eyelid comprises layers of skin and mucous membrane (palpebral conjunctiva) separated by muscle and specialized glands, particularly of the sebaceous type. Lesions of the eyelids for which cytologic evaluation is useful include ulcerative and exudative lesions of the epidermal surface (blepharitis) and discrete masses on either the epidermal or conjunctival surface. Conjunctivitis and conjunctival cytology are described later.

Fine-needle aspiration (FNA) of ulcerated lesions and discrete masses usually provides diagnostic specimens. Frequently, specimens from eyelid lesions contain abundant blood. Scraping may be a reasonable means of sample collection for diffuse exudative epidermal lesions of the eyelid such as parasitic blepharitis. Touch imprints of exudative skin lesions may reflect the cause of the lesion or may contain only surface debris. Therefore, both touch imprints of the exudate and samples collected after cleaning the surface of the lesion should be examined.

Blepharitis

Blepharitis may be focal or diffuse and acute or chronic; bacterial, mycotic, parasitic, allergic, or immune-mediated blepharitis may occur. The objectives in cytologic examination of lesions of blepharitis are to characterize the type of exudate (neutrophilic, lymphocytic–plasmacytic, eosinophilic, or granulomatous) and search for the causative agent. Agents that may be encountered in scrapings are *Sarcoptes* spp., *Demodex* spp., dermatophytic yeast, and bacteria. *Demodex folliculorum* causes minimal exudation. Bacterial blepharitis, particularly staphylococcal blepharitis, has a neutrophilic exudate. Certain fungi,

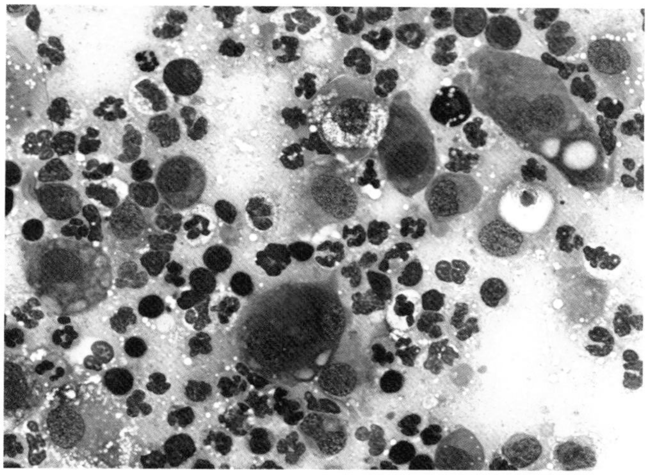

Figure 9-2 Pyogranulomatous inflammation in the eyelid of a dog. Note neutrophils and epithelioid macrophages, including binucleate forms. Lymphocytes and low numbers of red blood cells also are present. (Wright stain, original magnification 600×.)

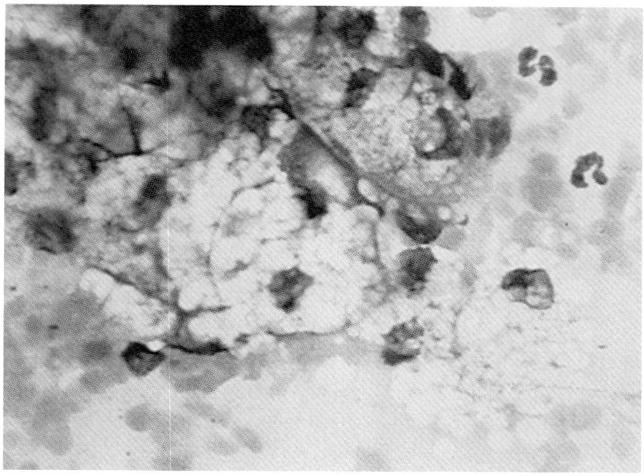

Figure 9-3 Sebaceous gland epithelial cells from a well-differentiated sebaceous gland tumor on a canine eyelid. (Romanowsky-type stain, original magnification 1000×.)

such as *Blastomyces dermatitidis*, cause either a primarily neutrophilic or a pyogranulomatous exudate, whereas others cause a granulomatous exudate composed of macrophages, including epithelioid forms, and giant cells. Foreign bodies may elicit a pyogranulomatous or granulomatous response (Figure 9-2).

Immune-mediated disease usually is characterized by a neutrophilic exudate, but eosinophilic types also occur. The presence of either bacteria or a primarily neutrophilic exudate does not exclude allergic and immune-mediated causes, especially if the lesion is ulcerated. In cats, eosinophilic plaques may manifest as periocular blepharitis. A fine-needle aspirate contains primarily eosinophils, some mast cells, and a mixture of other white blood cell (WBC) types.

Discrete Masses

Discrete masses on the eyelids may be neoplastic (benign or malignant) or nonneoplastic. Among neoplasms, benign sebaceous gland tumors (sebaceous adenoma, sebaceous epithelioma) are the most common type on canine eyelids. The glands of Zeis and Moll at the eyelid margin and the meibomian glands, which lie beneath the palpebral conjunctiva and open at the lid margin, are all of the sebaceous type; tumors arising from them are similar to cutaneous sebaceous gland tumors. The cells are readily recognized by their voluminous vacuolated cytoplasm that nearly obscures small rounded nuclei (Figure 9-3). The malignant counterpart of these tumors is rare on the eyelids.

Other tumors frequently encountered on the eyelids and readily diagnosed by cytologic examination include melanoma (benign and malignant), histiocytoma (Figure 9-4), lymphoma, mast cell tumor (low and high grade) (Figure 9-5), papilloma, and squamous cell carcinoma. Squamous cell carcinomas are frequently ulcerated. In mast cell tumors, mast cell granules sometimes are not visible if quick stains are used (see Figure 9-5, *B*). Other carcinomas and connective tissue tumors (fibrosarcoma, hemangiosarcoma, histiocytic sarcoma) occur less frequently and are discussed in Chapter 2.

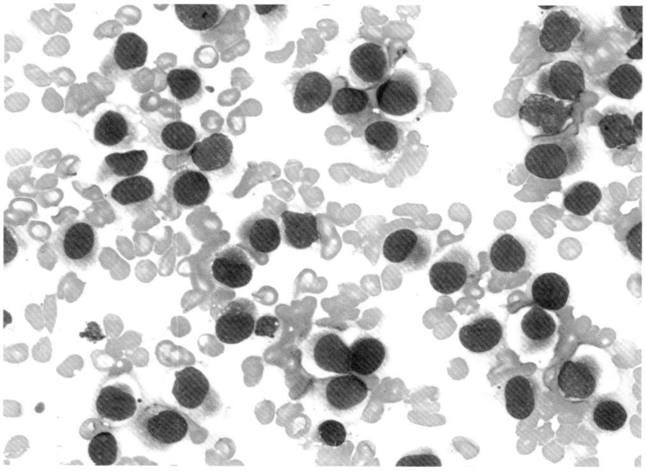

Figure 9-4 Discrete round cell tumor with cytologic characteristics of a histiocytoma on the eyelid of a dog. (Wright stain, original magnification 600×.)

Nonneoplastic discrete masses unique to the eyelid include the hordeolum, a localized purulent lesion of sebaceous glands, and the chalazion, a lipogranuloma of the meibomian gland. FNA of these lesions yields numerous foamy macrophages and a few giant cells and lymphocytes. The macrophages are apparently phagocytosing glandular secretory product; cytophagia is not prominent. Variable numbers of sebaceous epithelial cells also are found. Differentiating a hordeolum or chalazion from sebaceous gland adenoma by cytologic examination may be difficult if the latter has ruptured internally and caused secondary inflammation. A hordeolum or a chalazion may contain inspissated secretory product or mineralized debris that appears as amorphous granular material on cytologic preparations.

Ocular idiopathic adnexal granulomas may simulate neoplasms, be bilateral, and be a component of systemic

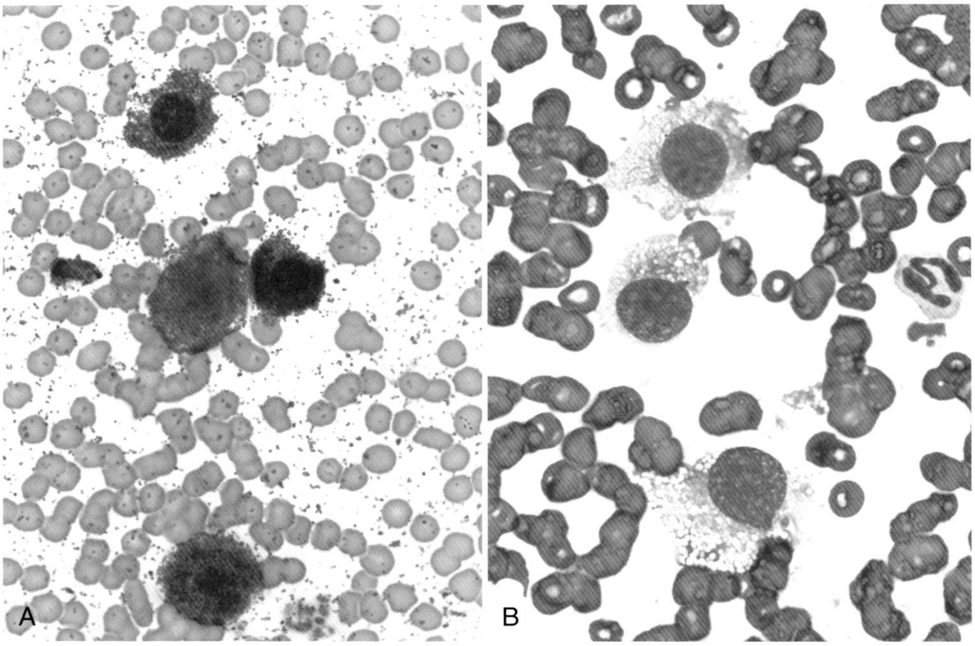

Figure 9-5 **A,** Well-granulated mast cell tumor on the eyelid of a dog. (Wright stain, original magnification 600×.) **B,** The same specimen stained with a quick stain. Note that mast cell granules did not stain. (Diff-Quik stain, original magnification 600×.)

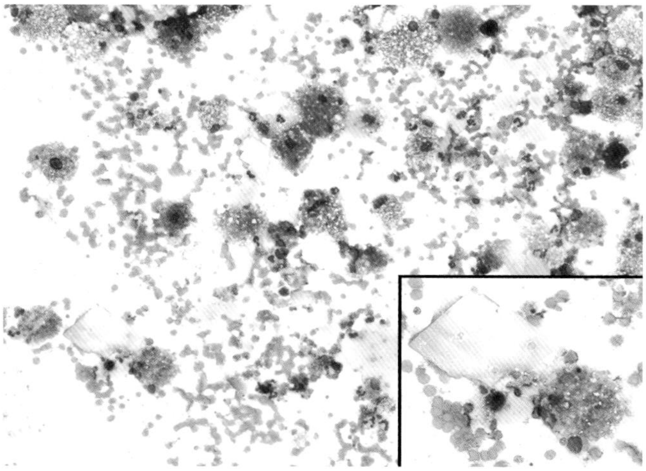

Figure 9-6 Cytocentrifuged material from a cyst on the eyelid of a dog. Note the foamy macrophages and cholesterol crystals. (Wright stain, original magnification 200×, inset 600×.)

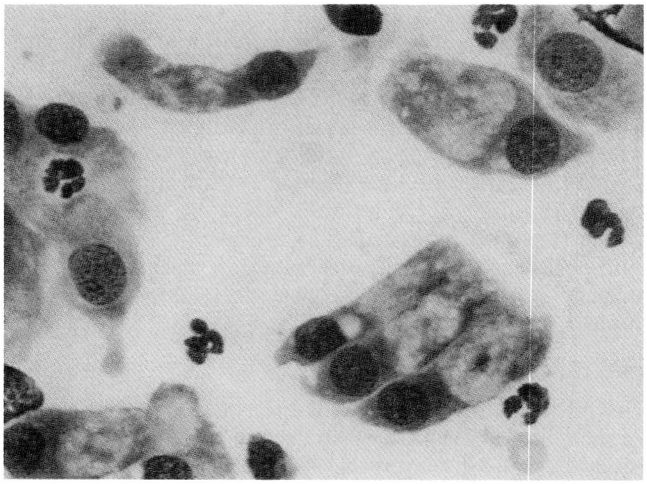

Figure 9-7 Canine conjunctival scraping contains palpebral columnar ciliated cells and goblet cells. (Romanowsky-type stain, original magnification 1000×.)

granulomatous disease.[3] Systemic histiocytosis of Bernese Mountain Dogs causes periocular granulomatous masses.[4,5] True cysts can occur on the eyelids and typically contain foamy macrophages and cholesterol crystals from epithelial degeneration (Figure 9-6).

CONJUNCTIVA

The primary goals for conjunctival cytologic evaluation are characterization of an exudate and identification of the cause of conjunctivitis. Certain anatomic structures affect the types of cells found on all preparations from normal and diseased eyes. The conjunctiva is composed of two continuous layers of epithelium that lie in apposition. The inner epithelial layer of the eyelid, called the palpebral conjunctiva, is composed of pseudostratified columnar epithelium and interspersed goblet cells (Figure 9-7). Cilia may be found on the columnar cells. At the fornix, deep within the conjunctival sac, the epithelium reflects back over the globe. This bulbar conjunctiva is composed of stratified squamous epithelium (Figure 9-8). Bulbar conjunctiva is continuous with the corneal epithelium at the limbus. The squamous cells are noncornified and often contain melanin granules (Figure 9-9). In most conjunctival scrapings, squamous cells are more numerous than columnar cells. In animals treated with topical ophthalmic

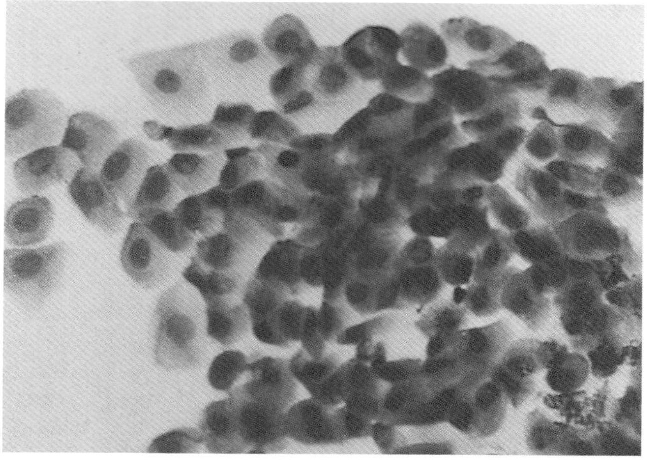

Figure 9-8 Basal, intermediate, and mature noncornified squamous cells typical of bulbar conjunctival epithelium from a canine conjunctival scraping. (Romanowsky-type stain, original magnification 400×.)

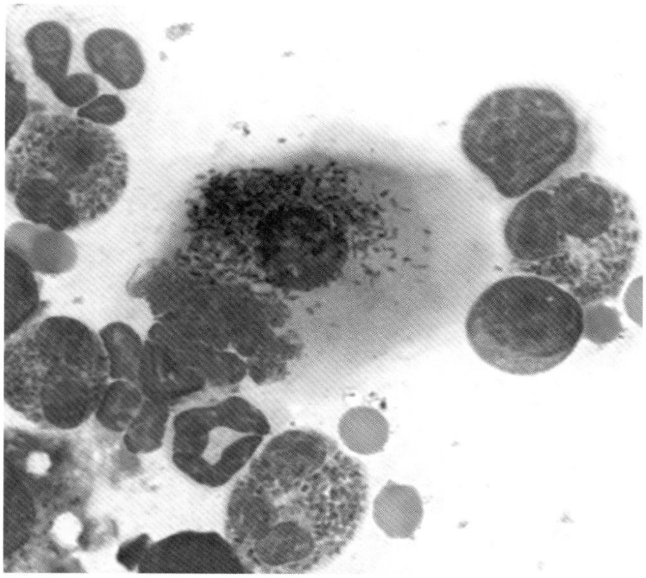

Figure 9-9 Conjunctival scraping from a cat. An epithelial cell contains numerous melanin granules. (Wright stain, original magnification 1000×.) (From Young KM, Taylor J: Laboratory medicine: yesterday-today-tomorrow. Eye on the cytoplasm, *Vet Clin Pathol* 35:141, 2006. Reprinted with permission of the American Society for Veterinary Clinical Pathology.)

ointments (particularly neomycin), epithelial cells may contain dense basophilic homogeneous cytoplasmic inclusions (Figure 9-10).[6] Such inclusions must be differentiated from infectious agents. At the fornix, conjunctival lamina propria contains lymphoid tissue; various types of lymphoid cells may be found in any conjunctival scraping. Without clinical signs of conjunctivitis, little emphasis should be placed on the observation of lymphocytes or plasma cells among epithelial cells.

Cytologic preparations from the conjunctiva should include freshly derived cells. If external debris within the conjunctival sac is present, imprints of the debris should

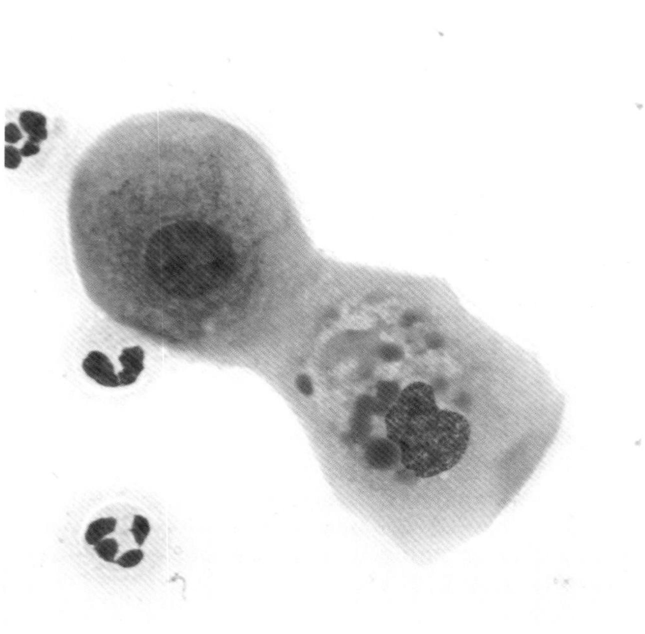

Figure 9-10 A corneal scrape contains squamous cells with dense, homogeneous, blue cytoplasmic inclusions believed to be a consequence of treatment with ophthalmic ointment. (Wright stain, original magnification 600×.) (From Young KM, Taylor J: Laboratory medicine: yesterday-today-tomorrow. Eye on the cytoplasm, *Vet Clin Pathol* 35:141, 2006. Reprinted with permission of the American Society for Veterinary Clinical Pathology.)

be made because this material may contain the etiologic agent such as *Blastomyces* spp. More often, the debris obscures the primary lesion; therefore, after imprints are made, the debris should be removed and conjunctival scraping performed with a flat, round-tipped spatula. Preparation of bulbar conjunctival imprints using filter strips following topical anesthesia has been reported in dogs.[7]

Neutrophilic Conjunctivitis

Canine and feline conjunctivitis frequently is neutrophilic and results from bacterial or viral infections, allergic disease, or other causes. Pseudomembranous (ligneous) conjunctivitis is neutrophilic.[8] Cytologic evaluation may not reveal the cause. Neutrophils may be nondegenerate or degenerate (Figure 9-11); in cats, the latter are rarely encountered. In both dogs and cats, intact neutrophils may be found within squamous cells, and the significance of this finding is unknown. Mucus is a common component of neutrophilic exudates and may cause cells to be aligned in rows on the smear.

The exudate of canine neutrophilic conjunctivitis often contains bacteria, regardless of the primary cause. Bacteria are often large or small cocci and less frequently rods (Figure 9-12). The dilemma is determining whether the bacteria are of primary importance or are merely opportunistic. Normal bacterial flora of the canine conjunctival sac have been described.[9] Keratoconjunctivitis sicca is a common canine disorder causing neutrophilic exudate in which bacteria frequently are encountered. The disease is diagnosed readily by the Schirmer tear test. In contrast to

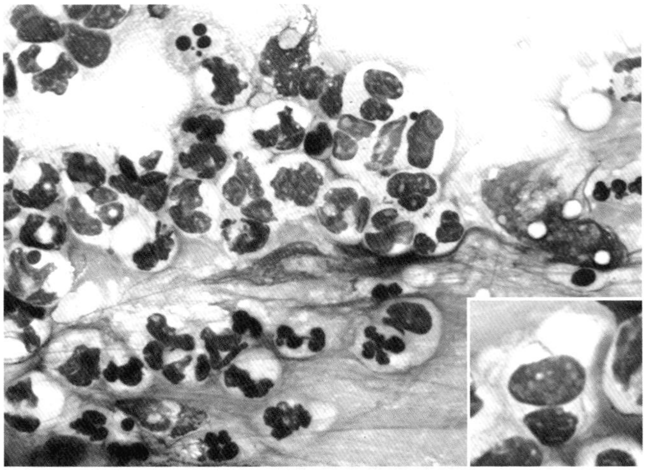

Figure 9-11 Conjunctival scrape from a dog with neutrophilic bacterial conjunctivitis. Both well-segmented nondegenerate neutrophils and degenerate neutrophils with swollen nuclei are present. (Wright stain, original magnification 600×.) *Inset,* A degenerate neutrophil with two thin bacterial rods. (Wright stain, original magnification 1000×.)

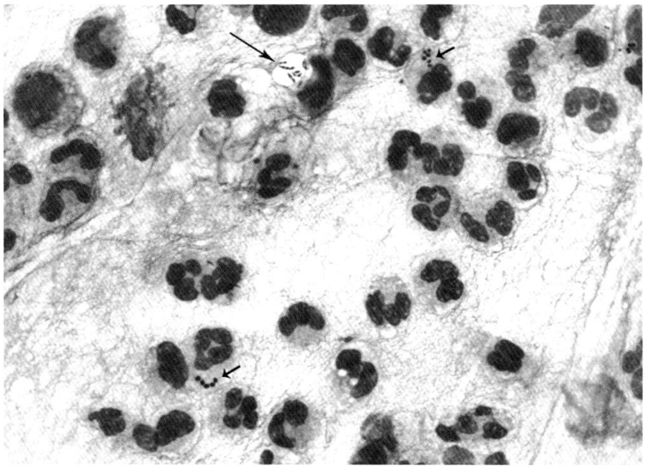

Figure 9-12 Conjunctival scrape from a dog. Note many neutrophils and bacterial rods (*long arrow*) and cocci (*short arrows*). (Wright stain, original magnification 1000×.)

that of dogs, the exudate of feline neutrophilic conjunctivitis rarely contains bacteria. When observed, bacteria should be considered clinically significant in feline conjunctivitis.

Distemper is the most important viral cause of canine neutrophilic conjunctivitis. Canine distemper is diagnosed on the basis of its classic clinical signs and fluorescent antibody staining of conjunctival smears. Canine distemper inclusion bodies in epithelial cells are found rarely (Figure 9-13), and a search for them has limited diagnostic value.

A common cause of feline neutrophilic conjunctivitis is herpesvirus infection. Diagnosis is confirmed by PCR analysis, fluorescent antibody staining of conjunctival smears, or viral isolation. Multinucleate epithelial cells may be found, but intranuclear inclusion bodies are seen rarely, if ever, cytologically.

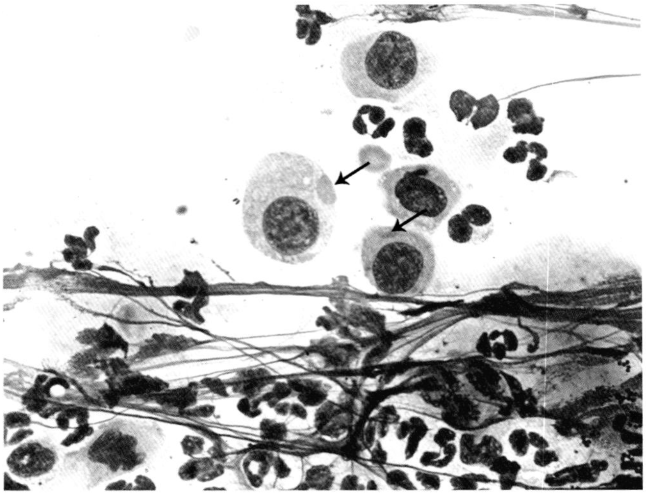

Figure 9-13 Conjunctival scrape from a dog. Variably sized distemper viral inclusions (*arrows*) are found within epithelial cells. Note neutrophils and small bacterial rods and cocci. (Wright stain, original magnification 1000×.) (Photomicrograph by Judith Taylor; from Young KM, Taylor J: Laboratory medicine: yesterday-today-tomorrow. Eye on the cytoplasm, *Vet Clin Pathol* 35:141, 2006. Reprinted with permission of the American Society for Veterinary Clinical Pathology.)

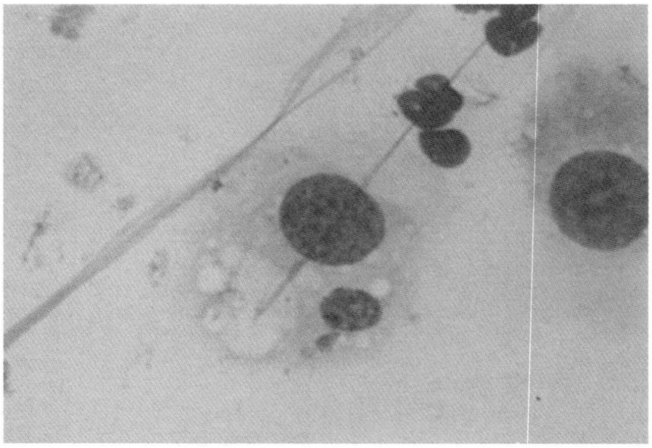

Figure 9-14 Initial body of *Chlamydophila felis* in the cytoplasm of a squamous cell in a conjunctival scrape from a cat. (Romanowsky-type stain, original magnification 1000×.)

Neutrophils also predominate in the conjunctival exudate of feline chlamydial infection. In experimental *Chlamydophila felis* infections, organisms were found on day 6 postinoculation, after clinical signs first appeared.[10] Solitary, large (3 to 5 micrometers [μm]), basophilic particulate forms initially are found in the cytoplasm of squamous epithelial cells (Figure 9-14). The particulate nature of the initial body is an important observation to distinguish *C. felis* from incidental foci of homogeneous cytoplasmic basophilia found in squamous epithelial cells (Figure 9-10); organisms also may appear as aggregates of coccoid basophilic bodies (elementary bodies), measuring 0.5 to 1 μm in diameter (Figure 9-15).[11] In experimental infections, organisms rarely were found by day 14 after inoculation, and in chronic conjunctivitis, intracytoplasmic

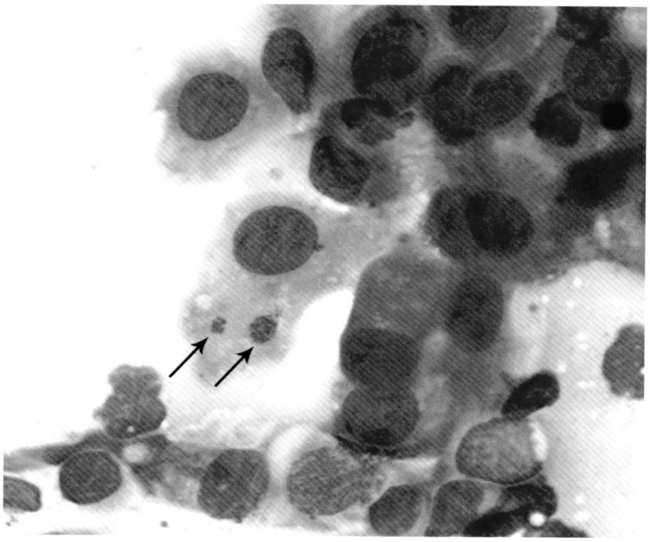

Figure 9-15 Conjunctival scraping from a cat with chlamydial conjunctivitis. Elementary bodies of *Chlamydophila felis* are found in an epithelial cell (*arrows*). (Wright stain, original magnification 1000×.) (From Young KM, Taylor J: Laboratory medicine: yesterday-today-tomorrow. Eye on the cytoplasm, *Vet Clin Pathol* 35:141, 2006. Reprinted with permission of the American Society for Veterinary Clinical Pathology.)

organisms are present only infrequently.[10,12] Chlamydial conjunctivitis may be confirmed by PCR analysis or fluorescent antibody staining. Chlamydiae other than *C. felis* also may play a role in ocular disease in cats.[13]

Feline mycoplasmosis, another cause of neutrophilic conjunctivitis, may be diagnosed by finding the organisms on epithelial cells on routinely stained smears. In one study, mycoplasmosis was diagnosed in nine naturally infected cats by isolation and identification of *Mycoplasma* spp. Of samples from 16 eyes, the organisms were found on Romanowsky-stained smears from 15 eyes, suggesting a high degree of diagnostic sensitivity for routine cytologic evaluation in *Mycoplasma* infection.[14] Other studies have found cytologic examination to be less reliable in the diagnosis of mycoplasmosis.[11] The basophilic organisms, 0.2 to 0.8 μm long, may be found in clusters adherent to the outer limits of the plasma membrane or over the flattened surface of squamous epithelial cells (Figure 9-16). They also may be seen in clusters between cells. *Mycoplasma* organisms should not be confused with melanin granules (Figure 9-9).

Lymphocytic–Plasmacytic Conjunctivitis

Conjunctivitis in which lymphoid cells predominate is less common than purulent conjunctivitis. Lymphocytic–plasmacytic conjunctivitis occurs in allergic and chronic infectious conjunctivitis (Figure 9-17). Follicular conjunctivitis yields cells typical of reactive lymphoid hyperplasia (see the section "Nictitating Membrane").

Eosinophilic and Mast Cell Conjunctivitis

Eosinophilic conjunctivitis is encountered in dogs and cats (Figure 9-18). It has been observed in cats as a sole entity and concomitant with eosinophilic keratitis. In conjunctival

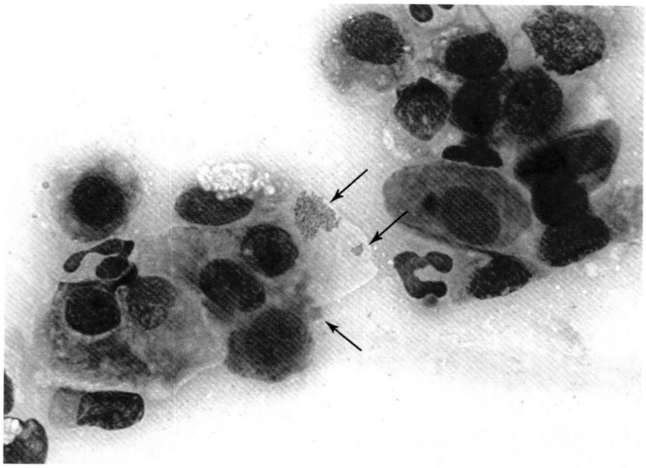

Figure 9-16 Conjunctival scraping from a cat with mycoplasmal conjunctivitis. *Mycoplasma felis* organisms (*arrows*) are visible on the surface of and adjacent to an epithelial cell. Note neutrophilic inflammation. (Wright stain, original magnification 1000×.) (From Young KM, Taylor J: Laboratory medicine: yesterday-today-tomorrow. Eye on the cytoplasm, *Vet Clin Pathol* 35:141, 2006. Reprinted with permission of the American Society for Veterinary Clinical Pathology.)

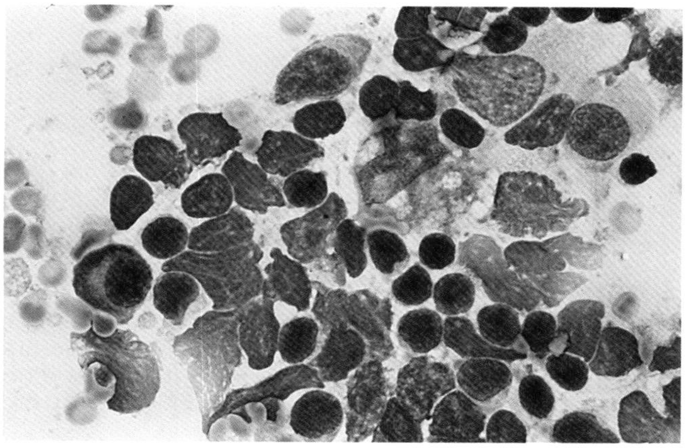

Figure 9-17 Conjunctival scraping from a cat with lymphocytic–plasmacytic conjunctivitis. Note numerous lymphocytes, a plasma cell (*left margin*), and a macrophage (*top right center*). (Romanowsky-type stain, original magnification 1000×.)

smears from both dogs and cats, mast cells also may be present. Some cases test positive for feline herpesvirus by PCR. In preparations stained with quick stains, sometimes neither eosinophil granules nor mast cell granules stain well, and eosinophils may be mistaken for neutrophils. In addition, free eosinophil granules, which are rod-shaped in cats, and mast cell granules from ruptured cells should not be mistaken for bacterial rods and cocci, respectively (see the section "Eosinophilic Keratitis").

Noninflammatory Lesions of Conjunctiva

Neoplasms of the conjunctiva include papilloma, squamous cell carcinoma, melanoma, lipoma, lymphoma (Figure 9-19), mast cell tumors, and others.[15] A unique form of mast cell neoplasia occurs in canine conjunctiva and

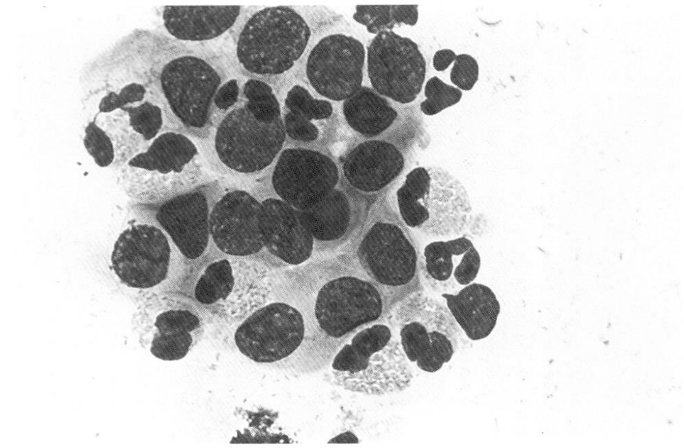

Figure 9-18 Eosinophils and squamous cells in a conjunctival scraping from a cat with eosinophilic conjunctivitis. (Romanowsky-type stain, original magnification 1000×.)

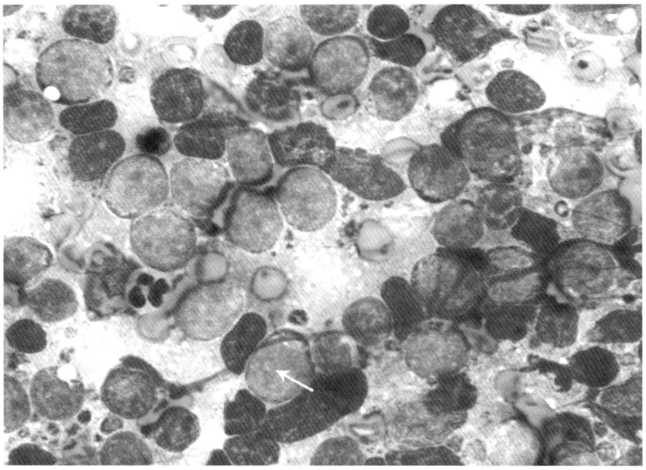

Figure 9-19 Conjunctival lymphoma from a dog. Note the predominance of large lymphoid cells with visible nucleoli (*arrow*). Free nuclei and cytoplasmic fragments from ruptured cells are present in the background. (Wright stain, original magnification 1000×.)

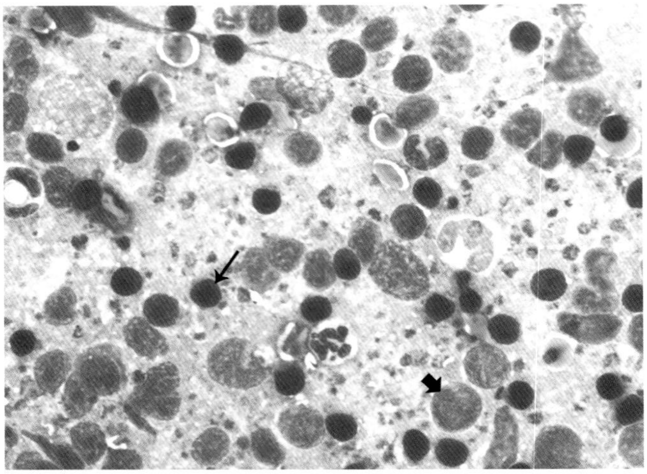

Figure 9-20 Corneal scrape from a dog with follicular conjunctivitis. Small lymphocytes (*thin arrow*) are numerous, and large lymphoid cells (*thick arrow*) also are present. Again, free nuclei and cytoplasmic fragments from ruptured cells are present in the background. (Wright stain, original magnification 1000×.)

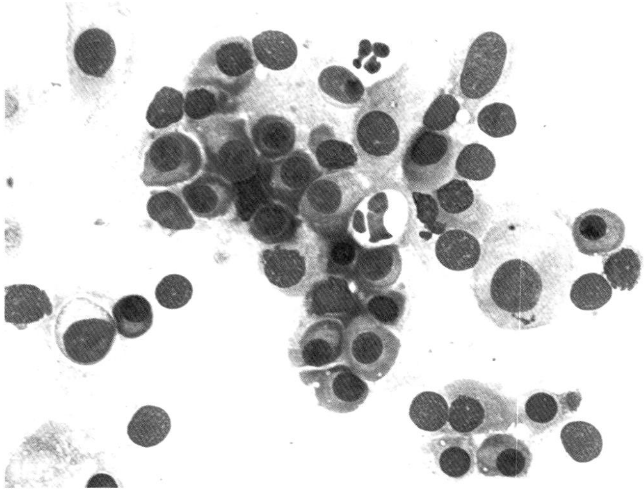

Figure 9-21 Numerous plasma cells in a scraping of the third eyelid from a German Shepherd with plasmacytic conjunctivitis. (Wright stain, original magnification 600×.)

manifests as severe diffuse swelling of the conjunctiva.[16] Cytologic examination of mast cell tumors is discussed in Chapters 2 and 4. Conjunctival hemangioma and hemangiosarcoma occur most frequently within the nonpigmented epithelium of the temporal bulbar conjunctiva in dogs or the nictitating membrane in dogs and cats.[17,18]

Cystlike swellings of the conjunctiva are uncommon and include dacryops (see discussion of nasolacrimal apparatus later in this chapter), zygomatic mucocele, deposteroid granuloma, tumors, staphyloma, and inclusion cysts. The cytologic findings for a mucocele are identical to salivary cysts described in Chapter 6.

NICTITATING MEMBRANE

The nictitating membrane, or third eyelid, is composed of T-shaped cartilage covered by conjunctiva that is continuous with the bulbar and palpebral conjunctiva on its inner and outer surfaces. The gland of the third eyelid, a seromucous gland, envelops the base of the cartilage. Lymphoid tissue is located on the bulbar surface superior to the gland. Consequently, cells found on nictitans scrapings depend on which surface is sampled. Scrapings of the bulbar surface of the membrane in normal or diseased eyes may resemble cytologic preparations from lymph nodes, with all expected types of lymphoid cells.

As a conjunctival surface, the nictitating membrane may be affected by most of the diseases of the conjunctiva described in the previous section. Only a few specific lesions of the membrane require cytologic evaluation for differential diagnosis. Cytologic evaluation of follicular hyperplasia reveals lymphoid hyperplasia (Figure 9-20). A specific lesion in German Shepherds is plasmacytic conjunctivitis, in which scrapings of the third eyelid reveal many plasma cells and some lymphocytes (Figure 9-21).

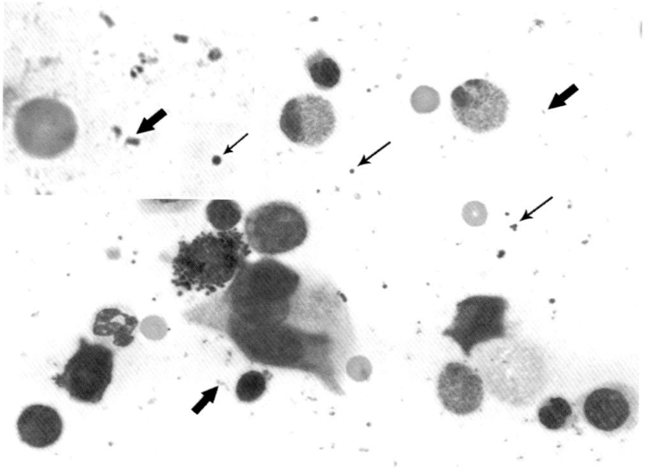

Figure 9-31 Numerous free rod-shaped eosinophil (*thick arrows*) and round mast cell (*thin arrows*) granules are found in a corneal scrape from a cat with eosinophilic keratitis. (Wright stain, original magnification 1000×.)

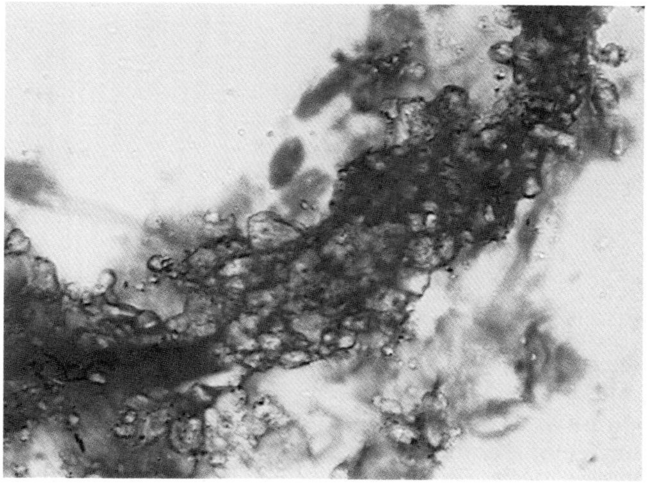

Figure 9-32 Amorphous nonstaining crystalline material and cell debris in a corneal scraping from a dog with mineralizing corneal degeneration. (Romanowsky-type stain, original magnification 1000×.)

the choroid, termed the posterior uvea. The diagnosis of anterior uveitis is made clinically, and aspiration of aqueous humor from the anterior chamber is performed in some cases with the goal of achieving a specific diagnosis. Posterior uveal disease is indicated by changes in the vitreous, which also can be aspirated for diagnostic purposes.

Aqueous Humor

Aspiration of aqueous humor for cytodiagnostic purposes may be indicated when the fluid is cloudy or opaque. However, clinical examination without cytologic examination is sufficient to discern hyphema, hypopyon, flare, and the presence of lipid. In feline anterior uveitis, no distinguishing cytologic features exist among various causes such as toxoplasmosis and infection with feline infectious peritonitis virus. Lymphoma may be diagnosed by examination of aqueous or iris aspirates; however, most other

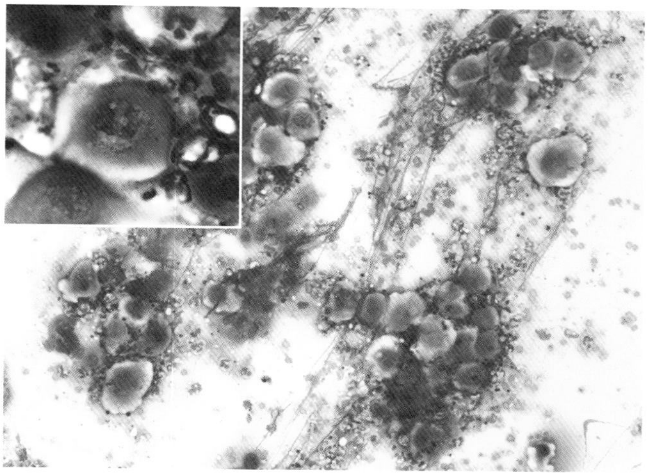

Figure 9-33 Squamous cell carcinoma on the cornea of a dog. Note the monolayer sheets of neoplastic squamous cells and numerous neutrophils. (Wright stain, original magnification 600×.) *Inset,* Perinuclear vacuolation in a neoplastic squamous cell. (Wright stain, original magnification 1000×.)

intraocular tumors, either primary or secondary, do not exfoliate into aqueous humor (see the following section "Iris and Ciliary Body"). In most cases of infectious endophthalmitis, identification of organisms from aspirates of vitreous is more productive than examining aqueous humor (see later discussion).

Under general anesthesia, aspiration of the anterior chamber is done with a 25-gauge or smaller needle attached to a 3-milliliter (mL) syringe. Except in hyphema, the protein content of aqueous humor is very low; consequently, in vitro disintegration of cells may be rapid. Sediment smears or cytocentrifuged preparations should be made soon after aspiration. Total cell counts and protein concentration may be determined if enough volume is obtained.

Neutrophilic infiltration of aqueous humor is characteristic of most causes of anterior uveitis, including lens-induced uveitis and viral infections. A few lymphocytes and monocytes may be found. In cases of hypopyon, bacteria may or may not be found among the neutrophils. Infection with *Bartonella* spp. was suspected as a cause of anterior uveitis in cats and of anterior uveitis and choroiditis in a dog on the basis of positive serologic titers.[26,27] *Blastomyces dermatitidis*, *Prototheca* spp., and *Leishmania donovani* may be found in aqueous humor. Ocular toxoplasmosis in cats with anterior uveitis is diagnosed on the basis of serologic testing, and its definitive diagnosis remains challenging.[28] Phagocytosis of melanin by neutrophils is an infrequent finding of unknown significance. Hyphema is characterized by either cells typical of fresh blood or, in protracted cases, blood with macrophages containing RBCs and hemosiderin. Tumors metastatic to the anterior uvea include carcinomas, sarcomas, lymphoma, canine transmissible venereal tumor, and feline myeloproliferative neoplasms. Cytologic examination of aqueous humor is most helpful for diagnosing lymphoma (Figure 9-34).

Iris and Ciliary Body

Space-occupying masses on the anterior uvea may be an indication for cytologic examination of fine-needle

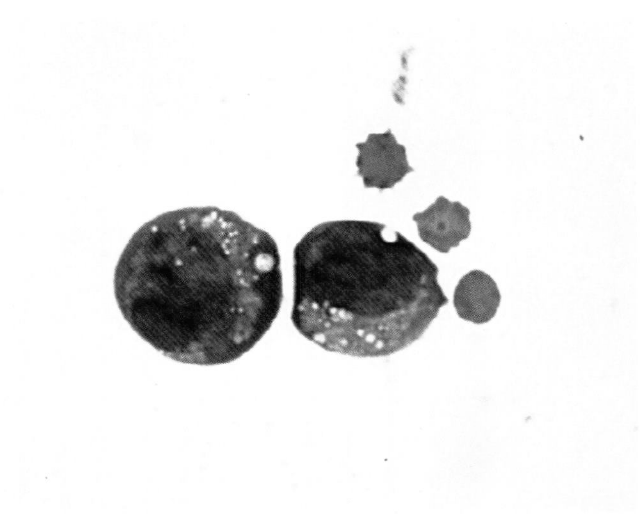

Figure 9-34 Aqueous humor aspirate from a dog with lymphoma. Note the large lymphoid cells with bizarre nucleoli and basophilic cytoplasm. (Wright-Giemsa stain, original magnification 1000×.)

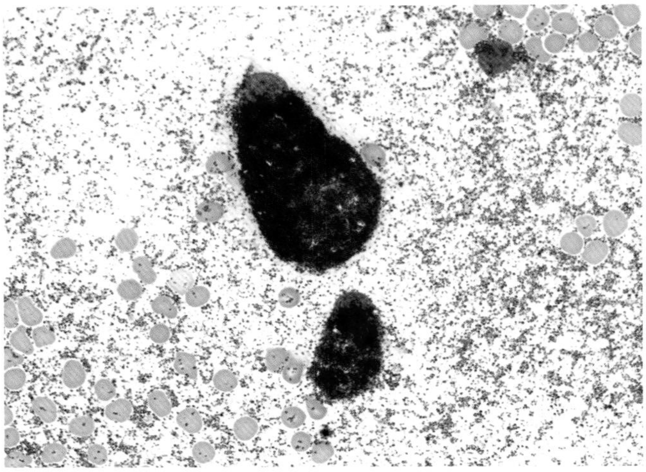

Figure 9-35 Fine-needle aspirate of an iris freckle from a cat. Abundant melanin is found within melanocytes and extracellularly. (Wright stain, original magnification 600×.)

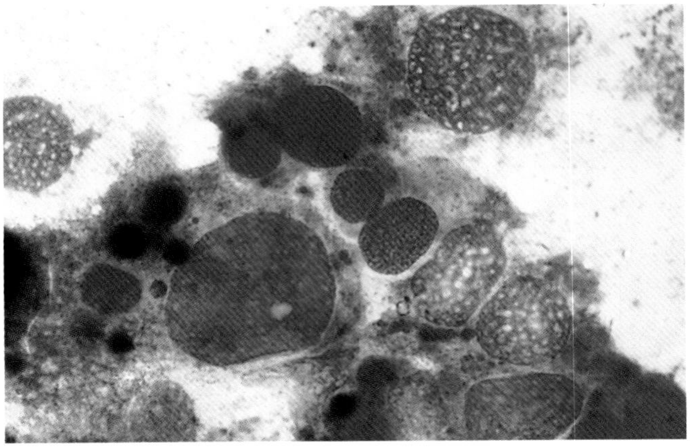

Figure 9-36 Fine-needle aspirate of the surface of a pigmented lesion on a feline iris. Cells have marked anisocytosis and anisokaryosis and contain melanin pigment. The diagnosis is feline iris melanoma. (Romanowsky-type stain, original magnification 1000×.)

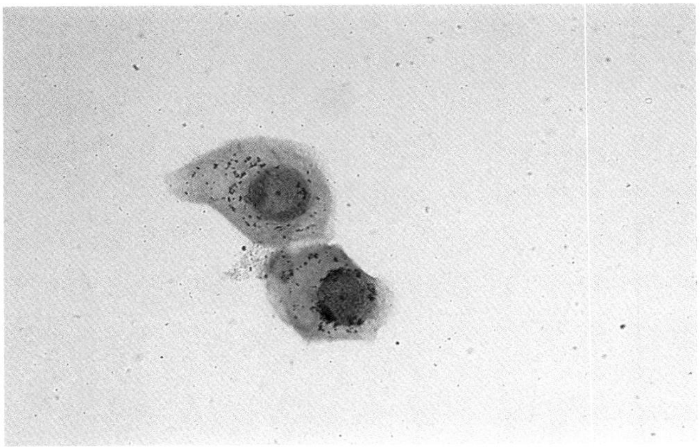

Figure 9-37 Normal melanocytes aspirated from the iris surface of a normal feline eye. Note the uniform size and shape of nuclei and cytoplasmic melanin. (Romanowsky-type stain, original magnification 1000×.)

aspirates. Direct aspiration of the iris nodule is accomplished under general anesthesia as described in the previous section on aqueous humor.

Melanoma: Melanoma is the most common primary intraocular tumor. The preparation should contain melanocytes that exhibit cytomorphologic features of malignancy to be diagnostic because free melanin and some melanocytes are a component of all uveal aspirates. In cats, progressive iris hyperpigmentation may represent diffuse iris melanoma. Melanosis (Figure 9-35), with accumulation of melanocytes forming a freckle, may undergo a transition to iris melanoma, a diagnosis that can be challenging to make. FNA (with a 25-gauge or smaller needle) of the anterior surface of the iris lesion, without needle penetration of the iris, may yield diagnostic cells.[29] Dilution of the sample with aqueous should be avoided. In iris melanoma, the most consistent cytologic findings are variability in the size and shape of nuclei and nucleoli (Figure 9-36). Binucleate cells may be found. Both normal and tumor cells are pigmented. Normal cells have uniform nuclei and small uniform nucleoli (Figure 9-37).

Lymphoproliferative Diseases: Lymphoma also occurs as a diffuse or nodular iris lesion. Large lymphocytes with visible nucleoli, lymphoid cells with broad pseudopodia, and mitotic figures often are present, and small lymphocytes and plasma cells also may be seen (see Chapter 11 for discussion and additional photomicrographs of lymphoma). Ocular lymphoma is usually part of multicentric disease. When it is suspected, the disease should be staged by evaluating the animal for systemic lesions that may be more easily sampled for diagnostic purposes. Extramedullary plasmacytoma in the iris of a cat with mandibular lymph node involvement but no other evidence of disease has been reported.[30]

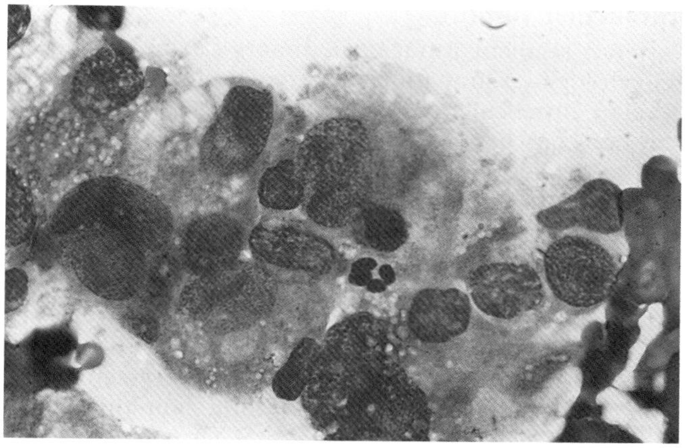

Figure 9-38 Fine-needle aspirate of an iridociliary carcinoma in a cat. Cells exhibit anisokaryosis, irregularly shaped nuclei, nuclear molding, and distinct cytoplasmic vacuoles of variable size. (Romanowsky-type stain, original magnification 1000×.)

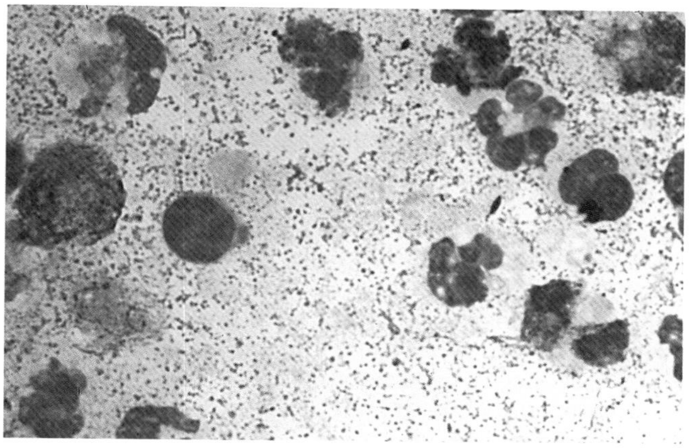

Figure 9-39 Vitreous smear from a dog. Background granular precipitate is characteristic of all vitreous smears. Note the oblong melanin granule (*right center*) and neutrophils. (Romanowsky-type stain, original magnification 1000×.)

Epithelial Tumors: Adenomas and adenocarcinomas may originate from the iris or ciliary body epithelium (Figure 9-38). Among primary intraocular tumors, these are second to melanomas in frequency. The anterior uvea also is a site for metastasis of systemic carcinomas.[31] Cytologic features of benign and malignant epithelial tumors are described in Chapter 2.

VITREOUS BODY

Opacity in the vitreous body is an indication for aspiration and cytologic examination. However, aspiration of the vitreous body is not an innocuous procedure. If a potentially visual eye is aspirated, care must be taken not to cause hemorrhage or other sequelae that could jeopardize vision. Under general anesthesia, a 23-gauge or smaller needle is used to penetrate the eye 6 to 8 millimeters (mm) caudal to the limbus: the needle is directed into the middle of the vitreous toward the optic nerve. The lens must be avoided to prevent disruption of the lens capsule and induction of lens-induced uveitis. Aspiration of 0.5 to 1.0 mL of fluid is recommended. Sediment smears or cytocentrifuged preparations should be made immediately after aspiration. After air-drying and before staining, the underside of the glass slide should be heated by passing it through the tip of a small flame two or three times. Heat fixation helps vitreous body material adhere to the slide.

Vitreous body material is normally acellular, although most samples contain a few RBCs and scattered melanin granules, which, in this location in dogs, are oblong with pointed ends (Figure 9-39). The background on stained smears is an eosinophilic granular precipitate. Lens fibers may be found in sediment smears in cases of pars planitis (snowbanking) (Figure 9-40). Microfilariae may be found in samples that contain blood from microfilaremic dogs, but they are not associated with ocular disease. Melanin-laden cells may be found in samples from normal or diseased eyes. Asteroid hyalosis is a degenerative disease of the vitreous consisting of calcium and lipid complexes. It is not an indication for cytologic examination.

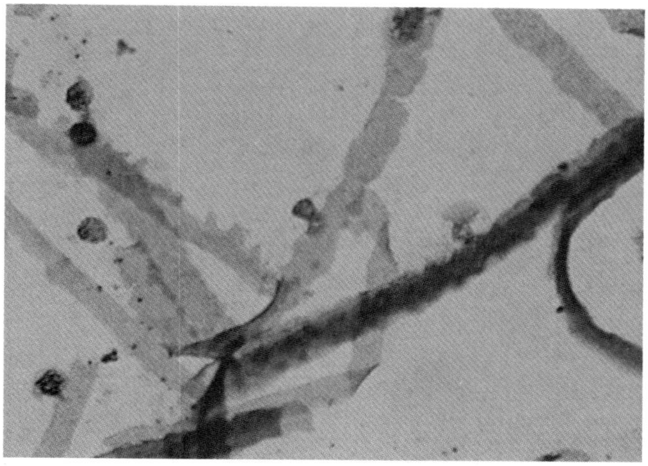

Figure 9-40 Lens fibers in the sediment of a vitreous body aspirate from a dog. Several red blood cells provide a size reference. (Romanowsky-type stain, original magnification 400×.)

Endophthalmitis

Bacterial endophthalmitis is purulent, and organisms are usually demonstrable in the exudate on vitreous smears. Neutrophilic exudate without organisms may be seen in lens-induced endophthalmitis and trauma. Mycotic endophthalmitis with opacification of the vitreous body is relatively common in dogs. Ocular lesions were found in 41% of dogs with blastomycosis.[32] Affected dogs had a neutrophilic exudate and *B. dermatitidis* yeast in vitreous body smears (Figure 9-41). Sometimes the organisms are found in the absence of inflammatory cells. Other fungi that may be found in the vitreous body include *Cryptococcus neoformans* (Figure 9-42), *Coccidioides immitis* (Figure 9-43), and *Histoplasma capsulatum*. In cryptococcal infection, in particular, little to no inflammation may be present owing to the protective mechanisms associated with the capsule, and care must be taken not to overlook the yeast forms. The use of India ink to highlight the yeast of *Cryptococcus* is sometimes suggested but is unnecessary and may even result in misinterpretation of a sample. The clear capsule around the yeast can be seen even in the presence of a pale background (Figure 9-42, *left*), and lipid droplets coated by India ink may be mistaken for organisms. Protothecosis also may affect the vitreous body. The organisms are usually systemic, although ocular manifestations because of chorioretinitis may be the initial clinical problem. A neutrophilic exudate and *Prototheca* organisms may be found on vitreous smears.

Hemorrhage

Cytologic findings in vitreous smears are similar to those in hematomas or other sites of hemorrhage. In addition to RBCs, monocytes and macrophages exhibiting erythrophagia and containing hemosiderin predominate. Causes of hemorrhage can be systemic or local, for example, bleeding disorders, retinal detachment, intraocular tumor, hypertension, or rickettsial disease.

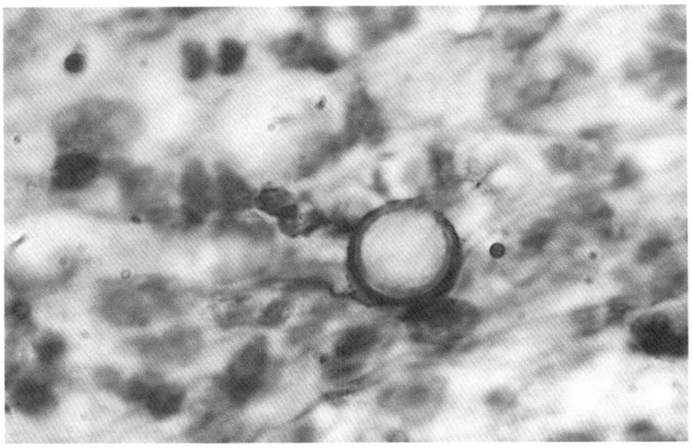

Figure 9-41 Vitreous aspirate from a dog. Note the broad-based budding yeast of *Blastomyces dermatitidis* surrounded by neutrophils. (Romanowsky-type stain, original magnification 1000×.)

Intraocular Tumors

Posterior segment intraocular tumors can be diagnosed on cytologic examination of vitreous smears. Cats may develop intraocular sarcomas following trauma.[33] This may be a consequence of metaplasia of the lens epithelium and subsequent proliferation and migration.[34] Primary intraocular osteosarcoma has been reported in a dog.[35] Absence of neoplastic cells does not exclude intraocular tumor from consideration.

RETINA

Rarely, cells from the retina are obtained accidentally if retinal detachment has occurred or if the subretinal space is aspirated when cloudy material is visualized in that location. Nuclei of photoreceptor cells from the outer nuclear layer and retinal pigmented epithelial cells were identified in an aspirate of subretinal fluid (Figure 9-44). Hypothetically, inflammatory cells could be identified if retinitis were present, but cytologic examination of the retina is rare.

ORBIT

Exophthalmos

Exophthalmos results from a space-occupying lesion in the orbit. Causes include tumors, abscesses, hematomas, foreign bodies, osteomyelitis, mucoceles, or extensions of inflammatory or neoplastic diseases from the sinus or oral cavity. Retrobulbar FNA and cytologic examination are indicated. Orbital cellulitis caused by retrobulbar *Toxocara canis* infection with larval migration has been reported in a dog.[36] Traumatic proptosis is not an indication for retrobulbar aspiration.

Imaging by survey radiography or ultrasonography and orbital palpation can help localize the lesion. Aspiration is done from the orbit or the mouth, caudal to the last

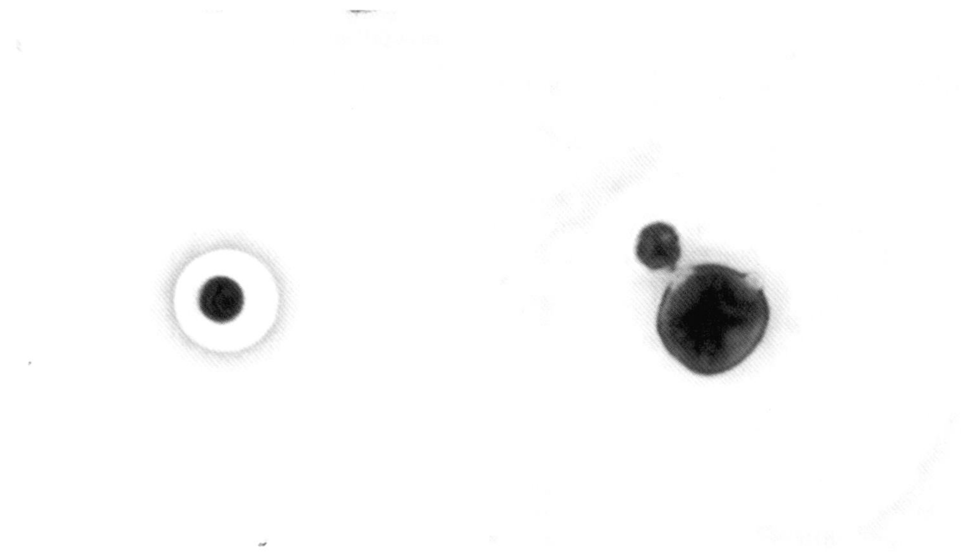

Figure 9-42 Vitreous aspirates from a cat with cryptococcosis. *Cryptococcus* organisms have a capsule and exhibit narrow-based budding (*right*). The clear capsule is evident even though the background material is pale (*left*), and staining with India ink is unnecessary. Inflammatory cells may be absent. (Wright strain, original magnification 1000×.)

molar. The critical structures to avoid are the optic nerve and globe. Principles of diagnostic cytology described throughout the text and in detail in the beginning chapters are applicable in differentiation of the various lesions.

Orbital Tumors

Dogs or cats with orbital tumors are presented with either exophthalmos or enophthalmos. The quantity of material obtained from retrobulbar tumors is sparse compared with an abscess or mucocele. Orbital neoplasms include lymphoma, plasmacytoma, squamous cell carcinoma, salivary adenocarcinoma, osteoma and osteosarcoma, chondroma and chondrosarcoma, hemangioma, melanoma, fibrosarcoma, meningioma (Figure 9-45), peripheral nerve sheath tumors (Figure 9-46), and carcinomas and sarcomas of unknown type. In dogs, a unique neoplasm in the orbit is canine lobular orbital adenoma, thought to be of lacrimal or salivary gland origin (Figure 9-47).[37] In most cases, the tumor is friable and difficult to excise completely but is typically a benign neoplasm. The most common orbital tumor in cats is squamous cell carcinoma.[38]

Postenucleation Orbital Lesions

Cysts are an infrequent complication of enucleation. A possible mechanism of cyst formation is implantation or incarceration of conjunctival epithelium or the gland of the third eyelid at the time of enucleation. Cytologic examination reveals basal, intermediate, and mature noncornified squamous cells, large foamy macrophages, and abundant mucus (Figure 9-48).

Frontal sinus osteomyelitis may extend into the orbit after enucleation. Osteoclasts, osteoblasts, and leukocytes are found. Mucocele and emphysema may affect the orbit following enucleation.

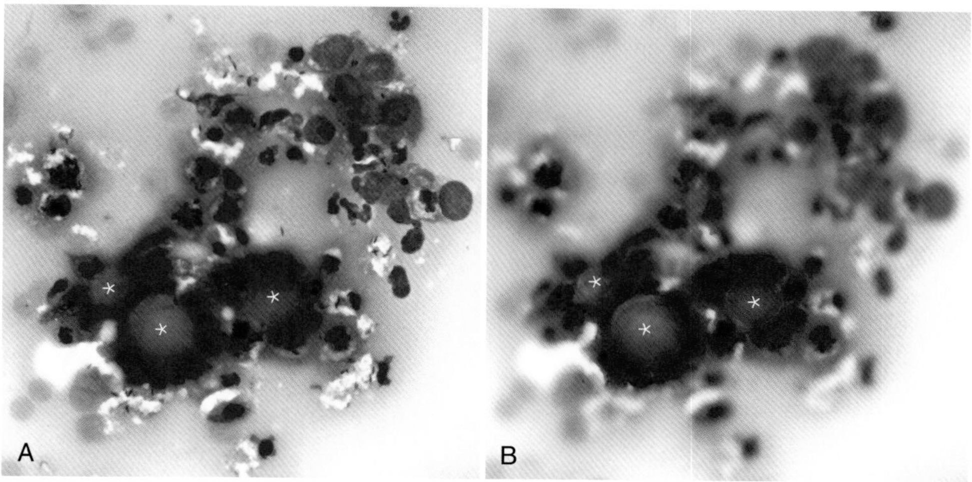

Figure 9-43 Yeast of *Coccidioides* spp. (*) in a vitreous aspirate from a dog. These large yeast forms appear out of focus when the inflammatory cells are in focus (*A*); conversely, the inflammatory cells are blurred when the yeast wall is in focus (*B*). (Wright-Giemsa stain, original magnification 600×.)

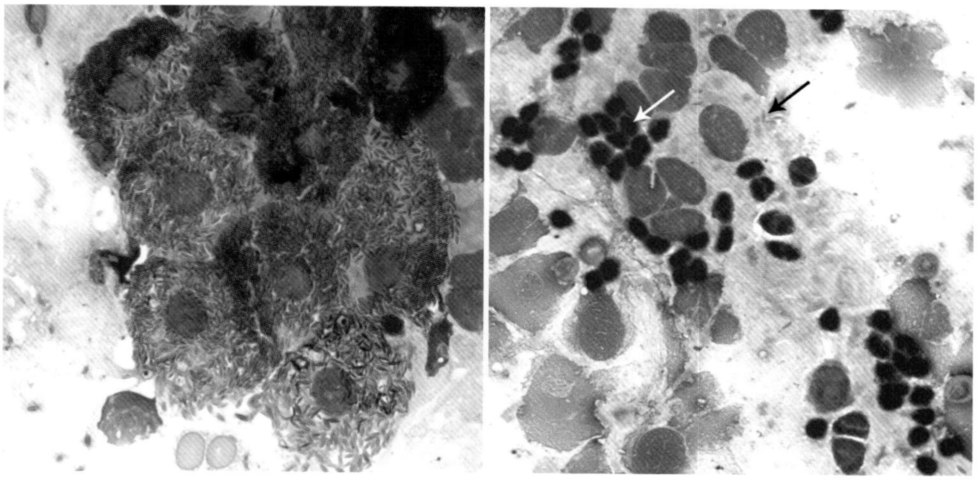

Figure 9-44 Retinal tissue in an aspirate of subretinal fluid from a dog. Note the retinal pigmented epithelial (RPE) cells (*left*), nuclei of photoreceptor cells (*right, white arrow*), and free spiculate melanin granules (*right, black arrow*) from RPE cells. (Wright-Giemsa stain, original magnification 1000×.)

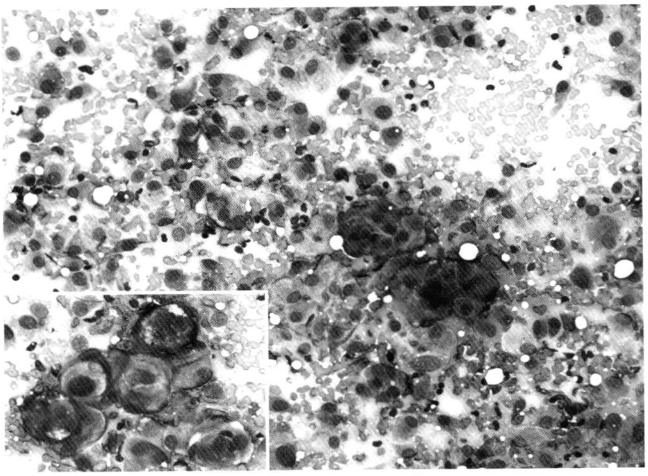

Figure 9-45 Fine-needle aspirate of an orbital mass from a dog with an orbital meningioma. Note the large cells with abundant cytoplasm that sometimes form whorls (*inset*). (Wright stain, original magnification 200×, inset 600×.)

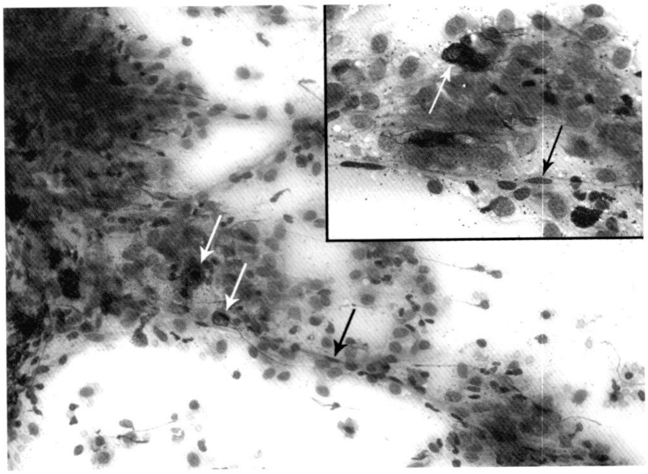

Figure 9-46 Fine-needle aspirate of an orbital mass from a dog with an orbital peripheral nerve sheath tumor. An endothelial-lined vessel (*black arrows*) courses through the polyhedral tumor cells that aggregate around vessels. Mast cells (*white arrows*) are sometimes found in these tumors. (Wright stain, original magnification 200×, inset 600×.)

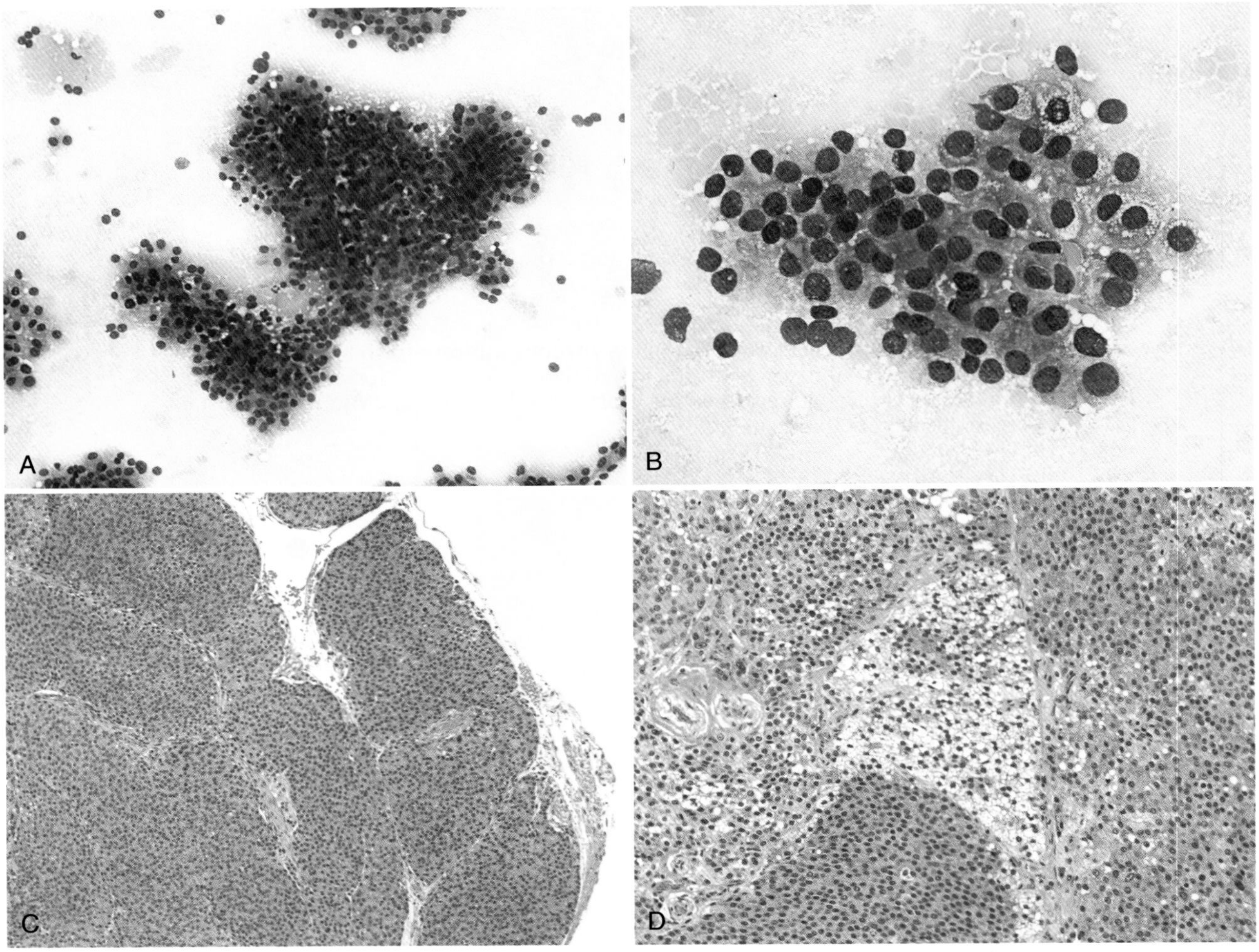

Figure 9-47 Canine lobular orbital adenoma. A and **B,** Fine-needle aspirate (Wright-Giemsa stain, original magnification 200× [*A*] and 600× [*B*]). Note cohesive clusters of monomorphic epithelial cells, some of which contain secretory vacuoles. **C** and **D,** Histologic section (H&E, original magnification 100× [*C*] and 200× [*D*]). Note neoplastic cells arranged in lobules; some cells are vacuolated.

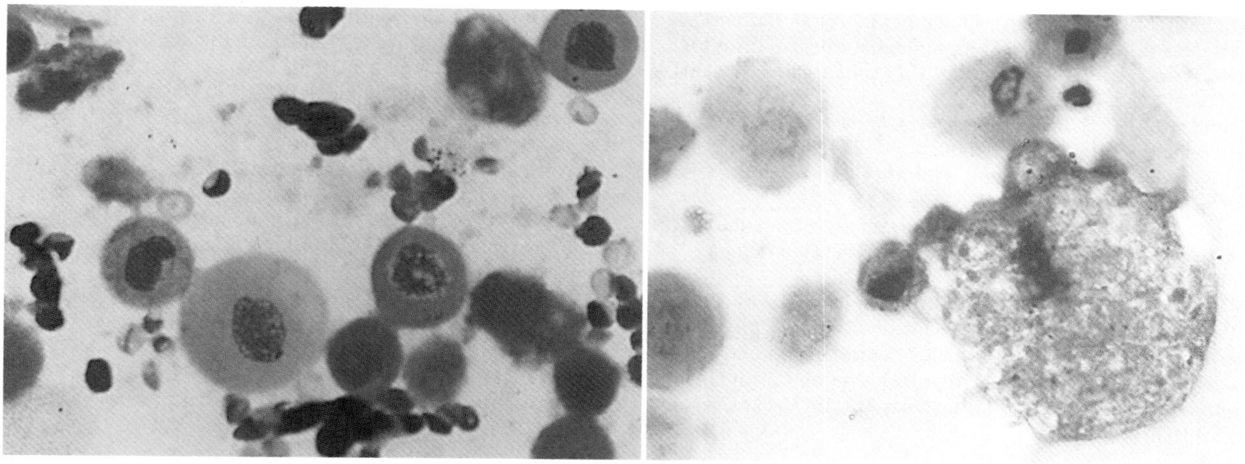

Figure 9-48 **Postenucleation orbital cyst in a dog.** Note the variably sized noncornified squamous cells, red blood cells, and cellular debris (*left*) as well as the degenerating squamous cells and a large foamy macrophage (*right*). (Romanowsky-type stain, original magnification 1000×.)

ACKNOWLEDGMENT

Thanks to Dr. Ellison Bentley, University of Wisconsin, for valuable input, and to Dr. Keith Prasse, Dean Emeritus, University of Georgia, one of the original authors of this chapter, for use of some of his original images.

References

1. Dubielzig RR, Ketring KL, McLellan GJ, et al: *Veterinary ocular pathology. A comparative review*, St. Louis, MO, 2010, Saunders.
2. Ketring KL, Glaze MB: *Atlas of feline ophthalmology*, ed 2, Ames, IA, 2012, Blackwell Publishing.
3. Collins BK, MacEwen EG, Dubielzig RR, et al: Idiopathic granulomatous disease with ocular adnexal and cutaneous involvement in a dog, *J Am Vet Med Assoc* 201:313–316, 1992.
4. Scherlie PH Jr, Smedes SL, Feltz T, et al: Ocular manifestation of systemic histiocytosis in a dog, *J Am Vet Med Assoc* 201:1229–1232, 1992.
5. Rosin A, Moore P, Dubielzig R: Malignant histiocytosis in Bernese mountain dogs, *J Am Vet Med Assoc* 188:1041–1045, 1986.
6. Streeten BW, Streeten EA: "Blue body" epithelial cell inclusions in conjunctivitis, *Ophthalmology* 92:575–579, 1985.
7. Bolzan AA, Brunelli AT, Castro MB, et al: Conjunctival impression cytology in dogs, *Vet Ophthalmol* 8:401–405, 2005.
8. Ramsey DT, Ketring KL, Glaze MB, et al: Ligneous conjunctivitis in four Doberman pinschers, *J Am Anim Hosp Assoc* 32:439–447, 1996.
9. Gelatt KN: Ophthalmic examination and diagnostic procedures. In Gelatt KN, editor: *Textbook of veterinary ophthalmology*, Philadelphia, PA, 1981, Lea & Febiger, pp 206–261.
10. Hoover EA, Kahn DE, Langloss JM: Experimentally induced feline chlamydial infection (feline pneumonitis), *Am J Vet Res* 39:541–547, 1978.
11. Hillström A, Tvedten H, Källberg M, et al: Evaluation of cytologic finings in feline conjunctivitis, *Vet Clin Pathol* 41:283–290, 2012.
12. Nasisse MP, Guy JS, Stevens JB: Clinical and laboratory findings in chronic conjunctivitis in cats: 91 cases (1983-1991), *J Am Vet Med Assoc* 203:834–837, 1993.
13. von Bomhard W, Polkinghorne A, Lu ZH, et al: Detection of novel chlamydiae in cats with ocular disease, *Am J Vet Res* 64:1421–1428, 2003.
14. Campbell LH, Snyder SB, Reed C, et al: Mycoplasma felis-associated conjunctivitis in cats, *J Am Vet Med Assoc* 163:991–995, 1973.
15. Fife M, Blocker T, Fife T, et al: Canine conjunctival mast cell tumors: a retrospective study, *Vet Ophthalmol* 14:153–160, 2011.
16. Johnson BW, Brightman AH, Whiteley HE: Conjunctival mast cell tumor in two dogs, *J Am Anim Hosp Assoc* 24:439–442, 1988.
17. Pirie CG, Knollinger AM, Thomas CB, et al: Canine conjunctival hemangioma and hemangiosarcoma: a retrospective evaluation of 108 cases (1989-2004), *Vet Ophthalmol* 9:215–226, 2006.
18. Pirie CG, Dubielzig RR: Feline conjunctival hemangioma and hemangiosarcoma: a retrospective evaluation of 8 cases (1993-2004), *Vet Ophthalmol* 9:227–231, 2005.
19. Hirayama K, Kagawa Y, Tsuzuki K, et al: A pleomorphic adenoma of the lacrimal gland in a dog, *Vet Pathol* 37:353–356, 2000.
20. Zarfoss MK, Dubielzig RR, Eberhard ML, et al: Canine ocular onchocerciasis in the United States: two new cases and a review of the literature, *Vet Ophthalmol* 8:51–57, 2005.
21. Massa KL, Murphy CJ, Hartmann FA, et al: Usefulness of aerobic microbial culture and cytologic evaluation of corneal specimens in the diagnosis of infectious ulcerative keratitis in animals, *J Am Vet Med Assoc* 215:1671–1674, 1999.
22. Ledbetter EC, Riis RC, Kern TJ, et al: Corneal ulceration associated with naturally occurring canine herpesvirus-1 infection in two adult dogs, *J Am Vet Med Assoc* 229:376–384, 2006.
23. Bernays ME, Peiffer RL Jr: Ocular infections with dematiaceous fungi in two cats and a dog, *J Am Vet Med Assoc* 213:507–509, 1998.
24. Nasisse MP, Glover TL, Moore CP, et al: Detection of feline herpesvirus 1 DNA in corneas of cats with eosinophilic keratitis or corneal sequestration, *Am J Vet Res* 59:856–858, 1998.
25. Schmidt GM, Prasse KW: Corneal epithelial inclusion cyst in a dog, *J Am Vet Med Assoc* 168:144, 1976.
26. Lappin MR, Black JC: *Bartonella* spp. infection as a possible cause of uveitis in a cat, *J Am Vet Med Assoc* 214:1205–1207, 1999.

27. Michau TM, Breitschwerdt EB, Gilger BC, et al: *Bartonella vinsonii* subspecies *berkhoffi* as a possible cause of anterior uveitis and choroiditis in a dog, *Vet Ophthalmol* 6:299–304, 2003.
28. Davidson MG: Toxoplasmosis, *Vet Clin North Am Small Anim Pract* 30:1051–1062, 2000.
29. Grossniklaus HE: Fine-needle aspiration biopsy of the iris, *Arch Ophthalmol* 110:969–976, 1992.
30. Michau TM, Proulx DR, Rushton SD, et al: Intraocular extramedullary plasmacytoma in a cat, *Vet Ophthalmol* 6:177–181, 2003.
31. Miller PE, Dubielzig RR: Ocular tumors. In Withrow SJ, Vail DM, editors: *Withrow & MacEwen's small animal clinical oncology*, ed 4, St. Louis, MO, 2007, Saunders, pp 686–698.
32. Legendre AM, Walker M, Buyukmihci N, et al: Canine blastomycosis: a review of 47 clinical cases, *J Am Vet Med Assoc* 178:1163–1168, 1981.
33. Dubielzig RR, Everitt J, Shadduck JA, et al: Clinical and morphologic features of post-traumatic ocular sarcomas in cats, *Vet Pathol* 27:62–65, 1990.
34. Zeiss CJ, Johnson EM, Dubielzi RR: Feline intraocular tumors may arise from transformation of lens epithelium, *Vet Pathol* 40:355–362, 2003.
35. Heath S, Rankin AJ, Dubielzig RR: Primary ocular osteosarcoma in a dog, *Vet Ophthalmol* 6:85–87, 2003.
36. Laus JL, Canola JC, Mamede FV, et al: Orbital cellulitis associated with *Toxocara canis* in a dog, *Vet Ophthalmol* 6:333–336, 2003.
37. Headrick JF, Bentley E, Dubielzig RR: Canine lobular orbital adenoma: a report of 15 cases with distinctive features, *Vet Ophthalmol* 7:47–51, 2004.
38. Gilger BC, McLaughlin SA, Whitley RD, et al: Orbital neoplasms in cats: 21 cases (1974-1990), *J Am Vet Med Assoc* 201:1083–1086, 1992.

CHAPTER 10

The External Ear Canal

Koranda A. Wallace, Heather L. DeHeer and Reema T. Patel

ANATOMY OF THE EXTERNAL EAR

The external ear consists of cartilage and the overlying skin, which create the pinna and external acoustic meatus (between the base of the pinna to the tympanic membrane). The auricular cartilage determines the shape and appearance of the pinnae and supports the vertical ear canal. The annular cartilage, found at the base of the auricular cartilage, supports the horizontal and external ear canal. The skin covering the cartilage within the canal contains sebaceous glands, tubular ceruminous glands, and small hair follicles (Figure 10-1).[1]

ETIOLOGY AND PATHOGENESIS OF OTITIS EXTERNA

Otitis externa, inflammation of the skin and adnexal structures of the ear canal, is commonly encountered in veterinary patients. It is estimated to affect 10% to 20% of canines and 2% to 6% of felines presented for veterinary care.[2,3]

Causes of otitis externa are multifactorial and are commonly divided into primary, predisposing, and perpetuating factors, which are discussed briefly below.

Primary Factors

Primary factors are those which initiate the inflammation of the external ear canal and include parasites, allergic skin disease, foreign bodies, disorders of keratinization, autoimmune diseases, trauma, sebaceous adenitis, zinc-responsive dermatoses, juvenile cellulitis, and certain endocrine disorders (Box 10-1).[4-6]

Predisposing Factors

Predisposing factors facilitate the development of otitis externa by promoting an environment suitable for the survival of the perpetuating factors. Predisposing factors not only include factors such as ear conformation, hypertrichosis of the ear canal; and breed predispositions, which are congenital, environmental, or both, but also iatrogenic trauma, excessive moisture, and obstructive ear disease (Box 10-2).[3,4]

Perpetuating Factors

Rather than initiating the otitis externa, perpetuating factors sustain the established disease; once the ear canal has been altered by primary and predisposing factors, opportunistic infections and progressive changes occur to prevent resolution of disease. These factors include bacteria, yeast, otitis media, and progressive hyperplastic changes of the ear canal caused by disease (Box 10-3).[3,4]

DIAGNOSIS OF OTITIS EXTERNA

Most cases of acute otitis externa can be readily managed by using the information gained from a thorough history, physical examination, otoscopic examination, and cytologic evaluation of the ear canal secretions. More advanced or chronic cases may require culture and susceptibility testing, biopsy, diagnostic imaging, endocrine testing, and assessment of allergic skin disease.

CYTOLOGIC EVALUATION OF EAR CANAL SECRETIONS

Cytologic examination of otic secretions is a simple, inexpensive, and rapid test to assist in the diagnosis and treatment of otitis externa. Physical characteristics, if not guided by cytology, may be misleading and unreliable. The primary goal of cytology of the external ear is to identify overgrowth or infection that may contribute to otitis externa. Cytology should be performed at recheck examinations as a means to monitoring and adjusting therapy.

Collection and Staining of Samples

Samples of the ear canal secretions for cytologic evaluation are collected using separate cotton-tipped swabs for each ear canal. Samples should be collected after performing otoscopic examination, to avoid obscuring the tympanic membrane with compressed debris, and prior to introduction of any cleaning agents or medication. The most clinically relevant samples are obtained from the deeper horizontal canal rather than the superficial vertical canal.[3] This can be accomplished in larger patients with insertion of a cotton-tipped swab through an otoscopic cone (Figure 10-2). However, surrounding circumstances such as painful ears, stenosis, and inflammation may make acquisition in this manner difficult without sedation. Another method to obtain samples is to carefully pass a swab into the ear canal, without the

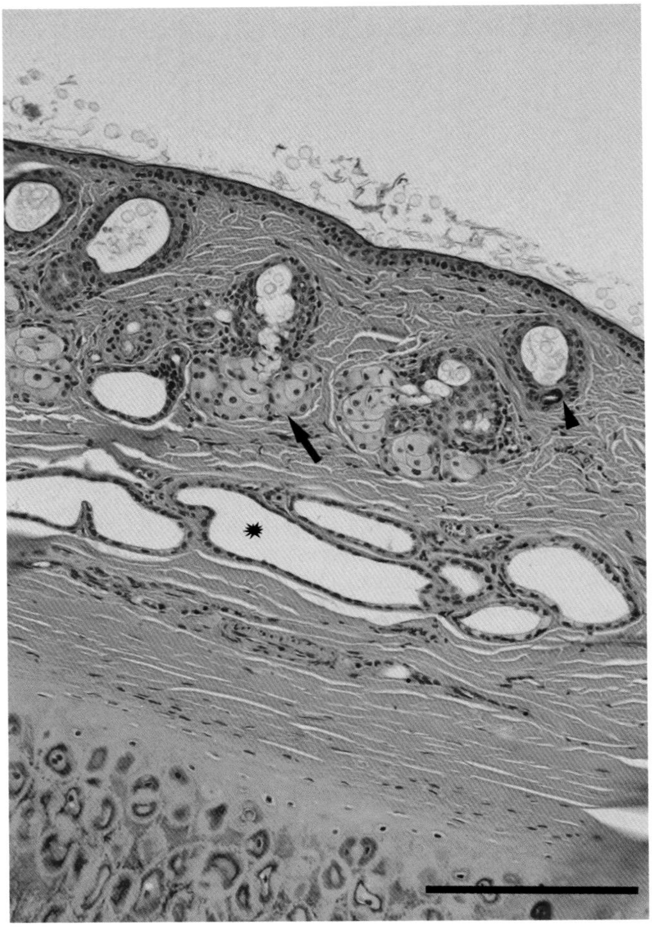

Figure 10-1 Hematoxylin and eosin (H&E) section of the normal feline vertical ear canal with hair follicle (*arrowhead*), sebaceous glands (*arrow*), and ceruminous glands (*asterisk*). (Magnification 200×, Bar = 100 um.)

BOX 10-1

Primary Causes of Otitis Externa

- Parasites
  - *Otodectes cynotis* (common)
  - *Otobius megnini* (found in southwest U.S.)
  - *Demodex* and other mites (rare)
- Allergic skin diseases
  - Atopy
  - Food allergy
  - Contact hypersensitivity
- Foreign bodies
  - Plant material (especially grass awns)
  - Dirt
  - Other debris
- Other skin disease
  - Pemphigus
  - Seborrhea
  - Sebaceous adenitis
- Endocrinopathies
  - Hypothyroidism

BOX 10-2

Predisposing Causes of Otitis Externa

- Ear conformation
  - Pendulous ears
  - Long narrow ear canal
  - Excessive hair in canal
- Iatrogenic trauma
  - Excessive ear cleaning
- Excessive moisture
  - Frequent swimming or bathing
- Obstructive ear disease
  - Hyperplasia
- Benign or malignant neoplasia causing obstruction of the ear canal

BOX 10-3

Perpetuating Causes of Otitis Externa

Bacteria

- Bacterial cocci
  - *Staphylococcus* (common)
  - *Enterococcus* (occasionally found)
  - *Streptococcus* (occasionally found)
- Bacterial rods
  - *Pseudomonas* (common)
  - *Proteus* (occasionally found)
  - *Escherichia coli* (occasionally found)

Fungi

- *Malassezia* (common)
- *Candida* (rarely found)

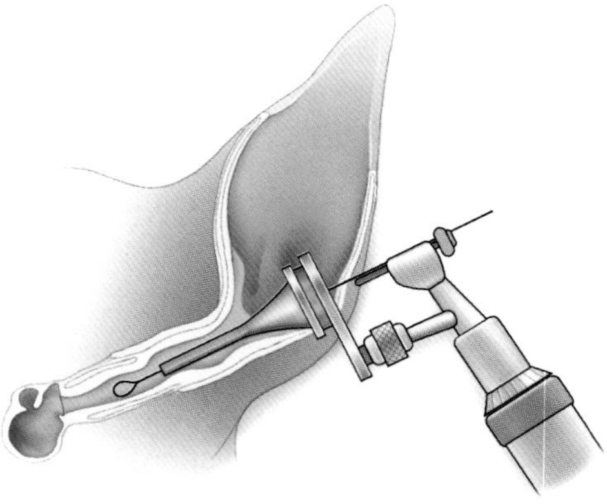

Figure 10-2 Smears of horizontal ear canal secretions may be collected by passing a cotton-tipped swab through the cone of an otoscope after otoscopic examination.

aid of an otoscope, aiming for the junction of the vertical and horizontal canal. Avoid straightening of the ear canal to avoid damage to the tympanic membrane.[3] If the patient requires anesthesia or sedation, ostoscopy and ear flushing, among other techniques, can be used to acquire samples. Samples should always be collected from both ears as animals that appear to have unilateral otitis may also have mild, less apparent disease in the other ear.[7-9]

After secretion from each canal has been collected, separate slides should be prepared for parasite identification and for routine staining. The slides must be labeled to indicate which ear was sampled. Slides for parasite identification should remain unstained, and the otic exudate should be mixed with a small amount of mineral oil, cover-slipped, and microscopically viewed on low power with the condenser down.

To prepare slides for routine staining, the swab is gently rolled onto a clean, dry slide in a thin layer, as thick smears are difficult to evaluate. Heat fixing neither systematically increases nor decreases numbers of yeast on specimens; although it is recommended by many to prevent loss of high lipid content, it is not necessary.[3,10,11] After the material on the slide is allowed to air-dry, it is stained with any of the usual hematologic stains (e.g., Diff-Quik or Wright stain). It is recommended to have two sets of staining jars, one reserved for ear cytology and one reserved for other samples (e.g., blood smears, mass aspirates) as yeast and bacteria from ear cytologies may overgrow in the stain solution and contaminate other slides.

Gram staining can be used for additional information on bacterial type; however, it is more time consuming and may be unnecessary, given that most bacterial cocci are gram positive and most bacterial rods are gram negative.

Cytologic Examination

Cerumen: Cerumen, with its high lipid content, does not take up stain and provides the background for many normal ear swab cytologies (Figure 10-3).

Keratinocytes: Keratinocytes, including occasional nucleated forms, are noted in normal ears of both dogs and cats. Normal dogs were noted to have 3.9 keratinocytes per 40× high-power field (hpf) and normal cats were noted to have 8 per 40× hpf.[13] The finding of nucleated forms should not be mistaken for a pathologic process (parakaratotic hyperkeratosis).

Bacteria: The ear canals of clinically normal dogs often contain small numbers of bacteria. The bacterial concentration typically is low enough that one sees only occasional or no bacteria on cytologic preparations (Figure 10-4). Many of these bacteria are potentially pathogenic and may colonize the ear canal when normal conditions are altered.[3,6,8,14] In animals with bacterial otitis, cytologic evaluation of ear canal secretions often reveals large numbers of bacteria free in the smear (Figure 10-5). Unfortunately, no definitive rule exists for deciding if the bacteria are clinically relevant and warrant treatment. The decision should be based on severity of clinical signs and cytologic findings. Semiquantitative criteria to assess relevance of bacterial populations have been proposed on the basis of their numbers per 40× hpf as follows (Table 10-1): Bacterial counts expected in normal dogs vary among studies and have been reported as a median of 0 cocci (to averaging 5 cocci or fewer).[14 12,13] Abnormal numbers have been reported to be an average of 25 or more organisms, with 6 to 24 organisms being in the "gray zone." Bacterial counts expected in normal cats vary among studies and have been reported as a median of 0.3 cocci per 40× hpf in one study[13] and an average of 4 or fewer cocci in a second study.[12] Abnormal numbers have been reported to be 15 or more organisms, with 5 to 14 organisms being in the "gray zone." Neither study identified bacterial rods as part of the normal ear cytology of dogs or cats.

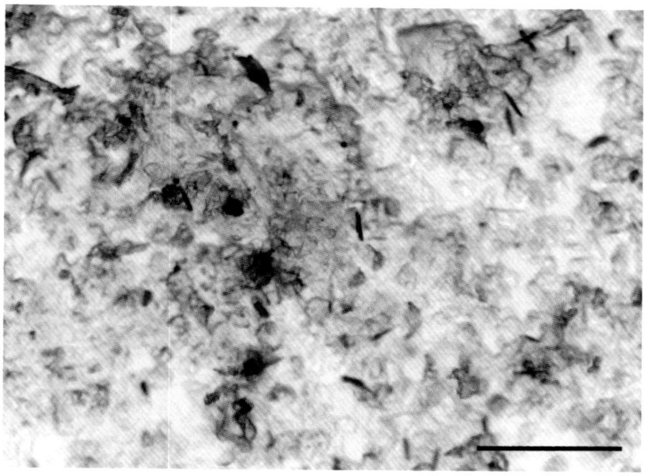

Figure 10-3 Ear swab from a normal dog shows some staining and nonstaining epithelial cells and ceruminous debris. (Wright-Giemsa stain. Magnification 100×, Bar = 200 μm.)

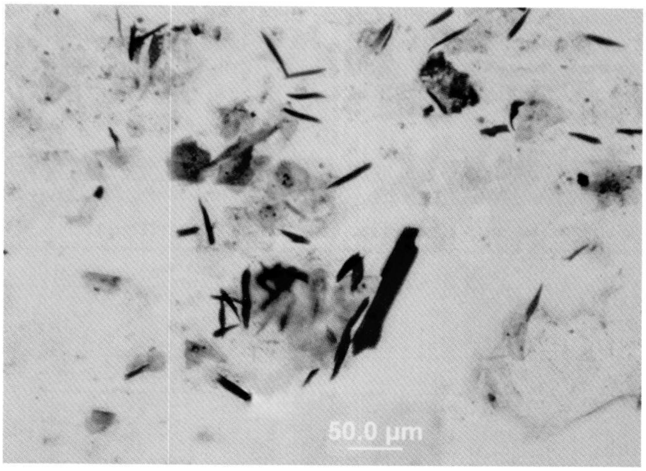

Figure 10-4 Ear swab from a normal dog shows some staining and nonstaining epithelial cells and debris. Note the absence of inflammatory cells and bacteria. (Wright stain. Magnification 200×.)

When secretions are viewed cytologically, neutrophilic inflammation may or may not be present, and bacteria may be observed phagocytized within neutrophils (Figure 10-6). Identifying whether the bacterial infection

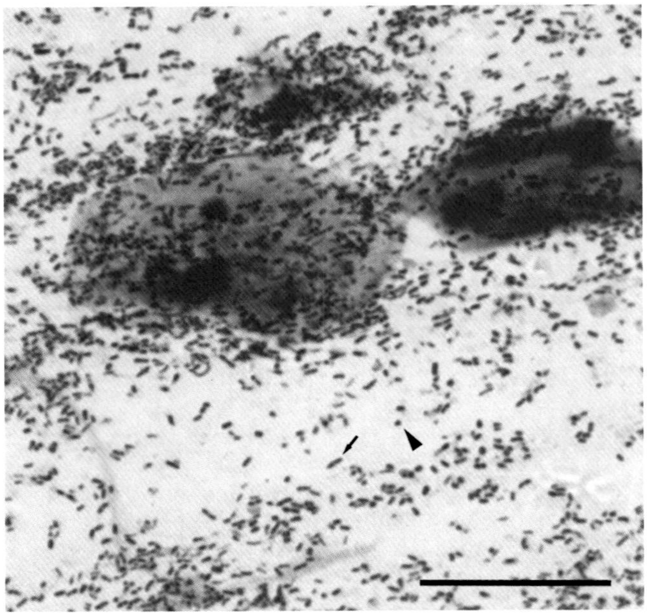

Figure 10-5 Mixed bacterial infection characterized by large numbers of bacterial cocci (*arrowhead*) and rods (*arrow*). Note the absence of neutrophils. (Wright-Giemsa stain, Magnification 1000×, Bar = 20 μm.)

TABLE 10-1

***Malassezia* and Bacteria: Expected Quantities**

	Normal	Gray zone	Abnormal
Malassezia			
Dog	0.2*or ≤2	3-4	≥5
Cat	0.2*or ≤2	3-11	≥12
Bacteria			
Dog	0*or ≤5	6-24	≥25
Cat	0.3*or ≤4	5-14	≥15

Proposed semiquantitative criteria for assessing organisms present in otic cytology based on median number (*)per 40× hpf; or average numbers of organisms per 40× hpf.

Tater KC, Scott DW, Miller jr WH, Erb HN: The cytology of the external ear canal in the normal dog and cat, *J Vet Med* 50:370-374, 2003. Ginel PJ, Lucena R, Rodriguez JC, Ortega J: A semiquantitative cytological evaluation of normal and pathological samples from the external ear canal of dogs and cats, *Vet Dermatol* 13: 151-156, 2002. Angus JC: Otic cytology in health and disease, *Vet Clin North Am Small Anim Pract* 34:411-424, 2004.

involves cocci, rods, or a mixture of both, assists with the initial selection of antibiotics.

Infections involving cocci usually represent *Staphylococcus* spp. or occasionally other species such as *Streptococcus*.[3,8] For infections containing bacterial rods, *Pseudomonas* is the most common species cultured but other species are occasionally found including *Proteus* and *Escherichia coli*.[3,6,8,9,14,15,16] When routine therapy is ineffective, culture and sensitivity testing are indicated because of the high incidence of antimicrobial resistance associated with otitis externa, especially when considering *Pseudomonas* spp.[16]

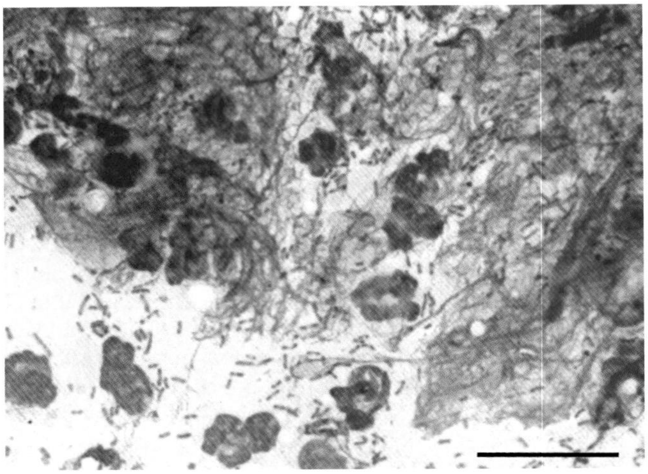

Figure 10-6 Ear swab from a dog with a bacterial infection. Numerous bacterial rods are present phagocytized within degenerate neutrophils and free in the background. (Wright-Giemsa stain. Magnification 1000×, Bar = 20 μm.)

Fungi

Malassezia: *Malassezia pachydermatis* is, by far, the most common yeast associated with otitis externa in dogs and cats, but it may also be found in the normal ear. *M. pachydermatis* may be found in up to 83% of dogs with otitis externa and in 15% to 49% of normal ear canals.[17,18] *Malassezia* infections may occur with or without bacterial coinfection.[3,6,7,8,9,14,15,16] In pure *Malassezia* infections, neutrophilic inflammation is not a common feature.[3,7,19]

The decision to treat *Malassezia* infection ultimately depends on cytologic findings, severity of clinical signs, and past history of otitis and response to treatment. The decision may, however, be guided by semiquantitive guidelines, which were proposed on the basis of numbers of organisms per 40× hpf as follows (see Table 10-1): Amounts in normal dogs have been reported as a median of 0.2 yeasts to an average of 2 or fewer yeast cells, with abnormal numbers reported as 5 or more, with 3 to 4 being in the "gray zone."[12] Amounts in normal cats have been reported as a median of 0.2 yeast cells, whereas another study had an average count of 2 or fewer yeast cells.[12] Abnormal numbers in cats have been reported as an average of 12 or more yeast cells, with 3 to 11 being in the "gray zone."[12]

Cytologically, yeast cells identified from normal dogs and cats were broad-based unipolar budding cells. *Malassezia* (Figure 10-7) is a broad-based budding, basophilic-staining, oval yeast that has a characteristic peanut or footprint shape when observed during budding. These yeast are fairly small, ranging from 2 micrometers (μm) × 4 μm up to 6 μm × 7 μm.[3,7,9]

Other: Although uncommon, *Candida* and *Microsporum* have been reported in cases of otitis externa.[6,12,20,21] In addition, saprophytes, including *Penicillium* and *Aspergillus*, have been cultured from normal dogs, atopic dogs, and dogs with otitis externa. No cytologic evidence of saprophytic fungal colonization or infection of the ear, however, was identified in any of the samples.[22]

Overall, when unidentified yeasts or hyphae are observed cytologically, culture is indicated for identification.

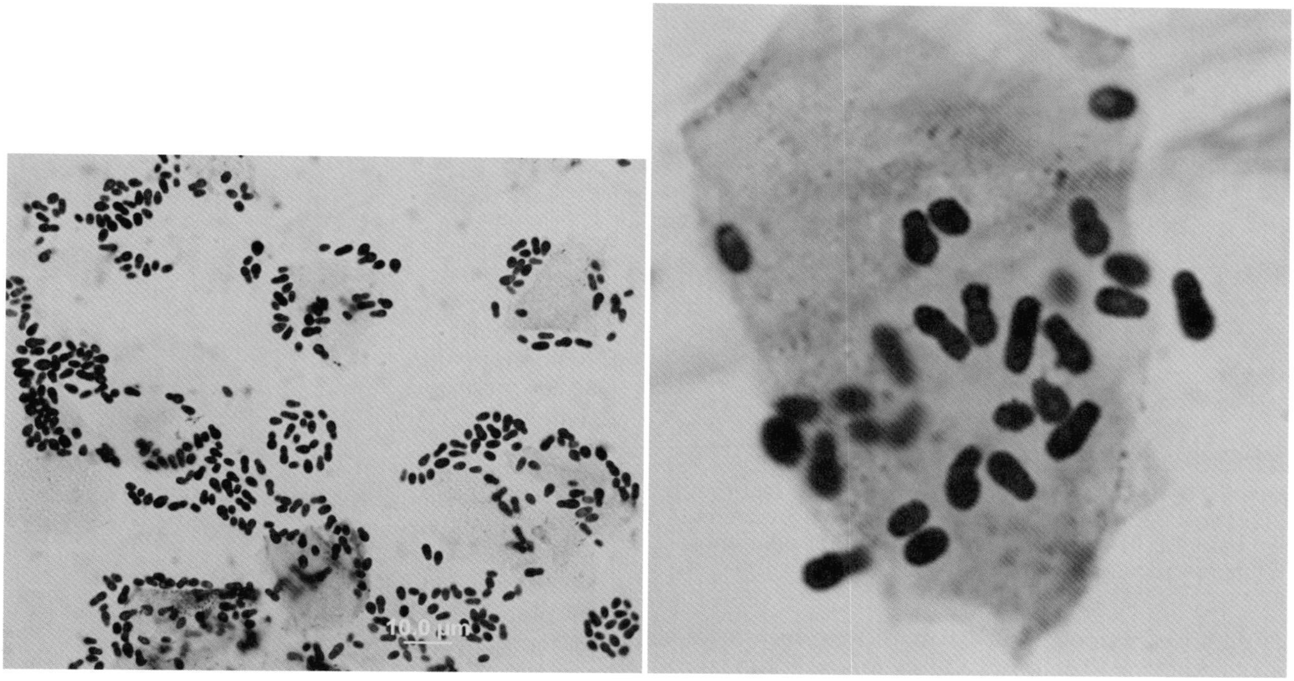

Figure 10-7 *Malassezia* infections are characterized by large numbers of broad-based, budding yeast organisms. Image on the right displays a magnified area. (Wright stain. Magnification 1000×.)

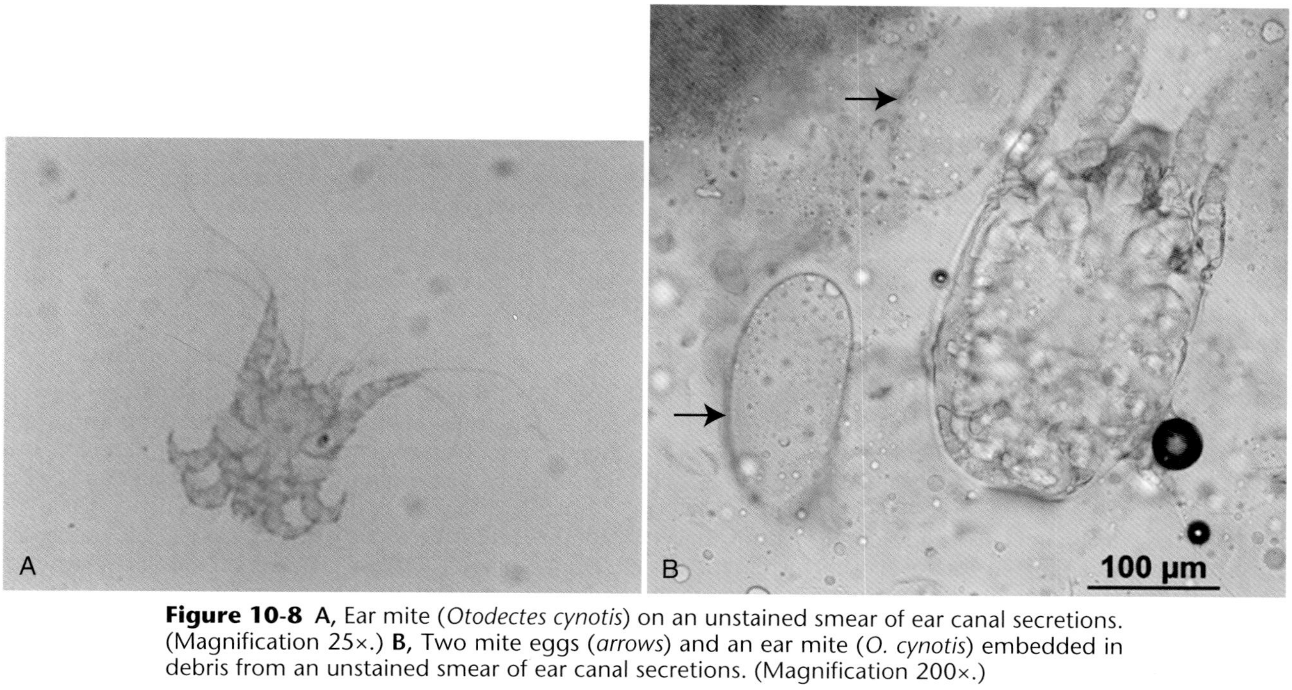

Figure 10-8 **A,** Ear mite (*Otodectes cynotis*) on an unstained smear of ear canal secretions. (Magnification 25×.) **B,** Two mite eggs (*arrows*) and an ear mite (*O. cynotis*) embedded in debris from an unstained smear of ear canal secretions. (Magnification 200×.)

Mites: Ear mites are a primary cause of otitis externa and are especially common in cats. *Otodectes cynotis* reportedly accounts for at least 50% of feline and at least 5% to 10% of canine cases of otitis externa (Figure 10-8).[6,7,9] In animals hypersensitized to mite antigens, clinical signs of otitis externa may develop with as few as two to three mites in the ear canal.[3,7,9,14] Typically, a dry, black, granular discharge is seen. Secondary bacterial infection, yeast infection, or both often coexist and may cause the discharge to become moist.[3,6] Larval and nymph stages of the spinous ear tick, *Otobius megnini*, found in southwest United States, may cause acute otitis externa, most commonly in dogs and infrequently in cats.[2,4] *Demodex canis* in dogs and *Demodex cati* in cats are rare causes of otitis externa, which may or may not be associated with lesions on other areas of the skin (Figure 10-9). In these rare cases,

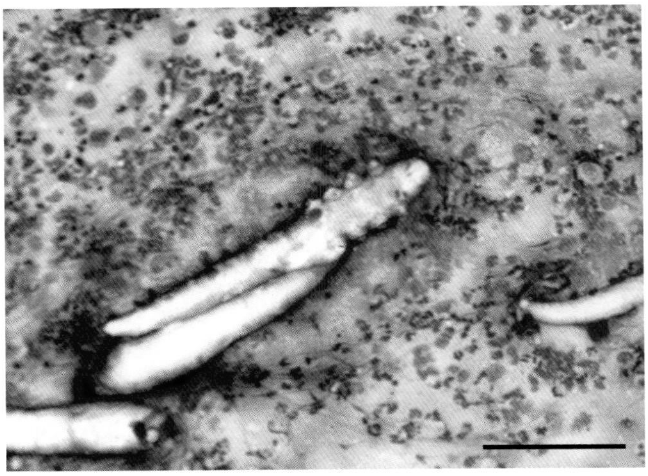

Figure 10-9 Aspirate of lesion on canine pinna. Note several unstained *Demodex* spp. mites surrounded by numerous inflammatory cells consisting predominantly of neutrophils with rare macrophages (Magnification 200×. Bar = 100 μm.)

large numbers of adult *Demodex* mites were seen in cerumen smears.[6,15,23,24] *Sarcoptes scabiei, Notoedres cati,* and *Eutrombicula alfreddugesi* or *Neotrobicula autumnalis* (chiggers) are other parasites that infrequently infest the ear canal and may be observed on cytology.[3,6,14]

Because small numbers of mites may not be visualized on otoscopic examination, careful cytologic evaluation of unstained exudate for eggs, larvae, or adult mites should be undertaken (see Figure 10-8). Both unstained and stained slides of ear canal secretions should always be evaluated. Mites readily wash off slides during the staining process and are seldom seen on stained slides. Hence, unstained slides are best for finding mites, and stained slides are best for recognizing increased numbers of bacteria, yeast, or both. Finding mites may be challenging, especially in hypersensitive patients with a low mite burden. Failure to find mites on cytologic examination should not definitively exclude the possibility of a mite infestation.

Inflammatory Cells: Normal ears do not contain inflammatory cells, and their presence is always associated with clinical signs of otitis externa.[12] Yet, conversely, not all forms of otitis contain inflammatory cells.[12]

If identified, cells may consist of neutrophils and macrophages. These cells generally gain access to the canal because of ulceration or extension from otitis media; their presence may indicate more severe disease.[3] However, rarely, white blood cells may be associated with noninfectious disease such as pemphigus foliaceous, in which sterile pustules may rupture and exude nondegenerative neutrophils along with acantholytic cells.

Finding bacterial phagocytosis indicates infection rather than overgrowth and may warrant systemic antibiotics (see Figure 10-6).[3]

Neoplasia: The ear canal can potentially develop any of the tumors that occur in skin, as well as ceruminous gland changes, including hyperplasia, adenoma, and adenocarcinoma.[7,25] In one large study of ear canal tumors in dogs and cats, the most common benign neoplasms were polyps, papillomas, basal cell tumors, and ceruminous gland adenomas. The most common malignant neoplasms were ceruminous gland adenocarcinomas, squamous cell carcinomas, and carcinomas of undetermined origin (Box 10-4).[26] Unfortunately, neoplastic cells are rarely seen on cytologic evaluation of external ear canal secretions. Many tumors are covered by normal epithelium, and their neoplastic cells are not available for collection with an ear swab. These tumors may alter the ear canal condition and allow secondary infection to develop.[14]

Cytologically, inflammation may be all that is observed from an ear swab. If a mass is observed on otoscopic examination of the ear canal and cytologic examination of an ear swab does not establish the cause of the mass, fine-needle aspiration or biopsy should be performed to help identify the mass (Figure 10-10).[15] In cats, fine-needle aspirates have been shown to be useful in distinguishing inflammatory polyps from neoplasia. However, benign and malignant neoplasia may be difficult to distinguish

BOX 10-4

Ear Canal Tumors in Dogs and Cats*

Dogs

***Benign tumors* (n = 33)**

Benign polyps: 8
Papillomas: 6
Sebaceous gland adenomas: 5
Basal cell tumor: 5
Ceruminous gland adenoma: 4
Histiocytoma: 2
Plasmacytoma: 1
Benign melanoma: 1
Fibroma: 1

***Malignant tumors* (n = 48)**

Ceruminous gland adenocarcinoma: 23
Carcinoma of undetermined origin: 9
Squamous cell carcinoma: 8
Round cell tumor: 3
Sarcoma: 2
Malignant melanoma: 2
Hemangiosarcoma: 1

Cats

***Benign tumors* (n = 8)**

Benign polyp: 4
Ceruminous gland adenoma: 3
Papilloma: 1

***Malignant tumors* (n = 56)**

Ceruminous gland adenocarcinoma: 22
Squamous cell carcinoma: 20
Carcinoma of undetermined origin: 13
Sebaceous gland adenocarcinoma: 1

From Greene CE: *Infectious diseases of the dog and cat.* St. Louis, MO, 2006, Saunders, (pp. 602-606, 885-891).
*Study of 145 cases.

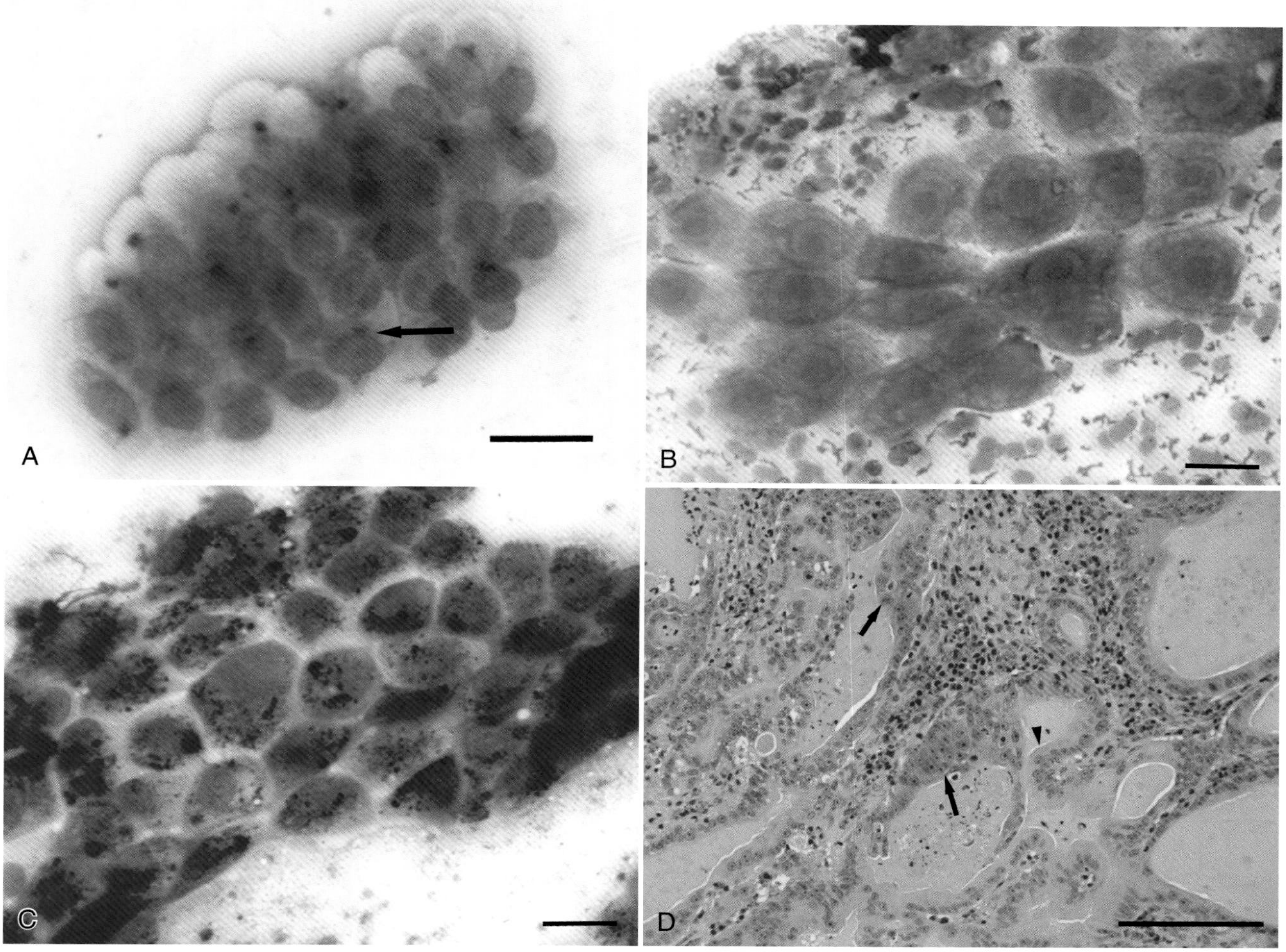

Figure 10-10 **A,** Ceruminous gland hyperplasia. Note the low columnar cells with a basally located nucleus with several cells containing globular to fine, dark-green pigment consistent with cerumen (*arrow*) (Magnification 500×. Bar = 20 μm.) **B,** Ceruminous gland adenocarcinoma. Note the loss of columnar shape, very large prominent single nucleolus, anisocytosis and anisokaryosis. (Magnification 500×. Bar = 20 μm.) **C,** Ceruminous gland adenocarcinoma with similar pleomorphism to *B*; however, these cells also contain globular to fine, dark-green pigment consistent with cerumen (Magnification 500×. Bar = 20 μm.) **D,** Ceruminous gland adenocarcinoma. Note the piling and stacking of neoplastic epithelial cells (*arrow*) displaying anisocytosis and anisokaryosis in addition to papilliferous projections into the glandular lumen (*arrowhead*) (H&E stain. Magnification 200×. Bar = 100 μm.)

on cytology, and histopathologic confirmation is recommended.[27] (See earlier chapters for further discussion on the evaluation of cutaneous and subcutaneous masses.)

Proliferative and Necrotizing Otitis Externa of Felines: Proliferative and necrotizing feline otitis externa is an uncommon and unique proliferative dermatitis with distinct histopathologic and clinical findings that affect the concave pinnae and vertical ear canal of young to middle-aged cats. The etiology is unknown but may be associated with T-cell–mediated apoptosis directed against keratinocytes.[28] Patients often respond to topical tacrolimus, although some patients, especially kittens, may show spontaneous regression.[29]

Grossly, the lesion is characterized by large, tan to dark brown-black, coalescing, slightly verrucous plaques that cover the concave pinnae and external ear canal (Figure 10-11).[28] Gentle manipulation of the plaques may result in their breaking off to reveal underlying ulcers and erosions.[29] Often, thick plugs of material within the ear canal and concurrent bacterial or yeast infection are present.[29]

Cytologically, the disease has not been well characterized. However, the ear canal exudate may often reveal bacterial and yeast infection, and treatment fails to alleviate all of the clinical and gross findings (Figure 10-12).

Histologically, the lesion is characterized by scattered and shrunken keratinocytes with hypereosinophilic and pyknotic nuclei and severe acanthosis of the outer follicular root sheath (Figure 10-13). The lumina of the hair follicles display mild hyperkeratosis and retained corneocyte nuclei, cell debris, and neutrophils. The inflammatory infiltrates within the dermis were often mixed

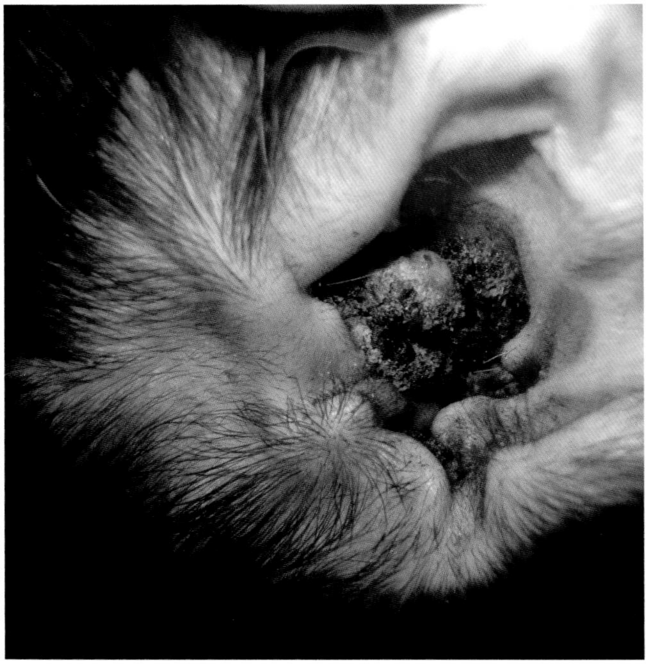

Figure 10-11 Gross image of feline external ear canal with dark brown to black coalescing plaques. (Photo courtesy of Dr. Andrea Lam.)

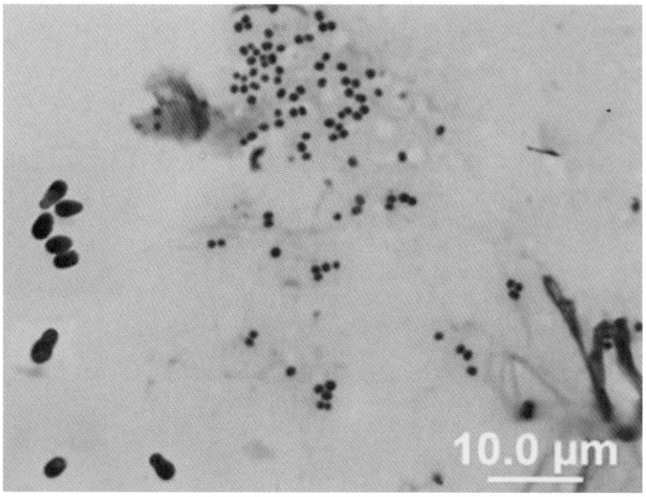

Figure 10-12 Mixed infection characterized by large numbers of bacterial cocci. Some *Malassezia* organisms are also present. (Wright stain. Magnification 1000×.)

(neutrophilic, plasmacytic, or eosinophilic, mastocytic) but varied between cases.[29]

Miscellaneous: Ceruminous otitis externa is associated with some seborrheic diseases.[6,7] The characteristic oily, yellow discharge may grossly resemble purulent exudate. However, because these secretions contain very few inflammatory cells and cerumen fails to take stain, very little material may be visible on microscopic examination of the discharge.[3]

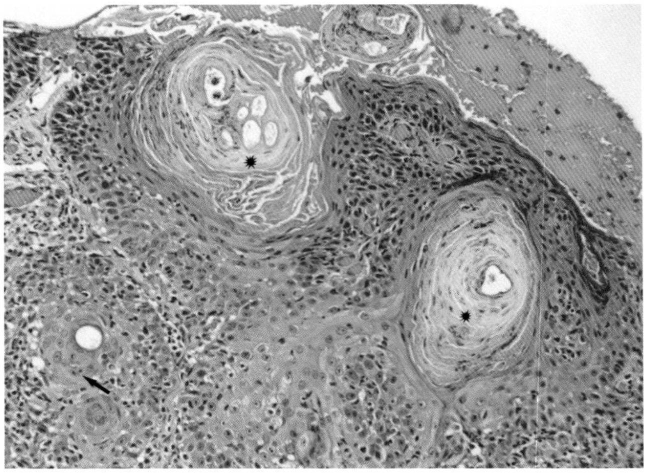

Figure 10-13 Feline external ear canal diagnosed with proliferative and necrotizing otitis externa. Scattered and shrunken keratinocytes with hypereosinophilic cytoplasm and pyknotic nuclei (*arrowhead*) and follicular lumen with parakeratosis and cell debris (*asterisk*) are seen. The epidermis is also covered by a hemorrhagic and cellular crust. (H&E stain. Magnification 200×, Bar = 100 µm.)

References and Suggested Reading

1. Dyce KM, Sack WO, Wensing CJ: *Veterinary anatomy*, ed 2, Philadelphia, PA, 1996, Saunders, pp 339–340.
2. Saridomichelakis MN, et al: Aetiology of canine otitis externa: a retrospective study of 100 cases, *Vet Dermatol* 18:341–347, 2007.
3. Angus JC: Otic cytology in health and disease, *Vet Clin North Am Small Anim Pract* 34:411–424, 2004.
4. Kahn CM, Line S: *The Merck veterinary manual*ed 10, Whitehouse Station, NJ, 2010, Merck and Co, Inc, pp 482–483.
5. Noxon JO: Chapter 59 Otitis externa. In Brichard SJ, Sherding RG, editors: *Saunders manual of small animal practice*, St Louis, 2006, MO. Elsevier Health Sciences, pp 574–581.
6. Rosser EJ Jr: Causes of otitis externa, *Vet Clin North Am Small Anim Pract* 34:459–468, 2004.
7. Scott DW, Miller WH: *Griffin CE Muller & Kirk's small animal dermatology*, ed 6, Philadelphia, PA, 2001, Saunders, pp 1204–1235.
8. Greene CE: *Infectious diseases of the dog and cat*St. Louis, MO, 2006, Saunders. (pp. 602–606, 885-891).
9. McKeever PJ, Globus H: In Bonagura JD, editor: *Kirk's current veterinary therapy XII*, Philadelphia, PA, 1995, Saunders, pp 647–655.
10. Griffin JS, Scott DW, Erb HN: Malassezia otitis externa in the dog: the effect of heat fixing otic exudate for cytological analysis, *J Vet Med* 54:424–427, 2007.
11. Toma S, et al: Comparison of 4 fixation and staining methods for the cytologic evaluation of ear canals with clinical evidence of ceruminous otitis externa, *Vet Clin Pathol* 35:194–198, 2006.
12. Ginel PJ, et al: A semiquantitative cytological evaluation of normal and pathological samples from the external ear canal of dogs and cats, *Vet Dermatol* 13:151–156, 2002.
13. Tater KC, et al: The cytology of the external ear canal in the normal dog and cat, *J Vet Med* 50:370–374, 2003.
14. Logas DB: Diseases of the ear canal, *Vet Clin North Am Small Anim Pract* 24:905–919, 1994.
15. Rosychuk RA: Management of otitis externa, *Vet Clin North Am Small Anim Pract* 24:921–952, 1994.

16. Graham-Mize CA, Rosser EJ Jr: Comparison of microbial isolates and susceptibility patterns from the external ear canal of dogs with otitis externa, *J Am Anim Hosp Assoc* 40:102–108, 2004.
17. Bond R, Saijonmaa-Koulumies LE, Lloyd DH: Population sizes and frequency of *Malassezia pachydermatis* at skin and mucosal sites on healthy dogs, *J Small Anim Pract* 36:147–150, 1995.
18. Crespo MJ, Abarca ML, Cabañes FJ: Occurrence of *Malassezia* spp. in the external ear canal of dogs and cats with and without otitis externa, *Med Mycol* 40:115–121, 2002.
19. Harvey RG, Harari J, Delauch AJ: Diagnostic procedure. *Ear disease of the dog and cat,* Ames, IO, 2001, Iowa state University Press, pp 43–80.
20. Guedeja-Marron J, Blanco JL, Garcia ME: A case of feline otitis externa due to *Microsporum canis, Med Mycol* 39:229–232, 2001.
21. Godfrey D: Microsporum canis associated with otitis externa in a Persian cat, *Vet Rec* 147:50–51, 2000.
22. Campbell JJ, et al: Evaluation of fungal flora in normal and diseased canine ears, *Vet Dermatol* 21:619–625, 2010.
23. Knottenbelt MK: Chronic otitis externa due to *Demodex canis* in a Tibetan spaniel, *Vet Rec* 135:409–410, 1994.
24. van Poucke S: Ceruminous otitis externa due to *Demodex cati* in a cat, *Vet Rec* 149:651–652, 2001.
25. Fan TM, de Lorimier LP: Inflammatory polyps and aural neoplasia, *Vet Clin North Am Small Anim Pract* 34:489–509, 2004.
26. London CA, Dubilzeig RR, Vail DM, et al: Evaluation of dogs and cats with tumors of the ear canal: 145 cases: 1978-1992, *J Am Vet Med Assoc* 208:1413–1418, 1996.
27. de Lorenzi D, Bonfanti U, Masserdotti C, et al: Fine-needle biopsy of external ear canal masses in the cat: cytologic results and histologic correlations in 27 cases, *Vet Clin Pathol* 34:100–105, 2005.
28. Videmont E, Pin D: Proliferative and necrotizing otitis in a kitten: first demonstration of T-cell-mediated apoptosis, *J Small Anim Pract* 51:599–603, 2010.
29. Mauldin EA, Ness TA, Goldschmidt MH: Proliferative and necrotizing otitis externa in four cats, *Vet Dermatol* 18:370–377, 2007.

Additional Reading

Cafarchia C, Gallo S, Capelli G, Otranto D: Occurrence and population size of *Malassezia* spp. in the external ear canal of dogs and cats both healthy and with otitis, *Mycopathologia* 160:143–149, 2005.

CHAPTER 11

The Lymph Nodes

Joanne B. Messick

ARCHITECTURE

When interpreting a cytologic specimen of the lymph node, it is useful to keep in mind the histologic structure and different cell types that are found in this tissue. The node is composed of a capsule, cortex, medulla, and sinuses (subcapsular, cortical, and medullary).[1] The cortex, or the more peripheral area of the node, is divided into follicular and diffuse (parafollicular cortex or paracortex) regions, and the medulla, or the more central area, is divided into the medullary cords and sinuses (Figure 11-1).

Within the parafollicular cortex are high endothelial venules through which both B- and T-lymphocytes from the blood enter the node. This region is also rich in interdigitating reticulum cells (IDCs), a specialized antigen-presenting cell. The initial immune response requires that the antigen presented by IDCs be recognized by T-lymphocytes and early B-lymphocytes in the parafollicular cortex, whereas the differentiation of B-lymphocytes in response to antigen occurs in the follicular cortex.

Follicles contain predominantly B-lineage lymphocytes. The primary follicles are composed of small, dark-staining lymphocytes. In contrast, secondary follicles have a peripheral rim or mantle zone of small, dark lymphoid cells similar to those in primary follicles and a central germinal center. In the germinal center, specialized cells of the mononuclear phagocytic system (MPS), the follicular dendritic cells (FDCs), capture antigen on their surfaces to promote B-lymphocyte differentiation. Thus, small resting B-cells undergo mitosis and divide to become the larger, more irregular small-cleaved, intermediate and large blast cells in the germinal center of a reactive node (follicular hyperplasia). T-cells (mainly CD4+ helper cells) that play a role in stimulating B-cells are also found in the follicles. Surviving B-cells may eventually differentiate into plasma cells, migrating to the medullary cords or leaving the node.

The parafollicular zone of the lymph node gradually transforms into medullary cords that are populated by B-cells and plasma cells. Sinuses containing macrophages surround these cords. A reactive process in the lymph node may also result in hyperplasia of the parafollicular region, of sinus cells (sinus histiocytosis), or of plasma cells (plasma cell hyperplasia). These different types of hyperplasia may occur either by themselves or in combination.

Lymph nodes are strategically located at sites throughout the body and are involved in a variety of local and systemic disease processes. Antigen reaches the node via the afferent lymphatics. The lymph percolates through the sinus and sinusoidal walls into the parenchyma (Figure 11-2), where foreign substances (antigens) are taken up and processed by specialized cells of the MPS. The sinuses (subcapsular, cortical, and medullary) form a network of branching channels that converge at the hilus of the node to exit by the efferent lymphatics. The primary functions of the lymph nodes include filtering particles and microorganisms, exposing antigens to circulating lymphocytes, and activating B- and T-lymphocytes. The superficial, subcutaneous location of some lymph nodes (mandibular, superficial cervical, inguinal, and popliteal) allows easy detection of enlargement and access for fine-needle aspiration (FNA) cytology. It is appropriate to aspirate any node that is enlarged, and in the case of lymph nodes draining areas affected by neoplasia, even in the absence of enlargement, aspiration may be justified.[2]

GENERAL CONSIDERATIONS

Lymph node aspiration cytology has become a popular procedure in human medicine in recent years, because of its great convenience.[3] Similarly, this high-yield diagnostic technique is frequently used in veterinary medicine.[4-7] A few points need to be considered when obtaining nodal samples for cytologic evaluation.

A normal lymph node is small and often difficult to aspirate. It is not uncommon for the cytology of a normal node to contain mostly perinodal adipose tissue and only a few or no lymphocytes. If multiple nodes are enlarged, then sampling from several nodes is recommended. Because the submandibular nodes drain the oral cavity, they often become enlarged, reactive, inflamed, or all of these may occur. A confusing mixture of malignant, reactive, and inflammatory cells may limit the accuracy of cytologic diagnosis of lymphoma based on FNA of these nodes. Thus, sampling of submandibular nodes should be avoided in cases where generalized lymph node enlargement exists. The prescapular and popliteal nodes are often a better choice. The mandibular salivary gland is quite frequently mistaken for a node and aspirated. However, the

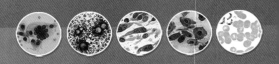

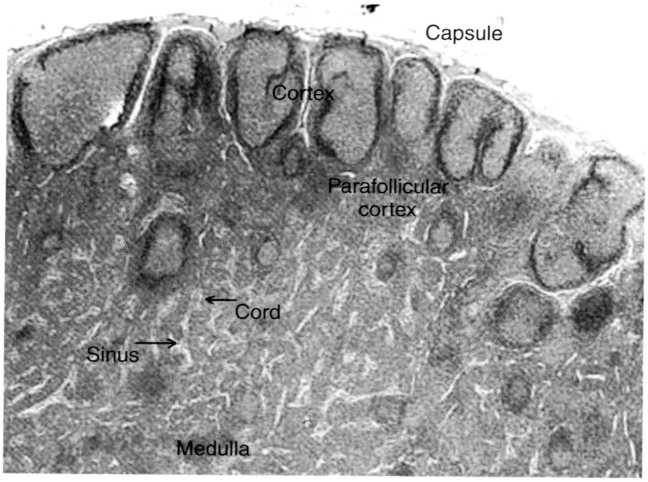

Figure 11-1 The lymph node has two basic parts: the cortex and the medulla. The cortex has both follicular and diffuse or parafollicular regions. The parafollicular region gradually transforms into medullary cords of B-lymphocytes and plasma cells, which are surround by sinuses containing macrophages attached to reticular fibers. Different populations of lymphocytes in these areas and other cells are found in nodal aspirates. (H&E stain.)

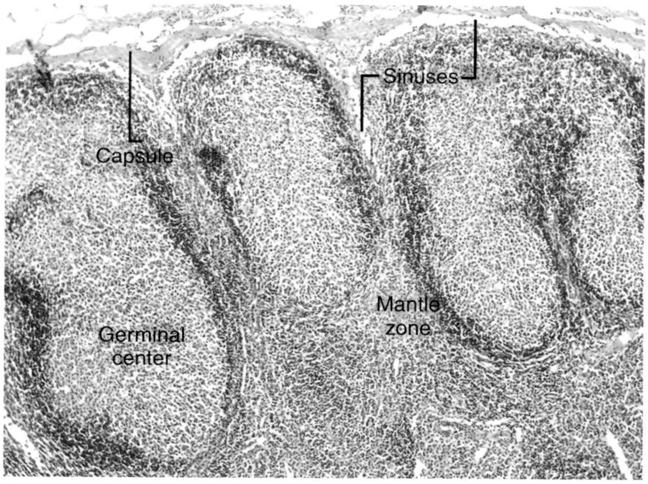

Figure 11-2 Lymph enters the node via the afferent lymphatics, percolating through subcapsular sinuses and sinusoids, where foreign substances (antigens) are taken up and processed. The secondary follicles in this node have a peripheral rim or mantle zone and a pale-staining, central germinal center. The differentiation of B-lymphocytes in response to antigen occurs in the germinal center of the follicular cortex. (H&E stain.)

presence of large, foamy epithelial cells, either individually or in clusters, and mucus in the background allows the salivary tissue to be easily identified.

Consideration also should be given to the size of the lymph node when deciding which node to aspirate —very large nodes may have areas of hemorrhage or necrosis. If the node must be sampled, the needle should be directed tangentially, avoiding the more central portions.[8] Finally, when obtaining a sample for cytologic evaluation, it is important to remember that the lymph node is a heterogeneous tissue, and multiple areas within the node should be sampled to be certain that what has been obtained is representative. While keeping the needle in the node, the needle should be repeatedly advanced and withdrawn in multiple directions until a small amount of aspirate appears in the hub of the needle. This procedure may be done using a syringe to apply gentle suction or with only the needle. If the former technique is used, the suction should be released before removing the needle from the node. Overly vigorous aspiration of the lymph node produces significant hemodilution and cells may rupture, limiting the interpretation of the sample. A large volume of aspirate is not required; the material within the hub of the needle is sufficient for making cytologic preparations. Because the lymphocytes are fragile, care must be taken to apply only minimal pressure when making slide preparations to prevent excessive rupturing of cells. The slides are air-dried (not heat-fixed) and stained for evaluation.

BOX 11-1

The Role of Fine-Needle Aspiration Cytology of Lymph Nodes

1. Diagnosis of infectious disease
2. Diagnosis of hyperplasia or reactive lymphadenopathy and recognition of specific conditions (i.e., lymph node hyperplasia of young cats) (If a cause for the change is not apparent, resolution does not occur, or both, follow-up and subsequent biopsy are indicated.)
3. Diagnosis of metastatic neoplasia and indication of possible primary site
4. Diagnosis of lymphoma that is optimally followed by a biopsy for confirmation and accurate subtyping
5. If known malignancy such as lymphoma or a metastatic mast cell tumor, staging and monitoring for relapse or effects of chemotherapy
6. For sampling of multiple sites as well as for obtaining samples from surgically inaccessible sites or from medically unfit patients
7. Obtaining material for clonality and research studies

FINE-NEEDLE ASPIRATION

FNA is a relatively safe and painless procedure, allowing for rapid and inexpensive sampling of peripheral lymph nodes. It does not require hospital admission or anesthesia of the pet. The role of this procedure is summarized in Box 11-1.

CYTOLOGIC FINDINGS

Normal Lymph Node

In the absence of architectural features that can be appreciated in a histologic section of a lymph node, the interpretation of cytology relies on proportions of different cell types and an understanding of what proportions are normal versus abnormal for these cell types. Small, well-differentiated lymphocytes compose greater than 75% to 85% of the total nucleated cell population (Figure 11-3

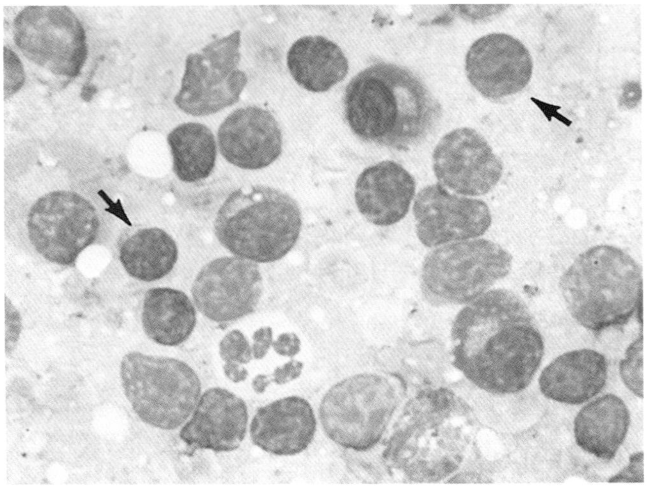

Figure 11-3 Aspirate from a hyperplastic lymph node. Small lymphocytes (*arrows*) and plasma cells characterize the reaction. Note that the small lymphocytes are smaller than the neutrophils and their nuclei are about the size of a red blood cell. Many free nuclei, identified by pink, homogeneous chromatin and an absence of cytoplasm, are evident. (Wright stain.)

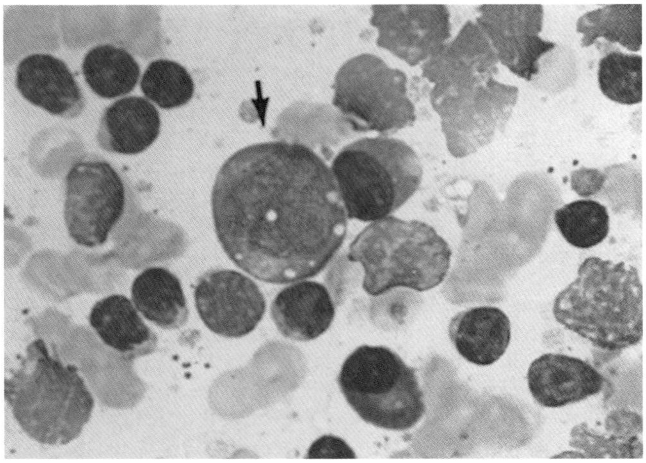

Figure 11-4 Small lymphocytes, plasma cells, and a large transformed lymphocyte (*arrow*) characterize this aspirate from a hyperplastic lymph node. Irregular, pink nuclei from lysed cells are seen. (Wright stain.)

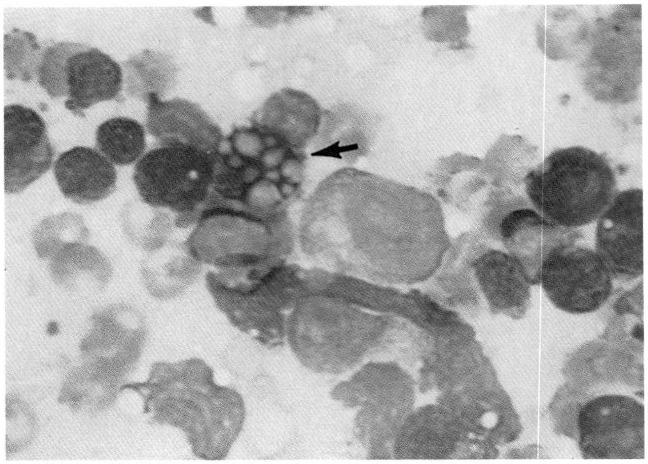

Figure 11-5 Plasma cells, small lymphocytes, and two large lymphocytes (lymphoblasts) characterize this aspirate from a hyperplastic lymph node. The plasma cell with the vacuolated cytoplasm is a Mott cell containing Russell bodies (*arrow*). The pink, amorphous structures are free nuclear material. (Wright stain.)

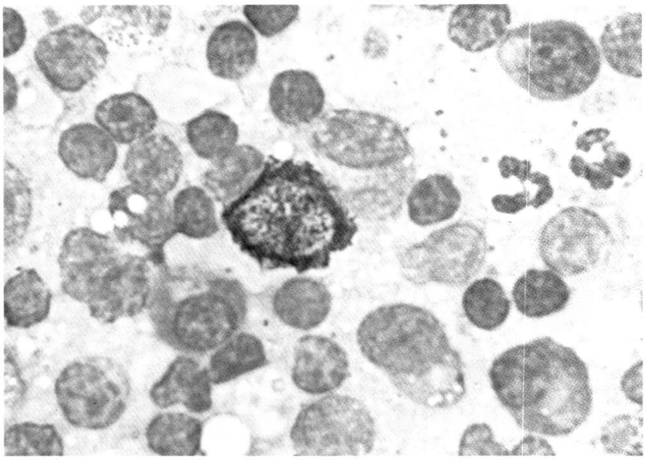

Figure 11-6 Small lymphocytes, plasma cells, neutrophils, and a single mast cell are present in this aspirate from a hyperplastic lymph node. (Wright stain.)

to Figure 11-7).[4-7] They have round nuclei that are about 1 to less than 1.5 times the size of a mature red blood cell (RBC), with an overall cell size that is smaller than that of a neutrophil. Their chromatin is densely clumped, and nucleoli are not visible. The nucleus-to-cytoplasm (N:C) ratio is high, with a narrow rim of basophilic cytoplasm. In addition to small lymphocytes, a normal node should have low numbers (<10% to 15%) of lymphocytes that are intermediate to large (often called *lymphoblasts*) in size; their nuclei are 1.5 to 3 times the size of an RBC, with an overall size ranging from about that of a neutrophil or larger to up to 4 times the size of an RBC (see Figure 11-5). Their chromatin is less clumped, and nucleoli may be visible and even multiple, prominent, or both. The cytoplasm is pale blue and more abundant than in small lymphocytes.

Plasma cells have small, round, eccentric nuclei with condensed chromatin (see Figures 11-3 to 11-6). Their abundant cytoplasm is deep blue and has a prominent, clear Golgi zone. Immature plasma cells (transformed B-lymphocytes) are larger and have less aggregated chromatin and a higher N:C ratio (see Figure 11-4). Their very blue cytoplasm may contain discrete vacuoles. Plasma cells in various stages of development are seen in small numbers in normal lymph nodes, but typically represent less than 3% of the total nucleated cell population.

Macrophages, characterized by abundant cytoplasm often containing vacuoles and granular debris, also are found in small numbers (see Figure 11-7). Macrophages from areas of intense lymphopoiesis and cellular turnover may contain prominent basophilic nuclear debris (tingible

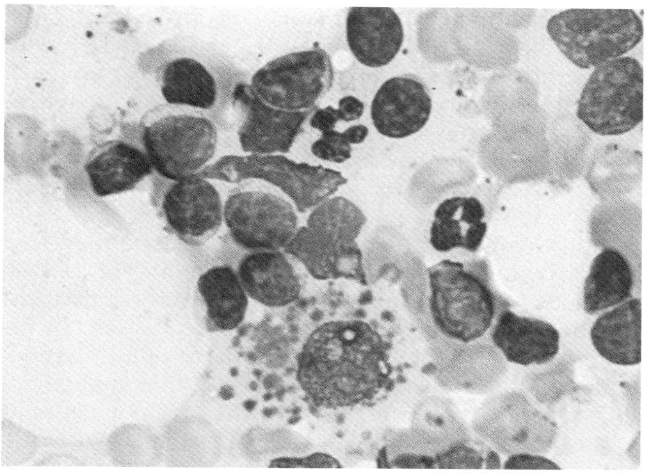

Figure 11-7 Seen among small and medium-sized lymphocytes is a large macrophage containing phagocytized debris. (Wright stain.)

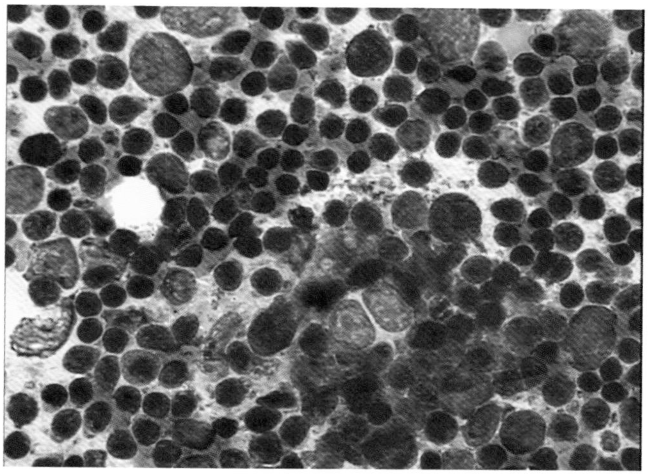

Figure 11-9 Several reticuloendothelial cells are seen in this lymph node aspiration cytology. Their nuclei are swollen, and they are devoid of cytoplasm. Small lymphocytes are the predominant cell type in this mildly hyperplastic node.

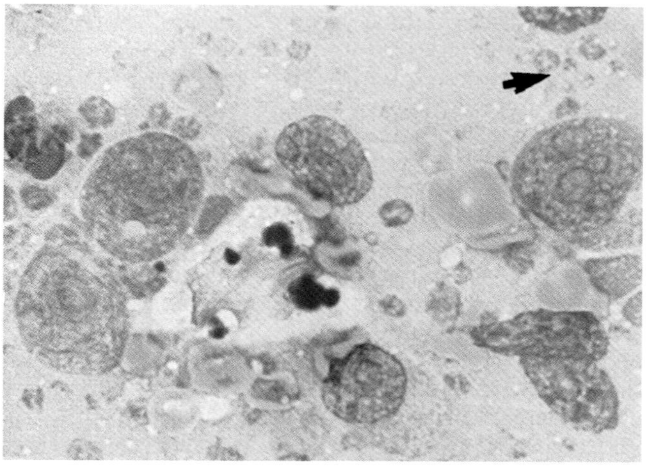

Figure 11-8 In this aspirate from a lymphomatous lymph node are large immature lymphocytes with prominent nucleoli, dispersed chromatin, and abundant blue cytoplasm. The large cell in the center with bluish cytoplasmic globules is a tingible-body macrophage. The small blue structures (*arrow*) are lymphoglandular bodies. (Wright stain.)

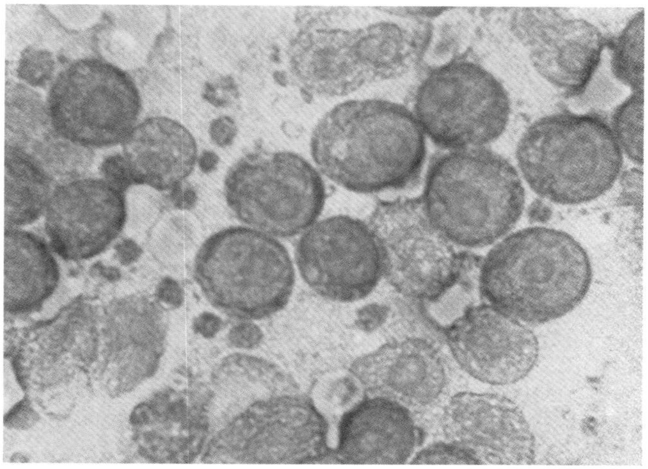

Figure 11-10 Immature, neoplastic lymphocytes characterize this smear from a dog with malignant lymphoma. Note that the cells are much larger than red blood cells. The pink structures lacking cytoplasm and containing prominent nucleoli are nuclei from lysed cells. Small blue lymphoglandular bodies are numerous. (Wright stain.)

bodies) (Figure 11-8). Occasionally, small numbers of neutrophils, eosinophils, and mast cells are observed in a normal node (see Figure 11-6). Each of these cell types should represent less than 1% of the cell populations in a normal node. It is important to consider the amount of blood contamination when making this assessment. Reticular cells and endothelial cells are common in lymph nodes, but these tissue-bound cells are rarely aspirated intact. They usually appear as large swollen nuclei, often devoid of cytoplasm (Figure 11-9).

Because of the pressures of the aspiration technique, lymphocytes, which are very fragile, may rupture and release their nuclei. Free nuclei are swollen and uniformly pink in contrast to the blue blocky or granular pattern of intact lymphocyte nuclei (see Figures 11-3 to Figure 11-5). Blue nucleoli are often exposed in the nuclear chromatin of ruptured cells. These free nuclei carry no diagnostic significance and should not be confused with large immature lymphocytes. Lymphoglandular bodies are cytoplasmic fragments and are highly characteristic of lymphoid tissue (see Figure 11-8; Figure 11-10). They are round, homogeneous, basophilic structures that are similar in size to platelets.

LYMPHADENOPATHY

One of the most common indications for performing aspiration cytology is enlargement of one or more lymph nodes. Three general processes cause lymph node enlargement: (1) inflammation (lymphadenitis—suppurative, pyogranulomatous, granulomatous, and eosinophilic), (2) immune

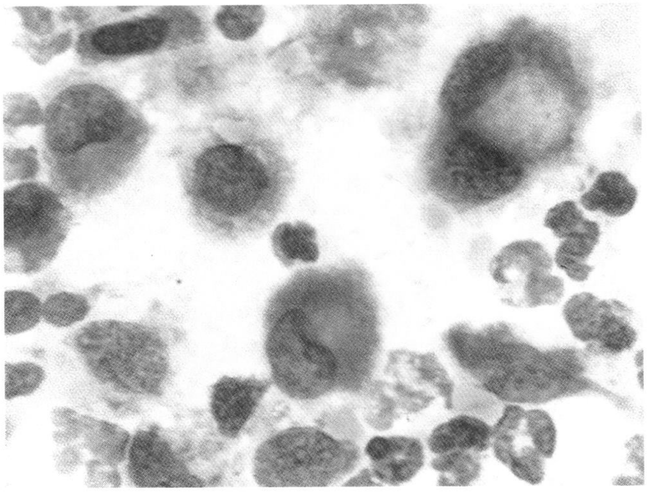

Figure 11-11 This aspirate from an animal with blastomycosis is characterized by pyogranulomatous inflammation. Neutrophils, epithelioid macrophages, and a single multinucleate giant cell are present. (Wright stain)

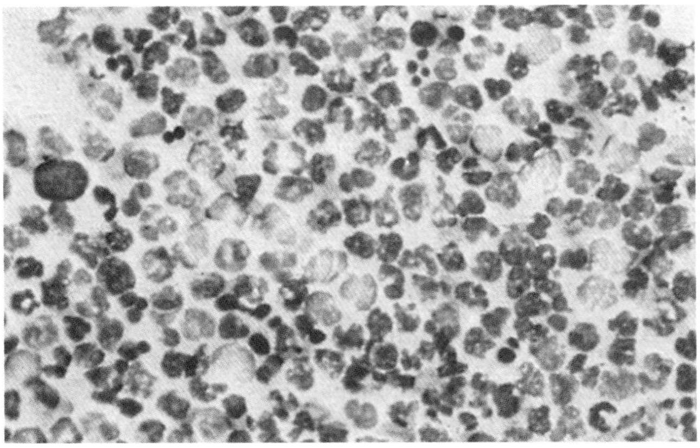

Figure 11-12 Purulent inflammation is characterized by the predominance of neutrophils. (Wright stain.)

stimulation (hyperplasia or reactive lymphadenopathy), and (3) neoplasia (lymphoma or metastatic). The cytologic evaluation of a sample obtained by FNA or touch imprint from the excised node usually allows differentiation of these processes. However, these processes are not mutually exclusive and may occur simultaneously.

Lymphadenitis

Lymphadenitis or inflammation of the node may be a primary (node itself is inflamed or necrotic) or secondary (node is draining an area of inflammation or necrosis) finding. This process is characterized cytologically by accumulation of inflammatory cells. Neutrophils, eosinophils, and macrophages occur singly or in combination. Inflammation is probably present when the population is greater than 5% neutrophils or greater than 3% eosinophils, provided no significant blood contamination has occurred. Macrophage numbers may increase in inflammation but also in hyperplasia and sometimes in neoplasia. Macrophages also may appear as epithelioid cells and multinucleated giant cells in granulomatous inflammation. Epithelioid macrophages are characterized by blue cytoplasm with minimal vacuolization and contain very little phagocytic debris (Figure 11-11). Organisms may, however, be present within the cytoplasm. These cells may occur in aggregates. Inflammatory cells may represent only a small portion of the total cell population, which otherwise suggests lymphoid hyperplasia, or they may completely replace the normal cell population.

Most bacterial infections elicit a neutrophilic or purulent response (Figure 11-12) but *Mycobacterium* spp. (Figure 11-13) may cause a granulomatous response. An eosinophilic exudate of varying degrees is common in lymph nodes draining allergic inflammation of skin, respiratory tract, and digestive tract. Systemic fungal infections such as histoplasmosis (Figure 11-14), blastomycosis (Figure 11-15), coccidioidomycosis (Figure 11-16), and cryptococcosis (Figure 11-17); protozoal infections such as cytauxzoonosis (Figure 11-18), toxoplasmosis

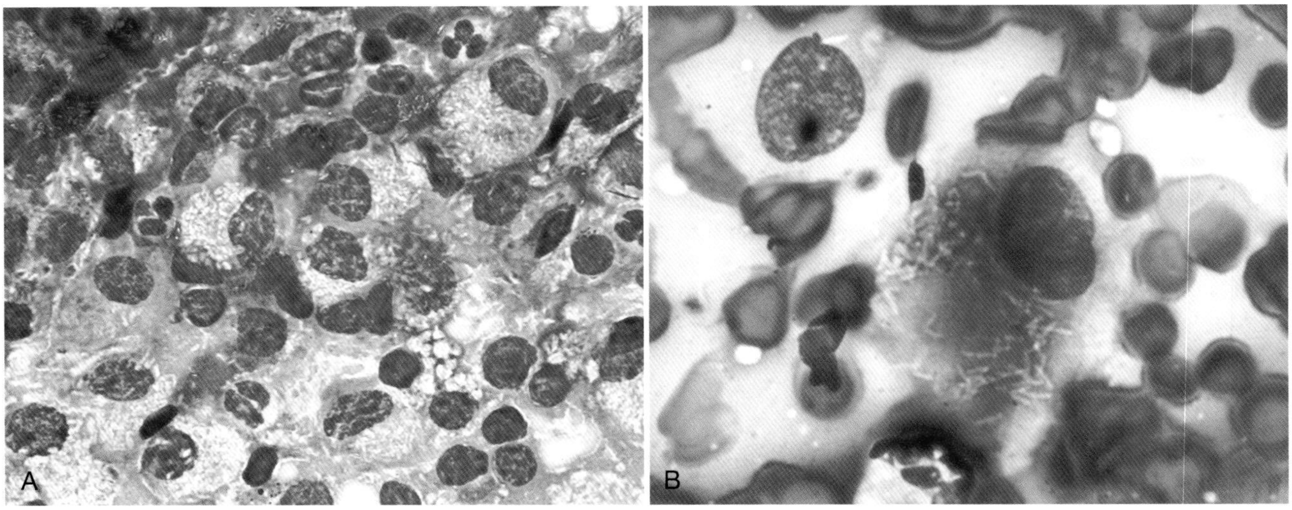

Figure 11-13 **A,** Lymph node aspirates showing a high number of macrophages containing nonstaining bacterial rods indicative of a *Mycobacterium* infection. **B,** Higher magnification of a single macrophage containing nonstaining bacterial rods identified as clear streaks through the cell. (Wright stain.) (Courtesy of Dr. R.L. Cowell)

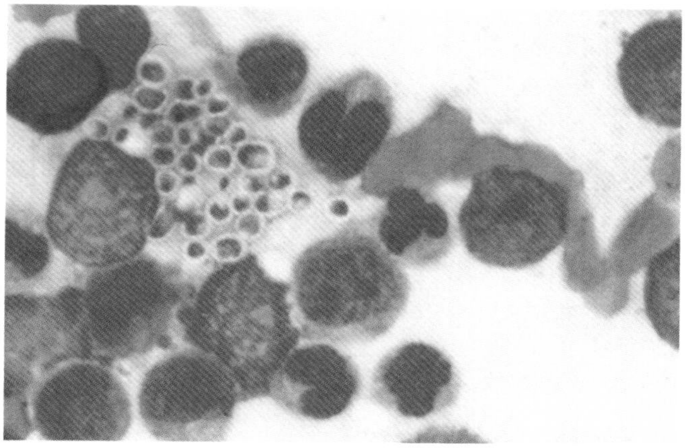

Figure 11-14 Macrophage containing numerous Histoplasma organisms. *Histoplasma* organisms are small, round to oval, yeast-like organisms that have a nucleus that stains dark purple and a thin clear halo. (Wright stain.) (Courtesy of Oklahoma State University.)

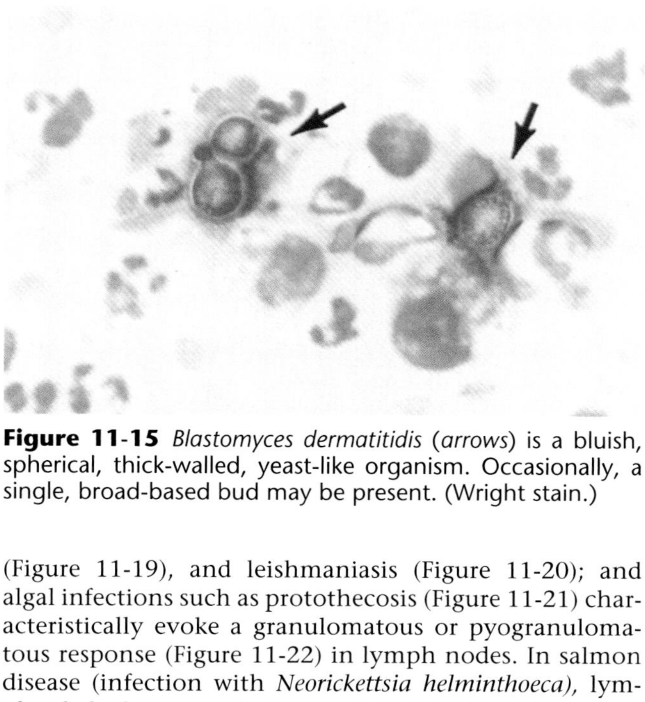

Figure 11-15 *Blastomyces dermatitidis* (*arrows*) is a bluish, spherical, thick-walled, yeast-like organism. Occasionally, a single, broad-based bud may be present. (Wright stain.)

(Figure 11-19), and leishmaniasis (Figure 11-20); and algal infections such as protothecosis (Figure 11-21) characteristically evoke a granulomatous or pyogranulomatous response (Figure 11-22) in lymph nodes. In salmon disease (infection with *Neorickettsia helminthoeca),* lymphoid depletion and sinus macrophage hyperplasia or sinus histiocytosis occur (Figure 11-23).

Reactive or Hyperplastic Node

No clear line of separation between a normal and a hyperplastic lymph node is evident on the basis of cytology alone. Differentiation, however, is probably a moot point because enlarged lymph nodes are reactive to some degree. Typically, a heterogeneous cell population is usually obtained as the needle is directed through follicular centers, the paracortical area, medullary cords, and medullary sinuses. If the reactive pattern is principally follicular hyperplasia, intermediate and large lymphocytes from expanding germinal centers are found in increased numbers. These cells may constitute up to 15% to 25% or more of the total cell population (Figure 11-24).[4-7] However, small lymphocytes are still the predominant cell type in hyperplastic as well as normal lymph nodes. Plasma cell numbers may vary from none to greater than 5% to 10% of the population in some areas of the smear. They occasionally are filled with vacuoles (Russell bodies) (see Figure 11-5). Immature plasma cells or transformed lymphocytes, which are medium to large in size, also may be observed. Macrophages may on occasion represent greater than 2% of the population, particularly with hyperplasia of sinus macrophages. An aspirate from a node with parafollicular hyperplasia is also heterogeneous; however, immunoblasts

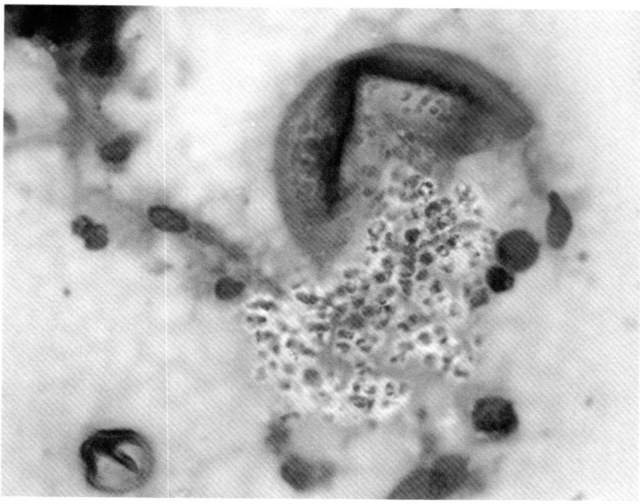

Figure 11-16 *Coccidioides immitis* organisms are large, double-contoured, clear to blue-staining, spherical bodies that range in size from 10 micrometers (μm) to greater than 100 μm. Occasionally, endospores varying from 2 to 5 μm in diameter may be seen within some of the larger spherules. (Wright stain.) (Courtesy of Dr. R.L. Cowell.)

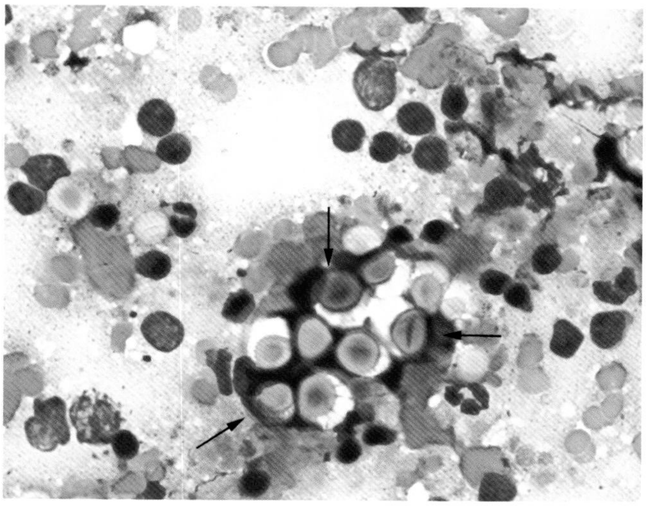

Figure 11-17 Lymph node aspirate from a cat with cryptococcosis. Scattered red blood cells, small lymphocytes, and a group of *Cryptococcus* organisms (*arrows*) are shown. *Cryptococcus* organisms stain eosinophilic to clear and may be the smooth form (large clear capsule) or rough form (small clear capsule) as shown here. (Wright stain.) (Courtesy of Dr. R.L. Cowell.)

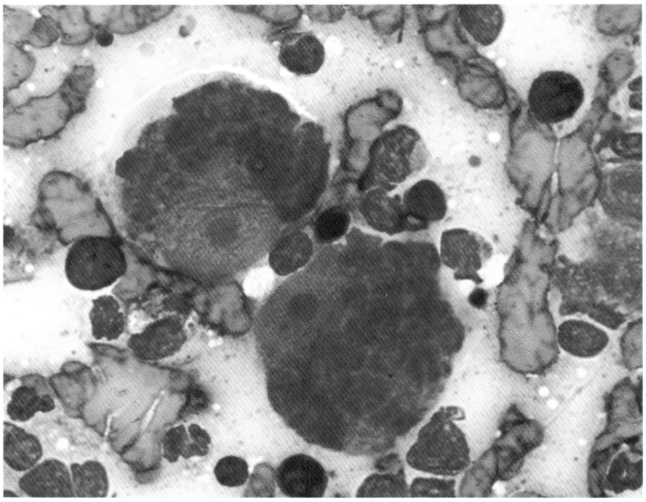

Figure 11-18 Lymph node aspirate from a cat showing two huge mononuclear cells with abundant cytoplasm, eccentric nuclei, and prominent nucleoli. These cells contain developing cytauxzoon merozoites, which appear as either small, dark-staining bodies or larger, irregularly defined clusters. (Wright stain.) (Courtesy of Dr. R.L. Cowell.)

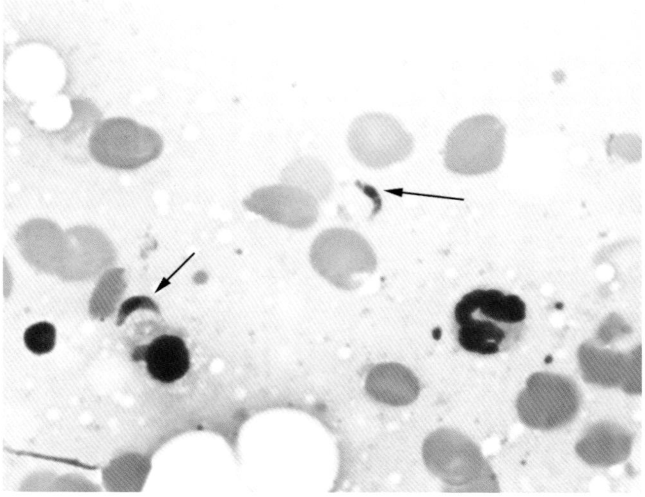

Figure 11-19 *Toxoplasma gondii* tachyzoites (*arrows*) appear as small, crescent-shaped bodies with a light blue cytoplasm and a dark-staining pericentral nucleus. (Wright stain.) (Courtesy of Dr. R.L. Cowell.)

are prominent in association with plasma cell hyperplasia, and tingible-body macrophages are lacking. The main cytologic characteristics of the immunoblasts (parafollicular zone cells) are their medium size, fine chromatin, and large centrally located nucleolus. In reactive lymph nodes of dogs associated with mammary tumor lymphadenopathies, systemic lupus erythematosus, and leishmaniasis, these cells may be found in high numbers.[9] Any enlarged lymph node with the aforementioned cytologic findings should be considered hyperplastic, since a normal node should not be enlarged.

Hyperplasia occurs when antigens in high concentration reach the draining lymph node and stimulate the immune system. In some instances, these antigens also cause

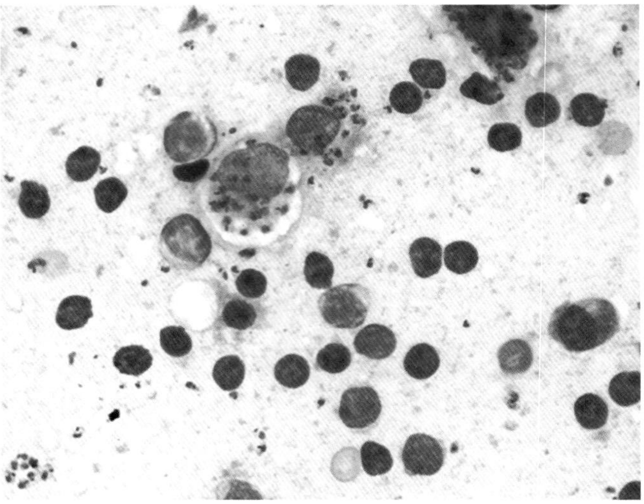

Figure 11-20 Lymph node aspirate from a dog showing many lymphocytes and two macrophages containing numerous *Leishmania donovani* organisms. *L. donovani* organisms are small, round to oval organisms with a clear to very-light-blue cytoplasm, an oval nucleus, and a small, dark, ventral kinetoplast. (Wright stain.) (Courtesy of Dr. R.L. Cowell.)

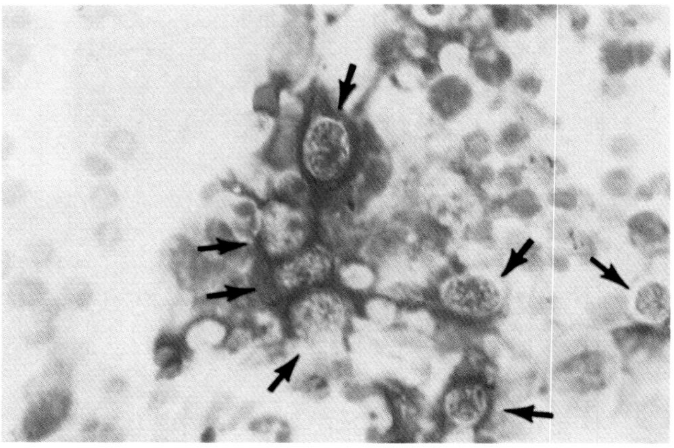

Figure 11-21 *Prototheca* organisms (*arrows*) are round to oval and have a granular basophilic cytoplasm and a clear cell wall. (Wright stain.)

inflammation and attract inflammatory cells to the node (lymphadenitis). In many cases, reactions causing hyperplasia are localized, but they may be systemic and affect all nodes. Generalized lymphadenopathy with a hyperplastic cytologic picture may occur in feline leukemia virus (FeLV) infection, feline immunodeficiency virus (FIV) infection, bartonellosis, Rocky Mountain spotted fever, and ehrlichiosis. It may occasionally be especially difficult to distinguish reactive nodal hyperplasia from lymphoma in cats. In these cases, additional testing is needed, such as histopathology, immunophenotyping, and polymerase chain reaction (PCR) for the assessment of clonality.[10-15]

Malignant Lymphoma

FNA is often sufficient for establishing a diagnosis of lymphoma in dogs and cats. This is caused by the predominance

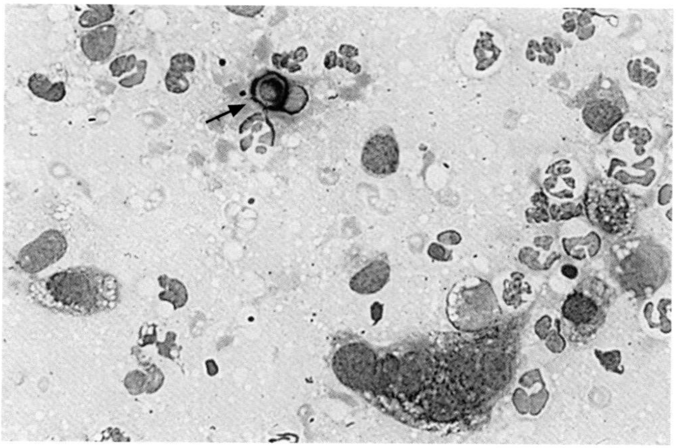

Figure 11-22 **Pyogranulomatous inflammation from a dog with blastomycosis.** A *Blastomyces dermatitidis* organism (*arrow*) is in the center of the field. Neutrophils, macrophages, and an inflammatory giant cell are present. (Wright stain.)

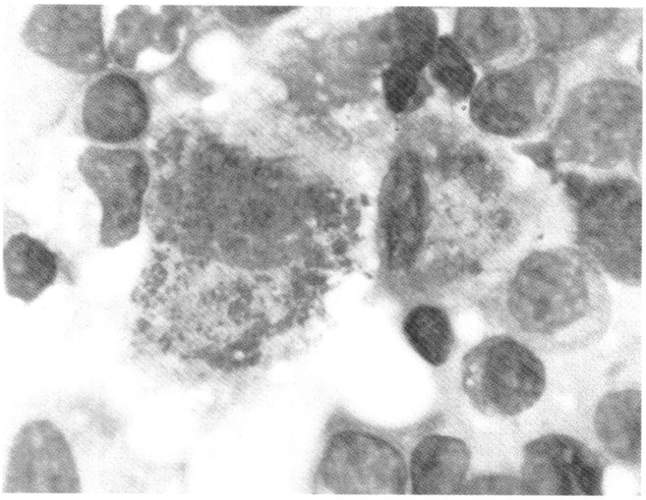

Figure 11-23 Aspirate of a lymph node from a dog with salmon disease. Large macrophages contain the causative agent, *Neorickettsia helminthoeca*. (Wright stain.)

of monomorphic lymphoid cells that lack the polymorphism of a reactive population. Still the opportunity must not be missed at the outset of the disease process to also obtain nodal tissue for histologic, immunocytochemical, and molecular evaluations. This will allow for the diagnosis to be confirmed and accurate subtyping performed, as well as providing archival materials that may be of use to further advances in diagnosis, treatment, or both.

Malignant lymphoma is characterized by lymphocytes that eventually replace the entire normal cell population (Figure 11-25 and Figure 11-26). However, not all lymphomas are the same; they are a diverse group of lymphoid neoplasms. Each of these neoplasms represents a clonal expansion of an anatomic or developmental compartment of lymphoid cells in the node, which have distinct morphologic and immunophenotypic characteristics.[16-18] When immature cells compose greater than 50% of the cell population, a diagnosis of malignant lymphoma may be reliably made, but smaller numbers may be present in early stages, making a diagnosis by cytologic examination

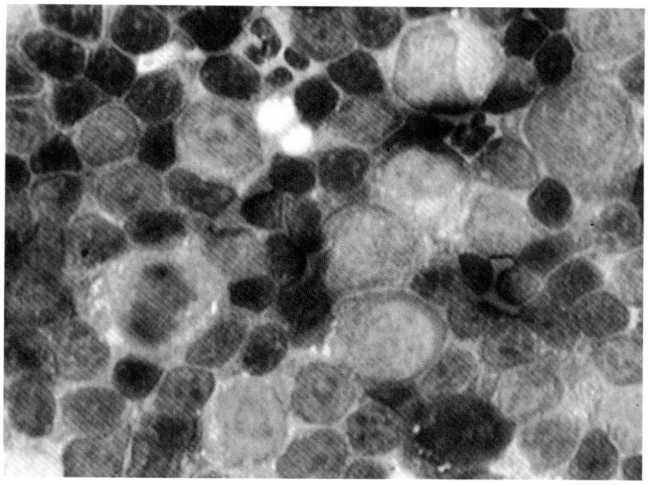

Figure 11-24 Intermediate and large lymphocytes from expanded germinal centers are found in increased numbers in this hyperplastic node (follicular hyperplasia). However, small lymphocytes are still the predominant cell type.

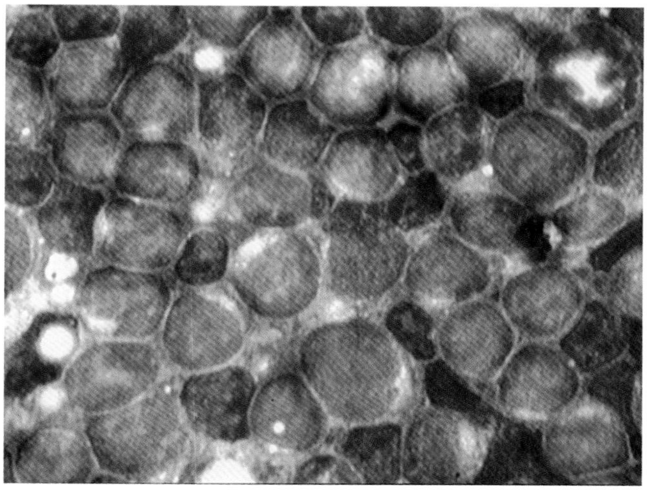

Figure 11-25 In this aspirate from an enlarged node of a dog, a monomorphic population of immature lymphocytes that are intermediate in size is seen. Some of the nuclei in these cells are indented (clefted) and uniformly have a fine, diffuse chromatin pattern; however, nucleoli are inapparent. The mitotic rate is high. This is a high-grade, aggressive T-cell lymphoblastic lymphoma with an associated paraneoplastic hypercalcemia. The cells of B- and T-cell lymphoblastic lymphoma are not distinguishable by cytology alone but are different morphologically from other high-grade lymphomas. Immunophenotyping was done to establish the T-cell type. (Wright stain.)

alone more difficult. Usually, these neoplastic lymphocytes are larger than neutrophils and have finely granular dispersed chromatin, nucleoli, a lower N:C ratio, and basophilic cytoplasm. The lymphocytes are considered medium and large if their nuclei are 1.5 to 2 times or more than 2 to 3 times the size of RBCs, respectively. Frequently, the percentage of the medium to large lymphocytes exceeds 80%, making the diagnosis more certain. Mitoses may be more numerous than in hyperplasia and tingible-body macrophages may indicate intense lymphopoiesis

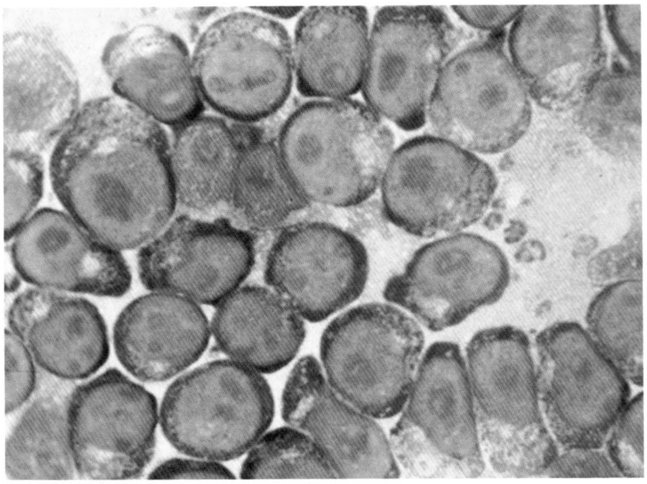

Figure 11-26 In this nodal aspirate from a cat, a monomorphic population of immature lymphocytes that are large in size is shown. These cells have a high nucleus-to-cytoplasm ratio and often a single prominent nucleolus or several in a paracentral location. The cytoplasm is deeply basophilic. The histopathology showed a mitotic rate that was high with a diffuse nodal involvement. Although these high-grade lymphomas are often B-cell phenotype, the T-cell counterpart cannot be distinguished by morphology alone. (Wright stain.)

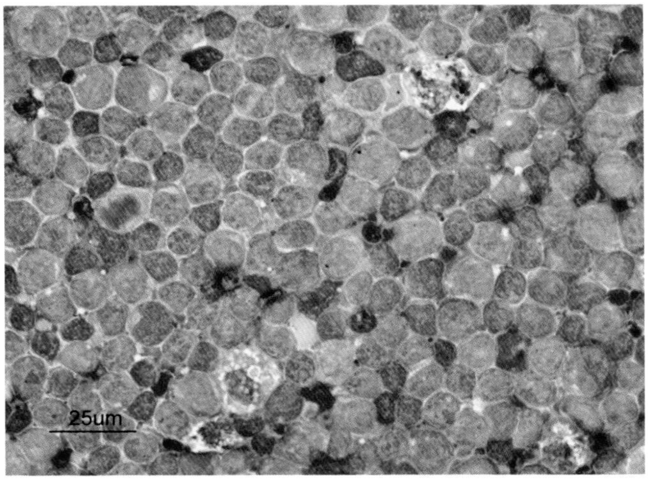

Figure 11-27 In this aspirate from a lymphomatous lymph node, many tingible-body macrophages were present, an indication of intense lymphopoiesis and cell turnover. (Wright stain.)

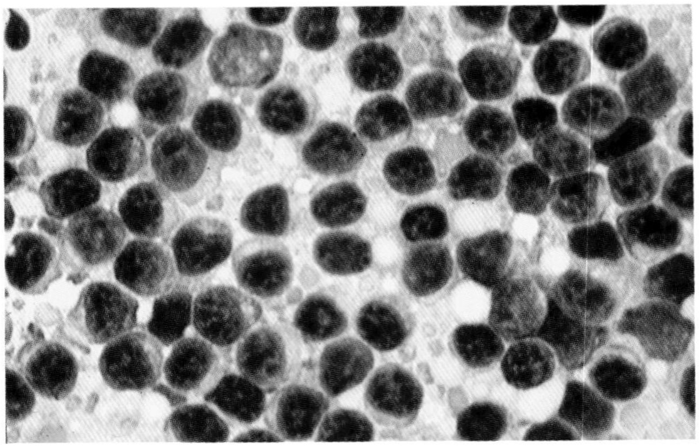

Figure 11-28 A monotonous population of small, well-differentiated lymphocytes is seen in this nodal aspirate from a dog. Mitoses are not observed. Their chromatin pattern is densely clumped, nucleoli are not visible, and mitotic figures are not observed. The presence of a generalized lymphadenopathy and monomorphic lymphoid cells that lack the polymorphism of a normal node or of a reactive population is a useful characteristic that supports this diagnosis. However, the effacement of normal nodal architecture by histopathology is needed to confirm this suspicion. The cells of B- and T-cell small cell lymphoma or chronic lymphocytic leukemia cannot be distinguished by morphology alone. The cells of this low-grade lymphoma are a T-cell type. (Wright stain.)

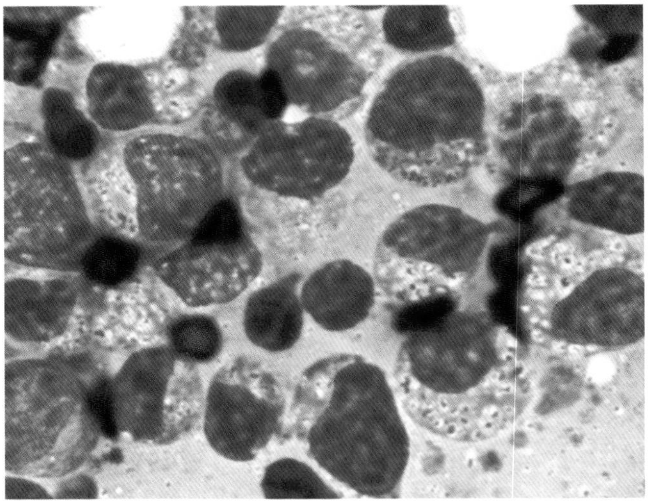

Figure 11-29 An aspirate from an alimentary lymph node in a cat with large granular lymphoma. Most of the lymphocytes are large and contain magenta intracytoplasmic granules. (Wright stain.) (Courtesy of Dr. R.L. Cowell.)

and cell turnover (Figure 11-27), but neither alone is a reliable indicator of neoplasia. Lymphoglandular bodies are more numerous than in hyperplasia.

Occasionally, lymphoma is manifested as the small, well-differentiated lymphocyte type (Figure 11-28). Diagnosis of these lymphomas, which may comprise up to 20% of all canine lymphomas, is based on recognizing a monotonous or restricted population of small, rather normal-appearing lymphoid cells in the FNA. Mitoses are extremely rare. A recent retrospective study describing the clinical characteristics, histopathologic and immunohistochemical features of indolent lymphomas in the dog, reported that a T-zone, small cell subtype comprises 61.7% of the lymphomas in this group.[19] This form is very difficult to distinguish from hyperplasia, especially in cytologic preparations, because small lymphocytes predominate in each. In some cases, small cell lymphoma is not diagnosed until significant blood involvement occurs.

Alimentary lymphoma occasionally consists of neoplastic lymphocytes that contain magenta intracytoplasmic granules and is referred to as a *large granular lymphoma*. However, neither the granules nor lymphocytes are consistently large (Figure 11-29).

Several classification schemes have been adapted in an attempt to characterize canine and feline lymphomas.[16-22] The most recent iteration of the World Health Organization (WHO) system of lymphoma classification identifies these neoplasms as disease entities and not as cell types. A study testing the accuracy and consistency of veterinary pathologists in applying this system of classification to canine lymphomas was recently published.[23] Diagnostic criteria, including cellular morphology, cell lineage, and topography and general biology of the neoplasm, were used to define specific disease entities. A high degree of accuracy was achieved by veterinary pathologists in applying these criteria; however, only 6 lymphoma categories (diffuse large B-cell, marginal zone, peripheral T-cell, T-zone, T-cell-lymphoblastic, and follicular lymphomas) were included in the study (Figures 11-30, *A-E* and 11-31, *A-B*). Nevertheless, these entities represent about 80% of all canine lymphomas. A future publication will address the prognostic significance of each of these morphologic entities.

The ultimate goals for classification are to correlate the variety of cell subtypes and architectural features of lymphoma to clinical behavior in terms of responsiveness to therapy and outlook for the patient. For the dog, cytomorphologic classification into low (small cells and low mitotic rate) or high (large cells and high mitotic rate) grades of lymphoma has been shown to have prognostic importance.[24-25] Although low-grade lymphomas permit long survivals, they are virtually incurable and may not be treated initially. In contrast, the high-grade lymphomas initially respond well to chemotherapy, and disease remission is achieved; yet, if left untreated, they are rapidly progressive and deadly. A predominance of high-grade lymphomas is seen in dogs and cats. Within the high-grade lymphomas, lymphoblastic and Burkitt-type lymphomas in dogs have poorer prognoses.[24]

Immunohistochemistry of histologic preparations have been used to classify lymphomas. Approximately 70% to 80% of canine lymphomas are of B-cell origin. T-cell lymphomas in the dog that are high grade have a worse prognosis than B-cell lymphomas of the same grade.[24] Cytospin preparations from FNAs also have been used in immunophenotypic analysis of canine malignant lymphomas.[25] Assessment of the immunophenotype does not appear to be of prognostic significance in cats.[26] Other biomarkers such as vascular endothelial growth factor (VEGF) and metalloproteinase (MMP) 9, are promising adjuncts for staging and may be useful for monitoring the effectiveness of chemotherapy.[27] The application of flow cytometry for identifying cell clonality and blood and marrow involvement and for determining the amount of minimal residual disease have added to our abilities to classify and monitor lymphomas in dogs and cats.[28]

If a diagnosis is equivocal, the entire lymph node should be removed, keeping the capsule intact and fixed in 10% buffered formalin. A complete cross-section is then examined to determine if a homogeneous population of neoplastic cells has obliterated the normal nodal architecture. A confusing mixture of malignant and reactive elements may limit the accuracy of both the histologic and cytologic diagnoses of lymphoma. This may be attributed to partial nodal involvement and is intrinsic to some lymphomas such as Hodgkin's disease and T-cell rich B-cell lymphomas.[15,17] Ancillary techniques, including immunophenotypic assessment of smears and histologic sections, quantitative immunophenotyping using flow cytometry, and PCR to determine clonality and cell lineage, also may be used to confirm a diagnosis.[14,15,18] To exclude the possibility of a primary leukemia that has infiltrated the node, a complete blood count should always be performed concurrently as part of the routine workup.

Metastatic Neoplasia

The presence of cells not normally found in lymph nodes or an increase in numbers of certain cell types normally present (i.e., mast cells) may suggest metastatic neoplasia (Figure 11-32 to Figure 11-37). Carcinomas frequently metastasize to lymph nodes. Metastatic epithelial cells (see Figures 11-32 and 11-33) may occur singly or in groups. They are very large and bear no resemblance to cellular constituents of normal or hyperplastic nodes. Epithelial cells of any type in a lymph node aspirate indicate neoplasia, but these cells must be differentiated from epithelioid cells of granulomatous inflammation, as described previously. Salivary epithelial cells (Figure 11-34) from the submandibular salivary gland may be accidentally aspirated. These cells are uniform in size and have round to oval nuclei and abundant blue foamy cytoplasm and should not be confused with carcinoma cells.

Malignant melanomas metastasize to lymph nodes. The melanocyte usually is identified by its granular brown-black cytoplasmic pigment (see Figure 11-35). Pigment in melanocytes should not be confused with that in melanophages that have phagocytized melanin originating from pigmented structures or lesions in the area drained by the node. Melanophages also phagocytize pigment released by melanocytes. Differentiation may be difficult, but melanocytes usually have more attenuated and less vacuolated cytoplasm. Hemosiderin, carbon, bile, and other pigments in macrophages must not be confused with melanin.

Although sarcomas do not metastasize to lymph nodes as frequently as carcinomas do, spindle cells in significant numbers should suggest a sarcoma of some type. Malignant mast cell tumors can metastasize to lymph nodes (see Figure 11-36). The tumor cells may be well differentiated and distinguished from normal mast cells only by the large number of cells present. More than 3% mast cells should raise the suspicion of neoplasia. However, the presence of foci or nests of mast cells is more supportive of metastatic disease compared with mildly increased numbers of single cells. Undifferentiated mast cell tumors have larger cells with fewer, less prominent granules. The presence of matching internal tandem duplication of the c-kit gene may be a more sensitive method for confirming the presence of metastasis in the node.[29-30] Transmissible venereal tumors (see Figure 11-37) may metastasize to lymph nodes.

In cases of neoplasia, usually metastatic neoplastic cells are specifically looked for because the justification for lymph node aspiration was a malignant tumor identified in the area drained by the particular node. Tumor cells are usually obtained if metastasis has progressed to cause clinically evident enlarged nodes; however, small

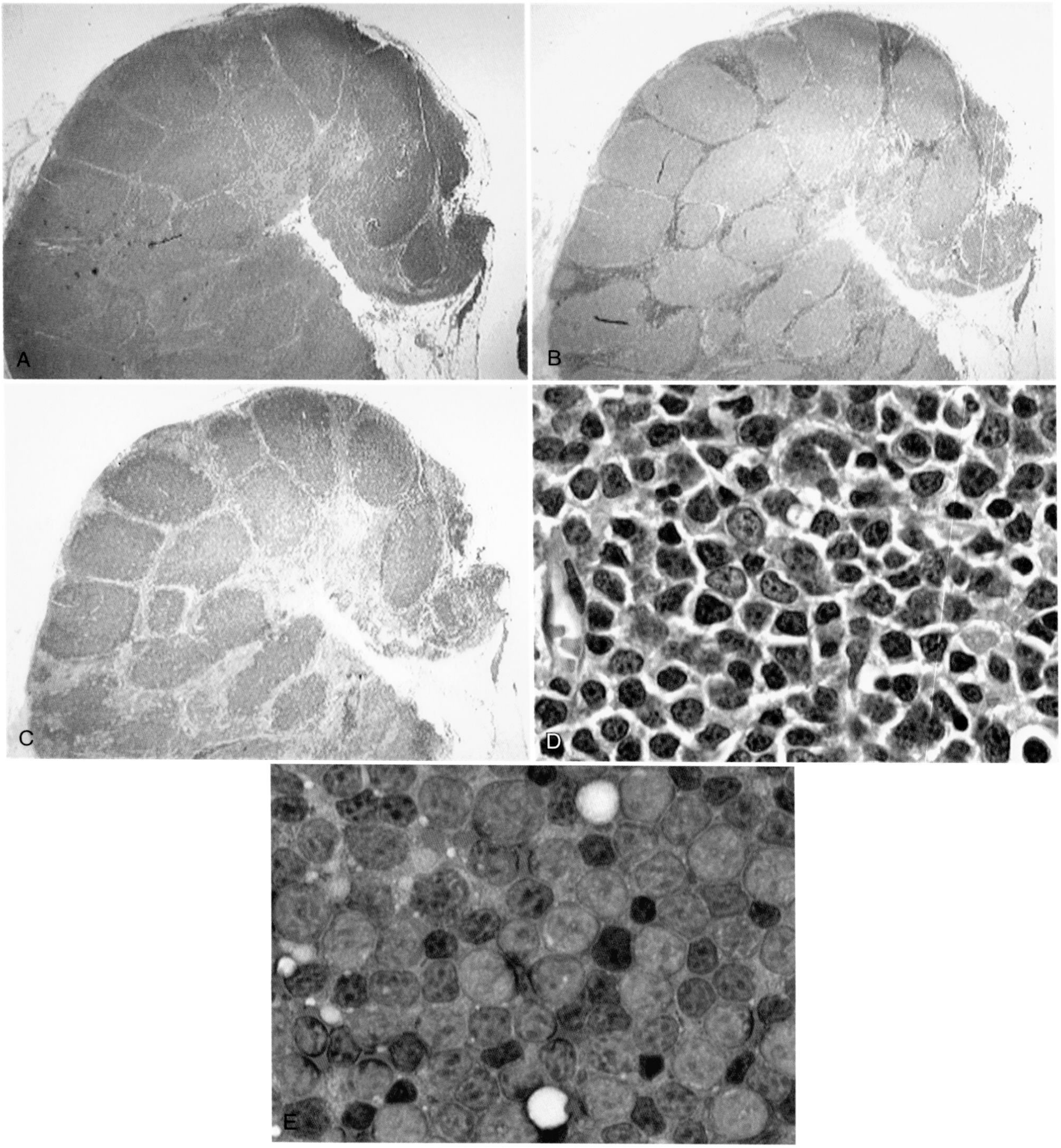

Figure 11-30 A to D, Canine lymph node, mixed intermediate (centrocytes) and large B-cell (centroblasts) follicular lymphoma. *Top left:* Histopathology mosaic photomicrograph. (H&E stain.) *Top right:* With CD3 staining, the interfollicular areas show residual paracortical T-cells. *Bottom left:* CD79a staining distinctly marks the proliferating B-cells with the interfollicular areas largely unlabeled. *Bottom right:* Cells in the follicular areas are intermediate to large in size with irregularly indented nuclei; nucleoli are multiple but often inconspicuous and sometimes impinge on the nuclear membrane. **E,** Wright-Giemsa–stained fine-needle aspiration cytology from same lymph node. Neoplastic B-lymphocytes showing variability in size and multiple, inconspicuous nucleoli. A few residual small lymphocytes are also seen.

CHAPTER 12

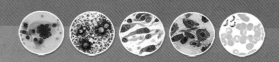

Synovial Fluid Analysis

Peter J. Fernandes

Synovium is essentially a living ultrafiltration membrane with fenestrated capillaries just below an intimal surface that contains wide intercellular gaps, but unlike true membranes, has no epithelial cells and no basement membrane. The fenestrated synovial capillaries, up to 50 times more permeable to water compared with continuous capillaries, allow water and small solutes into the subintima but exclude varied proportions of albumin and larger proteins such as fibrinogen and clotting factors.

As fluid enters and leaves the joint cavity, its diffusion and composition is regulated by connective tissue of the subintima and cells of the intima, or synovial lining. The intima is made-up mostly of secretory, fibroblast-related, synoviocytes (type B cell) and fewer macrophages (type A cell). The type B cells, which constitute 70% to 90% of intimal cells, secrete components for tissue interstitium and synovial fluid that include collagens, fibronectin, hyaluronan, and lubricin.[1,2] Type A are derived from bloodborne mononuclear cells and are considered resident tissue macrophages, much like hepatic Kupffer cells (Figure 12-1 and Figure 12-2). Type B cells and type A cells demonstrate immunohistochemical reactivity to heat shock protein 25 (HSP25) and CD18, respectively.[1]

ARTHROCENTESIS

In the verification, localization, diagnosis, and management of arthritis, synovial fluid examination is a key component of an initial medical database that includes clinical history, physical examination, radiographs, complete blood count, biochemical profile, and urinalysis. See Box 12-1 and Box 12-2 for indications and contraindications for arthrocentesis.

RESTRAINT

As temperament under physical immobilization and tolerance for discomfort of each individual is different, the clinician must judge which method of restraint is appropriate to allow for controlled manipulation and centesis of the joint. Complications of inadequate restraint may include damage to blood vessels, nerves, synovial membrane, and articular cartilage surfaces, along with blood contamination and retrieving a diagnostically insufficient volume of synovial fluid.

ASEPSIS

Routine aseptic technique should be followed. Normal joint spaces are sterile.

EQUIPMENT

Sterile disposable 3-milliliter (mL) syringes and 1-inch, 22-gauge or 25-gauge (for small dogs and cats), hypodermic needle are recommended. In large-breed dogs, sampling of the elbow or shoulder joints may require a 1½-inch needle and the hip joint may necessitate a 3-inch spinal needle. Microscope glass slides with frosted ends, red-top tubes, and ethylenetetraacetic acid (EDTA) blood tubes should be readied and labeled with the patient's name and the joint sampled. See Box 12-3 for a complete list of materials.

APPROACHES

In most cases, arthrocentesis is performed with the patient in lateral recumbency and the joint to be sampled uppermost. Palpation of the joint during manual flexion and extension helps identify the space to be entered. In all cases, the needle should be advanced gently toward and through the joint capsule to avoid damaging the articular cartilage. Once the needle is inside the joint space, the volume of fluid obtained depends on the particular joint and the disorder. Ordinarily, some synovial fluid is readily collected from the stifle joint, but it is most difficult to obtain from the carpal and tarsal joints. Obviously, when joint spaces are swollen, fluid is more easily aspirated. The plunger of the syringe should be released before the needle is removed from the joint space. This minimizes blood contamination of the sample as the needle is withdrawn.

Carpal Joint

Entry is obtained via the antebrachiocarpal joint or the middle carpal joint. In either case, the carpus is flexed to increase access to the joint's spaces. The needle is introduced from the dorsal aspect, just medial of center,

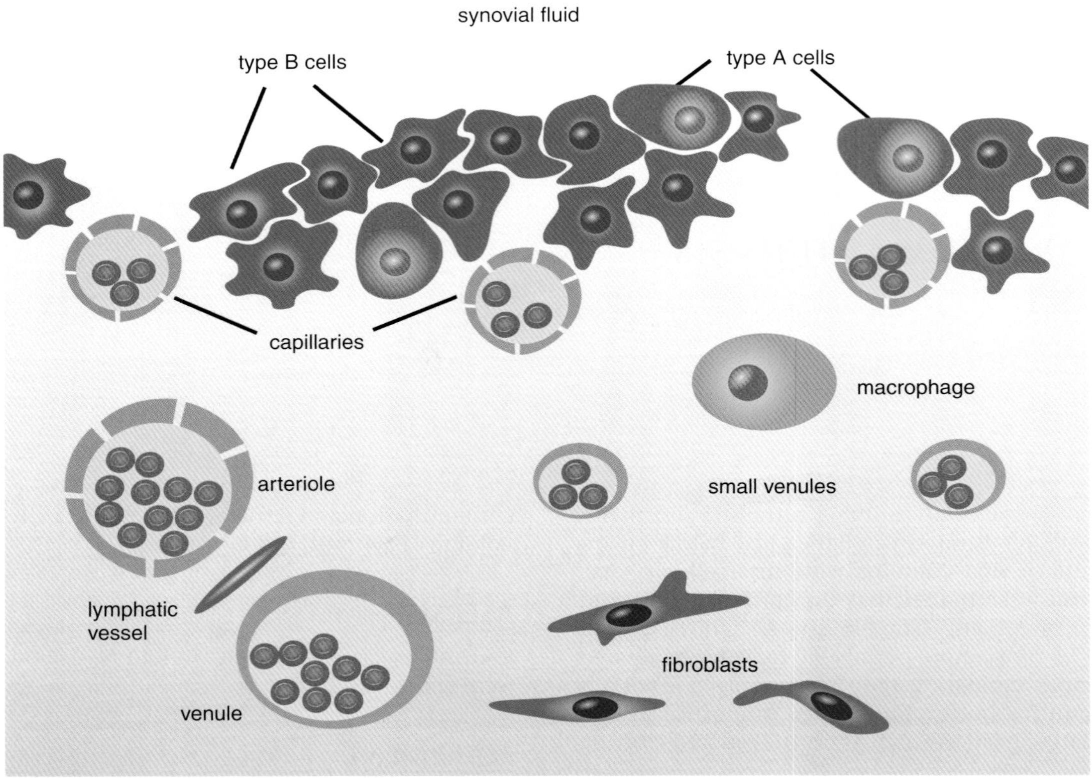

Figure 12-1 Schematic representation of normal synovium.

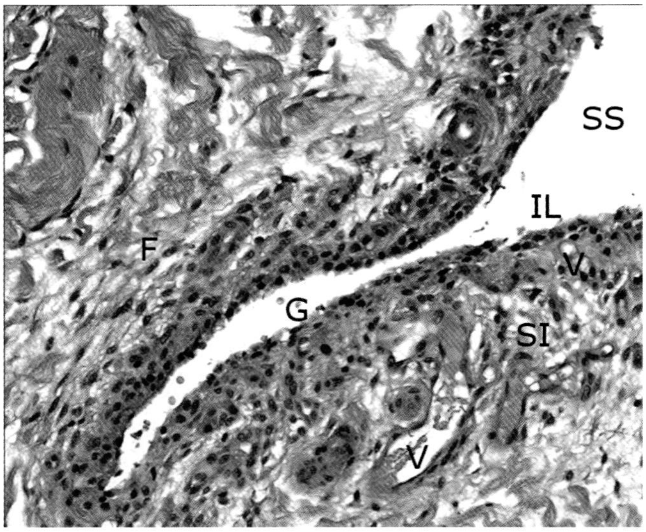

Figure 12-2 Histologic specimen of synovial membrane showing details within the valley of a normal fold in the lining. Directly interfacing with the synovial space (*SS*) is a sparse intimal layer (*IL*), only one to two cells thick, with underlying vessels (*V*) embedded among fibrous subintima (*SI*). Note the normal acellular gap in the intimal lining (*G*) and fibrocytes (*F*) within the subintima. (H&E stain. original magnification 20×.) (Courtesy of Dr. Dave Getzy.)

then inserted perpendicular to the joint. Landmarks for the antebrachiocarpal joint are the distal radius and the proximal radial carpal bone (Figure 12-3). The middle carpal joint is between the distal portion of the radial carpal bone and the second and third carpal bones.

BOX 12-1

Indications for Arthrocentesis

- Fever of unknown origin
- Unexplained lameness
- Generalized pain
- Joint swelling or effusion
- Weakness
- Acute monoarthropathy
- Abnormal limb function or gait
- Shifting leg lameness or polyarthropathy

BOX 12-2

Contraindications for Arthrocentesis

Absolute: Cellulitis or dermatitis over arthrocentesis site
Relative: Bacteremia or severe coagulopathy

Elbow Joint

Entry to the elbow may be attained with the joint in extension or flexion. Hyperextension of the elbow allows the needle to be introduced medial to the lateral epicondyle of the humerus and lateral to the olecranon. Once in the joint space the needle is guided cranially toward the humeral condyle (Figure 12-4). With the elbow in a 90-degree angle of flexion, the needle can be introduced just proximal to the olecranon and medial to the lateral

BOX 12-3

Materials for Arthrocentesis

- 1-inch, 25-gauge needles (small dogs and cats)
- ½-inch, 22-gauge needles (large to medium dogs)
- 3-mL syringes
- 3-mL ethylenetetraacetic acid blood tubes (lavender top)
- 3-mL no additive blood tubes (red top)
- 20-mL blood culture bottle (for 1 to 3 mL of fluid)
- Glass slides
- Clippers
- Sterile gloves
- Sterile scrub solution and alcohol

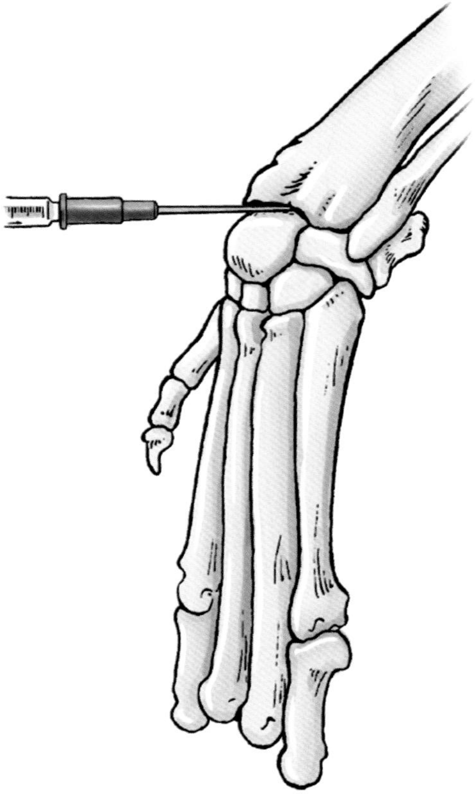

Figure 12-3 Arthrocentesis of the carpus joint. The joint may be located by applying fingertip pressure just distal to the radius during flexion and extension. The needle is introduced between the distal radius and proximal to the radial carpal bone. (From Piermattei DL, Flo G, DeCamp C: Chapter 1 - Orthopedic Examination and Diagnostic Tools. In: *Brinker, Piermattei, and Flo's Handbook of small animal orthopedics and fracture repair*, ed 4, St. Louis, MO, 2006, Saunders [p. 24].)

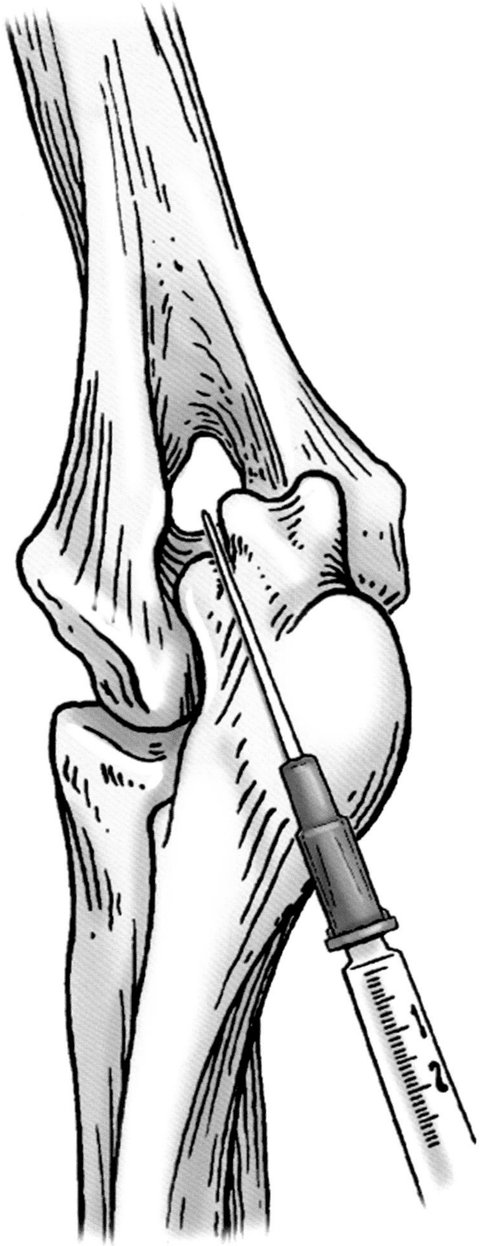

Figure 12-4 Arthrocentesis of the elbow joint. With the elbow in hyperextension, the needle is introduced medial to the lateral epicondyle of the humerus and lateral to the olecranon. (From Piermattei DL, Flo G, DeCamp C: Chapter 1 - Orthopedic Examination and Diagnostic Tools. In: *Brinker, Piermattei, and Flo's Handbook of small animal orthopedics and fracture repair*, ed 4, St. Louis, MO, 2006, Saunders [p. 23].)

epicondylar crest. The needle will be inserted parallel to the olecranon and the long axis of the ulna.

Shoulder Joint

Access is gained from the lateral aspect, with the needle introduced distal to the acromion of the scapula and caudal to the greater tubercle of the humerus. The needle is directed medially toward the greater tubercle and distal to the supraglenoid tubercle of the scapula (Figure 12-5).

Tarsal Joint

Access is gained via a cranial or caudal approach. In the cranial approach, the tarsus is slightly flexed, and the needle is introduced at the space palpated between the tibia and talus (tibiotarsal) bones, just lateral to the tendon bundle. For the caudal approach, the joint is extended and the needle can be inserted medial or lateral to the calcaneus (fibular tarsal bone) with a cranial and slightly plantar path (Figure 12-6).

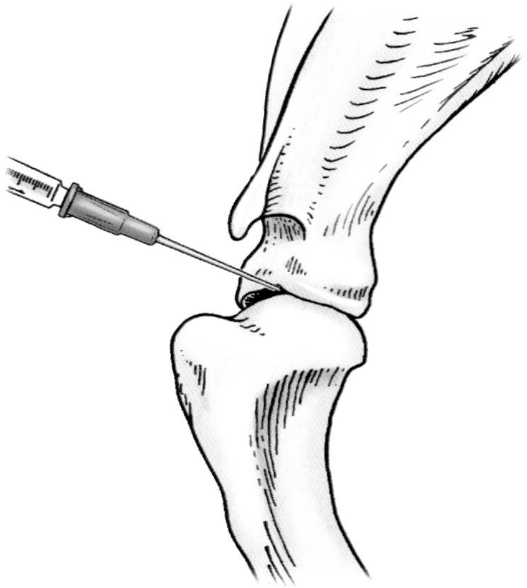

Figure 12-5 Arthrocentesis of the shoulder joint. The needle is introduced distal to the acromion of the scapula and caudal to the greater tubercle of the humerus and then directed medially towards the greater tubercle and just distal to the supraglenoid tubercle of the scapula. (From Piermattei DL, Flo G, DeCamp C: Chapter 1 - Orthopedic Examination and Diagnostic Tools. In: *Brinker, Piermattei, and Flo's Handbook of small animal orthopedics and fracture repair*, ed 4, St. Louis, MO, 2006, Saunders [p. 23].)

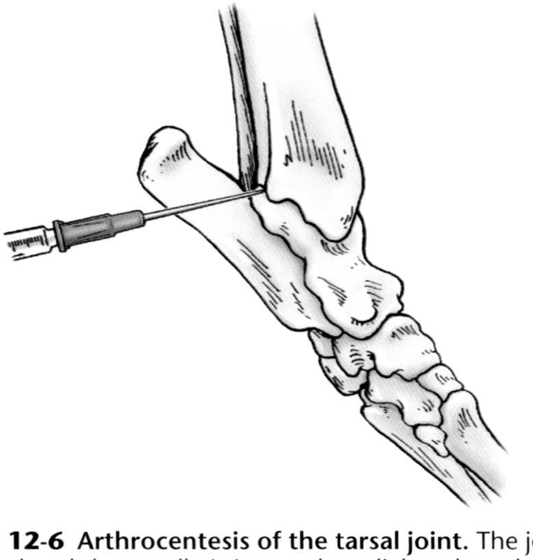

Figure 12-6 Arthrocentesis of the tarsal joint. The joint is extended and the needle is inserted medial to the calcaneus in a cranial path. (From Piermattei DL, Flo G, DeCamp C: Chapter 1 - Orthopedic Examination and Diagnostic Tools. In: *Brinker, Piermattei, and Flo's Handbook of small animal orthopedics and fracture repair*, ed 4, St. Louis, MO, 2006, Saunders [p. 22].)

Stifle Joint

The stifle is flexed, and the needle is introduced just lateral to the patellar ligament and distal to the patella. The needle is advanced in a medial and proximal direction pointing toward the medial condyle of the femur (Figure 12-7).

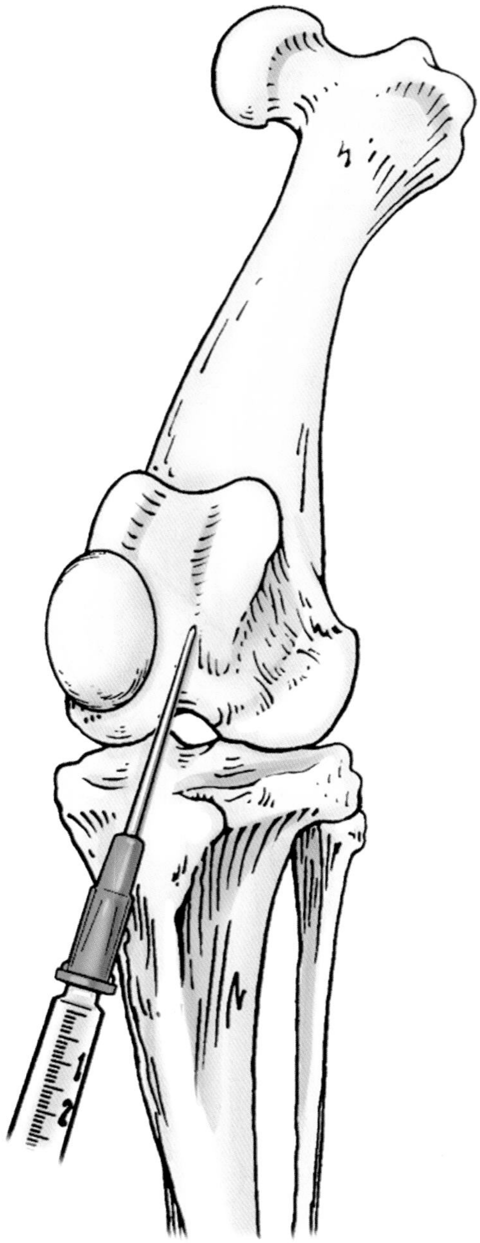

Figure 12-7 Arthrocentesis of the stifle joint. The stifle is flexed and the needle introduced lateral to the patellar ligament and distal to the patella and advanced in a medial and proximal direction toward the medial condyle of the femur. (From Piermattei DL, Flo G, DeCamp C: Chapter 1 - Orthopedic Examination and Diagnostic Tools. In: *Brinker, Piermattei, and Flo's Handbook of small animal orthopedics and fracture repair*, ed 4, St. Louis, MO, 2006, Saunders [p. 22].)

Hip Joint

The femur is abducted and the leg extended caudally. The needle is introduced cranial to the greater trochanter of the femur and inserted caudal and distal or ventral toward the joint (Figure 12-8).

SAMPLE HANDLING AND TEST PRIORITIES

Laboratory tests performed may be limited by volume of synovial fluid collected. While the sample is in the

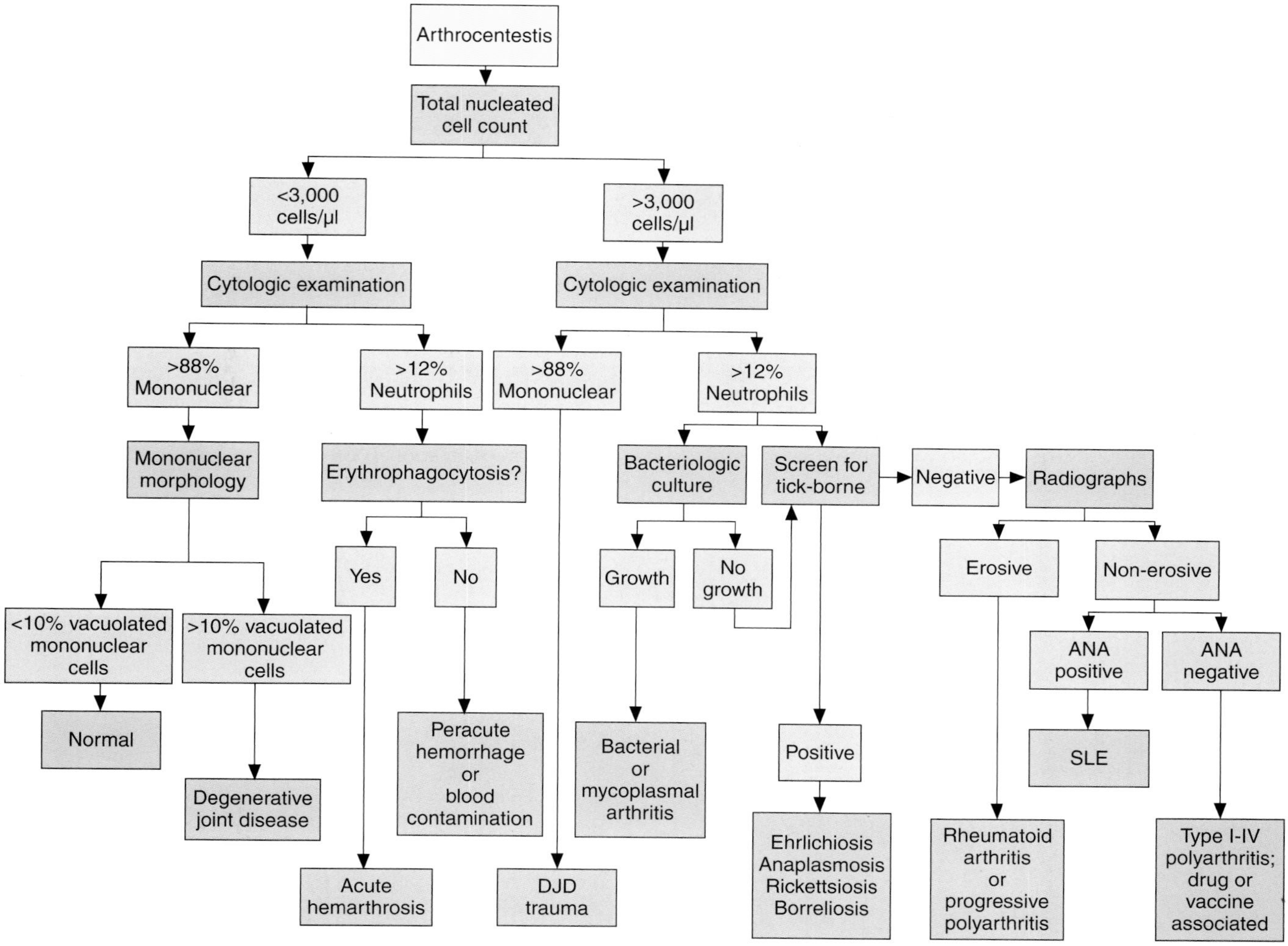

Figure 12-15 Diagnostic plan for cytologic evaluation of canine synovial fluid. *ANA*, antinuclear antibodies; *DJD*, degenerative joint disease; *SLE*, systemic lupus erythematosus.

TABLE 12-5

CHARACTERISTICS OF SYNOVIAL FLUID RESPONSES TO ARTICULAR INJURY

					NUCLEATED CELL DENSITY		
Category	Color	Turbidity	Viscosity	Mucin Clot	Total	Differential	Causes
Acute hemarthrosis	Red	Increased proportional to amount of blood	Mild to marked decrease	Fair to poor	Increased proportional to amount of blood	Differential may be similar to peripheral blood with platelets	Coagulopathies, like factor deficiency; severe blunt force trauma
Degenerative arthropathy	Normal	Usually normal	Normal to mildly decreased	Fair to poor	Likely increased	Mo: Normal to increased with vacuolation and phagocytic activity PMN: Increased	Osteoarthrosis or degenerative joint diseases; trauma; neoplasia
Inflammatory arthropathy	Yellow to off-white or red-brown	Increased in relation to the amount of inflammation and hemorrhage	Mildly to markedly decreased	Fair to very poor	Increased	Mo: normal to increased PMN: Increased	Infection; immune-mediated arthropathies

Mo, large mononuclear cells; *PMN*, neutrophils.

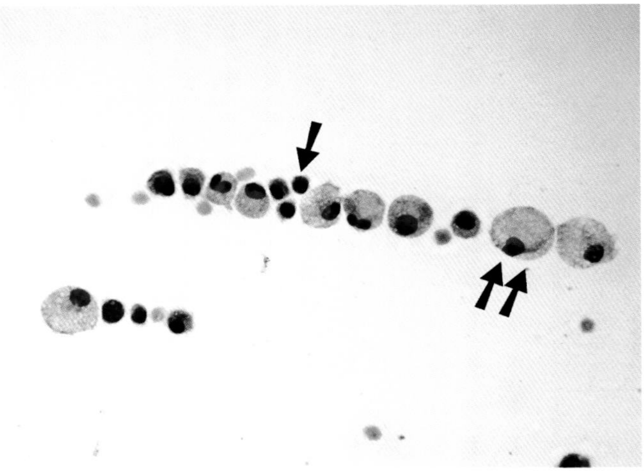

Figure 12-16 Synovial fluid from a dog with degenerative arthropathy, showing large mononuclear cells (*double arrow*) or macrophage-type cells mingled with lymphocytes (*arrow*). (Wright stain. Original magnification 500×.)

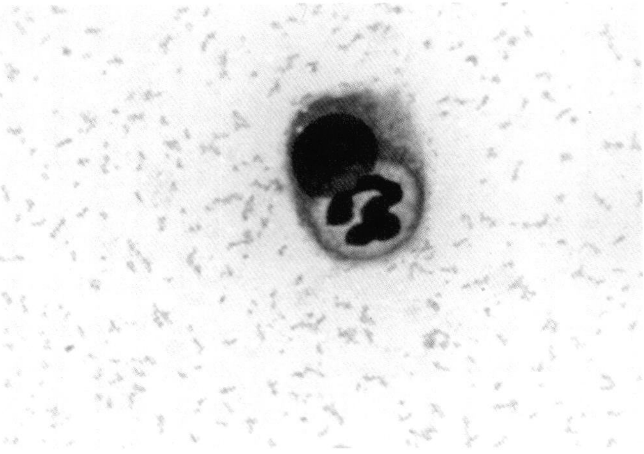

Figure 12-17 Synovial fluid from a dog with degenerative arthropathy. Note the leukophagocytic macrophage, indicating ongoing inflammation. (Wright-Giemsa stain. Original magnification 1000×.)

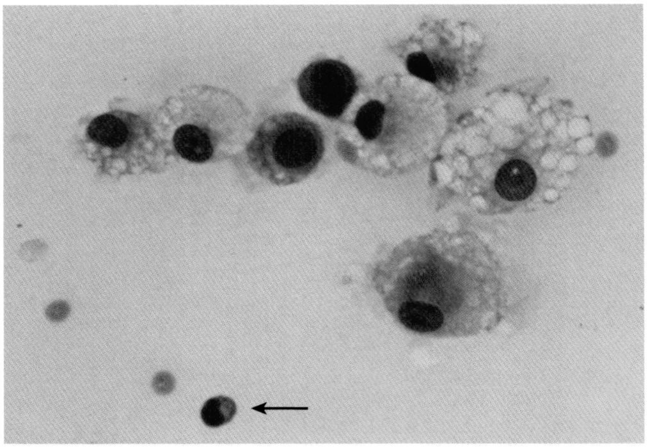

Figure 12-18 Synovial fluid from the stifle joint of a dog with a partially ruptured cranial cruciate ligament. The majority of nucleated cells are large mononuclear, among which most show a moderate to marked density of variable sized, colorless, clear, cytoplasmic vacuoles. A single lymphocyte is present (*arrow*). (Wright-Giemsa stain. Original magnification 500×.)

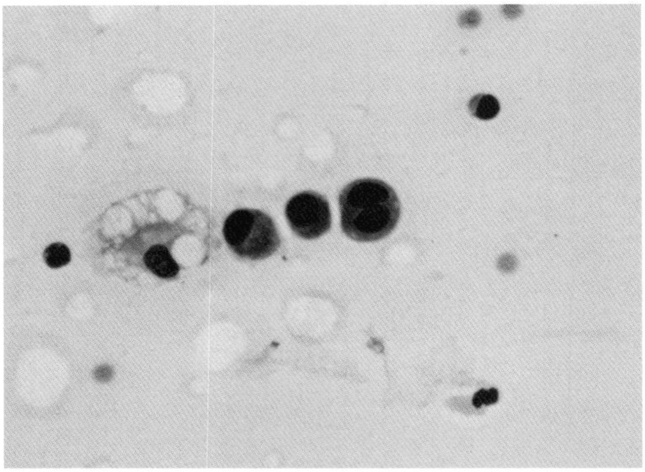

Figure 12-19 Synovial fluid from the stifle joint of a dog with a partially ruptured cranial cruciate ligament. The array of large mononuclear cells includes a binucleate form that is suggestive of hyperplasia of the intimal cell lining. (Wright-Giemsa stain. Original magnification 500×.)

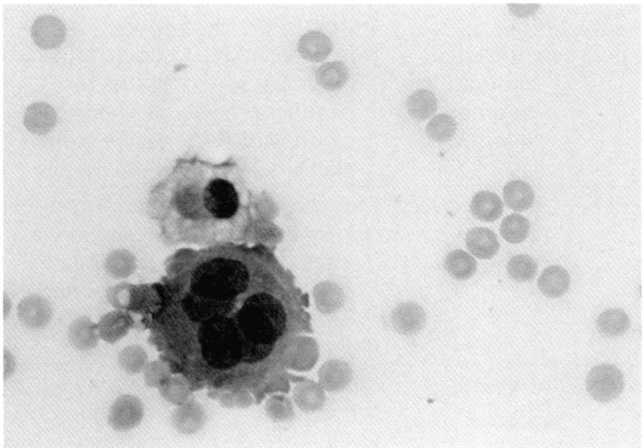

Figure 12-20 Synovial fluid from a dog with degenerative arthropathy. Note the multinucleate large mononuclear cell, an osteoclast, that indicates articular cartilage erosion to subchondral bone. (Wright-Giemsa stain. Original magnification 500×.)

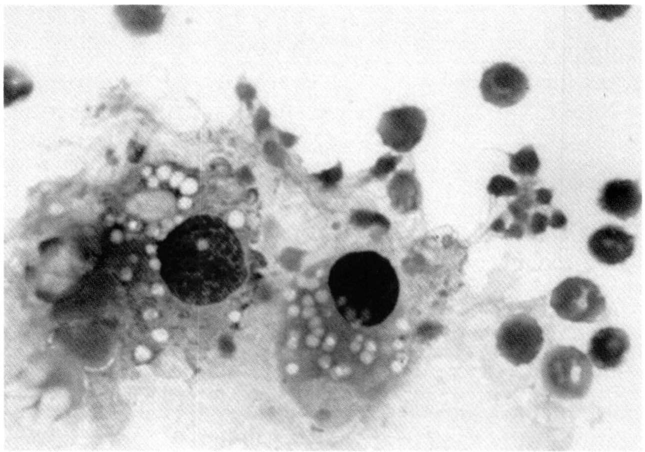

Figure 12-21 Direct smear of synovial fluid from a dog. Note the platelet clump, indicating recent hemorrhage. The large mononuclear cell, on the far left, is not intact and the erythrocytes along its edge are not convincing evidence of erythrophagocytosis. In this case, hemorrhage was caused by iatrogenic contamination. (Wright-Giemsa stain. Original magnification 1000×.)

sarcoma, chondrosarcoma, osteosarcoma, fibrosarcoma, metastatic bronchial carcinoma, and lymphoma.[2, 25-27] Diagnosis is made by obtaining a biopsy of the lesion for histopathologic examination. Cytologic examination of such biopsies is described in other chapters throughout this textbook. Synovial fluid changes are poorly described, but conceivably, characteristics of a degenerative or inflammatory arthropathy could be present. Neoplastic cells are infrequently evident in these fluids (Figure 12-23).

INFLAMMATORY ARTHROPATHIES

Inflammatory arthropathies are either infectious or noninfectious and immune mediated (see Box 12-4) and associated with an exudate showing increased neutrophil numbers and variable increases in the number of large mononuclear cells, which may be vacuolated or have engulfed debris. Concurrent and often mild hemorrhagic diapedesis is common. Other findings are listed in Table 12-5.

Fundamentally, the greater the inflammatory reaction, the more discolored and turbid is the fluid, and the poorer is the viscosity. Mucin clot test results often parallel sample viscosity. The total protein concentration is increased, and the sample may readily clot. Fibrin strands often cause clumping of inflammatory cells in the smear. If not apparent on a routinely stained smear, fibrin strands may be demonstrated by staining with new methylene blue (Figure 12-24, Figure 12-25, and Figure 12-26).

Infectious Arthritides

Infectious arthritis is an inflammatory arthropathy, in which the causative infectious agent might be cultured or isolated from synovial membrane or joint fluid. This is not to be confused with infectious diseases remote from the joint that cause arthritis via a hypersensitivity disorder. Although infectious arthritides are uncommon among dogs and cats, bacteria are the most frequently isolated cause, with far fewer cases attributed

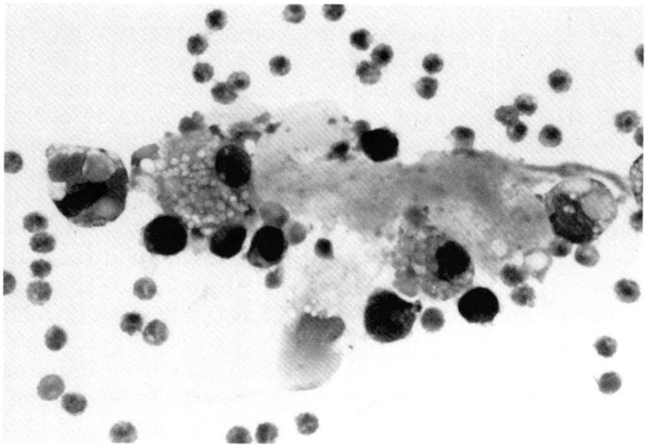

Figure 12-22 Synovial fluid from a dog with degenerative arthropathy. Note the erythrophagocytic macrophage, on the far left, that indicates concurrent hemorrhage and in spite of the large platelet clump this is not iatrogenic contamination. (Wright-Giemsa stain. Original magnification 500×.)

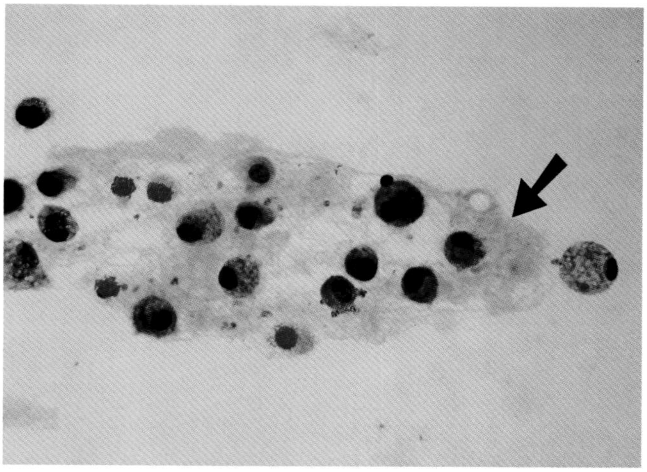

Figure 12-24 Synovial fluid from a dog with degenerative arthropathy. Note the large clump of fibrin with enmeshed cells (*arrow*). This is more often seen in inflammatory arthropathies. (Wright stain. Original magnification, 500×.)

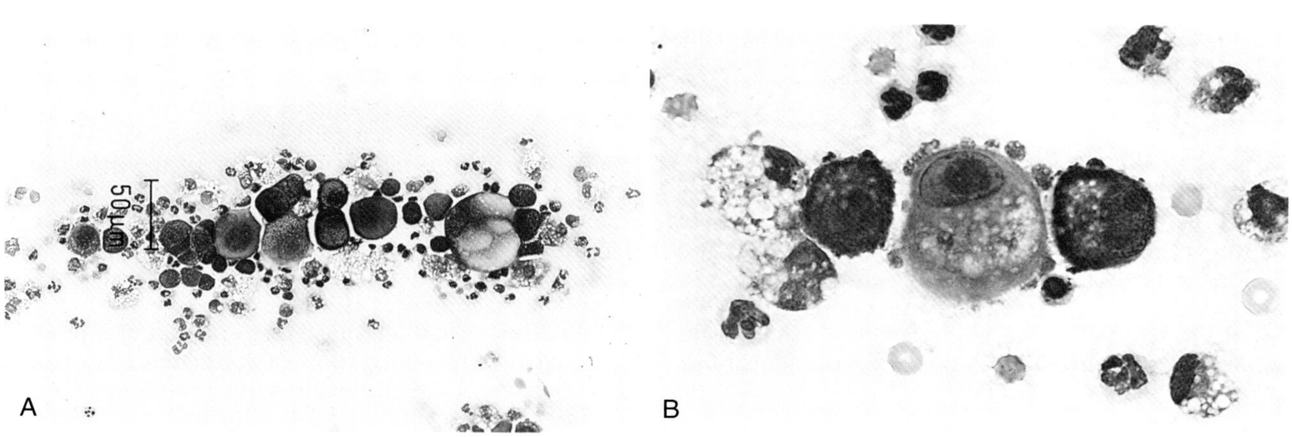

Figure 12-23 Synovial fluid from a dog with a metastatic bronchiolar-alveolar carcinoma. A, Low-magnification view showing a mixture of cells that includes metastatic carcinoma cells with many criteria of malignancy, including large prominent nucleoli. (Wright stain. Original magnification 100×.) **B,** Higher magnification showing metastatic carcinoma cells. (Wright stain. Original magnification 250×.)

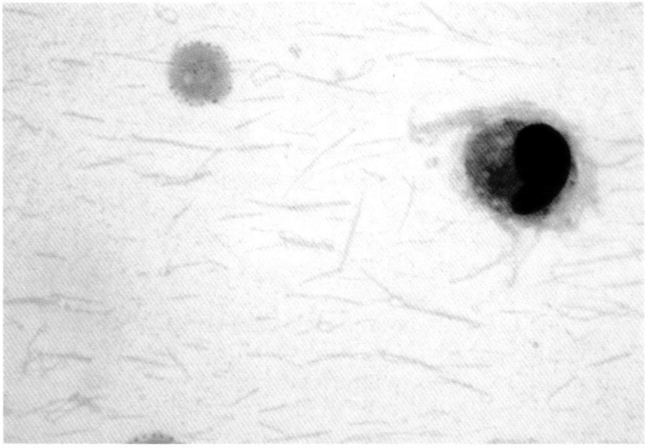

Figure 12-25 Synovial fluid from a dog with degenerative arthropathy. The background contains numerous individualized strands of fibrin and is clumped around the right most edge of the large mononuclear cell. This is not to be mistaken for an infectious agent (Wright stain. Original magnification, 1000×.)

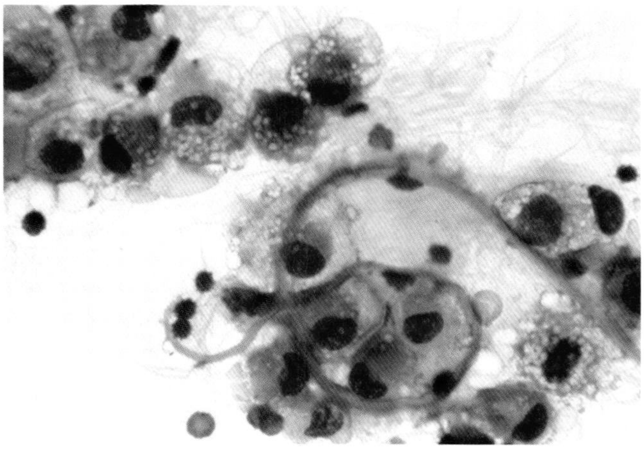

Figure 12-26 Synovial fluid from the stifle joint of a dog with a partially ruptured cranial cruciate ligament. The large mononuclear cells and thin band of pink-staining collagen are trapped by a clump of fibrin, which is noted in the upper right corner. (Wright-Giemsa stain. Original magnification 500×.)

to rickettsiae, spirochetes, mycoplasma, fungus, virus, and protozoa. Clinical presentation and history may be quite helpful because most infectious arthritides of a mature animal are monoarticular, acute in onset, and often the result of a percutaneous penetrating or surgical wound. When polyarticular infectious arthritides do occur, they are likely of hematogenous origin, as in omphalophlebitis in neonates or bacterial endocarditis in mature animals.

Bacterial Arthritides

Bacterial infectious arthritides demonstrate a markedly increased total nucleated cell count, usually greater than 50,000 cells/μL, with a predominance of neutrophils that are often greater than 75% of all nucleated cells.[28] Neutrophils are often intact and inconsistently show karyolysis or pyknosis and karyorrhexis (Figure 12-27). Karyolytic degeneration of cells suggests a septic process; however, in many infected joints, degenerative leukocyte changes or microorganisms are not observed. When clinical observations and intuition dictate, joint fluid should be reflexively cultured. Organisms commonly cultured from dogs with an infected joint include *S. intermedius*, *S. aureus*, or β-hemolytic *Streptococcus* spp.[29] Among cats with bacterial arthritis, hemolytic strains of *Escherichia coli* or *Pasteurella multocida* are most common.[30] Failure to isolate organisms on culture does not necessarily exclude a bacterial cause. The absence of bacteria on cytologic specimens may represent prior antibiotic therapy or an exuberant inflammatory response. Caution is warranted when attributing favorable clinical response to empiric antibiotic therapy with tetracyclines (e.g., doxycycline) because some of these drugs have immune modulatory, antiinflammatory, and chondroprotective properties.[31,32]

Rickettsial Arthritides

Granulocytic morulae have been observed in joint fluid of dogs infected with *Ehrlichia ewingii*.[33] Polymerase chain reaction (PCR) amplification of *E. ewingii* deoxyribonucleic acid (DNA) was used to differentiate it from infection with *Anaplasma phagocytophila*, formerly called *E. equi*. Patients presented with fever, lameness, thrombocytopenia, and, on occasion, central nervous system signs (i.e., proprioceptive deficits, neck pain, paraparesis, or ataxia). Neutrophilic polyarthritis was diagnosed in dogs with lameness and joint fluid contained a total nucleated cell count ranging from 16,000 to 125,000 cells/μL, of which neutrophils made up 63% to 99%. As with other rickettsial infections, polyarthritis is likely caused by immune complex–mediated disease or hemarthrosis.[34] Reports suggest that granulocytic morulae might be observed in 1% to 7% of neutrophils in synovial fluid and 0.1% to 26% of neutrophils in peripheral blood (Figure 12-28).[35,36] Tentative identification of granulocytic morulae as *A. phagocytophila* may be based on geographic distribution because the tick vectors for this organism are found in western United States and Canada and upper midwestern and northeastern United States.[37]

Spirochetal Arthritides

Arthritis is the most common clinical sign in dogs with Lyme disease, which is caused by the spirochete *Borrelia burgdorferi*. Joints closest to the site of the infecting tick bite are often involved in the first episodes of lameness and demonstrate the most extreme synovial fluid abnormalities. Although not observed on routine microscopy, live spirochetes are most frequently cultured from synovial membranes closest to the bite site.[38] Chronic oligoarthritis can be transient to persistent and may be caused by wider migration of spirochetes or antibody-mediated and T-lymphocyte–driven responses.[39] Because acute Lyme arthritis presents with monoarthritis or oligoarthritis, synovial fluid changes may be varied from joint to joint within the same dog. Joints of limbs that demonstrate lameness may have total nucleated cell counts that range between 1,400 and 76,200 cells/μL (median 12,700 cells/μL), with neutrophils composing

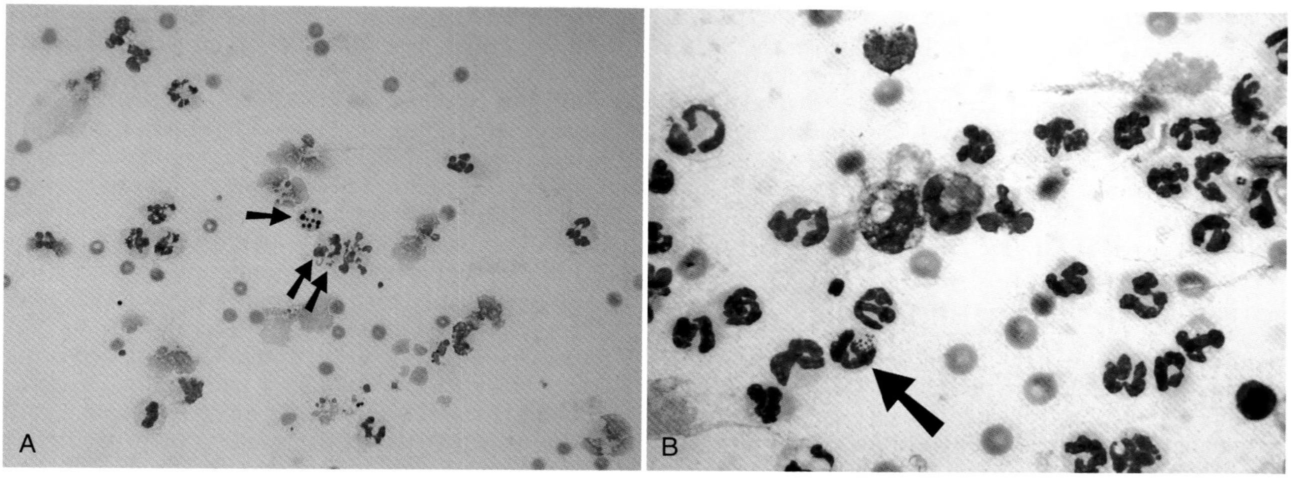

Figure 12-27 Synovial fluid from a dog with septic suppurative (neutrophilic) arthritis. A, Note nucleated cell with pyknotic nuclear material (*arrow*) and neutrophil with engulfed bacteria (*double arrow*). Background contains other neutrophils with hydropic degeneration (degenerative neutrophils) along with nuclear debris and erythrocytes (Wright stain. Original magnification 500×.) **B,** Note neutrophil with engulfed bacteria (*arrow*). (Wright stain. Original magnification 1000×.)

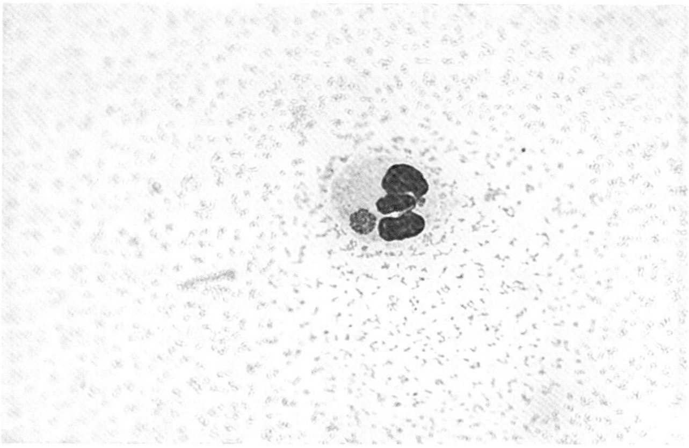

Figure 12-28 Synovial fluid from a dog with ehrlichial polyarthritis. Note the *Ehrlichia morula* in the neutrophil and the normal granular, eosinophilic proteinaceous background. (Wright stain. Original magnification 1250×.)

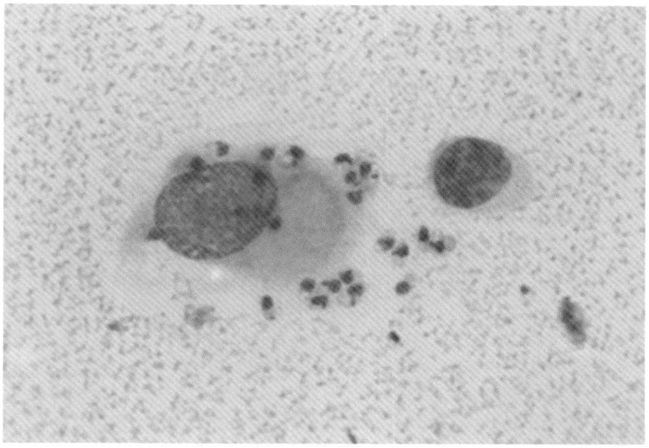

Figure 12-29 Synovial fluid specimen showing *Leishmania* spp. amastigotes engulfed by a macrophage and free in the background. (Wright stain. Original magnification 1000×.)

up to 97% of all nucleated cells (median 54%). In the same dog with monoarthritis or oligoarthritis, other joints may be quite dissimilar, with total nucleated cell counts ranging between 100 and 3,300 cells/μL (median 710 cells/μL) and sometimes include up to 19% neutrophils (median 0%). Dogs without lameness that are culture positive and seropositive for *B. burgdorferi* typically have total nucleated cell counts ranging between 100 and 3,000 cells/μL (median 600 cells/μL) but do not contain more that 15% neutrophils (median 0%).[38]

Fungal Arthritides

Fungal arthritides are uncommon but have been reported as a sequela of osteomyelitis or disseminated infection by *Blastomyces dermatitidis*, *Cryptococcus neoformans*, *Aspergillus* spp., *Coccidioides immitis*, *Histoplasma capsulatum*, and *Sporothrix schenckii*.[40,41] On occasion, fungal elements might be visible in synovial fluid.

Mycoplasmal Arithritides

Mycoplasmal arthritis has been diagnosed as a few rare cases in dogs and cats. The inflammatory reaction is neutrophilic with good cell morphology. Organisms may be observed on Romanowsky-stained smears or on mycoplasmal culture. Erosive polyarthritis of young Greyhounds has been associated with *Mycoplasma spumans*.[42] *Mycoplasma gateae* and *M. felis* have been isolated from synovial fluid of immuncompromised cats with polyarthritis.[30,43]

Protozoal Arthritides

Polyarthritis has been documented with canine visceral leishmaniasis that is caused by geographic variants of the *Leishmania donovani* complex, *L. donovani*, or *L. infantum*. Synovial fluid sometimes shows mononuclear inflammation and *Leishmania* spp. amastigotes in synovial fluid macrophages (Figure 12-29).[44,45]

Viral Arthritides

Feline calicivirus infection has been associated with lameness in kittens.[46] However, synovial fluid changes in experimental infections were minimal, with synovial fluid macrophage numbers subjectively increased to a moderate degree, and some leukophagocytosis exhibited.[47] Occasionally, cellularity may be markedly increased, but a predominance of macrophages with many exhibiting leukophagocytosis will still be present.[48]

IMMUNE-MEDIATED ARTHROPATHIES

Immune-mediated arthritides of dogs and cats are generally considered to be a type III hypersensitivity phenomenon.[49,50] Emerging evidence suggests concurrent cell-mediated or genetic mechanisms.[51,52] Arthritis is caused by immune complexes that are composed of circulating antigen and immunoglobulin G (IgG) or IgM antibodies. Much like renal glomeruli, synovial capillaries ultrafilter plasma, and as a result, immune complexes commonly deposit at these locations. Deposited immune complexes activate inflammatory cells to secrete cytokines that increase vascular permeability, augmenting immune complex deposition and further accelerating tissue and vessel damage via complement and Fc (Fragment, crystallizable) receptor–mediated pathways. Clinicopathologic features of immune-mediated arthritides are a reflection of immune complex predisposition for certain sites and are not determined by the primary source of the antigen. Because antibodies involved in immune-mediated arthropathies are not usually against fixed cell or tissue antigen, these immune complex–mediated diseases tend to have a systemic component, affecting multiple joints either concurrently or consecutively. Signals of systemic disease in patients with immune-mediated arthritis include fever, generalized stiffness, peripheral blood cytopenias, difficult to localize pain, neck or back pain, lymphadenopathy, or proteinuria.[53] Polyarthritis, associated with systemic immune-complex disease, is sometimes subclinical, and a patient may not demonstrate joint swelling or pain; therefore, four or more joints should be sampled with sufficient volume for complete fluid analysis.[41,54] See Box 12-5 and Box 12-6 for summaries of diagnostic features.

NONEROSIVE ARTHROPATHIES

Idiopathic (Type I) Polyarthritis

Idiopathic, or immune-mediated, polyarthritis is diagnosed by exclusion of other possible causes or specific

BOX 12-5

Diagnostic Features of Nonerosive, Immune-Mediated Arthritides

Idiopathic Polyarthritides for Which Other Causes of Inflammatory Arthropathy Have Been Ruled Out

- Type I – no evidence of types II, III, or IV
- Type II – Concurrent inflammatory process distant from joint (i.e., respiratory, urogenital, or integumentary systems)
- Type III – Associated with gastroenteritis of various causes or hepatopathy
- Type IV – Polyarthritis associated with malignancy remote from joint

Drug-Associated Reaction

- Arthritis develops in association with drug administration
- Previous exposure or long-term therapy
- Most commonly antibiotics such as potentiated sulfonamides, penicillins, and cephalosporins
- Signs resolve within 7 days of discontinuation

Vaccine Reaction

- 5 to 7 days after first dose of primary immunization
- Self-limiting, lasting 1 to 3 days
- Noted with feline calicivirus and canine polyvalent modified live virus vaccines

Polyarthritis-Meningitis Syndrome

- Concurrent signs of polyarthritis and neck pain
- Cerebrospinal fluid pleocytosis
- Reported with Bernese Mountain Dog, Boxer, Corgi, German Shorthair Pointer, Newfoundland, or Weimaraner
- Negative antinuclear antibody test

Polyarthritis-Polymyositis Syndrome

- Exercise intolerance and stiffness
- Myositis diagnosed in at least two muscle biopsies

Systemic Lupus Erythematosus

- Positive antinuclear antibody test
- Diagnosis of multisystemic immune-mediated disease (three of the following, serially or concurrently):
  - Polyarthritis
  - Mucosal or cutaneous lesions
  - Anemia, leukopenia, or thrombocytopenia
  - Glomerulonephritis or persistent proteinuria
  - Polymyositis
  - Serositis

Lymphoplasmacytic Gonitis

- Linked to subset of dogs with cranial cruciate ligament rupture

Juvenile-Onset Polyarthritis of Akitas

- Clinical signs before 8 months of age, most before 1-year-old
- Neutrophilic arthritis noted with:
  - Cyclic pain
  - Generalized lymphadenopathy
  - Nonregenerative anemia
  - Rarely concurrent meningitis

Synovitis-Amyloidosis of Shar-Peis

- Swollen joints with recurrent fever
- Glomerular disease from amyloidosis (proteinuria)

54. Center SA: Fluid accumulation disorders. In Willard MD, Tvedten H, Turnwald GH, editors: *Small animal clinical diagnosis by laboratory methods*, ed 4, St. Louis, MO, 2004, Saunders, pp 263–266.
55. Clements DN, Gear RN, Tattersall J, et al: Type I immune-mediated polyarthritis in dogs: 39 cases (1997-2002), *J Am Vet Med Assoc* 224(8):1323–1327, 2004.
56. Rondeau MP, Walton RM, Bissett S, et al: Suppurative, nonseptic polyarthropathy in dogs, *J Vet Intern Med* 19(5):654–662, 2005.
57. Sibilia J, Limbach FX: Reactive arthritis or chronic infectious arthritis? *Ann Rheum Dis* 61(7):580–587, 2002.
58. MacDonald KA, Chomel BB, Kittleson MD, et al: A prospective study of canine infective endocarditis in northern California (1999-2001): emergence of *Bartonella* as a prevalent etiologic agent, *J Vet Intern Med* 18(1):56–64, 2004.
59. Goodman RA, Breitschwerdt EB: Clinicopathologic findings in dogs seroreactive to *Bartonella henselae* antigens, *Am J Vet Res* 66(12):2060–2064, 2005.
60. Summers BA, Straubinger AF, Jacobson RH, et al: Histopathological studies of experimental Lyme disease in the dog, *J Comp Pathol* 133(1):1–13, 2005.
61. Greene CE, Breitschwerdt EB: Rocky Mountain spotted fever, murine typhuslike disease, rickettsial pox, typhus, and Q fever. In Greene CE, editor: *Infectious diseases of the dog and cat*, ed 3, St. Louis, MO, 2006, Saunders, pp 232–245.
62. Breitschwerdt EB: Obligate Intracellular bacterial pathogens. In Ettinger SJ, Feldman EC, editors: *Textbook of veterinary internal medicine*, St. Louis, MO, 2005, Saunders, pp 631–636.
63. Tarello W: Microscopic and clinical evidence for *Anaplasma (Ehrlichia) phagocytophilum* infection in Italian cats, *Vet Rec* 156(24):772–774, 2005.
64. Guilford WG: Idiopathic inflammatory bowel diseases. In Guilford WG, Center SA, Strombeck DR, et al: *Strombeck's small animal gastroenterology*, ed 3, Philadelphia, PA, 1996, Saunders, pp 451–486.
65. Webb AA, Taylor SM, Muir GD: Steroid-responsive meningitis-arteritis in dogs with noninfectious, nonerosive, idiopathic, immune-mediated polyarthritis, *J Vet Intern Med* 16(3):269–273, 2002.
66. Bennett D, Kelly DF: Immune-based non-erosive inflammatory joint disease of the dog. II. Polyarthritis/polymyositis syndrome, *J Small Anim Pract* 28:891–908, 1987.
67. Trepanier LA, Danhof R, Toll J, et al: Clinical findings in 40 dogs with hypersensitivity associated with administration of potentiated sulfonamides, *J Vet Intern Med* 17(5):647–652, 2003.
68. Couto CG, Krakowka S, Johnson G, et al: In vitro immunologic features of Weimaraner dogs with neutrophil abnormalities and recurrent infections, *Vet Immunol Immunopathol* 23(1-2):103–112, 1989.
69. Foale RD, Herrtage ME, Day MJ: Retrospective study of 25 young Weimaraners with low serum immunoglobulin concentrations and inflammatory disease, *Vet Rec* 153(18): 553–558, 2003.
70. Gaskell RM, Dawson S, Radford AW: Feline respiratory disease. In Greene CE, editor: *Infectious diseases of the dog and cat*, ed 3, St. Louis, MO, 2006, Saunders, pp 145–154.
71. Stone M: Systemic lupus erythematosus. In Ettinger SJ, Feldman EC, editors: *Textbook of veterinary internal medicine*, ed 6, St. Louis, MO, 2005, Saunders, pp 1952–1957.
72. Monier JC, Ritter J, Caux C, et al: Canine systemic lupus erythematosus. II. Antinuclear antibodies, *Lupus* 1(5):287–293, 1992.
73. Erne JB, Goring RL, Kennedy FA, et al: Prevalence of lymphoplasmacytic synovitis in dogs with naturally occurring cranial cruciate ligament rupture, *J Am Vet Med Asssoc* 235:386–390, 2009.
74. Dougherty SA, Center SA, Shaw EE, et al: Juvenile-onset polyarthritis syndrome in Akitas, *J Am Vet Med Assoc* 198(5):849–856, 1991.
75. Vaden SL: Glomerular disease. In Ettinger SJ, Feldman EC, editors: *Textbook of veterinary internal medicine*, ed 6, St. Louis, MO, 2005, Saunders, pp 1786–1800.
76. May C, Hammill J, Bennett D: Chinese Shar Pei fever syndrome: a preliminary report, *Vet Rec* 131(25-26):586–587, 1992.
77. Allan G: Radiographic signs of joint disease. In Thrall DE, editor: *Textbook of veterinary diagnostic radiology*, ed 4, Philadelphia, PA, 2002, Saunders, pp 187–207.
78. Bennett D: Immune-based erosive inflammatory joint disease of the dog: canine rheumatoid arthritis. I. Clinical, radiological and laboratory investigations, *J Small Anim Pract* 28:779–797, 1987.
79. Pedersen NC, Pool RR, O'Brien T: Feline chronic progressive polyarthritis, *Am J Vet Res* 41(4):522–535, 1980.

CHAPTER 13

The Musculoskeletal System

Susan E. Fielder

Although cytologic techniques have not been used extensively in evaluating diseases of the musculoskeletal system, they may be valuable aids in the diagnosis of certain important diseases affecting this system.

BONE

Diseases of bone yield diagnostic cytology specimens more often than do diseases of muscle. Although healthy bone tissue is difficult to sample and contains few cells and abundant matrix, both inflammatory and neoplastic bone diseases are usually accompanied by bone lysis and increased cellularity. Both lytic and proliferative bone lesions are often easily aspirated.

Sample Collection

Collection of material from bone lesions for cytologic examination may be complicated by the hardness of cortical bone. Lesions that have a major soft tissue component can be aspirated by techniques similar to those for any soft tissue mass. Even heavily mineralized masses can often be aspirated with a fine needle by careful palpation and exploration of the lesion surface. Examination of radiographs may reveal portions of the lesion that are less heavily mineralized and more likely to produce useful aspirates. Some lesions in which cortical bone remains intact will not yield to fine-needle aspiration (FNA). In such instances, the best way to obtain diagnostic material is to use a trephine to obtain a core biopsy specimen. Imprints can be made for cytologic evaluation before the specimen is fixed in formalin for histologic processing. It is important to keep cytology smears away from formalin fumes because these will inactivate cellular enzymes and interfere with cytologic staining and evaluation.

Inflammatory Diseases

Inflammatory lesions of the skeleton are important causes of disease in domestic animals, and cytology is a valuable diagnostic tool in identifying certain lesions. Cytologic specimens from inflammatory lesions of bone are generally similar to exudates from other organs. Neutrophils typically predominate in specimens from animals with osteomyelitis, although activated macrophages and multinucleate giant cells are a significant component of some exudates. Inflammatory lesions that are accompanied by new bone proliferation may yield cytologic specimens that also contain small numbers of osteoblasts, which typically range from plump and ovoid to fusiform with round to ovoid eccentric nuclei and dark-blue cytoplasm. They differ from neoplastic osteoblasts in that they are smaller and more uniform and lack nuclear manifestations of malignancy.

Osteoclasts may also be found in small numbers in specimens from inflammatory lesions. These cells resemble multinucleate giant cells and arise from precursor cells of the monocyte–macrophage cell line. They are very large and irregularly shaped with variable numbers (typically 6 to 10) of uniform, round nuclei arranged randomly throughout the cell and abundant, light blue cytoplasm (Figure 13-1).

Bacterial osteomyelitis typically results in a neutrophilic or suppurative inflammatory response. Some specific causes of bacterial osteomyelitis include *Actinomyces* spp. and *Nocardia* spp., and these are often seen as branching, filamentous rods. Staphylococcal, streptococcal, and gram-negative aerobic bacterial infections are common and may be identified on cytology.[1]

Osteomyelitis may also be seen with fungal infection, and the organisms may be detected in the exudate. The exudate with fungal infections is typically more mixed than that in bacterial infections and often contains a much larger component of activated macrophages and multinucleate giant cells. Fungal organisms include *Coccidioides immitis*, *Blastomyces dermatitidis*, and *Histoplasma capsulatum*. Hyphating fungal organisms such as *Aspergillus* spp. and *Geomyces* spp. may also be seen and appear as staining or nonstaining fungal hyphae (Figure 13-2 and Figure 13-3).[2] Rarely, protozoal organisms such as *Hepatozoon* spp. may be seen as gamonts within the neutrophils in inflammatory aspirates of bone.[3]

Neoplastic Diseases

Neoplasms of bone are relatively common in domestic animals, and cytologic examination is useful in establishing the diagnosis in some of these diseases. As with the interpretation of histologic sections of bone, evaluation of cytologic specimens from bone requires knowledge of

The author wishes to acknowledge the contribution of Dr. Edward A. Mahaffey, DVM, PhD, DACVP, who authored this chapter for previous editions of the book. His contribution served as the foundation for the material appearing in this edition.

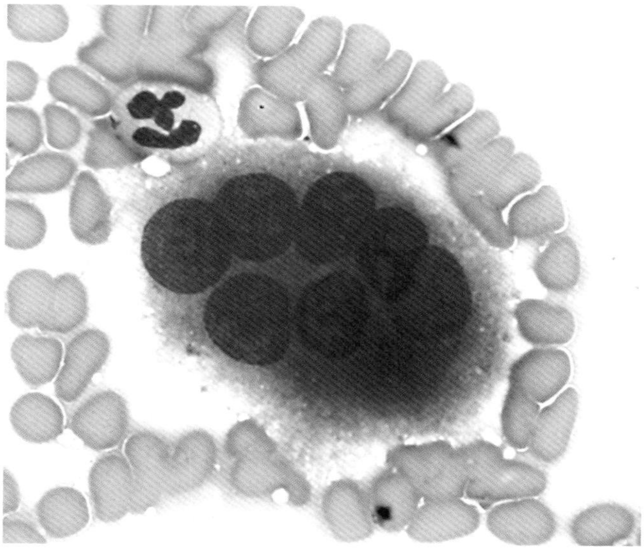

Figure 13-1 Osteoclast with multiple, relatively uniform nuclei and abundant cytoplasm from a lytic bone lesion. (Wright stain.)

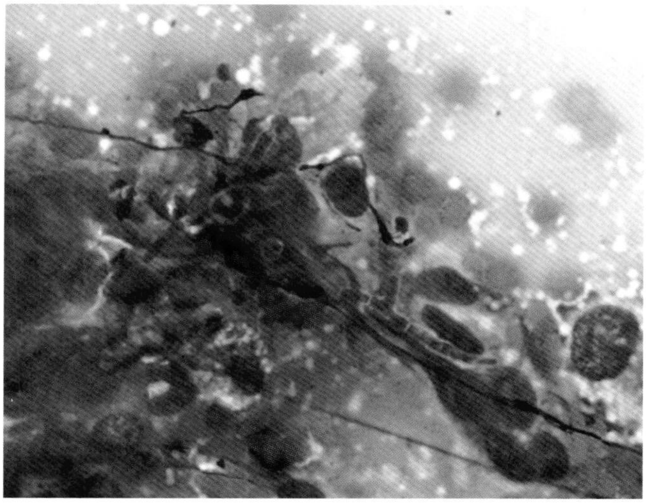

Figure 13-2 Fungal hyphae from lytic bone lesion in a dog. *Aspergillus* was cultured from this lesion. (Wright stain.)

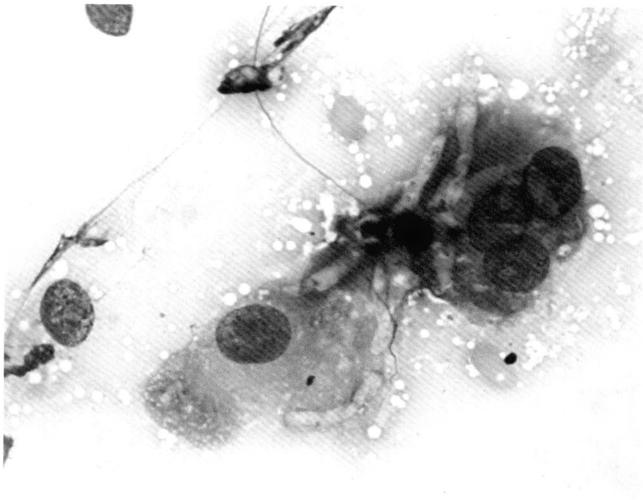

Figure 13-3 Nonstaining fungal hyphae from a lytic bone lesion. (Wright stain.)

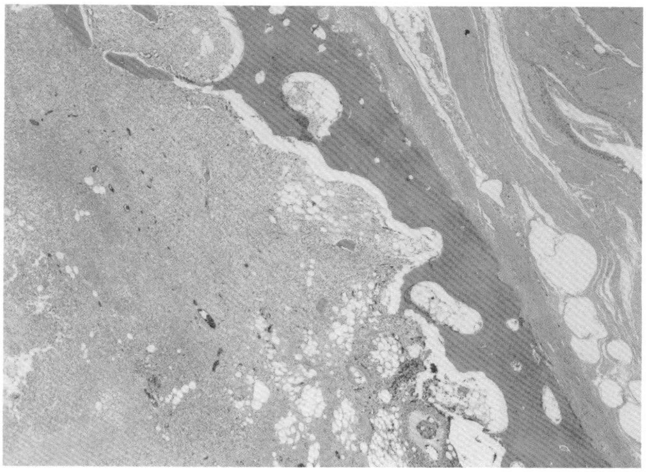

Figure 13-4 Mass from the radius of a dog. Within the cortex is a neoplasm that replaces marrow elements, and partially effaces cortical and trabecular bone. (H&E stain. Courtesy of Fabiano Oliveira.)

the clinical and radiographic features of a specific lesion. Cytology is probably more useful in distinguishing inflammatory bone disease from neoplasia than in identifying specific bone tumors; however, osteosarcomas and chondrosarcomas do have characteristic cytologic features that aid in diagnosis.

Special stains are available to differentiate osteosarcoma from other mesenchymal neoplasms of the bone. Nitroblue tetrazolium chloride/5-bromo-4-chloro-3-indolyl phosphate toluidine salt (NBT/BCIP) may be used to detect alkaline phosphatase activity in osteoblasts.[4] Because both reactive and neoplastic osteoblasts will stain positive, previous diagnosis of malignancy based on identification of criteria of malignancy on cytologic exam is necessary. Both unstained slides and prestained slides (aqueous Romanowsky method only) may be used.[5]

Osteosarcoma: Osteosarcoma is the most common primary bone tumor typically affecting the appendicular skeleton. In the dog, osteosarcoma occurs more commonly in the front limbs with the distal radius and proximal humerus as the most common sites (Figure 13-4).[6] Aspirates of osteosarcomas are often more highly cellular compared with aspirates of soft tissue sarcomas. Cells may occur individually or in aggregates. One characteristic feature that may be evident on low-power examination of the slide is the presence of islands of osteoid surrounded by tumor cells. Osteoid (Figure 13-5 and Figure 13-6) appears as a somewhat fibrillar, bright-pink material on Wright-stained slides. These structures are not found in most aspirates from osteosarcomas; however, when found, their presence provides strong evidence that the origin of a tumor is bone. Individual tumor cells vary from round to plump to fusiform and often vary greatly in size (Figure 13-7). They often have

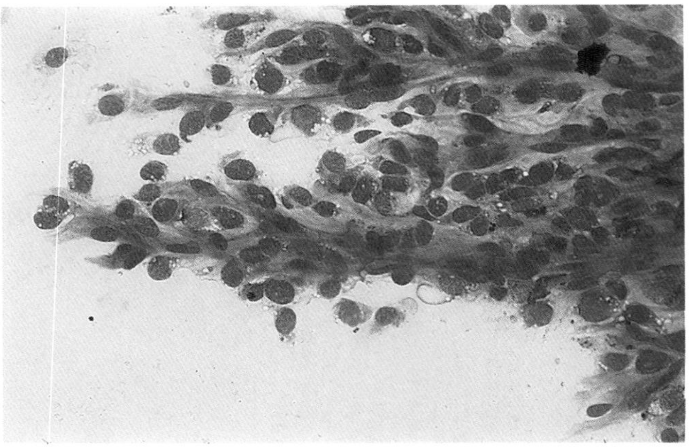

Figure 13-5 Osteoblasts interspersed with pink-staining intercellular matrix (osteoid) from an osteosarcoma. (Wright stain.)

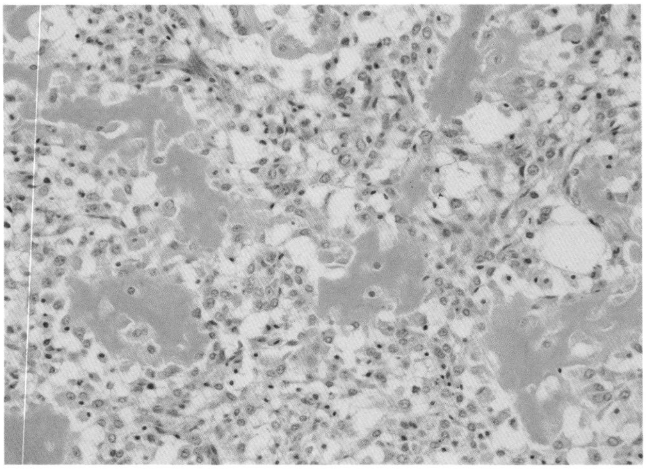

Figure 13-6 Mass from the radius of a dog. Detail of neoplastic cells of Figure 13-4. Neoplastic cells are round to spindle shaped, have oval to angulated nuclei, and surround an irregularly shaped, eosinophilic, and homogeneous material (tumor osteoid). (H&E stain. Courtesy of Fabiano Oliveira.)

many of the classic cytologic features of malignancy such as karyomegaly, anisokaryosis, large nucleoli, and multiple nucleoli that differ in size. The cytoplasm is typically dark blue and may contain several clear vacuoles (Figure 13-8). A proportion of the cells from most osteosarcomas contain scattered, pink cytoplasmic granules (Figure 13-9). These granules are not specific to osteosarcomas; similar granules may also occur in cells from chondrosarcomas and, less commonly, from fibrosarcomas. Cells from more differentiated osteosarcomas (Figure 13-10) are more uniform and may be difficult to distinguish from normal osteoblasts. Small numbers of inflammatory cells, nonneoplastic osteoblasts, and osteoclasts similar to those described in the previous section on inflammation may also be found in aspirates from osteosarcomas.

Chondrosarcoma: These tumors are the second most common sarcoma of bone. The ribs, turbinates, and pelvis are the most common sites for chondrosarcomas of dogs,

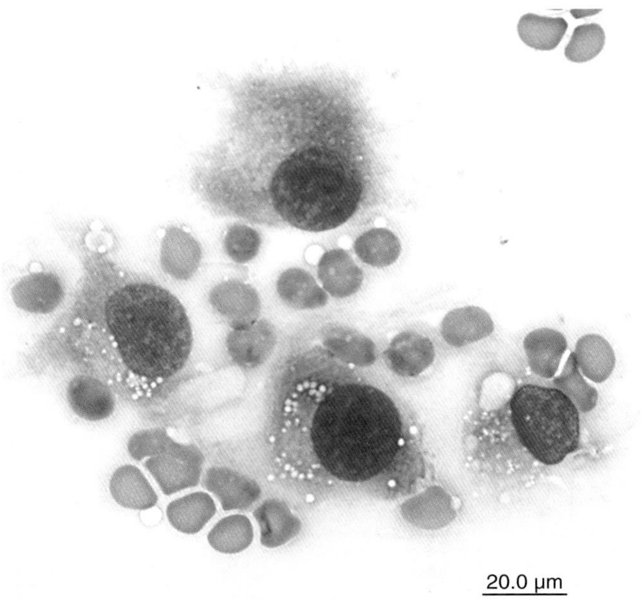

Figure 13-7 Aspirate of an osteosarcoma showing marked variation in cell size and shape. (Wright stain.)

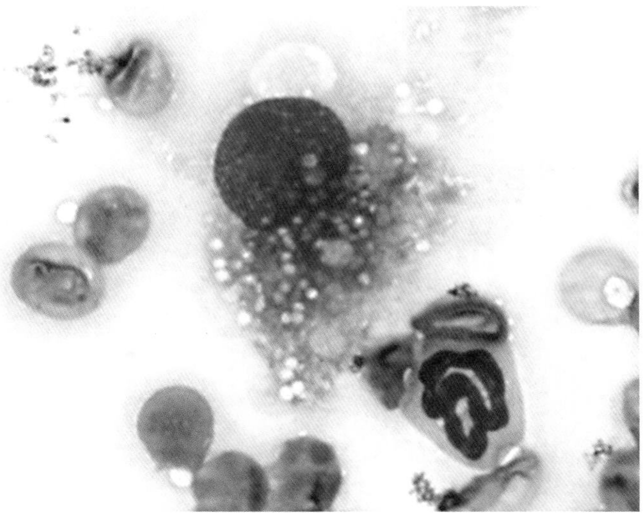

Figure 13-8 Osteoblast from an osteosarcoma with vacuolated cytoplasm and fine pink cytoplasmic granules. (Wright stain.)

and the scapulae, vertebrae, and ribs are more common sites in cats.[6,7] One useful cytologic feature of chondrosarcomas that may be evident on low-power examination of aspirates is the presence of chondroid. This is seen as lakes of bright pink, smooth or slightly granular material, in which cells may be embedded (Figure 13-11). Although the presence of this material suggests the possibility of a cartilaginous origin of a tumor, it is not a consistent finding in aspirates of chondrosarcomas. Individual chondroblasts from chondrosarcomas have cytologic features that are similar to those of malignant osteoblasts. They vary from round to fusiform, with large nuclei and dark-blue cytoplasm (Figure 13-12). Anisokaryosis is prominent and multinucleate tumor cells may be found. The cytoplasm

documented CSF production within the ventricular system and the SAS.[2]

Contraindications to Acquisition of Cerebrospinal Fluid

CSF should not be collected from patients with unacceptable anesthetic risk or with suspected coagulopathy, severe cervical trauma, or increased intracranial pressure secondary to edema, hemorrhage, hydrocephalus, or a large neoplasm.[9] CSF collection in the presence of elevated intracranial pressure may cause brain herniation and death secondary to compression of respiratory centers.[10] Signs of increased intracranial pressure may include: stupor, coma, bradycardia, systemic hypertension, cranial nerve deficits, rigid paresis, or all of these.[11,12] Mannitol and hypertonic saline are the first-line medical therapies for elevated intracranial pressure. Head elevation, modest hyperventilation, administration of drugs to slow brain metabolism, and craniectomy with durectomy are sometimes used in cases refractory to traditional treatments. Advanced imaging before CSF collection, especially in patients presenting with intracranial neurologic signs, may be useful in identifying contraindications. Imaging, in particular MRI, is exquisitely helpful in providing structural data which may be correlated to CSF results.

Collection Techniques

Collection Sites: CSF can be collected from the cerebromedullary cistern (at the atlanto-occipital space) or from the lumbar cistern in the L5-L6 interarcuate space. The cerebromedullary cistern is utilized more commonly because a larger volume of CSF with lower risk of blood contamination can be reliably collected.

Cerebromedullary Cistern versus Lumbar Cistern: A study of 158 dogs with focal, noninflammatory disease showed that in cases of spinal lesions, CSF was more likely to be abnormal if collected from the lumbar cistern, that is, caudal to the lesion.[13] This observation may be explained by presupposing cranial to caudal flow of CSF, but the traditionally held theory of CSF flow has recently been contested.[8] In canines, CSF collected from the cerebromedullary cistern generally has lower microprotein concentrations compared with samples collected from the lumbar cistern.[14] Blood contamination may be more pronounced in lumbar collection, as the desired subarachnoid space is more difficult to enter and yields a smaller volume of fluid that tends to flow more slowly.[10,11] Moreover, hemodilution may contribute to increased measured protein concentration.[14]

Rare instances of CSF contamination with hematopoietic precursors have only been reported from lumbar sites.[15] A low, but potentially catastrophic, risk of puncturing the cervical spinal cord or caudal brainstem exists during cerebromedullary collection. Because the spinal cord length is variable, spinal cord puncture is a possibility during lumbar collection, but it is associated with less severe adverse effects compared with injury following cisternal puncture. In a case series of 4 accidental cisternal parenchymal punctures (documented by MRI), 3 out of the 4 patients suffered neurologic decompensation and subsequently had to be euthanized.[16]

Equipment: The following equipment should be assembled: anesthesia and monitoring equipment, clippers, aseptic preparation materials for the skin, sterile gloves, and a spinal needle with stylet. For cerebromedullary cistern collection in dogs weighing less than 25 kg and for cats, a 22-gauge, 1.5″ spinal needle is usually adequate, and a 22-gauge, 2.5″ spinal needle is recommended for dogs weighing greater than 25 kg. For lumbar puncture, a 22-gauge spinal needle up to 6″ long may be required for obese or extremely large patients. If available, fluoroscopic equipment may aid in the acquisition of cisternal or lumbar CSF. At the chapter authors' institution, fluoroscopy is often used prior to cisternal CSF acquisition in toy-breed dogs to exclude the possibility of subclinical atlantoaxial subluxation.

Cerebrospinal Fluid Acquisition: The anesthetized patient is placed in lateral recumbency (it is generally easier for a right-handed clinician to have the patient in right-lateral recumbency, and vice versa), with the neck and back flush to the edge of a sturdy table. For collection from the cerebromedullary cistern, the neck is flexed such that the dorsum of the muzzle is 90 degrees to the long axis of the body (stabilizing the endotracheal tube, if needed, to prevent kinking and deflating the cuff, if necessary, to prevent tracheal trauma), and the snout is propped up slightly, if necessary, to keep it parallel with the table and not angulated from the sagittal plane.[11] A wide area (3 to 5 cm) around the atlanto-occipital joint (beyond atlas wings and axis spinous process and to the external occipital protuberance) is shaved and aseptically prepared, and landmarks are palpated with a gloved, nondominant hand.[10] The needle is inserted at the intersection of two imaginary perpendicular lines that run (1) along the dorsal midline (dividing the patient sagitally) from the occipital protuberance to the cranial spinous process of the axis (C2) and (2) across the craniolateral aspects of the wings of the atlas (C1) (dividing the patient craniocaudally).

For lumbar collection, the pelvic limbs are brought forward into full flexion, and the needle is inserted cranial and parallel to the dorsal spinous process of L6 for dogs and L7 for cats advancing the needle until the ventral aspect of the vertebral canal is encountered; the needle is then retracted slightly and CSF is collected from the ventral SAS.[11,17] The pelvic limbs may kick or twitch slightly during collection because of irritation of the cauda equina or spinal cord parenchyma.

For either location, once landmarks are palpated, the needle is held stably with the dominant hand and very slowly advanced, stylet in place. The heel of the dominant hand may be supported against the table. For cisternal collection, it is important to advance the needle toward the point of the nose without angulation. The stylet is removed with the nondominant hand every 2 to 3 mm to check for fluid within the needle hub, waiting a few seconds. It is common to feel a decrease in resistance to forward needle movement once the thecal space is entered. If bone is hit or frank hemorrhage is observed from the needle, it should be withdrawn slowly and collection reattempted.[10] If clear or slightly blood-tinged fluid is observed, advancement of the needle ceases and open tubes are placed directly under the needle hub to collect freely falling drops.

No significant objective data exist regarding the maximal amount of CSF that may be collected in dogs. Several authors claim that it is safe to collect 0.2 milliliters (mL) of CSF per kilogram of body weight (1 mL/5 kg); in other species much higher volumes of CSF per body weight are acquired standardly.[18] In general, 0.5 to 1 mL of CSF is adequate for routine diagnostic tests, including cell counts, protein concentration, and cytologic analysis. Larger volumes are necessary for additional diagnostics (cultures, titers, polymerase chain reaction [PCR], protein electrophoresis, etc.).

CSF is collected passively and should not be aspirated. Free drops are allowed to fall from the hub of the needle into an open tube placed just below. Two sets of tubes should be readied and ideally handled by an assistant. An ethylenediaminetetraacetic acid (EDTA)–treated (purple top) tube is used for cell counts and PCR testing for organisms, and plain (red top) tubes are used for protein concentration, culture, or immunologic assays.[11] Some sources indicate that plain tubes are recommended, as EDTA could increase protein concentration. If CSF analysis will occur rapidly (within 1 hour), collection into a plain tube is adequate, whereas preservation of cells may be improved with collection into EDTA if analysis will be delayed. If low volume is present, priority is given to the EDTA tube. If CSF appears red, then iatrogenic hemorrhage (puncture of a dural vessel) or actual CNS hemorrhage has occurred. In this instance, the first few drops are allowed to collect into the first set of tubes, and the second set of tubes are reserved for the latter portion of the sample, as iatrogenic hemorrhage tends to clear over time. If the hemorrhage does clear, a decision may be made about discarding the first set of tubes or keeping them for ancillary testing not affected by the hemorrhage. After collection, the needle is withdrawn without the stylet, and the CSF within the needle is allowed to drip into one of the tubes or is placed in an additional plain tube and saved for culture.

CEREBROSPINAL FLUID PROCESSING AND ANALYSIS

As with other clincopathologic and cytologic samples, evaluation of a fresh specimen is preferred to minimize cellular degradation, to which CSF is particularly vulnerable because of its relatively low protein concentration. Sample degradation will affect cell differential count to a greater extent than the total nucleated cell count or the protein concentration.[19] A study of 30 canine CSF samples with pleocytosis concluded that delay of analysis up to 8 hours was unlikely to alter interpretation, especially in samples with protein concentrations above 50 milligrams per deciliter (mg/dL).[19] Preservative should be added to low protein samples unless analysis is to be completed within 60 minutes (see next section), and a dilutional effect must then be factored into cell counts.[19] Samples to be shipped to a reference laboratory overnight should be kept at refrigeration temperature and shipped with ice packs for analysis within 48 hours.[10,17] The reference laboratory should be prenotified to ensure prompt analysis.

If analysis is to be delayed by more than 1 hour and the CSF sample has a protein concentration less than 50 mg/dL, one of the following may be added as a protein source to maintain cellular integrity: (1) hetastarch (add 1:1 volume), (2) fetal calf serum (3.7 g/dL protein; add 20% by volume), or (3) autologous plasma or serum (fresh or frozen; 11% by volume = one drop from 25-gauge needle (approximately 0.03 mL) mixed into 0.25 mL CSF).[11,20,21] One study demonstrated better preservation of mononuclear cells in canine samples when fetal calf serum was used instead of hetastarch.[19] All samples should be refrigerated at 4°C to minimize cellular degradation.

Cell Counts

A hemocytometer may be employed in practice to count nucleated cells and erythrocytes. Both sides of the coverslipped hemocytometer are loaded with unstained CSF, which is then placed in a humidified container for 10 to 15 minutes to allow cells to settle on the glass. Because the fluid is unstained, the microscope condenser is lowered to improve contrast. Erythrocytes and nucleated cells are differentiated by size, refraction, granularity, and smoothness of plasma membrane.[22] Some laboratories stain CSF samples with new methylene blue (NMB), as leukocytes will take up stain while erythrocytes remain unstained, making differentiation of leukocytes and erythrocytes easier (Figure 14-1).[23] A small volume of CSF is drawn into a capillary tube coated with NMB or a tube which has a small volume of NMB followed by an air pocket.[23] The tube containing NMB and CSF is gently rocked back and forth, allowing the cells to take up some stain without diluting the CSF with a volume of NMB.[23] The hemocytometer is then loaded, and each population is counted and totals are calculated, as follows: Neubauer chamber: (1) Count both areas of large nine squares, and find the average of the number of leukocytes and erythrocytes; (2) multiply the average by $^{10}/_{9}$ to get the cells per microliter (cells/μL).[11]

The ADVIA 120 (Siemens Medical Solution, Fernwald, Germany) hematology instrument has been validated for

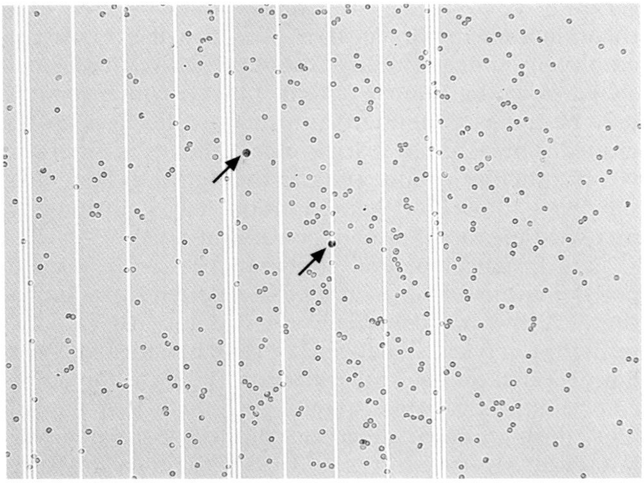

Figure 14-1 Numerous erythrocytes and two leukocytes present on a hemacytometer. The two nuclei of the two leukocytes in the center of the field stain dark purple (*arrows*). (New methylene blue stain. Original magnification 50×.)

analyzing canine CSF samples and shows excellent correlation with manual methods used in dogs with increased total cell counts (pleocytosis), but the instrument may overestimate the cell count in samples without pleocytoses and has not been validated for the identification of eosinophils.[24] The automated differential count is also more accurate at higher cell numbers and, thus, should be compared with a traditional manual differential. The ADVIA 2120 hematology analyzer displayed satisfactory agreement with the standard hemocytometer method.[25] Validation experiments using 67 canine samples showed a sensitivity of 100% and specificity of 89% for accurately identifying samples with pleocytosis when manual counting was considered the gold standard (>5 cells/μL).[25] The instrument tended to be less accurate at lower (within reference interval) nucleated cell counts.[25] Erythrocytes may be a source of interference, as a red blood cell (RBC) count of 250 cells/μL was shown to elevate the nucleated cell count. With regard to differential cell count, the instrument performed better in the presence of pleocytosis, whereas monocytes were overcounted at lower nucleated cell counts.[25] Automated cell counts should, thus, not replace a manual differential but may be used as another level of quality control. Automated instruments cannot recognize altered cell types such as atypical neoplastic cells.

Measurement of Microprotein Concentration

Measurement of CSF specific gravity is not considered to be helpful because of low sensitivity for detecting abnormalities.[12] CSF microprotein may be semiquantitatively measured by using urine dipsticks that detect albumin. This assay has a lower detection limit of 100 mg/dL; therefore, it has low sensitivity for mild to moderate CSF protein concentration elevations (30 mg/dL to 100 mg/dL). False-positive or false-negative reactions may occur if the dipstick reads at trace or 1+, but this method is useful if other techniques are not available.[11] Reference laboratories apply a similar, but more sensitive, methodology to measurement of CSF microprotein as serum protein, using the trichloroacetic acid method, the Ponceau S red dye binding method, or the Coomassie brilliant blue method.[22]

Screening tests for CSF globulins include the Nonne-Apelt (also called *Ross-Jones*) test and Pandy's reaction. In the Nonne-Apelt test, CSF is added to the top of 1 mL saturated ammonium sulfate and left standing for 3 minutes at room temperature. The presence of a white-gray ring at the interface is a positive reaction. In Pandy's reaction, a few drops of CSF are added to 1 mL of 10% carbolic acid solution and the resulting turbidity is graded 0 to 4. Any Pandy score above zero is considered elevated. Globulin concentration below 50 mg/dL will be undetectable with either test.[11,22]

Protein electrophoresis and immunoelectrophoresis may be performed on CSF as well as serum for maximum fractionation.[26] The utility of protein electrophoresis or immunoelectrophoresis of CSF lies in discriminating altered blood–brain barrier (BBB) permeability from increased localized production of immunoglobulin, which may be suggestive of (but not specific for) a disease entity for which an electrophoretic pattern has been established.

Cytologic Slide Preparation

Cytologic analysis is a critical component of CSF evaluation because the differential count (percentages) of cells may be abnormal, even if the total nucleated count is within reference interval. Cytology also enables examination for neoplastic cells, infectious agents, and evidence of prior hemorrhage. It may also serve as a quality control point, allowing for correlation between observed cellularity and the total count generated by a hemocytometer or an automated analyzer. Because of its low cellularity, CSF must be concentrated before cytologic smear preparation.

Use of an in-house sedimentation chamber (Sörnäs procedure) may be very useful and preserves cell-free fluid for ancillary testing.[11] This technique will recover approximately 60% of total cells, which is sufficient for analysis.[17] A syringe barrel (with the tip and needle aseptically removed with a scalpel blade) is turned upside down and the smooth, top side is placed in warm petroleum jelly and then onto a clean slide. Once a seal has formed, fresh CSF (at least 0.5 mL) is placed in the syringe and allowed to sit for 30 minutes.[17,22] Then, the supernatant is aspirated carefully with a pipette so as not to disturb the bottom layer contacting the slide. The syringe barrel is removed, and any excess CSF is carefully absorbed with a small piece of filter paper or paper towel. The slide is completely and rapidly air-dried without heat (inadequate drying results in cellular distortion), excess petroleum jelly removed with a scalpel blade, and the slide is stained with routine Romanowsky stains (e.g., Diff-Quik).

If CSF is sent to a reference laboratory, a cytologic slide will likely be prepared using cytocentrifugation (500 to 1000 revolutions per minute [rev/min] for 5 to 10 minutes, either onto a slide coated with albumin or with the addition of 0.05 mL of 30% albumin for improved cell capture) for maximal concentration of nucleated cells onto one slide.[17] Cytocentrifuged cytologies have excellent cellular detail, but the preparation may enlarge cells slightly and create an artifactual foamy or vacuolated appearance.[17] Slides are air-dried and stained with conventional Romanowsky stains. Multiple cytospin preparations may be made to yield 200 intact nucleated cells for classification.

Additional Cerebrospinal Fluid Testing

Culture: As it is rare for etiologic agents to localize only within the CNS, all cases of suspected infection may be aided diagnostically by fine-needle aspiration (FNA) cytology, biopsy with histopathology, culture of nonneural lesions, or all of these.[21] Bacterial culture and sensitivity testing of CSF is recommended for most cases of neutrophilic pleocytosis given appropriate clinical index of suspicion for a septic lesion. Even when organisms are visualized on CSF cytology, speciation and sensitivity testing may guide prognostic and treatment decisions. Alternatively, bacterial or fungal culture may be negative regardless of cytologic observation of organisms.[11,21] It must be remembered that bacterial CNS infection is highly uncommon in dogs and cats compared with other domestic animal species.[27]

Titers and Polymerase Chain Reaction Testing for Infectious Agents: Advanced techniques for neurologic disease diagnosis are expanding rapidly. Enzyme-linked immunosorbent assay (ELISA)–based assays for antibody detection and PCR-based assays for nucleic acid detection of several medically important microbes have been developed for use on CSF and may be instructive in the diagnosis of viral, rickettsial, protozoal, or fungal diseases.[21] A large canine study that included a subset of 16 dogs with neoplastic or inflammatory disease showed that CSF titer provided diagnosis in 25% of cases.[3] Antibody assays should be interpreted cautiously, as the presence of antibody may indicate prior exposure rather than active infection. Moreover, compromise to the BBB in states of inflammation may translate to the presence of antibodies within the CSF without local production. Occasionally cross-reactive antibodies may be present that do not represent presence of the disease agent under assessment. Similarly, specimens for PCR should be submitted to a laboratory with strict quality control to minimize false-negative and false-positive results. Poor collection technique may result in false-positive results, especially for bacterial species that are ubiquitous in the environment.[28] As with other aspects of CSF analysis, a negative PCR result does not definitively rule out the presence of a pathogen because of the sampling limitation of a small portion of the extracellular space.[21]

Enzymes, Neurotransmitters, and Other Molecules: CSF contains glucose, electrolytes, neurotransmitters, and enzymes, but these substances are not measured routinely, although this measurement represents a rapidly expanding area of research in the effort to give clinicians better tools for diagnosing patients as well as determining prognoses. CSF enzymes originate from the bloodstream, the CNS, or cells within CSF.[11] One study of 34 cats with non-inflammatory CNS disease showed that measurement of CSF activities of lactate dehydrogenase (LDH), aspartate aminotransferase (AST), and creatine kinase (CK) were not diagnostically sensitive but may be useful in detection of acute injury.[29] Multiple studies have correlated elevations in CSF CK activity with poor prognosis in dogs with neurologic disease or spinal cord injury.[30,31] Immunoassays for vascular endothelial growth factor (VEGF) and S-100 calcium-binding protein have shown elevations of both molecules in the CSF of experimentally induced hypothyroid dogs, suggesting endothelial and glial contribution to increased BBB permeability in this population.[32] Myelin basic protein (MBP) has been found to be elevated in lumbar CSF in dogs with degenerative myelopathy, supporting the conclusion that it is a demyelinating lesion.[33] Myelin basic protein concentration is elevated in the CSF of dogs affected by intervertebral disc herniation (IVDH) and has been found to be an independent predictor of poor prognosis.[34] Beta-2-microglobulin, a major histocompatibility complex I (MHC-I)–associated molecule, has been assayed by using ELISA and found to be elevated in the CSF of dogs with IVDH and inflammatory disease and also positively correlated with normal total nucleated cell count (TNCC).[35] The amino acids tryptophan and glutamine have been found to be elevated in the CSF of dogs with portosystemic shunts because of abnormal ammonia metabolism.[36] One study found increased oxytocin in the CSF of dogs with spinal cord compression, where it is believed to have an analgesic effect.[37] Gamma-aminobutyric acid (GABA) and glutamate neurotransmitter concentrations have been measured in dogs with epilepsy.[38]

NORMAL CEREBROSPINAL FLUID PARAMETERS

Gross Examination

Normal CSF is clear and colorless, with few cellular elements and a protein concentration approximately 200 to 300 times less than that of plasma or serum. Red or yellowish coloration indicates prior lesional hemorrhage or iatrogenic hemorrhage during collection. In the latter case, a pellet of red cells will be present after centrifugation. True xanthochromia (yellowish color of hemoglobin breakdown products) that does not clear on centrifugation, cytologic evidence of erythrophagia, or both, indicate prior hemorrhage into the subarachnoid space.[21] Increased bilirubin leakage into the SAS or high concentrations of CSF protein (>100 to 150 mg/dL) may cause xanthrochromia.[22] Increased turbidity of the sample may be caused by increased number of cells present (>400 RBCs/µL or >200 nucleated cells/µL) but is usually not affected by mild changes.[11,12]

Cell Counts

TNCC is fewer than 5 cells/µL in the dog and fewer than 8 cells/µL in the cat, and elevation above this range is termed *pleocytosis*.[11] Grading of pleocytosis is somewhat subjective: In one reference, "mild" was defined as 6 to 50 cells/µL; "moderate" as 51 to 1000 cells/µL; and "marked" as more than 1000 cells/µL.[4]

Microprotein Concentration

Depending on laboratory-specific reference intervals, normal protein concentration is usually less than 25 to 30 mg/dL for cisternal CSF and less than 45 mg/dL for lumbar CSF.[11,21] Approximately 80% to 95% of CSF protein is albumin, and 5% to 12% of CSF total protein comprises gammaglobulins.[2] Eighty percent of CSF protein is transferred from plasma, with the remainder produced within the CNS. The latter population includes molecules also produced by other organs and proteins unique to the CSF that may potentially be used as markers of CNS tissue damage. Experimental evidence and earlier literature support a gradient of increasing protein concentration from cranial to caudal within the subarachnoid space, which has been attributed to slower flow and greater blood–CSF permeability caudally.[13]

Normal Cytology

Normal CSF is acellular or contains small numbers of small lymphocytes (Figure 14-2 and Figure 14-3) and large mononuclear cells (macrophages, ependymal lining cells, meningothelial lining cells, choroid plexus cells) (Figure 14-4 and Figure 14-5). Large mononuclear cells may be vacuolated and contain phagocytized material (Figure 14-6). A low frequency of nondegenerate neutrophils (< 25%), which are usually indicative of blood contamination during collection, may be present.[39] A study of 359 samples of canine CSF found a 7.5% incidence of meningeal, choroid plexus, ependymal, endothelial cells, or all of these. No correlation existed between the presence of these cells and the presence of pleocytosis, elevated protein concentration, or the primary disease etiology.[40] Thus, it is postulated that the presence of

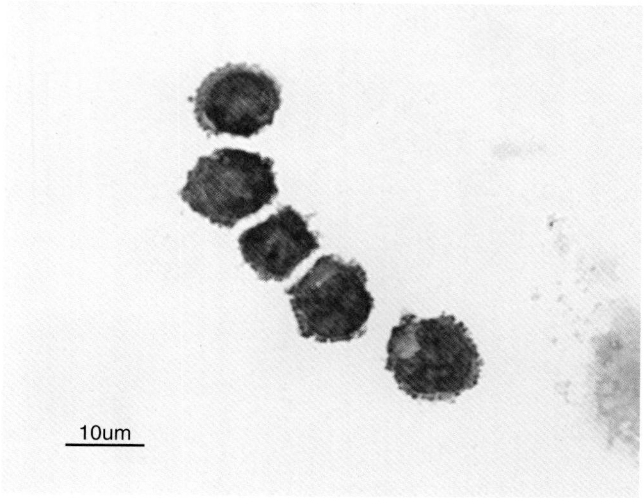

Figure 14-2 Small lymphocytes in a cerebrospinal fluid sample. (Wright-Giemsa stain.)

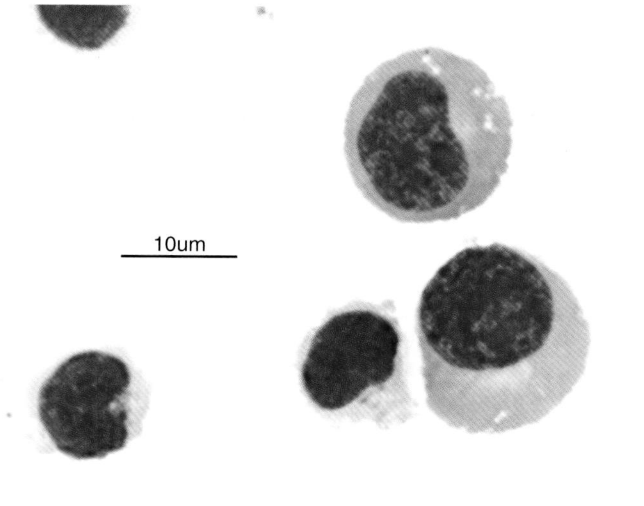

Figure 14-3 Small lymphocytes in a cerebrospinal fluid sample. The two cells to the right have slightly increased amounts of cytoplasm. (Wright-Giemsa stain.)

these cells is an artifact of collection and should not be overinterpreted. The authors recommended the term "surface epithelial cells" for the combined grouping (which cannot be distinguished cytologically), although not all of these cells (meningeal, endothelial) are of epithelial origin.[40] Occasionally, anucleate superficial squamous epithelial cells may be seen; these may be caused by contamination from the skin (Figure 14-7).

Other Parameters

Occasionally, small amounts of granular, foamy extracellular material are present and are consistent with myelin or myelin-like material, which will stain positively with Luxol fast blue. This material may consist of myelin fragments, which are generated from demyelination, or may consist of *myelin figures* (a nonspecific term for layered phospholipids exfoliated from damaged cells).[41] The two cannot be distinguished with light microscopy. The significance of this material remains unclear, as it may be observed in samples from patients with no discernible cause. A study of 98 canine cerebromedullary and lumbar CSF samples showed 20% incidence of myelin-like material, with a higher percentage in samples from the lumbar cistern or from small dogs (<10 kg).[42] The presence of the material was not correlated with case outcome.[42] Similarly, in a study of 61 Cavalier King Charles Spaniels with Chiari-like malformations, myelin-like material was observed in 57% of lumbar CSF collections and 12% of cerebromedullary collections.[43] Thus, myelin-like material may be a procedural artifact or may be consistent with a demyelinating (e.g., canine distemper virus, degenerative myelopathy) or potentially necrotizing disorder (e.g., IVDH, other spinal trauma, or a necrotic neoplasm).[41,42]

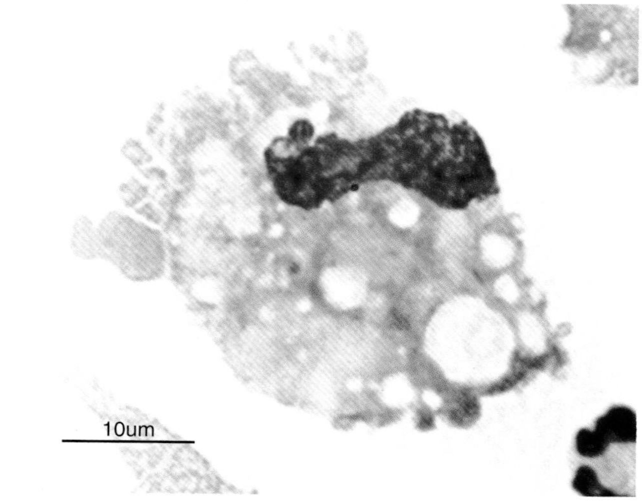

Figure 14-4 Large mononuclear cell with cytoplasmic vacuolation in a cerebrospinal fluid sample. (Wright-Giemsa stain.)

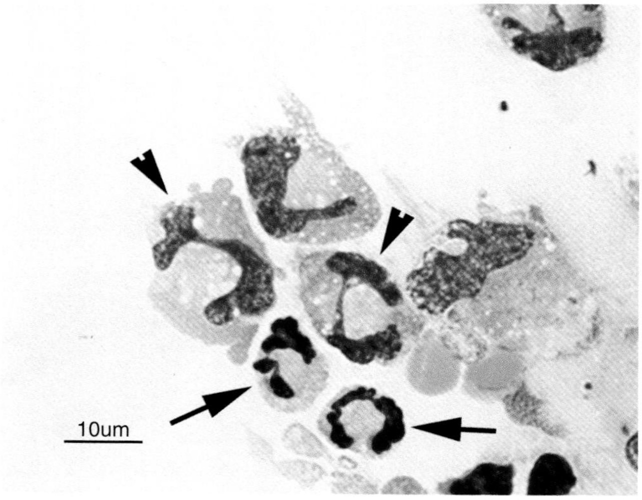

Figure 14-5 Numerous large foamy mononuclear cells and two neutrophils (*arrows*) in a sample of cerebrospinal fluid. Large mononuclear cells may have nuclei that are similar in shape to band cells or neutrophils, only larger (*arrowheads*). (Wright-Giemsa stain.)

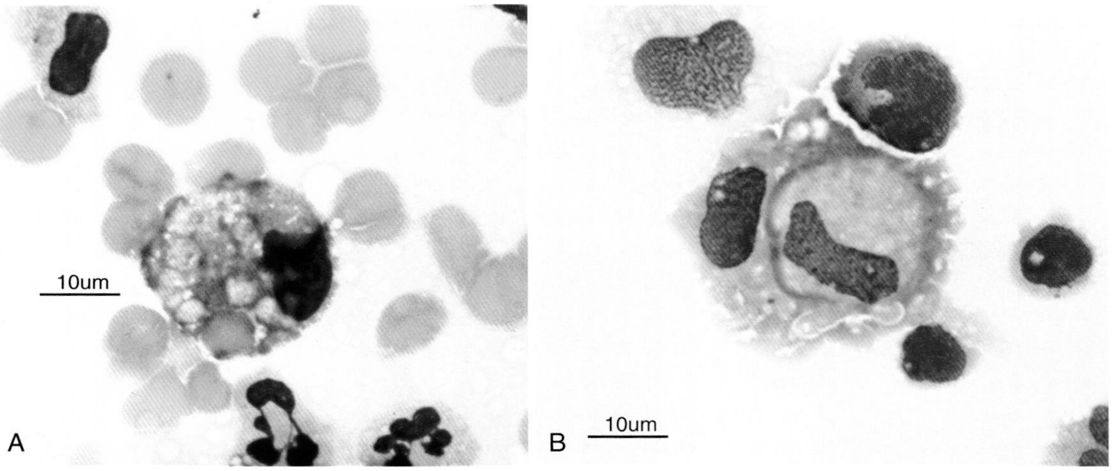

Figure 14-6 Large mononuclear cells in cerebrospinal fluid showing evidence of (*A*) erythrophagia and (*B*) leukocytophagia. (Wright-Giemsa stain.)

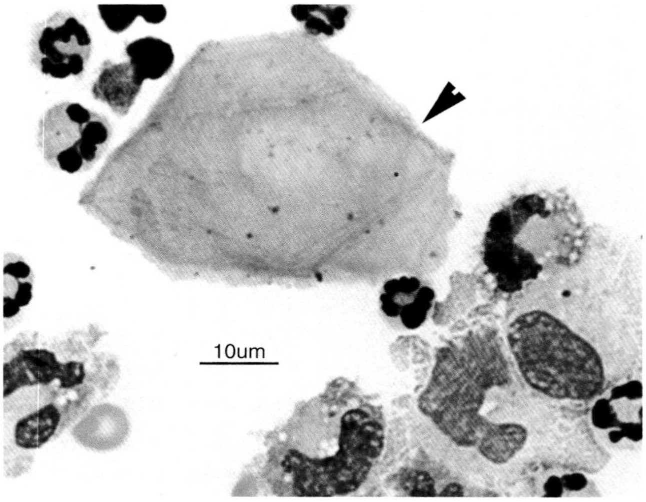

Figure 14-7 Cerebrospinal fluid sample from a dog. A single large keratinized epithelial cell is present (*arrowhead*). Squamous epithelial cells represent cutaneous contamination. (Wright-Giemsa stain.)

INTERPRETATION OF ABNORMAL CEREBROSPINAL FLUID

Blood Contamination and Hemorrhage

Normal CSF should not contain erythrocytes, but hemodilution is a common occurrence. Varying reports on the effect of blood contamination on TNCC, leukocyte differential, and protein concentration have been published.[44-47] Deciding whether increased TNCC or protein concentration is the result of hemodilution alone or a significant change concurrent with hemodilution necessarily remains, to an extent, a subjective assessment and must be critically evaluated in light of the magnitude of CSF findings along with the other pertinent facts of the case. One study in dogs determined that up to 13,200 erythrocytes/μL should not significantly affect TNCC or microprotein concentration, but feline CSF may be more sensitive to blood-induced changes.[44,45] Correction formulas for CSF parameters in the face of hemodilution (e.g., adding 1 nucleated cell/μL per 100 or 500 RBCs/μL) are unreliable.[46,47] In a recent study of 106 canine CSF samples without pleocytosis (TNCC <5/μL) but containing at least 500 RBC/μL, the mean percentage of neutrophils (45.2% versus 5.7%), percentage of samples with eosinophils present (36.8% versus 6.8%), and mean protein concentration (40 mg/dL versus 26 mg/dL) were found to be significantly increased in the samples with blood contamination compared with controls.[48] Significant RBC contamination warrants repeat sampling, if possible. Marked hemorrhage or evidence of prior hemorrhage (erythrophagocytosis, xanthochromia, hemosiderin-laden macrophages) may be useful in the diagnosis of CNS trauma, which may be accompanied by neutrophilic to mixed cell pleocytosis and mild increase in protein concentration.[4]

Elevated Microprotein Concentration

Elevated protein concentration in CSF (>30 mg/dL) may occur with or without pleocytosis, and in the absence of pleocytosis, is termed *albuminocytologic dissociation (ACD)*. High protein concentration may be the result of leakage of plasma or cellular proteins across the BBB, localized production of immunoglobulin, localized tissue damage or necrosis, decreased clearance of protein into the venous sinuses, obstruction of CSF circulation, or all of the above. As such, it is a nonspecific change that indicates CNS damage or hyperproteinemic disease and is consistent with disease of any etiology (e.g., trauma, metabolic, infectious, inflammatory, degenerative, or neoplastic). Caution should be exercised when diagnosing ACD if the sample is hemodiluted (> 500 RBC/μL).[48] As is true for pleocytosis, inflammation of the meninges and superficial regions of parenchyma will result in greater CSF protein elevations than for lesions that are more remote from the SAS.

Alterations of Leukocyte Percentages without a Pleocytosis

Occasionally, an abnormal leukocyte differential (shifted from mononuclear predominance to neutrophil predominance) without pleocytosis occurs. This may only be detected if cytologic analysis (after sedimentation

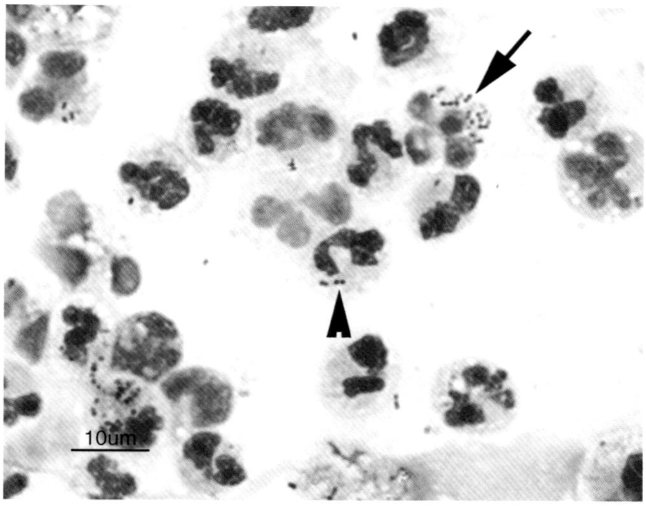

Figure 14-8 Septic meningoencephalitis. Note the degenerate neutrophils and the presence of bacteria (*arrow*). (Wright-Giemsa stain.)

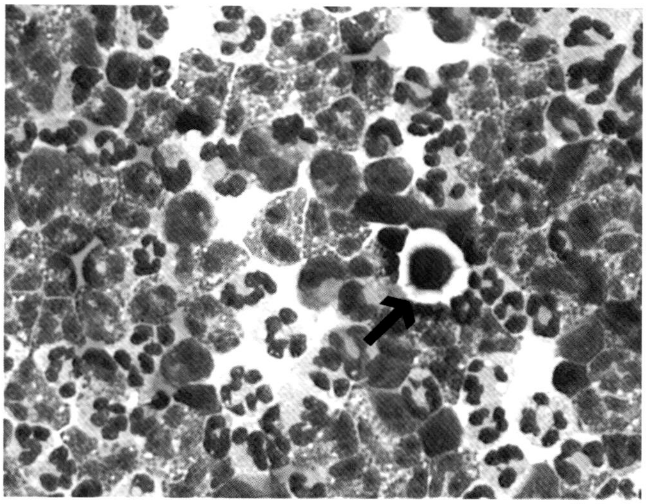

Figure 14-9 Cryptococcosis. Note the presence of Cryptococcus sp. (*arrow*) and the presence of numerous eosinophils. (Modified Wright stain. Original magnification 500x.)

or cytocentrifugation of CSF) is performed. Increased percentages of neutrophils may occur in early or mild inflammatory disease, noninflammatory CNS disease, disease that is remote from the SAS or sampling site, or in cases of hemodilution. An increased proportion of neutrophils is present when neutrophils comprise greater than 25% of all nucleated cells, and increased percentage of eosinophils occurs when eosinophils comprise greater than 1% of the differential.[11]

Increased Neutrophil Percentage: When present (with or without increased TNCC), neutrophils should be evaluated for toxic change, degenerative change, and intracellular organisms or other inclusions (Figure 14-8). Increased percentage of neutrophils without pleocytosis has been associated with healthy dogs, blood contamination, degenerative disc disease, neoplasia, cerebrovascular accident, fracture, and fibrocartilagenous embolism (FCE).[11,43] A study of 61 Cavalier King Charles Spaniels with Chiari-like malformation documented that those with syringomyelia were more likely to have an increased percentage of neutrophils, but it was not reported whether this subpopulation also had a concurrent pleocytosis.[43] In another study, cats with CNS neoplasia had increased percentage of neutrophils or lymphocytes without a pleocytosis.[29] Although not a classic pattern, infectious or inflammatory disease should not be ruled out if increased neutrophils are visualized without pleocytosis.

Increased Eosinophil Percentage: Increased percentage of eosinophils has been reported in parasitic and protozoal diseases such as *Neospora caninum* infection.[39] One cat with eosinophilic meningoencephalitis (EME) of unknown etiology had an increased percentage of eosinophils and lymphocytes without pleocytosis.[49]

Increased Nucleated Cell Counts (Pleocytoses)

The specific diseases mentioned in the next section on various categories of pleocytosis are a survey of the current literature and meant to be a helpful starting point in the generation of particular differential diagnoses. Thus, disease entities are listed in the section under which they are most commonly present, but it is important to note that for all disease entities, variability in the nature and the magnitude of pleocytosis may emerge in a particular patient at a particular point in time. Wherever possible, other categories of pleocytosis that have been reported for a disease have been mentioned. Generally, pleocytoses are defined by the cell type that comprises 70% or more of the nucleated cell population. If all cell types are 50% or less, the pleocytosis is classified as a *mixed cell pleocytosis*. And if, for example, lymphocytes are greater than 50% but less than 70%, some pathologists will classify the pleocytosis as *mixed cell, lymphocyte predominant.* A pleocytosis will be classified as eosinophilic if eosinophils compose at least 10% to 20% of the nucleated cell population.[12]

Neutrophilic Pleocytosis

Infectious Conditions

Bacterial Meningoencephalomyelitis: Bacterial infections of the CNS are unusual and represent a small portion of neutrophilic pleocytoses. Typically, this pleocytosis is severe (could be over 1000 cells/μL), neutrophilic, and accompanied by significantly elevated protein concentration, but the cell population may change to mononuclear during the course of treatment.[11,21,50] Rare instances of brain abscessation secondary to sepsis (which may be a sequela of iatrogenic immunosuppression) may result in marked neutrophilic pleocytosis, markedly elevated protein concentration, visualization of bacterial organisms (Figure 14-8), and abnormal MRI findings.[51] *Staphylococcus intermedius* was cultured from the CSF of a dog presenting with a retrobulbar abscess and neurologic signs.[52] The CSF showed a moderate neutrophilic pleocytosis (75 cells/μL) and borderline elevation in protein concentration (30 mg/dL).[52] *Pasteurella multocida* meningoencephalomyelitis in a kitten was characterized by marked neutrophilic pleocytosis (981 cells/μL) with mild protein elevation (31 mg/dL) and rare extracellular and intracellular bacterial rods.[53]

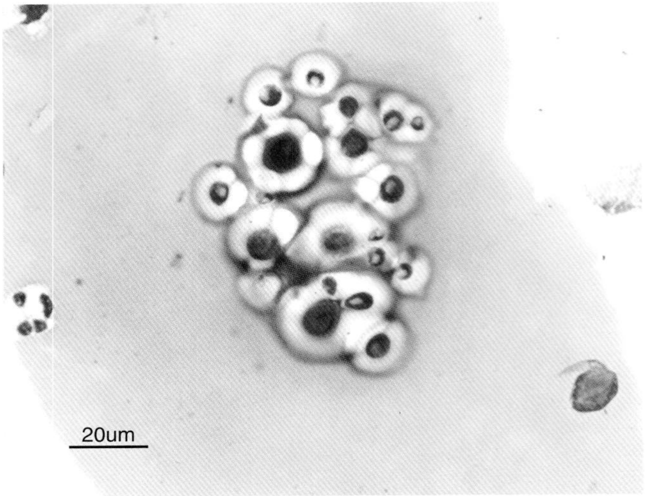

Figure 14-10 Cryptococcosis. Numerous yeasts show a thick clear capsule. Narrow-based budding is also evident. (Wright-Giemsa stain.)

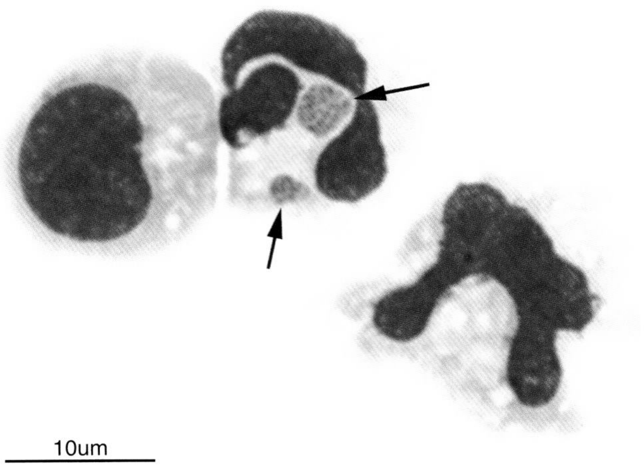

Figure 14-11 Cerebrospinal fluid from a dog with ehrlichiosis. Two ehrlichia morulae are evident in the central cell (*arrows*).

Bacterial culture and sensitivity testing are recommended but may have false-negative results if organisms are not circulating in the extracellular space or if prior antibiotic therapy had been given. Serology and CSF-PCR (using organism-specific or universal bacterial [UB] PCR), are recommended.[28,53]

Cryptococcosis in Dogs: *Cryptococcus* spp. are a large genus of systemic dimorphic fungi with a predilection for CNS tissue, which is infected hematogenously or via direct penetration of the cribriform plate. Only two species at this time are medically important: (1) *Cryptococcus neoformans* (var. *neoformans* and var. *grubii*) and (2) *Cryptococcus gattii*. In a recent study of 31 dogs with cryptococcosis, 68% had CNS infection, with neurologic signs being the most common reason for presentation.[54] Dogs and cats with cryptococcosis typically have pleocytoses and elevated protein concentrations, but pleocytoses may be variably neutrophilic, eosinophilic, mononuclear, or mixed. In a recent study of 15 dogs with CNS cryptococcosis, organisms were found in 11 of 15 CSF samples (see Figure 14-9 and Figure 14-10).[55] All affected dogs had pleocytoses that were mixed to mononuclear, whereas cats tended to have neutrophilic pleocytoses.[55] Of the samples, 11 of 12 also had increased protein concentrations (mean 494 mg/dL), which were significantly higher than in cats of the same study (mean 45 mg/dL).[55] Capsular antigen latex agglutination testing on serum or CSF is highly sensitive and specific and is recommended if cryptococcosis is suspected but organisms are not visualized cytologically.[56] This test may be negative if disease is present but localized (i.e., within the respiratory tract), so appropriate clinical signs should guide testing. Culture of CSF may also be helpful and may distinguish *C. neoformans* from *C. gattii* with the use of selective media. The finding of inflammatory foci on MRI may be supportive of the presence of fungal disease; cryptococcosis may result in mass lesions, meningitis, or pseudocyst formation.

Cryptococcosis in Cats: Cryptococcosis is the most common systemic fungal disease of cats and is believed to infect the CNS less frequently than in the dog. A recent study found that 42% of 62 cats with cryptococcosis had CNS infection, but respiratory signs were still a more common reason for presentation.[54] Mild to marked neutrophilic or mononuclear pleocytosis may occur, with variable and occasionally normal protein concentrations.[4] A study of cats with CNS cryptococcosis showed organisms in 9 of 11 of the CSF samples and a majority of cases (9 of 10) had neutrophilic pleocytosis and increased protein concentration (8 of 10).[55] Eosinophilic pleocytosis may also occur. Capsular antigen latex agglutination testing on serum or CSF is recommended for confirmation of *Cryptococcus* spp. infection, with rare false-negative reactions if disease is highly localized.

Histoplasmosis: *Histoplasma capsulatum* is a systemic dimorphic fungus that has been visualized in canine CSF and may be extracellular or within leukocytes.[57] A case report of an extradural *H. capsulatum* granuloma overlying spinal segments T11-L1 in a cat was associated with no cisternal CSF abnormalities.[58]

Aspergillosis: A study of dogs with systemic aspergillosis reported 4 of 8 CSF samples with neutrophilic pleocytosis (magnitude unspecified) and 1 of 8 with mononuclear reactivity.[59] Protein concentrations were not reported.[59]

Phaeohyphomycosis: *Phaeohyphomycosis* represents a group of darkly pigmented (typically brown, using routine stains) hyphal fungi, including neurotropic *Cladophialophora* spp. (formerly named *Cladosporidium* spp.) and *Xylohypha* spp. Acute infection may be characterized by mild to moderate neutrophilic pleocytosis and mild to moderately elevated protein concentration.[56]

Ehrlichiosis: Neutrophilic pleocytosis has been reported in cases of granulocytic *Ehrlichia* spp. in dogs (Figure 14-11).[60] Neurologic signs are uncommon in this disease, and affected dogs may display features ranging from ataxia to seizures.

Feline Infectious Peritonitis: Feline infectious peritonitis (FIP) has been traditionally linked to marked CSF changes, but current literature paints a somewhat more varied picture. One study of natural FIP infection showed

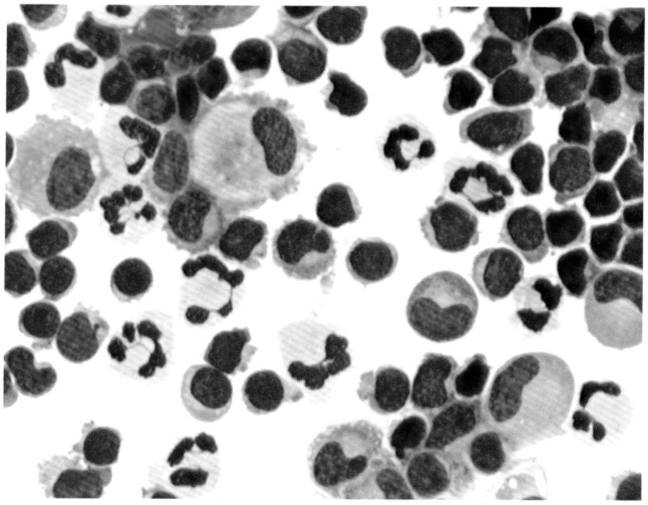

Figure 14-14 Granulomatous meningoencephalitis. Mixed mononuclear and neutrophilic inflammation. (Modified Wright stain. Original magnification 500×.)

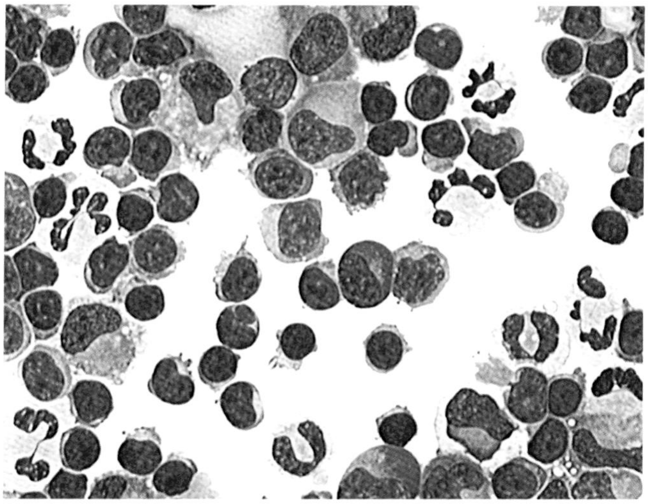

Figure 14-15 Granulomatous meningoencephalitis. Mixed mononuclear and neutrophilic inflammation. Note the presence of a plasma cell in the center. (Modified Wright stain. Original magnification 500×.)

Figure 14-15). In a study of 188 CSF samples from dogs with inflammatory neurologic diseases, marked pleocytosis (>1000 cells/μL) was found in cases of SRMA, bacterial encephalitis, or GME.[84] Pleocytosis may also be lymphocytic or neutrophilic.[11] CSF protein electrophoresis may be helpful, as several cases have been shown with increased β-globulin and γ-globulin fractions.[107]

Mixed Cell Pleocytosis: Most of the diseases described previously in this chapter may manifest as mixed cell pleocytoses, depending on the time interval between disease onset and CSF sampling, disease severity, and previous treatment administered. A mixed cell pleocytosis would be expected to occur during transition between different phases of the inflammatory response, where certain cells may predominate at specific times after injury.

Blastomycosis: Infection of the CNS by *Blastomyces dermatiditis* is typically rare and may involve chorioretinitis or focal cerebral granuloma in the cat.[108] A study of two dogs with systemic blastomycosis and neurologic signs showed mild mixed cell pleocytosis (8 cells/μL, mononuclear predominant; and 15 cells/μL, lymphocytic predominant).[109] Using CSF cytologic examination or culture to diagnose the organism may be unrewarding. Agar-gel immunodiffusion serologic testing has high sensitivity and specificity for canine antibodies and is recommended if appropriate clinical signs (respiratory signs or lymphadenopathy) are present.[56] Agar-gel immunodiffusion testing is less sensitive (25%–33%) in the cat based on a limited number of reports.[56] Urine antigen enzyme immunoassay (EIA) has good sensitivity for dogs and has been used successfully on at least one cat.[108] The EIA may also be performed on CSF. Cytology of nasal, pulmonary, or dermal lesions is more likely to yield direct visualization of organisms.

Neoplasia

Lymphoma: Lymphocytic pleocytosis of inflammatory origin may be difficult to distinguish from lymphoma exfoliating into the CSF (Figure 14-16). The size of lymphocytes and morphologic atypia may be helpful, although these may be challenging to differentiate from artifactual morphologic changes secondary to cytospin preparation. Cats with neoplasia may have lymphocytic pleocytoses (suggestive of lymphoma), mild to moderate mononuclear to mixed cell pleocytoses (suggestive of nonlymphoma tumors), or normal CSF. One study examined 6 cases of feline CNS or multifocal lymphoma which displayed pleocytoses of variable magnitude, absent to mildly elevated protein concentrations, and neoplastic cells visualized in 5 of 6 of the CSF samples.[4] In this study, 8 cats with CNS signs that were ultimately diagnosed with nonlymphoma tumors (e.g., meningioma, carcinoma, nerve sheath tumor) had mild CSF protein elevations and either normal TNCC (1 of 8) or mild to moderate mononuclear or mixed cell pleocytosis (7 of 8).[4] Another study of 11 cats with spinal lymphoma showed neoplastic cells visualized in one case, and hemodilution, ACD, or neutrophilic pleocytosis in the remainder of cases.[80] A case report of feline multiple myeloma involving lumbar vertebrae and associated soft tissues exhibited cisternal CSF with an elevated protein concentration of 290 mg/dL and mild pleocytosis (8 cells/μL) consisting of a majority of neoplastic plasma cells.[110] Diagnosis was further confirmed by abnormal urine protein electrophoresis and bone marrow aspiration.[110]

Histiocytic Malignancies: Malignant histiocytosis or histiocytic sarcoma tumor cells in canine CSF have been documented in two recent case reports; CSF cytology displayed marked mononuclear pleocytoses (>500 cells/μL) and mild to moderately elevated protein concentrations (<135 mg/dL).[111,112] Tumor cells phenotypically resembled macrophages, displayed multiple criteria of malignancy, and reacted positively to CD1c on immunocytochemistry, compatible with interstitial dendritic cell origin.[111,112] Necropsy was confirmatory and found no evidence of neoplasia outside of the CNS.[111,112] A case report of a gliomatosis cerebri (GC) neoplasm in a middle-aged poodle showed CSF with a mild lymphocytic pleocytosis (20 cells/μL) and protein

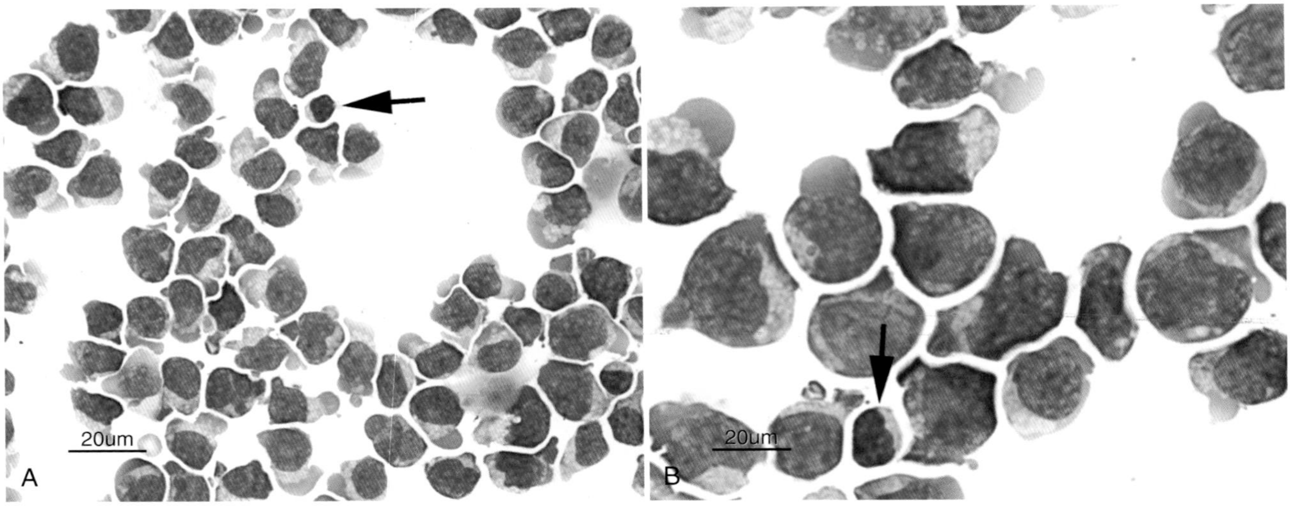

Figure 14-16 Cerebrospinal fluid samples from a dog with central nervous system lymphoma. A, Low magnification shows a cellular slide consisting almost entirely of large, pleomorphic lymphoid cells. A mature lymphocyte with condensed, mature chromatin is present (*arrow*). **B,** Higher magnification of the same slide. Lymphoid cells are large with pleomorphic nuclei and immature chromatin. Some cells have distinct nucleoli. A mature lymphocyte with condensed chromatin is present (*arrow*). (Wright-Giemsa stain.)

concentration elevation.[113] On histopathology, lymphocyte-like perivascular cuffing and meningitis were noted. Other case studies of canine GC have reported normal CSF or mild ACD.[114]

Meningioma: In a study of 56 dogs with intracranial meningioma, in which CSF analysis was performed, 29% had normal CSF, 45% had ACD, 27% had pleocytosis (2 of 3 of these neutrophilic pleocytosis; 1 of 3 unspecified), with the overall incidence of neutrophilic pleocytosis at 18%.[115] In this study, a positive correlation existed between elevated TNCC and anatomic localization of the lesion to the caudal (versus middle or rostral) portion of the cranial fossa, and no association between pleocytosis and necrosis within the lesion was found.[115] These findings contradict prior reports of a high percentage of abnormal CSF findings in meningioma, and the authors discuss that concurrent glucocorticoid therapy in some of the patients may have negatively biased the data.[12,115] A study of 26 dogs with spinal meningioma showed no cases with exfoliating tumor cells, 62% with mild pleocytosis up to 47 cells/μL (mean 11 cells/μL), and normal or variably elevated protein concentrations up to 836 mg/dL (mean 212 mg/dL).[116] Both cisternal and lumbar CSF samples were evaluated in this study and not found to be significantly different.[116] Interestingly, tumors of the lumbar region displayed higher mean TNCC and protein concentrations than did tumors of the cervical area (24 versus 4 cells/μL and 158 versus 98 mg/dL, respectively), which the authors postulate may be reflective of a higher number of lumbar CSF samples with proximity to the lesion.[116]

Other Neoplasms: A case report of canine CSF with 240 cells/μL was characterized by atypical neoplastic round cells that were confirmed on immunocytochemistry and immunohistochemistry to be from a metastatic mammary carcinoma.[117] Inflammatory cells were of low number and were of a mixed population.[117] A study of CSF from 25 dogs with choroid plexus tumors showed direct observation of tumor cells in 47% of the cases of carcinoma.[118] Mild to moderate mixed-cell pleocytosis was present in all cases of papilloma and in half of the carcinomas; when pleocytosis was present, no difference in magnitude existed between benign and malignant tumors.[118] All cases had elevated protein concentrations, with median concentration for carcinoma being significantly higher (108 mg/dL) than median concentration for papilloma (34 mg/dl).[118] A cutoff protein concentration of 80 mg/dL yielded a sensitivity of 67% and a specificity of 100% for detection of choroid plexus carcinomas.[118] Another case report of canine choroid plexus carcinoma had a mononuclear pleocytosis of 165 cells/μL, mildly elevated protein concentration of 30 mg/dL, and numerous tumor cells visualized.[119]

CENTRAL NERVOUS SYSTEM CYTOLOGIC EVALUATION

A rise in the availability of stereotactic brain biopsy has facilitated increased cytologic assessments of CNS lesions. This technique offers several advantages, although significant equipment investment and time to perfect techniques is required. Stereotactic biopsy often offers application accuracy for targeting lesions that approximate 3 mm or less in all directions. In one study, diagnostic accuracy of stereotactic biopsy specimens submitted for histopathology (i.e., agreement with specimens obtained via open approaches) exceeded 90%.[120] In experienced hands, stereotactic biopsy is believed to be a relatively low morbidity procedure. Cytologic interpretation of brain biopsy specimens acquired via stereotaxy or open approaches may be challenging and does require a tumor that exfoliates well, a surgeon willing to provide multiple samples, and a cytologist with expertise in this area.[121] A study of 42 canine and feline cases of biopsy or necropsy-confirmed CNS lesions showed squash-prep smear cytology to have 76% sensitivity in accurately determining

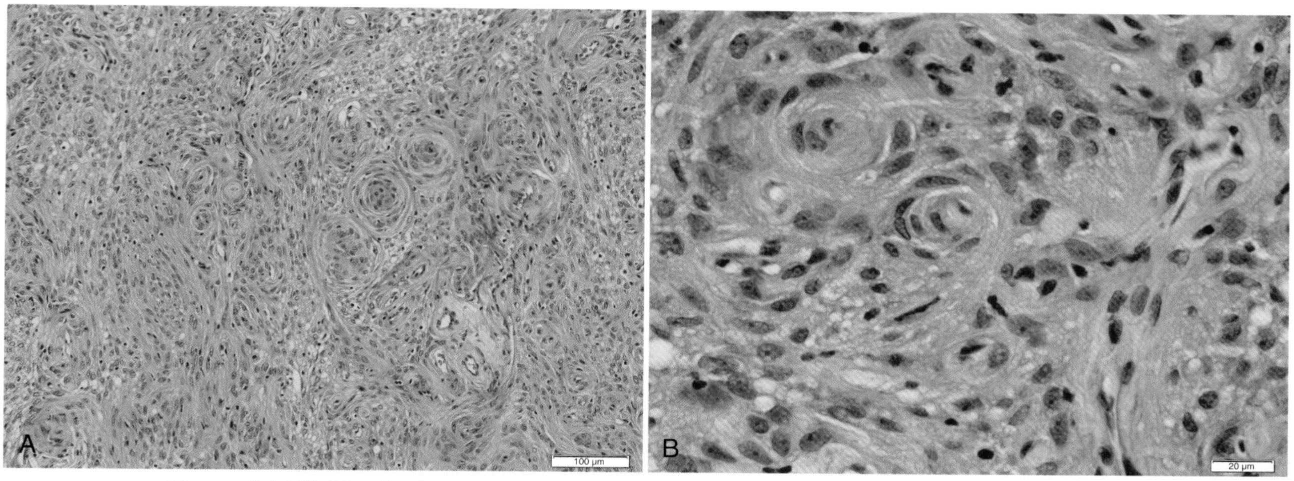

Figure 14-17 Meningioma. A, Low magnification shows spindle-shaped cells arranged in whorls and interweaving bundles. (Hematoxylin and eosin stain [H&E]. Original magnification 100×.) **B,** High magnification of spindle-shaped cells whorling around and weaving through bright pink supporting matrix. (H&E. Original magnification 400×.)

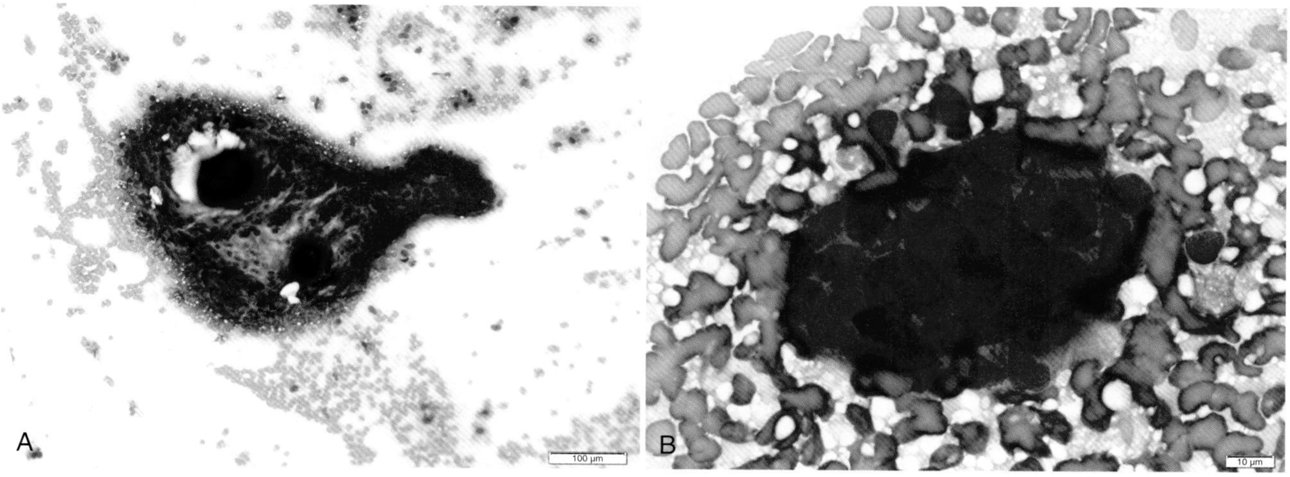

Figure 14-18 Meningioma. A, Low magnification view of spindle-shaped cells arranged in whorls around centrally located mineralized material (presumed psammoma body). (Diff-Quik. Original magnification 100×.) **B,** Spindle cells appear to pile up on one another. (Diff-Quik. Original magnification 600×.)

diagnosis, with an additional 14% of cases having partial correlation between cytology and histopathology. For the remaining 10% of cases, cytologic interpretation did not correlate with final diagnosis.[122] Cytologic interpretation of CNS lesions may be very difficult, and biopsy with histopathologic examination is recommended to confirm all diagnoses.

It is important for cytologic samples to be prepared in the same manner each time to avoid introducing additional cytologic variation for the pathologist to read through. Some authors recommend wet-fixation of tissues followed by staining with hematoxylin and eosin (H&E).[121] At the authors' institution, CNS cytologic samples are air-dried and stained with Diff-Quik or a modified Wright stain. The reader is referred elsewhere for a complete discussion of normal CNS cytology.[123] Clinical imaging findings, as well as signalment, should be considered carefully and may help the pathologist to formulate a list of potential differential diagnoses. It must be kept in mind that primary tumors may metastasize to the CNS, and these should be included on a differential list where appropriate.

Meningioma

Meningiomas are composed of neoplastic cells arising from the meningothelial cells of the leptomeninges of the CNS.[124] These tumors are the most common primary CNS tumors of dogs and cats.[125] Histologically, these neoplasms are classified into at least nine subtypes based on appearance and some tumors may be characterized by more than one pattern (Figure 14-17).[124] Cytologically, smears are often characterized by spindle-shaped cells draped around vessels and arranged in large whorling structures (Figure 14-18). Some

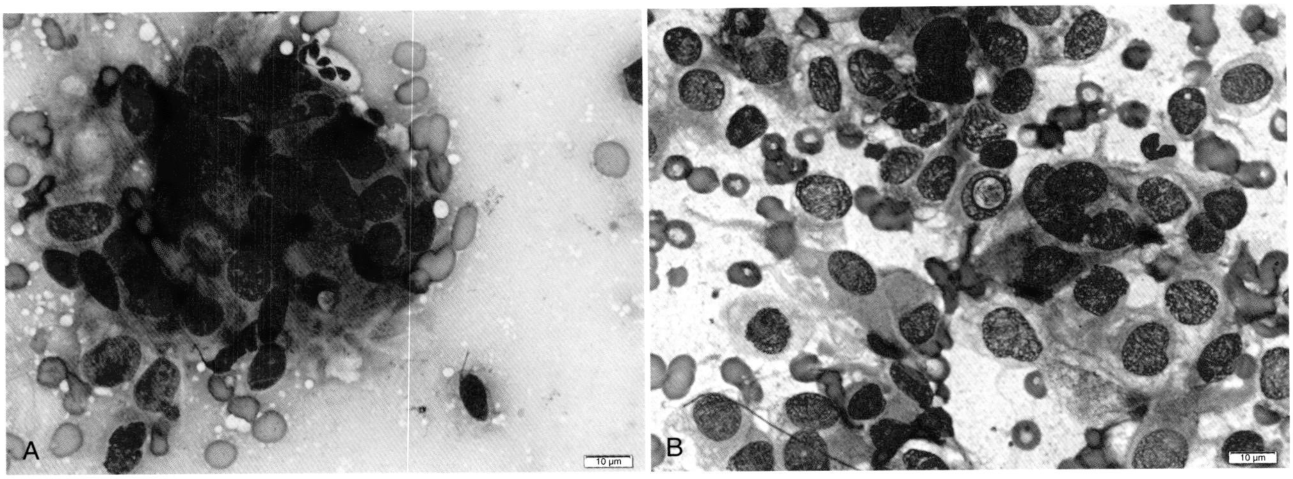

Figure 14-19 **Meningioma. A,** Cells contain plump oval to elongate nuclei and neutrophils are occasionally observed adjacent to cell aggregates. (Diff-Quik. Original magnification 600×.) **B,** Infrequent cells (*center*) display intranuclear cytoplasmic pseudoinclusions. (Diff-Quik. Original magnification 600×.)

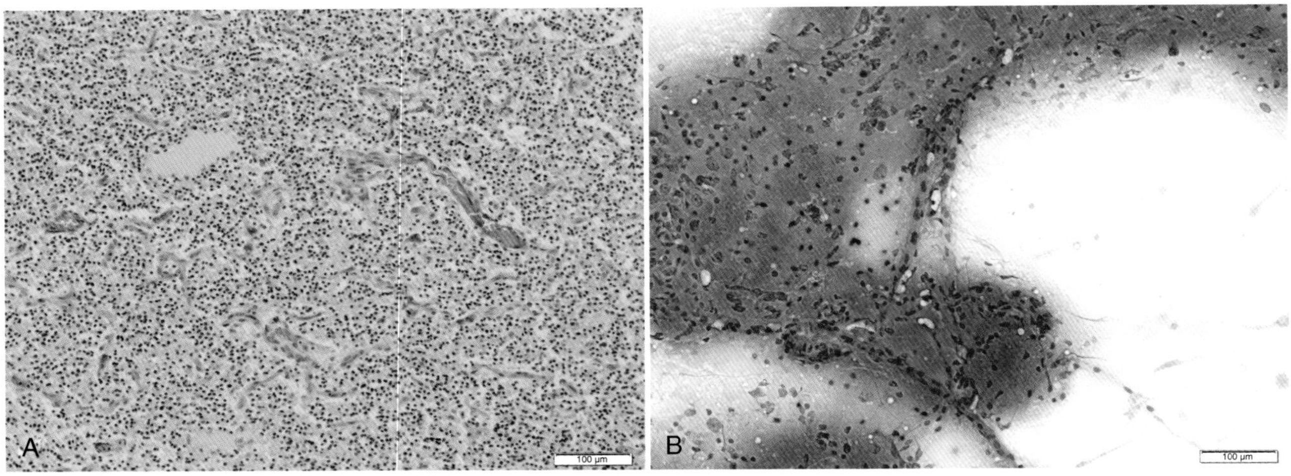

Figure 14-20 **Oligodendroglioma. A,** Tissue section showing round hyperchromatic nuclei surrounded by clear space admixed with branching capillaries and occasional lakes of basophilic mucin. (H&E. Original magnification 100×.) **B,** Numerous bare nuclei are seen admixed with purple fibrillar background material and branching capillary structures. (Diff-Quik. Original magnification 100×.)

cells may contain nuclei that display intranuclear cytoplasmic pseudoinclusions, but this is not a feature reliably seen on a majority of tumors (Figure 14-19).[126]

Glial Tumors

As a whole, this group represents the second most common primary CNS neoplasm seen in dogs and cats.[125] Glial tumors are more common than meningiomas in brachycephalic breeds.[125] Glial tumors arise from the supporting cells of the CNS. Astrocytomas are found most frequently in the cerebral hemispheres, although they have been reported to occur in various locations throughout the CNS.[124]

Astrocytoma: Astrocytomas arise from transformed astrocytes and are characterized cytologically by high cellularity, a high degree of nuclear pleomorphism, and fibrillar cytoplasmic processes.[124] Tumor cells will stain positively for glial fibrillary acid protein (GFAP).[124]

Oligodendroglioma: Oligodendrogliomas are derived from transformed oligodendrocytes and are found within the gray or white matter of the CNS, with the highest incidence in the cerebral hemispheres.[124] Cytologic preparations are characterized by large numbers of blood vessels surrounded by neoplastic cells (Figure 14-20).[124] Neoplastic oligodendrocytes have small amounts of eosinophilic cytoplasm surrounding uniformly round nuclei.[124]

Ependymoma

Ependymomas are derived from the ependymal lining cells found on the surface of the ventricular system of

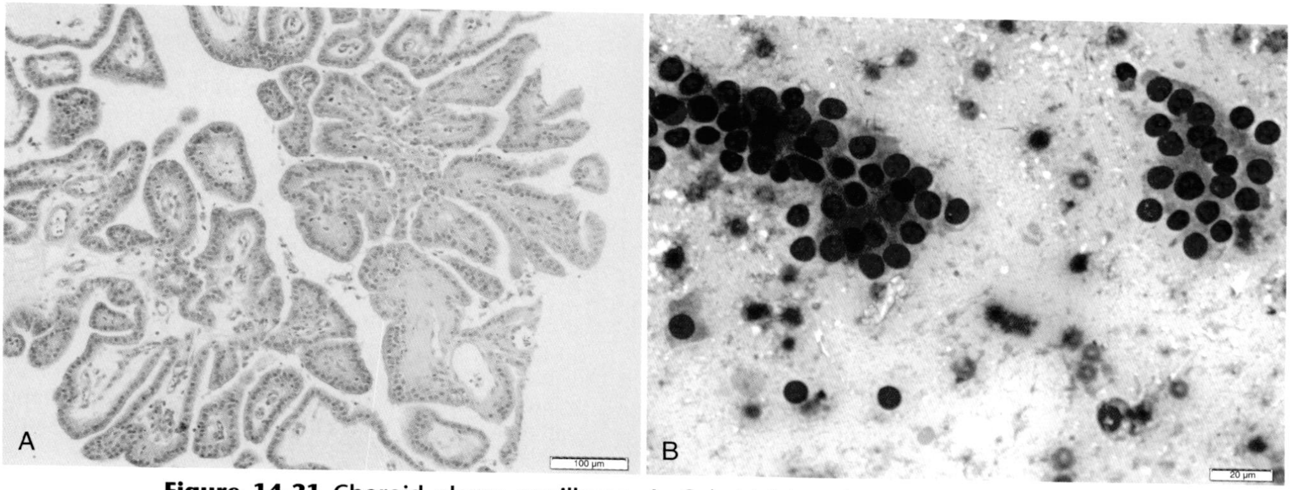

Figure 14-21 Choroid plexus papilloma. A, Cuboidal to columnar epithelial cells are arranged in papillary projections, which often contain small vessels. (H&E. Original magnification 100×.) **B,** Cuboidal epithelial cells are arranged in small sheets and papillary-like projections. (Diff-Quik. Original magnification 400×.)

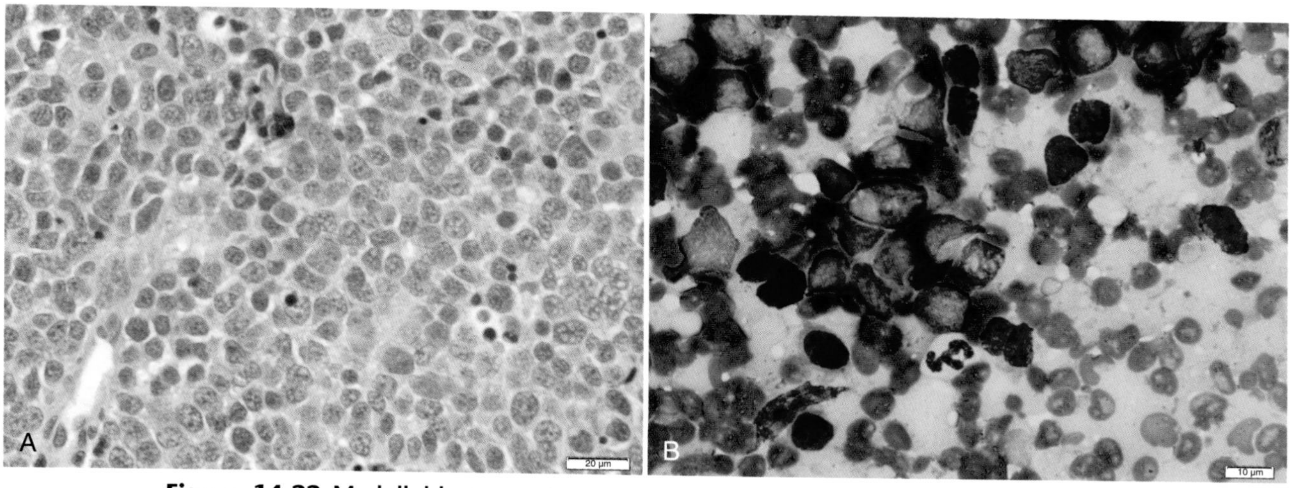

Figure 14-22 Medulloblastoma. A, Round cells are arranged in sheets. (H&E. Original magnification 400×.) **B,** Cells are large and round in shape with a high nucleus-to-cytoplasm (N:C) ratio and distinct cell borders. (Diff-Quik. Original magnification 600×.)

the brain and central canal of the spinal cord.[124] These tumors are rare and are found most often in the lateral ventricles.[124] Cytologically, smears are characterized by neoplastic cells palisading around branching vascular structures.[124] Cells are cuboidal to columnar in shape with high nucleus-to-cytoplasm (N:C) ratios and eccentrically placed nuclei.[124]

Choroid Plexus Tumor

Choroid plexus tumors arise from the modified ependymal lining cells that contribute to the production of CSF. They are more common in dogs than in cats.[124] Papillomas and carcinomas will have a very similar cytologic appearance and may only be reliably differentiated on the basis of histopathologic examination.[122] Cytologic preparations contain polygonal cells arranged in rafts, columns, or papillary projections around capillary structures (Figure 14-21).[124]

Medulloblastoma

Medulloblastoma arises within the cerebellum and is a type of primitive neuroectodermal tumor derived from a germinal neuroepithelial cell.[124] Cytologically, preparations are highly cellular, composed of individual round cells which are large in size and have moderate to high N:C ratios. The appearance of these cells is reminiscent of large lymphocytes or histiocytes (Figure 14-22).

Nephroblastoma

Nephroblastoma is a unique tumor arising in the spinal cord of young dogs (under 4 years of age), usually between the T10 and L2 spinal cord segments.[124] The cytologic appearance of this tumor has been described in a recent report and is characterized by three populations of cells: (1) high N:C ratio blastemal cells, (2) spindle-shaped mesenchymal cells, and (3) cuboidal epithelial cells.[127]

References

1. de Lahunta A, Glass E: *Veterinary neuroanatomy and clinical neurology*3 ed, St. Louis, MO, 2009, Saunders. 540.
2. Di Terlizzi R, Platt S: The function, composition and analysis of cerebrospinal fluid in companion animals: part I - function and composition, *Vet J* 172:422–431, 2006.
3. Bohn AA, Wills TB, West CL, et al: Cerebrospinal fluid analysis and magnetic resonance imaging in the diagnosis of neurologic disease in dogs: a retrospective study, *Vet Clin Pathol* 35:315–320, 2006.
4. Singh M, Foster DJ, Child G, et al: Inflammatory cerebrospinal fluid analysis in cats: Clinical diagnosis and outcome, *J Feline Med Surg* 7:77–93, 2005.
5. Gonçalves R, Platt SR, Llabrés-Díaz FJ, et al: Clinical and magnetic resonance imaging findings in 92 cats with clinical signs of spinal cord disease, *J Feline Med Surg* 11:53–59, 2009.
6. Lamb CR, Croson PJ, Cappello R, et al: Magnetic resonance imaging findings in 25 dogs with inflammatory cerebrospinal fluid, *Vet Radiol Ultrasound* 46:17–22, 2005.
7. Lester SJ, Malik R, Bartlett KH, et al: Cryptococcosis: update and emergence of *Cryptococcus gattii*, *Vet Clin Pathol* 40:4–17, 2011.
8. Oreskovic D, Klarica M: The formation of cerebrospinal fluid: nearly a hundred years of interpretations and misinterpretations, *Brain Res Rev* 64:241–262, 2010.
9. Kornegay JN: Cerebrospinal fluid collection, examination, and interpretation in dogs and cats, *Compend Contin Edu Practic Veterinarian* 3:85–90, 1981.
10. Elias A, Brown C: Cerebellomedullary cerebrospinal fluid collection in the dog, *Lab Anim* 37:457–458, 2008.
11. Di Terlizzi R, Platt SR: The function, composition and analysis of cerebrospinal fluid in companion animals: part II - analysis, *Vet J* 180:15–32, 2009.
12. Meinkoth JH, Crystal MA: Cerebrospinal Fluid Analysis. In Cowell RL, Tyler RD, Meinkoth JH, editors: *Diagnostic cytology and hematology of the dog and cat*, 2 ed, St. Louis, MO, 1999, Mosby.
13. Thomson CE, Kornegay JN, Stevens JB: Analysis of cerebrospinal fluid from the cerebellomedullary and lumbar cisterns of dogs with focal neurologic disease: 145 cases (1985-1987), *J Am Vet Med Assoc* 196:1841–1844, 1990.
14. Bailey CS, Higgins RJ: Comparison of total white blood cell count and total protein content of lumbar and cisternal cerebrospinal fluid of healthy dogs, *Am J Vet Res* 46:1162–1165, 1985.
15. Christopher MM: Bone marrow contamination of canine cerebrospinal fluid, *Vet Clin Pathol* 21:95–98, 1992.
16. Lujan Feliu-Pascual A, Garosi L, Dennis R, et al: Iatrogenic brainstem injury during cerebellomedullary cistern puncture, *Vet Radiol Ultrasound* 49:467–471, 2008.
17. Cellio BC: Collecting, processing, and preparing cerebrospinal fluid in dogs and cats, *Compend Continuing Edu Practic Veterinarian* 23:786–792, 2001.
18. Hoerlein BF: *Canine neurology: diagnosis and treatment*, St. Louis, MO, 1978, Saunders.
19. Fry MM, Vernau W, Kass PH, et al: Effects of time, initial composition, and stabilizing agents on the results of canine cerebrospinal fluid analysis, *Vet Clin Pathol* 35: 72–77, 2006.
20. Bienzle D, McDonnell JJ, Stanton JB: Analysis of cerebrospinal fluid from dogs and cats after 24 and 48 hours of storage, *J Am Vet Med Assoc* 216:1761–1764, 2000.
21. Nghiem PP, Schatzberg SJ: Conventional and molecular diagnostic testing for the acute neurologic patient, *J Vet Emerg Crit Care (San Antonio)* 20:46–61, 2010.
22. Jamison EM, Lumsden JH: Cerebrospinal fluid analysis in the dog: methodology and interpretation, *Semin Vet Med Surg (Small Animal)* 3:122–132, 1988.
23. Desnoyers M, Bedard C, Meinkoth JH, et al: Cerebrospinal fluid analysis. In Cowell RL, Tyler RD, Meinkoth JH, editors: *Diagnostic cytology and hematology of the dog and cat*, 3 ed, St. Louis, MO, 2008, Mosby, pp 215–234.
24. Ruotsalo K, Poma R, da Costa RC, et al: Evaluation of the ADVIA 120 for analysis of canine cerebrospinal fluid, *Vet Clin Pathol* 37:242–248, 2008.
25. Becker M, Bauer N, Moritz A: Automated flow cytometric cell count and differentiation of canine cerebrospinal fluid cells using the ADVIA 2120, *Vet Clin Pathol* 37:344–352, 2008.
26. Behr S, Trumel C, Cauzinille L, et al: High resolution protein electrophoresis of 100 paired canine cerebrospinal fluid and serum, *J Vet Intern Med/Am Coll Vet Intern Med* 20:657–662, 2006.
27. Radaelli ST, Platt SR: Bacterial meningoencephalomyelitis in dogs: a retrospective study of 23 cases (1990-1999), *J Vet Intern Med* 16:159–163, 2002.
28. Messer JS, Wagner SO, Baumwart RD, et al: A case of canine streptococcal meningoencephalitis diagnosed using universal bacterial polymerase chain reaction assay, *J Am Anim Hosp Assoc* 44:205–209, 2008.
29. Rand JS, Parent J, Percy D, et al: Clinical, cerebrospinal fluid, and histological data from thirty-four cats with primary noninflammatory disease of the central nervous system, *Can Vet J /La revue veterinaire canadienne* 35:174–181, 1994.
30. Indrieri RJ, Holliday TA, Keen CL: Critical evaluation of creatine phosphokinase in cerebrospinal fluid of dogs with neurologic disease, *Am J Vet Res* 41:1299–1303, 1980.
31. Witsberger TH, Levine JM, Fosgate GT, et al: Associations between cerebrospinal fluid biomarkers and long-term neurologic outcome in dogs with acute intervertebral disk herniation, *J Am Vet Med Assoc* 240:555–562, 2012.
32. Pancotto T, Rossmeisl JH Jr, Panciera DL, et al: Blood-brain-barrier disruption in chronic canine hypothyroidism, *Vet Clin Pathol* 39:485–493, 2010.
33. Oji T, Kamishina H, Cheeseman JA, et al: Measurement of myelin basic protein in the cerebrospinal fluid of dogs with degenerative myelopathy, *Vet Clin Pathol* 36:281–284, 2007.
34. Levine GJ, Levine JM, Witsberger TH, et al: Cerebrospinal fluid myelin basic protein as a prognostic biomarker in dogs with thoracolumbar intervertebral disk herniation, *J Vet Intern Med* 24:890–896, 2010.
35. Munana KR, Saito M, Hoshi F: Beta-2-microglobulin levels in the cerebrospinal fluid of normal dogs and dogs with neurological disease, *Vet Clin Pathol* 36:173–178, 2007.
36. Holt DE, Washabau RJ, Djali S, et al: Cerebrospinal fluid glutamine, tryptophan, and tryptophan metabolite concentrations in dogs with portosystemic shunts, *Am J Vet Res* 63:1167–1171, 2002.
37. Brown DC, Perkowski S: Oxytocin content of the cerebrospinal fluid of dogs and its relationship to pain induced by spinal cord compression, *Vet Surg* 27:607–611, 1998.
38. Podell M, Hadjiconstantinou M: Cerebrospinal fluid gamma-aminobutyric acid and glutamate values in dogs with epilepsy, *Am J Vet Res* 58:451–456, 1997.
39. Chrisman CL: Cerebrospinal fluid analysis, *Vet Clin North Am Small Anim Pract* 22:781–810, 1992.
40. Wessmann A, Volk HA, Chandler K, et al: Significance of surface epithelial cells in canine cerebrospinal fluid and relationship to central nervous system disease, *Vet Clin Pathol* 39:358–364, 2010.

41. Bauer NB, Bassett H, O'Neill EJ, et al: Cerebrospinal fluid from a 6-year-old dog with severe neck pain, *Vet Clin Pathol* 35:123–125, 2006.
42. Zabolotzky SM, Vernau KM, Kass PH, et al: Prevalence and significance of extracellular myelin-like material in canine cerebrospinal fluid, *Vet Clin Pathol* 39:90–95, 2010.
43. Whittaker DE, English K, McGonnell IM, et al: Evaluation of cerebrospinal fluid in Cavalier King Charles Spaniel dogs diagnosed with Chiari-like malformation with or without concurrent syringomyelia, *J Vet Diagn* 23:302–307, 2011.
44. Hurtt AE, Smith MO: Effects of iatrogenic blood contamination on results of cerebrospinal fluid analysis in clinically normal dogs and dogs with neurologic disease, *J Am Vet Med Assoc* 211:866–867, 1997.
45. Rand JS, Parent J, Jacobs R, et al: Reference intervals for feline cerebrospinal fluid: cell counts and cytologic features, *Am J Vet Res* 51:1044–1048, 1990.
46. Sweeney CR, Russell GE: Differences in total protein concentration, nucleated cell count, and red blood cell count among sequential samples of cerebrospinal fluid from horses, *J Am Vet Med Assoc* 217:54–57, 2000.
47. Wilson JW, Stevens JB: Effects of blood contamination on cerebrospinal fluid analysis, *J Am Vet Med Assoc* 171:256–258, 1977.
48. Doyle C, Solano-Gallego L: Cytologic interpretation of canine cerebrospinal fluid samples with low total nucleated cell concentration, with and without blood contamination, *Vet Clin Pathol* 38:392–396, 2009.
49. Rand JS, Parent J, Percy D, et al: Clinical, cerebrospinal fluid, and histological data from twenty-seven cats with primary inflammatory disease of the central nervous system, *Can Vet J / La revue veterinaire canadienne* 35:103–110, 1994.
50. Tipold A, Stein VM: Inflammatory diseases of the spine in small animals, *Vet Clin North Am Small Anim Pract* 40:871–879, 2010.
51. Bach JF, Mahony OM, Tidwell AS, et al: Brain abscess and bacterial endocarditis in a Kerry Blue Terrier with a history of immune-mediated thrombocytopenia, *J Vet Emerg Crit Care* 17:409–415, 2007.
52. Oliver JA, Llabres-Diaz FJ, Gould DJ, et al: Central nervous system infection with *Staphylococcus intermedius* secondary to retrobulbar abscessation in a dog, *Vet Ophthalmol* 12:333–337, 2009.
53. Messer JS, Kegge SJ, Cooper ES, et al: Meningoencephalomyelitis caused by *Pasteurella multocida* in a cat, *J Vet Intern Med* 20:1033–1036, 2006.
54. Trivedi SR, Sykes JE, Cannon MS, et al: Clinical features and epidemiology of cryptococcosis in cats and dogs in California: 93 cases (1988-2010), *J Am Vet Med Assoc* 239:357–369, 2011.
55. Sykes JE, Sturges BK, Cannon MS, et al: Clinical signs, imaging features, neuropathology, and outcome in cats and dogs with central nervous system cryptococcosis from California, *J Vet Intern Med* 24:1427–1438, 2010.
56. Lavely J, Lipsitz D: Fungal infections of the central nervous system in the dog and cat, *Clin Tech Small Anim Pract* 20:212–219, 2005.
57. Clinkenbeard KD, Cowell RL, Tyler RD: Disseminated histoplasmosis in cats: 12 cases (1981-1986), *J Am Vet Med Assoc* 190:1445–1448, 1987.
58. Vinayak A, Kerwin SC, Pool RR: Treatment of thoracolumbar spinal cord compression associated with Histoplasma capsulatum infection in a cat, *J Am Vet Med Assoc* 230:1018–1023, 2007.
59. Schultz RM, Johnson EG, Wisner ER, et al: Clinicopathologic and diagnostic imaging characteristics of systemic aspergillosis in 30 dogs, *J Vet Intern Med* 22:851–859, 2008.
60. Meinkoth JH, Hoover JP, Cowell RL, et al: Ehrlichiosis in a dog with seizures and nonregenerative anemia, *J Am Vet Med Assoc* 195:1754–1755, 1989.
61. Foley JE, Lapointe JM, Koblik P, et al: Diagnostic features of clinical neurologic feline infectious peritonitis, *J Vet Intern Med* 12:415–423, 1998.
62. Boettcher IC, Steinberg T, Matiasek K, et al: Use of anti-coronavirus antibody testing of cerebrospinal fluid for diagnosis of feline infectious peritonitis involving the central nervous system in cats, *J Am Vet Med Assoc* 230:199–205, 2007.
63. Steinberg TA, Boettcher IC, Matiasek K, et al: Use of albumin quotient and IgG index to differentiate blood- vs brain-derived proteins in the cerebrospinal fluid of cats with feline infectious peritonitis, *Vet Clin Pathol* 37:207–216, 2008.
64. Kent M: The cat with neurological manifestations of systemic disease. Key conditions impacting on the CNS, *J Feline Med Surg* 11:395–407, 2009.
65. Lappin MR: Feline toxoplasmosis: interpretation of diagnostic test results, *Semin Vet Med Surg (Small Anim)* 11:154–160, 1996.
66. Lavely JA, Vernau KM, Vernau W, et al: Spinal epidural empyema in seven dogs, *Vet Surg* 35:176–185, 2006.
67. Bisby TM, Holman PJ, Pitoc GA, et al: *Sarcocystis* sp. encephalomyelitis in a cat, *Vet Clin Pathol* 39:105–112, 2010.
68. Kent M, Platt SR, Rech RR, et al: Multisystemic infection with an *Acanthamoeba* sp. in a dog, *J Am Vet Med Assoc* 238:1476–1481, 2011.
69. Hodge PJ, Kelers K, Gasser RB, et al: Another case of canine amoebic meningoencephalitis—the challenges of reaching a rapid diagnosis, *Parasitol Res* 108:1069–1073, 2011.
70. Dvir E, Perl S, Loeb E, et al: Spinal intramedullary aberrant *Spirocerca lupi* migration in 3 dogs, *J Vet Intern Med* 21:860–864, 2007.
71. Lowrie M, Penderis J, McLaughlin M, et al: Steroid responsive meningitis-arteritis: a prospective study of potential disease markers, prednisolone treatment, and long-term outcome in 20 dogs (2006-2008), *J Vet Intern Med* 23:862–870, 2009.
72. Schwartz M, Puff C, Stein VM, et al: Pathogenetic factors for excessive IgA production: Th2-dominated immune response in canine steroid-responsive meningitis-arteritis, *Vet J* 187:260–266, 2011.
73. Lowrie M, Penderis J, Eckersall PD, et al: The role of acute phase proteins in diagnosis and management of steroid-responsive meningitis arteritis in dogs, *Vet J* 182:125–130, 2009.
74. Bathen-Noethen A, Carlson R, Menzel D, et al: Concentrations of acute-phase proteins in dogs with steroid responsive meningitis-arteritis, *J Vet Intern Med* 22:1149–1156, 2008.
75. Windsor RC, Vernau KM, Sturges BK, et al: Lumbar cerebrospinal fluid in dogs with type I intervertebral disc herniation, *J Vet Intern Med / Am Coll Vet Intern Med* 22:954–960, 2008.
76. De Risio L, Adams V, Dennis R, et al: Magnetic resonance imaging findings and clinical associations in 52 dogs with suspected ischemic myelopathy, *J Vet Intern Med* 21:1290–1298, 2007.
77. Cauzinille L: Fibrocartilaginous embolism in dogs, *Vet Clin North Am Small Anim Pract* 30:155–167, 2000. vii.
78. Mikszewski JS, Van Winkle TJ, Troxel MT: Fibrocartilaginous embolic myelopathy in five cats, *J Am Anim Hosp Assoc* 42:226–233, 2006.
79. Marks SL, Lipsitz D, Vernau KM, et al: Reversible encephalopathy secondary to thiamine deficiency in 3 cats

ingesting commercial diets, *J Vet Intern Med* 25:949–953, 2011.
80. Marioni-Henry K, Van Winkle TJ, Smith SH, et al: Tumors affecting the spinal cord of cats: 85 cases (1980-2005), *J Am Vet Med Assoc* 232:237–243, 2008.
81. Shiel RE, Mooney CT, Brennan SF, et al: Clinical and clinicopathological features of non-suppurative meningoencephalitis in young greyhounds in Ireland, *Vet Rec* 167:333–337, 2010.
82. Windsor RC, Sturges BK, Vernau KM, et al: Cerebrospinal fluid eosinophilia in dogs, *J Vet Intern Med / Am Coll Vet Intern Med* 23:275–281, 2009.
83. Gupta A, Gumber S, Bauer RW, et al: What is your diagnosis? Cerebrospinal fluid from a dog. Eosinophilic pleocytosis due to protothecosis, *Vet Clin Pathol* 40:105–106, 2011.
84. Tipold A: Diagnosis of inflammatory and infectious diseases of the central nervous system in dogs: a retrospective study, *J Vet Intern Med* 9:304–314, 1995.
85. Tarlow JM, Rudloff E, Lichtenberger M, et al: Emergency presentations of 4 dogs with suspected neurologic toxoplasmosis, *J Vet Emerg Crit Care* 15:119–127, 2005.
86. Schatzberg SJ, Haley NJ, Barr SC, et al: Use of a multiplex polymerase chain reaction assay in the antemortem diagnosis of toxoplasmosis and neosporosis in the central nervous system of cats and dogs, *Am J Vet Res* 64:1507–1513, 2003.
87. Saengseesom W, Mitmoonpitak C, Kasempimolporn S, et al: Real-time PCR analysis of dog cerebrospinal fluid and saliva samples for ante-mortem diagnosis of rabies, *Southeast Asian J Tropic Med Public Health* 38:53–57, 2007.
88. Amude AM, Alfieri AA, Balarin MR, et al: Cerebrospinal fluid from a 7-month-old dog with seizure-like episodes, *Vet Clin Pathol* 35:119–122, 2006.
89. Amude AM, Alfieri AA, Alfieri AF: Clinicopathological findings in dogs with distemper encephalomyelitis presented without characteristic signs of the disease, *Res Vet Sci* 82:416–422, 2007.
90. Haines DM, Martin KM, Chelack BJ, et al: Immunohistochemical detection of canine distemper virus in haired skin, nasal mucosa, and footpad epithelium: a method for antemortem diagnosis of infection, *J Vet Diagn Invest* 11:396–399, 1999.
91. Johnson GC, Fenner WR, Krakowka S: Production of immunoglobulin G and increased antiviral antibody in cerebrospinal fluid of dogs with delayed-onset canine distemper viral encephalitis, *J Neuroimmunol* 17:237–251, 1988.
92. Greer KA, Wong AK, Liu H, et al: Necrotizing meningoencephalitis of Pug dogs associates with dog leukocyte antigen class II and resembles acute variant forms of multiple sclerosis, *Tissue Antigens* 76:110–118, 2010.
93. Higgins RJ, Dickinson PJ, Kube SA, et al: Necrotizing meningoencephalitis in five Chihuahua dogs, *Vet Pathol* 45:336–346, 2008.
94. Levine JM, Fosgate GT, Porter B, et al: Epidemiology of necrotizing meningoencephalitis in Pug dogs, *J Vet Intern Med* 22:961–968, 2008.
95. Williams KJ, Summers BA, de Lahunta A: Cerebrospinal cuterebriasis in cats and its association with feline ischemic encephalopathy, *Vet Pathol* 35:330–343, 1998.
96. Altay UM, Skerritt GC, Hilbe M, et al: Feline cerebrovascular disease: clinical and histopathologic findings in 16 cats, *J Am Anim Hosp Assoc* 47:89–97, 2011.
97. Coates JR, March PA, Oglesbee M, et al: Clinical characterization of a familial degenerative myelopathy in Pembroke Welsh Corgi dogs, *J Vet Intern Med* 21: 1323–1331, 2007.
98. Gaitero L, Anor S, Montoliu P, et al: Detection of *Neospora caninum* tachyzoites in canine cerebrospinal fluid, *J Vet Intern Med* 20:410–414, 2006.
99. Galgut BI, Janardhan KS, Grondin TM, et al: Detection of Neospora caninum tachyzoites in cerebrospinal fluid of a dog following prednisone and cyclosporine therapy, *Vet Clin Pathol* 39:386–390, 2010.
100. Garosi L, Dawson A, Couturier J, et al: Necrotizing cerebellitis and cerebellar atrophy caused by *Neospora caninum* infection: magnetic resonance imaging and clinicopathologic findings in seven dogs, *J Vet Intern Med* 24:571–578, 2010.
101. Negrin A, Cherubini GB, Steeves E: Angiostrongylus vasorum causing meningitis and detection of parasite larvae in the cerebrospinal fluid of a pug dog, *J Small Anim Pract* 49:468–471, 2008.
102. Cross JR, Rossmeisl JH, Maggi RG, et al: *Bartonella*-associated meningoradiculoneuritis and dermatitis or panniculitis in 3 dogs, *J Vet Intern Med* 22:674–678, 2008.
103. Marchetti V, Lubas G, Baneth G, et al: Hepatozoonosis in a dog with skeletal involvement and meningoencephalomyelitis, *Vet Clin Pathol* 38:121–125, 2009.
104. Widmer WR, Blevins WE, Cantwell HD, et al: Cerebrospinal fluid response following metrizamide myelography in normal dogs: effects of routine myelography and postmyelographic removal of contrast medium, *Vet Clin Pathol* 19:66–76, 1990.
105. Widmer WR, DeNicola DB, Blevins WE, et al: Cerebrospinal fluid changes after iopamidol and metrizamide myelography in clinically normal dogs, *Am J Vet Res* 53:396–401, 1992.
106. Johnson GC, Fuciu DM, Fenner WR, et al: Transient leakage across the blood-cerebrospinal fluid barrier after intrathecal metrizamide administration to dogs, *Am J Vet Res* 46:1303–1308, 1985.
107. Sorjonen DC, Golden DL, Levesque DC, et al: Cerebrospinal fluid protein electrophoresis: a clinical evaluation of a previously reported diagnostic technique, *Prog Vet Neurol* 2:261–267, 1991.
108. Smith JR, Legendre AM, Thomas WB, et al: Cerebral *Blastomyces dermatitidis* infection in a cat, *J Am Vet Med Assoc* 231:1210–1214, 2007.
109. Lipitz L, Rylander H, Forrest LJ, et al: Clinical and magnetic resonance imaging features of central nervous system blastomycosis in 4 dogs, *J Vet Intern Med* 24:1509–1514, 2010.
110. Appel SL, Moens NM, Abrams-Ogg AC, et al: Multiple myeloma with central nervous system involvement in a cat, *J Am Vet Med Assoc* 233:743–747, 2008.
111. Tzipory L, Vernau KM, Sturges BK, et al: Antemortem diagnosis of localized central nervous system histiocytic sarcoma in 2 dogs, *J Vet Intern Med / Am Coll Vet Intern Med* 23:369–374, 2009.
112. Zimmerman K, Almy F, Carter L, et al: Cerebrospinal fluid from a 10-year-old dog with a single seizure episode, *Vet Clin Pathol* 35:127–131, 2006.
113. Galan A, Guil-Luna S, Millan Y, et al: Oligodendroglial gliomatosis cerebri in a poodle, *Vet Comparat Oncol* 8:254–262, 2010.
114. Porter B, de Lahunta A, Summers B: Gliomatosis cerebri in six dogs, *Vet Pathol* 40:97–102, 2003.
115. Dickinson PJ, Sturges BK, Kass PH, et al: Characteristics of cisternal cerebrospinal fluid associated with intracranial meningiomas in dogs: 56 cases (1985-2004), *J Am Vet Med Assoc* 228:564–567, 2006.
116. Petersen SA, Sturges BK, Dickinson PJ, et al: Canine intraspinal meningiomas: imaging features,

histopathologic classification, and long-term outcome in 34 dogs, *J Vet Intern Med* 22:946–953, 2008.
117. Behling-Kelly E, Petersen S, Muthuswamy A, et al: Neoplastic pleocytosis in a dog with metastatic mammary carcinoma and meningeal carcinomatosis, *Vet Clin Pathol* 39:247–252, 2010.
118. Westworth DR, Dickinson PJ, Vernau W, et al: Choroid plexus tumors in 56 dogs (1985-2007), *J Vet Intern Med* 22:1157–1165, 2008.
119. Pastorello A, Constantino-Casas F, Archer J: Choroid plexus carcinoma cells in the cerebrospinal fluid of a Staffordshire Bull Terrier, *Vet Clin Pathol* 39:505–510, 2010.
120. Koblik PD, LeCouteur RA, Higgins RJ, et al: CT-guided brain biopsy using a modified Pelorus Mark III stereotactic system: experience with 50 dogs, *Vet Radiol Ultrasound* 40:434–440, 1999.
121. Vernau KM, Higgins RJ, Bollen AW, et al: Primary canine and feline nervous system tumors: intraoperative diagnosis using the smear technique, *Vet Pathol* 38:47–57, 2001.
122. De Lorenzi D, Mandara MT, Tranquillo M, et al: Squash-prep cytology in the diagnosis of canine and feline nervous system lesions: a study of 42 cases, *Vet Clin Pathol* 35:208–214, 2006.
123. Raskin RE, Meyer D: *Canine and feline cytology—E-Book: a color atlas and interpretation guide*, Philadelphia, PA, 2009, Elsevier Health Sciences.
124. Meuten DJ: *Tumors in domestic animals*, Ames, IA, 2002, Iowa State University Press.
125. Summers BA, Cummings JF, DeLahunta A: *Veterinary neuropathology*, St. Louis, MO, 1995, Mosby.
126. Harms NJ, Dickinson RM, Nibblett BM, et al: What is your diagnosis? Intracranial mass in a dog, *Vet Clin Pathol* 38:537–540, 2009.
127. De Lorenzi D, Baroni M, Mandara MT: A true "triphasic" pattern: thoracolumbar spinal tumor in a young dog, *Vet Clin Pathol* 36:200–203, 2007.

CHAPTER 15

Effusions: Abdominal, Thoracic, and Pericardial

Amy C. Valenciano, Tara P. Arndt and Theresa E. Rizzi

The three primary body cavities are (1) thoracic (pleural), (2) abdominal (peritoneal), and (3) pericardial. In health, these cavities contain a small amount of fluid that acts as a lubricant allowing the free motion of internal organs against one another and body cavity walls. The body cavities are lined by mesothelial cells, which are specialized cells that play an active role in the homeostasis of these potential spaces. *Body cavity effusion* is defined as the abnormal accumulation of fluid of any type.

An effusion is not a disease in itself but, rather, an indication of a pathologic process in the fluid production and removal system or an accumulation from an ectopic source. Fluid analysis, including cytologic evaluation and classification, is a quick, easy, inexpensive, and relatively safe way to obtain useful information in the diagnosis, prognosis, and treatment of diseases resulting in thoracic, abdominal, and pericardial fluid accumulations. Common causes of body cavity effusions include trauma, neoplasia, cardiovascular compromise, metabolic disorders, altered Starling's forces, ruptured urinary or gall bladder, ruptured vessels or lymphatics, and bleeding diathesis, as well as infectious and inflammatory diseases.

The numerous etiologies of thoracic, abdominal, and pericardial effusions will be categorized in the section titled "General Classification of Effusions" and explored in detail in the section titled "Specific Disorders Causing Effusions."

THORACIC AND ABDOMINAL EFFUSIONS

Dogs and cats with thoracic effusions often show dyspnea as the most common clinical sign.[1,2] Other clinical signs include a crouched, sternal recumbent position with extension of the head and neck; open-mouth breathing; tachypnea; and forceful abdominal respiration. Cyanosis may be present. With milder effusions, lethargy and lack of stamina may be the only clinical signs. Animals, especially cats, with mild to moderately severe effusions often adapt by decreasing their activity, thus concealing their illness until it is severe. With chronic pleural effusion, dogs and cats may present with coughing as the only clinical sign.[1] Physical findings with pleural effusion depend on the amount of fluid present but include muffled heart and lung sounds.

Patients with abdominal effusions may present for lethargy, weakness, and abdominal distension—the latter may be mistaken by pet owners as weight gain, gas, or ingesta. Physical findings with abdominal effusions include a fluid wave during ballottement in high-volume effusions and pain if peritonitis is present.

PERICARDIAL EFFUSIONS

Pericardial effusions in the cat are often secondary to congestive heart failure or feline infectious peritonitis but may be caused by primary cardiac neoplasia such as lymphoma.[3] The most common causes of pericardial effusion in the dog include cardiac neoplasia and idiopathic pericardial effusion.[4,5] Hemangiosarcoma is the most common cardiac neoplasm reported, but other reported neoplasms include chemodectoma, lymphoma, and thyroid carcinoma.[4] Other less common causes include cardiac disease, inflammatory or infectious diseases, trauma, coagulopathy, and congenital defects.

Clinical signs include weakness, lethargy, exercise intolerance, collapse, and coughing. Physical findings with pericardial effusion vary with the volume of fluid present but include muffled heart sounds, weak pulses, and pallor.

COLLECTION TECHNIQUES

For all fluids collected, a portion of the fluid (2–3 milliliters [mL]) should be placed in a sterile EDTA lavender top Vacutainer (Becton Dickinson Vacutainer Systems, Franklin Lakes, NJ) tube for cell counts, protein analysis, and cytologic evaluation. Ethylenediaminetetraacetic acid (EDTA) prevents blood clots from forming in the fluid in the event of iatrogenic blood contamination. A second portion (2–3 mL) should be placed in a sterile red top Vacutainer tube without anticoagulant to assess for clot formation and to have on hand if aerobic or anaerobic bacterial cultures are required or biochemical analyses are desired (bilirubin, cholesterol, triglyceride, creatinine, etc.).

Thoracocentesis

Pleural effusions are typically abundant and bilateral but may be mild, unilateral, compartmentalized, or both.

Radiography and ultrasonography help determine the extent and location of the effusion and guide thoracocentesis. If the fluid is not compartmentalized, thoracocentesis is performed approximately two thirds down the chest, near the costochondral junction at the sixth, seventh, or eighth intercostal space.

The animal is restrained in the sternal recumbent or standing position. The site of needle insertion is shaved and aseptically prepared. Tranquilization and local anesthesia are generally not necessary for collecting a small sample for analysis but may be needed if a large amount of fluid must be drained from the chest. Large dogs may require a 1½-inch, 18- to 20-gauge needle or over-the-needle catheter, but a ⅞-inch, 19- or 21-gauge butterfly needle is preferred for cats and small dogs. The catheter unit allows the needle to be withdrawn after the catheter is introduced into the thoracic cavity, decreasing the chances of injury to intrathoracic organs.

The needle should be inserted next to the cranial surface of the rib to minimize the risk of lacerating the vessels on the rib's caudal border. As long as the needle or catheter is below the fluid line, air will not be aspirated into the thoracic cavity. If only a single syringe of fluid is to be collected, the syringe may be attached to the catheter, the fluid aspirated, and the catheter withdrawn with the syringe attached. If a larger volume of fluid is to be removed or the syringe is to be repeatedly filled, extension tubing and a three-way stopcock should be attached (Figure 15-1).

Abdominocentesis

The ventral midline of the abdomen, 1 to 2 centimeters (cm) caudal to the umbilicus, is the usual site of needle insertion. This site avoids the falciform fat, which may block the needle barrel. The urinary bladder is emptied to help avoid accidental cystocentesis. The site of needle insertion is shaved and aseptically prepared. Neither local nor general anesthesia is usually needed. With the animal in lateral recumbency, a ventral midline puncture is made using a 1- to 1½-inch, 20- to 22-gauge needle, or a 16- to 20-gauge, 1½- to 2-inch plain or fenestrated over-the-needle catheter without the syringe attached. Free-flowing fluid should be collected into appropriate collection tubes. The needle may be rotated if fluid is not visible in the needle hub or a syringe may be attached and gentle negative pressure applied.[6] If a previous surgical incision is present, the needle should be inserted at least 1.5 cm away from the site to avoid abdominal viscera that may have adhered to the abdominal wall in the area of the scar. To enhance fluid collection, abdominal compression may be applied when an over-the-needle catheter is used after the stylet has been removed, leaving only the catheter in the abdominal cavity. Although the catheter may kink, sufficient fluid can usually be collected for analysis.

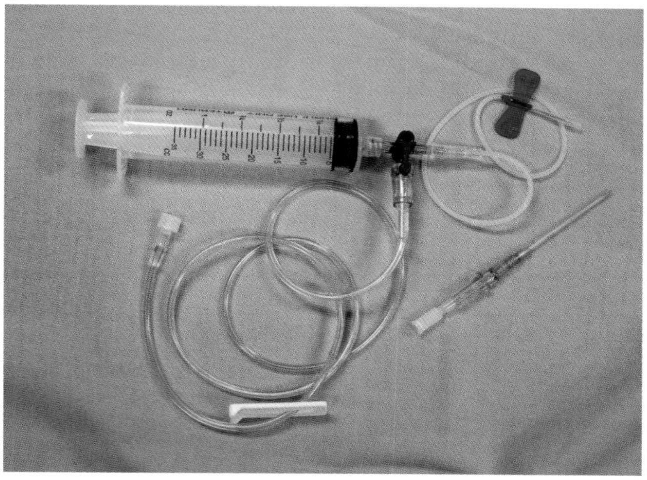

Figure 15-1 Basic equipment for thoracocentesis, abdominocentesis, or pericardiocentesis: Syringe, three-way stopcock, extension tubing, butterfly catheter, and over-the-needle catheter.

If the technique described above fails to yield fluid, four-quadrant paracentesis or diagnostic peritoneal lavage (DPL) may be performed. In four-quadrant paracentesis, the umbilicus serves as a central point, and centesis, as previously described, is performed in the right and left cranial and caudal quadrants.[7] If DPL is performed, the animal is placed in dorsal recumbency, the area clipped and aseptically prepared, and a small 2-cm incision caudal to the umbilicus is made. A peritoneal lavage catheter without the trocar is inserted into the abdominal cavity and directed caudally into the pelvis. A syringe is attached and gentle suction applied. If no fluid is obtained, 20 mL/kg of warm sterile saline may be infused into the abdominal cavity. The patient is then rolled from side to side and the fluid collected via gravity drainage.[6,7]

Pericardiocentesis

Pericardiocentesis may be performed with the animal in the standing position or in sternal or left lateral recumbency. Adequate restraint is needed to avoid cardiac puncture, coronary artery laceration, or pulmonary laceration. Sedation is used as necessary. Electrocardiogram (ECG) monitoring is recommended but not essential. Cardiac contact with the catheter or needle usually causes an arrhythmia. A large area of the right hemithorax from the third to the eighth rib is shaved and aseptically prepared. Local anesthesia, including infiltration of the pleura with lidocaine, may be used to minimize discomfort associated with pleura penetration. Puncture is generally made between the fourth and fifth intercostal spaces at the costochondral junction. The needle is attached to a three-way stopcock, extension tubing, and syringe, and gentle negative pressure is applied.[5,8]

SLIDE PREPARATION AND STAINING

Preparation of the sample for cytologic evaluation depends on the character and quantity of the fluid, the type of stain used, and whether the cytologic evaluation will be performed in the hospital or sent to a diagnostic laboratory.

Clear, colorless fluids are usually transudates (low protein content and low cellularity). Preparation of sedimented or cytospin concentrated slides from low cellularity fluids aid in cytologic evaluation. Clear-amber and mildly opaque fluids are often modified transudates of low to moderate cellularity. Moderately to markedly opaque fluids, however, are usually exudates of moderate to very high cellularity. Slide preparation and staining techniques for various types of fluids are additionally presented in Chapter 1.

Sediment smears should be made on all nonturbid fluid specimens. This is done by centrifuging the fluid for 5 minutes at 165 to 360 gravity (G). This may be achieved in a centrifuge with a radial arm length of 14.6 cm by centrifuging the fluid at 1000 to 1500 revolutions per minute (rpm). After centrifugation, nearly all of the supernatant is poured off, leaving only about 0.5 mL of fluid with the pellet in the bottom of the tube. The supernatant may be used for total protein and chemical analysis (avoid EDTA samples which interfere with chemical analyses). The pellet is then resuspended in the remaining 0.5 mL of fluid by gentle agitation, a drop of the suspension is placed on a glass slide, and a routine pull smear or squash prep is made (see Chapter 1). The smear is air-dried and then stained with an appropriate hematologic stain.

Opaque fluids may need only a direct smear because of high cellularity. Direct smears may be made by making either pull smears or squash preps on well-mixed, uncentrifuged fluid.

LABORATORY DATA

Cell Counts and Counting Techniques

Accurate nucleated cell counts may be determined at commercial laboratories on many modern automated cell counters or by manual methods using a hemacytometer, however, cell clumping, cell fragmentation, and noncellular debris may cause counting errors with automated and manual techniques.[10] Determination of nucleated cell counts should be performed on EDTA-preserved fluid to prevent clot formation or clumping of the sample. Serum separator tubes may introduce artifact to the count and therefore should not be used. A nucleated cell differential may be made on cytology preparations and often aids in classification of the effusion type.

Automated red blood cell (RBC) counts may help determine the amount of blood in the effusion. If grossly bloody fluid is obtained, a packed cell volume (PCV) may be performed. The RBC count, together with cytologic assessment (identification of platelets, erythrophagocytosis, intracellular and extracellular heme pigments such as hemosiderin and hematoidin), may aid in determination of the origin of the blood as far as iatrogenic blood contamination, per-acute hemorrhage, chronic hemorrhage, and increased capillary permeability with diapedesis of RBC into the cavity.[10]

Total Protein Measurement and Techniques

Fluid total protein concentration is used with the nucleated cell count to classify effusions as transudates, modified transudates, or exudates and to estimate the severity of inflammation, if present. The total protein content may be determined biochemically or estimated by refractometry. For ease and accuracy, the method of choice for determining total protein concentrations in effusions is refractometry. If the fluid is opaque, it is best to determine the refractive index of the supernatant after centrifugation, as the refraction of light by suspended nonprotein particles (i.e., lipoproteins, urea, cholesterol, and glucose) may result in an erroneous total protein reading.[10,11] It must be kept in mind that chylous or lipemic fluids may not separate sufficiently to allow total protein to be estimated by refractometry or chemical methods.

Biochemical Analysis

In conjunction with fluid analysis, measurement of abdominal effusion supernatant bilirubin and creatinine and comparison with serum values may be performed to diagnose bile peritonitis and uroperitoneum, respectively. Additionally, when a white, opaque effusion is obtained, measurement and comparison of effusion supernatant and serum triglyceride and cholesterol values may be used to distinguish between pseudochylous and chylous effusions (Table 15-1). Specific biochemical analyses performed on effusions will be highlighted in the section titled "Specific Disorders Causing Effusions."

Microbiologic Cultures

Effusion fluid may be submitted for either bacterial or fungal cultures. It is best to contact the laboratory for specific information regarding submission protocol, types of transport containers and media, as many laboratories will provide special transport tubes and, in the case of anaerobic bacterial culture, special anaerobic tubes or media. In general, if the cytologic evaluation of an effusion suggests bacterial infection caused by the presence of large numbers of neutrophils, or if definitive bacteria are identified, the fluid should be cultured for both aerobic and anaerobic bacteria. Fluid samples for aerobic and anaerobic cultures should be collected using aseptic technique to avoid

TABLE 15-1

Ancillary Tests: Biochemical Analysis of Effusion Fluid

Biochemical Test	Indications	Interpretation
Bilirubin	Bile peritonitis	Two-fold or greater concentration in effusion fluid than serum supports bile peritonitis.
Creatinine	Uroperitoneum	Two-fold or greater concentration in effusion fluid versus serum supports uroperitoneum.
Triglyceride	Chylous effusion	Triglyceride level greater than 100 milligrams per deciliter (mg/dL) in fluid supports chylous effusion.
Cholesterol	Nonchylous effusion	Higher concentration of cholesterol in effusion fluid versus serum supports nonchylous effusion.

contamination. Fluid should be placed into a sterile tube (i.e., sterile red top tube) without EDTA, which may be bacteriostatic or bactericidal. Note that some transport systems support both aerobic and anaerobic bacteria. Submission of fluid for fungal culture should be performed as in the case of fluid submitted for aerobic bacterial culture. Chapter 1 contains a detailed discussion of methods for collection and transportation of samples for microbiologic culture.

CELLS AND STRUCTURES SEEN IN EFFUSIONS

Neutrophils

Neutrophils are present to some degree in most effusions and tend to predominate in effusions associated with inflammation. Cytologically, two general classes of neutrophils exist: (1) degenerate and (2) nondegenerate. Degenerate neutrophils are neutrophils that have undergone hydropic degeneration. This is a morphologic change that occurs in tissue and effusion neutrophils secondary to bacterial toxins that alter cell membrane permeability. The toxins allow water to diffuse into the cell and through the nuclear pores, causing the nucleus to swell, fill more of the cytoplasm, and stain homogeneously eosinophilic. This swollen, loose, homogeneous, eosinophilic nuclear chromatin pattern characterizes the degenerate neutrophil (Figure 15-2). Although all cell types are exposed to the same toxin, degenerative change is evaluated only in neutrophils.

Nondegenerate neutrophils such as peripheral blood neutrophils are those with tightly clumped, basophilic nuclear chromatin (Figure 15-3). Some neutrophils in effusions may be hypersegmented. Hypersegmentation is an age-related change; the nuclear chromatin condenses and eventually breaks into round, tightly clumped spheres (pyknosis) (Figure 15-4). These aged neutrophils are often seen phagocytized by macrophages (cytophagia) (Figure 15-5). The presence of nondegenerate neutrophils suggests that the fluid is not septic; however, bacteria that are not strong toxin producers, for example, *Actinomyces* spp., may be associated with nondegenerate neutrophils. Also, some infectious agents such as *Ehrlichia* and *Toxoplasma* spp. and various fungi may be associated with nondegenerate neutrophils.

Effusions may also contain toxic neutrophils. Toxic changes (i.e., Döhle bodies, toxic granulation, diffuse cytoplasmic basophilia, foamy cytoplasm) develop in the bone marrow in response to accelerated granulopoiesis caused by inflammation. Toxic neutrophils in the peripheral blood migrate into the body cavity and are observed in effusions of the cavity.[10] Although foamy cytoplasm is considered a toxic change, cytoplasmic vacuolation may be seen in neutrophils of peritoneal or thoracic fluid smears because of age-related change or EDTA-induced artifact.

Mesothelial Cells

Mesothelial cells line pleural, peritoneal, and pericardial cavities as well as visceral surfaces, and are present in variable numbers in most effusions. Mesothelium easily

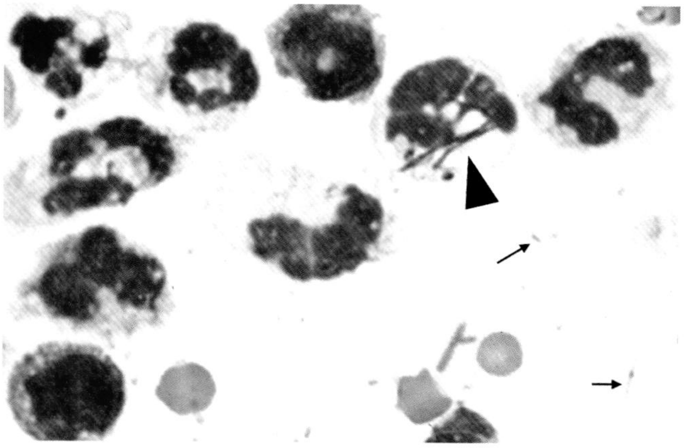

Figure 15-2 Numerous degenerate neutrophils with swollen nuclear chromatin. Phagocytized bacterial rods *(arrowhead)* and extracellular bacteria are in the background *(arrows)*.

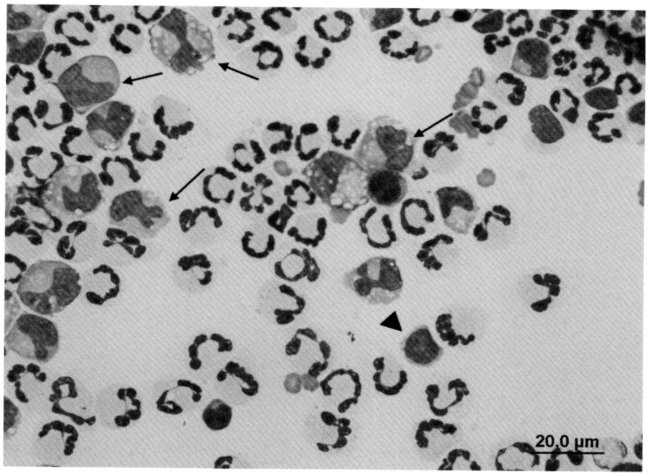

Figure 15-3 Feline abdominal fluid. Numerous nondegenerate neutrophils. The chromatin is clumped and segmented. Also present are macrophages *(arrows)* and a small lymphocyte *(arrowhead)*.

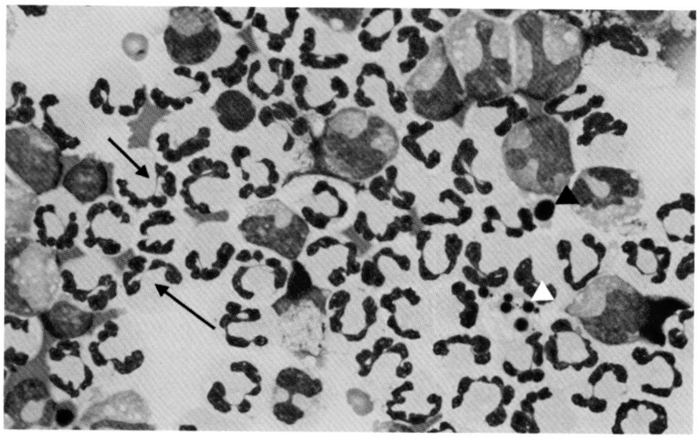

Figure 15-4 Feline abdominal fluid. Numerous nondegenerate neutrophils are present; some are hypersegmented with only thin chromatin strands connecting the segments *(small arrows)*. Pyknotic nuclei *(arrowheads)* are also present.

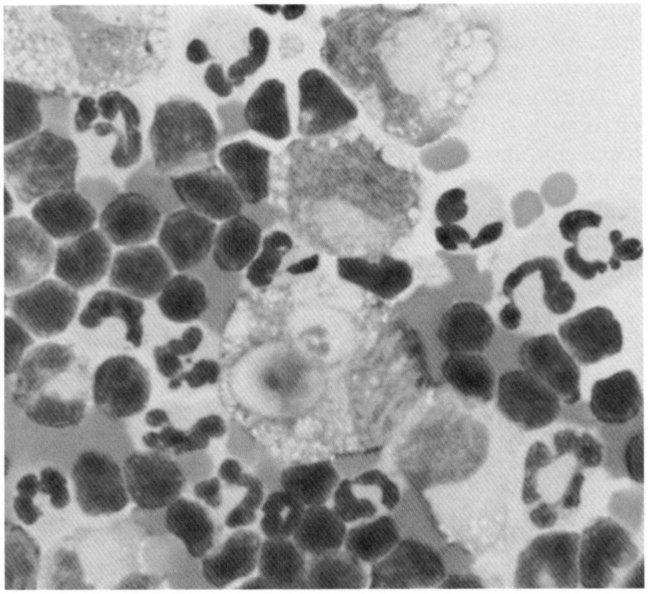

Figure 15-5 Abdominal fluid from a cat. A large macrophage is present in the center, with a phagocytized remnant of a neutrophil. Numerous small lymphocytes and macrophages are present.

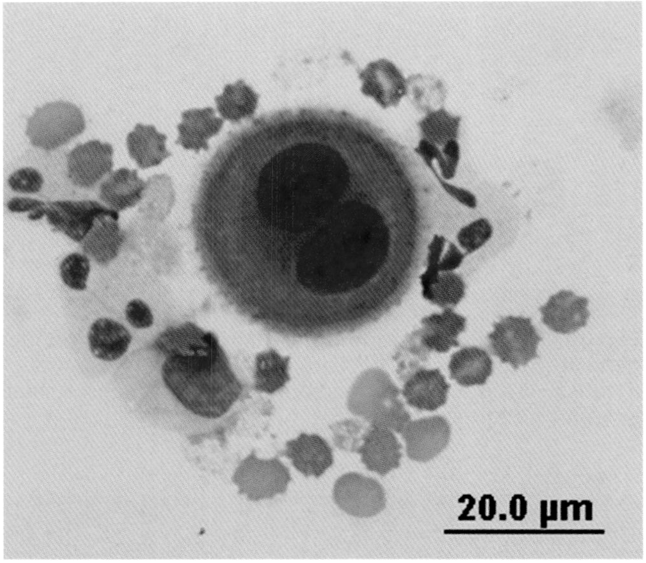

Figure 15-6 A binucleate mesothelial cell with deeply basophilic cytoplasm and an encircling eosinophilic fringe border.

becomes activated and reactive or hyperplastic in the face of inflammation or fluid accumulation of any type. In effusions, mesothelial cells are large, round cells present singly or in clusters, with singular, round central nuclei. Multinucleation occurs when cells are reactive (Figure 15-6). The nuclear chromatin has a fine reticular pattern and nucleoli may be present. Normal mesothelial cells are often noted to have moderate amounts of pale blue cytoplasm, and a pronounced pink cytoplasmic coronal fringe is often present in reactive cells (Figure 15-7). Mesothelial cells may be present in low or moderate numbers, as individual cells, in small clusters, and sometimes

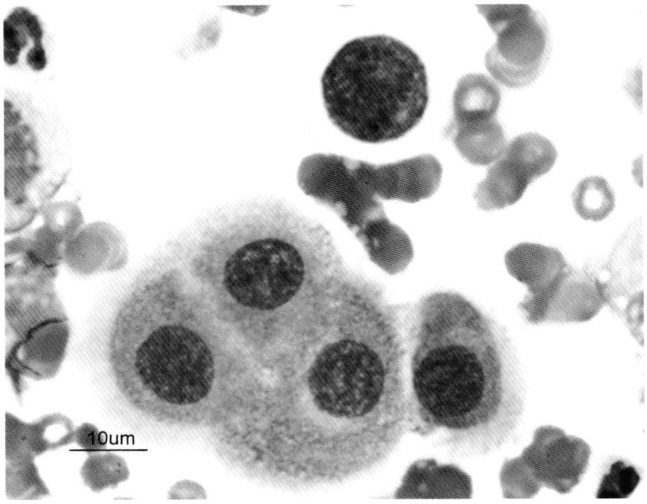

Figure 15-7 A small cluster of mesothelial cells.

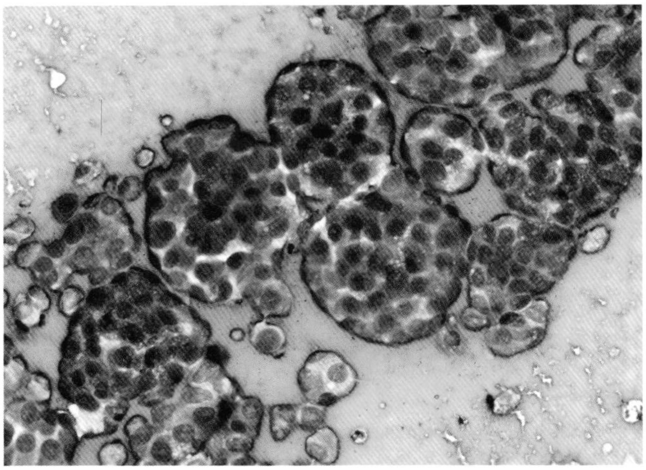

Figure 15-8 Pericardial fluid from a dog. In a concentrated cytospin specimen, several three-dimensional aggregates of mildly pleomorphic mesothelial cells are present in a hemodilute background. The high numbers might suggest mesothelial hyperplasia.

in large, three-dimensional balls (Figure 15-8). Reactive mesothelial cells may have several morphologic characteristics of malignancy and may be easily confused with neoplastic cells.

Macrophages

Macrophages found in effusions generally have a single oval to bean-shaped nucleus and resemble tissue macrophages. The nuclear chromatin is lacy and cytoplasm is frequently vacuolated and may contain phagocytized debris or degenerate cells (Figure 15-9 and Figure 15-10).

Lymphocytes

Lymphocytes are commonly seen in effusions and are often the predominant cell type in chylous effusions (Figure 15-11) and neoplastic effusions secondary to lymphoid malignancy (Figure 15-12 and Figure 15-13). Small

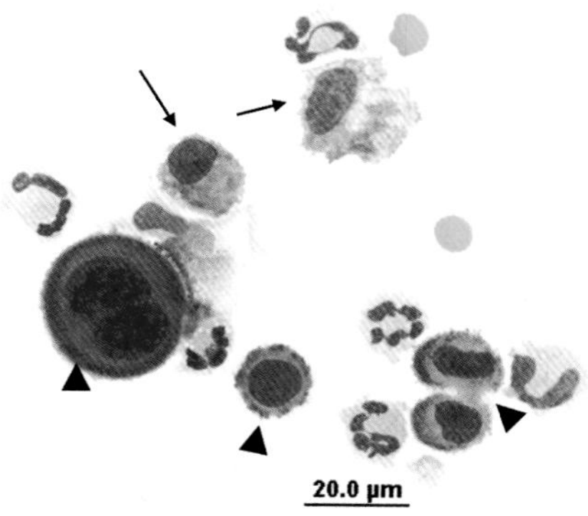

Figure 15-9 Macrophages (*arrows*), mesothelial cells (*arrowheads*), and nondegenerate neutrophils.

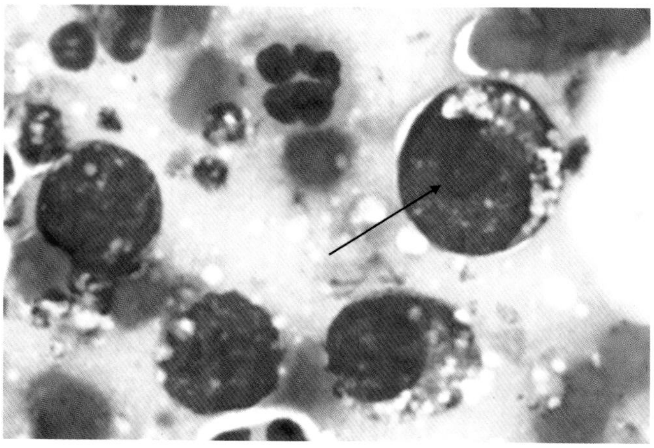

Figure 15-12 Lymphoblast with visible nucleolus *(arrow)*. Small vacuoles are present in the cytoplasm.

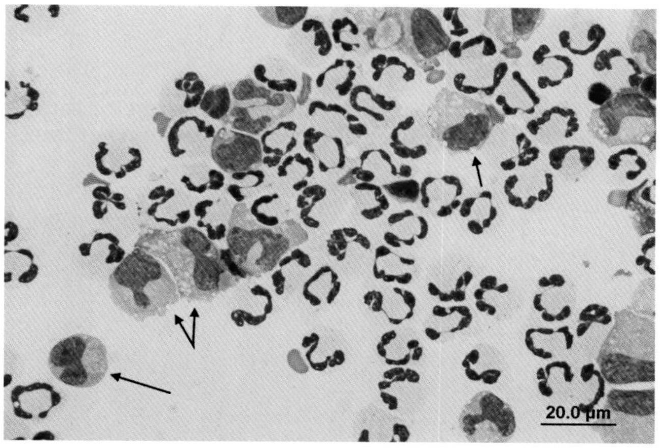

Figure 15-10 Numerous nondegenerate neutrophils and macrophages with variable nuclear morphologies (*arrows*).

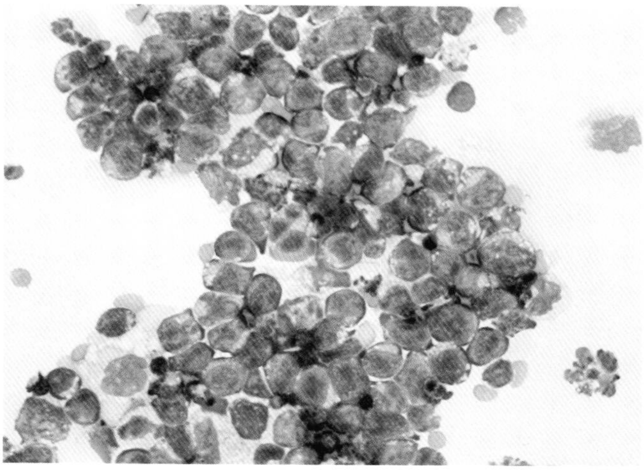

Figure 15-13 Pleural fluid from a cat with lymphoma. Numerous lymphoblasts with visible nucleoli are present.

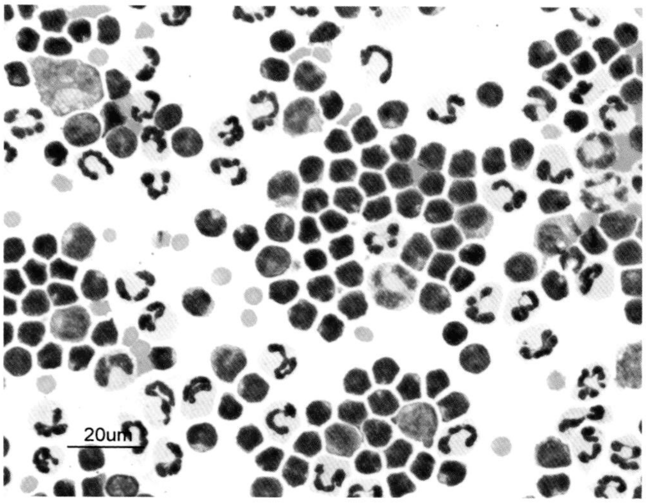

Figure 15-11 Chylous effusion from a cat. Small lymphocytes are the predominant cells. The small lymphocytes are typically smaller than neutrophils. They have round or indented nuclei and a small amount of cytoplasm.

to intermediate or medium-sized lymphocytes present in body cavity fluids will appear similar to peripheral lymphocytes, with a scant rim of blue cytoplasm, round nucleus with evenly clumped to coarse chromatin, and no apparent nucleoli. Normal fluids will have low numbers of lymphocytes. Reactive lymphocytes may be seen in inflammatory effusions and are slightly larger than small lymphocytes, with deeply basophilic cytoplasm imparting a plasmacytoid appearance (Figure 15-14).

Eosinophils

Eosinophils (Figure 15-15) are readily recognized by their rod-shaped (in cats) or variably sized round (in dogs) eosinophilic granules. When present in moderate to high numbers in effusions, eosinophils are indicative of an underlying pathologic process such as heartworm disease, allergic reactions, hypersensitivity, and neoplasia (mast cell neoplasia, occult lymphoma) (Figure 15-16).[12]

Mast Cells

Mast cells (Figure 15-17 and Figure 15-18) are readily identified by their numerous, round, red-purple cytoplasmic granules. Mast cells may be found in low numbers in effusions in dogs and cats with many different inflammatory disorders. Mast cell tumors within body cavities may be associated with effusions and frequently exfoliate large numbers of mast cells into the effusion. Visceral forms of mast cell neoplasia are rare in the dog.[12,13] Visceral forms of mast cell tumors are more common in cats than in dogs and may involve the spleen, liver, gastrointestinal tract, or all of these.[13]

Erythrocytes

Erythrocytes may be seen cytologically within effusions secondary to overt hemorrhage or contamination with peripheral blood. It is important to differentiate iatrogenic causes from true intracavity hemorrhage, based on clinical signs, laboratory data, and the presence or absence of erythrophagia, hemosiderin or hematoidin pigments, and platelets in the effusion, as described in the discussion of hemorrhagic effusions later in this chapter.

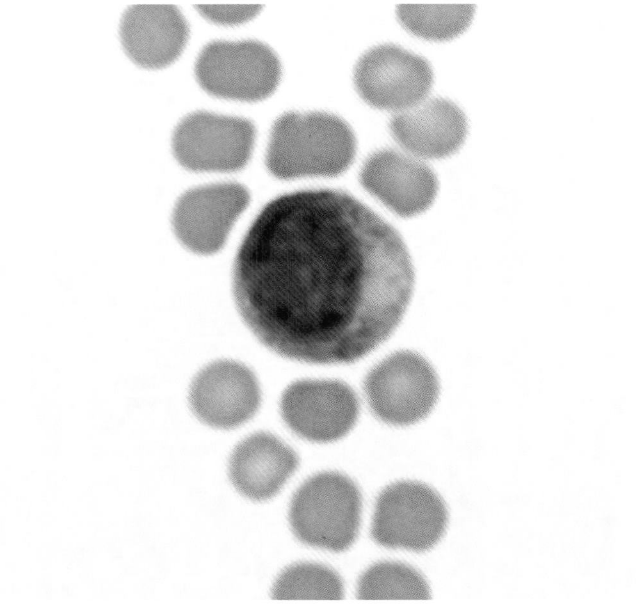

Figure 15-14 Reactive lymphocyte.

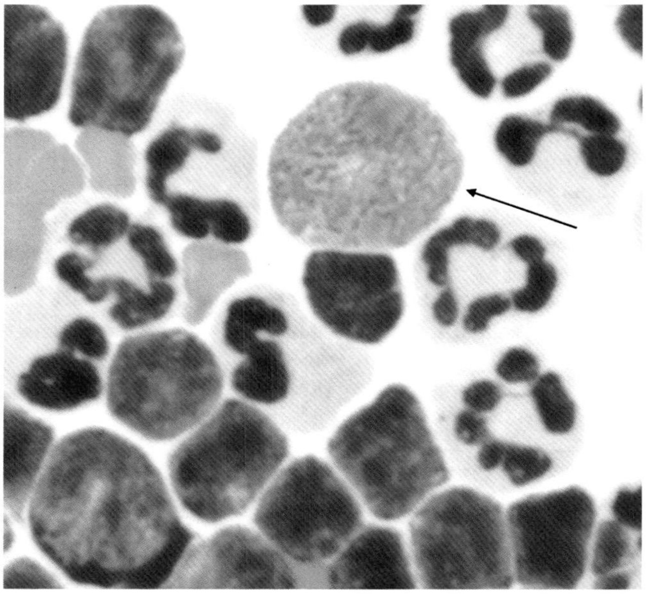

Figure 15-15 Eosinophil *(arrow)* in pleural fluid from a cat.

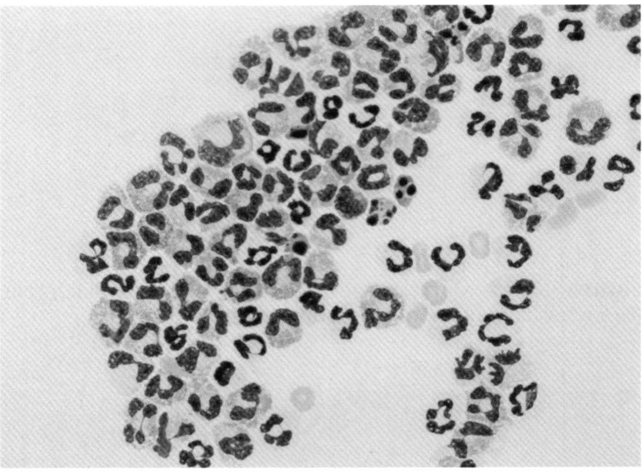

Figure 15-16 Canine pleural effusion with numerous eosinophils and fewer pyknotic cells, nondegenerate neutrophils, one monocyte, and few red blood cells.

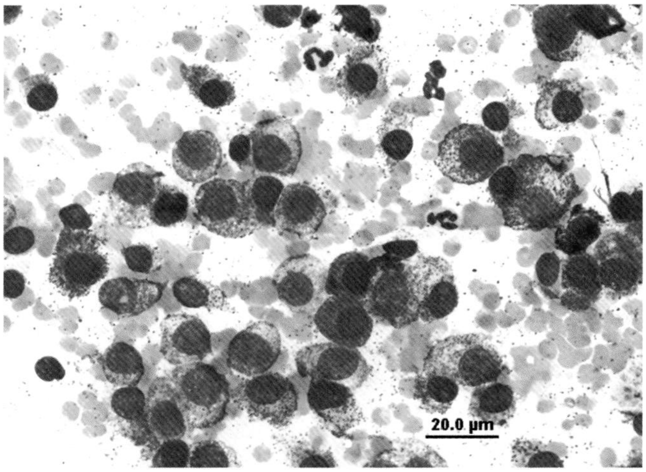

Figure 15-17 Many heavily granulated mast cells.

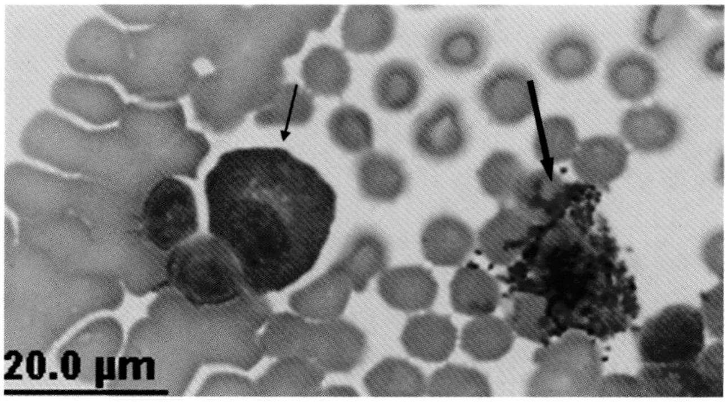

Figure 15-18 Mast cell *(arrow)*, plasma cell *(small arrow)*, and three small lymphocytes in abdominal fluid from a dog.

Neoplastic Cells

Neoplastic cells may be observed in low to high numbers in effusions secondary to many different types of neoplasia. Various carcinomas and adenocarcinomas (epithelial cell tumors), lymphoma and mast cell tumors (discrete cell tumors), hemangiosarcomas (vascular endothelial-derived neoplasia), and mesotheliomas may exfoliate neoplastic cells into the pleural, peritoneal, or pericardial cavity. Identification of the neoplastic cells depends on the viewer's ability to recognize the cell type and signs of malignancy. (See the discussion of neoplasia later in this chapter and the general criteria of malignancy in Chapter 1.)

Miscellaneous Findings

Glove Powder: Cornstarch (glove powder) may be seen on slides made from effusion fluid (Figure 15-19). Typically, it is a clear-staining, large, round to hexagonal structure with a central fissure and may be slightly refractile. Glove powder is a contaminant and should not be confused with an organism or cell.

Microfilariae: Microfilariae may occasionally be seen within hemorrhagic effusions. These are generally *Dirofilaria* or *Acanthocheilonema* (formerly *Dipetalonema)* larvae that have entered the cavity with the peripheral blood (see Figure 15-39).

Basket Cells: Basket cells are free cell nuclei from ruptured nucleated cells. When cells rupture, the nuclear chromatin spreads out and stains eosinophilic. Nucleated cells may rupture because of the stresses induced in slide preparation; however, certain effusions (i.e., chylous effusions and septic exudates) cause increased cell fragility and may result in increased numbers of ruptured cells. Neoplastic effusions may contain fragile neoplastic cells and increased cellular rupture may be seen (especially true for neoplastic lymphoblasts).

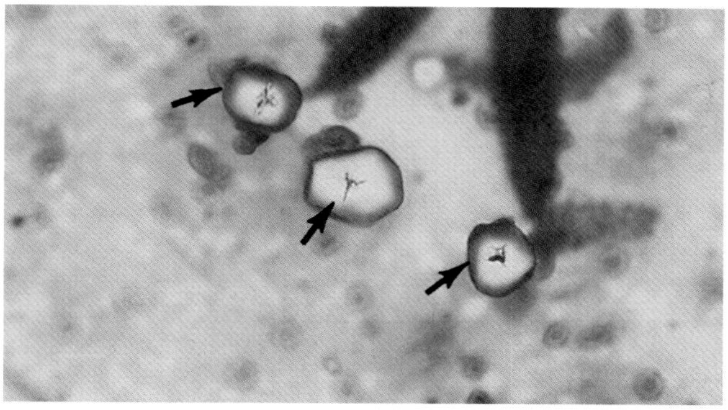

Figure 15-19 Glove powder artifact *(arrows)*.

GENERAL CLASSIFICATION OF EFFUSIONS

Generally, abdominal, thoracic, and pericardial fluid accumulations are classified as transudates, modified transudates, or exudates, based on the total nucleated cell count (TNCC), total protein (TP) concentration, and cellular content. Classifying the effusion helps direct the clinician to the general mechanism of fluid accumulation and should be interpreted in light of clinical signs and other relevant data. Occasionally, some overlap may occur in these classifications (i.e., a fluid may have a TNCC in the transudate range and a TP in the modified transudate range). If a disparity exists, TP is the more important criterion in separating transudates from modified transudates, and cellularity is more important in separating modified transudates from exudates. Although evaluation of an effusion may be diagnostic for such conditions as neoplasia or infection, many effusions simply indicate a process. Historical, physical, and clinical information and imaging studies may aid in achieving a definitive diagnosis. Figure 15-20 shows an algorithm for the classification of effusions based on cell counts and total protein.

Transudates

Transudative effusions are generally clear and colorless, with low TP concentrations (<2.5 grams per deciliter [g/dL]) and low TNCC (<1500 cells per microliter [cells/μL]). Most transudates have protein concentrations <1.5 g/dL; however, 2.5 g/dL is used as the cutoff point, as this is the lowest protein concentration at which refractometry is reliable. Cells found in transudative effusions consist primarily of mononuclear cells (macrophages and small lymphocytes), mesothelial cells, and few nondegenerate neutrophils. The general mechanism for a transudative fluid to accumulate is passive fluid shifting caused by decreased oncotic pressure or increased hydrostatic pressure. Conditions associated with these mechanisms include severe hypoalbuminemia (<1.0 g/dL) caused by renal glomerular disease, hepatic insufficiency, protein-losing enteropathy, malnutrition or malabsorption and portal hypertension or portosystemic shunt, hepatic insufficiency, and early myocardial insufficiency (more common in cats). Early bladder rupture may result in a fluid classified as a transudate; however, the nature of the effusion will change rapidly as

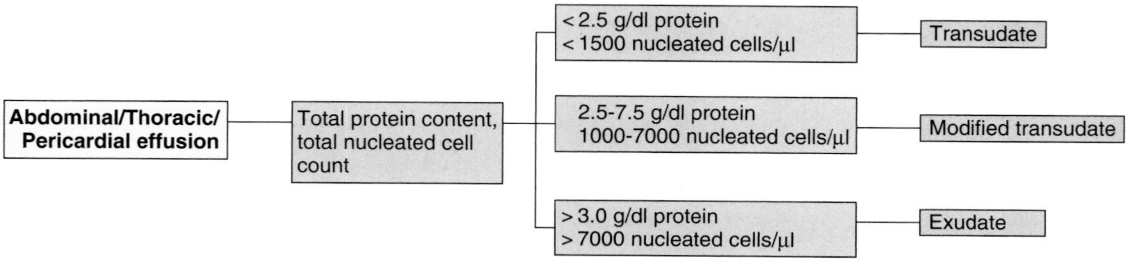

Figure 15-20 An algorithm to classify effusions as transudates, modified transudates, or exudates, based on total protein content and nucleated cell count.

uroperitoneum often induces a rapid chemical peritonitis. Overzealous intravenous fluid administration may also cause a transudative process by dilution of the peripheral albumin concentration. Figure 15-21 is a flow chart of the more common causes of transudative effusions.

Modified Transudates

Modified transudates are essentially transudates that have been modified by the addition of protein, cells, or both and are predominantly noninflammatory or mildly inflammatory. Most modified transudates generally occur as a result of leakage from blood vessels or lymphatics carrying high-protein fluid and are commonly a sequela to cardiovascular disease or neoplasia.

Modified transudates have low to moderate cellularity ranging from 1000 to 7000 cells/μL and protein concentration in the range of 2.5 to 7.5 g/dL. Modified transudates vary in color from amber to red or white and are variably turbid. Mesothelial cells (often reactive or hyperplastic), nondegenerate neutrophils (up to 30%), macrophages, small lymphocytes, and other cells will vary in number, depending on the cause of the effusion.

Modified transudates often are the least specific from a diagnostic standpoint. In general, they are caused by conditions that produce an increase in vascular hydrostatic pressure, permeability within capillaries or lymphatics, or both. A flow chart of the more common causes of modified transudates is outlined in Figure 15-22.

Cardiovascular disease (right-sided or biventricular failure) is one of the more common causes of modified transudates in dogs and cats. Either abdominal or thoracic effusion may develop; however, ascites is more common in dogs, and pleural effusion (often chylous) is typical in cats. Physical examination findings, thoracic radiography, and echocardiography often confirm functional abnormalities.

Neoplastic disease may result in a modified transudate, presumably by obstruction of lymphatics. Neoplastic cells may or may not be present in the effusion. Cytologic examination of effusion is most likely to be diagnostic in animals with round cell tumor and epithelial tumors. In contrast, mesenchymal tumors rarely exfoliate neoplastic cells into an effusion. In cases of hemorrhagic (or serosanguinous) modified transudates, nonexfoliating or poorly exfoliating neoplasia (i.e., hemangiosarcoma) should be considered if no history of trauma or coagulopathy exists.[14]

Feline infectious peritonitis (FIP) is a common cause of abdominal or thoracic effusion and occasionally pericardial effusion in cats. Although FIP may produce an exudative effusion, modified transudates are also common. In most cases, the fluid has a very high protein concentration (>4 g/dL). Nondegenerate neutrophils and macrophages are the primary cell types and may be present in low to high numbers. Unfortunately, no conclusive cytologic feature is diagnostic of FIP. Other physical examination or laboratory findings consistent with FIP (i.e., serum hyperglobulinemia or polyclonal gammopathy, serum albumin-to-globulin ratio (A:G) <0.8 g/dL, ocular lesions, neurologic abnormalities, nonregenerative anemia, fever, lymphopenia, positive coronavirus antibody titer) may strengthen a clinical suspicion. Histopathology (vasculitis and pyogranulomatous inflammation of affected tissue) is considered the gold standard for definitive diagnosis of FIP.

Rupture of the urinary bladder initially results in an effusion classified as a transudate or modified transudate at the time of diagnosis as the amount of fluid released into the peritoneal cavity dilutes out accumulated cells and protein. This effusion may quickly become exudative.

Chylous effusions are usually easily recognized by their milky appearance and predominance of small lymphocytes; however, in some cases, recognition is not so

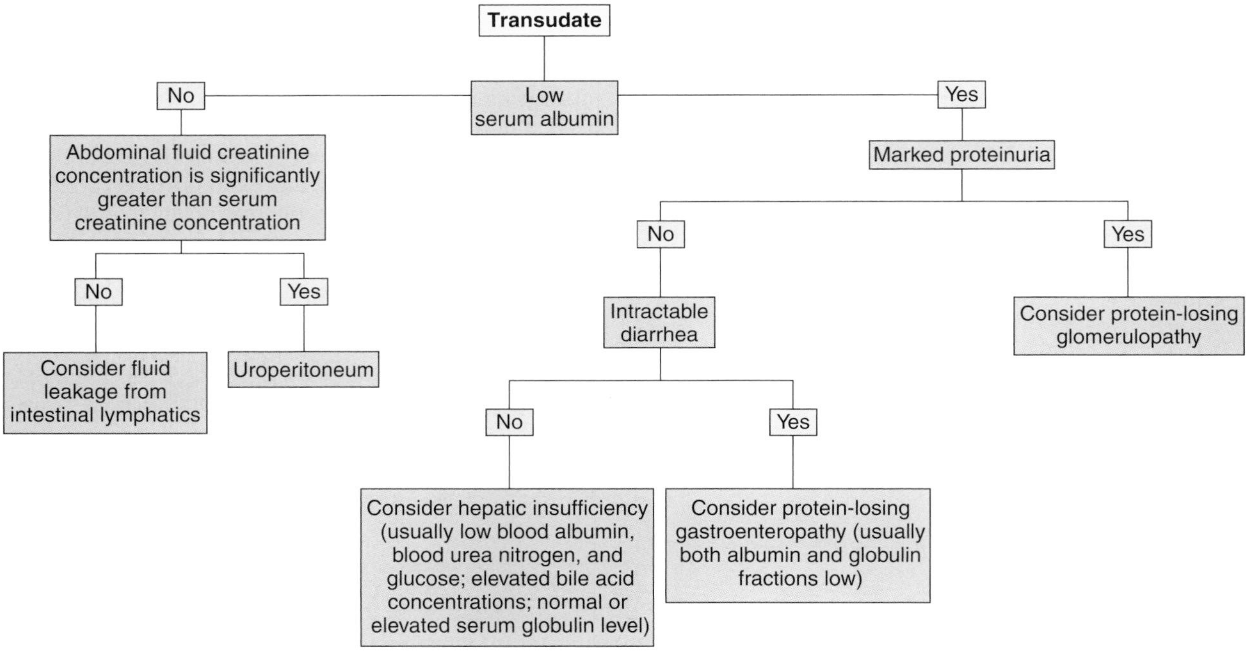

Figure 15-21 An algorithmic approach to the more common causes of transudative effusions.

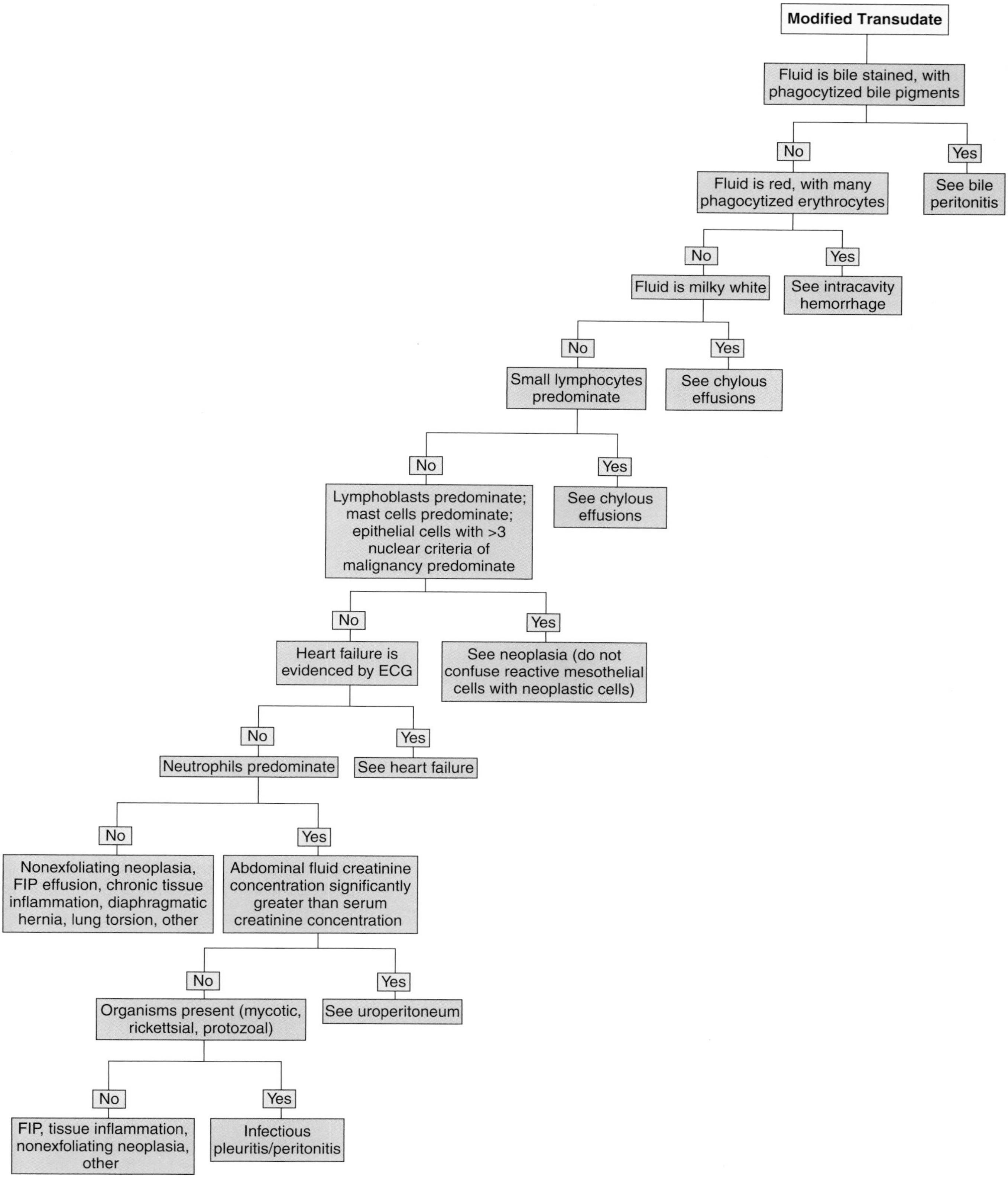

Figure 15-22 An algorithmic approach to some common causes of modified transudates.

clear-cut. The cytology of such effusions may be variable, with neutrophils predominating in some instances, especially if previous centesis procedures have resulted in inflammation or if the chylous effusion is chronic in nature. Also, the fluid may appear opaque rather than milky white in animals that are anorectic and not ingesting lipids. In such instances, comparing serum and fluid levels of triglycerides and cholesterol may help determine the nature of the fluid.

Effusions containing peripheral blood, as a result of either intracavitary hemorrhage or blood contamination during collection, are often classified as modified transudates because of added cells and serum proteins. Such effusions are easily recognized by their reddish appearance and the presence of numerous erythrocytes on cytologic examination. The presence of erythrophagocytosis, macrophages containing RBC-breakdown products (hemosiderin and hematoidin), or a combination of both helps differentiate true intracavitary hemorrhage from blood contamination.

Hepatic disease is a common cause of ascites and may also cause pleural effusion. If the serum albumin is significantly decreased because of hepatic disease and lack of production, a transudate secondary to hypoalbuminemia with loss of oncotic pressure may occur. If mild to moderate hypoalbuminemia is complicated with systemic venous hypertension or portal hypertension, it may produce a modified transudate.

Other miscellaneous causes of modified transudates include lung lobe torsion, diaphragmatic hernia, hyperthyroidism, and glomerulonephritis. The etiology of many of these effusions is multifactoral and the nature of the effusion is variable, depending on the circumstances present in each individual case.

Exudates

Exudates have high protein concentrations (>3.0 g/dL) and a nucleated cell count generally greater than 7,000 cells/μL. Exudates may vary from amber to red or white and are often turbid to cloudy. A flow chart of the more common causes of exudative effusions is outlined in Figure 15-23. Exudates are commonly inflammatory in nature and associated with a wide range of pathologic conditions, including infectious disease (i.e., bacterial, protozoal, viral, parasitic, fungal) and noninfectious conditions (i.e., pancreatitis, steatitis, neoplasia, chemical irritants).

Exudates occur most commonly in response to the presence of chemoattractants in the respective body cavity making neutrophils the predominant cell type in most exudates, especially in septic exudates. In the case of a predominantly neutrophilic exudate, a thorough investigation for an infectious agent is warranted. Typically, degenerate neutrophils are present in cases of sepsis, and nondegenerate neutrophils are seen in nonseptic exudates caused by other sterile inflammatory processes. However, not finding organisms cytologically does not rule out an infectious cause. Previous or concurrent antibiotic use may reduce bacterial numbers and as not all bacteria produce strong or large amounts of toxin, the lack of degenerate neutrophils does not rule out the possibility of bacterial infection. Whenever a significant neutrophilic inflammatory component is present, regardless of the cytological presence of bacteria, bacterial culture should be considered.

Occasionally, an exudate develops because of abundant exfoliation of neoplastic cells or secondary to a chronic chylous effusion, in which case neoplastic cells or small lymphocytes, respectively, may predominate. In these instances, the effusions are generally called *neoplastic* or *chylous effusions,* rather than *exudate,* to reflect the cytologic findings.

SPECIFIC DISORDERS CAUSING EFFUSIONS

Septic Exudates

Inflammation of the body cavities is associated with the production of chemotactants and vasoactive substances. Chemotactants cause increased neutrophil and monocyte or macrophage numbers, and the vasoactive substances cause an influx of high-protein fluid. This results in an exudative effusion because of increased capillary permeability, with a massive outpouring of peripheral blood neutrophils and high-protein plasma filtrate into the cavity. A septic effusion may result from systemic sepsis via hematogenous or lymphatic spread or from a focal source such as extension of pleuropneumonia or gastrointestinal compromise or intestinal perforation and also by introduction of organisms via penetration of the body cavity (i.e., trauma, foreign body, surgery, and prior centesis).

Degenerate neutrophils typically predominate in bacterial infections (Figure 15-24); organisms may be seen intracellularly and extracellulary (Figure 15-25 and Figure 15-26). The presence of long, slender, filamentous rods in a fluid with "tomato soup" characteristics is highly suggestive of *Actinomyces* spp., *Nocardia* spp., *Fusobacterium* spp., or all three (Figure 15-27). Spirochetes are occasionally seen in association with bacterial peritonitis and pleuritis, especially secondary to bite wounds. Although bacterial infections are the most common causes of septic exudates, mycotic infections associated with *Histoplasma* spp., *Blastomyces* spp., *and Coccidioides* spp., may occur (Figure 15-28, Figure 15-29, and Figure 15-30). Additionally, effusions secondary to protozoal (*Neospora* spp.) (Figure 15-31), and rickettsial (*Leishmania* spp.) infections have been reported.[15,16]

Tissue Inflammation

Inflammation of an intracavity organ (liver, pancreas, lungs), or a walled-off abscess may cause an effusion. Inflammatory processes release chemotactants that cause an influx of neutrophils and monocytes into the area of inflammation, and vasoactive products that increase vascular permeability, causing an influx of high-protein fluid. When the inflammatory process extends into the cavity or inflammatory products are released into it, the cavity becomes inflamed and inflammatory cells tend to accumulate in large numbers. Many factors, including duration and whether an accompanying pleuritis, peritonitis, or pericarditis has occurred, determine whether the effusion is a modified transudate or exudate.

In effusions subsequent to tissue inflammation, nondegenerate neutrophils generally predominate, but macrophages, mesothelial cells, and some lymphocytes are

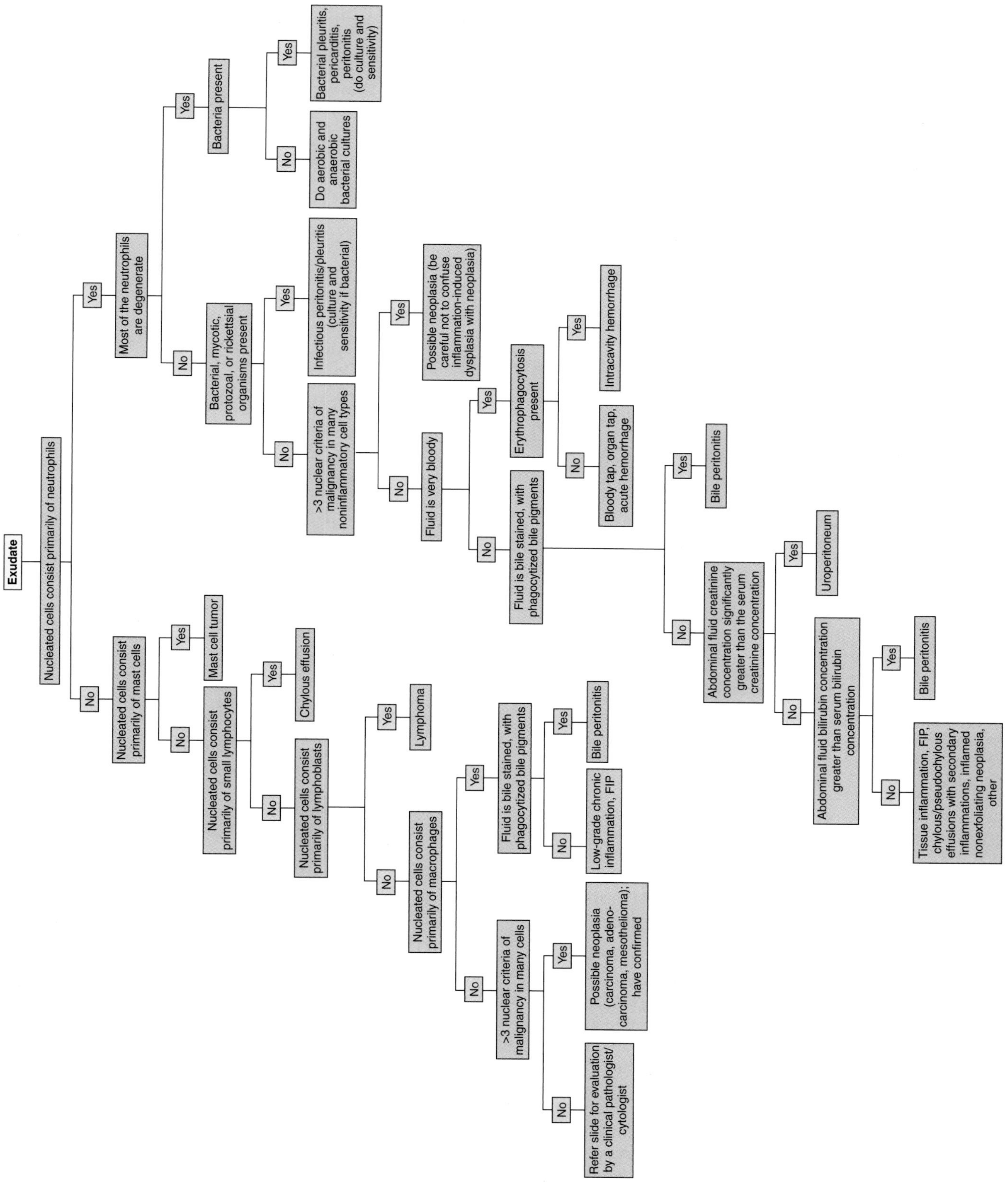

Figure 15-23 An algorithmic approach to the more common causes of exudative effusions.

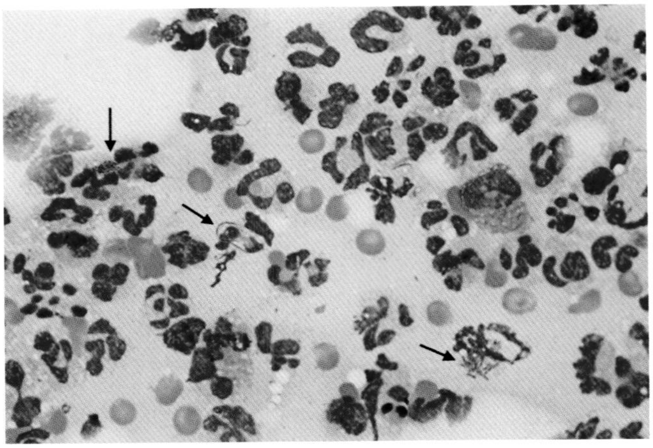

Figure 15-24 Septic exudates showing degenerate neutrophils and phagocytized bacteria (*arrow*).

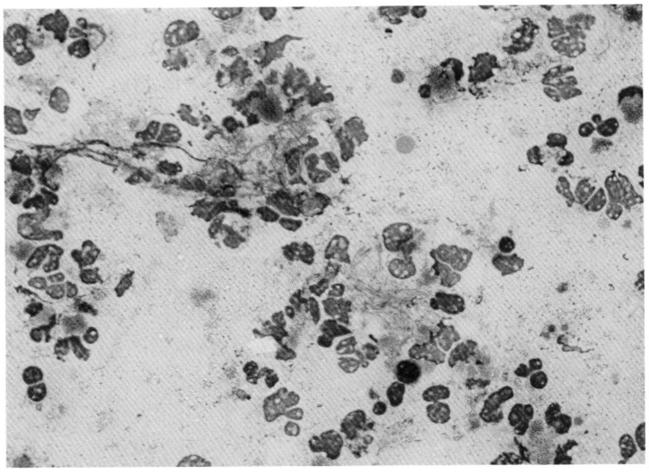

Figure 15-25 Feline pyothorax. Large numbers of severely degenerate neutrophils and many phagocytized and extracellular mixed bacteria consisting of cocci and long strands of bacilli.

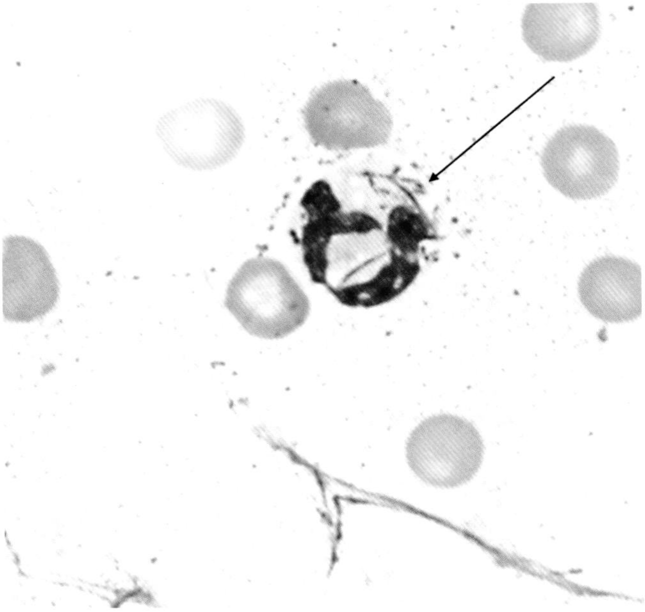

Figure 15-26 Phagocytized filamentous bacterial rod (*arrow*).

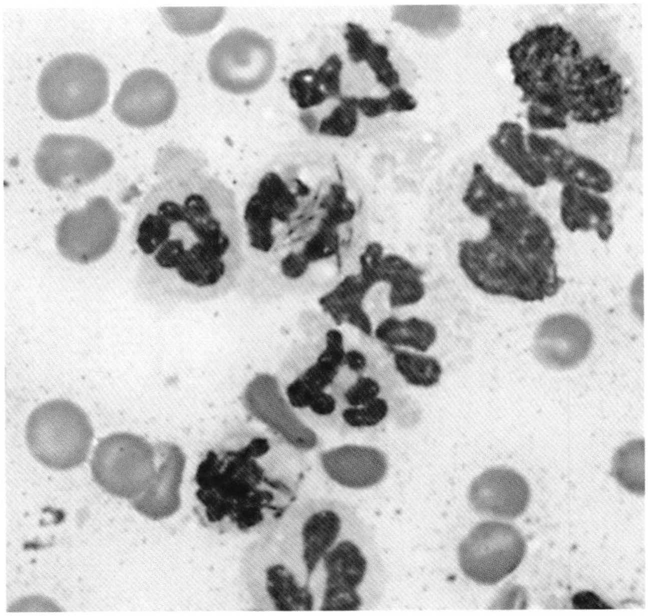

Figure 15-27 Filamentous bacterial rods.

also present. Macrophages, however, may become the predominant cell type in some chronic inflammatory processes. Cytologic evaluation of these effusions readily identifies the process but is typically nondiagnostic as to etiology and must be correlated with physical findings, history, and other diagnostic test results.

Feline Infectious Peritonitis

Effusive or wet FIP is the classic nonseptic exudate in the cat. Clinical FIP may occur in cats of all ages, but in a recent study, the proportion of cats with FIP between the ages of 6 months and 2 years was significantly higher compared with the control cats in similar age groups.[17] In effusive FIP, fluid may accumulate in the abdomen, thorax, pericardium, or in all of these areas. Evaluation of fluid may lend significant support to a diagnosis of FIP. The effusion is odorless, straw colored to golden in color, tenacious, and may contain flecks or fibrin strands, and foams upon agitation because of the high protein content, which is often greater than 4 g/dL. Cell counts may be variable but are typically low to moderate (2000 to 6000 cells/μL), and typically, hemodilution is minimal.

Cytologically, the typical FIP effusion has a prominent stippled proteinaceous basophilic background (Figure 15-32) and consists primarily (60% to 80%) of nondegenerate to mildly degenerate neutrophils and lesser numbers of macrophages, small lymphocytes, and occasionally plasma cells. Effusions consisting primarily of neutrophils but with large numbers of macrophages are referred to as *pyogranulomatous* and are also common in effusions associated with FIP. Although these findings are not diagnostic of FIP, when associated with clinical

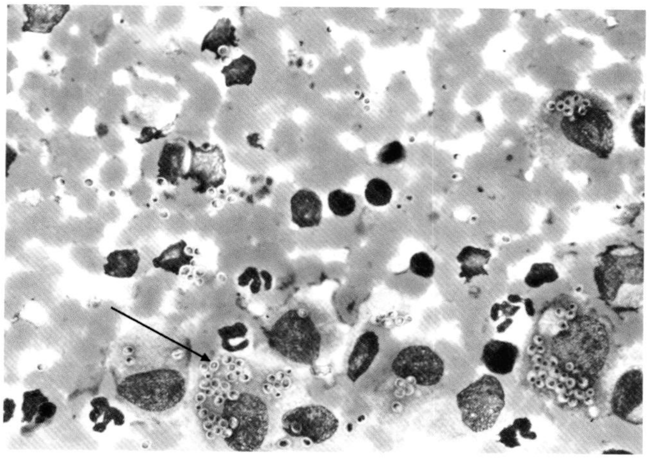

Figure 15-28 Numerous ***Histoplasma capsulatum*** **organisms** *(arrow)*. Numerous organisms are both phagocytized by macrophages and present extracellularly.

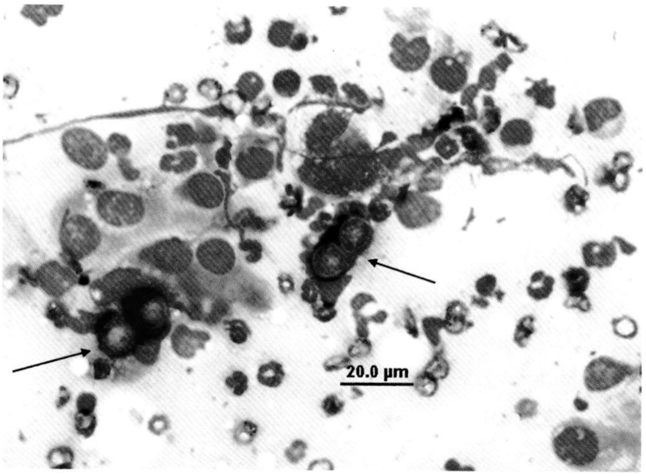

Figure 15-29 Pleural fluid from a cat. Several *Blastomyces* spp. organisms (*arrows*) are present.

findings, a presumptive diagnosis of FIP may be made. Other diagnostic tests are often used collaboratively to rule in or rule out FIP. These include determining the A:G in serum and fluid. Serum A:G less than 0.8 g/dL and effusion A:G less than 0.9 g/dL are often present with FIP. Antifeline corona virus (FCoV) antibodies in serum should be interpreted with caution because many healthy cats are FCoV antibody positive.[17,18] In a study by Hartmann et al., low to medium titers (1:25, 1:100, 1:400) of FCoV antibodies were of no diagnostic value in determining FIP infection; however, antibody titers of 1:1600 increased the probability of FIP.[18] A negative test does not rule out the possibility of FIP infection. In this study, the anti-FCoV antibody test was negative in 10% of the cats that did, in fact, have FIP.[18] Tests that show promise include reverse transcriptase-polymerase chain reaction (RT-PCR) performed on effusion fluids and an RT-PCR for the detection of FCoV messenger ribonucleic acid (mRNA) in peripheral blood mononuclear cells. Thus far, histologic examination of affected tissue samples remains the gold standard for diagnosing FIP.

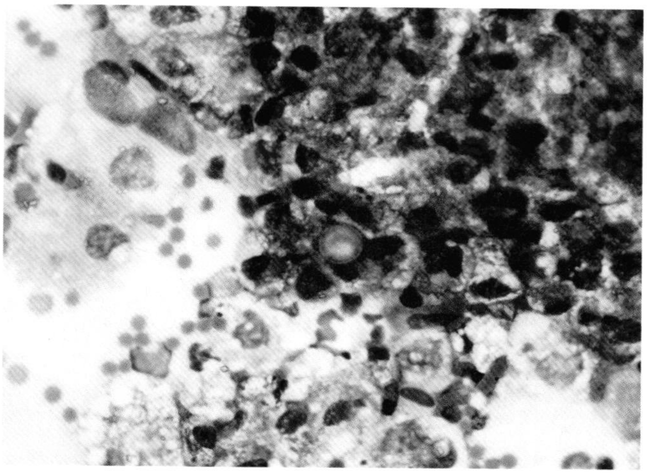

Figure 15-30 Pericardial fluid from a dog. In the center of the picture, a singular, large, pale blue, round yeast with a cell wall, consistent with *Coccidioides* spp., is present. The yeast is surrounded by macrophages containing intracellular hemosiderin and hematoidin. Extracellular rhomboid, golden hematoidin crystals are also evident.

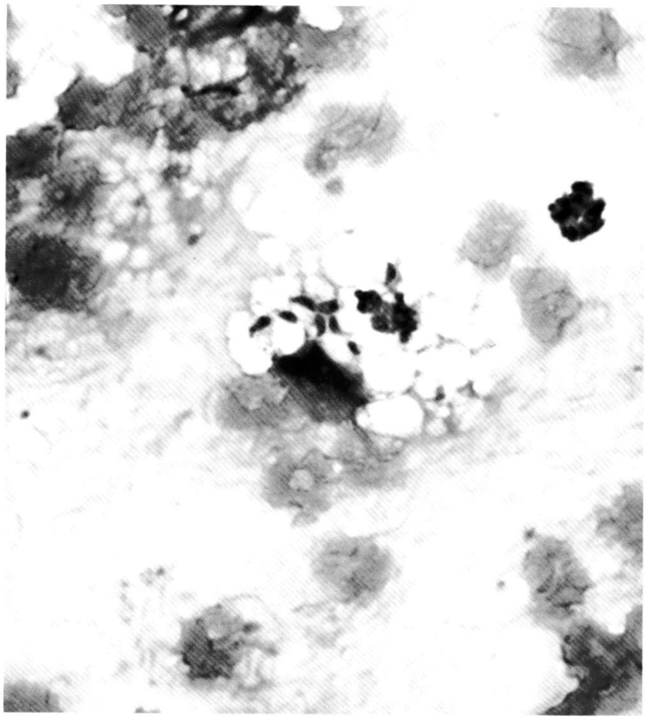

Figure 15-31 *Toxoplasma* organisms within a macrophage. (Courtesy of Susan Fielder, Oklahoma State University.)

Bile Peritonitis

Release of bile into the abdominal cavity secondary to gallbladder or bile duct rupture produces peritonitis. Rupture of the biliary system may occur secondary to bile duct obstruction, trauma, mucocele formation, biliary tract inflammation, and percutaneous biopsy of the liver. Bile in the peritoneal cavity causes a chemical peritonitis that is typically exudative. The effusion fluid color is typically

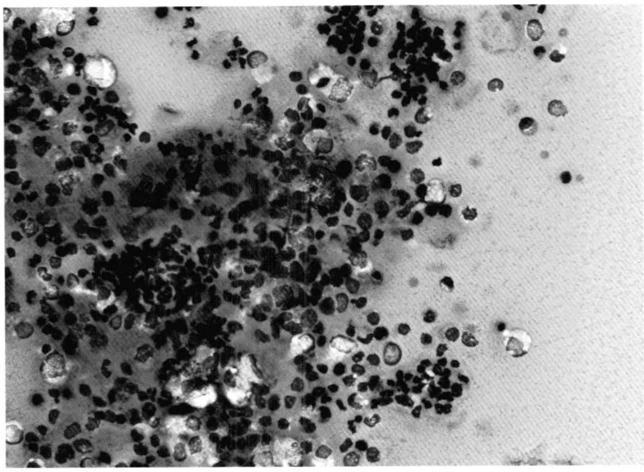

Figure 15-32 Abdominal fluid from a cat with effusive feline infectious peritonitis. Note the nondegenerate neutrophils, macrophages, and rare small lymphocytes within a granular, stippled, proteinaceous background.

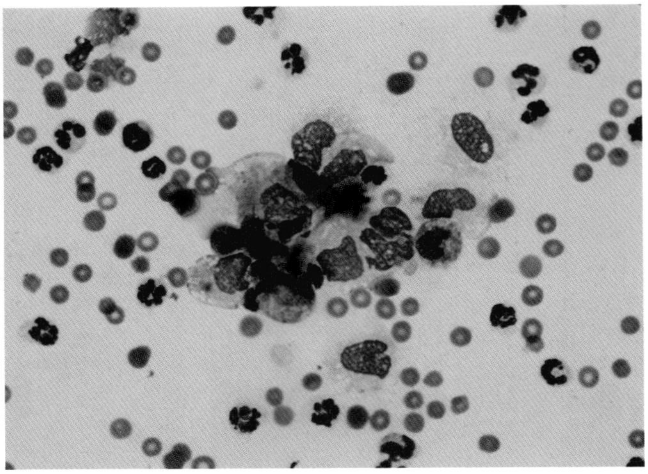

Figure 15-34 Abdominal fluid from a dog. Dark, yellow-green, amorphous extracellular and phagocytized bile pigment, with several mildly degenerate neutrophils and macrophages.

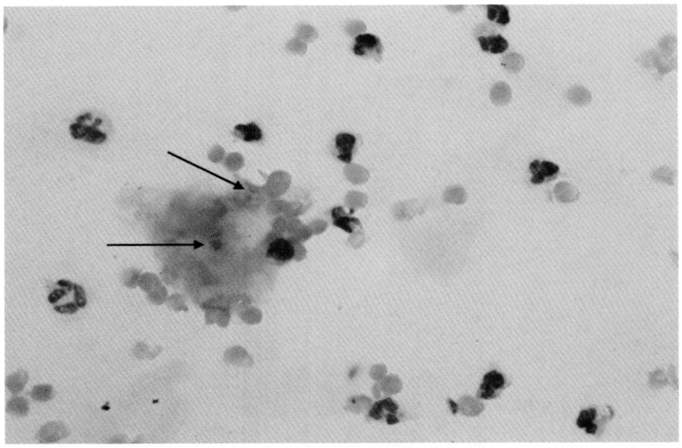

Figure 15-33 Abdominal fluid from a dog. Extracellular bile pigment (*arrows*) and many nondegenerate neutrophils.

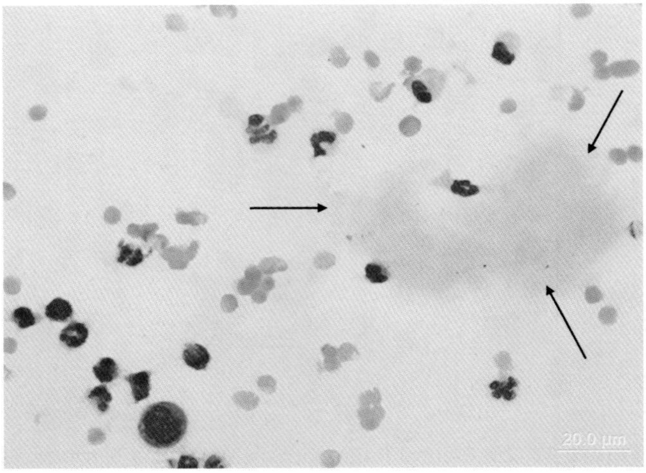

Figure 15-35 Abdominal fluid from a dog. Extracellular homogeneous basophilic material, or "white bile" (*arrows*).

green tinged to yellow-orange. Amorphous to slightly spiculated, blue-green to yellow-green bile pigment may be seen within macrophages and extracellularly (Figure 15-33 and Figure 15-34). These pigments may resemble hemosiderin seen in hemorrhagic effusions, and caution should be used during interpretation. If definitive differentiation is necessary, Prussian blue staining may be used to highlight the iron in hemosiderin. Bilirubin concentration may also readily be measured in the abdominal fluid and serum and compared: If the abdominal fluid bilirubin level is at least twofold greater than concurrent serum bilirubin levels, bile peritonitis is likely.

A mucocele (mucinous cystic hyperplasia) of biliary and gallbladder epithelial cells may occur secondary to inflammation and cholelithiasis. In one retrospective study of 30 dogs, the histologic findings suggested that mucoceles resulted from dysfunction of mucus-secreting cells within the gallbladder mucosa, leading to accumulation of bile and potential rupture.[19] Rupture of a biliary mucocele may cause atypical bile peritonitis, and the effusion fluid color may be yellow or red. The cellularity is exudative and composed of high numbers of nondegenerate to mildly degenerate neutrophils and low to moderate numbers of macrophages and reactive mesothelial cells. Varying amounts of mostly extracellular amorphous, homogeneous, mucinous, basophilic material is seen in small clumps and lakes. This material has been termed *white bile,* although this mucinous material does not contain bile constituents (Figure 15-35 and Figure 15-36). In these cases, abdominal fluid bilirubin concentrations are typically, but not always, higher than serum bilirubin concentrations.[20]

Uroperitoneum

Uroperitoneum may result from leakage of urine from the kidney, ureter, urinary bladder, or urethra. Urine released into the peritoneal cavity acts as a chemical irritant and causes inflammation that may lead to an exudative process. Uroperitoneum effusions will have varying numbers of inflammatory cells depending on the duration and

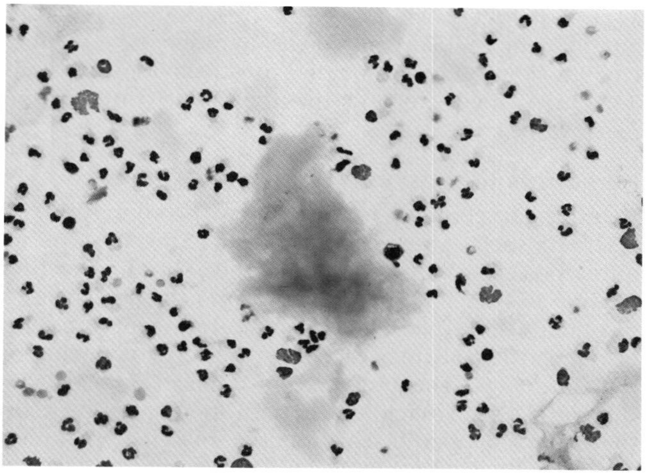

Figure 15-36 Abdominal fluid from a dog. "White bile" seen as a large accumulation of extracellular, homogeneous, pale basophilic, mucinous-type material, with large numbers of mildly degenerate neutrophils.

dilutional effect of urine; however, nucleated cell counts are typically less than 4000 cells/µL. the total protein content is generally low (<3 g/dL) because of the dilutional effect of urine volume. Neutrophils may be degenerate and ragged even in a nonseptic fluid because of the chemical irritant nature of urine. Bacteria and urinary crystals may also be found in the abdominal fluid if they were present in the bladder at the time of rupture. Comparing creatinine levels of the abdominal fluid to concurrent serum levels may confirm uroperitoneum. Creatinine of the abdominal fluid will generally be higher than the creatinine level of serum, as it equilibrates more slowly compared with blood urea nitrogen (BUN). Often, hyperkalemia and hyponatremia are present concurrently in serum. [21]

Heart Disease

Cats may develop a thoracic effusion secondary to cardiac insufficiency. These effusions are clear yellow to milky white and typically consist of greater than 50% (often >80%) small lymphocytes (see the following section titled "Chylous Effusions"). However, the proportion of neutrophils increases with repeated drainage of the effusion and also with the chronicity of the effusion.

Dogs may develop abdominal effusion secondary to right-sided heart failure. This effusion develops secondary to increased intrahepatic pressure and congestion with leakage of high-protein hepatic lymph. Nucleated cell counts and protein content are typically in the modified transudate range. Most of the nucleated cells consist of a mixture of mesothelial or macrophage-type cells, nondegenerate neutrophils, and lymphocytes. No cytologic finding in these effusions is pathognomonic for heart failure. Clinical signs, physical examination findings, radiography, echocardiography, and electrocardiography are usually necessary to establish a diagnosis of cardiovascular disease.

Chylous Effusions

Chylous effusions contain chylomicron-rich lymph fluid (chyle) that circulates in the lymphatic system.

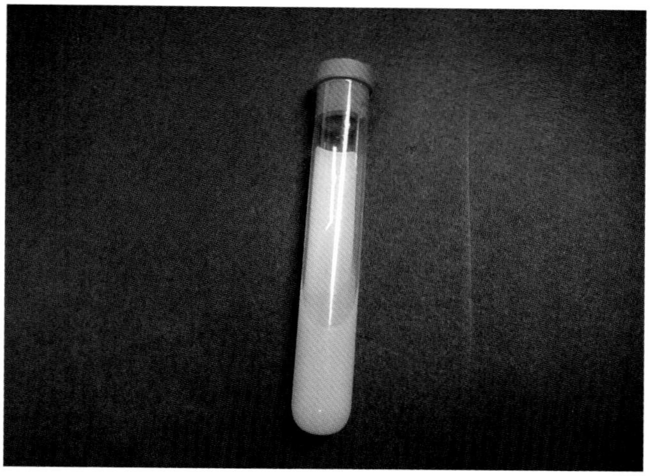

Figure 15-37 Milky white chylous pleural effusion from a cat.

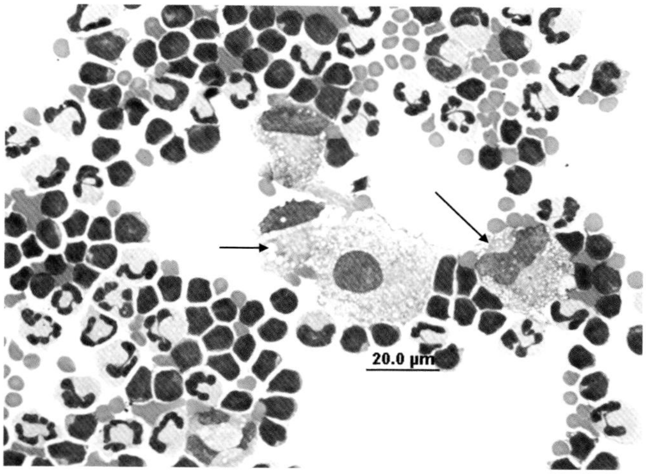

Figure 15-38 Chylous effusion. Numerous small lymphocytes and several macrophages containing small, distinct clear cytoplasmic vacuoles (*arrows*).

Chylomicrons are triglyceride-rich lipoproteins absorbed from the intestines after the ingestion of food containing lipids. Chylous effusions in dogs and cats occur most frequently as bilateral thoracic effusions, and chylous ascites occurs less frequently.[22]

The classic description of a chylous effusion is a milky fluid that does not clear after centrifugation and consists primarily of moderate to high numbers of small mature lymphocytes (Figure 15-37). Often, fewer macrophages are filled with small, punctate clear vacuoles and plasma cells (Figure 15-38). Chylous effusions are odorless and may vary in color from classic milky white to an opaque-yellow and an opaque-pink, depending on diet (i.e., thin or anorectic patients may not have the characteristic opaque white fluid because of lack of systemic lipids) and the number of RBCs in the fluid. Although small lymphocytes are typically thought of as the predominant cell type, chylous effusions may occur with predominating neutrophils, lipid-containing macrophages, or both.[23] Increased neutrophils occur secondary to inflammation induced by repeated thoracocentesis and the presence of chyle in the pleural cavity. Chyle is considered a nonirritant; however, it often causes an inflammatory reaction in some dogs and in most cats and may eventually lead to pleural fibrosis.[23] Bacterial infection in chylous effusions is uncommon because of the bacteriostatic effect of the fatty acids in chyle.[2,22,23] However, bacteria may be introduced as a result of repeated thoracocentesis.

If a chylous effusion that does not display the classic milky white color is suspected and if it is not predominated by mature lymphocytes, measurement and comparison of effusion and serum triglyceride and cholesterol concentrations may be performed.[2,22,23] With chylous effusions, the triglyceride concentration is higher in the effusion than in the serum, and the cholesterol concentration is higher in the serum than in the effusion.[2,22,23] The reverse is true for nonchylous effusions.[2,22] Identifying fat droplets cytologically on Sudan III–stained smears of the effusion aids in diagnosis of a chylous effusion; however, it is often unnecessary.[2,23]

Chyle normally drains from the thoracic duct into the venous system. Chylous effusions form when there is an obstruction (physical or functional) of lymphatic flow resulting in increased pressure within lymphatics and dilation of the thoracic duct (lymphangiectasia). Rupture of the thoracic duct (i.e., following surgery or blunt trauma) is a rare cause of chylous effusion in veterinary medicine and is usually self-limiting.[2,22] Physical obstructions of the thoracic duct may result from neoplasms (thymoma, lymphoma, lymphangiosarcoma), granulomas, or inflammatory reactions in the mediastinum that compress the thoracic duct or the vessels into which it drains, or secondary to obstruction of intralymphatic flow with neoplastic cells. Functional obstructions may occur with cardiovascular disease from increased central venous pressure (right-sided heart failure) or increased lymphatic flow from increased hepatic lymph production that exceeds drainage capability.[22,23] Cardiovascular disease (i.e., cardiomyopathy, heartworm disease, pericardial effusions) resulting in poor venous flow may also lead to chylous effusion as a functional effect.

Many other miscellaneous causes of chylous effusion, including coughing and vomiting, diaphragmatic herniation, congenital defects, trauma, and thrombosis of the thoracic duct, have been reported, and often, no underlying etiology can be determined despite extensive testing (idiopathic chylous effusion). [2,22,23]

Although most milky effusions are true chylous effusions, they may rarely be pseudochylous. True pseudochylous effusions are a debated entity; however, they are milky effusions that do not contain chyle. Instead, the white color is classically thought to be the result of cellular debris, lecithin globulin complex, cholesterol from cell membranes, or all of these. Pseudochylous effusions described in humans are most commonly the result of longstanding pleural effusions caused by tuberculosis, rheumatoid pleuritis, and malignant effusions, with resultant cell breakdown within the fluid. Despite much discussion about differentiating these two types of fluids, pseudochylous effusions are not well described in veterinary medicine and are rare in dogs and cats.[2,22] Cytologically, the presence of cellular breakdown material such as cholesterol crystals, as well as the lack of a significant lymphocytic cellular component, may suggest a pseudochylous effusion. Additionally, pseudochylous effusions have high cholesterol and low triglyceride content compared with serum.

Hemorrhagic Effusions

Hemorrhagic effusions may be seen with various primary disorders such as hemostatic defects (congenital or acquired coagulopathies), trauma, heartworm infection (Figure 15-39), and neoplasia. Hemorrhagic effusions secondary to neoplasia may contain no neoplastic cells, or neoplastic cells may be present in low, moderate, or high numbers. The presence or absence of neoplastic cells in a hemorrhagic effusion is often dependent on the type of neoplasm. For example, mesenchymal neoplasms such as hemangiosarcoma (splenic, hepatic, cardiac) often lack neoplastic cells or contain low numbers of neoplastic cells within the hemorrhagic effusion. In comparison, if mesothelioma is associated with a hemorrhagic effusion, often moderate to high numbers of neoplastic mesothelial cells are evident. Thus, determining the etiology of a hemorrhagic effusion, just as in the case of other effusion categories, requires not only cytological assessment of the fluid, but also correlation with clinical signs, history, laboratory data base, imaging analysis and often, fine-needle aspiration (FNA) or fine-needle aspiration biopsy (FNB) of abnormalities found in the respective body cavity.

Distinguishing hemorrhagic effusions from iatrogenic blood contamination or inadvertent aspiration of an organ (i.e., liver, spleen) is of diagnostic importance. Differentiating blood contamination from per-acute or acute hemorrhage may be difficult; however, assessment of clinical signs, physical examination findings, and laboratory data are helpful. Hemorrhage of more than 24 hours duration may be differentiated from blood contamination by identifying erythrophagocytosis in the sample (Figure 15-40) and noting the presence or absence of platelets and the RBC

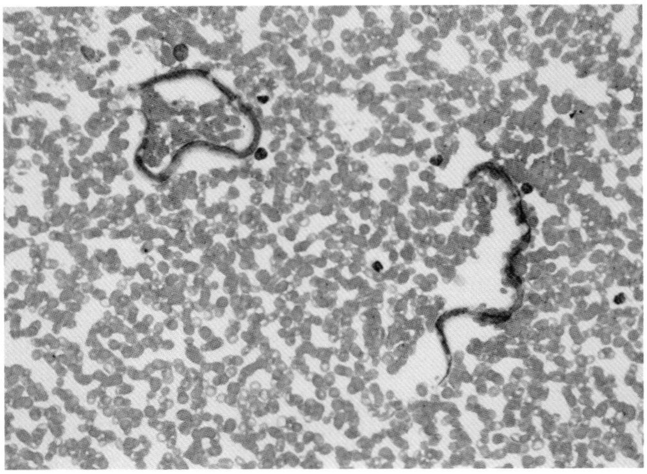

Figure 15-39 Hemodilute background with two large, basophilic microfilaria and few scattered blood leukocytes and few small platelet clumps. (Courtesy of Jennifer Neel, North Carolina State University.)

breakdown products, hemosiderin, and hematoidin (Figure 15-41, Figure 15-42, and Figure 15-43). When blood enters a body cavity, the platelets quickly aggregate, degranulate, and disappear. Also, RBCs are phagocytized and digested by macrophages. Therefore, the presence of platelets and lack of erythrophagocytosis or heme breakdown products suggests either per-acute hemorrhage or iatrogenic blood contamination. Concurrent identification of platelets and erythrophagocytosis, with or without heme breakdown products, suggests either chronic persistent hemorrhage or previous hemorrhage with iatrogenic contamination. The absence of platelets, with evidence of erythrophagocytosis, heme breakdown products, or a combination of both, supports chronic or previous hemorrhage.

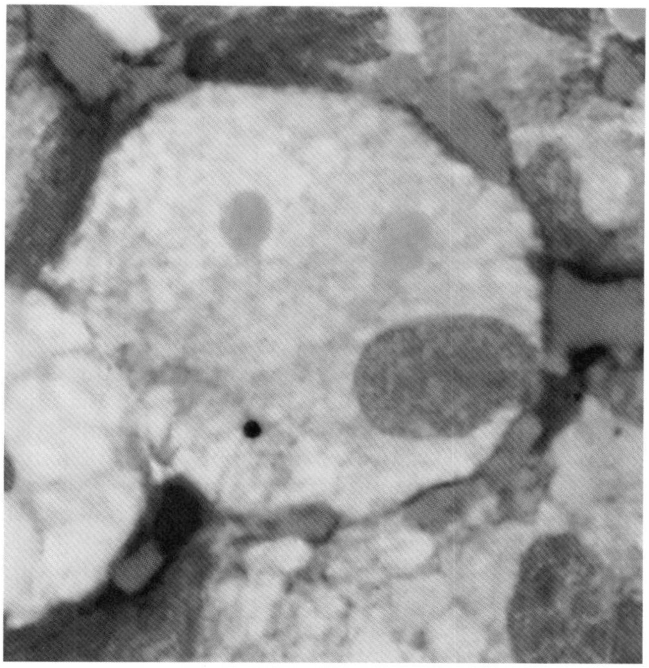

Figure 15-40 Erythrophagocytosis.

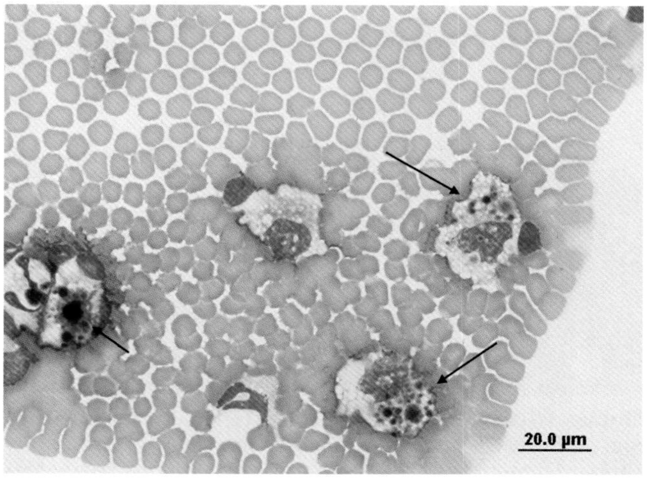

Figure 15-41 Numerous macrophages containing hemosiderin pigment (*arrows*).

In cases of inadvertent organ aspiration, inadvertent major vessel puncture, or frank intracavity hemorrhage, the fluid obtained will be grossly bloody. With a major vessel or splenic aspirate, the PCV of the fluid is generally equal to (vessel puncture) or greater than (splenic aspirate) the peripheral blood PCV. With severe intracavity hemorrhage, clinical signs of hemorrhagic shock are expected.

Neoplastic Effusions

Effusions may occur secondary to many forms of neoplasia (lymphoma, mast cell neoplasia, sarcoma, mesothelioma, carcinoma or adenocarcinoma, etc.) and may often be diagnosed by cytologic examination of the fluid. In one study, the sensitivity of cytologic examination of effusions to detect malignant neoplasms was 64% in dogs and 61% in cats.[24] Poorly exfoliating tumors will generally have effusions in the modified transudate range and may

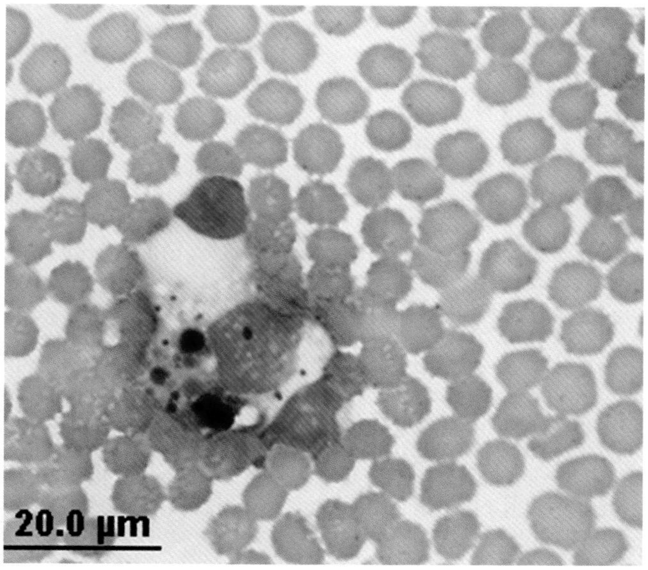

Figure 15-42 Macrophage containing hemosiderin pigment and numerous red blood cells.

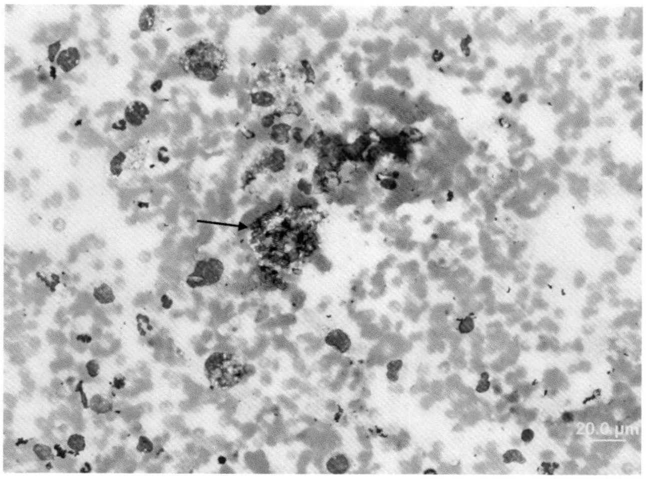

Figure 15-43 Hemorrhagic pericardial fluid and a macrophage containing hematoidin crystals (*arrow*).

have concurrent inflammation. As some tumors do not exfoliate neoplastic cells, the absence of neoplastic cells within effusions does not rule out neoplasia. Similar to tissue aspirates, neoplastic cells in an effusion must be distinguished from dysplastic cells secondary to inflammation. Thus, the presence of concurrent inflammation in the fluid may confound definitive diagnosis of neoplasia, especially if neoplastic cells are not in high numbers, do not exhibit significant cytologic criteria of malignancy, or both. Distinguishing neoplastic epithelial cells (exfoliative carcinoma or adenocarcinoma) from mesothelioma, and mesothelioma from hyperplastic and reactive mesothelial cells, which are frequently found in both neoplastic and non-neoplastic fluids, is of particular challenge in effusion cytology. This dilemma is discussed further in the section on mesothelioma below. Neoplastic effusions are inherently difficult samples to interpret for many of the reasons outlined above, and therefore, in-house samples interpreted as neoplastic, or suspected of being neoplastic, should be confirmed by a veterinary clinical pathologist.

Lymphoma: A neoplastic effusion secondary to high-grade lymphoma may occur with lymphoma of the intracavitary lymph nodes, spleen, liver gastrointestinal tract, kidneys, thymus, and mediastinum. Cytologically, low to high numbers of a monomorphic population of exfoliating lymphoblasts pay be present (see Figure 15-12 and Figure 15-13; Figure 15-44). Lymphoblasts are large cells, with a scant to moderate amount of basophilic cytoplasm, round to variably shaped eccentric nuclei, finely stippled nuclear chromatin, and prominent nucleoli.

Mast Cell Neoplasia: Mast cell tumors within body cavities (nodal, hepatic, splenic, gastrointestinal) may cause effusions and frequently exfoliate large numbers of mast cells into the effusion (see Figure 15-17). Mast cells are readily identified by large numbers of metachromatic (purple) cytoplasmic granules. In effusions, mast cells tend to have "packeted" granules, and because of the high affinity of granules for stain and stain exhaustion, the nucleus may stain poorly or not at all. Diff-Quik stain does not undergo the same metachromatic reaction as Wright-Giemsa or modified Wright stain and often does not stain mast cell granules well. Eosinophils are occasionally (but not reliably) present, as are few scattered nondegenerate neutrophils, mesothelial cells, and macrophages.

Sarcoma: Sarcomas involving intracavity organs often do not exfoliate neoplastic mesenchymal cells into effusions and are rarely diagnosed on fluid analysis alone. Often, effusions secondary to mesenchymal tumors are hemorrhagic secondary to rupture of the tumor (i.e., splenic and hepatic hemangiosarcoma) and of low nucleated cellularity. In this case, making concentrated specimens or buffy coat preparations may aid in concentrating low numbers of neoplastic cells. In the rare event that neoplastic cells are identified, the cells have a characteristic spindle appearance and malignant criteria (see Chapter 2). Recently, a myxosarcoma of the right auricle of a dog was identified on the basis of the presence of a myxoid, mucopurulent pleural fluid and atypical cell components together with histopathology of the tumor.[25]

Mesothelioma: Mesotheliomas are uncommon tumors in domestic species and are difficult to diagnose cytologically because of the pleomorphism exhibited by reactive mesothelial cells. Thus, when an effusion contains high numbers of mesothelial cells where significant cytologic criteria of malignancy is not evident, it is often impossible to differentiate mesothelial reactivity or hyperplasia from mesothelioma. When mesothelial cells exhibit marked criteria of malignancy—notably large clumps of cells, extreme macrocytosis, marked anisokaryosis, large variably shaped nucleoli, large numbers of mitotic figures, and aberrant mitoses—although diagnostic on cytology for an exfoliative neoplasm, it may be nearly impossible to differentiate mesothelioma from carcinoma or adenocarcinoma (Figure 15-45).[26] In the latter case, identification of a primary

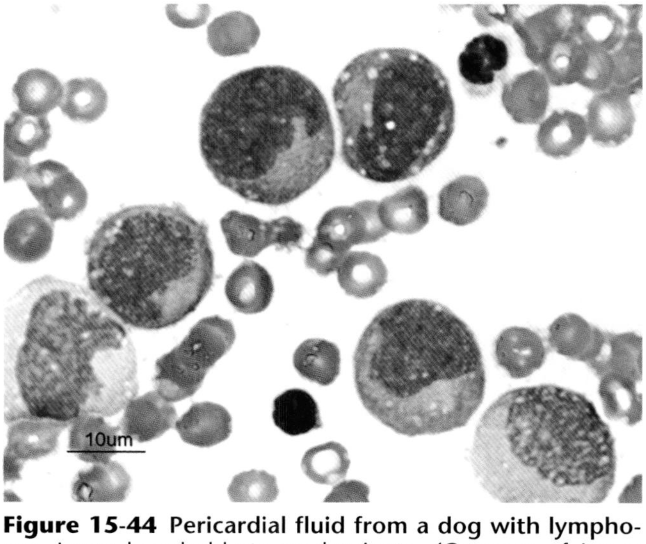

Figure 15-44 Pericardial fluid from a dog with lymphoma. Large lymphoblasts predominate. (Courtesy of James Meinkoth, Oklahoma State University.)

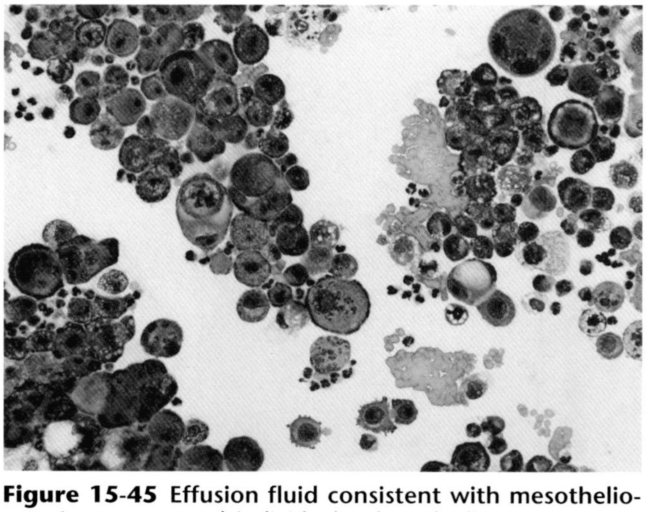

Figure 15-45 Effusion fluid consistent with mesothelioma. Aggregates and individualized markedly pleomorphic, neoplastic mesothelial cells are present. Note the many features of malignancy such as cell giganticism, multinucleation, macrokaryosis, macronucleoli, and multiple nucleoli.

tumor is helpful. If a primary tumor is not identified, histopathology of affected mesothelium is necessary, and as for cytology, sometimes histopathologic differentiation of reactive or hyperplastic mesothelial cells from neoplastic mesothelial cells may be challenging. Histopathologically, no single defined criterion to diagnose mesothelioma exists. Mesothelioma may be epitheliod (carcinoma-like), sarcomatoid (spindle-cell features), or both (biphasic).[27] Assessing for neoplastic invasion into the submesothelial tissues is helpful, and immunohistochemistry, electron microscopy, or both may be helpful.[26] Figure 15-46 demonstrates the histopathology of mesothelioma.

Carcinoma or Adenocarcinoma: Carcinomas and adenocarcinomas may often be diagnosed by cytologic evaluation of effusions on the basis of significant numbers of exfoliating cells and numerous criteria of malignancy. Neoplastic effusions may be inflammatory (Figure 15-47) or noninflammatory. Neoplastic epithelial cells often form aggregates, clusters, and sheets (see Figure 15-47). Occasional glandular (acinar) arrangements may be found. Significant anisokaryosis may exist, with cell giganticism and abundant basophilic cytoplasm that may be vacuolated or contain intracytoplasmic eosinophilic secretory material. Documenting strong nuclear criteria of malignancy is important in definitive diagnosis and may include anisokaryosis; nuclear gigantism; coarse nuclear chromatin; large, bizarre, or angular nucleoli; multiple nucleoli; nuclear molding; high nucleus-to-cytoplasm ratios; multinucleation (Figure 15-48); numerous mitotic figures; and aberrant mitoses (Figure 15-49 and Figure 15-50). When an effusion is diagnostic for epithelial neoplasia, imaging analysis of the respective body cavity may identify masses or organomegaly, prompting FNA or tissue biopsy to further characterize it.

Thymoma: Thymomas are neoplasms of the thymic epithelium and are a top differential for the presence of a cranial mediastinal mass. Thymomas may be benign or malignant, and invasive and noninvasive forms exist. Additionally, thymomas may be heterogeneous, cystic, and inflamed. A detailed description of the cytologic appearance of aspirates from thymomas is provided in Chapter 17. When thymomas are associated with a thoracic effusion, the effusion may be nondiagnostic or suggestive of thymoma but is rarely definitively diagnostic. An effusion associated with thymoma may contain large numbers of small mature lymphocytes, which are often a significant and occasionally predominant nonneoplastic cell population in thymomas. The presence of a prominent population of mature lymphocytes, together with low to

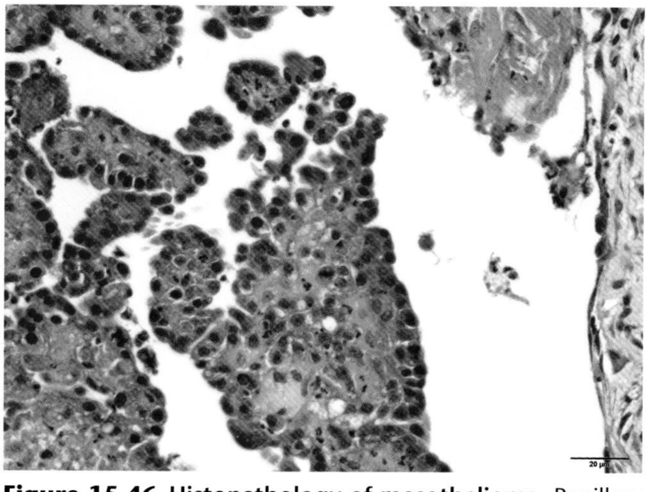

Figure 15-46 Histopathology of mesothelioma. Papillary projections of multilayer neoplastic mesothelium with significant cellular pleomorphism and frequent mitoses. (Courtesy of Luke Borst, North Carolina State University.)

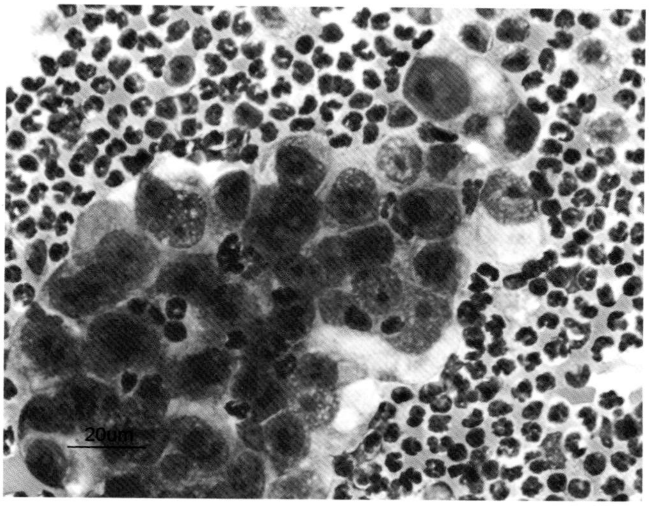

Figure 15-47 Pleural fluid from a dog with adenocarcinoma. A cluster of atypical cells and numerous nondegenerate neutrophils. (Courtesy of James Meinkoth, Oklahoma State University.)

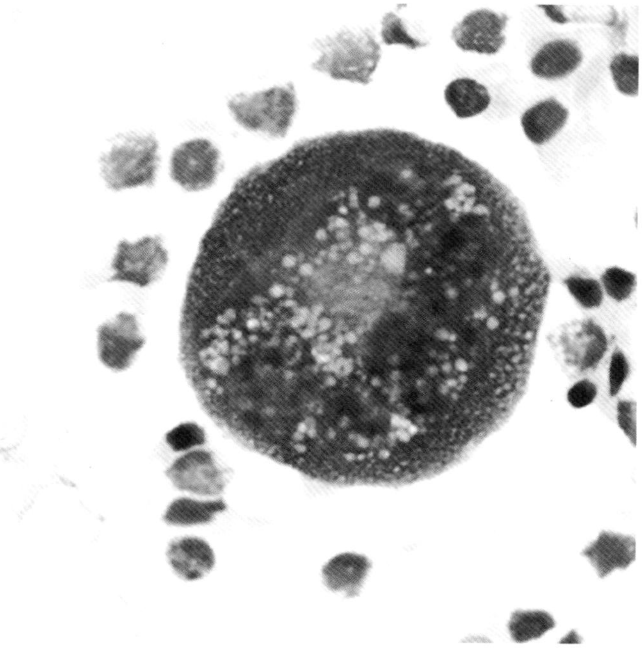

Figure 15-48 Note the large atypical multinucleate cell in pleural fluid from a dog with carcinoma.

moderate numbers of well-differentiated mast cells (also a prominent cell population in thymomas), helps lend support to a diagnosis of thymoma if a cranial mediastinal mass is evident. It is uncommon for the neoplastic epithelial component to exfoliate, and if it is present, it may be difficult to differentiate from mesothelial cells. The neoplastic epithelial cells have somewhat ill-defined borders, are found in aggregates and sheets, and contain small to moderate amounts of pale blue cytoplasm, round central nuclei, and indistinct nucleoli. The cells often are minimally pleomorphic. Usually, direct aspiration, tissue biopsy, or both are needed for definitive diagnosis of thymoma and to rule out thymic lymphoma.

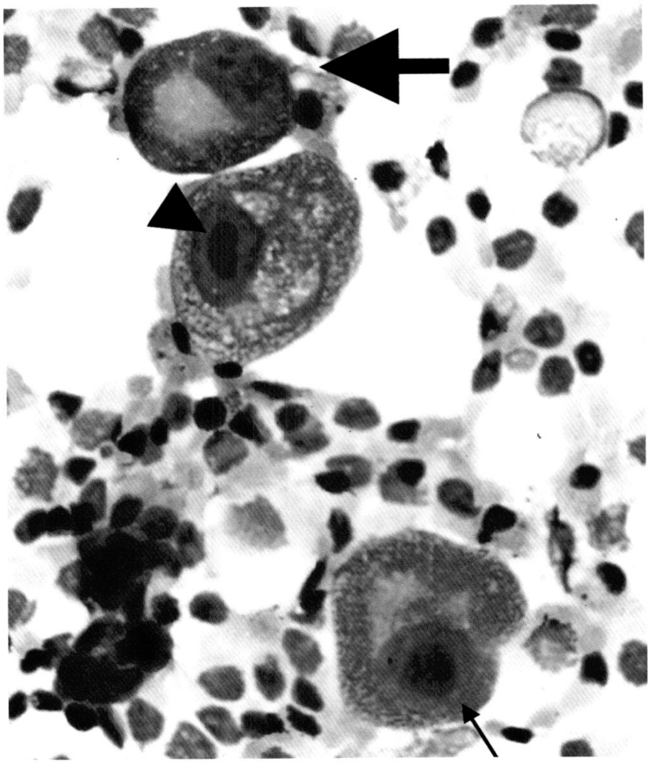

Figure 15-49 Several large atypical cells with large (*small arrow*), angular (*arrowhead*), and multiple (*large arrow*) nucleoli.

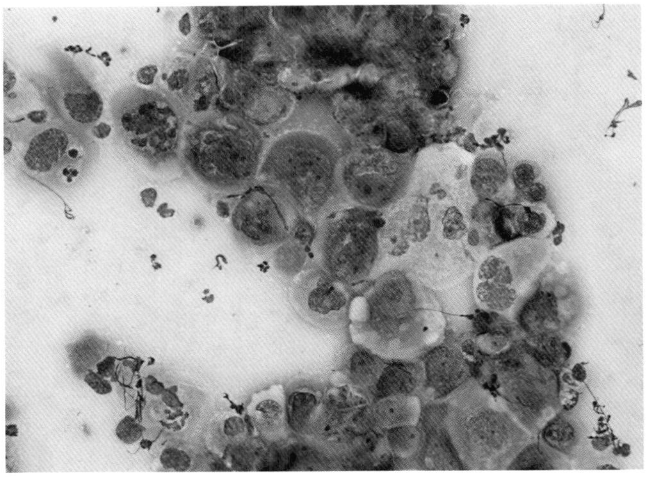

Figure 15-50 Pleural fluid from a cat with adenocarcinoma. Aggregates of haphazardly arranged, markedly pleomorphic, and extremely large neoplastic epithelial cells are present. Note the large size of cells, nuclei, and nucleoli compared with the few background neutrophils.

Parasitic Effusions

Abdominal effusion caused by aberrant larval migration of the tapeworm *Mesocestoides* spp. is uncommon. Cases of canine infection are reported in northwestern United States, particularly in California, with fewer cases in Washington.[28] Clinical signs may include anorexia, vomiting, weight loss, depression, and abdominal distension. In reported cases of parasitic effusions, the gross appearance of the fluid contains small opaque flecks which are the metacestodes.[28] Analysis of the aspirated fluid is in the exudative range. Cytologic features include numerous inflammatory cells, partial to intact metacestodes, and numerous round to angular, clear to pink refractile calcareous corpuscles (Figure 15-51 and Figure 15-52).

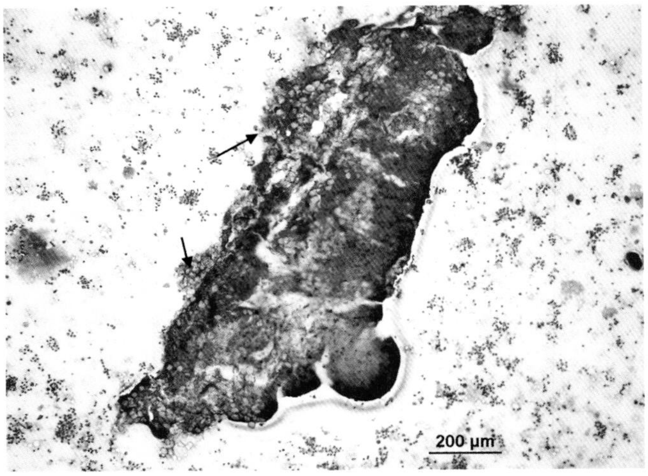

Figure 15-51 Remnant of metacestode. Note the size of the red blood cells and inflammatory cells in the background. The clear, nonstaining structures are calcareous corpuscles (*arrows*).

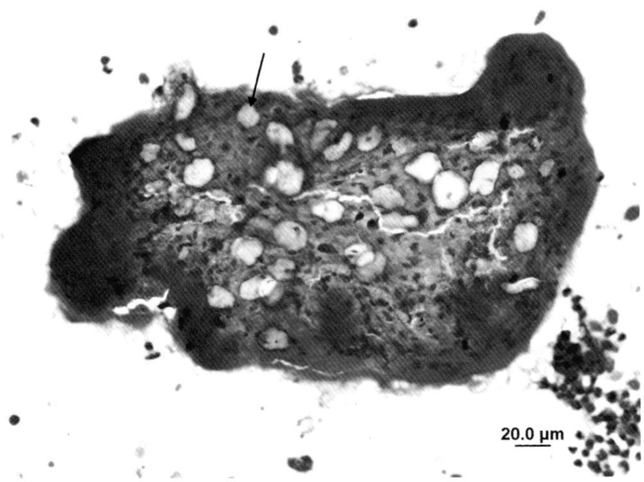

Figure 15-52 Remnant of a metacestode. The clear, nonstaining structures are calcareous corpuscles (*arrow*).

References

1. Nelson OL: Pleural effusion. In Ettinger SJ, Feldman EC, editors: *Textbook of veterinary internal medicine*, Philadelphia, PA, 2005, Saunders, pp 204–207.
2. Fossum TW: Surgery of the lower respiratory system: pleural cavity and diaphragm. In Fossum TW, editor: *Small animal surgery*, St Louis, MO, 2005, Mosby, pp 788–820.
3. Zoia A, Hughes D, Connolly DJ: Pericardial effusion and cardiac tamponade in a cat with extranodal lymphoma, *J Small Anim Pract* 45:467–471, 2004.
4. Tobias AH: Pericardial disorders. In Ettinger SJ, Feldman EC, editors: *Textbook of veterinary internal medicine*, Philadelphia, PA, 2005, Saunders, pp 1107–1111.
5. Gidlewski J, Petrie JP: Therapeutic pericardiocentesis in the dog and cat, *Clin Tech Small Anim Pract* 20:151–155, 2005.
6. Fossum TW: Surgery of the abdominal cavity. In Fossum TW, editor: *Small animal surgery*, St, Louis, MO, 2002, Mosby, pp 271–272.
7. Walters JM: Abdominal paracentesis and diagnostic peritoneal lavage, *Clin Tech Small Anim Pract* 18(1):32–38, 2003.
8. D'Urso L: Thoracic and pericardial taps and drains. In Ettinger SJ, Feldman EC, editors: *Textbook of veterinary internal medicine*, Philadelphia, PA, 2005, Saunders, pp 380–831.
9. Johnson M, et al: A retrospective study of clinical findings, treatment and outcome in 143 dogs with pericardial effusion, *J Small Anim Pract* 45:546–552, 2004.
10. Cowell RL, et al: Collection and evaluation of equine peritoneal and pleural effusions, *Vet Clin North Am (Equine Pract)* 3:543–561, 1987.
11. George JW: The usefulness and limitations of hand-held refractometers in veterinary laboratory medicine: an historical and technical review, *Vet Clin Path* 30(4):201–210, 2001.
12. Cowgill E, Neel J: Pleural fluid from a dog with marked eosinophilia, *Vet Clin Pathol* 32(4):147–149, 2003.
13. Takahashi T, et al: Visceral mast cell tumors in dogs: 10 cases (1982-1997), *J Am Vet Assoc* 216(2):222–226, 2000.
14. Barger A, Riensche M: What is your diagnosis? Hemorrhagic effusion in a dog, *Vet Clin Pathol* 38(4):529–531, 2009.
15. Arndt Holmberg T, Vernau W, Melli AC: Conrad PA: Neospora caninum associated with septic peritonitis in an adult dog, *Vet Clin Pathol* 35(2):235–238, 2006.
16. Dell'Orco M, Bertazzolo W, Paccioretti F: What is your diagnosis? Peritoneal effusion from a dog, *Vet Clin Pathol* 38(3):367–369, 2009.
17. Rohrbach BW, et al: Epidemiology of feline infectious peritonitis among cats examined at veterinary medical teaching hospitals, *J Am Vet Assoc* 218(7):1111–1115, 2001.
18. Hartmann K, et al: Comparison of different tests to diagnose feline infectious peritonitis, *J Vet Intern Med* 17:781–790, 2003.
19. Pike FS, et al: Gallbladder mucocele in dogs: 30 cases (2000-2002), *J Am Vet Assoc* 224(10):1615–1622, 2004.
20. Owens SD, et al: Three cases of canine bile peritonitis with mucinous material in abdominal fluid as the prominent cytologic finding, *Vet Clin Pathol* 32(3):114–120, 2003.
21. Aumann M, Worth LT, Drobatz KJ: Uroperitoneum in cats: 26 cases (1986-1995), *J Am Anim Hosp Assoc* 34(4):315–324, 1998.
22. Meadows RL, MacWilliams PS: Chylous effusions revisited, *Vet Clin Pathol* 23:54–62, 1994.
23. Mertens MM, Fossum TW: Pleural and extrapleural diseases. In Fossum TW, editor: *Small animal surgery*, St. Louis, MO, 2002, Mosby, pp 1281–1282.
24. Hirschberger J, et al: Sensitivity and specificity of cytologic evaluation in the diagnosis of neoplasia in body fluids from dogs and cats, *Vet Clin Path* 28(4):142–146, 1999.
25. Riegel CM, et al: What is your diagnosis? Muculent pleural effusion from a dog, *Vet Clin Pathol* 37(3):353–356, 2008.
26. Reggeti F, Brisson B, Ruotsalo K, et al: Invasive epithelial mesothelioma in a dog, *Vet Pathol* 42:77–81, 2005.
27. Head KW, Else RW, Dubielzig RR: Tumors of the alimentary tract. In Meuten DJ, editor: *Tumors of domestic animals*, ed 4, Ames, IA, 2002, Iowa State Press, pp 477–478.
28. Caruso KJ, et al: Cytologic diagnosis of peritoneal cestodiasis in dogs caused by *Mesocestoides* sp, *Vet Clin Pathol* 32(2):50–60, 2003.

CHAPTER 16

Transtracheal and Bronchoalveolar Washes

Kate English, Rick L. Cowell, Ronald D. Tyler and James H. Meinkoth

Respiratory flushes or washes sample the contents of the airways, the trachea, bronchi, and alveolar spaces. These samples frequently provide clinically useful information of the pulmonary disease process and may also provide definitive diagnosis in some patients. Pulmonary disease is often defined by the area that it affects (e.g., bronchitis) or by the changes that may occur as a result of the disease process (e.g., bronchiectasis); however, the underlying pathology may be variable with these disease presentations, and cytology and culture of a lower respiratory tract sample may be helpful in determining the etiology. In pathologies that solely involve abnormal structure or function of the airways or in diseases that do not have direct airway involvement, which may include some primary or metastatic neoplasms, the information obtained from a flush or wash sample may be limited.[1,2] Cytology of flush or wash samples may, however, be highly sensitive in cases of inflammatory airway disease.[3]

Tracheal wash or bronchoalveolar lavage (TW/BAL) samples are quick, easy, and inexpensive ways to obtain diagnostic samples from the respiratory tree. Although complications are rare, subcutaneous emphysema, pneumomediastinum, hemorrhage, resultant hypoxia, needle tract infection, transient hemoptysis, bronchoconstriction, and other complications have been reported.[4-7]

It is frequently helpful to perform radiography in conjunction with the wash procedure, although radiographic changes may not always be apparent in the early stages of respiratory disease.[8,9] Radiography prior to a flush or wash procedure may be invaluable if the disease is focal because this will indicate which lung lobe is most likely to provide a diagnostic yield and allow selective sampling, particularly if bronchoscope-guided lavage is used. If the disease is diffuse, sampling of any area of the lung may be representative, although sampling from multiple sites is more likely to provide a diagnostic yield.[10]

The cell types noted in the sample may vary, depending on the site of sampling (Table 16-1 and Table 16-2).

TECHNIQUE OF TRACHEAL WASH AND BRONCHOALVEOLAR LAVAGE

Approach to the lower respiratory tract may be transtracheal or endotracheal. If the endotracheal approach is used, sampling may be performed by bronchoscopic or nonbronchoscopic (blind) methods.

The advantage of the bronchoscope is that observation of the mucosa lining the airways and quantification of mucus or secretions present may provide additional information during patient assessment. More directed sampling of the individual lobes may also be performed. Nonbronchoscopic sampling, however, does not require expensive equipment and so may be more widely available in first opinion practice.

Many reviews of the sampling techniques exist.[11-14] However, a brief summary is outlined here.

TABLE 16-1

Lining Cells of the Lower Respiratory Tract That May Be Noted on Tracheal Wash or Bronchoalveolar Lavage Sampling

Airway	Lining cell
Large airway, trachea, and bronchi	Ciliated columnar epithelium, goblet cell
Bronchiole	Columnar to cuboidal epithelium, ciliated to nonciliated
Alveolus	Type I pneumocyte (not commonly observed on bronchoalveolar lavage cytology)

From Bacha WJ Jr., Bacha LM: Respiratory system. Anderson RC: **Nematode Parasites of Vertebrates. Their Development and Transmission.** 2nd Edition. CABI Publishing, Wallingford, Oxon (UK) 2000.

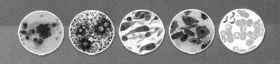

TABLE 16-2

Average of Mean Percentage Cell Differential of Nonepithelial Populations from a Number of Studies of Bronchoalveolar Lavage Samples from Healthy Dogs and Cats

	Macrophage	Neutrophil	Eosinophil	Lymphocyte	Mast Cell
Dogs	71%	5%	5%	17%	2%
Cats	70%	6%	18%	4%	1%

Transtracheal Sampling

The transtracheal or percutaneous method is optimal for patients who are a high anesthetic risk because it may be performed with local anesthesia only or with additional sedation, if required. This technique may also be less prone to oropharyngeal contamination and, therefore, may be preferred if obtaining a sample for culture. Small amounts of fluid are instilled, and a cough reflex is essential for fluid recovery.

- The skin over the cranioventral larynx is clipped and the site is prepared as for aseptic surgery. Surgical gloves should be worn.
- A small amount of 1% to 2% lidocaine is injected into subcutaneous tissue. Very light sedation may be helpful in cats and small dogs;[4] intravenous ketamine has been recommended for sedation of cats.[5]
- The animal is restrained in a sitting position or in sternal recumbency, with the neck extended. Overextension of the neck, however, may result in increased oropharyngeal contamination.
- A small, triangular depression is digitally palpated just cranial to the ridge of the cricoid cartilage. This is the location of the cricothyroid ligament and of needle insertion (Figure 16-1). Alternatively, the catheter may be inserted between two tracheal rings 1 to 3 cm below the larynx (e.g., C2 to C3, or C3 to C4).[15]
- Using a large commercial intravenous catheter set, "through the needle," or intravascular catheter and a 3.5-French (Fr) polyethylene urinary catheter, with the needle directed slightly caudad, the skin, subcutaneous tissue, and cricothyroid ligament of the larynx, or ligament between the tracheal rings, are penetrated.[5] Smaller catheters are recommended for cats and very small dogs.
- Once in the tracheal lumen, the needle is positioned parallel to the trachea, and the catheter is advanced through the needle and down the lumen of the trachea to a level just above the carina. Insertion of the needle and passage of the catheter induces coughing in most animals.[4,5]
- The catheter should pass easily; if it does not, it may have become embedded in the dorsal tracheal wall or failed to enter the trachea and may be embedded in the peritracheal tissue.[16] In either case, the needle and the entire catheter should be withdrawn and the procedure repeated. Also, the catheter may bend, causing it to advance toward the oropharynx, which results in the washing of the oropharynx, not the bronchial tree.
- Once the catheter is properly placed, the needle is withdrawn, leaving the catheter in place. With some severe pulmonary diseases, a sample may be obtained by simply aspirating after positioning the catheter. However, the infusion of saline into the bronchial tree is usually necessary before aspiration to obtain an adequate sample. A 12-mL (milliliter) or larger syringe containing 1 to 2 mL of nonbacteriostatic, sterile, buffered saline for every 5 kilogram (kg) of body weight is attached to the catheter. The saline is injected into the bronchial lumen until either the animal starts to cough or all of the fluid is injected.
- The animal will typically start coughing before all of the saline is injected, at which time aspiration must start. If coughing does not occur, coupage may be helpful. Only a small portion of the injected fluid will be retrieved. The injected fluid remaining in the tracheobronchial tree will be rapidly absorbed and is no cause for concern.[4]
- The operator aspirates for only a few seconds and then stops. Aspiration for a prolonged time results in more fluid being collected, but the chances of a contaminated wash are greatly increased because the animal will cough fluid into the oropharyngeal area and reaspirate the fluid, which now contains cellular and bacterial contaminants.

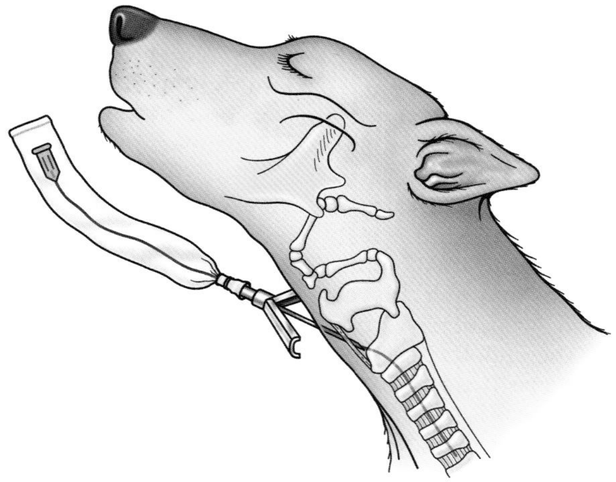

Figure 16-1 Diagrammatic representation of needle placement through the cricothyroid ligament of the larynx.

Maintaining gentle pressure on the puncture site for a few minutes generally inhibits the formation of subcutaneous emphysema.[15] Applying mild pressure to the puncture site with a gauze wrap for 12 to 24 hours also helps eliminate the formation of subcutaneous emphysema.

Endotracheal Tube Technique

Alternatively, samples are collected through an endotracheal tube (Figure 16-2). This procedure requires general anesthesia. This technique may be used to obtain either a TW or a BAL. For a tracheal sample, the sample catheter extends beyond the end of the endotracheal tube but does not extend past the carina. The location of the carina is externally assessed as approximately the level of the fourth intercostal space.[10] For a blind BAL, a sample tube of appropriate size for the patient (e.g., a 16-Fr polyvinyl chloride stomach tube in a medium- to large-sized dog, and a 5-Fr polypropylene urinary catheter in a cat) was shown to consistently maintain a snug fit between the external landmarks of the seventh and eleventh ribs, so the sample tubing should be a minimum length to reach the level of the eleventh rib.[17,18] Sterile tubing should be used. Pretreatment with bronchodilators is recommended by some authors prior to BAL.[7]

- Once the patient has reached a suitable plane of anesthesia, an endotracheal tube should be carefully placed with as minimal contact with the oropharynx and larynx as may be achieved.
- Preoxygenation is recommended. Fitting of a T- or Y-piece to the endotracheal tube will allow delivery of oxygen and anesthetic gas throughout the procedure. If the leakage of gas is a particular concern to the veterinary staff, anesthesia may be maintained by injectable anesthetic agents administered via an intravenous (IV) catheter.
- The patient is placed in sternal or lateral recumbency; if the lateral position is used, it is preferable to place the most affected side down.[14] In some cases, use of a foam wedge to elevate the cranial part of the thorax above that of the caudal part has been recommended.[19]
- A bronchoscope, tube, or catheter through which the sample will be obtained is introduced through the endotracheal tube, ensuring this does not contact the oropharynx.

The canine bronchial tree branches in an irregular manner and has been reviewed in detail.[20] Briefly, when the patient is orientated in sternal recumbency, from the bronchial tree, the entrance to the right principal bronchus appears as almost a direct continuation of the trachea, with the left principal bronchus seen at a more acute angle. The first lobar bronchus on the right is the right cranial lung lobe, in the lateral wall of the bronchus opposite the carina. The next lobar bronchus is the right middle lung lobe, in the ventral floor, usually between the 6 and 8 o'clock positions. The right accessory lobe is located in the ventromedial to medial aspect of the right principal bronchus, just beyond the origin of the middle lobe bronchus, extending in a ventromedial direction. Beyond this bronchus is the lobar bronchus for the right caudal lung lobe. On the left the left cranial lung lobe is accessed ventrolateral to the lateral aspect of the left cranial bronchus. Beyond this, the left principal bronchus becomes the left caudal lung lobe bronchus. Figure 16-3 shows a cast of a canine bronchial tree to provide an idea of the branching that may be seen in vivo.

The feline bronchial tree has also been reviewed.[21] The right principal bronchus is similarly a near continuation of the trachea, as in the dog, with the left principal bronchus at a slightly more acute angle. Entering the right principal bronchus, the right cranial bronchus

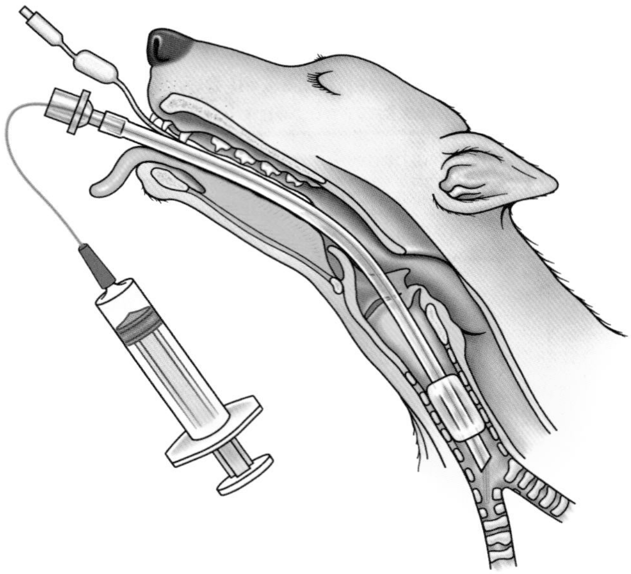

Figure 16-2 Diagrammatic representation of catheter placement and tracheal wash or bronchoalveolar lavage collection through an endotracheal tube.

is first encountered, arising lateral to the right principal bronchus and directly opposite the carina. Advancing caudally, the next lobar bronchus is the right middle lung lobe located ventrally. The right accessory lobe bronchus and the first segment of the right caudal lobar bronchus arise at approximately the same level, with the right accessory lobe bronchus being located ventromedially and the right caudal bronchus dorsally. The second segment of the right caudal lobe bronchus is more dorsal and located ventrally, with the third segment more caudal and dorsal. Entering the left principal bronchus, the left cranial lobar bronchus is lateral and slightly ventral. The continuation of the left principal bronchus enters the left caudal lobe bronchus, with the segmental bronchi branching alternately dorsally and ventrally as in the right caudal lobe. It may not be possible to enter all of the bronchi or even visualize the more caudal bronchi in all cats examined.

- If the patient is in lateral recumbency, the orientation and access to the lung for sampling may be altered.[22]
- When the desired level has been reached for a TW or a BAL (see previous), then fluid may be introduced. To optimize recovery of fluid from a BAL, the bronchoscope or tube should be wedged into the bronchi. This may be determined visually on a bronchoscope. If performing a blind BAL, then the tube should be advanced gently until it stops; it should then be withdrawn a few centimeters, rotated gently, and readvanced until resistance is felt at a consistent level.[17]
- Once a snug fit has been achieved, a syringe with an appropriate volume of fluid and an additional 5-mL of air to ensure complete delivery of the fluid is attached to the top of the sample tube. Volumes used may vary; however, a suitable volume in cats is reported to be aliquots of 5-mL/kg.[23] This volume may be used in dogs, but volumes of 2-mL/kg have been reported to be adequate.[24,25] Repeat aliquots may be administered until sufficient fluid is retrieved; however, no more than three aliquots are generally used.

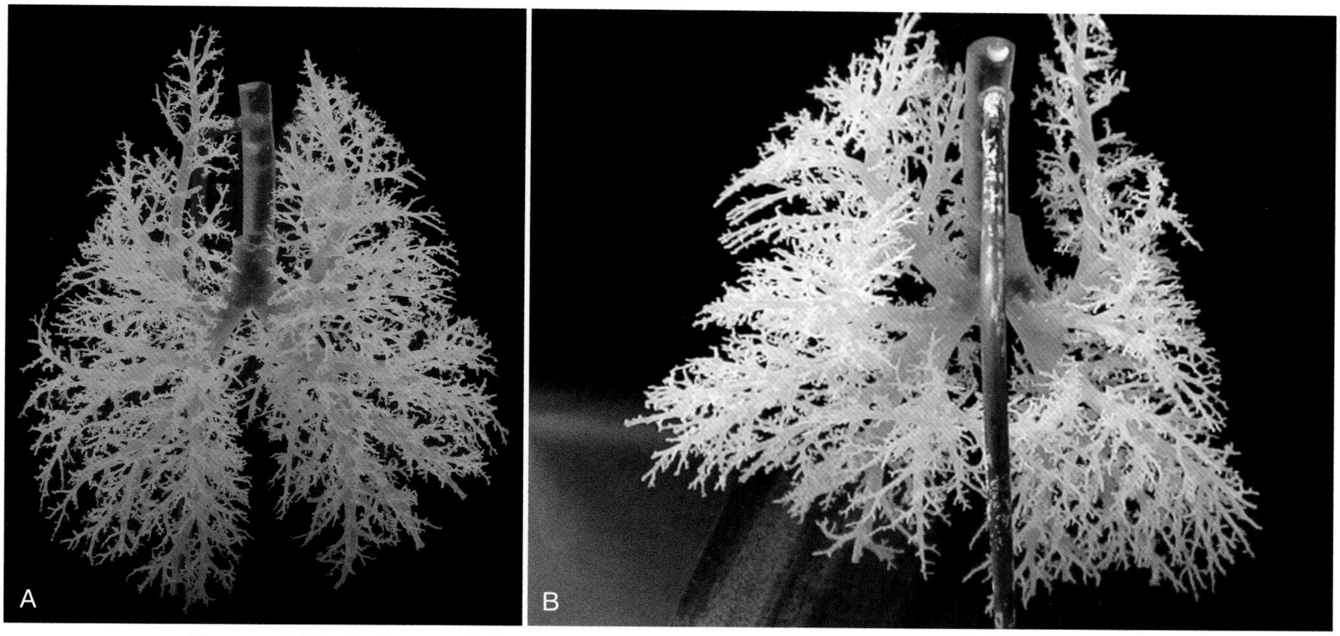

Figure 16-3 **A,** A cast of the canine bronchial tree. **B,** Close-up of the area of the bifurcation of the trachea to show the bronchial branching in more detail. (**A,** Courtesy of A. Crook, RVC, U.K.)

- Fluid recovery may be affected by the tightness of the fit of the bronchoscope or sample tubing in the airway. In the double catheter technique, the catheter to collect the sample is placed a few centimeters above the level of the catheter delivering the fluid aliquot; the authors describing this technique have reported good fluid recovery without the need for a snug fit.[26]

Other measures that may increase fluid retrieval include tilting the head of the patient downward and rotating the patient with the lavaged lung area uppermost to encourage fluid drainage.[27] This may be complicated in larger patients, and the risk of gastric dilation-volvulus in large, deep-chested dogs may also be a concern with rotation of these patients. Coupage may also be helpful.

Retrieved fluid should appear foamy if the sampling has been adequate and is reported to reflect the presence of surfactant.[14]

Other techniques that have been reported via bronchoscopic sampling are bronchial brushings and biopsy.[15] One study suggested that in some instances, bronchial brushing may be a more sensitive test to assess for inflammation, although in one patient, BAL was the more sensitive test.[28] However, the criteria to determine what constitutes inflammation from these types of samples alone is not clearly defined.

Bronchoscopy may also be used for treatment, as in the removal of tracheobronchial foreign bodies.[29] Therapeutic bronchoalveolar lavage has also been described in one dog affected by pulmonary alveolar proteinosis.[30]

SAMPLE SUBMISSION

Several studies in healthy patients have shown that no significant differences exist between different lobes of the lung lavaged either in overall cell numbers or differential counts.[19,31] Therefore, increases of cells will be interpreted similarly, no matter which area of the lung the samples are derived from. The first aliquot is reported to have fewer epithelial cells and higher numbers of polymorphonuclear cells, and some authors recommend discarding the first aliquot, although it is unlikely to significantly affect clinical interpretation if the first aliquot is combined with subsequent aliquots.[23]

It is recommended to prepare fresh smears at the time of sample collection, within 30 minutes because cell morphology is not well preserved in TW/BAL samples.[31] A direct smear of turbid fluid (or if mucous flecks are noted grossly), a smear of mucus material, and additional cytocentrifuged preparations are likely to provide the most information from the sample.

Recommendations for samples submitted to the laboratory are noted in Box 16-1. Guidelines for preparing smears from fluids are presented in Chapter 1.

If the TW/BAL is deemed unacceptable because of oropharyngeal contamination (or for any other reason) and is to be repeated, it should be repeated either immediately or after 48 hours. Even though a sterile saline solution is used for the wash, it induces a neutrophilic response that peaks about 24 hours after washing. If a TW/BAL is performed the next day (i.e., 24 hours after the first wash), an inflammatory response will be present, and it may be difficult to tell whether it is secondary to the prior wash or because of an inflammatory lung disease.[32-34] However, no significant difference may exist in samples collected 48 hours apart.[24,32,34] If a contaminated wash is obtained, it is ideal to wait at least 48 hours to collect a TW/BAL again because it allows the lungs time to clear the oropharyngeal contaminants. Sometimes, however, such a delay is not practical. Although some contaminants from the previous wash

BOX 16-1

Samples for Submission to the Pathology Laboratory

- Smears prepared from the flush or wash sample within 30 minutes of obtaining the sample
- Ethylenetetraacetic acid (EDTA) sample for further cytology preparations
- Plain sterile sample for culture
- Optional specific media preparations (e.g., for mycoplasma culture); contact laboratory before sampling

may be collected, if the TW/BAL is repeated immediately, the amount of oropharyngeal contamination should be minimal, and this may be preferable to waiting 48 hours.

CELL COUNTS

Cell counts are difficult to perform on TW/BAL fluids because of the mucous content, and the dilution factor may be variable.[35] The method of obtaining cell counts is also varied in many studies of TW/BAL in dogs and cats, so values may not be directly comparable, and diagnostic significance is often difficult to determine.[36] One study of cases of idiopathic pulmonary fibrosis found increased total cell counts in diseased individuals compared with controls, although differential cell counts were generally not altered.[37] Cell counts are recommended by some authors to determine whether an adequate sample has been obtained and to assess whether resampling is necessary. However, this may not be easily applicable in the practice setting. Qualitative estimates (normal or increased) of cellularity may be done on stained sediment smears and may be useful.

CYTOLOGIC EVALUATION

Mucus

A small amount of mucus may be present in TW/BAL specimens from clinically normal dogs and cats. Mucus appears as amorphous sheets ranging from blue to pink or as homogeneous strands that are frequently twisted or whorled (Figure 16-4; see also Figures 16-7, 16-12, 16-13, 16-17, and 16-18).[4,27] A granular appearance of the mucus is frequently associated with increased cellularity.[4] Inflammation, irritation, or upper airway damage, which may be a result of chronic airway disease, may result in increased numbers of goblet cells, and an increased amount of mucus is generally present, possibly with altered mucus properties.[4,32,38] In inflammatory conditions, mucus usually stains eosinophilic because of the incorporation of inflammatory proteins and material from lysed cells.[4]

Curschmann spirals (Figure 16-4) are mucous casts of small bronchioles that appear as spiral, twisted masses of mucus that may have perpendicular radiations, giving them a test tube-brush-like appearance.[39] They may be seen in TW/BAL specimens from patients with any disorder that results in chronic, excessive production of mucus and are an indication of bronchiolar obstruction.

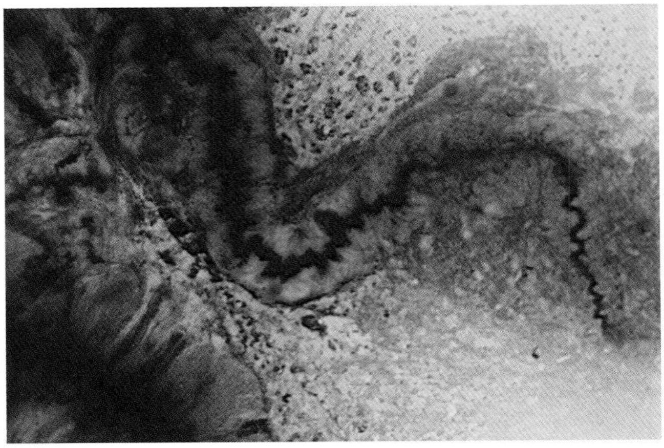

Figure 16-4 Tracheal wash or bronchoalveolar lavage from a dog with chronic bronchial disease. A large Curschmann's spiral and scattered alveolar macrophages are present in an eosinophilic mucous background. (Wright stain. Original magnification 50×.)

Cell Types

Many different types of cells (e.g., ciliated and nonciliated columnar cells, ciliated and nonciliated cuboidal cells, alveolar macrophages, neutrophils, eosinophils, lymphocytes, mast cells, erythrocytes, and dysplastic and neoplastic cells) may be seen in TW/BAL specimens (see Tables 16-1 and 16-2). Ciliated and nonciliated columnar and cuboidal cells and alveolar macrophages are the cell types seen in washings from normal dogs and cats. They are also seen in many disease states unless the washed area is filled with exudative secretions or the disease process has obliterated normal lung parenchyma. In one study in cats, storage of the bronchoalveolar lavage specimen for 24 hours or longer has been shown to result in decreased neutrophil percentages and increased eosinophil percentages. In a few individual cases, this change was sufficient to alter the cytologic interpretation.[40] One study in dogs reported that neutrophil and eosinophil percentages were both decreased on the smears prepared at 24 hours after sampling compared with those prepared 3 hours after sampling.[41] Cytocentrifugation has been reported to affect the cell populations, particularly reducing the number of small lymphocytes present.[42] However, in one canine study, neutrophils were found to be more represented on cytospin preparations compared with direct smears of pelleted cells.[43] One canine study suggested that age may influence differential cell counts, but the group size was small and the findings were at variance with a previous study, suggesting that further work may be needed to determine if age should be considered when assessing bronchoalveolar lavage cytology.[44,45] When determining differential cell counts, it is difficult to be consistent when assessing the epithelial population, and many do not consider this essential to assess the sample. When assessing macrophages, neutrophils and eosinophils, counting 200 cells from a cytospin preparation, if available, has been shown to provide repeatable results.[46]

Columnar and Cuboidal Cells: Ciliated columnar cells (Figure 16-5 and Figure 16-6) have an elongated or cone shape, with cilia on their flattened apical ends. The

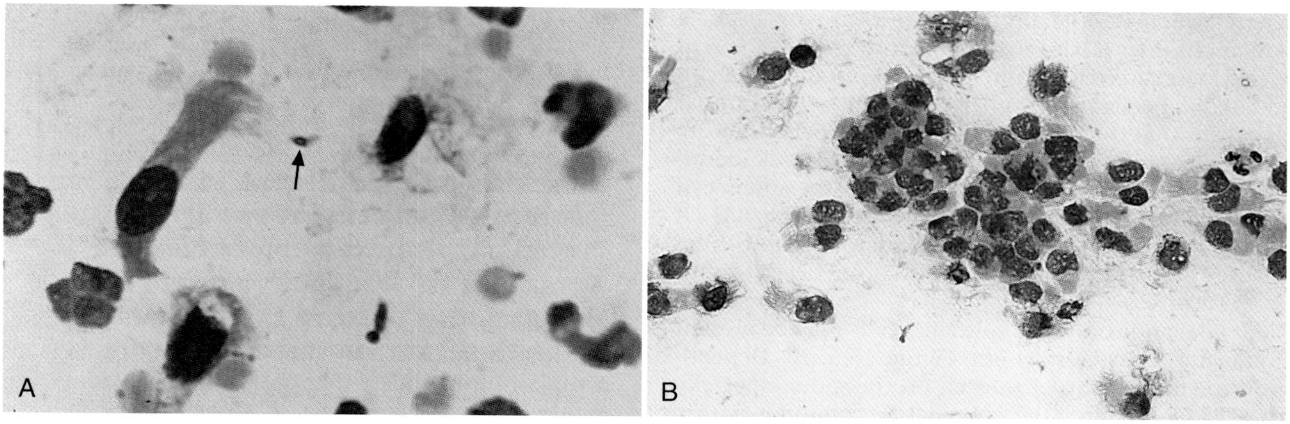

Figure 16-5 A, Tracheal wash or bronchoalveolar lavage from a dog with toxoplasmosis. A ciliated columnar cell, red blood cells, scattered neutrophils, and an extracellular *Toxoplasma gondii* organism (*arrow*) are shown. (Wright stain. Original magnification 250×.) **B,** Ciliated columnar cells are present both individually and in a cluster. The morphology of the cells in the cluster cannot be discerned. Cilia are evident on the cells that are well spread out. Many of the cells are traumatized as evidenced by their irregular nuclear outlines. (Wright stain. Original magnification 160×.)

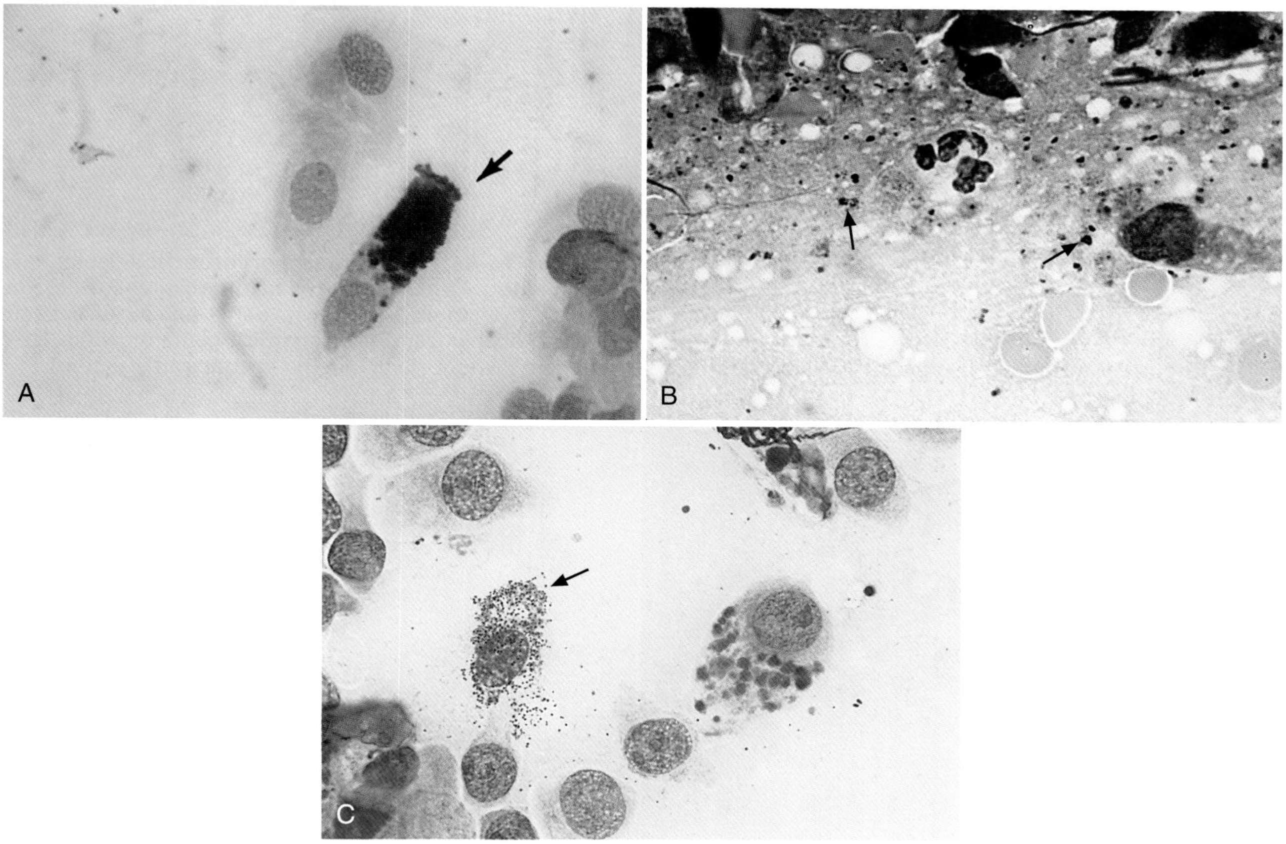

Figure 16-6 A, Tracheal wash or bronchoalveolar lavage from a dog. A goblet cell (*arrow*) and several ciliated columnar cells are present. (Wright stain, original magnification 250×). B, Granules from ruptured goblet cells are shown extracellularly (arrows) and must not be confused with bacterial cocci. (Wright stain. Original magnification 330×.) **C,** Goblet cells can be differentiated from mast cells (*arrow*), which have smaller granules.

nucleus, which is generally round to oval with a finely granular chromatin pattern, is present in the basal end of the cells, which often terminate in a thin tail.[39] The ciliated cuboidal cells look similar to the ciliated columnar cells except that the cuboidal cells are as wide as they are tall. Nonciliated columnar and cuboidal cells look identical to their ciliated counterparts except for the absence of cilia. These cell types are normal findings in TW/BAL. If these cell types are predominant in a sample, the washing procedure probably sampled mainly bronchi and bronchioles (as opposed to alveolar spaces).

Cuboidal and columnar epithelial cells may be present individually or in clusters (see Figure 16-5, *B*). Depending on the orientation of the cell on the slide (especially with cells in clusters), the cuboidal or columnar nature of the cells and cilia may be difficult to visualize. This is of little clinical significance, but these cells must not be interpreted as abnormal cell types.[39] Also, the majority of the columnar cells may be poorly preserved in many washes (see Figure 16-5, *B*) as a result of the low protein fluid in which they are collected. Cells traumatized during slide preparation may show irregular nuclear outlines or be overtly ruptured (e.g., smudge cells).

Goblet Cells: Goblet cells (see Figure 16-6) are mucus-producing bronchial cells that are generally elongated (i.e., columnar) with a basally placed nucleus and round granules of mucin, which frequently distend the cytoplasm.[39] Occasionally, the cytoplasm is so distended that the cell appears round. The granules stain from red to blue to clear with Romanowsky (e.g., Giemsa-Wright) stains. Free granules from ruptured goblet cells may be seen in the smear (see Figure 16-6, *B*). The shape of the cells and the large size of the granules are helpful in differentiating these cells from mast cells (see Figure 16-6, *C*). Goblet cells are not frequently seen; however, any chronic pulmonary irritant may result in increased numbers of goblet cells.

Macrophages: Alveolar macrophages (Figure 16-7) (see also Figures 16-9, 16-13, and 16-18) are readily found and are often the predominant cell type in TW/BAL samples from clinically normal animals. They are present in samples that have adequately washed the alveolar spaces and, therefore, are a useful indicator of sample adequacy. The nucleus is round to bean shaped and eccentrically positioned. A binucleate alveolar macrophage is rarely seen in clinically normal animals. Alveolar macrophages have abundant blue-gray granular cytoplasm. When they become activated, their cytoplasm becomes more abundant and vacuolated (i.e., foamy) and may contain phagocytized material (see Figure 16-7, *B*).[31]

Eosinophils: Eosinophils (Figures 16-8, 16-9, and 16-10) are polymorphonuclear granulocytes that contain intracytoplasmic granules, many of which have an affinity for the acid dye, eosin (i.e., eosinophilic), which stains them red with Romanowsky stains.[47] Increased numbers of eosinophils indicate a hypersensitivity reaction that is either allergic or parasitic;[4] see the discussion on hypersensitivity later in this chapter.

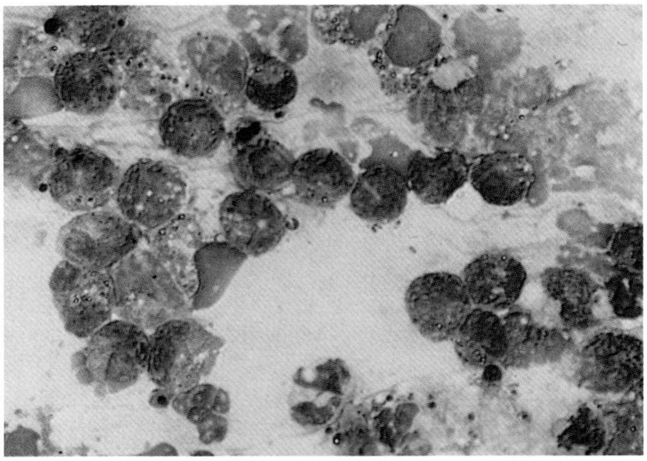

Figure 16-8 Tracheal wash or bronchoalveolar lavage from a dog. Mucus, scattered neutrophils, and a large number of eosinophils are shown. Some extracellular bacterial rods, probably from oropharyngeal contamination, are also present. (Wright stain. Original magnification 330×.)

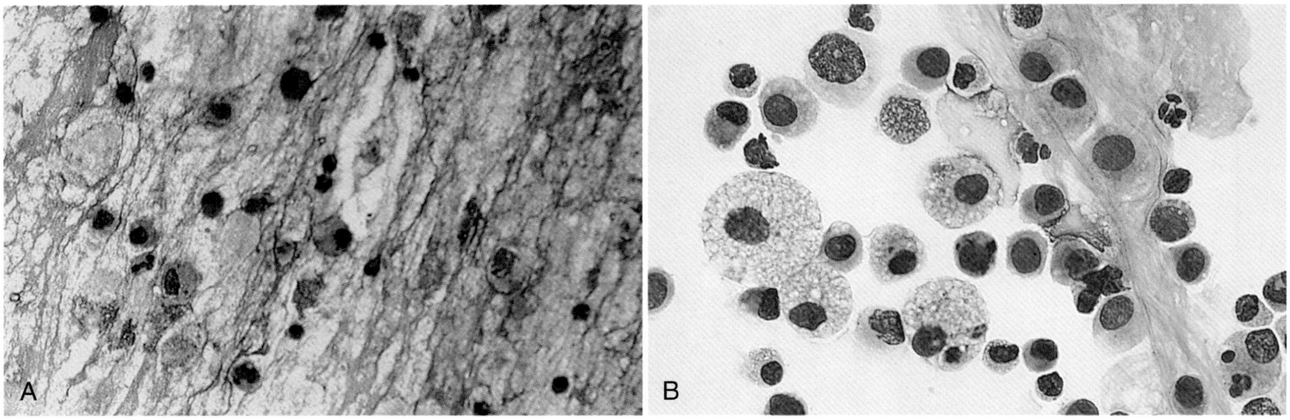

Figure 16-7 A, Tracheal wash or bronchoalveolar lavage (TW/BAL) from a dog. Many alveolar macrophages and some neutrophils are present in an eosinophilic mucous background. (Wright stain. Original magnification 132×.) **B,** TW/BAL from a dog. Numerous stimulated and unstimulated alveolar macrophages and scattered granulocytes and lymphocytes are present in strands of mucus. (Wright stain. Original magnification 250×.)

Careful examination is required to distinguish eosinophils from neutrophils in some wash specimens. In thick areas where the cells are not well spread out, individual granules may be hard to see. If normal neutrophils are present, the contrast in cytoplasmic color is usually evident; however, caution must be exercised because the cytoplasm of neutrophils, especially in exudative samples, sometimes stains a diffuse, uneven, eosinophilic color. When differentiating these two cells, it is best to search for well-spread-out cells with definitive cytoplasmic granules instead of diffuse eosinophilic coloration. Individual granules are most readily observed in partially ruptured cells that are spreading out and are also free in the background of the smear (see Figure 16-9, *B*). In cats, eosinophils may be difficult to recognize because they tend to be tightly packed with slender, rod-shaped granules that are not as pronounced in color as those in dogs (see Figure 16-9, *A*). Eosinophils tend to be slightly larger than neutrophils, and their nuclei are less segmented (often bilobed or trilobed), which may aid in their identification (see Figures 16-9, *A*, and 16-10, *B*).

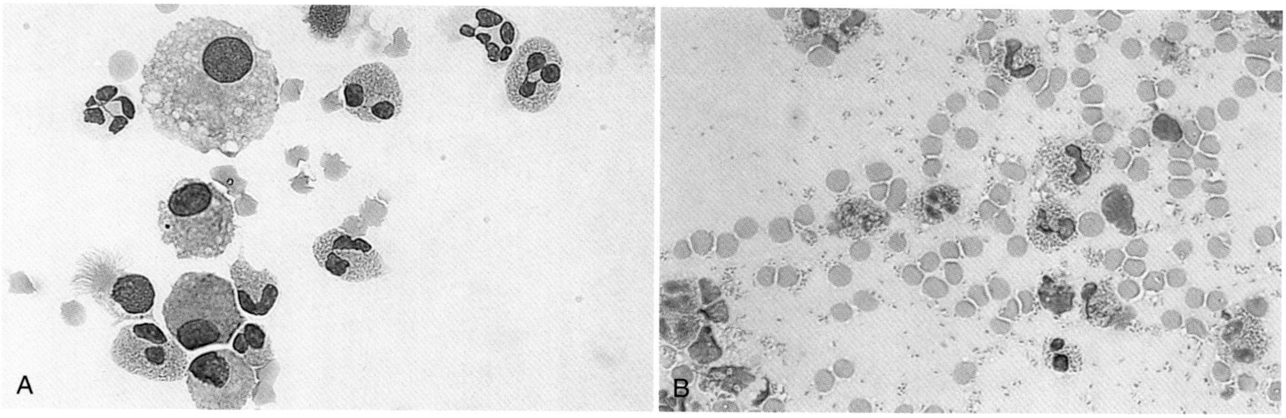

Figure 16-9 **A,** Tracheal wash or bronchoalveolar lavage specimen from a cat with a hypersensitivity reaction. Several eosinophils with bilobed and trilobed nuclei, scattered alveolar macrophages, two neutrophils with multilobulated nuclei, and a ciliated columnar epithelial cell are shown. The granules of the eosinophils are tightly packed, slender rods that may be easily overlooked. Note that the eosinophils are somewhat larger than the neutrophils and have less segmented nuclei. (Wright stain. Original magnification 250×.) **B,** Feline eosinophils. Granules are seen more easily in cells that are well spread out or partially ruptured. Many free eosinophil granules are seen in the background. (Wright stain. Original magnification 250×.)

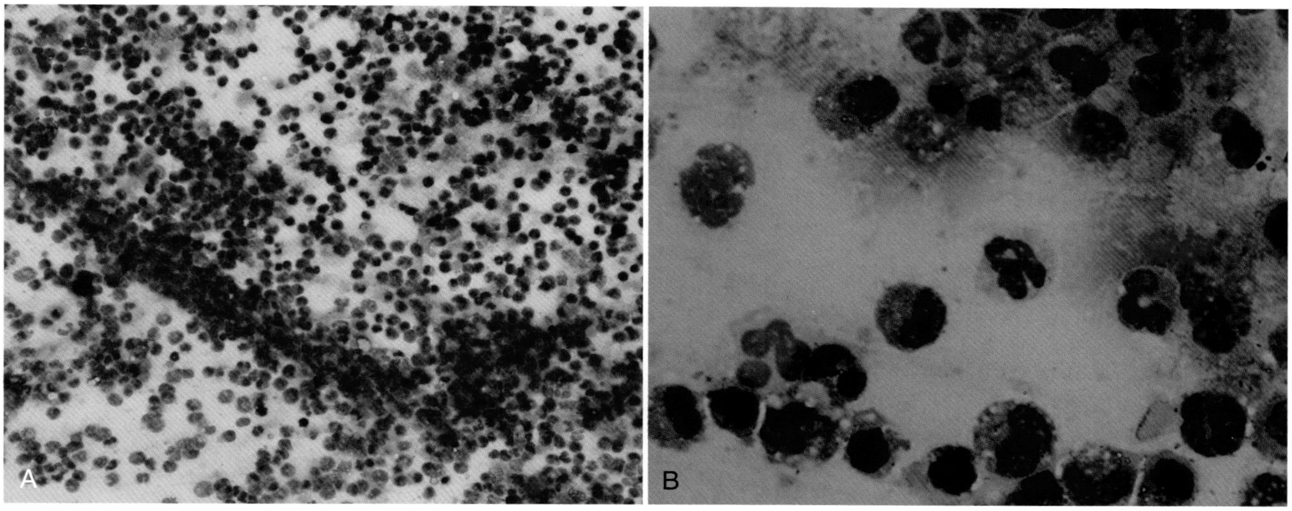

Figure 16-10 Bronchoalveolar lavage from a dog with a hypersensitivity reaction. A, Note the abundant brightly staining eosinophils, in conjunction with less prominently staining cells. (Wright stain. Original magnification 200×.) **B,** Higher magnification of slide shown in *A*. Note the central neutrophil with pale eosinophilic staining cytoplasm and multilobulated nucleus. The eosinophils possess brightly staining eosinophilic granules, to the left an unlobulated nucleus, presumptive globule leukocyte, and to the right a trilobed nucleus, typical of eosinophils. (Wright stain. Original magnification, 1000×.)

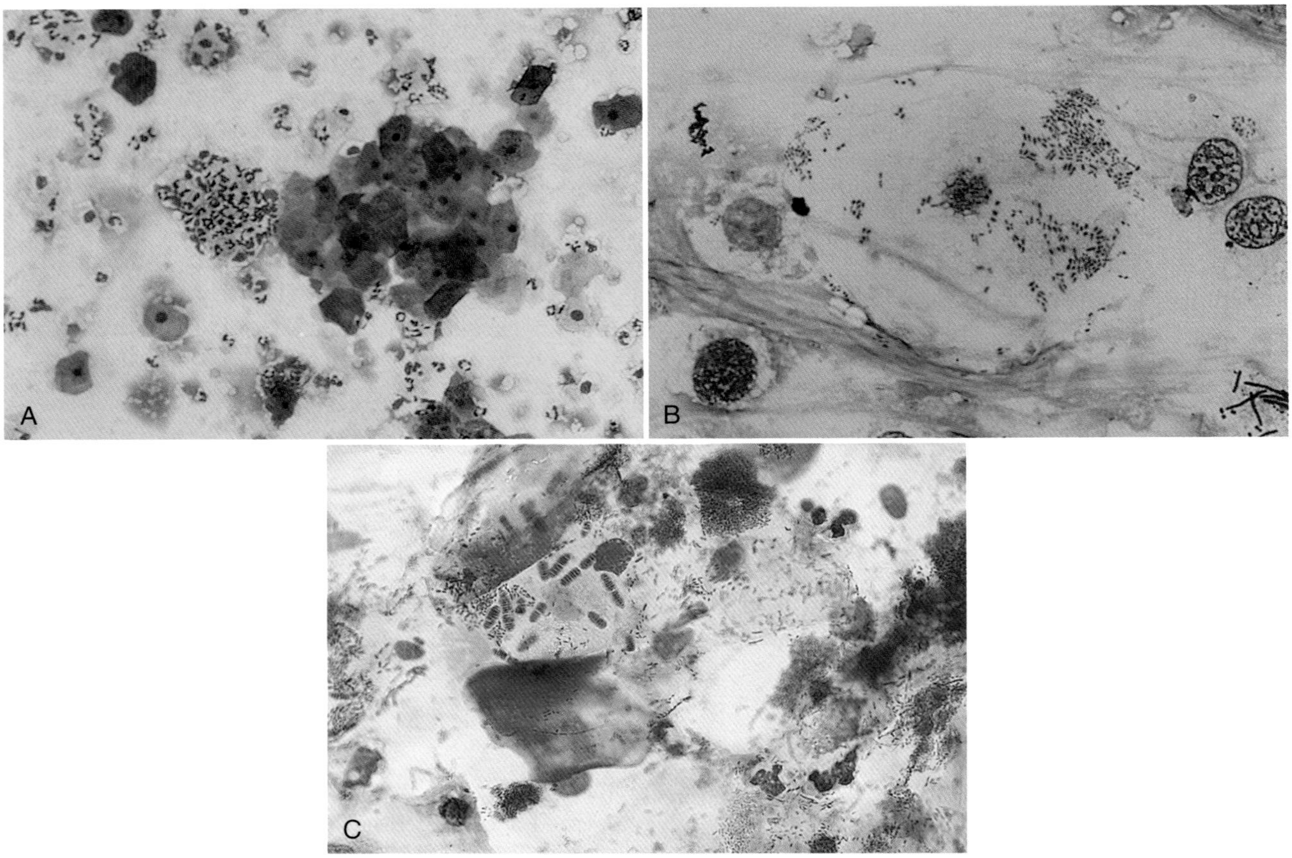

Figure 16-11 **A,** Tracheal wash or bronchoalveolar lavage (TW/BAL) from a dog. Superficial squamous cells, which denote oropharyngeal contamination, and neutrophils are shown. (Wright stain. Original magnification 50×.) **B,** Oropharyngeal contamination in a TW/BAL from a dog. Mucus, alveolar macrophages, and a large superficial squamous cell (with bacteria adhering to its surface) are present. Bacteria are also scattered throughout the slide. (Wright stain. Original magnification 250×.) **C,** TW/BAL from a cat. High numbers of bacteria, including some *Simonsiella* spp. organisms, are adhering to the surface of the squamous epithelial cells. *Simonsiella* spp. organisms are normal inhabitants of the oropharynx and indicate that the wash from this area is contaminated. (Wright stain. Original magnification 250×.)

Neutrophils: In TW/BAL samples, neutrophils look like peripheral blood neutrophils (Figures 16-11 and 16-12), although degenerative changes may be present. Increased numbers of neutrophils indicate inflammation; see the discussion on inflammation later in this chapter.

Globule Leukocytes: Another distinct population of cells containing eosinophilic cytoplasmic granules, but with round to oval, eccentric nuclei, have been seen in bronchial wash specimens (see Figure 16-10, *B*).[31] Although in one study, these cells have been identified as atypical-appearing eosinophils, because of identification of specific microgranules, they may also represent the rare globule leukocyte.[48] Globule leukocytes are cells which remain of uncertain origin but have been reported in the respiratory tract of dogs and cats.[49]

Lymphocytes or Plasma Cells: Lymphocytes (Figure 16-13) may represent a small percentage of the cells in TW/BAL samples from normal dogs and cats. Increased numbers of lymphocytes generally denote nonspecific

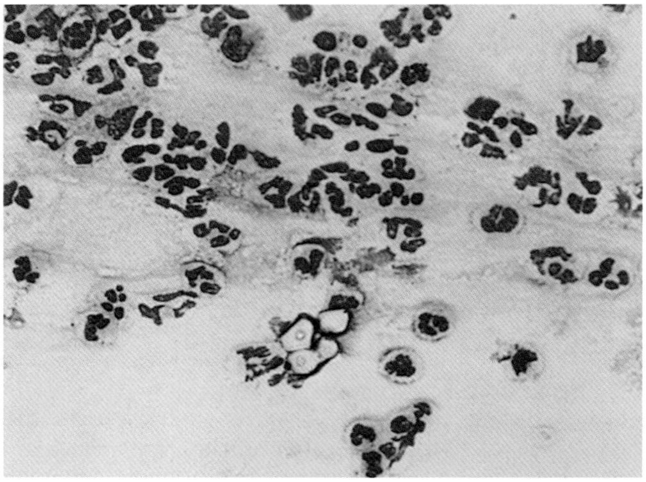

Figure 16-12 Tracheal wash or bronchoalveolar lavage from a dog. High numbers of neutrophils, an alveolar macrophage, and a cluster of four granules of cornstarch (glove powder) are present in an eosinophilic mucous background. (Wright stain. Original magnification 165×.)

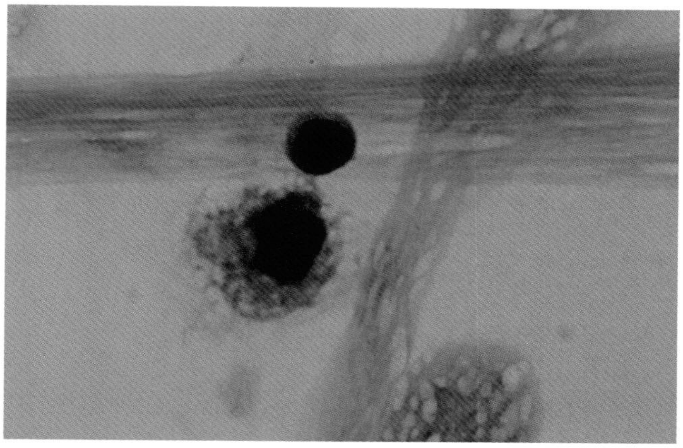

Figure 16-13 Small lymphocyte with scant cytoplasm trapped within mucin, and macrophage with vacuolated cytoplasm noted below. (Wright stain. Original magnification, 1000×.)

inflammation and are of limited diagnostic value. Lymphocytes may, on occasion, appear reactive with more abundant cytoplasm staining a deeper basophilic color. Plasmacytoid differentiation, where a perinuclear clearing may develop, or mature plasma cells may also be rarely seen. Mildly increased numbers of lymphocytes reportedly occur with airway hyperreactivity, viral diseases of the tracheobronchial tree, and chronic infections.[4,50] Marked increases in lymphocyte numbers, especially lymphoblasts, may suggest pulmonary lymphoma.

Mast Cells: Mast cells (see Figure 16-6, *C*), which are occasionally observed in TW/BAL samples from dogs and cats with many different inflammatory lung disorders, are usually present in low numbers and are of little diagnostic significance. They are readily identified by their small red-purple, intracytoplasmic granules, which are frequently present in high numbers and may obscure the nucleus. Free, scattered granules from ruptured mast cells may be present on the slide and must not be confused with bacteria. A mild increase in mast cell numbers has been reported to occur with airway hyperreactivity.[50]

Superficial Squamous Cells: Superficial squamous cells are large epithelial cells with abundant, angular cytoplasm and small, round nuclei. Their presence in a TW/BAL sample indicates oropharyngeal contamination (see Figure 16-11), either from endotracheal sampling, or accidental catheter misdirection in transtracheal wash sampling. A rare differential for their presence may be a bronchoesophageal fistula, congenital or acquired.[51] See the discussion on oropharyngeal contamination later in this chapter.

Erythrocytes: Erythrocytes may be present within macrophages or free on the slide. Erythrophagocytosis (see Figure 16-19) indicates intrapulmonary hemorrhage or diapedesis. See the discussion on hemorrhage later in this chapter.

Atypical Cell Types

Atypical cells may be seen with pulmonary metaplasia, dysplasia, or neoplasia (primary or metastatic). Mild dysplasia of the respiratory epithelium may be seen whenever inflammation is present. Anticancer therapy (i.e., irradiation and chemotherapy) may result in such severe atypia of the cells of the tracheobronchial epithelium, the terminal bronchial epithelium, and the alveolar epithelium that differentiation from neoplasia is not reliable.[39] When atypical cells are observed cytologically, they should be evaluated for malignant criteria (see Chapter 2). TW/BAL samples collected after cancer therapy should be interpreted with caution.

Metaplasia: Metaplasia is an adaptive response of epithelial cells to chronic irritation.[39] Replacement of normal pulmonary epithelial cells of the trachea, bronchi, and bronchioles with stratified squamous epithelium (i.e., squamous metaplasia) is an example of pulmonary metaplasia.[39] These metaplastic cells mimic maturing squamous epithelium and must not be confused with neoplasia.

Dysplasia: Dysplasia is, by definition, a nonneoplastic change; however, severely dysplastic changes are sometimes referred to as *carcinoma in situ*. Dysplastic changes include variation in cell size and shape, darker-staining cells, and increased nucleus-to-cytoplasm (N:C) ratio and numbers of immature cells. These changes can be difficult to differentiate from neoplasia and may progress to neoplasia.[52]

Neoplastic Cells: Neoplastic cells are not often seen on cytologic evaluation of TW/BAL samples. Unless the neoplasm has invaded the tracheobronchial tree and the invaded bronchiole is not blocked by a mucous plug, they are not accessible for collection by TW/BAL. Neoplastic cells, when observed, are generally from lymphoma or a carcinoma. High numbers of lymphoblasts may be seen in animals with lymphoma involving the respiratory system (see Figure 16-31). Carcinoma cells are large epithelial cells that may be present in clusters or as single cells (Figure 16-30). Their cytoplasm is generally basophilic and vacuolated, and they show marked variation in cellular and nuclear size, often with grossly enlarged nuclei. They have a high N:C ratio, coarse nuclear chromatin, and prominent nucleoli that are frequently large and angular. Care must be taken not to confuse inflammation-induced cell dysplasia with neoplasia.

Miscellaneous Findings

Corn Starch: Corn starch (glove powder) is occasionally seen cytologically on slides from TW/BAL. It is typically a large, round to hexagonal structure that stains clear or blue and has a central fissure (see Figure 16-12). Corn starch is an incidental finding and should not be confused with an organism or cell.

Plant Pollen: Plant pollen or plant cells may occasionally be present in TW/BAL samples and should not be confused with infectious organisms or cells.

Barium Sulfate: Aspirated barium sulfate has been reported to occur as greenish granular refractile material, most commonly noted in macrophages.[53]

CYTOLOGIC INTERPRETATION

Figure 16-14 presents an algorithm to aid in the evaluation of TW/BAL samples. Integrating historical, physical, and radiographic findings with the results of other diagnostic tests may allow for further diagnostic refinement. TW/BAL specimens are interpreted according to the type, quantity, and proportion of cells recovered. Cell proportions often differ between transtracheal aspirates and BAL samples.

Cellular patterns can generally be categorized as follows:

- *Insufficient sample*—no cells or an inadequate number of cells for evaluation
- *Oropharyngeal contamination*—superficial squamous cells, *Simonsiella* spp. of bacteria, or both (see the discussion on oropharyngeal contamination later in this chapter)
- *Eosinophilic infiltrate*—increased numbers of eosinophils (see the discussion on hypersensitivity later in this chapter)

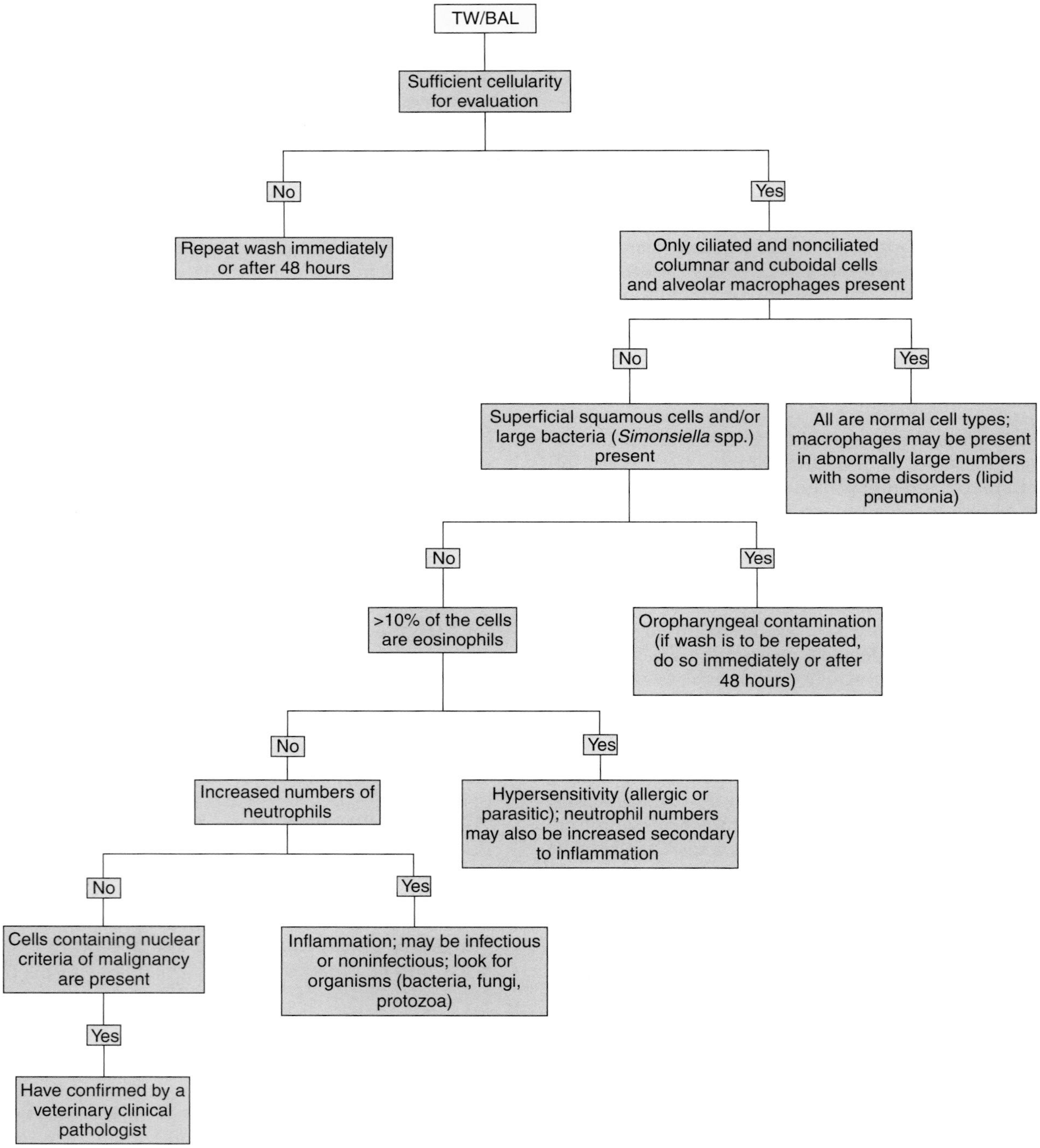

Figure 16-14 Flowchart for evaluation of tracheal wash or bronchoalveolar lavage specimens.

- *Neutrophilic infiltrate*—increased numbers of neutrophils (see the discussion on inflammation later in this chapter)
- *Macrophage (histiocytic or granulomatous) infiltrate*—very cellular sample of primarily macrophages (see the discussion on inflammation later in this chapter)
- *Presence of atypical cells*—evaluation for criteria of malignancy (see the discussion on neoplasia later in this chapter)

These categories, aside from insufficient samples, are not mutually exclusive. Classification of TW/BAL samples into one or more of these categories may allow the process or processes to be identified.

Insufficient Sample

The absence of cells on a smear or concentrated preparation may indicate that this sample is not truly representative of the cytology of the respiratory tract. Additionally, when assessing a BAL sample in which only columnar respiratory epithelial cells are noted, the absence of macrophages would indicate that only the airways and not the alveolar space had effectively been sampled.

Oropharyngeal Contamination

Oropharyngeal contamination is much more likely to occur when a TW/BAL sample is collected by passing a catheter through an endotracheal tube than when a transtracheal sample is taken and the oropharyngeal area is bypassed. Regardless of the procedure used, careful attention must be paid to technique to avoid oropharyngeal contamination.

Superficial squamous cells and certain large bacteria (e.g., *Simonsiella* spp.) are the hallmark of oropharyngeal contamination (see Figure 16-11).[54] Superficial squamous cells are large epithelial cells with abundant, angular cytoplasm and small, round nuclei. Many bacteria may adhere to the surface of squamous epithelial cells (see Figure 16-11, *B* and *C*). *Simonsiella* spp. organisms (see Figure 16-11, *C*) are bacteria that divide lengthwise, thus lining up in parallel rows that give the impression of a single large bacterium. These are nonpathogenic organisms that may adhere to superficial squamous cell surfaces or be free in smears. When superficial squamous cells or *Simonsiella* spp. organisms are present, indicating oropharyngeal contamination, whatever cellular constituents and bacterial organisms were present in the oropharyngeal area may also be present in the contaminated wash. Therefore, a variety of bacterial rods and cocci may be present in a contaminated wash (see Figure 16-11, *B*). Bacteria are generally present without neutrophils when the wash primarily consists of oropharyngeal contaminants. Neutrophils may occur in a TW/BAL sample secondary to oropharyngeal contamination if the animal has a purulent or ulcerative oropharyngeal lesion. Therefore, oropharyngeal contamination may significantly alter the cytologic evaluation and culture results.

Hypersensitivity

Increased numbers of eosinophils in a TW/BAL specimen indicate a hypersensitivity response. Normal animals of most species, including dogs, generally have very low numbers of eosinophils (<5%) in bronchial wash specimens, but clinically normal cats may have significantly higher numbers of eosinophils compared with other species.[23,55,56] In some studies, eosinophils comprised an average 20% to 25% of the cells present in bronchial wash specimens from asymptomatic cats with no evidence of pulmonary disease or parasitism. In a few of these animals, eosinophils were the predominant cell type present. Whether these findings are truly normal or merely represent a subclinical hypersensitivity response is not known, but these animals were asymptomatic throughout the observation periods; thus, the clinical significance of a cytologic diagnosis of hypersensitivity reaction, when based on relatively low numbers of eosinophils (10% to 25% of cells present), may depend on the clinical and radiographic findings of the case.

Clinically normal dogs typically have wash specimens of less than 5% eosinophils.[31,45,57] Many of the studies describing normal BAL cytology were done using dogs reared in closed environments. One study showed that random source dogs had significantly higher percentages of eosinophils (24%) compared with dogs reared in an isolated environment with routine prophylactic antihelminthic treatment (<5%).[58] It was suggested that previously heavy parasitic burdens may have been responsible for the high numbers of eosinophils in these animals; however, other studies have also found increased eosinophil percentages in apparently healthy dogs.[59,60] These authors' experience suggests that such a significant percentage of eosinophils is unusual in most clinically normal dogs. Specimens composed of more than 10% eosinophils are indicative of a significant hypersensitivity component of the disease process.

Increased numbers of neutrophils, macrophages, or both may be seen along with increased numbers of eosinophils if tissue irritation is sufficient to induce an inflammatory response. Cells are not always evenly distributed throughout wash specimens, especially if thick mucous strands are present. Eosinophils, trapped in strands of mucus, often predominate in certain areas of the slides, whereas other areas may be predominantly neutrophilic. A careful examination of the entire slide is necessary for an accurate evaluation.

Allergic bronchitis or pneumonitis, feline asthma, lungworm and heartworm infestations, and eosinophilic bronchopneumopathy (previously pulmonary infiltrates with eosinophils [PIE]) are some of the disorders that frequently cause the hypersensitivity responses seen in TW/BAL specimens.[61,62] Specimens should be scanned on low-power (10× objective) for parasitic larvae or ova (Figure 16-15). If present, parasitic larvae (e.g., *Filaroides* spp., *Aelurostrongylus abstrusus*, *Angiostronygulus vasorum*, and *Crenosoma vulpis*) and ova (e.g., *Eucoleus aerophilus* and *Paragonimus* spp.) are large and readily identified, but sometimes only an eosinophilic exudate is present. Multiple fecal examinations (including Baermann and zinc sulfate flotation techniques) may be helpful in identifying infestations. Even when not found in wash specimens, larvae may sometimes be identified in brushings or biopsies of parasitic nodules visible in the bronchi of affected animals.

Free eosinophil granules, which stain eosinophilic and should not be confused with bacteria, may be seen secondary to cell rupture in the smear. These granules may

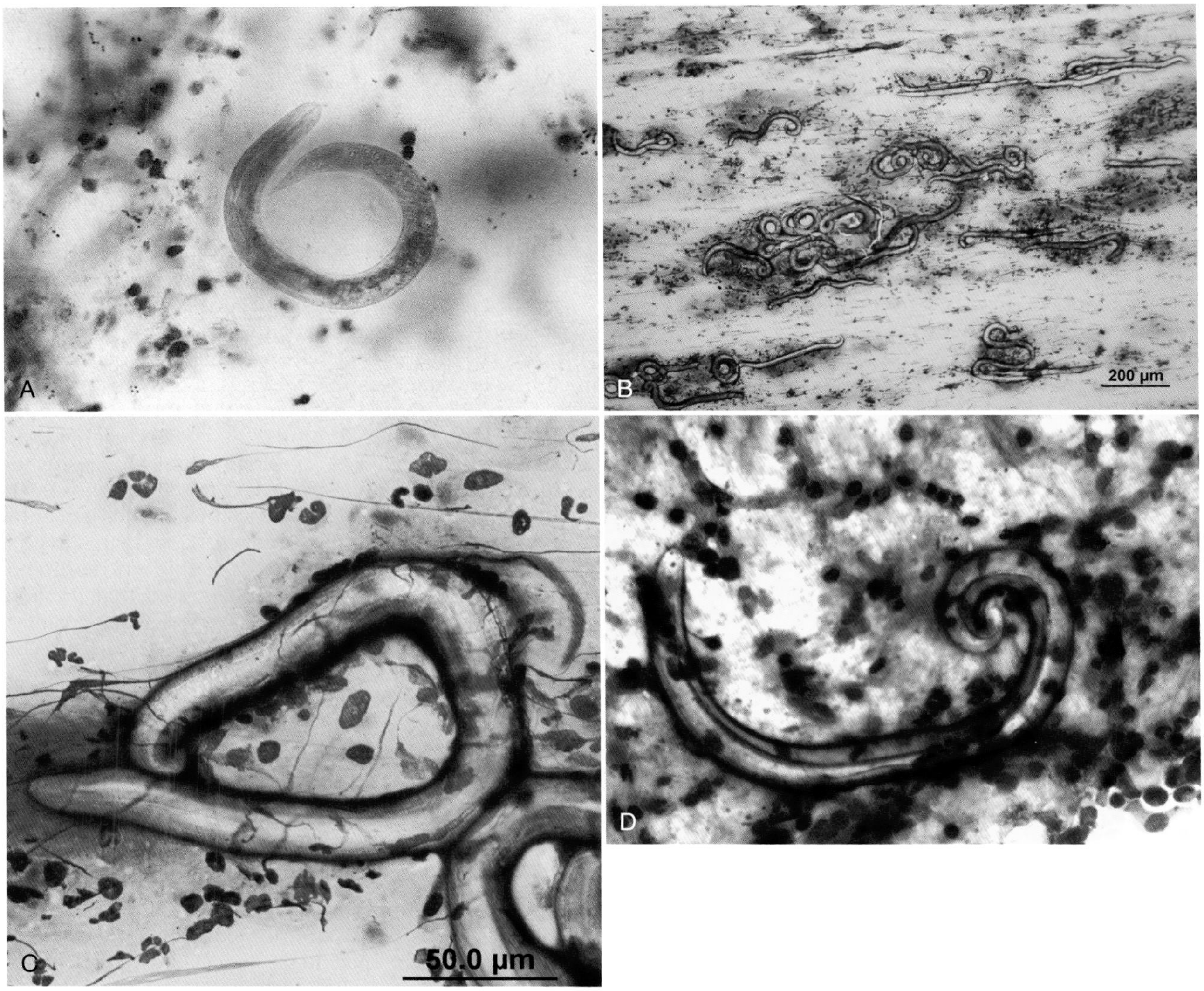

Figure 16-15 **A,** Tracheal wash or bronchoalveolar lavage (TW/BAL) from a dog. A large lungworm larva is present. (Wright stain. Original magnification, 100×.) **B,** TW/BAL from a cat. Low-power magnification showing large numbers of lungworm larvae (*Aelurostrongylus* spp.). (Wright stain.) **C,** Higher magnification from the same case shown in *B*. Lungworm larvae (*Aelurostrongylus* spp.) and scattered inflammatory cells are shown. (Wright stain.) **D,** TW/BAL from a dog. Although the tail of the lungworm larva (*Angiostrongylus vasorum*) may be observed on BAL cytology, it is not always possible to see enough detail to speciate. Wet preparations are preferred for identification. (Wright-Giemsa stain. Original magnification 400×.) (**B** and **C,** Courtesy of Dr. T. Rizzi. **D,** Slide courtesy of A. Leuschner, TDDS, U.K.)

coalesce into a large crystal known as a *Charcot-Leyden crystal* (Figure 16-16), which may occur in any condition that causes large numbers of eosinophils to accumulate.

Inflammation

Neutrophils are present only in very low numbers (generally <5%) in TW/BAL specimens from normal dogs and cats.[4,31] Cytologically, neutrophils in bronchial mucus look like peripheral blood neutrophils, but they may show degenerative changes because of bacterial toxins or be smudged (ruptured) secondary to trauma from collection and preparation. An influx of neutrophils occurs early in an inflammatory response, making neutrophils from TW/BAL a sensitive indicator of inflammation.[32] Even very mild insults such as sterile saline TW/BAL result in marked influxes of neutrophils. As a result, neutrophil numbers are increased in nearly all conditions (infectious and noninfectious) that cause inflammation. Infectious disorders include bacterial (Figure 16-17), mycotic (see Figure 16-25), viral, or protozoal (see Figure 16-28) diseases. Noninfectious disorders include tissue irritation or necrosis secondary to inhalation of a toxic substance (e.g., smoke), as well as neoplasia that has outgrown its blood supply and developed a necrotic center. Whenever neutrophil numbers are increased, one should look closely (and, especially, intracellularly) for bacteria and other microorganisms (see Figure 16-17). Organisms may be found cytologically in most bacterial infections, but

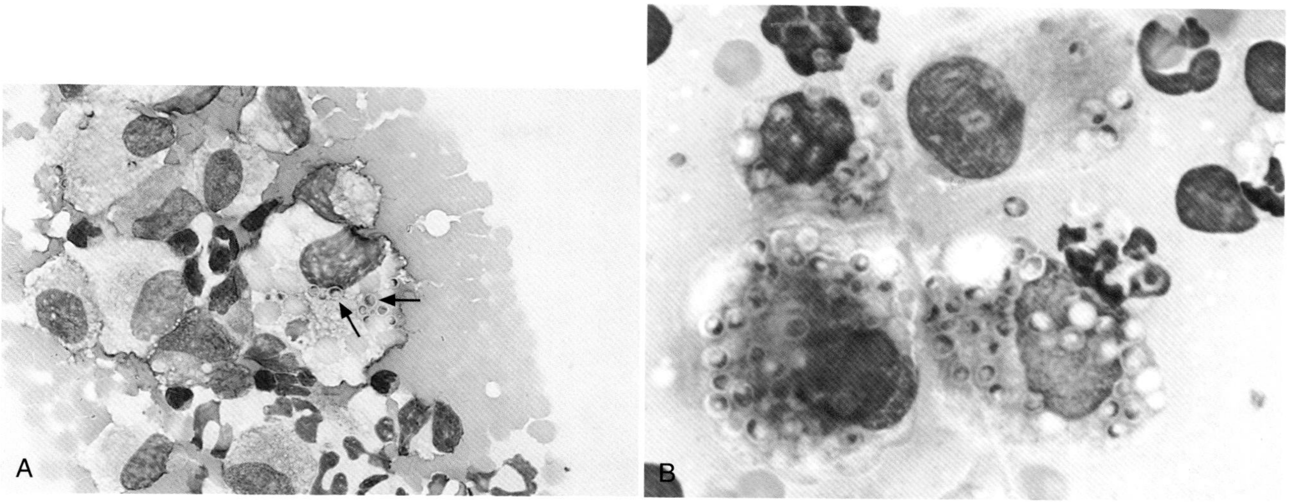

Figure 16-26 **A,** Tracheal wash or bronchoalveolar lavage from a cat with pulmonary histoplasmosis. Many macrophages, some of which show the yeast phase of *Histoplasma capsulatum* (*arrows*); scattered neutrophils and lymphocytes; and red blood cells are seen. A macrophage also displays erythrophagocytosis. (Wright stain. Original magnification 250×.) **B,** Fine-needle aspirate of lung showing large macrophages containing numerous *H. capsulatum* organisms. *Histoplasma* organisms are small (1 to 4 micrometers [μm] in diameter), round to oval, yeast-like organisms that have a dark blue to purple staining nucleus. The organism is often surrounded by a thin, clear halo. (Wright stain.) (Courtesy of Dr. R. L. Cowell, IDEXX Laboratories.)

Cryptococcus). These appear similar but have a thin clear capsule. Occasional organisms showing narrow-based budding may be found. A case report in a cat demonstrated organisms 3 to 15 μm diameter with a thick nonstaining wall in the BAL sample, although the organisms from the lymph node of the patient were reported as 8 to 12 μm in size with a 1 to 6 μm nonstaining capsule.[9] Pulmonary involvement is not the most frequent presentation of this disease.[83]

Histoplasma: *Histoplasma* organisms may be more likely to be noted in BAL in the acute presentation of the disease, compared with a more chronic presentation. These organisms are most commonly noted intracellularly, but extracellular organisms may be observed on smears because of cell rupturing.

Histoplasma organisms are small (approximately 2 to 4 μm diameter), with a thin, clear halo surrounding a darker staining, round-to-oval, yeastlike organism (Figure 16-26).[84] Coughing may not be reported in many patients with pulmonary lesions of histoplasmosis.[85]

Pneumocystis: *Pneumocystis* is an opportunistic fungal pulmonary pathogen, which may be observed in either cyst form (5 to 10 μm diameter with up to eight intracystic bodies) (Figure 16-27) or troph form (1 to 2 μm).[86] Cytologically, it may appear morphologically similar to a protozoal organism, and this led to misclassification in the past. Particular breeds have been overrepresented in the literature—the Miniature Dachshund in the southern hemisphere and the Cavalier King Charles Spaniel in the northern hemisphere.[87,88] However, this is likely related to the underlying immunodeficiencies that are reported in these breeds because any breed may be affected by this organism. It is not possible to culture this organism on media.

Parasites

When considering parasites of the lungs, nematodes (see Figure 16-15) and occasionally trematodes are most commonly considered, although *Toxoplasma* (Figure 16-28), a protozoal agent, is also classified as a parasitic organism.

An outline of the nematode and trematode parasites noted in dogs and cats is provided in Table 16-3, although the sizing of the larvae differs among authors. If specific identification is required, it is recommended that expert opinion be sought.

Although eosinophilic inflammation may be expected with these organisms, many patients will present with only neutrophilic inflammation.[89,90]

Oslerus osleri (*Filaroides osleri*) and *Filaroides hirthi* ova and larvae noted in respiratory washings are very similar in appearance (see Figure 16-15). Differentiation may be undertaken by identification of nodules formed by *O. osleri*, particularly at or in the area surrounding the bifurcation of the trachea, whereas *F. hirthi* organisms are more likely to form subpleural nodules.[89,91] The airway nodules may be noted on bronchoscopy, and either may be noted on radiography. In some instances, the nodules may be difficult to distinguish radiographically from neoplastic foci. *Filaroides milksi* is almost identical to *F. hirthi*, and whether these are two separate species is still being debated.[92]

Angiostrongylus vasorum is reported in many areas worldwide, including Europe, South America, North America (Newfoundland), and Africa, with the geographic range likely to continue to expand.[93] Associated clinical signs may include hypercalcemia and bleeding diatheses

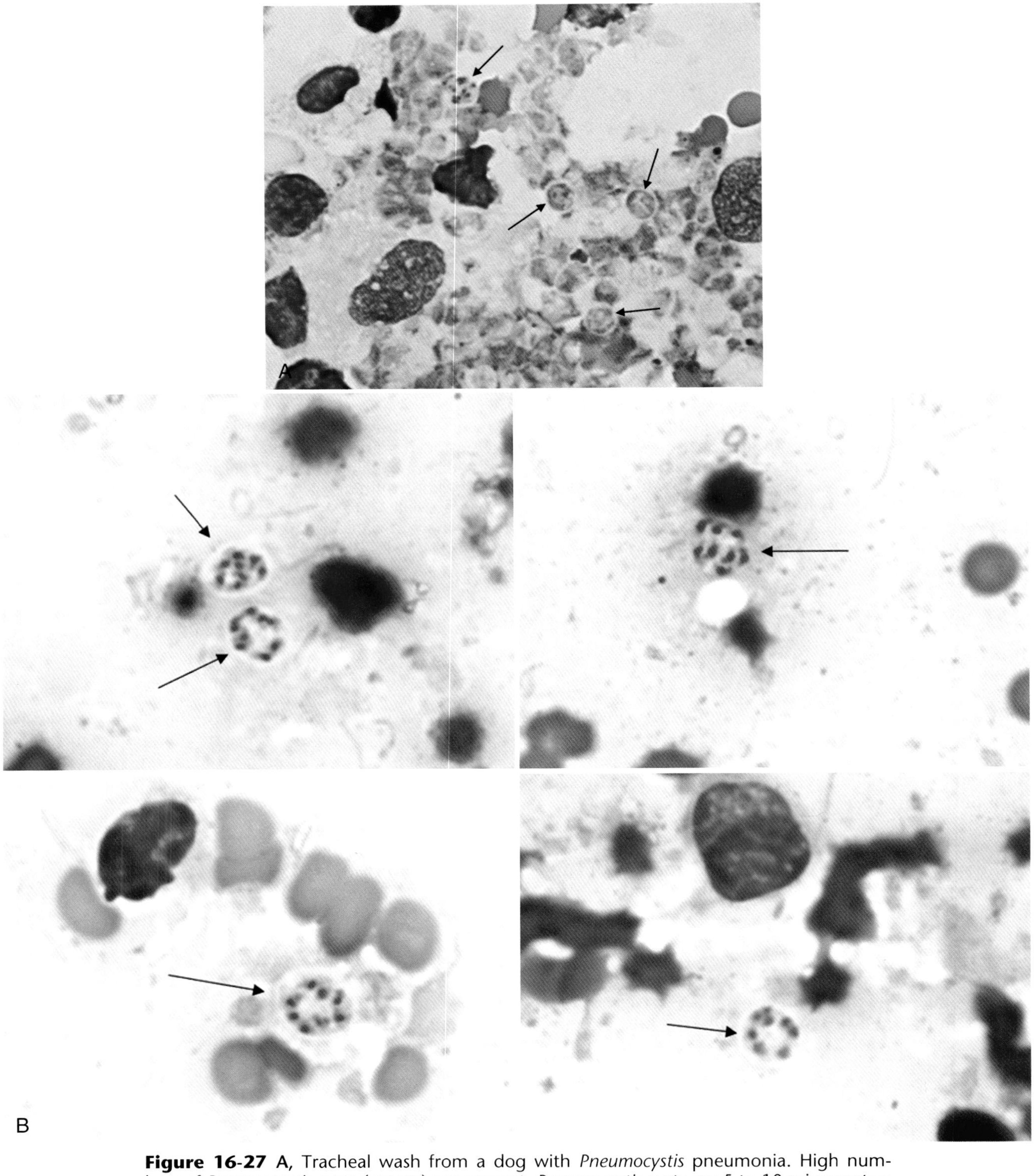

Figure 16-27 **A,** Tracheal wash from a dog with *Pneumocystis* pneumonia. High numbers of *Pneumocystis* cysts (*arrows*) are present. *Pneumocystis* cysts are 5 to 10 micrometers (μm) in diameter and usually contain four to eight intracystic bodies that are 1 to 2 μm in diameter. **B,** Composite showing high-magnification pictures of *Pneumocystis* cysts. (Wright stain.) (Courtesy of Dr. R. L. Cowell, IDEXX Laboratories.)

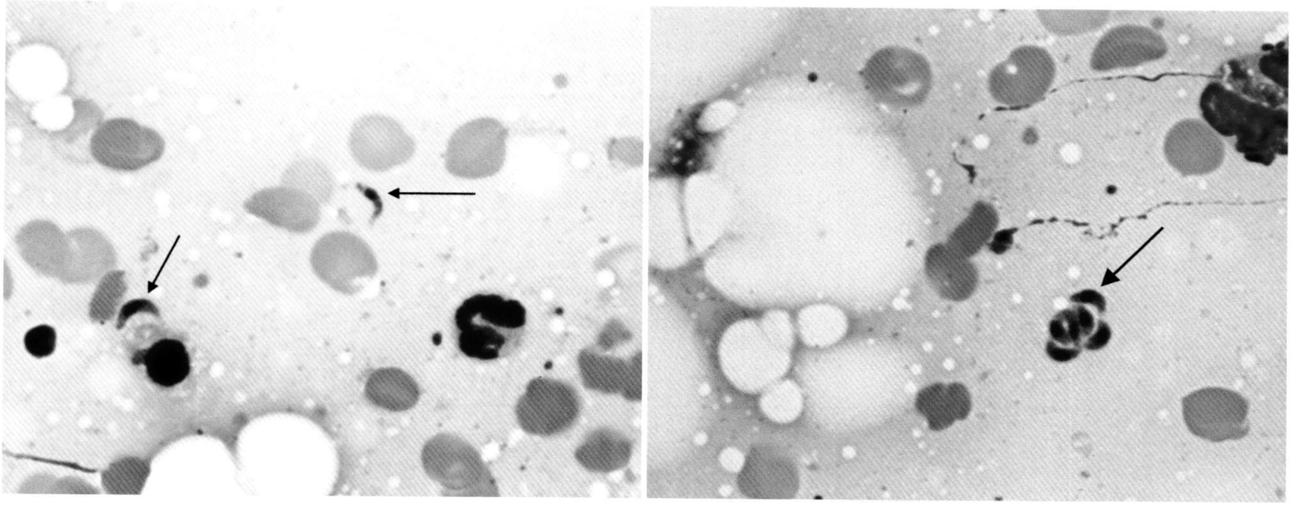

Figure 16-28 **Tracheal wash or bronchoalveolar lavage from a cat with toxoplasmosis.** *Toxoplasma gondii* tachyzoites (*arrows*) appear as small crescent-shaped bodies with a light blue cytoplasm and a dark-staining pericentral nucleus. (Courtesy of Dr. R. L. Cowell, IDEXX Laboratories.)

from prolongation of prothrombin time, activated partial thromboplastin time, or both, resolving on successful treatment of the worm burden.

Toxoplasma gondii infection in cats may frequently involve the lung. Identification of tachyzoites both extracellularly and within macrophages, which may be numerous, have been reported in the BAL samples of cats with both experimentally induced and spontaneous clinical disease.[94-96] *T. gondii* tachyzoites appear as small crescent-shaped bodies, with a light-blue cytoplasm and a dark-staining pericentral nucleus (see Figure 16-28).

Viral Diseases

Many viral respiratory diseases may cause lung damage and allow for secondary bacterial infection. Cytologically, increased numbers of neutrophils indicate inflammation. Lymphocytes may be increased, but the numbers are often low and nonspecific. If a secondary bacterial infection has occurred, bacterial organisms may be seen intracellularly and extracellularly on the slides. Viral agents are not usually identified on cytologic preparations of lavage fluids from the lungs of dogs and cats. Many papers describe immunhistochemical detection of various viral agents, but this is generally performed on postmortem lung samples. Viral pneumonia may be caused by viruses that are not commonly considered to affect the respiratory system[97] (Figure 16-29).

Neoplasia

Neoplasia may exist as single, solitary nodules or a diffuse infiltration. Solitary lesions are rare in metastatic lung tumors but common in primary lung tumors. Most solid tissue pulmonary neoplasms (i.e., not lymphoid) are metastatic nodules from malignant tumors at sites other than the lungs. Because metastatic lung tumors are generally interstitial, neoplastic cells are not collected with TW/BAL unless the tumor has invaded the bronchial tree and the affected portion of the bronchial tree is not clogged by secretions or is so peripherally located that its cells cannot be collected with TW/BAL. Primary lung tumors that involve the bronchial tree are more likely to exfoliate cells that are collected by routine washings (Figure 16-30).

Carcinomas comprise 80% or more of all primary lung tumors in dogs and cats.[98,99] Lung carcinomas tend to appear in the following three areas:[99]

- Hilus of the lungs
- Multifocal and often peripheral sites (most commonly)
- In an entire lobe or lobes

Carcinomas are epithelial cell tumors; when cytologic evidence of acini formation or secretory product production is seen, they are classified as adenocarcinomas. Lymphoma is a common neoplasm in both dogs and cats. It is typically multicentric and may involve the pulmonary parenchyma in dogs. Large numbers of lymphoblasts may be diagnostic of lymphoma. Scattered large lymphoid cells, when they are part of a generalized inflammatory reaction, are not sufficient for a diagnosis. TW/BAL specimens may be useful in diagnosing pulmonary involvement of lymphoma (Figure 16-31). In one study, 31 of 47 dogs with multicentric lymphoma (66%) had pulmonary involvement, as determined by examination of BAL fluid collected with a bronchoscope.[100] In the same group of dogs, examination of TW fluid (collected by passing a urinary catheter through a sterile endotracheal tube) was much less sensitive, documenting pulmonary involvement in only 4 of the 46 dogs tested.

TABLE 16-3

Overview of the Nematode and Trematode Parasites of the Dog and Cat Lung

	Host	Location in Lung	Stage in Lung Commonly Observed by Flush or Wash Sample
Nematode Parasite			
Aelurostrongylus abstrusus	Cat	Terminal and respiratory bronchioles, alveolar ducts	Ova and larvae
			Ova 70–80 micrometers (μm) by 50–75 μm, with thin shell, embryonated
			L1, 360–400 μm, short thick larvae with sinus wave shaped kink and dorsal spine on tail, granular contents
			L3, 460–530 μm
Angiostrongylus vasorum	Dog	Pulmonary arteries, right heart	L1
			310–400 μm length, sharply pointed tail with distinct notch on dorsal surface "dorsal notch" cephalic button on anterior end; not regularly identified in more recent studies
Eucoleus aerophilus (*Capillaria aerophila*)	Dog and cat	Trachea, bronchi, bronchioles	Ova
			Bipolar thick-walled, pigmented golden brown
			58–79 μm length, 29–40 μm width
Crenosoma vulpis	Dog	Trachea, bronchi, and bronchioles	L1 243–281 μm length L3, 458–549 μm length
			Slightly curved tail, no kink
			Adult worms, observed grossly, stout, white, ~0.5–1cm length
Filaroides hirthi	Dog	bronchioles alveoli, lung parenchyma	Embryonated ova and larvae
			Larvae 240–290 μm length ~10–14 μm width, slightly kinked tail
			Adults 2.3–13mm length ~30–100 μm width, both stages have prominent basophilic granules internally
Oslerus osleri	Dog	Trachea and bronchial nodules, particularly nodules at bifurcation of trachea	Ova and larvae practically identical to *Filaroides hirthi* L1 223–267 μm Adults 6.5–13.5mm length
Trematode Parasite			
Paragonimus spp.	Dog and cat	Primarily right caudal lung lobe	Ova 75–118 μm length, 42–67 μm width
			Ovoid with single flattened operculum, golden brown

Anderson RC: **Nematode Parasites of Vertebrates. Their Development and Transmission.** 2nd Edition. CABI Publishing, Wallingford, Oxon (UK) 2000.

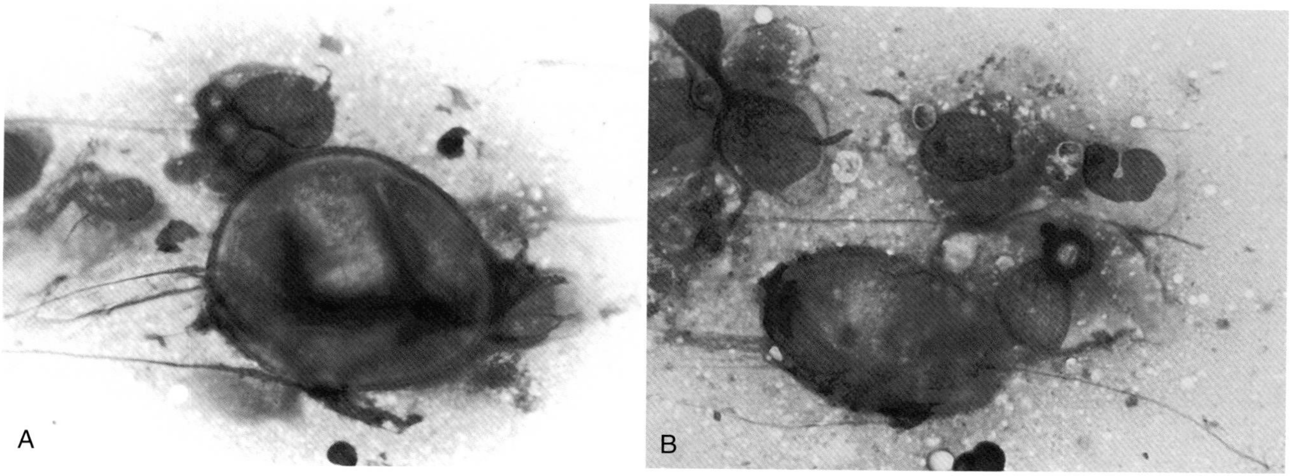

Figure 17-16 Skin, FNA, cat, coccidioidomycosis. A, One large extracellular spherule (measuring 35 μm in diameter) with a thick, well-demarcated wall is adjacent to a macrophage containing three smaller spherules. **B**, One large extracellular, partially folded spherule is adjacent to a macrophage containing one small spherule. Few small extracellular endospores (3-5 μm) are also present. (Wright stain. Original magnification 1000×.) (Glass slide courtesy of Sharon Dial).

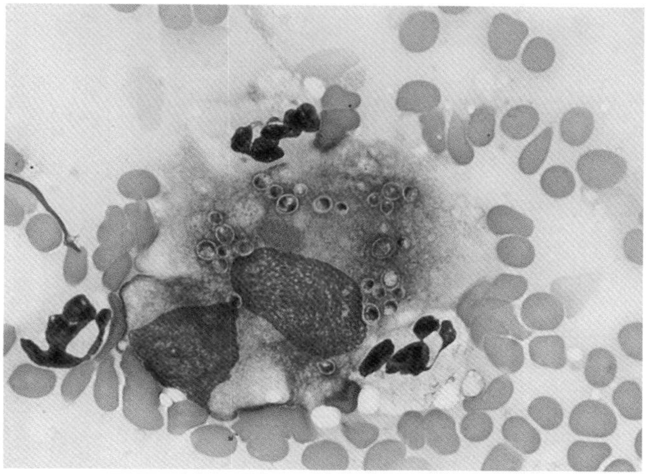

Figure 17-17 Lung, FNA, cat, histoplasmosis. A macrophage contains many small, round to oval yeast with an eccentric, often crescent-shaped nucleus consistent with *Histoplasma capsulatum.* (Wright stain. Original magnification 1000×.)

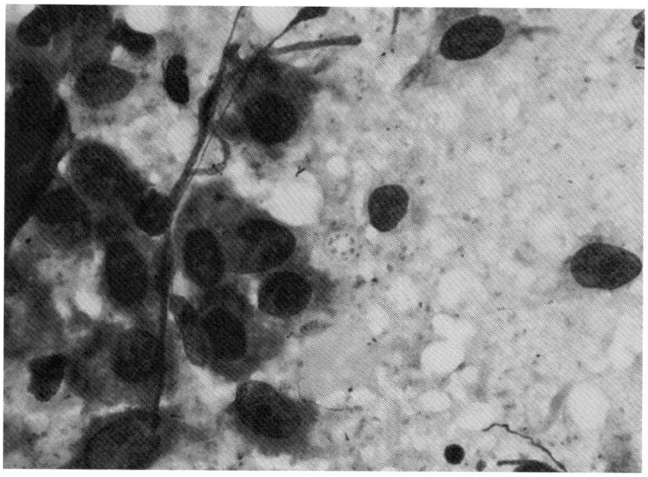

Figure 17-18 Lung, impression smear, dog, ***Pneumocystis.*** One extracellular, round cyst consisting of seven basophilic bodies arranged in a circular fashion is shown in the center of the photograph. Many small pleomorphic, poorly defined trophozoites are also found adjacent to many necrotic epithelial cells. (Wright stain. Original magnification 1000×.) (Glass slide from 2005 ASVCP case review session, submitted by Drs. Tara Holmberg and Sonjia Shelly).

results in a tissue phase characterized by large, distended macrophages that contain a cytoplasm-consuming schizont packed with many morphologically indistinct merozoites. The nuclei of the infected macrophages typically contain very large and prominent nucleoli. These cells may be found in tissues throughout the body but are most commonly identified on histopathologic samples from the spleen, liver, and lungs.[39,40] Protozoa of the genus *Acanthamoeba* may also infect the pulmonary parenchyma of cats and dogs;[41] trophozoites, cysts, or both may (rarely) be seen cytologically (Figure 17-21).

Helminthic Infection: Lung worms are uncommonly diagnosed by cytologic evaluation of bronchoalveolar lavage or transtracheal wash fluid. Very rarely, evaluation of pulmonary parenchymal aspirates results in the identification of helminthic infections (Figure 17-22).

Neoplasia

Hypertrophy (increased cell size), hyperplasia (increased number of cells), metaplasia (replacement of one cell type by another), and dysplasia (abnormal pattern of tissue growth with asynchronous nuclear and cytoplasmic maturation), are reversible, preneoplastic changes.[42] Distinguishing these changes from well-differentiated neoplasia with certainty is best accomplished histologically.

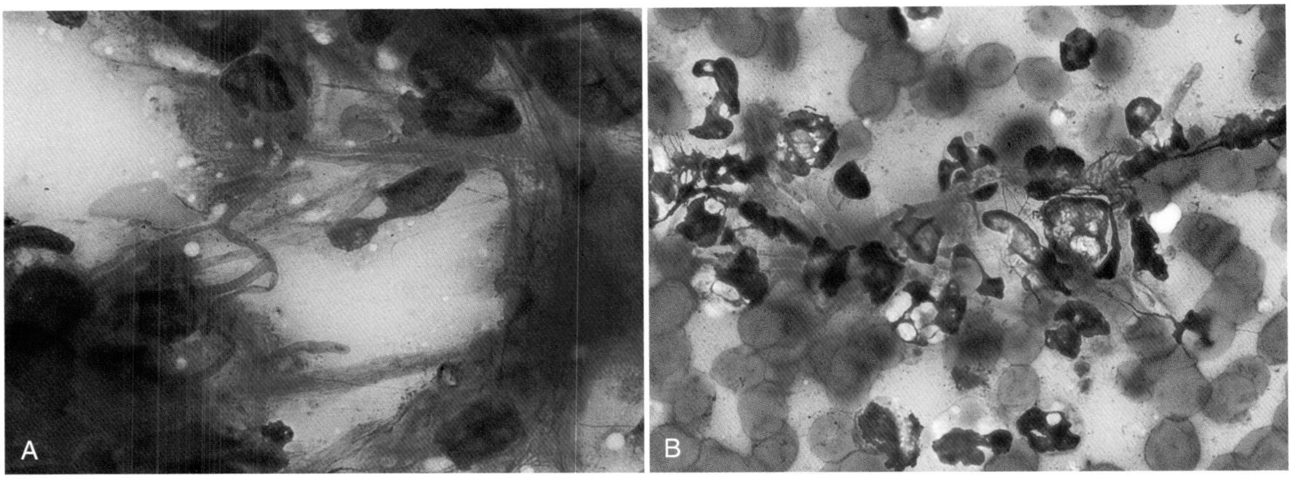

Figure 17-19 Nose, FNA, dog, aspergillosis. Lightly stained, branching fungal hyphae are seen admixed with respiratory epithelial cells (*A*) and poorly preserved neutrophils (*B*). (Wright stain. Original magnification 1000×.)

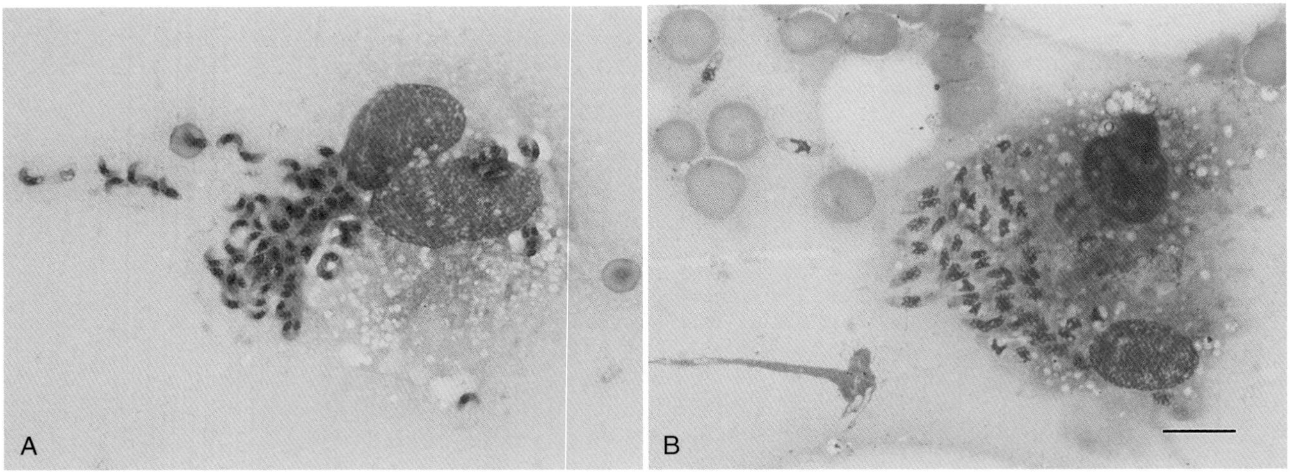

Figure 17-20 A, Lung, impression smear, cat, toxoplasmosis. **B,** Lung, FNA, dog, neosporosis. (Wright stain. Original magnification 1000×.) Both photomicrographs consist of vacuolated macrophages containing intracellular, banana- to cigar-shaped tachyzoites with centrally located oval nuclei. Extracellular tachyzoites are also seen in both cases. (Part A Glass slide from 2005 ASVCP case review session, submitted by Dr. Deborah Davis.)

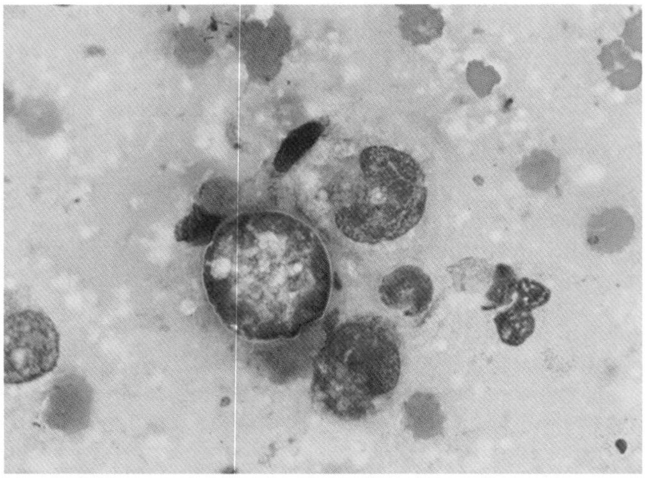

Figure 17-21 Lung, impression smear, dog, *Acanthamoeba*. A 28-μm–diameter cyst is seen adjacent to few macrophages and a small amount of cellular debris. Note the thin, nonstaining wall and the coarsely granular internal structure of the cyst. (Modified Wright stain.) (Glass slide from 2010 ASVCP case review session, submitted by Dr. Katie Boes).

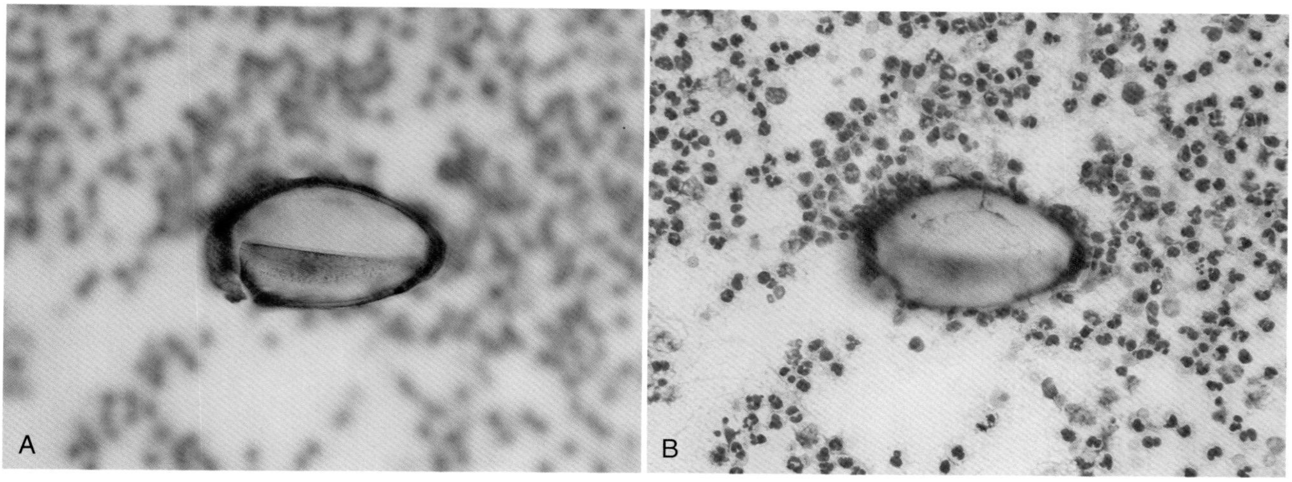

Figure 17-22 Lung, FNA, cat, paragonimiasis. A, Focused on ovum. **B,** Focused on background cellularity. A large (45 × 75 μm) single-operculated ovum is surrounded by many neutrophils, eosinophils, and few macrophages. (Wright-Giemsa stain. Original magnification 400×.)

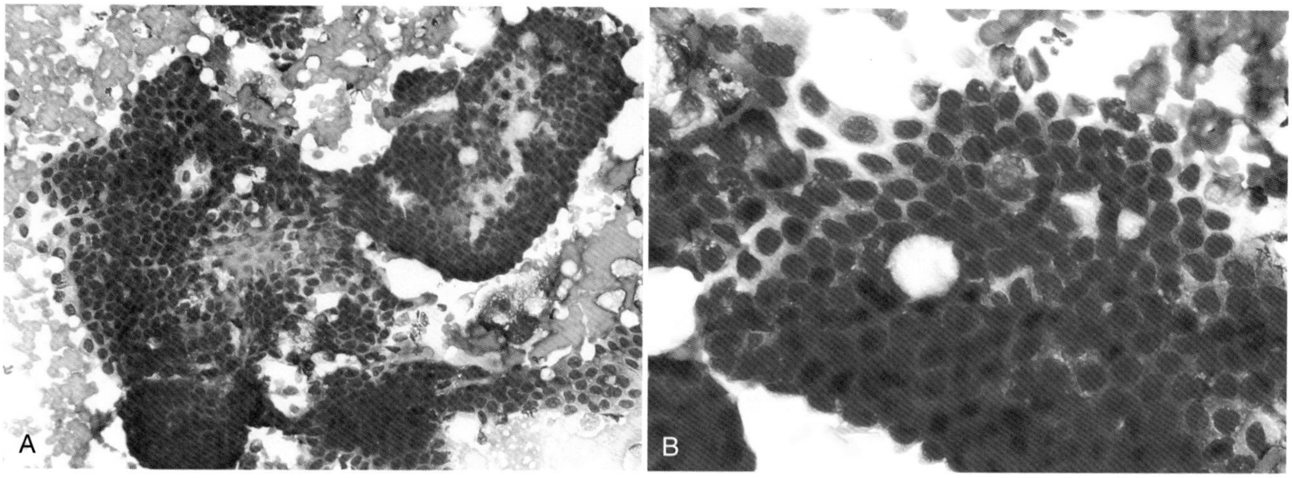

Figure 17-23 Lung, FNA, dog, carcinoma. A, Several clusters to sheets of very basophilic epithelial cells with high nuclear to cytoplasmic ratio. Anisokaryosis is minimal. (Wright stain. Original magnification 200×.) **B,** Although a benign lesion or a metastatic lesion cannot be ruled out, the cellularity and uniformity of this tumor is most consistent with primary pulmonary epithelial neoplasia. (Original magnification 500×).

Canine and feline primary tumors of the lung are most commonly epithelial in origin.[43-45] Histologic classification of primary pulmonary epithelial tumors may be complicated.[45] With the exception of squamous cell carcinoma, cytologic differentiation of various primary epithelial tumors is usually not possible (see Figures 17-11; Figure 17-23 and Figure 17-24). Observing acinar structures may suggest a glandular cell origin (adenoma, adenocarcinoma), but this arrangement of cells is often not apparent. Furthermore, differentiating a primary from a metastatic epithelial tumor in the lung is typically not achievable. Aspiration of primary malignant and metastatic epithelial lung tumors often yields highly cellular smears that consist of clusters of round to polygonal, basophilic cells with malignant criteria. However, primary malignant epithelial tumors may also appear quite uniform, exhibiting minimal anisokaryosis and nuclear atypia (see Figure 17-23). Lastly, any tumor may be associated with necrosis, inflammation (most often neutrophilic or pyogranulomatous), or both. Necrotic material appears cytologically as bluish-gray, amorphous, extracellular debris and, in the lung, is most commonly observed in association with primary epithelial tumors (see Figures 17-10; Figure 17-25).

Primary mesenchymal tumors of the lung are not common. Histiocytic sarcoma may manifest as a primary lung tumor or as a metastatic lesion in the disseminated variant of this malignancy.[46] Cytologically, histiocytic sarcomas may consist of individual round cells or spindle to pleomorphic cells. Typically, these cells have an abundant amount of lightly to moderately basophilic cytoplasm that is often, but not always, vacuolated (Figure 17-26). The nuclear to cytoplasmic ratio is variable. A common and often distinguishing feature of these tumors is the presence of large, multinucleate cells. Although other

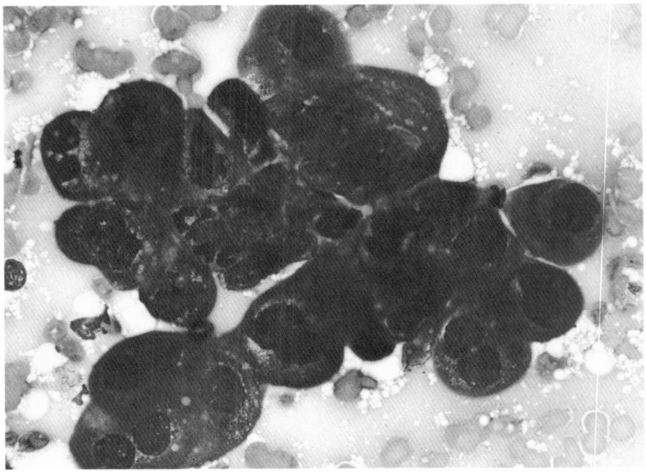

Figure 17-24 Lung, FNA, dog, carcinoma. Epithelial cells exhibiting many malignant criteria. (Wright stain. Original magnification 1000×.)

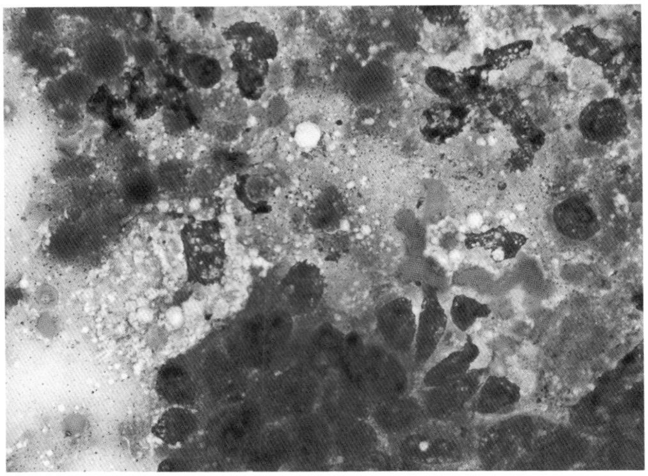

Figure 17-25 Lung, FNA, dog, carcinoma. A cluster of malignant epithelial cells is associated with few highly vacuolated macrophages and a large amount of amorphous cellular debris consistent with necrosis. (Wright stain. Original magnification 500×.)

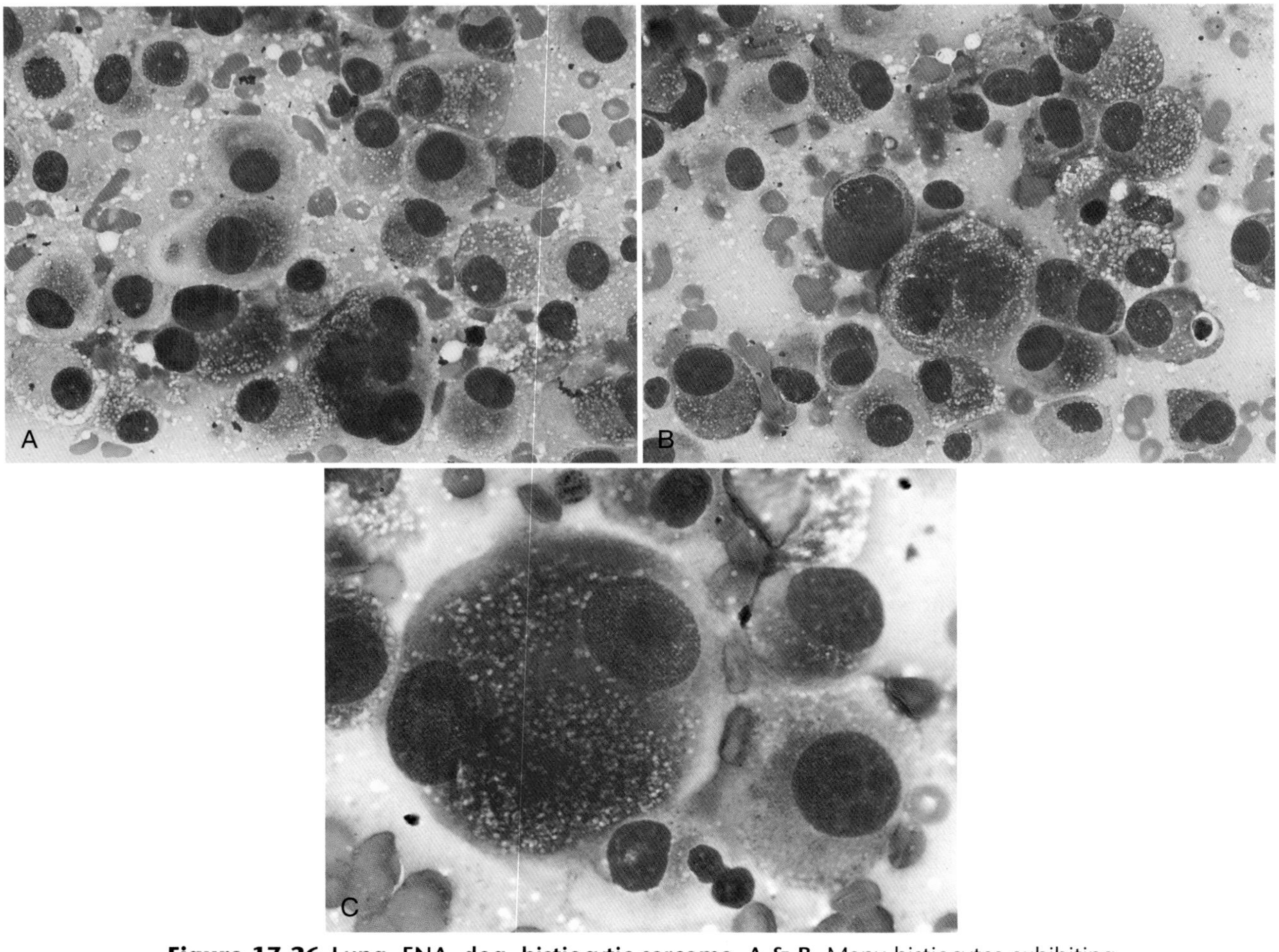

Figure 17-26 Lung, FNA, dog, histiocytic sarcoma. A & B, Many histiocytes exhibiting malignant criteria are seen. Occasional large multinucleated cells are also present. Phagocytic activity (*B*) is rarely noted. (Wright stain. Original magnification 500×.) **C,** Higher-power magnification of a large binucleate histiocyte with coarse chromatin and multiple prominent nucleoli. (Original magnification 1000×.)

tumors may contain multinucleate cells, when these cells are in the presence of the cells described above, histiocytic sarcoma should be a top differential.

Lymphomatoid granulomatosis is a term that has been used to describe a spectrum of pulmonary diseases, usually lymphomas, in which the neoplastic cells have an atypical morphology with histiocytic features. The term *lymphomatoid granulomatosis* is controversial because it has been applied to lesions with varying cytologic and molecular features. In dogs, the term has been applied to tumors consisting of large, pleomorphic, mononuclear cells admixed with few to many eosinophils and lower numbers of plasma cells and small lymphocytes.[47,48]

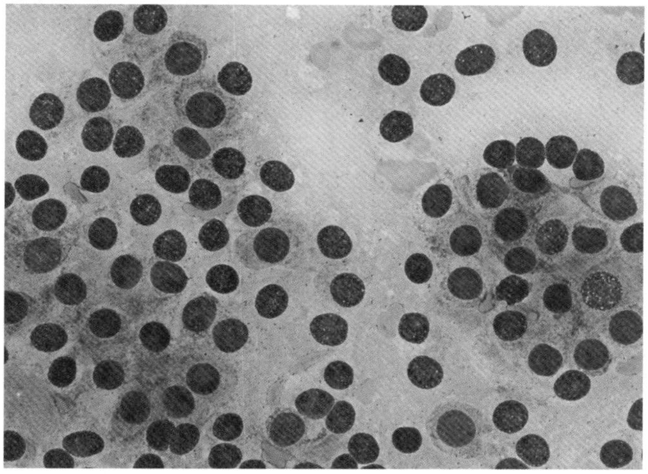

Figure 17-27 Lung, FNA, dog, endocrine or neuroendocrine carcinoma. Loosely cohesive clusters of uniform cells with indistinct cytoplasmic borders are consistent with a tumor of endocrine or neuroendocrine origin. The extracellular pink material is consistent with colloid, suggesting a metastatic thyroid carcinoma. (Wright stain. Original magnification 500×.)

Lung carcinoids are primary pulmonary tumors that arise from neuroendocrine cells in the airway epithelium. These tumors are also rare but have been presumptively diagnosed via FNA and cytologic evaluation.[49]

Because the pulmonary capillaries are the first filter met by many tumor emboli, secondary tumors in the lung are relatively common.[50] Common practices in monitoring veterinary patients with cancer allow pulmonary metastases to be readily identified and frequently aspirated. Essentially, any tumor may metastasize to the lungs, but tumors more likely to do so include oral and nail bed melanoma, thyroid carcinoma (Figure 17-27), osteosarcoma, mammary carcinoma, and high-grade soft tissue sarcoma (personal communication, Dr. Amy K. LeBlanc).[29]

Other

Hemorrhage: Hemorrhage is indicated by the presence of erythrophagia (consistent with acute hemorrhage, Figure 17-28, *A*), the presence of pigmented hemoglobin breakdown products (associated with chronic hemorrhage), or both. Hemoglobin breakdown products include hemosiderin (globular to irregular, bright-blue to black, pigmented material within macrophages; see Figure 17-28, *B*) and hematoidin (small, rhomboid, bright-orange crystals present extracellularly or within macrophages; see Figure 17-28, *B*). Hemorrhage may be secondary to another process (e.g., neoplasia, inflammation) or may be the primary pulmonary lesion (e.g., in patients with coagulopathy).

Benign Epithelial Cells: As cytology from normal lung tissue is typically of low cellularity, a sample with increased numbers of respiratory epitheliocytes that lack striking features of malignancy is suggestive of atelectasis or hyperplasia (a benign proliferation of epithelial cells secondary to chronic irritation or some other stimulus, discussed previously). A well-differentiated carcinoma

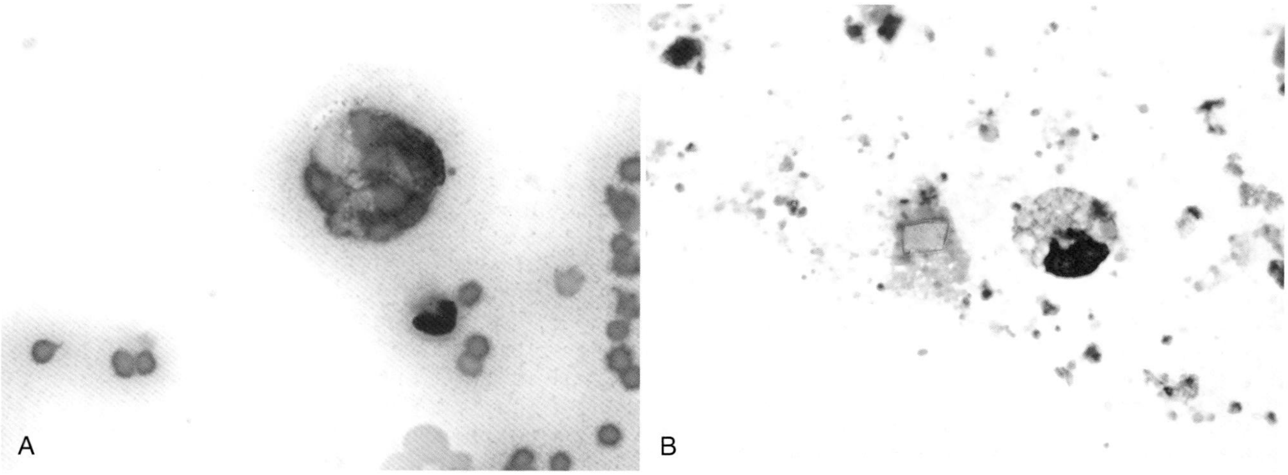

Figure 17-28 A, Subcutaneous mass, FNA, cat. A macrophage containing several phagocytized erythrocytes indicates acute hemorrhage. (Wright stain. Original magnification 1000×.) **B,** Subcutaneous mass, FNA, dog. Bright blue, irregular, pigmented material (hemosiderin) is present extracellularly and within macrophages, and a single, hematoidin crystal is present extracellulary, indicating chronic hemorrhage. (Wright stain. Original magnification 1000×.)

should be considered a differential in light of suggestive historical, clinical, or other findings.

Benign Mesenchymal Cells: When cytology reveals a predominance of fusiform (mesenchymal) cells that lack striking criteria of malignancy and which are sometimes associated with small amounts of amorphous, pink, extracellular matrix material, a benign mesenchymal proliferation should be considered. Fibroplasia and fibrosis are nonspecific, secondary changes wherein mesenchymal cells proliferate (most commonly) in response to chronic irritation. In such cases, evidence of the primary disease process (inflammation, neoplasia, necrosis, etc.) may not be seen. Fibrosis may also represent a specific clinical entity, for example, canine pulmonary fibrosis (CPF) in West Highland White Terriers.[51] CPF is, however, rarely diagnosed cytologically because of the tendency of these lesions to be poorly exfoliative. Benign mesenchymal neoplasms of the pulmonary parenchyma are rare.

CYTOLOGY OF THE MEDIASTINUM

The mediastinum is the structure of tissues and organs between the pleural spaces. It contains the heart, which separates the cranial and caudal portions of the mediastinum; lymphoid tissue, including thymus and lymph nodes; portions of trachea, bronchi, esophagus, and major blood vessels, lymphatic vessels, and nerves; fat; and loose connective tissue.[52,53]

FNA sampling of mediastinal lesions is feasible, but the deep intrathoracic location, presence of vital structures, and cardiorespiratory movement carry associated risks. Sampling should be performed under imaging guidance to minimize the likelihood of major complications. See the techniques section earlier in this chapter for more information on imaging-guided sample acquisition.

Indications for cytology of mediastinal lesions include the presence of masses, organomegaly, and abnormal accumulations of fluid. Contraindications for FNA of mediastinal lesions are similar to those previously described for pulmonary lesions. Cytology of many mediastinal lesions is covered below; lymph node and pericardial effusion cytology are covered in Chapters 11 and 15, respectively.

The expected cellularity of FNA samples of mediastinal lesions depends on the nature of the lesion. For example, lymphoid and epithelial lesions typically yield high-cellularity samples; by contrast, connective tissue lesions are often poorly exfoliative, and tend to yield low-cellularity samples. Potential contaminants in mediastinal samples include cells or other material from tissues pierced by the needle (e.g., skin, blood, fat, mesothelium, effusion fluid, mucus, microbes) and introduced contaminants (e.g., glove powder, ultrasound gel).

Thymus

The thymus is located principally in the cranial mediastinum. (The shape and exact location of the thymus varies among domestic animals.[53] Cats may have cervical and thoracic thymic lobes; the cervical lobe is usually small but may extend along the lateral surfaces of the cervical trachea. Dogs do not have a cervical lobe.) The normal size of the organ varies with age: It is largest in relation to body mass at birth, and involutes after sexual maturity. After involution, thymic tissue is replaced by loose connective tissue and fat, but microscopic remnants of the original tissue remain.[53]

In addition to being a primary lymphoid organ that is essential for normal development of T-lymphocytes, the thymus also has an epithelial component. Hassall's corpuscles, foci of epithelial cells in the thymic medulla, are a characteristic histologic feature of the organ.[53] Interactions between the thymic epithelial cells and lymphocytes are critical to normal thymic function and may also play a role in some diseases (see "Thymoma," below). Thymic lymphocytes (sometimes called *thymocytes*) have a characteristic CD4+CD8+ phenotype, which distinguishes them from lymphocytes in other organs.[54] Figure 17-29 shows normal thymic microanatomy.

Thymic lesions reported in dogs and cats include thymoma, lymphoma, cysts, and other disorders that occur more rarely (Box 17-1).[55]

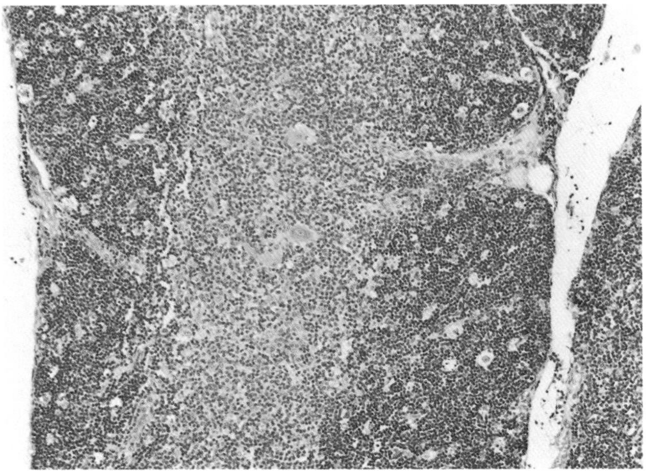

Figure 17-29 Normal thymus, juvenile dog. The cortex is darker because it contains a higher concentration of T-lymphocytes (thymocytes) than the medulla. Hassall's corpuscles, evident here as round, pink foci in the center of the image, are a characteristic feature of the medulla but are usually not detectable in thymic aspirates. The large cells with abundant pale cytoplasm that are scattered throughout the cortical areas are cytophagic ("tingible body") macrophages. (H&E.) (Image courtesy of Dr. Linden Craig.)

BOX 17-1

Thymic Lesions Reported in Dogs and Cats

- Neoplastic
  - Thymoma/Thymic carcinoma[54,55,63,64,104]
  - Thymic lymphoma[54,55]
  - Thymolipoma/Thymofibrolipoma[105,106]
  - Thymic carcinoid (in a Bengal tiger)[107]
  - Squamous cell carcinoma[108,109]
  - Lymphangiosarcoma[110]
- Non-neoplastic
  - Amyloidosis[104]
  - B lymphoid follicles[111]
  - Cysts[55,65-69]
  - Hematoma/Hemorrhage[55,86,112,113]
  - Hyperplasia[55,86]
  - Hypoplasia[55]

Thymoma: Thymoma is a major differential diagnosis for a cranial mediastinal mass; rare reports of ectopic thymomas in dogs and cats have been published.[56,57] Thymomas are thymic epithelial neoplasms that may be benign or malignant (malignant thymoma is also known as *thymic carcinoma*) and often have a nonneoplastic lymphoid component.[55] In vitro experiments have shown that neoplastic thymic epithelial cells induce differentiation of CD4-CD8- T-lymphocyte precursors to those with the CD4+CD8+ phenotype typical of cortical thymocytes.[58] In fact, in dogs and cats with thymomas, lymphocytes usually comprise the majority population of nucleated cells in FNA cytology samples, whereas epithelial cells are often absent or present in relatively low numbers. Presumably, lymphocytes predominate in these cases because the neoplastic thymic epithelial cells produce cytokines that promote lymphoid hyperplasia and because lymphocytes exfoliate readily. Classifying thymomas as benign or malignant or according to the predominant cell type is most reliably accomplished histologically.[59,60] The system proposed by the World Health Organization (WHO) has gained wide acceptance for histologic classification of thymomas and thymic carcinomas in people.[58,61]

Most lymphocytes in thymomas are well-differentiated, small, CD4+CD8+ lymphocytes. Relatively low numbers of larger lymphocytes may also be present. Flow cytometric immunophenotyping has been used to discriminate thymomas from aspirates of other lymphocyte-rich mediastinal lesions in dogs.[54] Another common feature of thymomas is the presence of low numbers of well-differentiated mast cells. Thymic epithelial cells may be variably shaped—from round or oval to polygonal to fusiform—and present individually and in more cohesive arrangements, or both. These cells typically have round to oval nuclei, inconspicuous nucleoli, and moderate amounts of lightly basophilic cytoplasm. They usually lack striking morphologic features of malignancy. Foci of pink extracellular material, perhaps originating from the capsule of the tumor or from intralesional septae, may also be present in aspirates of thymomas.[62] Figure 17-30

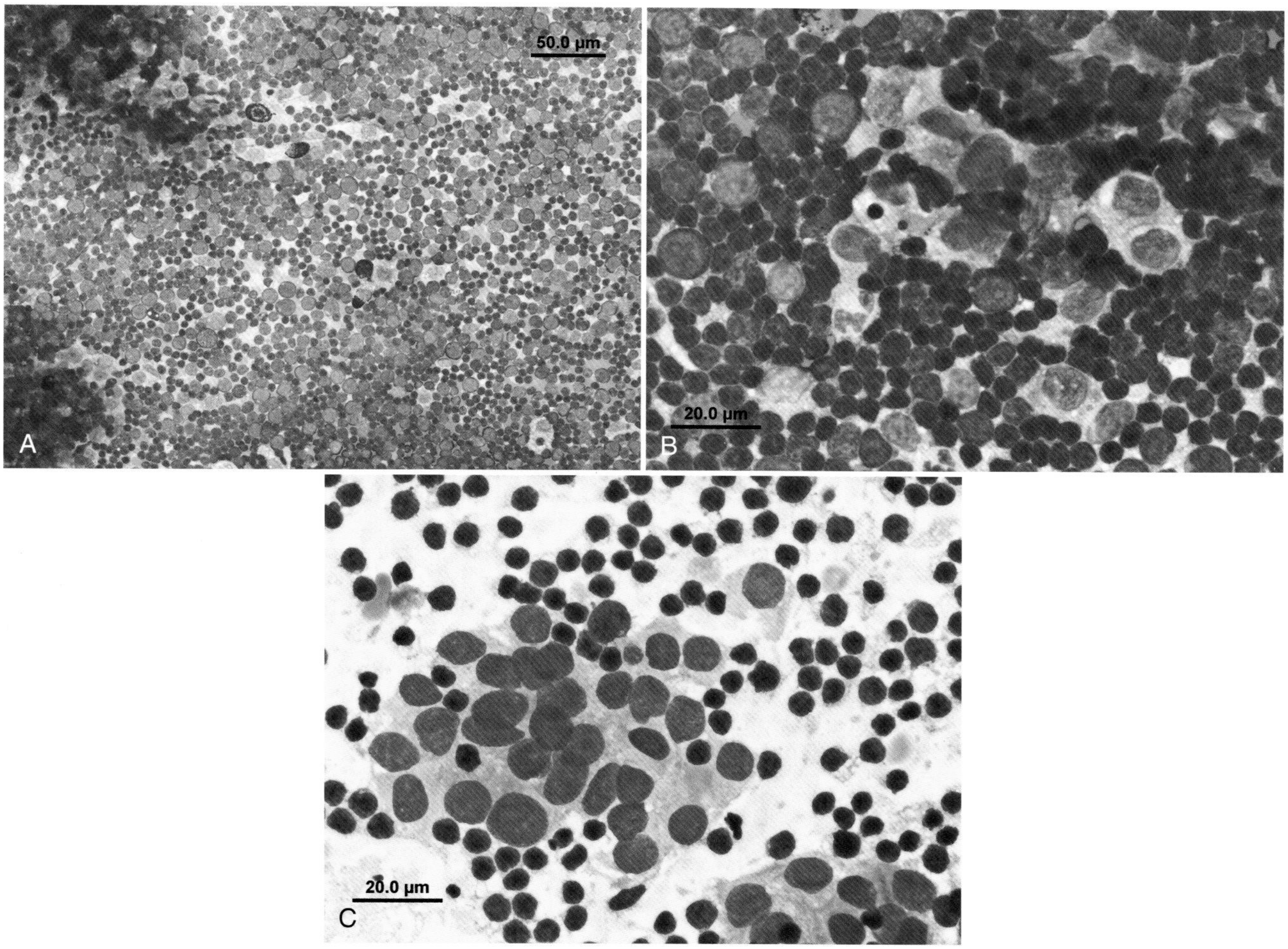

Figure 17-30 Cranial mediastinal mass, FNA, dog, thymoma. Low-magnification (*A*) and high-magnification (*B*) images. The sample consists mostly of a mixed population of lymphocytes, including many small lymphocytes. Also present are thymic epithelial cells, which in *A* are present mainly as poorly defined clusters (*in the upper and lower left corners*), and a few well-differentiated mast cells (*present near the center of A*). An aspirate from a different canine thymoma (*C*) shows a higher concentration of thymic epithelial cells. (Wright stain.) (Image C from slide courtesy of Dr. David F. Edwards.)

shows classic cytologic findings of a canine thymoma; Figure 17-30, *C*, shows an example of a sample containing high numbers of thymic epithelial cells.

Thymomas are often associated with the autoimmune disorder myasthenia gravis in people and in dogs and cats.[55,58,63] The exact mechanism responsible for this association is not clear but may involve development of altered T-lymphocyte repertoires.[58] Hypercalcemia and other paraneoplastic disorders have also been reported in dogs and cats with thymomas.[55,63,64]

Thymic Lymphoma: The interpretive principles that apply to cytologic diagnosis of lymphoma in lymph nodes and other organs also apply to diagnosis of lymphoma in the thymus, mediastinal lymph nodes, and other intrathoracic locations. Cytologic diagnosis of lymphoma is covered in detail in Chapter 11.

Other major differentials for mediastinal samples consisting mostly of lymphocytes include thymoma, as discussed above, and lymphoid hyperplasia (also covered in Chapter 11).

Thymic Cysts: The thymus originates during embryogenesis from pharyngeal (branchial) pouches, and remnants of these structures may be associated with cysts, neoplasms, or both. Thymic branchial cysts have been reported in dogs and cats, including some cases in which the cysts were associated with thymic neoplasia.[55,65-69] Histologically, they are lined with ciliated columnar epithelial cells, and some of these cells may be present in aspirates obtained for cytologic evaluation, but aspirates of these cystic lesions are likely to consist mostly of low-cellularity fluid. A publication on branchial cysts in people that included results of FNA biopsy in 36 patients found varying proportions of inflammatory cells, mature squamous epithelial cells, cholesterol crystals, and cellular debris.[70] Mediastinal cysts of nonthymic origin (e.g., parathyroid, thyroglossal, pleural) may also occur and are likely to have similarly low-cellularity fluid.[71,72] Figure 17-31 shows an aspirate of a cystic mediastinal lesion in a cat.

Other Thymic Lesions: Other thymic lesions reported in dogs, cats, or both are shown in Box 17-1.

Mediastinal Lymph Nodes

Clinically relevant thoracic lymph nodes are present in the mediastinum and include the sternal, cranial mediastinal, and tracheobronchial lymph nodes. The presence or absence and number of intrathoracic lymph nodes varies considerably between individuals.[73] Lymph node cytology is covered in Chapter 11.

Other Mediastinal Lesions

Cardiac and Chemoreceptor Tumors: FNA sampling of cardiac lesions for cytologic evaluation is uncommon. The lesions sampled most often are heart base tumors, particularly chemodectoma (a form of paraganglioma arising from aortic or carotid body chemoreceptor organs) and hemangiosarcoma.

Chemodectoma cytologic findings have been reported in dogs and cats.[74,75] Like other neuroendocrine tumors, chemodectomas are composed of cells that frequently lyse during sample collection, leaving many free nuclei among a background of free cytoplasm. Intact cells are often present both individually and in sheets or clusters. The cells are typically round to polygonal and have round to oval nuclei that are often eccentrically placed, and small to moderate amounts of lightly basophilic cytoplasm that often contains very fine pink granules (Figure 17-32, *A*); a report of a chemodectoma in a cat describes some cells with numerous round cytoplasmic vacuoles. Anisocytosis and anisokaryosis are usually mild to moderate. The nuclei typically have stippled chromatin and often have one to several discernible nucleoli. Special stains (e.g., Churukian-Schenk; see Figure 17-32, *B*) may be used to confirm the argyrophilia of the cytoplasmic granules.

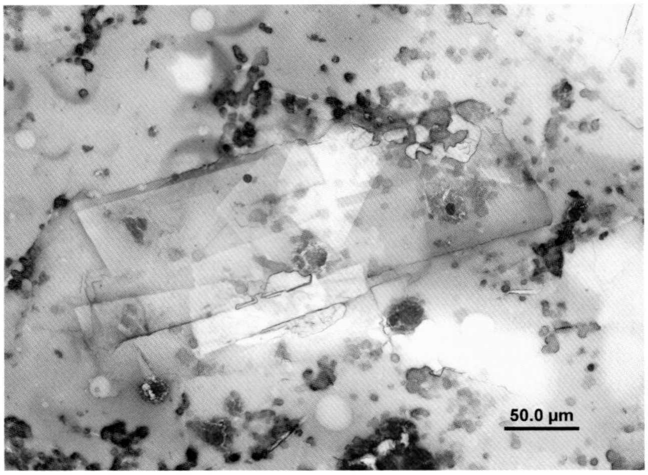

Figure 17-31 Cystic mediastinal lesion, FNA, cat. Some large cholesterol crystals and a few hemosiderin-laden macrophages are present, similar to what is often seen in aspirates of cystic fluid from other anatomic locations. It was not determined whether this lesion was associated with a tumor. (Wright stain.)

The right atrium is a site of predilection for hemangiosarcoma in dogs, but it is more common to sample hemangiosarcoma lesions for cytologic evaluation from abdominal organs (especially spleen or liver) than from the heart. The morphology of hemangiosarcoma cells does not tend to vary greatly, depending on the anatomic location of the tumor; regardless of location, cytologic samples of hemangiosarcomas are usually bloody and otherwise of relatively low cellularity. Hemangiosarcoma cytology is covered in more detail in Chapters 20 (Liver) and 21 (Spleen).

Pericardial Lesions: Mesothelioma, which may arise from or progress to involve the pericardial surface, is covered under pleural lesions (see below).

Other Neoplasms: A partial list of other neoplasms that may arise in the mediastinum (in addition to thymoma, lymphoma, chemodectoma, and hemangiosarcoma) but that are more often diagnosed in other anatomic locations, includes the following:

- Mesothelioma – usually diagnosed cytologically in effusion fluid (see Chapter 15)
- Neoplasms of ectopic thyroid or parathyroid tissue[76] (see Chapter 6)

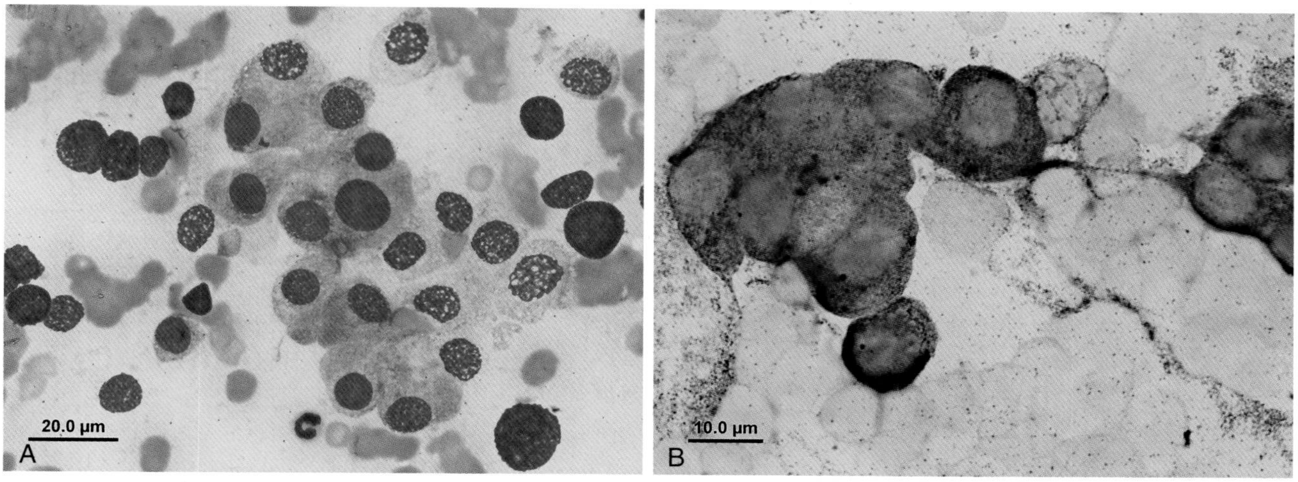

Figure 17-32 Cranial mediastinal mass, FNA, dog, chemodectoma. A, The neoplastic cells have a typical neuroendocrine morphology—round to polygonal in shape, present individually and in clusters, with lightly basophilic cytoplasm containing fine pink granules; the free nuclei are also a characteristic feature of neuroendocrine tumor aspirates. (Wright stain.) **B,** Another slide from the same aspirate, showing the argyrophilia of the cytoplasmic granules (also present in the background from lysed cells). (Churukian-Schenk stain.)

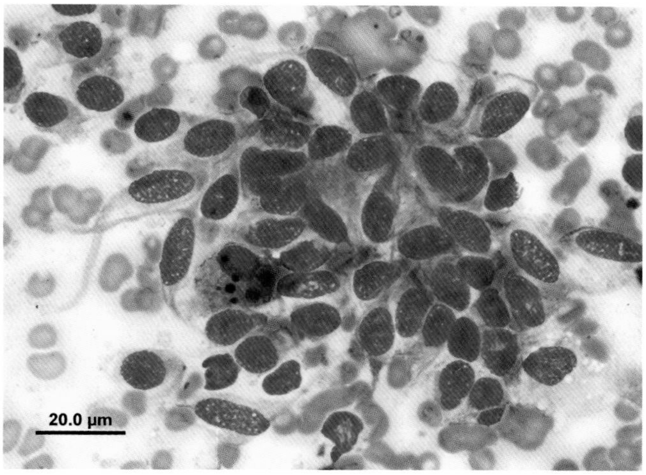

Figure 17-33 Mediastinal mass, FNA, dog, histologically diagnosed as anaplastic sarcoma. The fusiform cell morphology and loosely aggregated arrangement of the cells are characteristic of mesenchymal tumors. A cell to the left of center contains two intracytoplasmic (likely phagocytized) erythrocytes and some dark globular material that may be hemosiderin; it is not clear whether this cell is an activated macrophage or part of the neoplastic population. (Wright stain.) Immunohistochemical staining of the tumor for CD18 and von Willebrand factor (to identify histiocytic and endothelial cell origin, respectively) was negative.

- *Spirocerca lupi*–associated esophageal sarcoma (see below)
- Lipoma or liposarcoma[77,78]
- Histiocytic sarcoma[79,80]
- Chondrosarcoma[81,82]
- Leiomyoma or leiomyosarcoma[83,84]

Figure 17-33, Figure 17-34, and Figure 17-35 are examples of mediastinal sarcomas. Of course, many different tumor types have the potential to metastasize to mediastinal lymph nodes or other mediastinal locations.

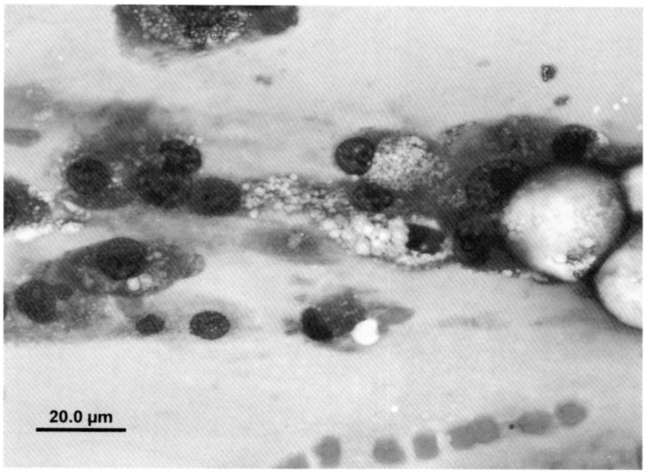

Figure 17-34 Mediastinal mass, FNA, dog, myxoid liposarcoma. These tumors produce a mucinous extracellular matrix that may cause the cells to form linear patterns ("windrows"), as shown affecting the erythrocytes at the bottom of this image. The vacuoles in liposarcoma cells will stain positive with cytochemical stains for lipid, such as Oil red O (*not shown here*). (Wright stain.)

Hemorrhage: Mediastinal hematomas have been reported in dogs with possible elastin dysplasia, and mediastinal hemorrhage was reported in a dog with rodenticide intoxication.[85,86] Cytologic features of hemorrhage are discussed in the earlier section on cytology of the lung.

Esophageal Lesions: Esophageal granulomas are among the classic lesions associated with canine spirocercosis, a disease with worldwide distribution in tropical and subtropical regions.[87,88] Cytologic preparations from these lesions are likely to show evidence of pyogranulomatous inflammation and may contain *Spirocerca lupi* ova (Figure 17-36).[89] Affected dogs are strongly predisposed

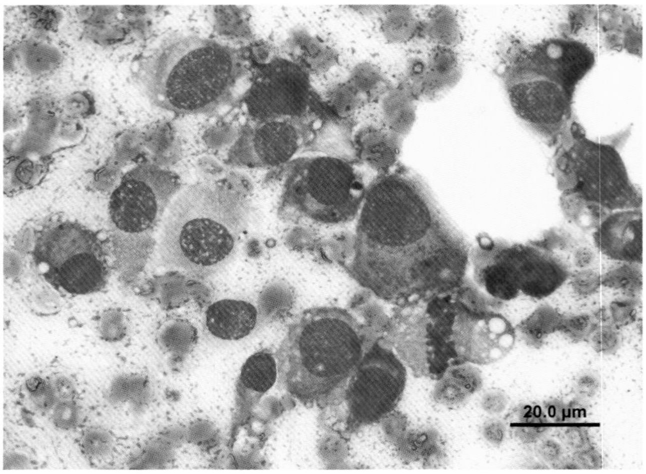

Figure 17-35 Cranial mediastinal mass, FNA, dog, sarcoma. This mass apparently originated from the manubrium. Findings were diagnostic for sarcoma based on the striking features of malignancy. Histopathologic confirmation of the cell type was unavailable in this case, but osteosarcoma was considered most likely based on the cytomorphology and extracellular matrix consistent with osteoid (see Chapter 13), and on the anatomic location. (Wright stain.)

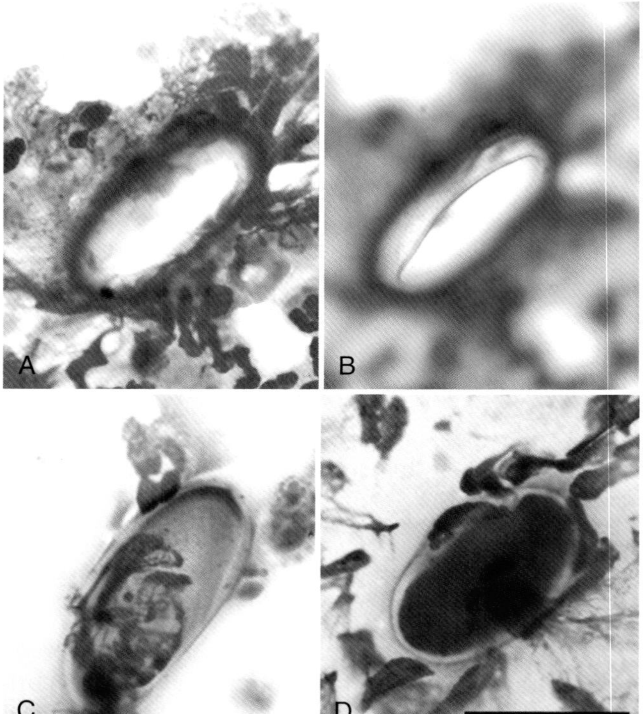

Figure 17-36 Esophageal nodule, FNA, dog, spirocercosis. *Spirocerca lupi* egg (*A*). Same egg, in a different plane of focus (*B*); note the longitudinal fold on egg surface. Note the filamentous (*C*) or homogeneous (*D*) material filling the eggs. (May-Grünwald–Giemsa stain. Bar = 20 mm.) (From De Lorenzi D, Furlanello T: What is your diagnosis? Esophageal nodules in a dog. *Vet Clin Pathol* 39(3),391-392, 2010. Used with permission.)

to developing esophageal sarcomas (especially osteosarcoma or fibrosarcoma).[90]

A case of a dog with a large, encapsulated, inflamed, cystlike (fluid-filled but not epithelial-lined), caudal mediastinal mass suspected to have originated from an esophageal perforation has been reported.[91]

Infectious Diseases: Although uncommon, certain infectious diseases may manifest as mediastinal lesions. A partial list includes cryptococcosis, blastomycosis, paecillomycosis, aspergillosis, bartonellosis, and oomycosis.[92-97]

CYTOLOGY OF OTHER INTRATHORACIC LESIONS

Pleural Lesions

The most common types of pleural lesions are reactive mesothelial lesions, malignancies (especially mesothelioma or carcinomatosis), and inflammatory lesions. Cytologic specimens of these lesions may be obtained directly by aspiration or by biopsy impression smears but are more often obtained indirectly by sampling of pleural effusion fluid (see Chapter 15).

Chest Wall Lesions

Nonpleural intrathoracic lesions include neoplasms and inflammatory lesions associated with the chest wall. More reports have been made of primary chest wall tumors in dogs than in cats. A partial list of cases reported in dogs includes osteosarcoma (see Figure 17-35), chondrosarcoma, hemangiosarcoma, and fibrosarcoma.[98-102]

Diaphragmatic Hernias

Diaphragmatic hernias may cause displacement of abdominal contents into the mediastinum or the pleural cavity. Therefore, cytologic features consistent with that of abdominal organs should prompt consideration of diaphragmatic hernia as a differential diagnosis. A report of ectopic hepatic parenchyma in the thorax of a cat has also been published.[103]

References

1. Cole SG: Fine needle aspirates. In King SG, editor: *Respiratory disease in dogs and cats*, St. Louis, 2004, Saunders.
2. Roudebush P, Green RA, Digilio KM: Percutaneous fine-needle aspiration biopsy of the lung in disseminated pulmonary disease, *J Am Anim Hosp Assoc* 17:109, 1981.
3. Teske E, Stokhof AA, Vandeningh TSGAM, et al: Transthoracic needle aspiration biopsy of the lung in dogs with pulmonic diseases, *J Am Anim Hosp Assoc* 27:289, 1991.
4. Smallwood LJ, Zenoble RD: Biopsy and cytological sampling of the respiratory tract, *Semin Vet Med Surg (Small Anim)* 8:250, 1993.
5. Finn-Bodner ST, Hathcock JT: Image-guided percutaneous needle biopsy: ultrasound, computed tomography, and magnetic resonance imaging, *Semin Vet Med Surg (Small Anim)* 8:258, 1993.
6. Hecht S: Thorax. In Penninck D, d'Anjou MA, editors: *Atlas of small animal ultrasonography*, Ames, IA, 2008, Blackwell Publishing.

7. Kirberger RM, Stander N: Interventional procedures. In Barr F, Gaschen L, editors: *BSAVA manual of canine and feline ultrasonography*, Gloucester, U.K., 2011, British Small Animal Veterinary Association.
8. Mcmillan MC, Kleine LJ, Carpenter JL: Fluoroscopically-guided percutaneous fine-needle aspiration biopsy of thoracic lesions in dogs and cats, *Vet Radiol* 29:194, 1988.
9. Nyland TG, et al: Ultrasound-guided biopsy. In Nyland TF, Mattoon JS, editors: *Small animal diagnostic ultrasound*, Philadelphia, PA, 1995, W.B. Saunders.
10. Tidwell AS, Johnson KL: Computed tomography-guided percutaneous biopsy in the dog and cat: description of technique and preliminary evaluation in 14 patients, *Vet Radiol Ultrasound* 35:445, 1994.
11. Wood EF, O'Brien RT, Young KM: Ultrasound-guided fine-needle aspiration of focal parenchymal lesions of the lung in dogs and cats, *J Vet Intern Med* 12:338, 1998.
12. Zekas LJ, Crawford JT, O'Brien RT: Computed tomography-guided fine-needle aspirate and tissue-core biopsy of intrathoracic lesions in thirty dogs and cats, *Vet Radiol Ultrasound* 46:200, 2005.
13. Menard M, Papageorges M: Ultrasound corner: technique for ultrasound-guided fine needle biopsies, *Vet Radiol Ultrasound* 36:137–138, 1995.
14. Papageorges M, et al: Ultrasound-guided fine-needle aspiration: an inexpensive modification of the technique, *Vet Radiol* 29:269, 1988.
15. Bigge LA, Brown DJ, Penninck DG: Correlation between coagulation profile findings and bleeding complications after ultrasound-guided biopsies: 434 cases (1993-1996), *J Am Anim Hosp Assoc* 37:228, 2001.
16. Vignoli M, Rossi F, Chierici C, et al: Needle tract implantation after fine needle aspiration biopsy (FNAB) of transitional cell carcinoma of the urinary bladder and adenocarcinoma of the lung, *Schweiz Arch Tierheilkd* 149:314, 2007.
17. Bonfanti U, Bussadori C, Zatelli A, et al: Percutaneous fine-needle biopsy of deep thoracic and abdominal masses in dogs and cats, *J Small Anim Pract* 45:191, 2004.
18. DeBerry JD, Norris CR, Samii VF, et al: Correlation between fine-needle aspiration cytopathology and histopathology of the lung in dogs and cats, *J Am Anim Hosp Assoc* 38:327, 2002.
19. Cowell RL, et al: The lung and intrathoracic structures. In Cowell RT, Tyler RD, Meinkoth JH, DeNicola D, editors: *Diagnostic cytology and hematology of the dog and cat*, ed 3, St. Louis, MO, 2008, Mosby.
20. Burkhard MJ, Millward LM: Respiratory tract. In Raskin RE, Meyer DJ, editors: *Canine and feline cytology: a color atlas and interpretation guide*, ed 2, St. Louis, MO, 2010, Saunders Elsevier.
21. Roudebush P, Green RA, Digilio KM: Percutaneous fine-needle aspiration biopsy of the lung in disseminated pulmonary disease, *J Am Anim Hosp Assoc* 17:109, 1981.
22. Jones DJ, et al: Endogenous lipid pneumonia in cats: 24 cases (1985-1998), *J Am Vet Med Assoc* 216:1437, 2000.
23. Raya AI, Fernandez-de Marco M, Nunez A, et al: Endogenous lipid pneumonia in a dog, *J Comp Pathol* 135:153, 2006.
24. Clercx C, Peeters D: Canine eosinophilic bronchopneumopathy, *Vet Clin North Am Small Anim Pract* 37:917, 2007.
25. Clercx C, Peeters D, Snaps F, et al: Eosinophilic bronchopneumopathy in dogs, *J Vet Intern Med* 14:282, 2000.
26. Calvert CA, et al: Pulmonary and disseminated eosinophilic granulomatosis in dogs, *J Am Anim Hosp Assoc* 24:311, 1988.
27. Von Rotz A, et al: Eosinophilic granulomatous pneumonia in a dog, *Vet Rec* 23:631, 1986.
28. Sauve V, Drobatz KJ, Shokek AB, et al: Clinical course, diagnostic findings and necropsy diagnosis in dyspneic cats with primary pulmonary parenchymal disease: 15 cats (1996-2002), *J Vet Emerg Crit Care* 15:38, 2005.
29. Cohn L: Pulmonary parenchymal disease. In Ettinger SJ, Feldman EC, editors: *Textbook of veterinary internal medicine*, ed 7, St. Louis, MO, 2010, Saunders.
30. Rufenacht S, Bogli-Stuber K, Bodmer T, et al: *Mycobacterium mycroti* infection in the cat: a case report, literature review and recent clinical experience, *J Feline Med Surg* 13:195, 2011.
31. Rodriguez-Tovar LE, Ramirez-Romero R, Valdez-Nava Y, et al: Combined distemper-adenoviral pneumonia in a dog, *Can Vet J* 48:632, 2007.
32. Crews LJ, Feeney DA, Jessen CR, et al: Utility of diagnostic tests for and medical treatment of pulmonary blastomycosis in dogs: 125 cases (1989-2006), *J Am Vet Med Assoc* 232:222, 2008.
33. Barron PM, Rose A: Cryptococcal pneumonia in a boxer without obvious extrapulmonary dissemination, *Aust Vet Pract* 38:108, 2008.
34. Graupmann-Kuzma A, Valentine BA, Shubitz LF, et al: Coccidioidomycosis in dogs and cats: a review, *J Am Anim Hosp Assoc* 44:226, 2008.
35. Kobayashi R, Tanaka F, Asai A, et al: First case report of histoplasmosis in a cat in Japan, *J Vet Med Sci* 71:1669, 2009.
36. Watson PJ, Wotton P, Eastwood J, et al: Immunoglobulin deficiency in Cavalier King Charles Spaniels with *Pneumocystis* pneumonia, *J Vet Int Med* 20:523, 2006.
37. Harkin KR: Aspergillosis: an overview in dogs and cats, *Vet Med* 98:602, 2003.
38. Dubey JP, Carpenter JL: Histologically confirmed clinical toxoplasmosis in cats: 100 cases (1952-1990), *J Am Vet Med Assoc* 203:1556, 1993.
39. Snider TA, Confer AW, Payton ME: Pulmonary histopathology of *Cytauxzoon felis* infections in the cat, *Vet Pathol* 47:698, 2010.
40. Meinkoth JH, Kocan AA: Feline cytauxzoonosis, *Vet Clin North Am Small Anim Pract* 35:89, 2005.
41. Greene CE, Howerth EW, Kent M: Nonenteric amebiasis: acanthamebiasis, hartmannelliasis, and balamuthiasis. In Greene CE, editor: *Infectious diseases of the dog and cat*, ed 3, St. Louis, MO, 2006, Saunders.
42. Kuseeit D: Neoplasia tumor and biology. In Zachary JF, McGavin MD, editor: *Pathologic basis of veterinary disease*, ed 5, St. Louis, MO, 2012, Mosby.
43. Ogilvie GK, Haschek WM, Withrow SJ, et al: Classification of primary lung tumors in dogs: 210 cases (1975-1985), *J Am Vet Med Assoc* 195:106, 1989.
44. Reichle JK, Wisner ER: Non-cardiac thoracic ultrasound in 75 feline and canine patients, *Vet Radiol Ultrasound* 41:154, 2000.
45. Wilson DW, Dungworth DL: Tumors of the respiratory tract. In Meuten DJ, editor: *Tumors in domestic animals*, ed 4, Ames, IA, 2002, Iowa State Press, Blackwell Publishing.
46. Affolter VK, Moore PF: Localized and disseminated histiocytic sarcoma of dendritic cell origin in dogs, *Vet Pathol* 39:74, 2002.
47. Bain PJ, et al: An 18-month-old spayed female boxer dog: lymphomatoid granulomatosis, *Vet Clin Pathol* 26:55, 1997.
48. Berry CR, Moore PF, Thomas WP, et al: Pulmonary lymphomatoid granulomatosis in 7 dogs (1976-1987), *J Vet Intern Med* 4:157, 1990.
49. Choi US, Alleman AR, Choi JH, et al: Cytologic and immunohistochemical characterization of a lung carcinoid in a dog, *Vet Clin Pathol* 37:249, 2008.

50. Lopez A: Respiratory system, mediastinum, and pleurae. In Zachary JF, McGavin MD, editors: *Pathologic basis of veterinary disease*, ed 5, St. Louis, MO, 2012, Mosby.
51. Norris AJ, Naydan DK, Wilson DW: Interstitial lung disease in West Highland White Terriers, *Vet Pathol* 42:35, 2005.
52. *Dorland's illustrated medical dictionary*, ed 27, Philadelphia, 1988, W.B. Saunders.
53. Zachary JF, McGavin MD: Diseases of white blood cells, lymph nodes, and thymus. In Zachary JG, McGavin MD, editors: *Pathologic basis of veterinary disease*, ed 5, St. Louis, MO, 2012, Elsevier.
54. Lana S, Plaza S, Hampe K, et al: Diagnosis of mediastinal masses in dogs by flow cytometry, *J Vet Intern Med* 20:1161, 2006.
55. Day MJ: Review of thymic pathology in 30 cats and 36 dogs, *J Small Anim Pract* 38:393, 1997.
56. Faisca P, Henriques J, Dias TM, et al: Ectopic cervical thymic carcinoma in a dog, *J Small Anim Pract* 52:266, 2011.
57. Lara-Garcia A, Wellman M, Burkhard MJ, et al: Cervical thymoma originating in ectopic thymic tissue in a cat, *Vet Clin Pathol* 37:397, 2008.
58. Okumura M, Fujii Y, Shiono H, et al: Immunological function of thymoma and pathogenesis of paraneoplastic myasthenia gravis, *Gen Thorac Cardiovasc Surg* 56:143, 2008.
59. Dell'Orco M, Bertazzolo W, Caniatti M, et al: Cytological features of 11 cases of canine and feline thymoma and correlation with a human histologic classification, *Veterinaria (Cremona)* 22:23, 2008.
60. Rae CA, Jacobs RM, Couto CG: A comparison between the cytological and histological characteristics in thirteen canine and feline thymomas, *Can Vet J* 30:497, 1989.
61. Ströbel P, et al: Thymoma and thymic carcinoma: an update of the WHO Classification 2004, *Surg Today* 35:805, 2005.
62. Andreasen CB, Mahaffey EA, Latimer KS: What is your diagnosis? Mediastinal mass aspirate from a 10-year-old dog, *Vet Clin Pathol* 20:15, 1991.
63. Atwater SW, Powers BE, Park RD, et al: Thymoma in dogs: 23 cases (1980-1991), *J Am Vet Med Assoc* 205:1007, 1994.
64. Zitz JC, Birchard SJ, Couto GC, et al: Results of excision of thymoma in cats and dogs: 20 cases (1984-2005), *J Am Vet Med Assoc* 232:1186, 2008.
65. Newman AJ: Cysts of branchial arch origin in the thymus of the Beagle, *J Small Anim Pract* 12:681, 1971.
66. Liu S, Patnaik AK, Burk RL: Thymic branchial cysts in the dog and cat, *J Am Vet Med Assoc* 182:1095, 1983.
67. Parnell PG, Andreasen CB: What is your diagnosis? Cranial mediastinal mass from a dog, *Vet Clin Pathol* 21:9, 1992.
68. Levien AS, Summers BA, Szladovits B, et al: Transformation of a thymic branchial cyst to a carcinoma with pulmonary metastasis in a dog, *J Small Anim Pract* 51:604, 2010.
69. Uchida K, Awamura Y, Nakamura T, et al: Thymoma and multiple thymic cysts in a dog with acquired myasthenia gravis, *J Vet Med Sci* 64:637, 2002.
70. Kadhim AL, et al: Pearls and pitfalls in the management of branchial cyst, *J Laryngol Otol* 118:946, 2004.
71. Zekas LJ, Adams WM: Cranial mediastinal cysts in nine cats, *Vet Radiol Ultrasound* 43:413, 2002.
72. Swainson SW, et al: Radiographic diagnosis: mediastinal parathyroid cyst in a cat, *Vet Radiol Ultrasound* 41:41, 2000.
73. Miller M, Evans H, editors: *Miller's anatomy of the dog*, ed 3, Philadelphia, PA, 1993, Saunders.
74. Zimmerman KL, et al: Mediastinal mass in a dog with syncope and abdominal distension, *Vet Clin Pathol* 29:19, 2000.
75. Caruso KJ, Cowell RL, Upton ML, et al: Intrathoracic mass in a cat, *Vet Clin Pathol* 31:193, 2002.
76. Patnaik AK, MacEwen EG, Erlandson RA, et al: Mediastinal parathyroid adenocarcinoma in a dog, *Vet Pathol* 15:55, 1978.
77. Messick JB, Radin MJ: Cytologic, histologic, and ultrastructural characteristics of a canine myxoid liposarcoma, *Vet Pathol* 26:520, 1989.
78. Woolfson JM, Dulisch ML, Tams TR: Intrathoracic lipoma in a dog, *J Am Vet Med Assoc* 185:1007, 1984.
79. Kohn B, Arnold P, Kaser-Hotz B, et al: Malignant histiocytosis of the dog: 26 cases (1989-1992), *Kleintierpraxis* 38:409, 1993.
80. Walton RM, Brown DE, Burkhard MJ, et al: Malignant histiocytosis in a domestic cat: cytomorphologic and immunohistochemical features, *Vet Clin Pathol* 26:56, 1997.
81. Cohen JA, Bulmer BJ, Patton KM, Sisson DD: Aortic dissection associated with an obstructive aortic chondrosarcoma in a dog, *J Vet Cardiol* 12:203, 2010.
82. Mellanby RJ, Holloway A, Woodger N, et al: Primary chondrosarcoma in the pulmonary artery of a dog, *Vet Radiol Ultrasound* 44:315, 2003.
83. Fews D, Scase TJ, Battersby IA: Leiomyosarcoma of the pericardium, with epicardial metastases and peripheral eosinophilia in a dog, *J Comp Pathol* 138:224, 2008.
84. Rollois M, Ruel Y, Besso JG: Passive liver congestion associated with caudal vena caval compression due to oesophageal leiomyoma, *J Small Anim Pract* 44:460, 2003.
85. Boulineau TM, Andrews-Jones L, Van Alstine W: Spontaneous aortic dissecting hematoma in two dogs, *J Vet Diagn Invest* 17:492, 2005.
86. Rickman BH, Gurfield N: Thymic cystic degeneration, pseudoepitheliomatous hyperplasia, and hemorrhage in a dog with brodifacoum toxicosis, *Vet Pathol* 46:449, 2009.
87. Van der Merwe LL, Kirberger RM, Clift S, et al: Spirocerca lupi infection in the dog: a review, *Vet J* 176:294, 2008.
88. Mylonakis ME, Rallis T, Koutinas AF, et al: Clinical signs and clinicopathologic abnormalities in dogs with clinical spirocercosis: 39 cases (1996-2004), *J Am Vet Med Assoc* 228:1063, 2006.
89. De Lorenzi D, Furlanello T: What is your diagnosis? esophageal nodules in a dog, *Vet Clin Pathol* 39:391, 2010.
90. Ranen E, Lavy E, Aizenberg I, et al: Spirocercosis-associated esophageal sarcomas in dogs: a retrospective study of 17 cases (1997-2003), *Vet Parasitol* 119:209, 2004.
91. Aulakh KS, et al: What is your diagnosis? A large soft tissue mass measuring approximately 15 X 12 X 13 cm is present in the caudodorsal aspect of the thorax, just right of midline, extending from the tracheal bifurcation to the diaphragm, *J Am Vet Med Assoc* 238:699, 2011.
92. Meadows RL, et al: Chylothorax associated with cryptococcal mediastinal granuloma in a cat, *Vet Clin Pathol* 22:109, 1993.
93. Schmiedt C, Kellum H, Legendre AM, et al: Cardiovascular involvement in 8 dogs with *Blastomyces dermatitidis* infection, *J Vet Intern Med* 20:1351, 2006.
94. Nakagawa Y, Mochizuki R, Iwasaki K, et al: A canine case of profound granulomatosis due to *Paecillomyces* fungus, *J Vet Med Sci* 58:157, 1996.
95. Wood GL, Hirsh DC, Selcer RR, et al: Disseminated aspergillosis in a dog, *J Am Vet Med Assoc* 172:704, 1978.
96. Saunders GK, Monroe WE: Systemic granulomatous disease and sialometaplasia in a dog with *Bartonella* infection, *Vet Pathol* 43:391, 2006.
97. Grooters AM, Hodgin EC, Bauer RW, et al: Clinicopathologic findings associated with *Lagenidium* sp. infection in 6 dogs: initial description of an emerging oomycosis, *J Vet Intern Med* 17:637, 2003.

TABLE 18-1—cont'd

Infectious Agents of the Gastrointestinal Tract

Category	Organism	Cytologic Description	Common Location for Diagnosis	Additional Diagnostic Tests (if applicable)
	Cyniclomyces guttulatus 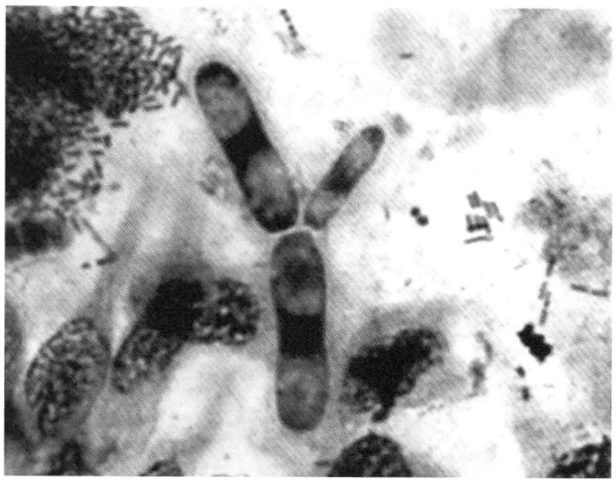	Individual or short branching or forking chains of cylindrical yeast, 5–7 × 15–20 μm in size, with a clear cell wall and an interior that stains uniformly purple, mottled or vacuolated, or has a broad, transverse, poorly staining central region	Feces	
Protozoa	*Cryptosporidium parvum*† 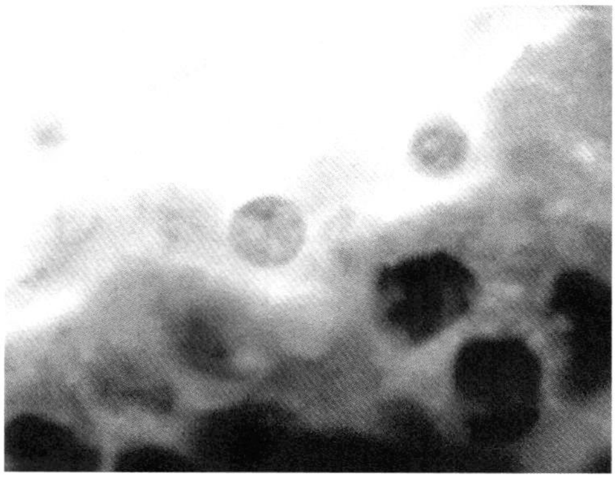	Small, 2- to 4-μm, oocysts or trophozoites on the surface of enterocytes, often with a stippled appearance with Romanowsky stains; typically only oocysts are seen in feces	Feces	Acid-fast staining (organisms stain red-pink), direct fluorescence antibody detection, PCR, concentration techniques such as Sheather sucrose flotation, zinc sulfate flotation, saturated sodium chlorine methods
	Giardia spp.* 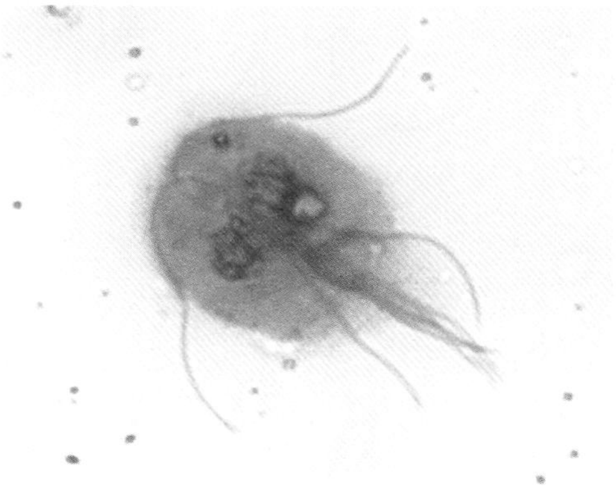	Pear-shaped, flagellated (four pairs: one anterior, two posterior, one caudal) trophozoites, 15 to 10 μm in length, "smiling face" appearance formed by two anterior nuclei, a longitudinal axioneme running between them and a transverse median body situated in the posterior portion of the cell	Feces	Multiple fecal exams may be required (shed intermittently), ELISA (IDEXX SNAP *Giardia* antigen detection test), PCR, zinc sulfate centrifugation float, direct fluorescent antibody test

Continued

TABLE 18-1—cont'd

Infectious Agents of the Gastrointestinal Tract

Category	Organism	Cytologic Description	Common Location for Diagnosis	Additional Diagnostic Tests (if applicable)
	Entamoeba histolytica 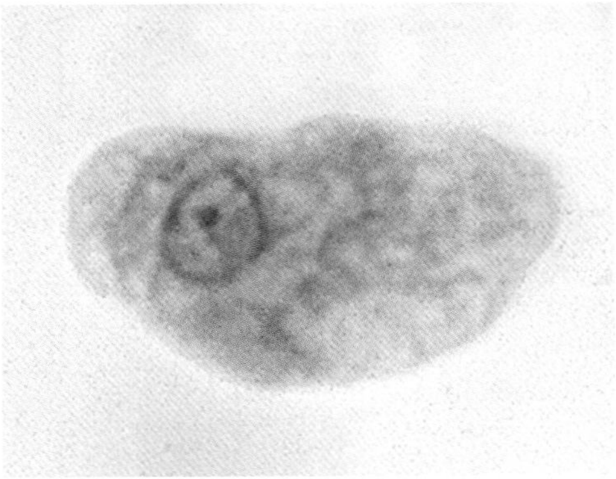	Large (12-50 μm) round to oval trophozoites with a small round, eccentrically placed nucleus with evenly distributed peripheral chromatin, a central compact karyosome and basophilic cytoplasm, with possible phagocytosis of RBCs	Large intestine, feces	Trichome or iron-hematoxylin stained fecal smears, methylene blue, specific culture media is available
	Pentatrichomonas hominis 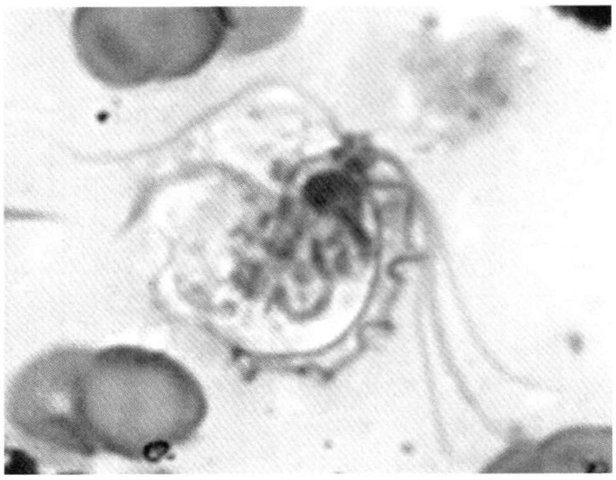	Spindle- to pear-shaped, highly motile, flagellated organism with five anteriorly directed flagella and a single posteriorly directed flagellum, and an undulating membrane	Feces	PCR
	Tritrichomonas foetus 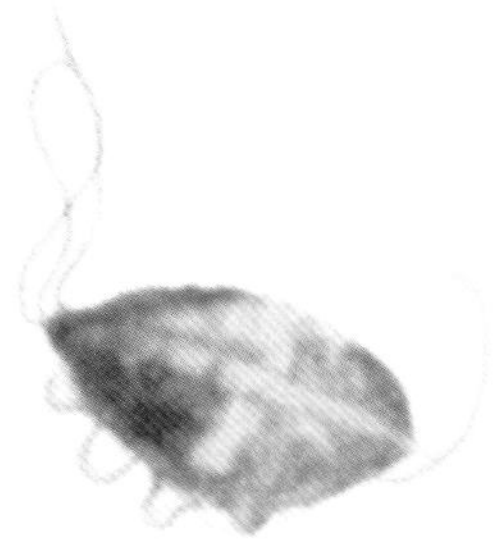	Oval to pear-shaped, 5-20 × 3-14 μm, highly motile, flagellated organism with three anteriorly directed flagella, a single posteriorly directed flagellum, an undulating membrane, oval anterior nucleus and an axostyle protruding from the posterior end	Large intestine, feces	Culture using the InPouch TF test (Biomed Diagnostics, White City, OR), PCR

TABLE **18-1**—cont'd

Infectious Agents of the Gastrointestinal Tract

Category	Organism	Cytologic Description	Common Location for Diagnosis	Additional Diagnostic Tests (if applicable)
Algae	*Prototheca* spp. 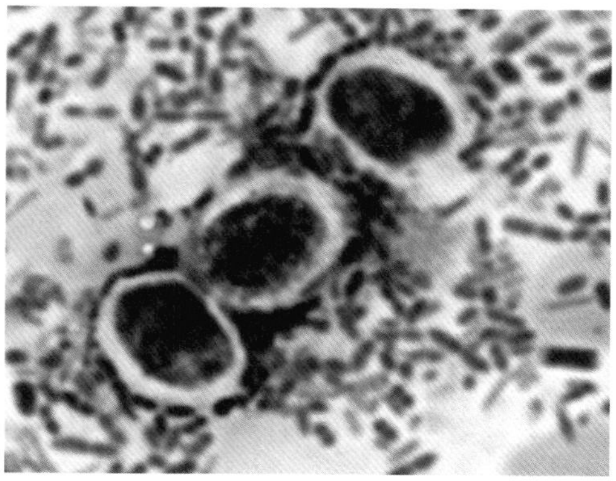	Oval algal organisms with granular basophilic to magenta internal structure surrounded by a clear capsule ("jelly bean" appearance) with internal endosporulation	Large intestine, feces	Culture
	Pythium insidiosum 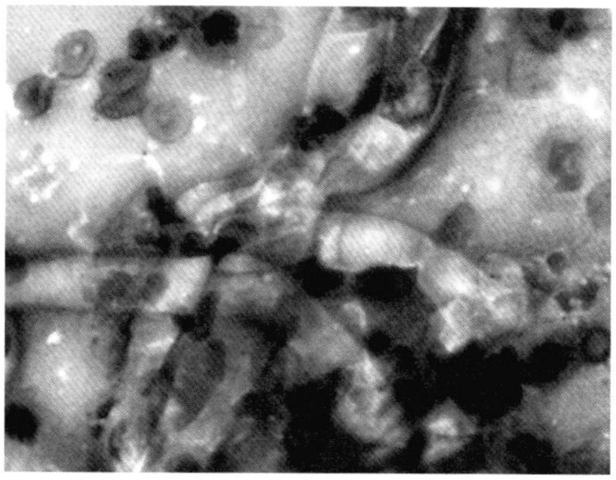	Wide, nonstaining to poorly staining, occasionally branching hyphal like structures with parallel cell walls and infrequent septation	Stomach, small intestine, and ileocolic junction	Culture, serology, PCR

*Image courtesy of Rick Cowell.
†Slide courtesy of Jody Gookin.
From Broussard JD: Optimal fecal assessment, *Clin Tech Small Anim Pract* 18:218, 2003; Greene CE: *Infectious diseases of the dog and cat*, ed 4, St. Louis, M, 2012, Saunders; Marks SL, Rankin SC, Byrne BA, et al: Enteropathogenic bacteria in dogs and cats: diagnosis, epidemiology, treatment, and control, *J Vet Int Med* 25:1195, 2011.

or definitive diagnosis before histopathology results are available. Although care must be taken to preserve the integrity of the biopsy sample, it is important to gently wipe or blot the blood and serum off of the tissue before making the touch imprints to allow proper adhesion of cells to the slide. It is also possible to make touch imprints of ultrasound-guided or endoscopically obtained tissue biopsies, but the smaller size and greater fragility of these types of samples makes this more difficult.

Fecal Examination

Fecal testing is a common diagnostic procedure in the clinical evaluation of GI disease. Timing of sample collection and preparation is very important. Feces are altered after stool is passed and significant degeneration of cells and some organisms such as *Giardia* spp. or *Tritrichomonas foetus* can occur rapidly making identification increasingly difficult with time (Figure 18-1).[1] With delayed processing of the fecal sample, some nematode eggs will release larvae, and bacterial overgrowth may occur. A fresh sample that can be processed immediately is best.

Several collection techniques are used for either the luminal contents or the surface mucosa of the rectum. Defecated feces and feces obtained during a digital rectal examination or with a fecal loop represent the rectal lumen, whereas rectal lavage or rectal scrape samples are representative of the mucosal surface. If defecated feces are used, it is critical that they be fresh and not heavily contaminated with debris. Additional fecal diagnostics include fecal flotation, fecal sedimentation, and the

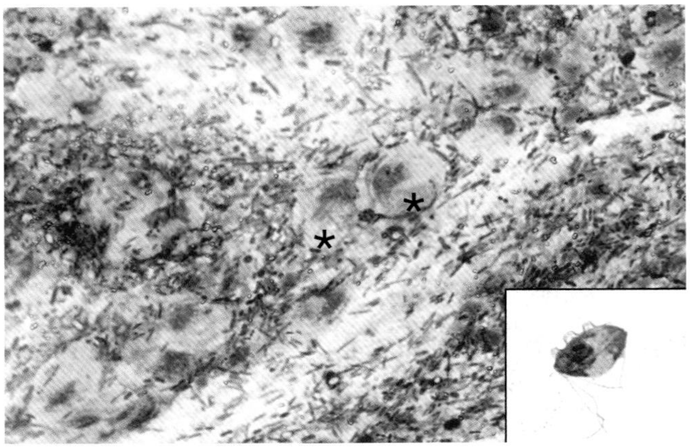

Figure 18-1 Feline fecal smear; degenerating ***Tritrichomonas foetus*** **organisms.** Many degenerating organisms are present (*two are indicated by asterisks [*]*) on a background of fecal material. The degenerating trophozoites are large round structures with round, dark, basophilic nuclei and an abundant amount of light basophilic cytoplasm. These could easily be mistaken for debris, degenerating tissue cells or histiocytes. *Tritrichomonas* degenerates quickly on exiting the body; thus, it is imperative that smears or wet mount preparations be made with fresh feces. The inset image is of a cytology preparation made from cultured *T. foetus* trophozoites. Typical morphologic features may be seen, including three anterior flagella, an undulating membrane, a longitudinal axostyle, an anterior nucleus, and a single posterior flagellum. (Modified Wright-Giemsa stain. Original magnification 50× objective. *Inset:* Wright-Giemsa stain. Original magnification 100× objective.). (*Tritrichomonas* culture courtesy of Katie Tolbert.)

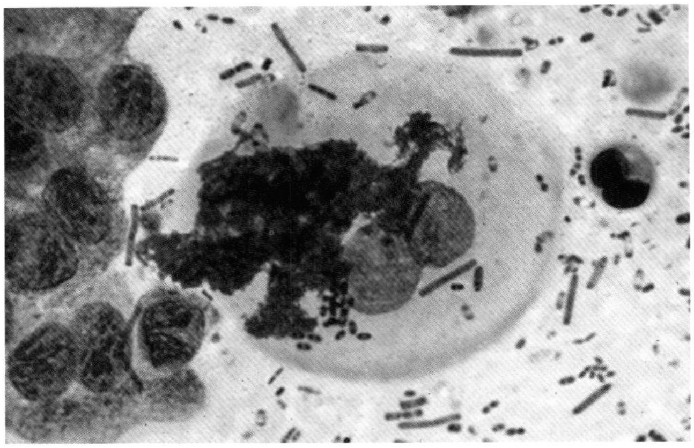

Figure 18-2 Fecal sample from a dog; abundant lubricant gel. Few columnar epithelial cells are present at the left of the image with two squamous epithelial cells in the center. The morphologic characteristics of the squamous epithelial cells are partially obscured by bright pink–magenta granular to globular lubricant material. (Wright-Leishman stain.)

Baermann technique; consultation of a veterinary parasitology text is recommended for additional information about these techniques.

When sampling the feces or rectal mucosa, lubricant gel should be used sparingly or avoided entirely, since the lubricant material could complicate evaluation of the cytologic specimen. Cytologically, lubricant has the appearance of thick extracellular magenta aggregates of material that may obscure the cells and organisms within the sample (Figure 18-2).

Direct Smears of Fecal Material: Direct smears from a luminal sample are made by spreading a small amount of feces thinly and evenly across the slide. The sample should not be heat-fixed; it is unnecessary and could cause significant damage to cells and organisms.[1] After air-drying, the slide may be stained with a standard Romanowsky-type stain (e.g. Wright stain, Giemsa stain, rapid stains) and evaluated like any cytologic sample. If using a rapid stain (i.e., Diff-Quik), it is recommended to have a separate "dirty" staining station for fecal and ear cytology so as not to contaminate the station where "clean" cytology and hematology samples are stained.

Rectal Lavage: To perform a rectal lavage, the end of a lubricated red rubber catheter is inserted into the rectum and approximately 6 to 12 milliliters (mL) of saline is infused and aspirated multiple times until the sample has a mudlike appearance.[1] Rectal lavage yields a small sample but allows the sample to be directly examined as an unstained wet mount preparation rather than as a stained dry fecal smear.

BOX 18-1

Tips for Performing a Rectal Scraping

1. Clear rectum of feces prior to sampling.
2. Avoid lubricant gel, or use it sparingly.
3. Use a rigid instrument to perform the scraping procedure (see Figure 18-3).
4. Sample far enough cranially to access the rectum while avoiding the anus.
5. Scrape firmly enough to sample the mucosa, but be careful not to cause perforation.
6. Protect the sample with a gloved finger when removing the sample.

Rectal Scraping: To obtain a sample by rectal scraping, the rectum is cleaned of feces, use of lubricant gel is minimized or avoided, and a rigid instrument such as a conjunctival scraper or chemistry spatula is used to obtain the specimen (Box 18-1 and Figure 18-3). The sample should be obtained cranially enough to reach the rectum, avoiding sampling of the anal mucosa; pressure should be applied firmly enough to sample the mucosa, rather than just the surface material, while being careful not to perforate the rectal wall. Slides are prepared, dried, and stained in a manner similar to the process for a fecal smear.

ESOPHAGUS

Normal Esophagus

The esophagus consists of a mucosal epithelium, submucosa, and a muscular wall. The esophageal mucosa is lined by nonkeratinizing stratified squamous epithelium. Submucosal mucous glands are present throughout the

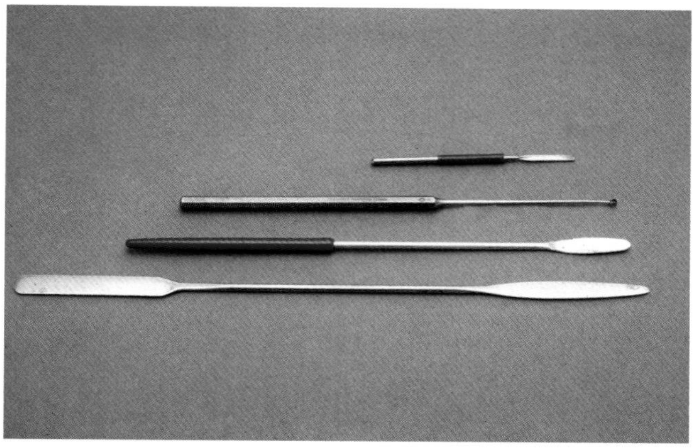

Figure 18-3 Various instruments used to perform rectal mucosal scrapings include (*top to bottom*) a conjunctival scraper, an ear curette, and two blunt chemistry spatulas.

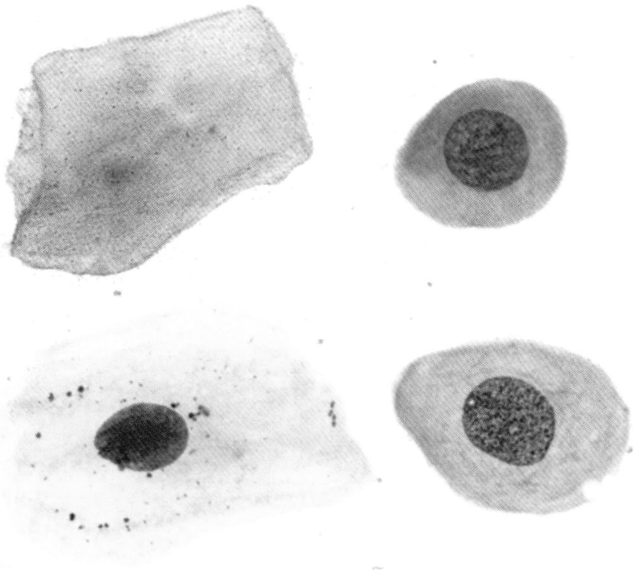

Figure 18-4 Esophageal brushings from normal dogs; various stages of esophageal squamous cells. *Beginning at the top right and moving clockwise:* A parabasal cell, a deep intermediate cell, an intermediate cell and a superficial cell. Intermediate cells are most numerous in normal esophageal samples and, compared with superficial cells, are characterized by a less angular shape, a similar amount abundant cytoplasm that is nonkeratinized and a round, medium-sized nucleus. (Wright-Giemsa stain. Original magnification 50× objective.) (Slides courtesy of Sally Bissett.)

esophagus in the dog and are located only at the pharyngeal–esophageal junction in the cat.[6]

Cells from multiple layers of the squamous epithelium may be identified in cytologic specimens (Figure 18-4). Progressing from superficial to deep, superficial squamous cells are angular with a pyknotic to absent nucleus, intermediate cells are somewhat angular with a larger nucleus, and deep intermediate and parabasal cells have a smaller volume of more deeply basophilic cytoplasm with rounded borders.[7] Cytology of normal esophageal brushings and washings consists of predominantly intermediate squamous cells with occasional superficial squamous cells. Cells from the deeper layers, including deep intermediate cells, parabasal cells, and rarely submucosal glandular epithelial cells, may also be seen cytologically, depending on the aggressiveness of the sampling technique, but this finding is typically an indicator of disease.[8] Oropharyngeal contamination may be seen in normal or abnormal esophageal samples and may consist of a mixed bacterial population including *Simonsiella*, and, rarely, respiratory epithelial cells. *Simonsiella* is a Gram-negative large (6-8 micrometers [μm] long and 2-3 μm wide) rod-shaped bacteria that contains segmented groups of cells aligned face-to-face in juxtaposition, giving it a barcode-like or stacked-disk appearance.

BOX 18-2

Causes of Esophagitis

- Foreign body
- Irritant (caustic agent, medication lodged)
- Thermal injury (radiation, hot ingesta)
- Gastroesophageal reflux
- Eosinophilic esophagitis
- Infectious etiology
- Neoplasia

Esophageal Inflammation

Esophagitis occurs with injury to the esophageal mucosa due to a variety of underlying causes, including foreign bodies, infectious etiologies, and mucosal irritants (Box 18-2). Although esophagitis often has an erosive or ulcerative component, lack of a discernible superficial lesion at endoscopy does not rule out underlying esophagitis.

In addition to ingestion of substances damaging to the esophageal mucosa, an important cause of esophagitis with mucosal injury is reflux esophagitis. This condition, which is most common in the distal esophagus, is the effect of gastric acid, pepsin, and possibly bile salts and pancreatic enzymes on the esophageal mucosa.[9] Reflux of these substances into the esophagus may occur with relaxation of the lower esophageal sphincter under anesthesia, a hiatal hernia, or chronic vomiting.[10] In addition to esophageal inflammation, a possible sequela of gastroesophageal reflux is metaplasia of the distal esophageal stratified squamous epithelium to a more acid-friendly simple columnar epithelium with interspersed goblet cells (Figure 18-5). This lesion has been reported in dogs and cats; grossly or endoscopically, these may range from a region of hyperemia to a polypoid mass, which could be mistaken for neoplasia (Table 18-2).[11] In humans, this condition is known as Barrett esophagus, and the lesion may progress and transform into a distal esophageal adenocarcinoma.

Cytologic findings with esophagitis are typically nonspecific with the presence of neutrophils amid the squamous epithelial cells. The presence of eosinophils in esophageal cytology may occur with neoplastic, parasitic, or fungal disease; with reflux esophagitis; as a part of eosinophilic gastroenteritis; or with eosinophilic esophagitis (Figure 18-6). Eosinophilic esophagitis has been reported in dogs, may be associated with allergic skin disease, and is a diagnosis of exclusion after eliminating the aforementioned causes of eosinophils within an esophageal sample.[12]

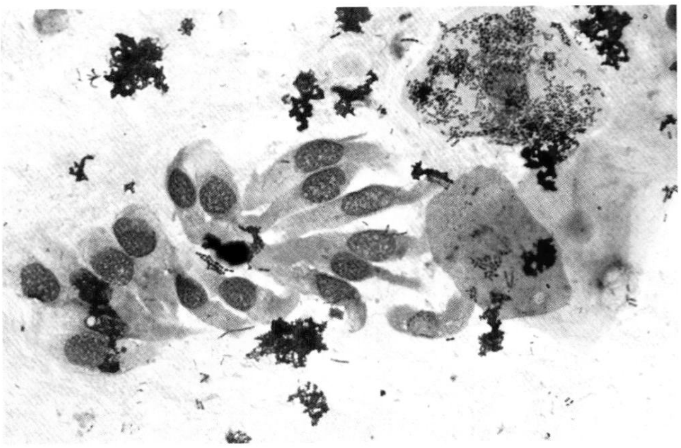

Figure 18-5 Canine brush cytology of a midesophogeal lesion; esophageal metaplasia. The presence of uniform columnar epithelial cells (*left side of image*) indicates metaplasia has occurred. Note (*in the right side of the image*) the three superficial squamous epithelial cells with adhered bacteria and free bacteria in the background, indicating oropharyngeal contamination, and the small scattered clumps of magenta extracellular material consistent with lubricant gel. This pet was suffering from chronic vomiting. (Wright-Giemsa stain. Original magnification 50× objective.)

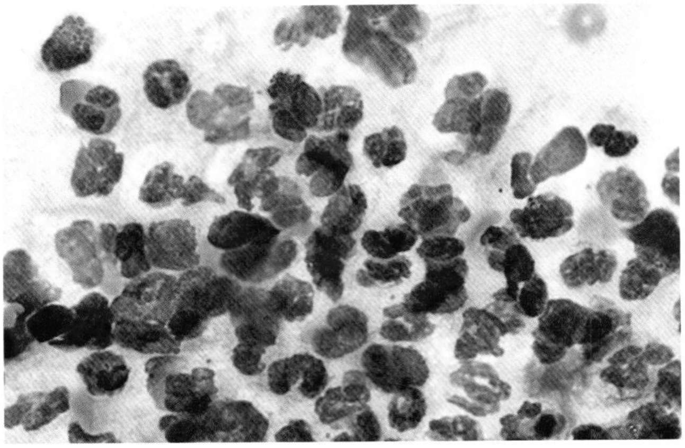

Figure 18-6 Esophageal brushing from a dog; eosinophilic esophagitis. The sample has a mix of eosinophils and neutrophils on a background of mucus. Eosinophilic inflammation of the esophagus is not specific for the entity of eosinophilic esophagitis and other causes such as neoplasia, parasitic or fungal disease, reflux esophagitis, and eosinophilic gastroenteritis must be ruled out. In this case, no improvement was seen following treatment with a proton pump inhibitor, but significant improvement occurred following corticosteroid administration. (Wright Giemsa stain. Original magnification 100× objective.)

TABLE 18-2

Benign Non-Neoplastic Lesions That May Be Confused for Neoplasia

Organ	Lesion
Esophagus	Barrett esophagus (metaplasia resulting from reflux esophagitis) Parasitic granuloma (*Spirocerca lupi*)
Stomach	Chronic hypertrophic gastropathy Chronic hypertrophic pyloric gastropathy Pyloric stenosis Granulomatous gastritis (pythiosis) Idiopathic eosinophilic gastrointestinal masses Schirrous eosinophilic gastritis Feline gastrointestinal eosinophilic sclerosing fibroplasia Gastric polyps
Intestine	Granulomatous enteritis or colitis (histoplasmosis, pythiosis, feline infectious peritonitis, protothecosis) Histiocytic ulcerative colitis of Boxers Idiopathic eosinophilic gastrointestinal masses Feline gastrointestinal eosinophilic sclerosing fibroplasia Intestinal polyps

Pyogranulomatous esophagitis may occur with pythiosis in dogs (see "Gastric Inflammation"). *Spirocerca lupi* infection causes a masslike granulomatous lesion in the distal esophagus of dogs because of the presence of adult nematodes in the esophageal submucosa. Typically, a single mass is present in the caudal thoracic portion of the esophagus, occasionally with surface ulceration or protrusion of adult worms into the esophageal lumen. An association exists between spirocercosis and the development of esophageal fibrosarcoma or osteosarcoma.

Esophageal Neoplasia

Primary esophageal neoplasia, which is rare in dogs and cats, includes squamous cell carcinoma and smooth muscle tumors, with rare reports of adenocarcinoma, neuroendocrine carcinoma, primary extraskeletal osteosarcoma, or plasma cell neoplasia.[13,14] Fibrosarcoma and osteosarcoma associated with *Spirocerca lupi* infection is discussed above (see "Esophageal Inflammation"). Rarely, esophageal involvement of canine oral papillomavirus infection may occur.[9]

Squamous cell carcinoma arising from the esophageal mucosal epithelium most commonly occurs in the middle third of the esophagus and is typically an ulcerated plaque with circumferential esophageal thickening.[13] Cytologically, this tumor resembles squamous cell carcinoma elsewhere in the body and often will have superimposed inflammation or evidence of superficial infection. Esophageal adenocarcinoma is rare but may arise from the submucosal esophageal glands or from regions of glandular metaplasia, as with reflux esophagitis. Leiomyomas in the esophagus are more common in dogs and are most commonly found in the outer muscular layer of the distal esophagus at the gastroesophageal junction.[14]

STOMACH

Normal Stomach

The stomach in dogs and cats is glandular, and, from proximal to distal, contains cardiac, fundic, and pyloric

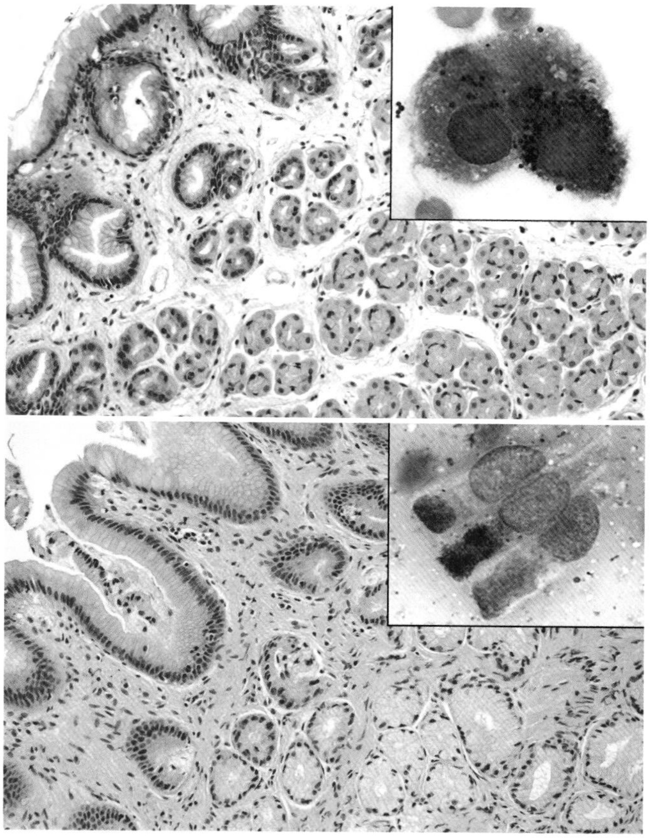

Figure 18-7 Stomach from a dog. *Top:* The mucosa of the fundus is covered by a simple columnar epithelium with vacuolated cytoplasm (foveolar epithelium) that invaginates to form gastric pits. Deeper within the mucosa, glandular structures are present, with an inner rim of cuboidal basophilic to vacuolated chief cells (pepsinogen-secreting cells) and an outer rim of round eosinophilic parietal cells (hydrochloric acid-secreting cells). (H&E stain. Original magnification 20× objective.) The inset of a cytologic specimen has a chief cell with basophilic to purple cytoplasmic granules (*right*) and likely a parietal cell with pink cytoplasmic granules (*left*) (Modified Wright stain) *Bottom:* The mucosa of the pylorus is covered by a similar epithelium to the fundus, but the deeper mucosa contains predominantly mucus-secreting glands lined by pale, highly vacuolated epithelial cells. (H&E stain. Original magnification 20× objective.) The inset of a cytologic specimen has few mucus-secreting columnar epithelial cells, which contain apical pink-magenta cytoplasmic mucus-containing granules. (Wright-Giemsa stain. Original magnification 100× objective.)

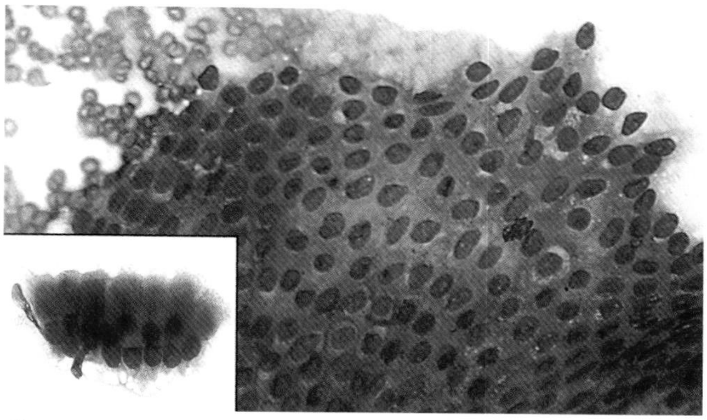

Figure 18-8 Normal gastric epithelium. A large cluster of normal epithelium is present. Cells are uniform and have a honeycombed appearance within the cluster. The inset image is of a smaller cluster in which the columnar appearance of the cells can be appreciated. Cells are uniform with basilar oriented small round nuclei and abundant cytoplasm. (Modified Wright stain.)

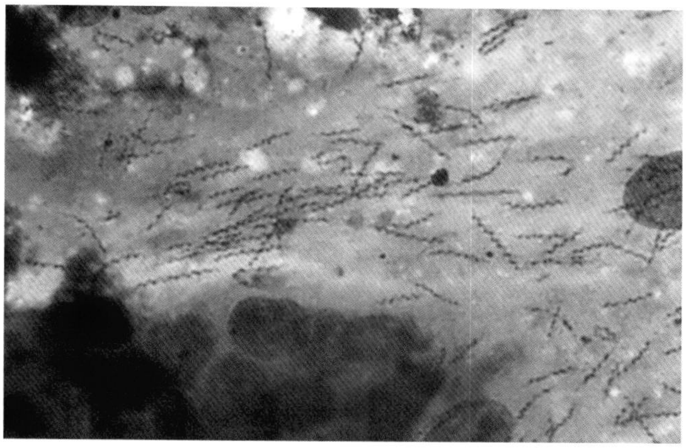

Figure 18-9 Pyloric region of the stomach of a dog; spiral bacteria consistent with *Helicobacter* spp. The S-shaped spiral bacteria are embedded in thick streaming clumps of mucus; note the gastric epithelial cells at the bottom of the image. The significance of this finding is unknown, since *Helicobacter* spp. is commonly found in the stomachs of dogs and cats and may or may not be associated with inflammation. (Wright-Giemsa stain. Original magnification 50× objective.)

regions and consists of the mucosa, muscularis mucosae, submucosa, and smooth muscle wall. The largest portion of the stomach is the fundus, which consists of a surface columnar foveolar epithelium with subjacent glandular cells, including parietal cells and chief cells, which secrete hydrochloric acid and pepsinogen, respectively (Figure 18-7). The pyloric region consists of a similar surface epithelium with predominantly mucous glands in the deeper mucosa (see Figure 18-7).

Normal gastric cytology usually consists of small, to rarely large, sheets of surface epithelium that has a characteristic honeycomb appearance (Figure 18-8). These columnar cells have round to oval basally oriented nuclei with an abundant amount of finely vacuolated cytoplasm.[7] Parietal and chief cells may be seen in gastric cytology samples collected from brushing techniques that access the deeper mucosal tissue (see Figure 18-7). Parietal cells have abundant granular eosinophilic to vacuolated cytoplasm, whereas chief cells have many well-staining basophilic cytoplasmic granules.[7,8] Particularly in the pyloric region, mucus-secreting cells may be identified in cytologic samples (see Figure 18-7).

Helicobacter spp. are spiral bacteria that are commonly identified in samples of the gastric surface of dogs and cats, often in close association with surface mucus (Figure 18-9). The possible clinical significance of finding *Helicobacter* organisms in the stomach is discussed below (see "Gastric Inflammation"). Gastric samples may be easily

BOX 18-3

Causes of Gastritis

- Inflammatory bowel disease
- Mechanical mucosal damage
- Chemical mucosal damage
- Drug administration
  - Nonsteroidal anti-inflammatory drugs (NSAIDs)
  - Corticosteroids
  - Antibiotics
  - Chemotherapeutic agents
- Gastric or gastroduodenal ulcers
- Hyperplastic, hypertrophic, or atrophic conditions
- Infectious etiology
- Neoplasia

From Webb C, Twedt DC: Canine gastritis, *Vet Clin N Am Small Anim Pract* 33:969, 2003.

contaminated by food material, or material from the oral cavity and esophagus, which is indicated by the presence of *Simonsiella* organisms and squamous epithelial cells. Ciliated columnar respiratory epithelium may be noted if the patient swallowed sputum, whereas red blood cells (RBCs) may be identified with traumatic sample collection and blood contamination.

Gastric Inflammation

Gastritis is a nonspecific finding that may occur with a variety of causes (Box 18-3).[15] The majority of gastritis cases in dogs and cats are likely a component of inflammatory bowel disease (IBD), which may have predominantly lymphoplasmacytic, eosinophilic or granulomatous inflammation, although the presence of inflammation is not specific for IBD. Normal endoscopic appearance of the gastric mucosa does not rule out underlying inflammation.

Neutrophilic Inflammation: Neutrophilic inflammation in gastric samples may occur with a variety of lesions but is seen most often with gastric ulcers; for a more complete list of common causes, see Table 18-3. Ulcers in the stomach or proximal small intestine may occur as a result of mechanical or chemical irritation, drug administration, or hormone secretion (i.e., gastrin hypersecretion or histamine release). Ulceration with nonsteroidal anti-inflammatory drug (NSAID) administration is secondary to compromise of mucosal protective mechanisms, whereas with excess exogenous or endogenous corticosteroids, mucosal perfusion is reduced.[9] Uremic gastropathy is not typically an inflammatory lesion histologically but may cause gastric congestion, hemorrhage, and edema, possibly with ulceration, necrosis, and mineralization of the mucosa.[9]

Lymphoplasmacytic Inflammation: Lymphoplasmacytic gastritis is the most common histopathologic finding in abnormal gastric biopsies in dogs and has a variety of causes and disease associations, including IBD, hyperplastic, hypertrophic, or atrophic conditions, and others (Figure 18-10).[16] For a more complete list of potential causes, see Table 18-3.

Several hyperplastic or hypertrophic gastric conditions occur in dogs (see Table 18-3). In addition to a lymphoplasmacytic inflammatory component, these conditions often have a component of mucosal epithelial proliferation, with or without thickening or muscular hypertrophy of the stomach wall; therefore, increased mucosal epithelium may be noted cytologically in these conditions. As a result of their gross or endoscopic appearance as a diffuse or regional masslike thickening of portions of the stomach, these hyperplastic and hypertrophic lesions may be confused with gastric adenocarcinoma (see Table 18-2).[13] For this reason, it is important to consider these benign conditions when increased mucosal epithelium is seen in cytology specimens.

Helicobacter spp. are highly prevalent spiral bacteria found in the stomach of dogs and cats; however, it is controversial whether a causal association exists between the presence of *Helicobacter* and the presence of gastritis in these species (see Figure 18-9 and Table 18-1). In cats, an association seems to exist between *Helicobacter* and lymphoid follicle formation or epithelial proliferation in the stomach, and possible associations have been made between *Helicobacter* infection and gastric mucosal-associated lymphoid tissue (MALT) lymphoma.[17,18] *Helicobacter* may be present in higher numbers and easier to identify in cytologic specimens than in histologic samples because of their presence in the surface mucus, which is readily sampled for cytologic evaluation.

Eosinophilic Inflammation: Eosinophilic inflammation in stomach samples may occur as a component of IBD or with other diseases typically associated with eosinophils (see Table 18-3). Other conditions with a predominance of eosinophils include idiopathic eosinophilic GI masses, scirrhous eosinophilic gastritis, and feline GI eosinophilic sclerosing fibroplasia; an important feature of these diseases is their tendency to form a thickened or masslike region in the stomach, giving the impression of neoplasia (see Table 18-2). The term *idiopathic eosinophilic gastrointestinal masses (IEGM)* refers to a condition in dogs, with a predisposition in Rottweiler dogs, in which one or multiple mass lesions consisting of eosinophilic inflammation are present in the GI tract, with intervening eosinophil-free regions.[19] *Scirrhous eosinophilic gastritis* in dogs is a thickening of the gastric wall with granulation tissue and eosinophils.[13] Feline *gastrointestinal eosinophilic sclerosing fibroplasia* is a masslike lesion, most commonly at the pyloric sphincter but also common at the ileocecocolic junction, and it may also involve the mesenteric lymph nodes. Cytologically, this lesion has either increased eosinophils, alone or in combination with large spindle cells amid pink, extracellular matrix, with neutrophils and intracellular and extracellular rod-shaped or coccoid bacteria with fewer lymphocytes, plasma cells, and mast cells (Figure 18-11).[20]

Granulomatous Inflammation: Granulomatous inflammation in stomach samples may occur as a component of IBD or with infectious etiologies (see Table 18-3). Because of the nature of granulomatous inflammation leading to a thickening of the gastric wall, these lesions may be mistaken for neoplasia grossly or endoscopically (see Table 18-2).

TABLE 18-3

Causes of Gastric Inflammation

Type of Inflammation	Disease Process	Potential Causes
Neutrophilic	Mechanical ulceration Chemical gastritis Gastric or gastrointestinal (GI) ulcers	Gastric foreign body, hairball Ingestion of irritating plants or chemicals Hypersecretion of acid (liver disease, gastrin-secreting tumor) Histamine release (mast cell tumor, medications and hormones) Drug therapy (nonsteroidal anti-inflammatory drugs [NSAIDs], corticosteroids) Sepsis, burns, hypoadrenocorticism, surgery
Lymphoplasmacytic	Inflammatory bowel disease	
	Hyperplastic or hypertrophic conditions	Chronic hypertrophic gastropathy of Drentsche Patrijshond and Basenji dogs Chronic hypertrophic pyloric gastropathy Pyloric stenosis Benign gastric polyps
	Atrophic conditions	Chronic atrophic gastritis of Norwegian Lundehund dogs
	Healing gastric ulcers	
	Helicobacter infection	
	Parasite infestation	*Physaloptera* and *Gnathostoma* in dogs and cats *Ollulanus* and *Cylicospirura* in cats
	Secondary to other conditions	Neoplasia
Eosinophilic	Inflammatory bowel disease	
	Allergy or hypersensitivity disorders	
	Neoplasia	Mast cell tumor, T-cell lymphoma
	Infectious agents	Pythiosis, *Toxocara canis* larval migration
	Miscellaneous	Feline hypereosinophilic syndrome Canine idiopathic eosinophilic gastrointestinal masses Scirrhous eosinophilic gastritis Feline gastrointestinal eosinophilic sclerosing fibroplasia
Granulomatous	Inflammatory bowel disease	
	Infectious etiologies	Mycobacteriosis, histoplasmosis, pythiosis

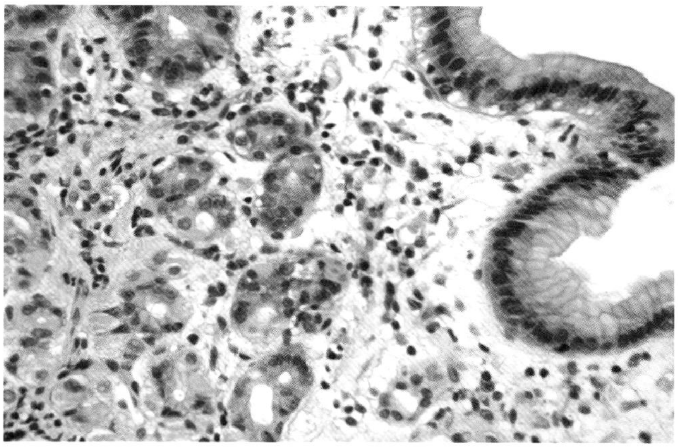

Figure 18-10 Stomach from a dog; lymphoplasmacytic gastritis as a component of inflammatory bowel disease. Within the lamina propria of the superficial gastric mucosa, increased numbers of lymphocytes and plasma cells are seen, with mild edema and increased connective tissue. (H&E stain. Original magnification 40× objective.)

Pythiosis, caused by the aquatic oomycete *Pythium insidiosum*, has been reported to cause GI lesions in dogs and cats and has been reported as a cause of hypercalcemia.[21] Typically, it causes a transmural masslike obstructive or nonobstructive thickening most commonly in the stomach, small intestine, or ileocolic junction; mesenteric lymph nodes are commonly involved. Cytologically, pyogranulomatous inflammation is seen along with eosinophils and nonstaining to poorly staining hyphal structures with fairly parallel walls that are 4 to 8 μm wide with infrequent septation (Figure 18-12). Cytology alone cannot definitively distinguish between *Pythium*, *Lagenidium* (another aquatic oomycete), and zygomycete organisms (fungi); therefore, additional diagnostics such as culture or polymerase chain reaction (PCR) may be required (see Table 18-1). *Candida* spp. are typically opportunistic invaders of the mucosal epithelium in immunocompromised patients. This organism has yeast, pseudohyphal, and true hyphal forms, and finding all three forms together is consistent with *Candida* spp. (Figure 18-13; also see Table 18-1).

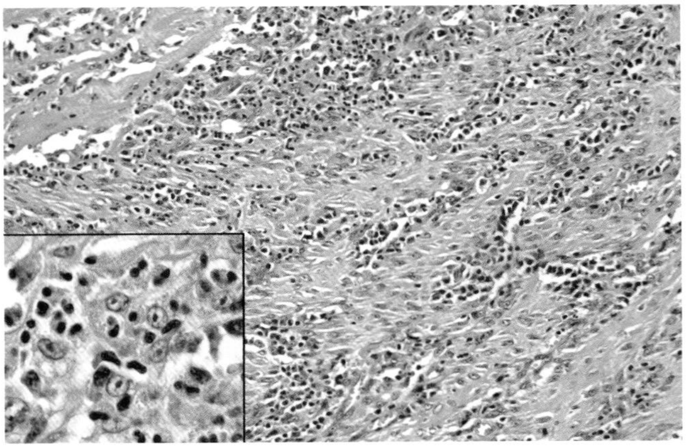

Figure 18-11 Pyloric region of the stomach from a cat; feline gastrointestinal eosinophilic sclerosing fibroplasia. The majority of the masslike lesion is composed of thick anastomosing bands of dense collagenous or fibrous stroma, with plump proliferating fibroblasts and intervening aggregates of numerous eosinophils. The inset is a closer view of the inflammatory cells and fibroblasts with predominantly eosinophils and fewer macrophages, lymphocytes, and plasma cells. (H&E stain. Original magnification 20× objective. *Inset:* H&E stain. Original magnification 100× objective.) (Case from Joint Pathology Center Veterinary Pathology Services: Wednesday Slide Conference 2011-12, Conference 15 Case 1.)

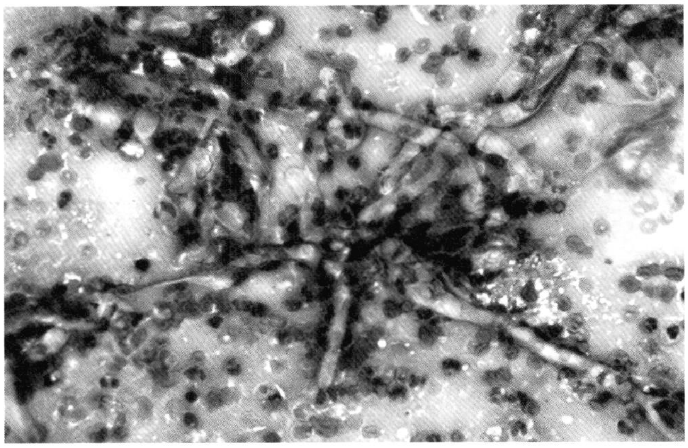

Figure 18-12 Tissue from a dog; pythiosis. A mat of wide, poorly staining hyphal structures with parallel walls and infrequent septation is present on a background of suppurative inflammation and blood. Cytologic appearance alone cannot be used to definitively distinguish between *Pythium*, *Lagenidium*, and zygomycete organisms (true fungi). In this case, culture of the lesion and immunohistochemistry performed on biopsy samples using anti–*P. insidiosum* specific antibodies confirmed infection with *P. insidiosum*. (Modified Wright stain. Original magnification 40× objective.) (American Society of Veterinary Clinical Pathology: Mystery Slide Conference, 1998 Case 10, submitted by Casey LeBlanc.)

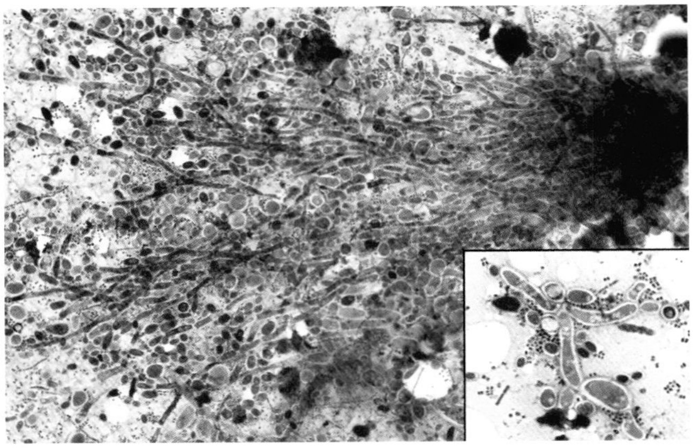

Figure 18-13 Gastric tube plaque from a dog; fungal and bacterial colonization and overgrowth. A large fungal plaque consisting of round yeast and long, slender, septated hyphae is present. The inset image consists of round to elongated chaining yeast (pseudohyphae) on a background of cocci and rod-shaped bacteria. Finding yeast, hyphae, and pseudohyphae together is consistent with *Candida* spp. In this case, the lack of inflammation and location of the plaque within the lumen of the gastric tube were consistent with colonization and overgrowth rather than a true infection. (Wright-Giemsa stain. Original magnification 10× objective. *Inset:* Wright-Giemsa stain. Original magnification 50× objective.).

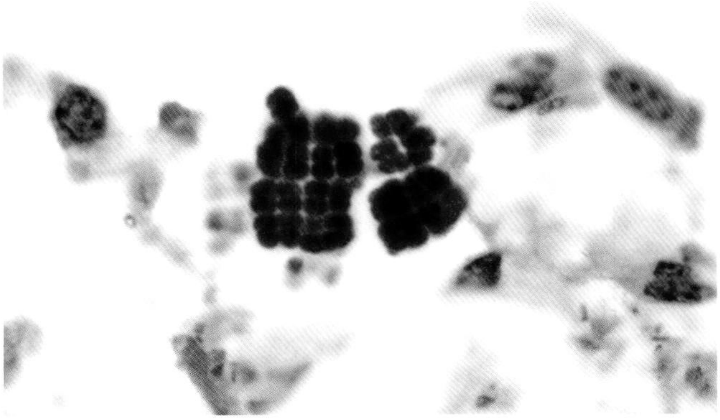

Figure 18-14 Gastric lumen. The organisms present are consistent with *Sarcina* spp. and are very large cocci arranged in characteristic packets and bundles. These organisms have been associated with abomasal bloat in calves and lambs and with gastric dilatation in dogs. (H&E stain. Original magnification 100× objective.) (Slide courtesy of Kara Corps.)

Although it is not known to cause significant inflammation, *Sarcina ventriculi*, a large Gram-positive coccoid bacterium, has been associated with abomasal bloat in small ruminants and calves and may be associated with acute gastric dilatation in dogs.[22] This organism has a characteristic appearance with formation of packets and bundles of very large cocci and is not a component of the normal gastric bacterial flora in dogs (Figure 18-14).

Gastric Neoplasia

Gastric tumors are uncommon in dogs and cats and include epithelial, mesenchymal, and round cell tumors (Table 18-4). In dogs, gastric carcinoma is most common, whereas in cats, lymphoma is most common.[23] On endoscopic examination, gastric neoplasia may appear as a mass, a polypoid lesion, an area of ulceration, or a regional or diffuse infiltrative process. The infiltrative endoscopic appearance or the presence of a stenotic lesion in the

TABLE 18-4

Types of Gastric or Intestinal Neoplasia

Category of Neoplasm	Most Common Neoplasms
Epithelial	Adenoma, adenocarcinoma, neuroendocrine carcinoma (carcinoid)
Mesenchymal	Leiomyoma, leiomyosarcoma, gastrointestinal stromal tumors
Round cell	Lymphoma, mast cell tumor, plasma cell tumor

pylorus with gastric neoplasia may be difficult to differentiate from hyperplastic or hypertrophic or eosinophilic gastric lesions (see Table 18-2). Neoplasia in the stomach may also be secondary to extension of neoplasia from an adjacent organ, metastasis from a distant site, or gastric involvement in carcinomatosis.

Epithelial Neoplasia: Epithelial proliferations include both benign and malignant lesions. In dogs, malignant epithelial tumors occur more commonly.[13] Gastric polyps (a nonneoplastic benign lesion) and adenomas typically are solitary lesions, most commonly arising from the pylorus, and it may be difficult to distinguish one from the other histologically.[13] Gastric adenocarcinomas are most common in the pylorus and may present as a plaque-like ulcerated thickening, diffuse nonulcerating thickening, or a raised polypoid mass and often have annular thickening and stenosis of the pyloric lumen caused by a scirrhous or fibrous response with contraction of the tissue. The neoplastic cells are typical of an adenocarcinoma with tubular or papillary structures; but they may be mucinous with abundant production of extracellular mucin or have a "signet ring" morphology, with intracellular mucin accumulation that displaces the nucleus to the periphery of the cell.[14] Gastric adenocarcinomas most commonly metastasize to the regional lymph nodes but also readily seed the abdomen with subsequent carcinomatosis and less often metastasize to the lungs.

Neuroendocrine carcinoma (carcinoid) of the stomach is rare and has a typical neuroendocrine cytologic appearance (Figure 18-15). In the rare chronic atrophic gastritis of Norwegian Lundehund dogs, the mild chronic inflammation with fundic gland atrophy may be associated with subsequent development of gastric neuroendocrine carcinoma (carcinoid).[24]

Mesenchymal Neoplasia: Mesenchymal neoplasia in the stomach primarily includes smooth muscle tumors and gastrointestinal stromal tumors (GISTs). These tumors have been associated with paraneoplastic hypoglycemia caused by tumor production of insulin-like growth factor II (IGF-II), or paraneoplastic erythrocytosis caused by tumor production of erythropoietin.[9] Leiomyomas and leiomyosarcomas arise from the smooth muscle wall of the stomach. In dogs, leiomyomas are more common, occur most typically in the outer muscle coat of the gastroesophageal region in older animals, and may

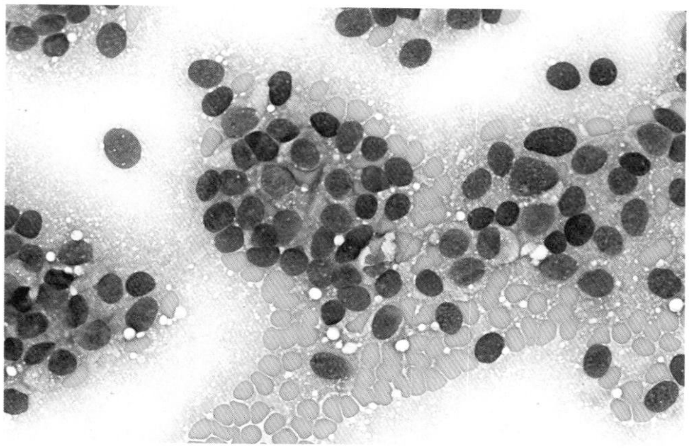

Figure 18-15 Touch imprints of the ileocecocecal junction at the serosal surface from a dog; gastrinoma. The population has a neuroendocrine appearance characterized by relatively uniform cell size, loosely cohesive clusters with many naked nuclei, pale, delicate, and mildly vacuolated cytoplasm, and round nuclei with finely stippled chromatin. These features are seen in many different neuroendocrine tumors; a diagnosis of gastrinoma in this case was supported by positive immunohistochemical staining for gastrin on the surgical biopsy specimen. (Modified Wright-Giemsa stain. Original magnification 50× objective.) (American Society of Veterinary Clinical Pathology: Mystery Slide Conference, 2011 Case 10, submitted by Sarah Colledge.)

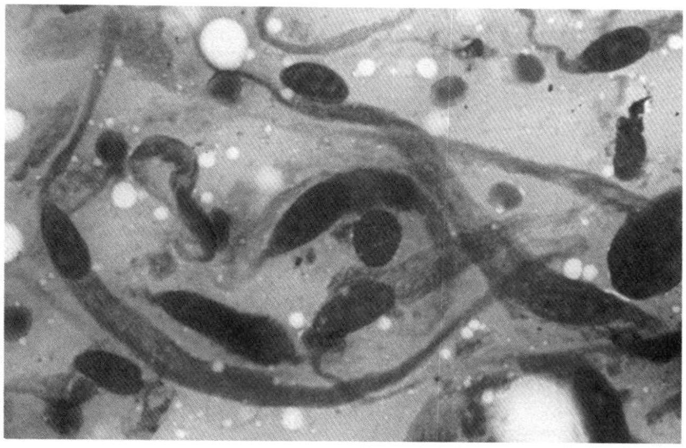

Figure 18-16 Gastric leiomyosarcoma in a dog. Spindle cells are elongated with extensive thin cytoplasmic projections and oval to flattened nuclei. The cytologic appearance is diagnostic for a spindle cell neoplasm; a definitive diagnosis of leiomyosarcoma was made with histopathology and immunohistochemistry in this case. (Wright stain.)

be single or multiple.[13] Leiomyosarcomas are typically single, larger symptomatic tumors and tend to be more pleomorphic compared with leiomyomas. These tumors are characterized by plump spindle cells with elongated, blunted, cigar-shaped nuclei (Figure 18-16). GISTs may have a similar morphology but often have a more haphazard arrangement with a looser, pale pink stroma histologically (Figure 18-17). Although leiomyosarcomas and GISTs may have slightly different features, significant overlap exists, so definitive differentiation requires immunohistochemistry (Table 18-5).[25] Metastasis of these malignant mesenchymal tumors is slow and occurs only

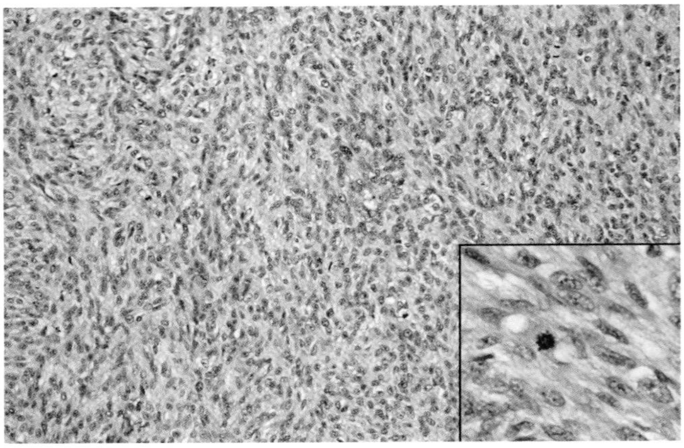

Figure 18-17 Gastrointestinal stromal tumor (GIST) in a dog. The neoplastic cells are arranged in haphazard interwoven fascicles in the middle of a loose, pale eosinophilic stroma. Cells are spindle shaped, with eosinophilic fibrillar cytoplasm and an oval nucleus with clumped chromatin and one to three prominent nucleoli. Pleomorphism is mild in this population, with occasional mitotic figures (*inset*). Immunohistochemistry was positive for c-kit, which is diagnostic for a GIST. (H&E stain. Original magnification 20× objective. *Inset:* H&E stain. Original magnification 100× objective.)

TABLE 18-5

Differentiating Leiomyosarcomas and Gastrointestinal Stromal Tumors

	Leiomyosarcoma	Gastrointestinal Stromal Tumors
Origin	Smooth muscle cells	Interstitial cells of Cajal (pacemaker cells of the GI tract)
Immunohistochemistry	C-kit negative, smooth muscle actin positive, +/- desmin positive	C-kit positive, +/– smooth muscle actin positive, desmin negative
Most common locations	Stomach (pylorus), small intestine	Large intestine

Russell KN, Mehler SJ, Skorupski KA, et al: Clinical and immunohistochemical differentiation of gastrointestinal stromal tumors from leiomyosarcomas in dogs: 42 cases (1990-2003), *J Am Vet Med Assoc* 230:1329, 2007.

late in the disease, with lymph node and liver as potential sites of spread.

Round Cell Neoplasia: Round cell neoplasia in the stomach includes gastric lymphoma, mast cell tumor, and, rarely, plasma cell tumor. Gastric lymphoma may present as a diffuse infiltrative process or as one to multiple transmural plaques or nodules and may be primary or a component of alimentary or multicentric lymphoma (Figure 18-18). In cats, gastric lymphoma is usually B-lymphocyte in origin.[26] Mast cell tumor is more common in the stomach than in other parts of the GI tract, and arises from mucosal mast cells, which is distinct from cutaneous mast cell tumors that arise from connective tissue mast cells (see "Intestinal Neoplasia" for further discussion). A rare variant of mast cell tumor in cats, known as *feline sclerosing mast cell tumor*, may occur in the stomach but is more often reported in the intestine (see "Intestinal Neoplasia").

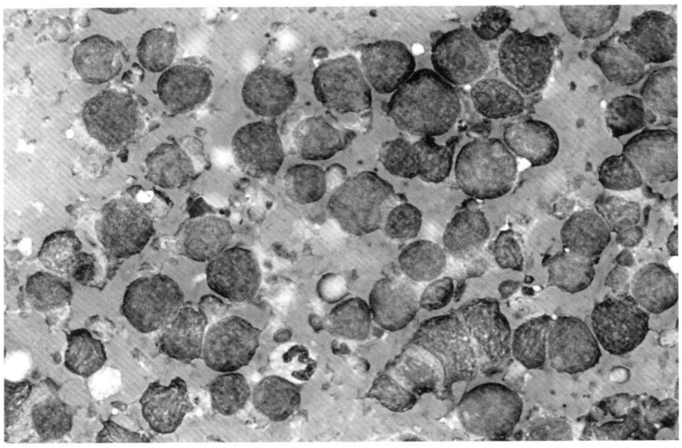

Figure 18-18 Stomach of a dog; lymphoma. Classic appearance of lymphoma. Cells are primarily large with open, dispersed chromatin, variably prominent nucleoli and have a thin rim of basophilic cytoplasm. Scattered lymphoglandular bodies are also present. (Wright-Giemsa stain. Original magnification 50× objective.)

SMALL AND LARGE INTESTINES

Normal Intestine

The intestinal tract consists of a mucosal epithelium with muscularis mucosae, submucosa and smooth muscle wall. Unremarkable small intestinal (duodenum, jejunum, and ileum) and large intestinal (cecum, colon, and rectum) mucosa consists of simple columnar epithelium with variable numbers of goblet cells, whereas unremarkable anal mucosa consists of squamous epithelial cells. The small intestine has villi projecting from the mucosal surface, whereas the large intestine lacks villi and has more numerous goblet cells (Figure 18-19).[6] Lymphoid nodules called Peyer patches are present in the submucosa throughout the intestinal tract, especially in the ileum.

The cytologic appearance of the small intestinal epithelial cells consists of honeycomb-like sheets of tall columnar cells, with basally located nuclei and a distinct striated microvillous border, or terminal bar, at the apical surface (absorptive enterocytes) and lesser numbers of goblet cells (mucus-secreting cells), which often appear as large pale or vacuolated cells (Figure 18-20).[7] Cytology of a Peyer patch, if sampled, will consist of a mixed lymphoid population, which includes small, intermediate, and large lymphocytes along with rare plasma cells. Given how large Peyer patches may be, even in health, this is an important consideration with intestinal aspirates yielding a lymphoid-predominant cell population (Figure 18-21).

The epithelium of the large intestine is similar to that of the small intestine with a honeycomb pattern of tall columnar glandular epithelial cells, with higher numbers of goblet cells compared with the small intestine. At any level of the intestinal tract, fine-needle aspirates of the intestines may contain rare spindle-shaped cells that may

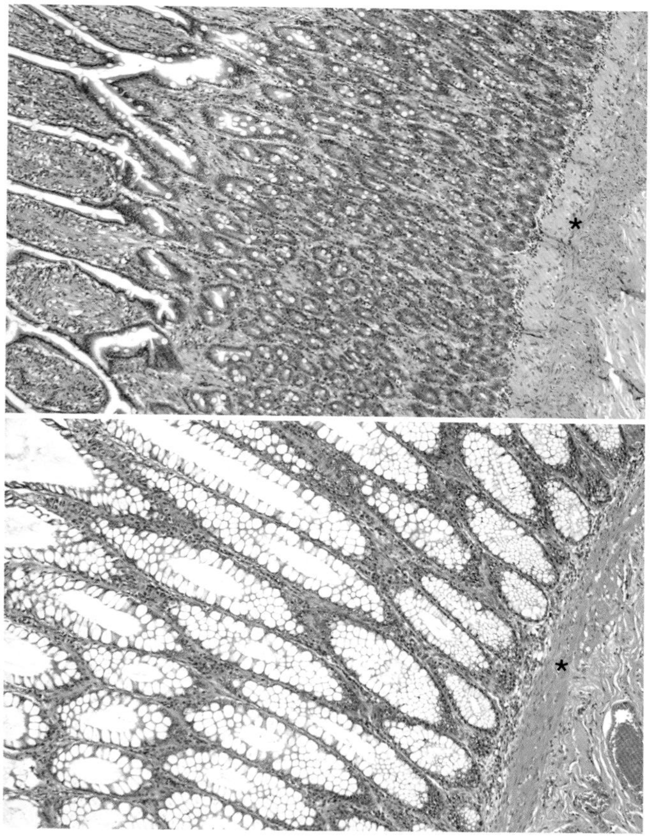

Figure 18-19 Small intestine (*top*) and large intestine (*bottom*) from a dog. The small intestinal mucosa (*top image*) has surface villi lined by absorptive enterocytes with few mucin-containing pale-gray goblet cells and has numerous tightly packed crypts in the deeper mucosa. The large intestinal mucosa (*bottom image*) lacks villi and has numerous tightly packed crypts containing more numerous goblet cells than in the small intestine. Both the small and large intestines have a muscularis mucosae composed of smooth muscle (*), which separates the mucosa from the submucosa. (H&E stain. Original magnification 20× objective.)

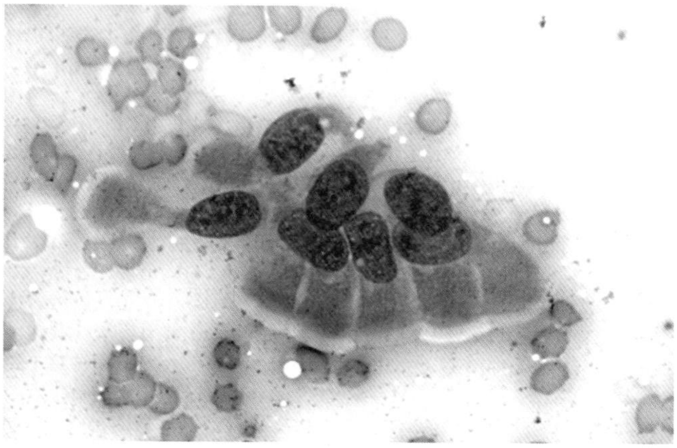

Figure 18-20 Intestinal aspirate from a cat. Uniform enterocytes characterized by a columnar shape, round basilar oriented nuclei, basophilic cytoplasm and a microvillus brush border (*terminal bar*) are present. (Wright-Giemsa stain. Original magnification 100× objective.) (Slide courtesy of Jaime Tarigo.)

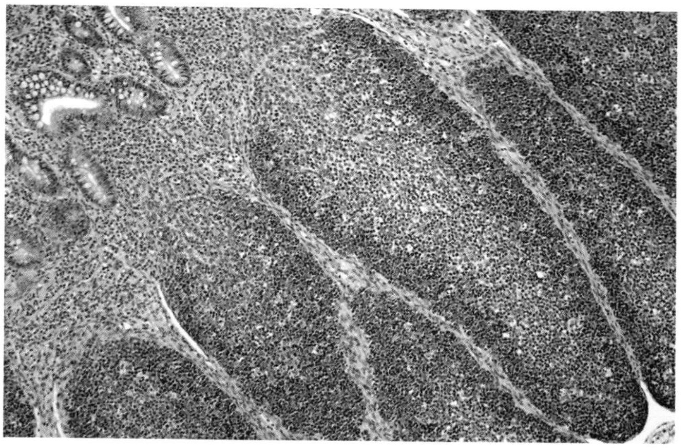

Figure 18-21 Ileum with Peyer patches in a young animal. The Peyer patches within the submucosa are very large and have prominent germinal centers, which are lighter-staining than the peripheral rim of smaller lymphocytes. It is feasible that on aspiration of the intestinal wall in this region, a robust lymphoid population would be identified. If the majority of the cells aspirated are from the germinal center, the presence of large lymphocytes could be confused with a diagnosis of lymphoid neoplasia. (H&E stain. Original magnification 10× objective.) (Slide courtesy of Jody Gookin.)

represent submucosal fibrocytes or smooth muscle cells from the muscularis layers.[7] Magenta-staining gel or lubricant products may be seen as a contaminant in intestinal samples, depending on method of sample collection (e.g., ultrasound-guided, rectal scraping) (see Figure 18-1).

Intestinal Inflammation

Enteritis, colitis, or enterocolitis may be idiopathic, immune mediated, or caused by infectious etiologies or neoplasia. Types of inflammation may include lymphoplasmacytic, neutrophilic, eosinophilic, or granulomatous inflammation, and the nature of the inflammation depends on the underlying etiology; for more specific details on causes for each type of inflammation, see Table 18-6.

Lymphoplasmacytic Inflammation: IBD is a common cause of enterocolitis in dogs and cats; it is often referred to as *inflammatory bowel disease* when it occurs in the small intestine and as *idiopathic mucosal colitis* when it affects the colon. The inflammation is most commonly lymphoplasmacytic, but eosinophilic and macrophage-predominant or granulomatous forms also occur (Figure 18-22). IBD is thought to be caused by dysregulation of mucosal immunity in predisposed animals with loss of tolerance to certain antigens; therefore, an immune-mediated component to the pathogenesis is likely.[27] The World Small Animal Veterinary Association (WSAVA) has published guidelines for the standardization of GI inflammation on histologic examination of biopsy specimens to help pathologists better categorize the severity and type of inflammatory disease.[28] Cytologic evidence of inflammation is a typical finding with IBD but is not specific for this disease process.

A rare cause of lymphocytic inflammation deep within the muscular wall of the intestinal tract is an entity known as *chronic intestinal pseudo-obstruction (CIPO)*, which is

TABLE 18-6

Causes of Intestinal Inflammation

Type of Inflammation	Disease Process	Specific Causes
Lymphoplasmacytic	Inflammatory bowel disease (IBD)	
	Chronic intestinal pseudo-obstruction (CIPO)	
Neutrophilic	IBD	
	Infectious agents	Bacterial (*Escherichia coli*, *Salmonella* spp., *Clostridium* spp.)
		Parasitic (typhlocolitis in dogs with *Trichuris vulpis* infection)
	Secondary	Erosions or ulcers of any cause
	Necrotizing colitis	Glucocorticoid administration, hyperadrenocorticism, spinal trauma, uremia
Eosinophilic	IBD	
	Allergic disease	Food allergies, gluten sensitivity
	Neoplasia	Mast cell tumor, T-cell lymphoma
	Infectious	Pythiosis, parasitism, *Toxocara canis* migration
	Miscellaneous	Feline hypereosinophilic syndrome, canine idiopathic eosinophilic gastrointestinal masses, feline gastrointestinal eosinophilic sclerosing fibroplasia
Granulomatous	Infectious	Histoplasmosis, cryptococcosis, protothecosis, schistosomiasis (*Heterobilharzia*), amoebiasis, feline infectious peritonitis (FIP), salmon poisoning disease in dogs, histiocytic ulcerative colitis of Boxers, pythiosis, mycobacteriosis, leishmaniasis, or mycotic infection
	Noninfectious	Intestinal lymphangiectasia with transmural lipogranulomatous lymphangitis

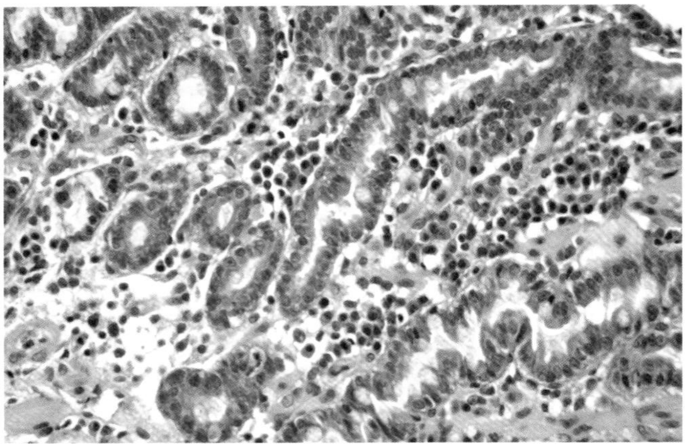

Figure 18-22 Small intestine from a dog; inflammatory bowel disease characterized by lymphoplasmacytic enteritis. The intestinal crypts are mildly separated by an increased amount of connective tissue and moderate numbers of lymphocytes and plasma cells, with a predominance of plasma cells. (H&E stain. Original magnification 40× objective.)

an immune-mediated lymphocytic intestinal leiomyositis (inflammation of the smooth muscle wall).[29] This lesion does not affect the mucosa but leads to a decrease in motility with marked dilation of the intestinal loops, which mimics an obstructive lesion.

Neutrophilic Inflammation: Although neutrophil transmigration into the GI lumen is the main route of neutrophil elimination from the body, finding numerous neutrophils in cytologic specimens from the intestine is abnormal. Similarly, on histologic examination, the presence of neutrophils in the intestinal mucosa is never considered a normal finding. Since neutrophilic inflammation in the intestines has various causes, finding a component of neutrophilic inflammation is a relatively nonspecific finding (see Table 18-6). If neutrophilic inflammation is identified as a component of IBD, it is likely secondary to epithelial damage (erosions or ulcers), whereas a primary neutrophilic inflammatory lesion is more likely with bacterial infection or other etiologic agents.

Eosinophilic Inflammation: Eosinophilic enterocolitis may occur as a component of IBD or may be associated with other causes (see Table 18-6). In hypereosinophilic syndrome in cats, the associated eosinophilic enteritis, if present, predominantly involves the small intestine and is accompanied by marked smooth muscle hypertrophy of the intestinal wall, which greatly expands the wall thickness. The eosinophilic infiltrate may also involve the mesenteric lymph nodes in these cases.[9] Canine idiopathic eosinophilic GI masses and feline GI eosinophilic sclerosing fibroplasia do occur in the intestine but are discussed elsewhere (see "Gastric Inflammation").

Granulomatous Inflammation: Granulomatous enteritis, colitis, or both are typically associated with a variety of infectious and some noninfectious diseases (see Table

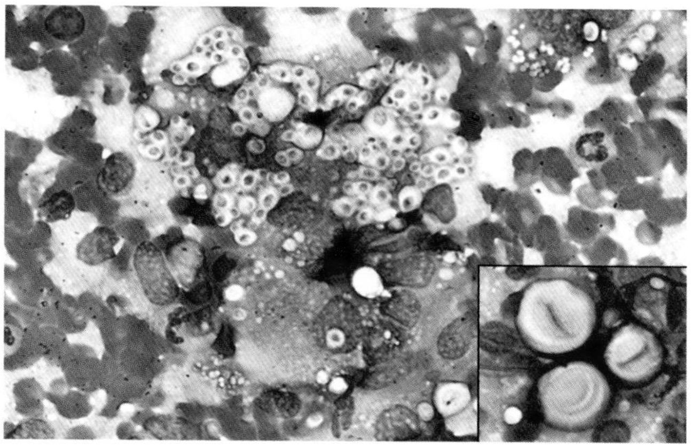

Figure 18-23 Intestinal aspirate from a dog; *Cryptococcus neoformans* infection. A cluster of epithelioid macrophages and few neutrophils are present, along with many small extracellular yeast organisms characterized by a pale interior and a variably wide nonstaining capsule. Because of the small size of the organisms and somewhat petite capsule, they could be confused with other fungal agents such as *Histoplasma capsulatum* or the yeast form of *Candida*. The inset is of organisms from a different region of the sample characterized by larger size and a distinctive fold in the cell wall giving the cell a partially deflated kick-ball or folded contact lens appearance. (Wright-Giemsa stain. Original magnification 50× objective. *Inset:* Wright-Giemsa stain. Original magnification 50× objective.)

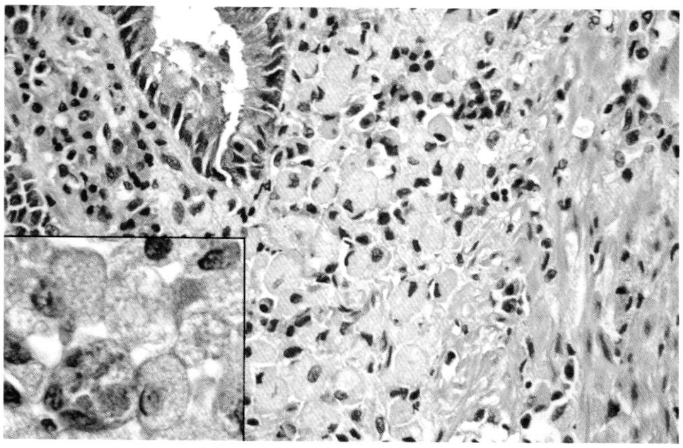

Figure 18-24 Colon from a Boxer; histiocytic ulcerative colitis. A dense infiltrate of foamy macrophages separates and elevates the colonic crypts. The macrophages contain granular eosinophilic to basophilic cytoplasmic material, which is suggested to be phagocytized membranous or cellular debris and stains positive with periodic acid-Schiff (PAS; *not pictured*). This condition is thought to be associated with, and is likely caused by, bacterial infection with *Escherichia coli*. (H&E stain. Original magnification 40× objective. *Inset*: H&E stain. Original magnification 100×.) (Case from Joint Pathology Center Veterinary Pathology Services (formerly AFIP): Wednesday Slide Conference 2010-11, Conference 7 Case 1.)

18-6). Many granulomatous intestinal diseases cause segmental thickening of the intestinal wall and may cause a masslike lesion, which may be radiographically or ultrasonographically confused with neoplasia (see Table 18-2).

Histoplasma capsulatum, a fungal organism, causes segmental transmural granulomatous inflammation in the stomach, small intestine, or large intestine (see Table 18-1). Infection with *Prototheca zopfii* or *P. wickerhamii* causes a hemorrhagic and ulcerative colitis with a mild lymphohistiocytic inflammatory response relative to the marked numbers of algal organisms present (see Table 18-1). Canine schistosomiasis, caused by the trematode *Heterobilharzia americana*, causes granulomatous enteritis in response to the transmigration of eggs across the intestinal wall. The adult trematodes live in the mesenteric vessels, release their eggs into the mucosal venules, and the eggs migrate to the intestinal lumen to pass in the feces. An association may exist between this infection and hypercalcemia (see Table 18-1).[30] *Entamoeba histolytica*, an amoeba, causes an ulcerative and granulomatous colitis with numerous trophozoites and cyst forms (see Table 18-1). Although rare in the intestinal tract, *Cryptococcus neoformans* infection may be associated with granulomatous enterocolitis (Figure 18-23; see Table 18-1).

Feline infectious peritonitis (FIP) may present as a regional granulomatous colitis and may also involve the colic lymph node. This presentation of FIP may be isolated to the colon and associated lymph node and may not be accompanied by more widespread FIP lesions. Salmon poisoning disease, caused by the rickettsial organism *Neorickettsia helminthoeca* transmitted to dogs by the trematode *Nanophyetus salmincola*, is associated with granulomatous enteritis resulting from the presence of the fluke and intralesional intrahistiocytic rickettsial organisms. The more damaging lesion associated with salmon poisoning disease occurs in lymphoid tissues.

Histiocytic ulcerative colitis (or *granulomatous colitis*) of Boxers is characterized by transmural thickening of the colon with mucosal and submucosal dense infiltrates of macrophages, which contain numerous periodic acid-Schiff (PAS)–positive granules in the cytoplasm (Figure 18-24). The inflammatory lesion may also affect the mesenteric lymph nodes. Originally thought to be an idiopathic or immune-mediated disease, it is now associated with, and likely caused by, bacterial infection with an adherent and invasive *Escherichia coli* organism.[31] The PAS-positive material in macrophages may consist of broken-down cell membranes and bacterial organisms.

Pythiosis (discussed in more detail earlier in "Gastric Inflammation") causes segmental transmural granulomatous inflammation (see Figure 18-12). Mycobacterial infection and leishmaniasis are uncommon causes of intestinal granulomatous inflammation and more commonly cause disease elsewhere in the body. An occasional cause of granulomatous colitis is a fungal infection such as with *Aspergillus*, *Candida*, or zygomycete organisms. Often, they represent a secondary infection from immunocompromise or other primary GI disease, as may occur with panleukopenia virus infection in cats.[9]

Other Inflammatory or Noninflammatory Conditions:

Other infectious agents associated with inflammation in the intestine include *Clostridium piliforme* colitis in cats, in which surface colonic epithelial cells contain multiple, fine, linear, rod-shaped bacteria in the cytoplasm, *Anaerobiospirillum* in cats, in which numerous spiral bacteria are associated with ileocolitis, and *Tritrichomonas foetus* in cats, which has many luminal organisms within colonic crypts and associated inflammation and is of the highest prevalence in cattery-housed cats (Table 18-1).[9,32]

Several infectious agents in dogs and cats are associated with diarrhea, although they do not always cause marked histologic inflammatory lesions. They include whipworms in the large intestine (*Trichuris vulpis* in dogs) and small intestinal protozoal infections (giardiasis, cryptosporidiosis, and coccidiosis caused by *Cystisospora* spp. in dogs and cats) (see Table 18-1). Infection with other nematodes in the small intestine may be associated with disease or ill-thrift, particularly in younger animals, including roundworms (*Toxocara canis* in dogs, *Toxocara cati* in cats, *Toxascaris leonina* in dogs and cats) and hookworms (*Ancylostoma caninum* in dogs, *Ancylostoma tubaeformae* in cats). *Toxoplasma gondii* is a protozoal organism with cats serving as the definitive host, so various stages of developing organisms may be found in the small intestine of cats.

Intestinal Neoplasia

Intestinal tumors in dogs and cats include epithelial, mesenchymal, and round cell tumors (see Table 18-4). In dogs, intestinal neoplasia is more often malignant than benign and is more likely of epithelial than nonepithelial origin; intestinal adenocarcinoma is the most common tumor. In cats, lymphoma is most common, and adenocarcinoma is second most common. In cats that do have epithelial neoplasia, malignant tumors are far more common than are benign lesions.[14] Besides primary neoplasia arising from the intestine, the intestine may be involved in secondary neoplasia caused by extension from an adjacent tissue, including the pancreas, urinary bladder, biliary system, or stomach, as part of carcinomatosis, which predominantly affects the serosal tissue, or with metastatic disease as a part of widespread metastasis from a distant site.

Epithelial Neoplasia: Epithelial proliferations in the intestine include hyperplastic or adenomatous polyps, adenomas, adenocarcinomas, and neuroendocrine carcinomas or carcinoids. Controversy exists in the literature with regard to the criteria for diagnosing a nonneoplastic polyp versus a benign epithelial neoplasm. Polypoid lesions in the intestine occur most commonly in the rectum, with most sources referring to the rectal lesions as *rectal papillary adenomas*. These tumors, which protrude into the rectal lumen, are composed of proliferative columnar epithelial cells. The cellular morphology may be somewhat pleomorphic; therefore, the tissue architecture on histopathology is required to differentiate an adenocarcinoma from a papillary adenoma (Figure 18-25 and Figure 18-26).[9,14] An adenocarcinoma is diagnosed if evidence of tissue invasion deeper into the rectal wall or into lymphatic vessels is present. Given the degree of pleomorphism that may be identified in the papillary adenoma, cytologic distinction between this benign lesion and an adenocarcinoma should be made with caution,

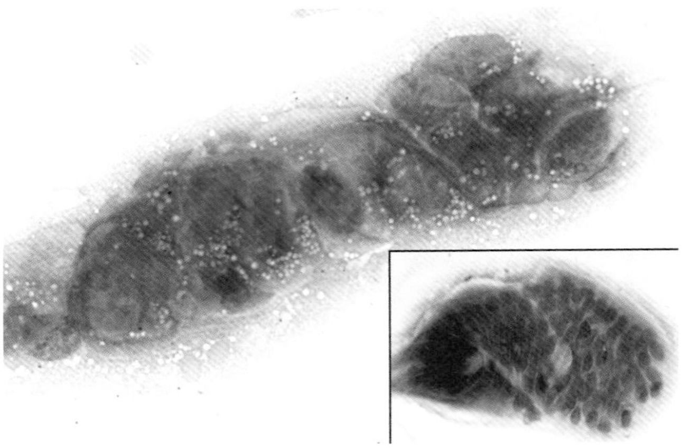

Figure 18-25 Aspirate from a polypoid rectal mass in a dog. The sample contained regions of moderately pleomorphic epithelial cells, characterized by anisocytosis, anisokaryosis, a jumbled and crowded appearance to the cell clusters, large nuclei, visible nucleoli and fine cytoplasmic vacuolization. Although these findings may suggest a malignant process, much of the sample consisted of uniform epithelial cells (*inset*). Caution should be exercised when evaluating apparent cytologic criteria of malignancy in polypoid rectal masses as papillary adenomas may have regions of moderate pleomorphism. In this case, histopathology showed that the vast majority of the tumor was well differentiated, with only one region of possible invasion into the rectal wall. (Wright-Giemsa stain. Original magnification 50× objective. *Inset:* Wright-Giemsa stain. Original magnification 50× objective.)

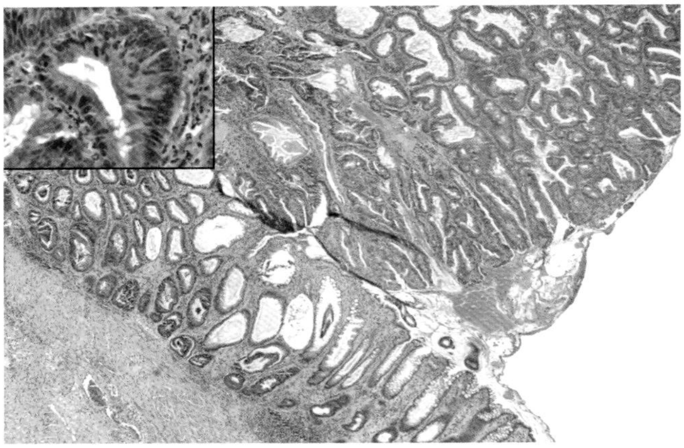

Figure 18-26 Rectum from a dog; rectal papillary adenoma. A polypoid mass arising from the rectal mucosa projects into the rectal lumen. The neoplastic cells are arranged in papilliferous projections and form tubules supported by a fibrovascular stroma. Cells are columnar with a basally located nucleus and eosinophilic cytoplasm. As identified in the inset, frequent piling of cells on one another occurs, with occasional mitotic figures. A diagnosis of a malignant neoplasm requires evidence of invasion of the neoplastic cells into the underlying submucosal tissue, which is not evident in this case despite the atypical morphologic features of the individual cells. For this reason, diagnosis of malignancy based on cytologic or individual cell features is not advised; histopathology with evaluation for submucosal invasion is required for more definitive diagnosis. (H&E stain. Original magnification 4× objective. *Inset:* H&E stain. Original magnification 40× objective.)

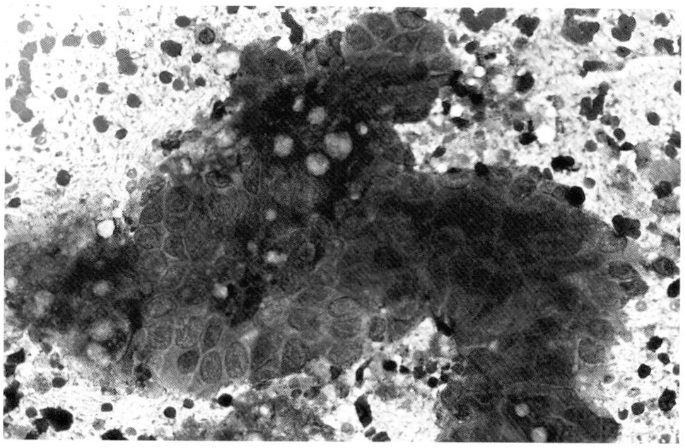

Figure 18-27 Jejunal aspirate from a cat; adenocarcinoma. A large cluster of carcinoma cells is present on a background of necrosis and cellular debris. Cells have features typical of a carcinoma with moderate pleomorphism. Note the clear vacuoles present in the cluster suggesting there may be mucin formation by the tumor cells. (Wright-Giemsa stain. Original magnification 50× objective.) (Slide courtesy of Jamie Tarigo.)

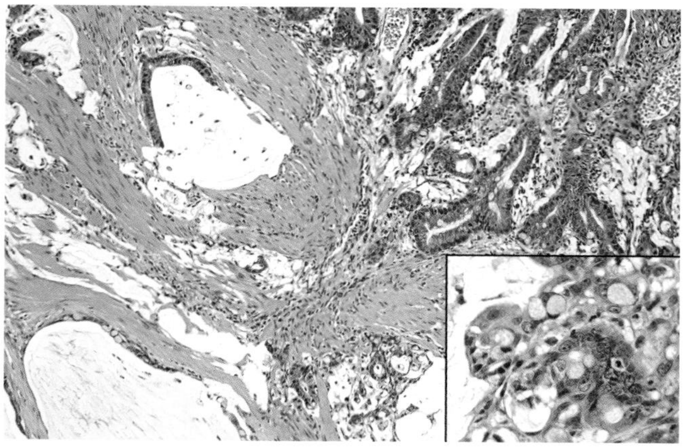

Figure 18-28 Small intestine from a dog; mucinous intestinal adenocarcinoma. The neoplastic epithelial cells form tubular and acinar structures within the mucosa and extend into the submucosal and muscularis layers of the intestinal wall. Large lakes of mucinous material accumulate within portions of the neoplasm, as depicted on the left side of the image. Individual neoplastic cells occasionally have a signet ring morphology with an intracytoplasmic accumulation of mucin material that peripheralizes the nucleus (*inset*). (H&E stain. Original magnification 10× objective. *Inset:* H&E stain. Original magnification 40× objective.) (Case from Joint Pathology Center Veterinary Pathology Services (formerly AFIP): Wednesday Slide Conference 2009-10, Conference 21 Case 2.)

and histopathology should be recommended for more definitive diagnosis.

Adenocarcinomas in the GI tract in dogs are more common in the stomach, whereas these are more common in the intestine in cats (Figure 18-27).[9] Grossly, intestinal adenocarcinomas may be intramural or intraluminal and may be plaquelike, ulcerated, or masslike. The intramural tumors are often annular or circumferential leading to stenosis as a result of the scirrhous response to the tumor. Because of the extensive mural involvement in some cases, sampling of the mucosal or surface component alone may miss the lesion, whether by endoscopic cytology or biopsy technique. Subtypes of adenocarcinoma are similar to the gastric carcinomas and may have acinar, tubular, or papillary structures, a mucinous variant with abundant production of extracellular mucin, or signet-ring morphology with intracellular mucin accumulation that displaces the nucleus to the periphery of the cell (Figure 18-28). Rare cases have adenosquamous morphology with both glandular and squamous differentiation. Cases with extensive desmoplasia may have a component of mesenchymal cells identified cytologically, which should not be mistaken for mesenchymal neoplasia (Figure 18-29 and Figure 18-30). Occasionally, in cats, intestinal adenocarcinomas have osseous or chondroid metaplasia within the stromal component of the tumor.[9] Metastasis occurs typically to the mesenteric lymph nodes or by seeding of the abdomen with carcinomatosis.

Neuroendocrine carcinomas (carcinoids) arise from enteroendocrine cells throughout the intestinal mucosa and have a typical neuroendocrine appearance cytologically (see Figure 18-15). These tumors are rare and are typically malignant and aggressive in their behavior with metastasis to the liver, which is the most common site of spread.[14]

Mesenchymal neoplasia: Mesenchymal neoplasia in the intestinal tract includes the more common leiomyoma, leiomyosarcoma, and GIST, with rare reports of other

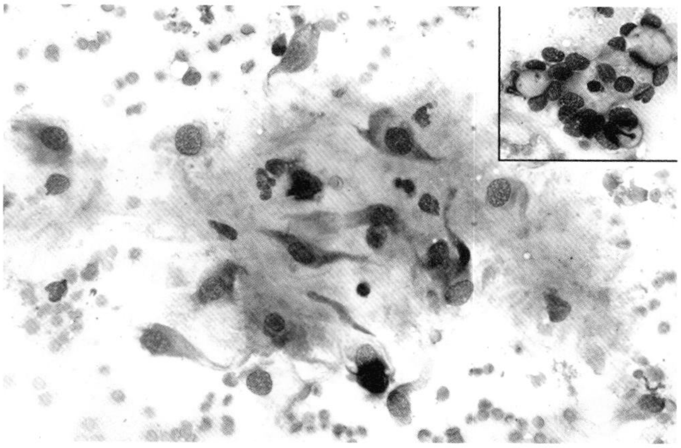

Figure 18-29 Abdominal mass aspirate from a dog; intestinal adenocarcinoma with a scirrhous response. Many immature mesenchymal cells are admixed with bright-pink, fibrillar, extracellular matrix material. Although the cells do not have strong nuclear criteria of malignancy, the presence of primarily immature mesenchymal cells could lead to an erroneous diagnosis of sarcoma; thus, it is important to keep nonneoplastic causes of mesenchymal cell proliferation in mind, especially when cells lack overt features of malignancy. The inset image is of one of the rare clusters of adenocarcinoma cells that were present in this sample. In this particular case, the cells have a prominent signet ring appearance. (Wright-Giemsa stain. Original magnification 40× objective. *Inset:* Wright-Giemsa stain. Original magnification 40× objective.)

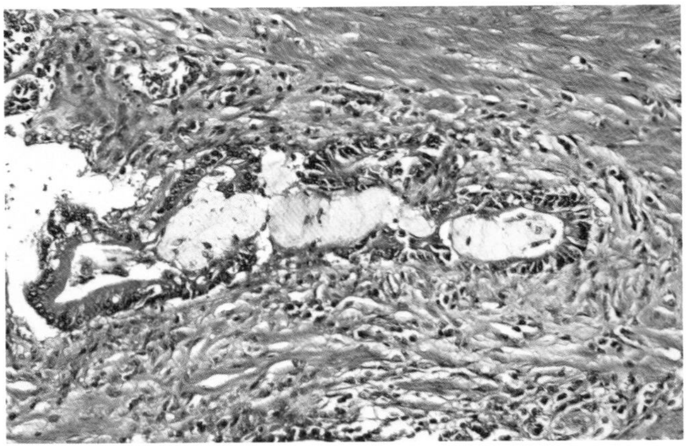

Figure 18-30 Small intestine from a dog; intestinal adenocarcinoma and desmoplasia. Within the tunica muscularis (*note the smooth muscle at the top right of the image*), an infiltrative group of neoplastic epithelial cells form a large tubular structure. Surrounding the carcinoma cells, concentric rings of loose collagenous tissue with plump fibroblasts are seen, consistent with a scirrhous host response to the neoplasm, also known as *desmoplasia*. (H&E stain. Original magnification 20× objective.)

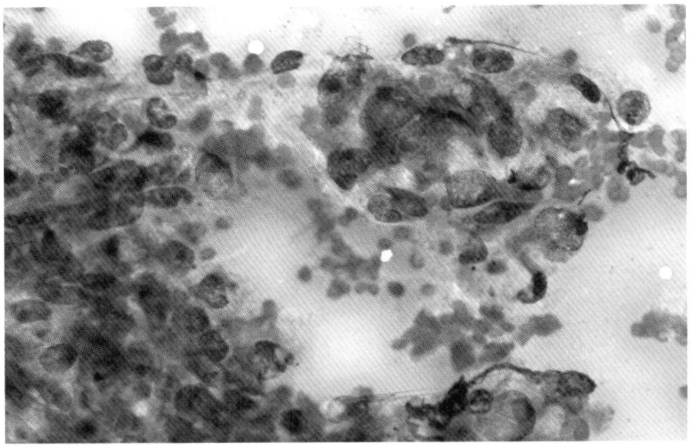

Figure 18-31 Mesenteric aspirate from a cat; hemangiosarcoma (HSA). Hemangiosarcoma of the gastrointestinal tract is an uncommon diagnosis. Although aspiration of HSA is often unrewarding due to poor exfoliation, occasionally, as this case demonstrates, a diagnostic specimen may be obtained. In this image, loose aggregates of overtly neoplastic spindle cells are present, indicating a sarcoma. Red blood cells are intercalated between tumor cells, which suggests vascular space formation and possible HSA. Tumor type was confirmed via histopathology. (Wright-Giemsa stain. Original magnification 50× objective.)

tumors (Figure 18-31 and Figure 18-32). Leiomyomas in dogs occur more commonly in the proximal duodenum near the pylorus and are less common in cats. Differentiation of leimyosarcoma and GISTs have been previous discussed (see Table 18-5; see Figure 18-16 and Figure 18-17). GISTs do have the potential to metastasize to the regional lymph nodes, mesentery, or liver but may carry a better prognosis compared with other malignant neoplasms of the intestinal tract.[9] Rare reports of extraskeletal osteosarcoma arising within the intestine at the site of a retained surgical sponge have been published.[33]

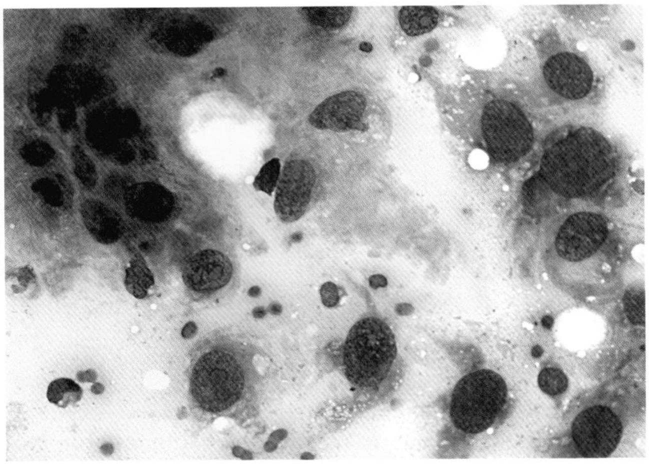

Figure 18-32 Small intestinal tissue imprint from a dog; sarcoma with evidence of smooth muscle differentiation. A pleomorphic population of plump sarcoma cells are admixed with pink, extracellular matrix material. Although the cells have clear mesenchymal features and criteria of malignancy, they do not have specific cytologic features that may allow tumor identification beyond sarcoma. In this case, histochemical or immunohistochemical staining revealed a vimentin-positive, c-kit-negative, desmin-positive (intracytoplasmic globules present in 10% of cells), smooth muscle actin-positive (10% of neoplastic cells) neoplasm suggestive of smooth muscle origin. (Wright-Giemsa stain. Original magnification 50× objective.) (American Society of Veterinary Clinical Pathology: Mystery Slide Conference, 2009 Case 23, submitted by Rebeccah Urbiztondo.)

Round Cell Neoplasia: Lymphoma, which is the most common round cell tumor of the intestinal tract, has varying morphologies (Figure 18-33). GI lymphoma may occur as a component of multicentric disease or, more commonly, as primary alimentary lymphoma. Alimentary lymphoma often spreads to the mesenteric lymph nodes and to the liver. The accuracy of cytology in diagnosing GI neoplasia has varying views, ranging from 72% to 89% correlation with histopathologic findings, but cytology is considered reasonably accurate for a diagnosis of GI lymphoma.[34]

In cats, overall, GI lymphoma occurs more commonly in the small intestine, followed by the stomach, and less often the large intestine. In the small intestine, T-cell lymphoma is more common, whereas in the stomach and large intestine, B-cell lymphoma is more common.[26] Usually, an association with feline leukemia virus (FeLV) infection in alimentary lymphoma does not exist. Cats have three main presentations of GI lymphoma: (1) diffuse small cell lymphocytic lymphoma, (2) large cell lymphoblastic lymphoma, and (3) granulated lymphoma; additional information comparing these types is found in Table 18-7. Cytologically, these types of lymphoma have different morphologic characteristics (see Figure 18-33). Histologically, it may be difficult to definitively differentiate between IBD and diffuse small cell lymphoma. Therefore, an algorithm using certain histologic criteria, then immunohistochemistry, and lastly PCR for antigen receptor rearrangement (PARR) has been proposed; this combination of tests increases the likelihood of successful

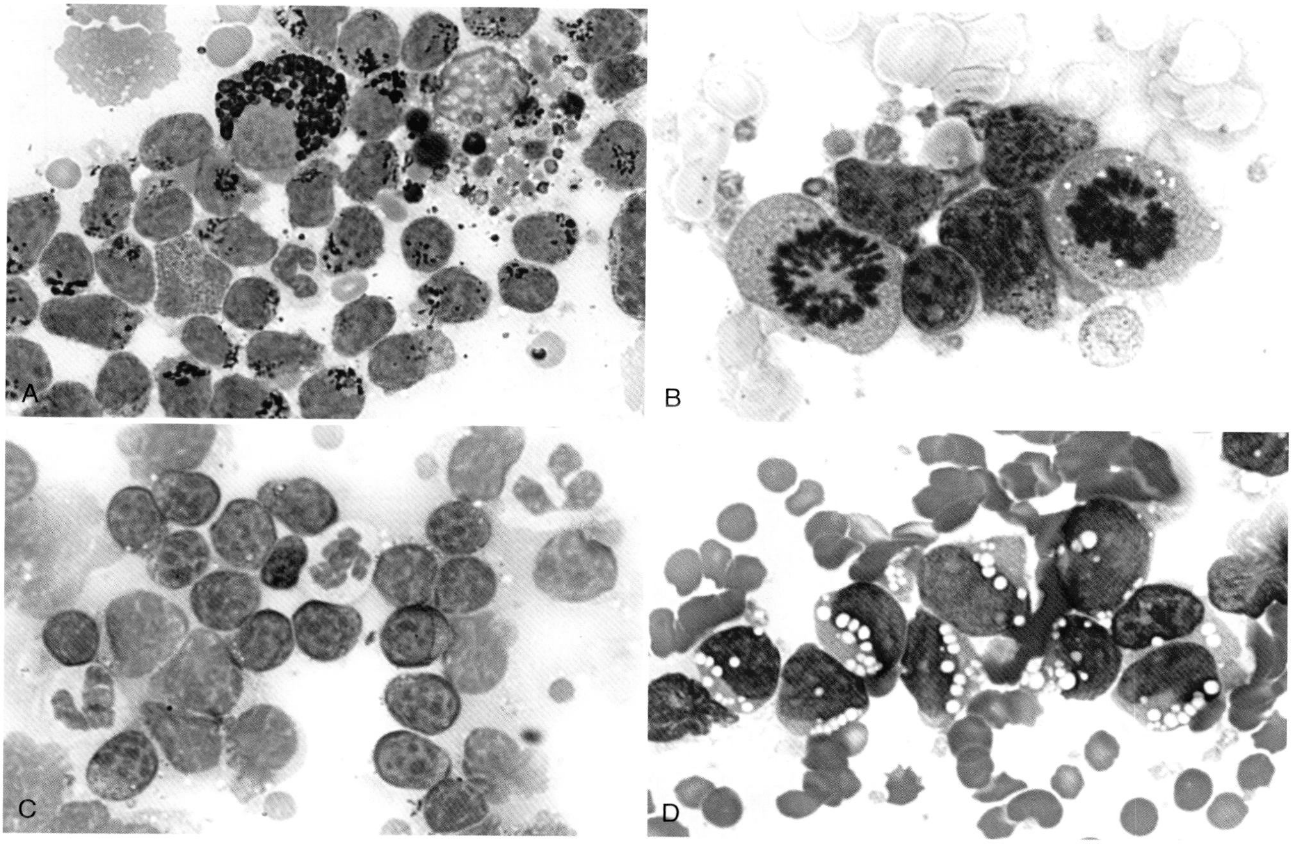

Figure 18-33 Morphologic comparison of four different intestinal lymphomas. **A**, Granular lymphoma from a cat. Cells are intermediate to large in size; nuclei contain smudged chromatin but do not have obvious nucleoli; and the cytoplasm contains large, chunky magenta granules. Note the single tumor cell in the top middle of the image with many extremely large granules. To the right of this cell is a slightly disrupted macrophage with phagocytized granules and debris, and below the granulated tumor cell are a neutrophil and an eosinophil. (Wright-Giemsa stain. Original magnification 100× objective.) **B**, Granular lymphoma from a cat. Cells are intermediate to large in size, with coarse chromatin and some visible nucleolar rings, and contain few very fine magenta granules. Note the two mitotic figures and the presence of granules in the lymphoglandular body in the lower right region of the slide. (Wright-Giemsa stain. Original magnification 100× objective.) **C**, Small cell lymphoma in a cat. Cells are smaller than the neutrophils with coarse, clumped chromatin and a thin rim of basophilic cytoplasm. Because of the well-differentiated appearance of these cells, a definitive diagnosis of lymphoma could be challenging on the basis of the cytology alone. (Wright-Giemsa stain. Original magnification 100× objective.) **D**, Lymphoma in a cat. Cells in this case have typical nuclear characteristics of lymphoma but the cytoplasm contains scattered, prominent, medium-sized vacuoles. (Wright-Giemsa stain. Original magnification 100× objective.) (**A**, Slide courtesy of Jaime Tarigo. **B**, Slide courtesy of Taryn Sibley. **D**, Slide courtesy of Jaime Tarigo.)

differentiation between these entities compared with any of these diagnostic tests alone.[35] Although not always clinically possible, full-thickness biopsy samples are preferred over endoscopic samples to allow for evaluation of mural invasion by the lymphocytes, which is central to the histologic diagnosis of lymphoma over IBD (Figure 18-34 and Figure 18-35). Other histologic criteria supportive of lymphoma include intraepithelial nests of lymphocytes, a monomorphic population of cells, intravascular infiltration, and a high mitotic index.[36] With regard to large granular lymphoma, additional diagnostic features include the classic immunohistochemical profile of perforin-positive cytoplasmic granules and CD3-positive, CD8$\alpha\alpha$-positive, and CD103-positive lymphocytes, which is consistent with intestinal intraepithelial lymphocyte origin in cats (see Figure 18-33, *A* and *B*). These cases may have concurrent involvement of the mesenteric lymph nodes, liver, peritoneal effusion, and peripheral blood.[36]

In dogs, alimentary lymphoma affects the small intestine more than it affects the stomach and less often involves the colon.[9] Lymphoma may present as mass lesions with possible ulceration or may be more a diffuse or regional infiltrative lesion. In dogs, GI lymphoma is most commonly of T-cell origin and is often epitheliotropic, that is, invasion of neoplastic lymphocytes into the mucosal epithelium occurs, and some T-cell lymphomas

TABLE 18-7

Types of Intestinal Lymphoma

Subtype of Lymphoma	Cell of Origin/ Immunophenotype	Cytologic Description	Gross/Ultrasonographic Appearance	Additional Findings
Small cell lymphocytic lymphoma	Epitheliotrophic T-cell, arising from mucosa associated lymphoid tissue MALT	Cells are small to intermediate in size, may appear well differentiated	Diffuse thickening (jejunum most common)	Ultrasound findings similar to inflammatory bowel disease (IBD); lymphomegaly more common with lymphoma than IBD
Large cell lymphoblastic lymphoma	High-grade B-cell neoplasm	Large, immature cells with visible nucleoli	One to multiple masses or transmural thickening	
Granulated lymphoma or large granular lymphoma	Intestinal intraepithelial lymphocyte origin (likely cytotoxic T cell or natural killer cell)	Variably sized (intermediate to large), variable nuclear features, magenta granules vary from fine to large and chunky	Segmental thickening of the intestinal wall or one to multiple mass lesions	Mesenteric lymph nodes, liver, peritoneal fluid and peripheral blood involvement may be seen

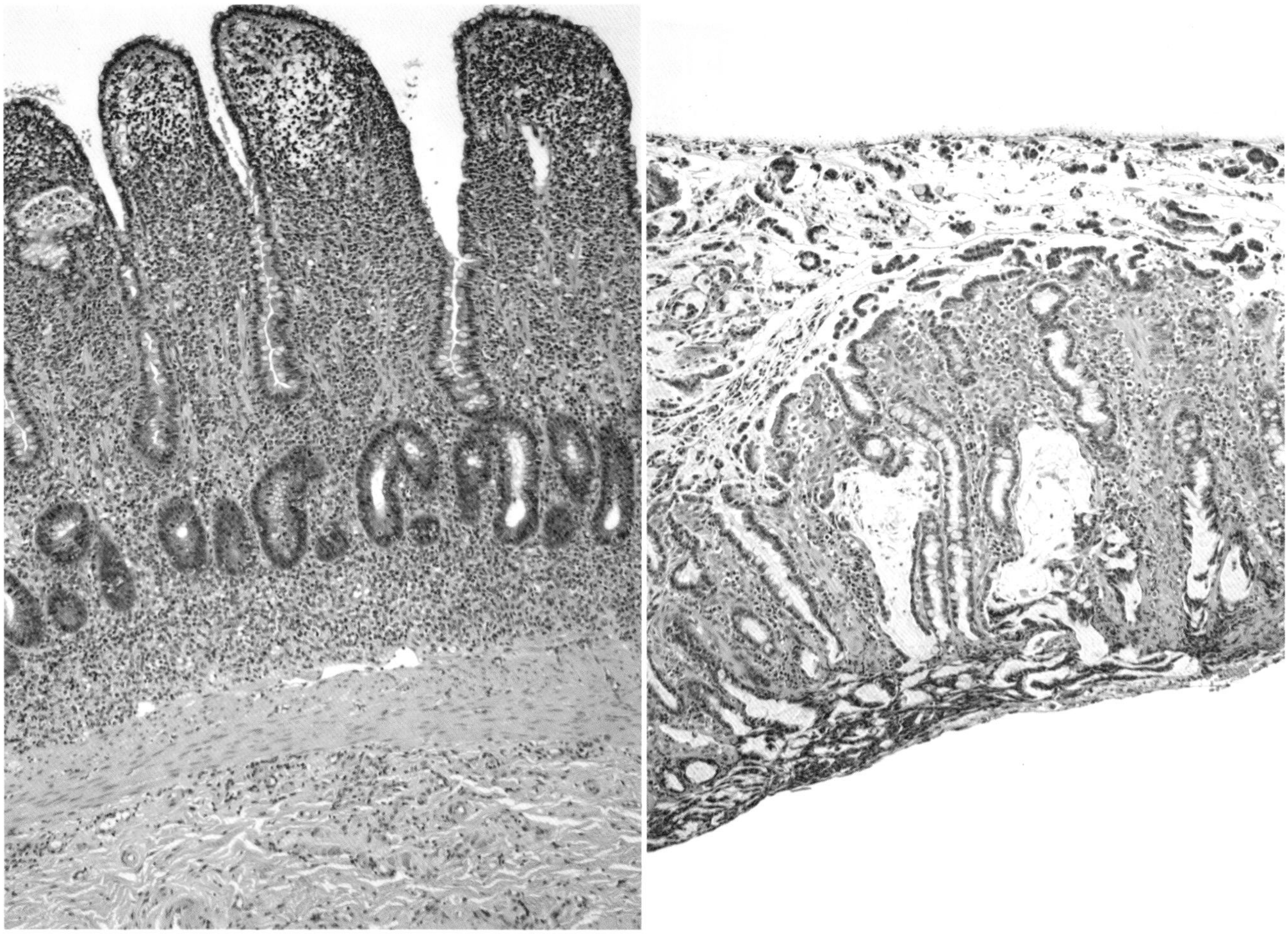

Figure 18-34 Small intestine from two dogs with intestinal lymphoma. *Left:* Full-thickness intestinal biopsy. Note the widened villi and loss of crypts with replacement by sheets of neoplastic lymphocytes, elevation of the crypts from the infiltrating neoplastic cells, and invasion of lymphocytes through the muscularis mucosae into the submucosa. (H&E stain. Original magnification 10× objective.) *Right:* Endoscopic mucosal biopsy with surface artifactual mucus and cellular debris. The volume of tissue available for evaluation is significantly smaller with endoscopic biopsies, often with only the superficial mucosa represented. Although this sample is still diagnostic for lymphoma, some criteria for the diagnosis of lymphoma cannot be evaluated on endoscopic biopsy samples. This includes transmural infiltration by the neoplastic cells, which is often an important criteria allowing for histologic distinction between lymphocytic inflammation and small cell lymphoma in dogs and cats. (H&E stain. Original magnification 10× objective.)

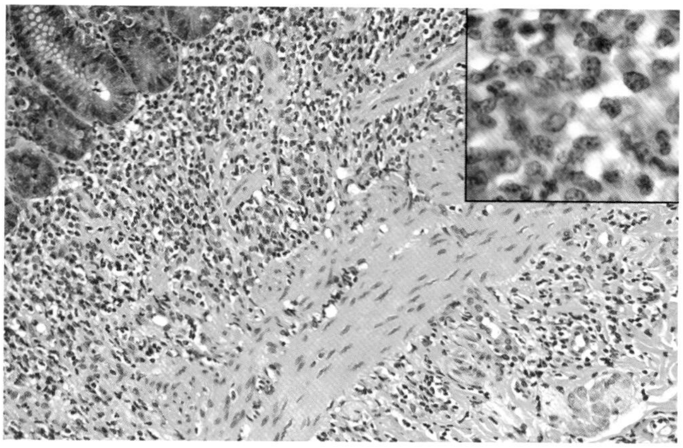

Figure 18-35 Small intestine from a dog; T-cell alimentary lymphoma. The infiltration of the neoplastic lymphocytes through the muscularis mucosae into the submucosa is a helpful feature in the diagnosis of lymphoma in this case. The neoplastic lymphocytes are small with moderate numbers of eosinophils (*inset*). With immunohistochemistry, the neoplastic cells were CD3-positive and CD79a-negative, which is consistent with a T-cell lymphoma. Eosinophilic infiltrates have been identified in association with T-cell lymphoma in dogs. (H&E stain. Original magnification 20× objective. *Inset:* H&E stain. Original magnification 100× objective.)

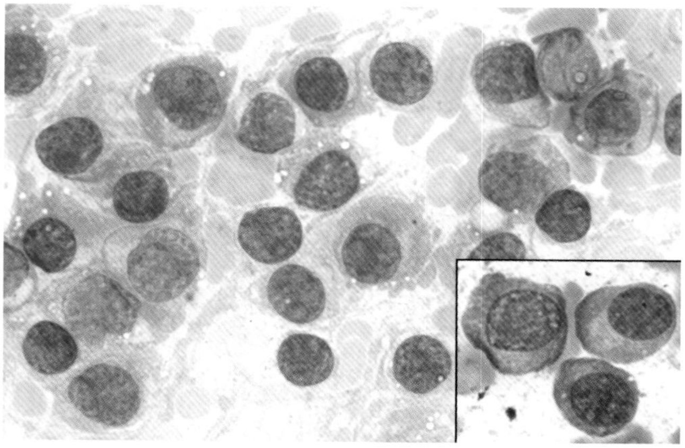

Figure 18-36 Rectal aspirate from a dog; plasma cell tumor. This tumor is moderately well differentiated with many variably intact cells. Cells are large and round with typical plasmacytoid features, including round eccentric nuclei, moderately coarse chromatin, deeply basophilic cytoplasm and a variably apparent perinuclear clear zone (Golgi apparatus). Cytoplasm from disrupted cells gives the background a basophilic swirling appearance. The inset is of a thicker region of the slide in which cells are better preserved. (Wright-Giemsa stain. Original magnification 100× objective. *Inset:* Wright-Giemsa stain. Original magnification 100× objective.)

have an intense infiltrate of eosinophils amid the neoplastic lymphocytes (see Figure 18-35).[37] Cytologic findings are not distinct from lymphoma in other sites (see Figure 18-18 and Figure 18-33). It may be very difficult to differentiate between lymphocytic enteritis and early alimentary lymphoma histologically, as previously discussed for cats, and full-thickness biopsies provide more tissue architecture to help make this distinction (see Figure 18-34 and Figure 18-35). In addition, PCR for antigen receptor rearrangement (PARR) may be considered for additional information on the clonality of neoplastic cells; however, the sensitivity of this test is lower (66.7%) compared with that for lymphoma in other sites.[38]

Plasma cell tumors are rare in the intestine and occur more in dogs than in cats, with the rectum being the most common site (Figure 18-36). They are most often considered benign lesions; however, rare reports of metastasis to the lymph nodes or distant sites have been published.[13] Mast cell tumors are more common in cats than in dogs and typically occur as distinct intestinal masses that are more often extraluminal in the outer layers of the intestinal wall but may have a varied gross appearance.[14] Similar to gastric mast cell tumors, intestinal mast cell tumors arise from the mucosal mast cells and, therefore, may be less well granulated and lack the associated GI ulceration typical for cutaneous mast cell tumors (Figure 18-37). Since they may be less well granulated, particularly histologically, tumors arising from these mucosal mast cells may be difficult to differentiate from lymphoma in a biopsy sample without the use of immunohistochemistry such as tryptase or c-kit (mast cell markers) or CD79a or CD3 (lymphocyte markers) (Figure 18-38).[37,39] The presence of eosinophils is variable in GI mast cell tumors and is not specific for this tumor. A variant of mast cell tumor in cats, known as *feline sclerosing mast cell tumor*, is a mass lesion composed of somewhat poorly granulated mast cells among a marked amount of sclerotic collagen with associated plump spindle cells and many eosinophils. Although these neoplastic mast cells have a low mitotic index, a high propensity to metastasize to the lymph nodes and liver does exist, so this tumor carries a guarded prognosis.[40] A differential diagnosis for this entity is *feline eosinophilic sclerosing fibroplasia*, a nonneoplastic lesion, which poses a diagnostic challenge on histopathology.

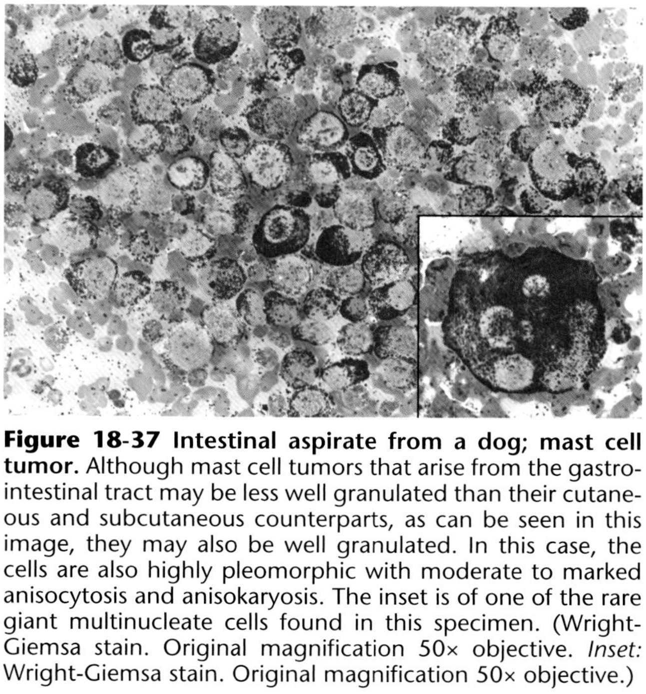

Figure 18-37 Intestinal aspirate from a dog; mast cell tumor. Although mast cell tumors that arise from the gastrointestinal tract may be less well granulated than their cutaneous and subcutaneous counterparts, as can be seen in this image, they may also be well granulated. In this case, the cells are also highly pleomorphic with moderate to marked anisocytosis and anisokaryosis. The inset is of one of the rare giant multinucleate cells found in this specimen. (Wright-Giemsa stain. Original magnification 50× objective. *Inset:* Wright-Giemsa stain. Original magnification 50× objective.)

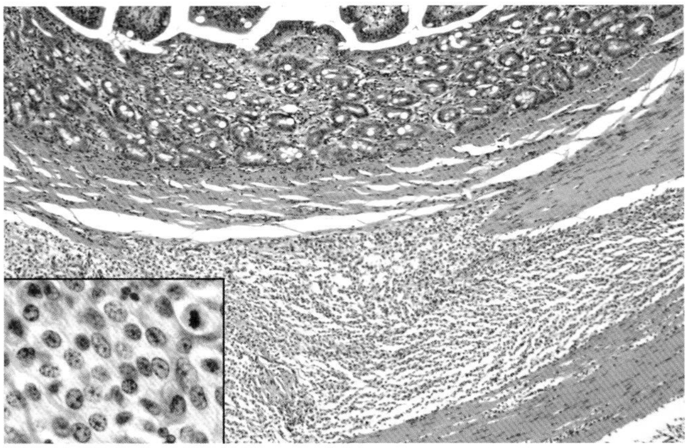

Figure 18-38 Small intestine from a cat; intestinal mast cell tumor. Within the wall of the small intestine, separating smooth muscle bundles of the tunica muscularis and extending into the submucosa, sheets of neoplastic mast cells are pale-staining and lack very obvious granularity. This morphology is typical for tumors arising from mucosal mast cells, compared with cutaneous mast cell tumors, which are often more obviously granulated. The relative lack of granularity may make diagnosis of mast cell tumor over other round cell tumors such as lymphoma difficult in some cases. In the inset, a mitotic figure is identified (*right aspect of image*) with few eosinophils (*left aspect of image*). (H&E stain. Original magnification 10× objective. *Inset:* H&E stain. Original magnification 100× objective.)

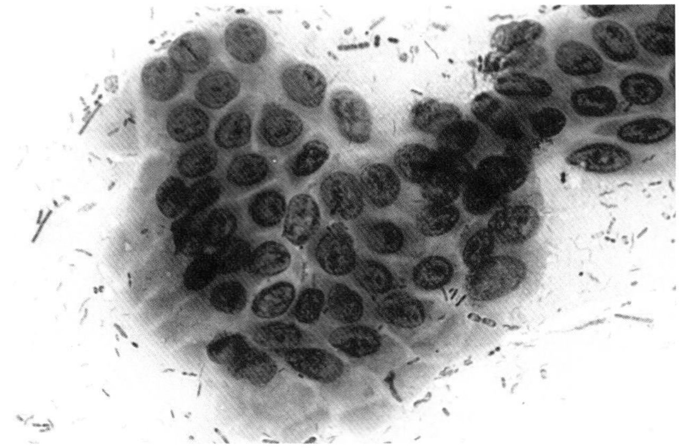

Figure 18-39 Rectal scraping from a dog; normal rectal mucosa. A medium-sized cluster of normal columnar epithelial cells is present. Cells are uniform in appearance with round basally oriented nuclei and moderate amounts of deeply basophilic cytoplasm. The columnar appearance is best appreciated on the left side of the cluster; in the center, the cells appear more cuboidal. (Wright-Giemsa stain. Original magnification 100× objective.)

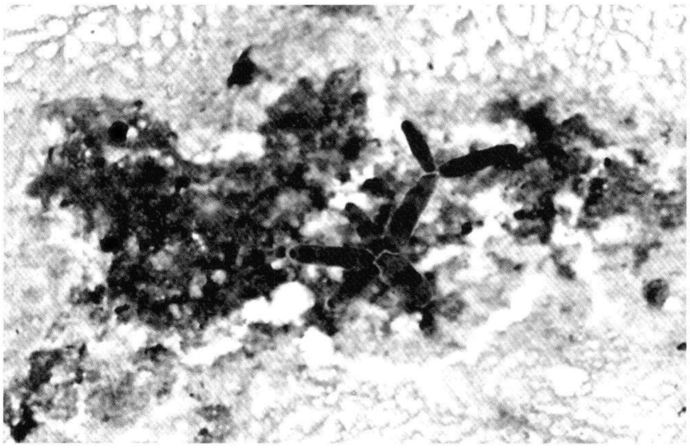

Figure 18-40 Aspirate of a peripancreatic mass in a dog; necrotic material and ***Cyniclomyces guttulatus*** **organisms.** The underlying lesion in this animal was a full thickness ulcer, which led to intestinal rupture and leakage of intestinal contents. Amorphous clumps of muted mauve material consistent with necrotic debris and large bacillus-shaped yeast organisms with branching or forked morphology and a banded, basophilic staining interior consistent with *C. guttulatus* were present. Organisms were considered incidental to the leakage of gastrointestinal contents and were not identified in tissue biopsy specimens. (Wright-Giemsa stain. Original magnification 50× objective.)

FECAL ANALYSIS

Normal Fecal Cytology

Normal fecal cytology consists of a polymorphic population of microbial flora that consists predominantly of rod-shaped bacteria with rare coccoid bacteria and occasional yeast structures with a background of mucus and debris.[1] Clusters of columnar epithelium may be noted occasionally on rectal scraping samples (Figure 18-39). Squamous epithelium may be noted as a result of contamination from the anus. *Cyniclomyces guttulatus* is a fungal agent that is part of the normal GI flora in rodents and lagomorphs (see Table 18-1). Occasionally, low numbers of *Cyniclomyces* organisms may be identified in canine feces and, rarely, feline feces; the significance of this organism is not well understood at this time. Cytologically, *Cyniclomyces* are large organisms present individually or as short, forked, or branching chains (Figure 18-40). Individual segments are approximately 5–7 × 15–20 μm, oval to cylindrical structures surrounded by a prominent clear cell wall, with an interior that stains uniformly purple, is mottled or vacuolated, or has a broad, transverse, poorly staining central region.[41]

Abnormal Fecal Cytology

Eosinophilic, neutrophilic, and lymphoplasmacytic inflammation may be noted and correspond to concurrent disease in the intestines such as IBD or infection (see "Intestinal Inflammation"). Since the normal flora identified in feces is a very mixed population of predominantly rod-shaped bacteria, alterations to this, including increased proportion of a bacterial subtype or a monomorphic bacterial proliferation, may indicate bacterial overgrowth. It is difficult to determine if overgrowth suggested cytologically is truly causing the clinical signs in a patient. Bacterial overgrowth may occur with a variety of disease processes or as a result of antibiotic therapy (Box 18-4).[42] In addition to bacterial overgrowth, overgrowth of yeast organisms may be identified in fecal samples (Figure 18-41). Occasionally, animals with diarrhea are found to have large numbers of *Cyniclomyces guttulatus* organisms on fecal examination or smears. It is not known whether the overgrowth of this organism may cause or contribute to diarrhea or if the organism is simply flourishing in an altered environment, but at least one report has suggested

Box 18-4

Causes of Microbial Overgrowth in the Gastrointestinal Tract

- Idiopathic (primary)
- Antibiotic administration
- Exocrine pancreatic insufficiency
- Inflammatory bowel disease
- Intestinal stagnation or abnormal motility
- Intestinal obstruction
- Neoplasia
- Lymphangiectasia
- Impaired mucosal defense mechanisms
- Decreased gastric acid secretion
- Gastric or enteric surgical procedures

From Tarpley HL, Bounous DI: Digestive system. In: Latimer KS, editor: *Duncan and Prasse's veterinary laboratory medicine clinical pathology*, ed 5, Ames, IA, 2011, Wiley-Blackwell.

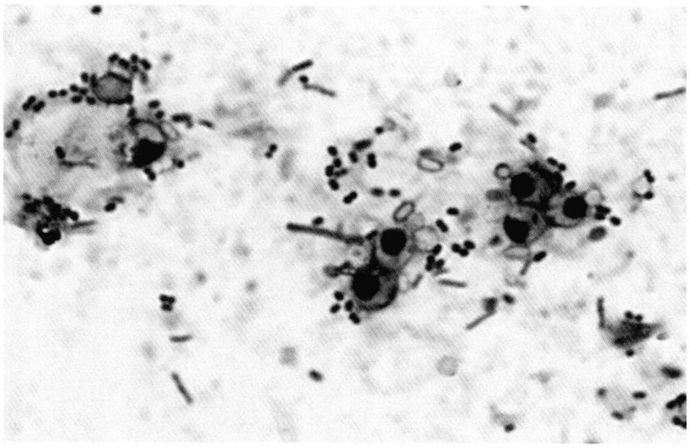

Figure 18-41 Fecal smear from a dog; yeast overgrowth. Multiple round yeast organisms with a basophilic round eccentric nucleus and light-blue cytoplasm are present on a background of mixed bacteria and fecal debris. Polymerase chain reaction sequencing and culture indicated the organism was likely *Pichia* spp., and findings were interpreted as overgrowth of this nonpathogenic yeast. (Wright-Giemsa stain. Original magnification 100× objective.) (American Society of Veterinary Clinical Pathology: Mystery Slide Conference, 2008 Case 14, submitted by Shir Gilor.)

that treating dogs with diarrhea, with high numbers of organisms on fecal floatation, with a short course of nystatin often results in resolution of clinical signs.[43]

Bacterial agents that have been associated with diarrhea include large sporulating rod-shaped bacteria such as *Clostridium* spp. and spirochetes such as *Campylobacter* spp. (Figure 18-42 and Figure 18-43). Although the presence of more than 3 to 5 sporulating cells per 100× field on cytologic examination has previously been used to suggest *Clostridium perfringens*–associated diarrhea, several studies have shown that fecal endospore counts do not correlate with the presence of diarrhea or detection of the enterotoxin in fecal specimens and that sporulation may be found in animals with and without diarrhea.[3] In general, it may be difficult to differentiate nonpathogenic bacteria from pathogenic bacteria on fecal cytology; therefore, additional diagnostics such as culture, PCR, or toxin identification (for clostridial agents) are required for definitive identification (see Table 18-1).

Other than the normal bacterial flora, infectious agents, including *Histoplasma capsulatum*, *Prototheca* spp., *Pentatrichomonas hominis* and *Tritrichomonas foetus*, may occasionally be identified in fecal samples (see Figure 18-1; Figure 18-44, Figure 18-45, Figure 18-46, and Figure 18-47).[44] Detailed descriptions, additional diagnostic testing, and images of the most common organisms in feces and throughout the GI tract are presented in Table 18-1.

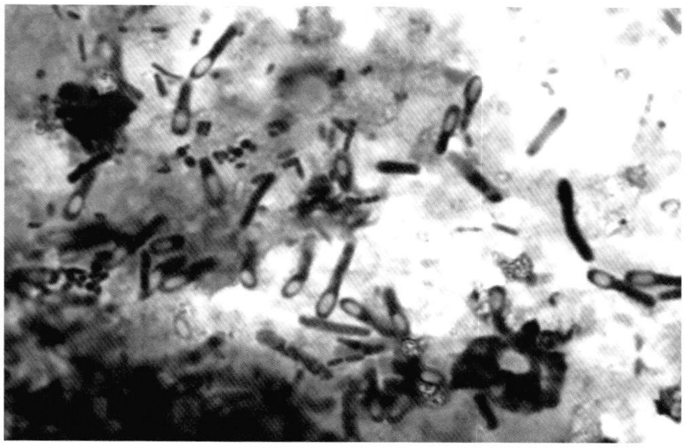

Figure 18-42 Fecal smear from a cat; overgrowth of sporulating rod bacteria. The bacteria are large and contain a single eccentric clear spore giving them a "tennis racket" appearance. Although the presence of sporulating cells in a diarrheal patient warrants concern about *Clostridium perfringens*–associated diarrhea, studies have shown that identification of fecal endospores does not correlate with the detection of the enterotoxin. In addition, sporulation may be found in animals with or without diarrhea, and other organisms such as *Bacillus* spp. may also sporulate. (Modified Wright-Giemsa stain. Original magnification 100× objective.)

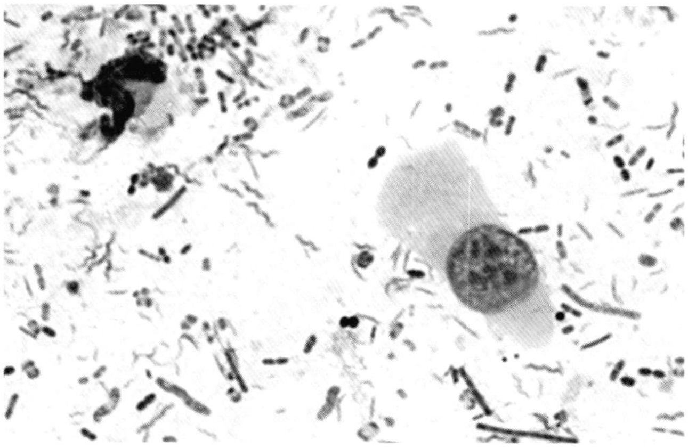

Figure 18-43 Rectal scraping from a dog; numerous *Campylobacter*-like organisms (CLOs). A single enterocyte surrounded by a mixed population of bacteria is present. Many of the bacteria have the distinctive "gull wing" appearance characteristic of CLOs. Because pathogenic *Campylobacter* spp., nonpathogenic *Campylobacter* spp., and other organisms such as *Arcobacter* may all share similar morphology, additional diagnostics such as culture and polymerase chain reaction should be used to diagnose campylobacteriosis. (Wright-Giemsa stain. Original magnification 100× objective.)

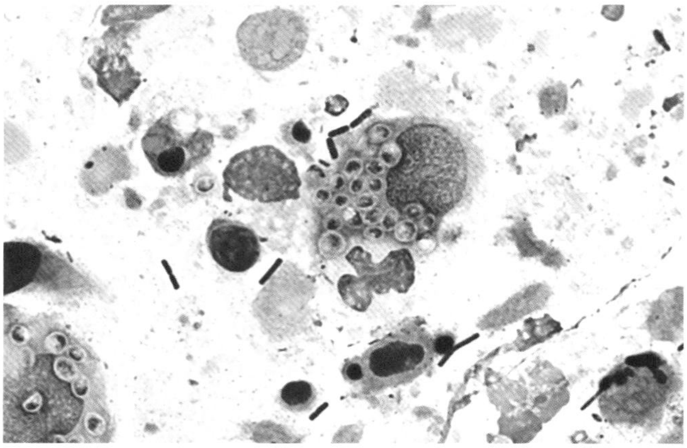

Figure 18-44 Rectal scraping from a cat; histoplasmosis. Two macrophages containing *Histoplasma capsulatum* yeast are present. *Histoplasma* yeast are small and round with a thin clear cell wall and an interior that stains part basophilic and part clear giving it a characteristic "half full, half empty" appearance. A monomorphic population of large rod bacteria is present suggesting there may be an abnormal overgrowth of bacteria as well. (Modified Wright-Giemsa stain. Original magnification 100× objective.)

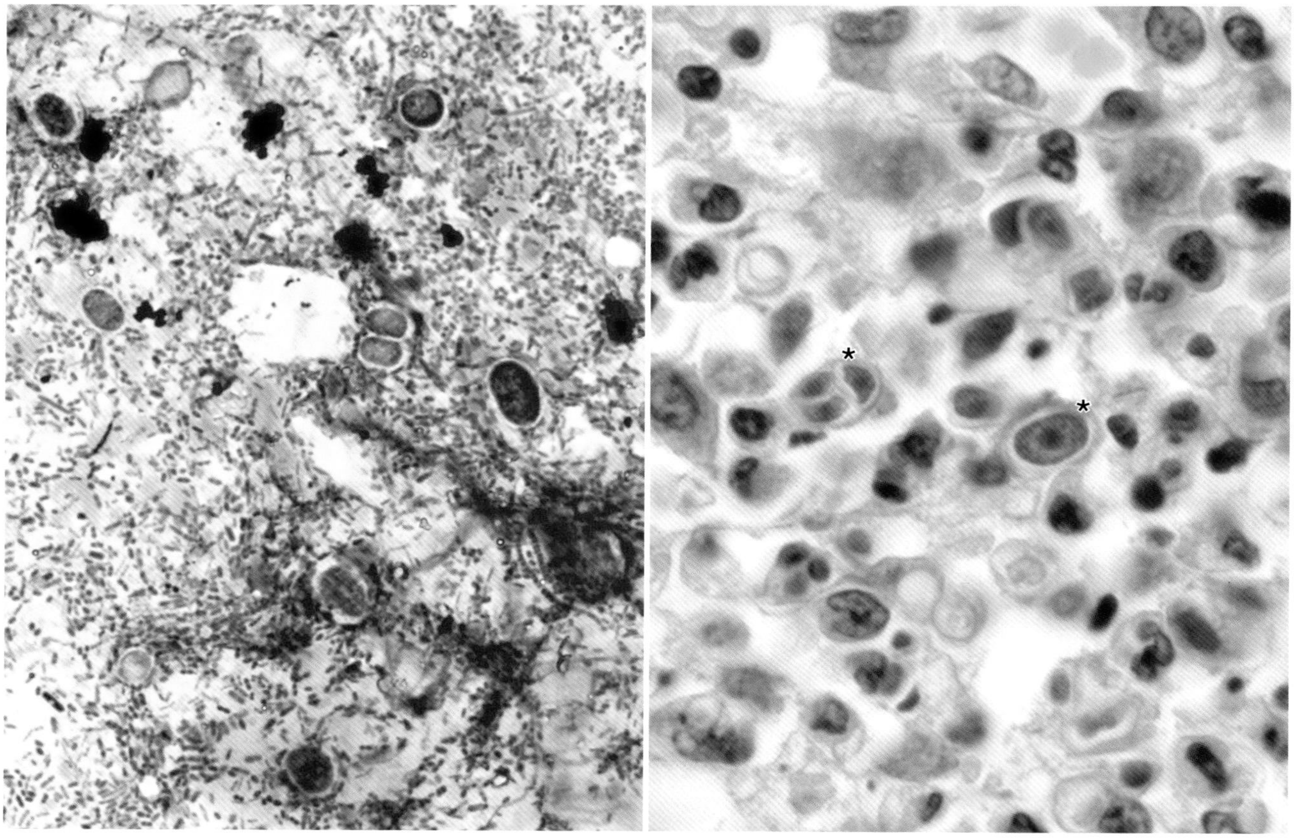

Figure 18-45 Fecal sample (*left*) and large intestinal biopsy (*right*) from a dog; *Prototheca* infection. *Left:* Scattered oval shaped organisms with a thin clear cell wall and deeply basophilic granular interiors are present ("jelly bean" appearance) on a background of mixed bacteria consistent with fecal flora. (Wright-Giemsa stain. Original magnification 50× objective.) *Right:* The inflammatory cells expanding the colonic wall consist mainly of epithelioid macrophages with fewer neutrophils and lymphocytes. Among the inflammatory cells, numerous empty cell walls of the *Prototheca* organisms are present. Several intact sporangia (*right**) are oval with a prominent magenta-purple nucleus and nucleolus and a clear halo of a cell wall, with occasional endosporulation (*left**). (H&E stain. Original magnification 100× objective.) (Case from Joint Pathology Center Veterinary Pathology Services (formerly AFIP): Wednesday Slide Conference 2002-03, Conference 16 Case 2.)

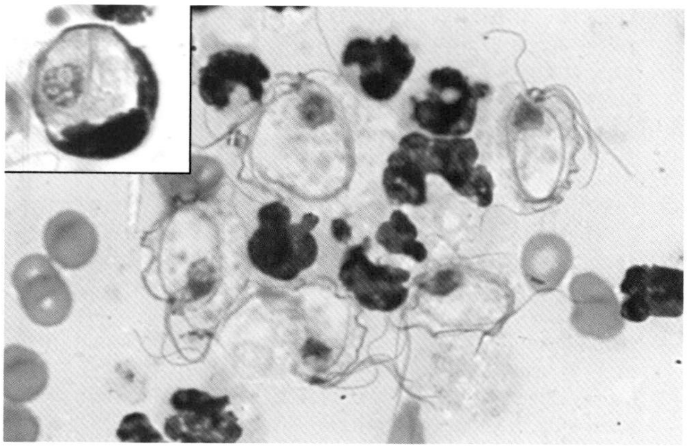

Figure 18-46 Intestinal mass aspirate from a dog; *Pentatrichomonas hominis* infection and a carcinoma (*not pictured*). A group of trophozoites admixed with degenerate neutrophils is present. The trophozoites are oval-shaped cells with five anterior flagella, a sixth recurrent flagellum associated with the undulating membrane, which runs the length of the cell, a single anterior nucleus, and a well-developed vertical axostyle. The inset image is of an organism that has been phagocytized by a neutrophil. (Modified Wright-Giemsa stain. Original magnification 100× objective.) (Slide courtesy of Valarie Pallatto.)

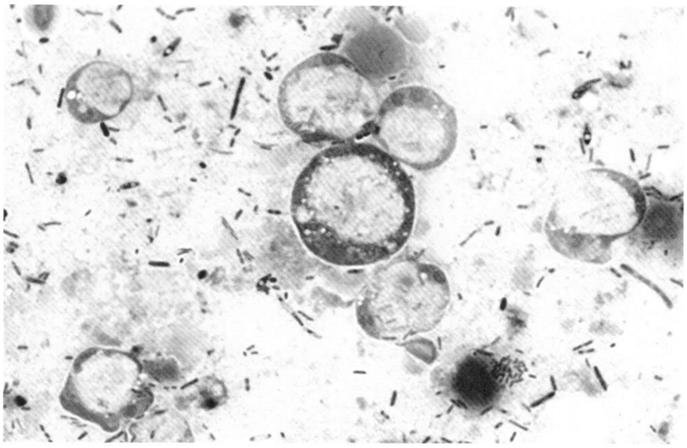

Figure 18-47 Fecal smear from a dog. Multiple large round parasitic organisms are present on a background of mixed primarily rod-shaped bacteria and are characterized by a central clear to pale staining area surrounded by a thin basophilic rim containing one to several round pink structures. The morphology is suggestive of the cyst form of *Iodamoeba butsclii*, a typically harmless organism that may cause amoebiasis in immune-compromised individuals; however, other organisms such as *Blastocystis* can have overlapping morphology. (Wright-Giemsa stain. Original magnification 100× objective.) (American Society of Veterinary Clinical Pathology: Mystery Slide Conference, 2004 Case 20, submitted by Craig Thompson.)

References

1. Broussard JD: Optimal fecal assessment, *Clin Tech Small Anim Pract* 18:218, 2003.
2. Greene CE: *Infectious diseases of the dog and cat*, ed 4, St. Louis, M, 2012, Saunders.
3. Marks SL, Rankin SC, Byrne BA, et al: Enteropathogenic bacteria in dogs and cats: diagnosis, epidemiology, treatment, and control, *J Vet Int Med* 25:1195, 2011.
4. Gaschen L: Ultrasonography of small intestinal inflammatory and neoplastic diseases in dogs and cats, *Vet Clin North Am Small Anim Pract* 41:329, 2011.
5. Tams TR: *Handbook of small animal gastroenterology*, ed 2, St. Louis, MO, 2003, Saunders.
6. Bacha WJ, Bacha LM: *Color atlas of veterinary histology*, ed 2, Philadelphia, PA, 2000, Lippincott Williams & Wilkins.
7. Atkinson BF: *Atlas of diagnostic cytopathology*, ed 2, Philadelphia, PA, 2004, Saunders.
8. Drake M: *Gastro-esophageal cytology*, Basel, Switzerland, 1985, Karger.
9. Brown CC, Baker DC, Barker IK: Alimentary system. In Maxie MG, editor: *Jubb, Kennedy, and Palmer's pathology of domestic animals*, ed 5, Philadelphia, PA, 2007, Saunders.
10. Sellon RK, Willard MD: Esophagitis and esophageal strictures, *Vet Clin North Am Small Anim Pract* 33:945, 2003.
11. Gibson CJ, Parry NMA, Jakowski RM, et al: Adenomatous polyp with intestinal metaplasia of the esophagus (Barrett esophagus) in a dog, *Vet Pathol* 41:116, 2010.
12. Mazzei MJ, Bissett SA, Murphy KM, et al: Eosinophilic esophagitis in a dog, *J Am Vet Med Assoc* 235:61, 2009.
13. Head KW, Else RW, Dubielzig RR: Tumors of the alimentary tract. In Meuten DJ, editor: *Tumors in domestic animals*, ed 4, Ames, IA, 2008, Iowa State Press.
14. Head KW, Cullen JM, Dubielzig RR, et al: *Histologic classification of the tumors of the alimentary system of domestic animals*. series 2, Washington, D.C, 2003, Armed Forces Institute of Pathology.
15. Webb C, Twedt DC: Canine gastritis, *Vet Clin N Am Small Anim Pract* 33:969, 2003.
16. Lidbury JA, Suchodolski JS, Steiner JM: Gastric histopathologic abnormalities in dogs: 67 cases (2002-2007), *J Am Vet Med Assoc* 234:1147, 2009.
17. Takemura LS, et al: *Helicobacter* spp. in cats: association between infecting species and epithelial proliferation within the gastric lamina propria, *J Comp Pathol* 141:127, 2009.
18. Bridgeford EC, Marini RP, Feng Y, et al: Gastric *Helicobacter* species as a cause of feline gastric lymphoma: a viable hypothesis, *Vet Immunol Immunop* 123:106, 2008.
19. Lyles SE, et al: Idiopathic eosinophilic masses of the gastrointestinal tract in dogs, *J Vet Int Med* 23:818, 2009.
20. Craig LE, Hardam EE, Hertzke EM, et al: Feline gastrointestinal eosinophilic sclerosing fibroplasia, *Vet Pathol* 46:63, 2009.
21. LeBlanc CJ, Echandi RL, Moore RR, et al: Hypercalcemia associated with gastric pythiosis in a dog, *Vet Clin Pathol* 37:115, 2008.
22. Vatn S, et al: Possible involvement of *Sarcina ventriculi* in canine and equine acute gastric dilatation, *Acta Vet Scand* 41:333, 2000.
23. Gualtieria M, Monzeglio MG, Scanziani E: Gastric neoplasms, *Vet Clin North Am Small Anim Pract* 29:415, 1999.
24. Qvigstad G, et al: Gastric neuroendocrine carcinoma associated with atrophic gastritis in the Norwegian Lundehund, *J Comp Pathol* 139:194, 2008.
25. Russell KN, Mehler SJ, Skorupski KA, et al: Clinical and immunohistochemical differentiation of gastrointestinal stromal tumors from leiomyosarcomas in dogs: 42 cases (1990-2003), *J Am Vet Med Assoc* 230:1329, 2007.
26. Pohlman LM, et al: Immunophenotypic and histologic classification of 50 cases of feline gastrointestinal lymphoma, *Vet Pathol* 46:259, 2009.
27. Cerquetella M, Spaterna A, Laus F: Inflammatory bowel disease in the dog: differences and similarities with humans, *World J Gastroenterol* 16:1050, 2010.

28. Day MJ, Bilzer T, Mansell J, et al: Histopathological standards for the diagnosis of gastrointestinal inflammation in endoscopic biopsy samples from the dog and cat: a report from the World Small Animal Veterinary Association Gastrointestinal Standardization Group, *J Comp Pathol* 138:S1, 2008.
29. Johnson CS, Fales-Williams AJ, Reimer SB, et al: Fibrosing gastrointestinal leiomyositis as a cause of chronic intestinal pseudo-obstruction in an 8-month-old dog, *Vet Pathol* 44:106, 2007.
30. Fabrick C, Bugbee A, Fosgate G: Clinical features and outcome of *Heterobilharzia Americana* infection in dogs, *J Vet Int Med* 24:140, 2010.
31. Craven M, Mansfield CS, Simpson KW: Granulomatous colitis of boxer dogs, *Vet Clin North Am Small Anim Pract* 41:433, 2011.
32. Yaeger MJ, Gookin JL: Histologic features associated with *Tritrichomonas foetus*-induced colitis in domestic cats, *Vet Pathol* 42:797, 2005.
33. Pardo AD, et al: Primary jejunal osteosarcoma associated with a surgical sponge in a dog, *J Am Vet Med Assoc* 196:935, 1990.
34. Frank JD, et al: Clinical outcomes of 30 cases (1997-2004) of canine gastrointestinal lymphoma, *J Am Anim Hosp Assoc* 43:313, 2007.
35. Kiupel M, Smedley RC, Pfent C, et al: Diagnostic algorithm to differentiate lymphoma from inflammation in feline small intestinal biopsy samples, *Vet Pathol* 48:212, 2011.
36. Krick EL, Little L, Patel R, et al: Description of clinical and pathological findings, treatment and outcome of feline large granular lymphocyte lymphoma (1996-2004), *Vet Comp Oncol* 6:102, 2008.
37. Ozaki K, et al: T-cell lymphoma with eosinophilic infiltration involving the intestinal tract in 11 dogs, *Vet Pathol* 43:339, 2006.
38. Fukushima K, Ohno K, Koshino-Goto Y, et al: Sensitivity for the detection of a clonally rearranged antigen receptor gene in endoscopically obtained biopsy specimens from canine alimentary lymphoma, *J Vet Med Sci* 71:1673, 2009.
39. Ozaki K, et al: Mast cell tumors of the gastrointestinal tract in 39 Dogs, *Vet Pathol* 39:557, 2002.
40. Halsey CHC, Powers BE, Kamstock DA: Feline intestinal sclerosing mast cell tumour: 50 cases (1997-2008), *Vet Comp Oncol* 8:72, 2010.
41. Neel JA, Tarigo J, Grindem CB: Gall bladder aspirate from a dog, *Vet Clin Pathol* 35:467, 2006.
42. Tarpley HL, Bounous DI: Digestive system. In Latimer KS, editor: *Duncan and Prasse's veterinary laboratory medicine clinical pathology*, ed 5, Ames, IA, 2011, Wiley-Blackwell.
43. Houwers DJ, Blankenstein B: *Cyniclomyces guttulatus* (brillendoosjesgist) en diarree bij honden [*Cyniclomyces guttulatus*{eyeglass box yeast} and diarrhea in dogs], *Tijdschr Diergeneesk* 126:502, 2001.
44. Raskin RE, Meyer DJ: *Canine and feline cytology: a color atlas and interpretation guide*, ed 2, St. Louis, MO, 2010, Saunders.

CHAPTER 19

The Pancreas

Dori L. Borjesson

Cytologic evaluation of the pancreas is becoming increasingly common as a tool to help clinicians distinguish between pancreatic disorders. This increase in pancreatic aspiration for cytologic evaluation may be related to an increase in clinician comfort with pancreatic manipulation and the ongoing utility of pancreatic aspiration with minimal complications in human medicine. Previous perceptions that pancreatic manipulation may result in secondary pancreatitis have largely been unsubstantiated. A recent study showed that fine-needle aspiration (FNA) of normal canine pancreas does not result in increased serum concentrations of trypsin-like immunoreactivity (TLI) or canine-specific pancreatic lipase (cPL).[1] However inter-operative biopsy was associated with increased serum TLI and sporadic, mild, peracute necrosis, inflammation, hemorrhage, and fibrin deposition.[1]

Currently, no single test conclusively differentiates inflammatory, cystic, neoplastic, and infectious diseases involving the pancreas. Patients with pancreatic disorders, with the exception of pancreatic insufficiency, often have similar histories and clinical signs. Clinicopathologic testing can frequently identify the presence of pancreatic disease in the dog.[2,3] However, in the cat, serum chemistry tests are often less useful.[4-8] In both dogs and cats, abdominal ultrasonography is a useful diagnostic tool to visualize and assess an abnormal pancreas, guide aspirates and biopsies, and monitor response to treatment.[6, 9-11] As with biochemical tests, however, the use of abdominal ultrasonography to definitively differentiate between pancreatic diseases has variable sensitivity and specificity, as ultrasonographic appearance in various pancreatic disorders overlap.[6, 9-11] Once visualized, ultrasound-guided FNA of the pancreas is a safe and effective adjunct to imaging in the diagnosis of pancreatic disorders. The pancreas exfoliates well, and cytologic examination of the pancreas in small animals has proved useful in the diagnosis of both neoplastic and nonneoplastic lesions, including abscesses, cysts, and pancreatitis.

NORMAL PANCREAS STRUCTURE

Anatomy and Histology

The pancreas consists of a right (duodenal) limb and a left (transverse or splenic) limb joined at the head. The number and position of the pancreatic duct(s) opening into the duodenum and the location of the duct(s) to the common bile duct varies among species and among individuals in each species.[12] The pancreas consists of endocrine and exocrine components. Numerous tubuloacinar secretory units form the exocrine component of the organ (Figure 19-1). These secretory units drain into long, narrow intercalated ducts lined by elongated, cuboidal cells. Intercalated ducts communicate directly with interlobular ducts.[13] Functionally, the tubuloacinar secretory units (exocrine pancreas) secrete digestive enzymes in an inactive proenzyme form. Pancreatic enzymes are activated by trypsin secreted by the duodenum.

The endocrine islets of Langerhans are clusters of epithelial cells scattered among the secretory units (Figure 19-2). Normal pancreatic islets contain four cell types, each secreting different pancreatic polypeptides:

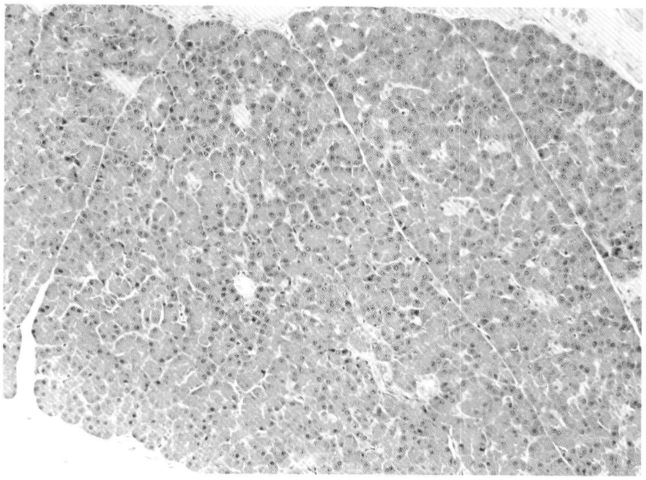

Figure 19-1 Histologic section of normal canine pancreas. Normal pancreas consists of numerous lobules separated by septa of connective tissue. Lobules are primarily composed of tubuloacinar secretory units which form the exocrine component of the organ. Acinar cells have small, dark, uniform nuclei with abundant bright-pink cytoplasm. Islets and scattered intercalated ducts are also present that drain the epithelial cells. (Hematoxylin and Eosin stain. Original magnification 100×.)

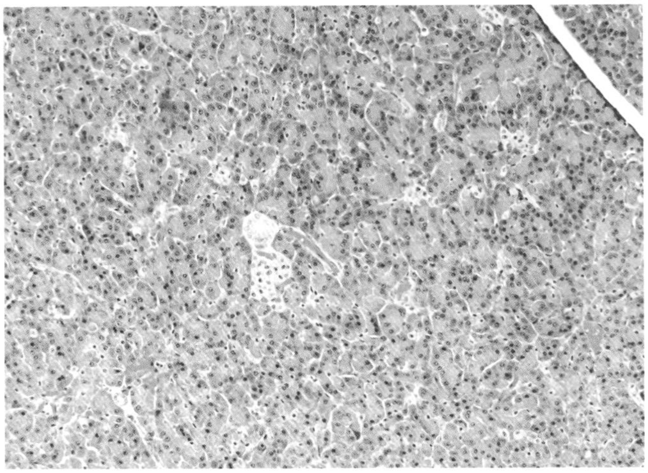

Figure 19-2 Histologic section of normal canine pancreas. A pancreatic lobule composed of exocrine tubuloacinar secretory units with a single duct and a single aggregate of pale pancreatic endocrine cells (islet of Langerhans cells) near the center of the section. Acinar cells have a distinct polarity with centrally located eosinophilia (zymogen granules) and basilar basophilia (nucleus and cytoplasm). Scattered small vessels and small intercalated ducts are also present. (Hematoxylin and Eosin stain. Original magnification 100×.)

(1) α-cells secrete glucagon; (2) β-cells secrete insulin, (3) D-cells secrete somatostatin, and (4) F-cells secrete pancreatic polypeptide. β-cells are the most numerous islet cells (constituting 60% to 70% of the islet cells), and they are generally concentrated in the central part of the islet. α-cells constitute about 20% of the islet cells and are generally located peripherally.[12]

SAMPLING TECHNIQUE

Methods

In veterinary medicine, percutaneous, ultrasound-guided FNA of the pancreas is the most common method of tissue sampling, although intraoperative sampling may also be performed.[14] FNA of the pancreas permits extensive sampling and, in humans, is associated with a low risk of morbidity and mortality. It is especially useful in discriminating between pancreatic neoplasia and inflammation. In human medicine, FNA is the diagnostic method of choice for patients with a pancreatic mass. The most common methods of sample procurement are computed tomography (CT)–guided or endoscopic ultrasonography–guided aspiration. The vast majority of human pancreatic masses are neoplastic; as such, FNA is used to establish a rapid tissue diagnosis before chemotherapy, surgery, or both. In dogs, dynamic CT has recently been used to assess normal and neoplastic lesions of the pancreas.[15]

Methods to obtain a FNA of the pancreas are outlined in Box 19-1. The described methods for sample procurement are closely based on methods originally published by Bjorneby and Kari.[14] In brief, the pancreas and surrounding abdominal structures should be thoroughly evaluated with ultrasonography to visualize the area to be aspirated. If a mass is present, multiple areas within the mass and surrounding tissue should be aspirated. In dogs, inflammation (purulent or lymphocytic) has been shown to occur in discrete areas throughout the pancreas (right and left limb).[14] Therefore, no site is considered preferential to sample the pancreas (and confirm pancreatitis) in the absence of a visible lesion. The following steps are then performed:

- Label clean, glass slides, preferably with frosted edges, with patient identification and site of aspiration.
- Draw 1 milliliter (mL) of air into a 3-mL syringe. Attach a 1½- to 3-inch 22-gauge needle to the syringe. This needle-and-syringe combination may permit more accurate needle placement and angle control.[16]
- Using an ultrasound biopsy guide or freehand technique, place the needle in the desired region for aspiration, and move the needle back and forth within the pancreas.
- Be sure to identify the location of the needle with ultrasonography at all times, and maintain the needle in the same tract. For sample procurement, no additional negative pressure is required. Do not attempt to redirect the needle because the tip of the needle may lacerate the tissue and cause excessive hemorrhage and leakage of pancreatic enzymes.[16]
- To minimize cell disruption, sample expulsion and smear preparation should be as gentle as possible.
- To ensure full evaluation of the cells present, expel the sample onto the middle of the slide where cells are most readily stained and visualized.
- Sample three to four different sites within the lesion, if possible.
- To ensure the best-quality sample (and, thus, enhance the likelihood of a cytologic diagnosis), make multiple smears using a variety of smear techniques that result in both thin and thick preparations.
- Slide preparation techniques include the squash smear (slide-over-slide) or blood smear technique. The smears should be air-dried and submitted to a veterinary clinical pathologist.[16]

BOX 19-1

Outline of Fine-Needle Biopsy Technique

- Use ultrasonography to visualize the area to be aspirated.
- Set out and label 6 to 10 clean glass slides.
- Draw 1 milliliter (mL) of air into a 3-mL syringe.
- Attach a 1½- to 3-inch 22-gauge needle to the syringe.
- Guide the needle attached to the syringe into the pancreas.
  - AVOID redirecting the needle; negative pressure is *not* needed.
- Quickly expel the sample onto a slide.
- Prepare multiple smears by using a variety of gentle techniques.
  - Include squash preparations and blood smear techniques.
- Sample multiple sites within the lesion.
- Rapidly air-dry the smears.
- Submit air-dried, labeled slides to a veterinary clinical pathologist.

Adapted from Bjorneby JM, Kari S: Cytology of the pancreas. *Vet Clin North Am Small Anim Pract* 32(6):1293-1312, 2002.

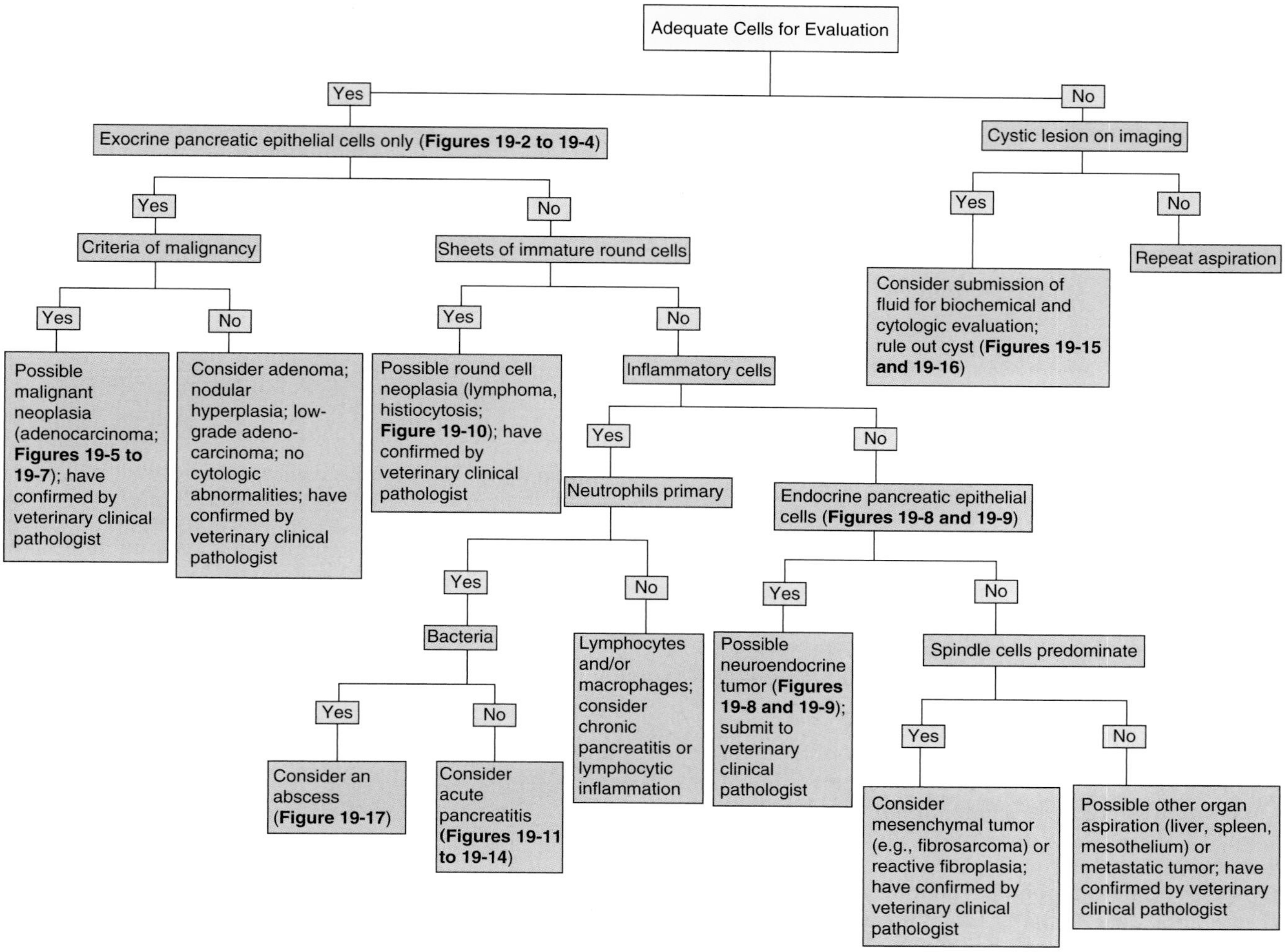

Figure 19-3 An algorithm to aid cytologic evaluation of pancreatic fine-needle aspirates.

Troubleshooting

In general, pancreatic tissue exfoliates well for FNA. In case of any concerns with regard to sample quality, a cytopathologist should be consulted about sample attainment and preparation. Ruptured cells may be the result of negative pressure in the syringe while aspirating or too much pressure on slides while making preparations.[16] Rapid drying of slides reduces refractile artifact on the slides. Hemodilution is common and generally will not confound diagnosis. However, if hemodilution is obscuring the diagnosis (especially distinguishing between blood contamination and inflammation), the number of times the needle is moved within the pancreas should be decreased. However, the tradeoff may be poor cytologic yield, which may occur if the needle biopsy technique is not aggressive enough. If clots tend to form, the needle and syringe should be flushed with an anticoagulant (i.e., ethylenediaminetetraacetic acid [EDTA]) prior to organ aspiration. Nondiagnostic samples because of poor cellularity may occur when lesions are fibrous or if the lesion was missed during aspiration. Nondiagnostic samples should be interpreted in light of imaging findings. Reaspiration may be attempted if the pancreas appears active and enlarged. However, if fibrosis is likely, intraoperative biopsy will likely be superior for obtaining a diagnosis. Cytologic findings should always be interpreted in light of imaging, physical examination, and biochemical findings. For example, if poorly cellular, proteinaceous fluid is obtained and the lesion on imaging is compatible with a cyst, then further diagnostics may not be warranted (Figure 19-3). However, if poorly cellular, proteinaceous fluid is obtained and the lesion is primarily solid or infiltrative with cystic or necrotic areas, reaspiration may be indicated because the primary lesion may not be represented.

Complications

Significant adverse effects secondary to percutaneous FNA of the pancreas in dogs or cats have not been reported. Rarely, FNA of the pancreas, in human beings, has been reported to cause complications, such as needle tract seeding of tumors, fistula formation, and ascites.[14] In one human study, complications arising from FNA of both solid and cystic lesions of the pancreas were noted in only 4 of 248 (1.2%) patients. These complications, which included acute pancreatitis and aspiration pneumonia, were noted only after aspiration of cystic lesions.[17] Recommendations from this study included avoiding needle

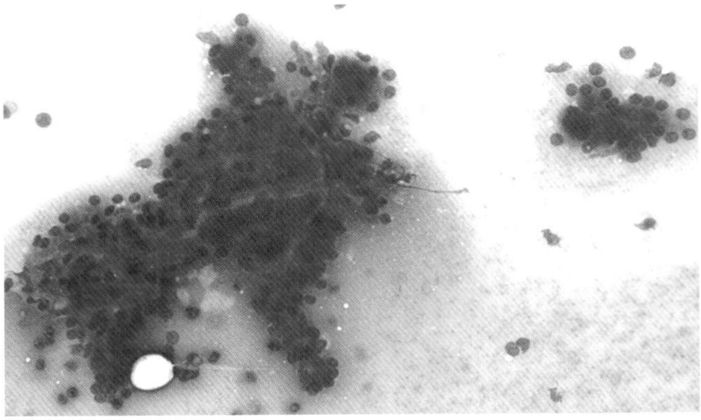

Figure 19-4 Fine-needle aspirate of normal canine pancreas. Exocrine epithelial cells predominate and often exfoliate in small sheets and large clusters with acinar and tubular formations. Cells are polyhedral, cytoplasm is abundant, nucleus-to-cytoplasm ratios are low, and nuclei are uniform. (Wright-Giemsa stain. Original magnification 200×.)

passage through the main pancreatic duct or branch ducts dilated proximal to an obstruction. In addition, aspiration was terminated if blood became visible in the syringe or if there was obvious hemorrhage within the target lesion.[17]

CYTOLOGIC EVALUATION

Normal

A decision tree to help guide initial cytologic evaluation of the pancreas is depicted in Figure 19-3. Exocrine epithelial cells are the most common cell type found on cytologic specimens from the pancreas. The background of the slide may contain blood from iatrogenic contamination, or it may be light pink, indicating a small amount of protein. Normal exocrine epithelial cells are found in small clusters to large sheets that may form tubular and acinar structures (Figure 19-4). On low magnification, the cytoplasm appears grainy with a pink hue because of the presence of small, pink zymogen granules. Unlike intestinal epithelial cells, cell-to-cell junctions are not prominent, giving cells a more indistinct, fluffy appearance (Figure 19-5). The cells are polyhedral, with abundant cytoplasm and a low nuclear-to-cytoplasmic ratio (Figure 19-4 Figure 19-5, and Figure 19-6). Nuclei are basilar in location, uniform, and round to oval. Chromatin is stippled to reticulate and a single, small, occasionally prominent nucleolus may be noted (Figure 19-5 and Figure 19-6). On high magnification, abundant pink, cytoplasmic granules, most consistent with membrane-bound zymogen granules, are noted. In preparations with abundant cell rupture, these granules may fill the background of the slide, giving a mottled blue-and-pink appearance (Figure 19-6). In a FNA of normal pancreas, no other cell populations will be present in high numbers. Occasionally, hematopoietic precursors, indicative of extramedullary hematopoiesis, small ductal cells, or uniform pancreatic endocrine cells, will be seen. The number of leukocytes present in the aspirate should be interpreted in light of peripheral blood cell counts to avoid interpreting peripheral neutrophilia or lymphocytosis as pancreatic inflammation.

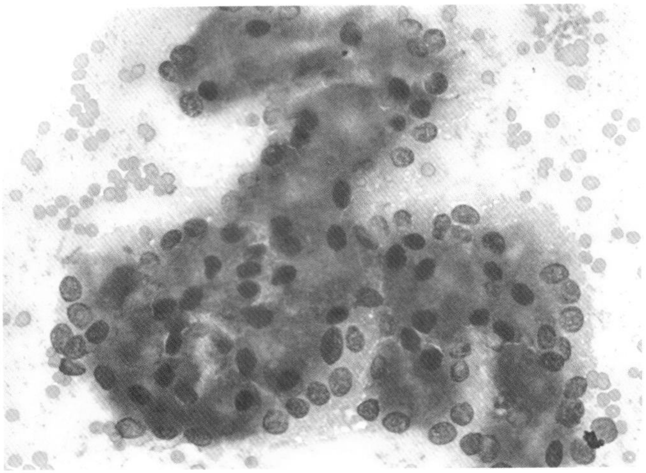

Figure 19-5 Fine-needle aspirate of normal feline pancreas. The nuclei of exocrine epithelial cells often show a basilar distribution. Clear cell-to-cell junctions are not apparent. Nuclei are round to oval, chromatin is stippled, and single, small, uniform nucleoli can be present. (Wright-Giemsa stain. Original magnification 500×.)

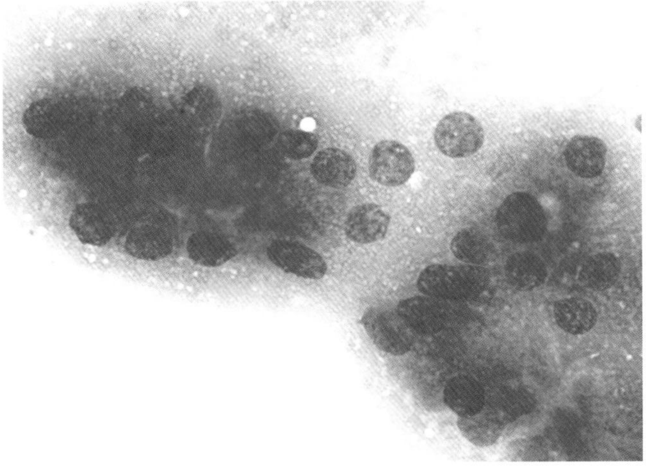

Figure 19-6 Fine-needle aspirate of normal canine pancreas. Exocrine epithelial cells are characterized by apical, abundant, small, pink cytoplasmic granules, most consistent with membrane-bound zymogen granules. These granules give densely packed pancreatic exocrine epithelial cells a pink hue at lower magnification. (Wright-Giemsa stain. Original magnification 1000×.)

Pancreatic Lesions

A summary of the World Health Organization (WHO) scheme for histologic classification of pancreatic lesions of domestic animals is summarized in Box 19-2.[18,19]

Neoplasia

Adenoma: Benign exocrine epithelial tumors (i.e., exocrine adenomas, ductal [tubular] adenomas, or acinar adenomas) are rare in small animals and far less common than their malignant counterparts. They are generally small, solitary lesions found incidentally on imaging or necropsy examination. Histologically, they are partially

BOX 19-2

Summary of World Health Organization Classification of Pancreatic Lesions in Small Animals

- Neoplastic lesions
- Exocrine epithelial tumors
  - Benign (e.g., adenoma)
  - Malignant (e.g., adenocarcinoma)
- Endocrine tumors (e.g., insulinoma, gastrinoma)
- Nonepithelial tumors (e.g., fibrosarcoma, metastatic lymphoma, hemangiosarcoma)
- Nonneoplastic lesions
- Nodular hyperplasia of acinar cells
- Acute pancreatitis
- Chronic pancreatitis
- Cyst (e.g., pseudocyst, congenital)
- Abscess

or totally encapsulated, distinguishing them from the more common lesion of nodular hyperplasia.[12,18,20] Cytologically, adenomas cannot be distinguished from normal or hyperplastic pancreatic tissue (Figure 19-3). If abundant, uniform, pancreatic exocrine epithelial cells are noted along with imaging findings suggestive of a solitary, solid lesion, differential diagnoses should include an adenoma, well-differentiated carcinoma, or a hyperplastic nodule (Figure 19-3).

Adenocarcinoma: Malignant tumors of the exocrine pancreas (i.e., adenocarcinomas, ductal [tubular] adenocarcinomas, or exocrine carcinomas) are rare in dogs and cats, with incidences of 17.8 in 100,000 patient years at risk in dogs and 12.6 in 100,000 patient years at risk in cats.[20,21] This is in contrast to human medicine, in which pancreatic malignant tumors are the fifth leading cause of cancer-related deaths in the United States, with ductal adenocarcinomas accounting for more than 90% of these malignancies.[21] The histiogenesis of adenocarcinomas in small animals remains uncertain. One author suggests that a ductular origin is likely based on tubular architecture, but ultrastructural analysis indicates that acinar cells may be the originator cell type, whereas other authors suggest that they may arise from either ductular or acinar epithelium, and often have features of both.[12,20]

In dogs, an increased incidence of pancreatic adenocarcinoma is seen with aging, and Airedale Terriers, Boxers, Labrador Retrievers, and Cocker Spaniels may be at increased risk.[21] In one study of 13 dogs and cats, the average age at diagnosis was 9 and 10 years of age for dogs and cats, respectively.[16] In another study, 85% of the dogs and cats with pancreatic adenocarcinoma had distant metastases at the time of diagnosis, and 88% of the patients had metastatic disease at the time of necropsy.[16] Common metastatic sites include abdominal or thoracic lymph nodes, mesentery, adjacent gastrointestinal (GI) organs (including liver, duodenum, and jejunum), lungs, and less frequently, spleen, kidney, and diaphragm.[16] Local, destructive infiltration may destroy the common bile duct.

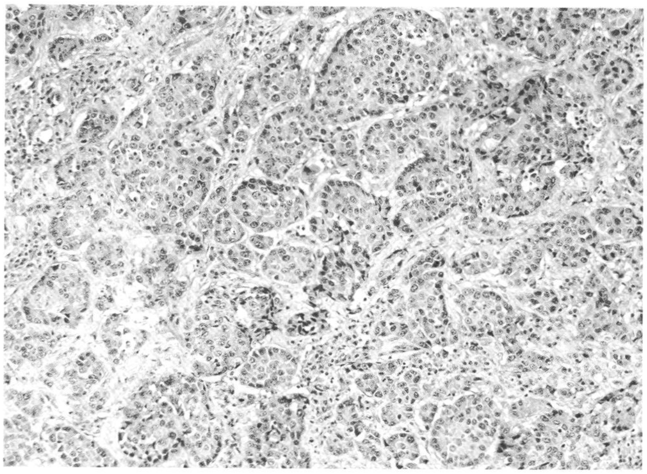

Figure 19-7 Histopathologic section of pancreatic carcinoma in a dog. The section is hypercellular and consists of variably disorganized acinar epithelial cells found in islands and primitive tubules. Neoplastic islands are separated by desmoplastic stroma (mesenchyme). A general loss of uniform acinar architecture occurs. Anisocytosis and anisokaryosis are noted along with increased nuclear to cytoplasmic ratio and large, pale nucleoli. (Hematoxylin and Eosin stain. Original magnification 100×.)

Clinical signs at the time of presentation are nonspecific, but weight loss, vomiting, abdominal pain, and anorexia are common. Jaundice and cholestasis may result from obstruction of the bile duct by tumor, secondary liver disease, or both. Clinicopathologic tests may show increases in pancreatic enzyme activity, but evidence of extrahepatic biliary obstruction, including elevations in alkaline phosphatase (ALP) and alanine aminotransferase (ALT) activities, is more frequently seen. A peripheral neutrophilia is often noted.[16] Described paraneoplastic syndromes include alopecia, exocrine pancreatic insufficiency, and cutaneous and visceral necrotizing panniculitis and steatitis.[22-24]

In dogs, pancreatic tumors frequently produce a mass, often in the midportion of the pancreas. In cats, tumors may be more diffuse and resemble nodular hyperplasia or chronic pancreatitis. Leakage of proteolytic enzymes from adenocarcinomas may be corrosive and result in cystic change in the primary tumor and necrotizing steatitis in the omental and peritoneal fat.[20] Histopathologically, pancreatic adenocarcinomas show a tremendous range of differentiation. Some are well-differentiated tubular adenocarcinomas that form acinar structures, whereas others may form more solid sheets of poorly differentiated cells that no longer resemble pancreatic acini (Figure 19-7). They may be associated with a dense supporting stroma with a resultant scirrhous reaction. Focal hemorrhage and necrosis may occur along with focal accumulations of inflammatory cells, including T-lymphocytes.[20]

Although pancreatic adenocarcinoma is far less common in dogs and cats than in humans, the majority of pancreatic neoplasms are malignant as in humans. Several studies of human pancreatic carcinoma have established objective cytologic criteria for the diagnosis of pancreatic carcinoma. The implementation of these criteria

BOX 19-3

Cytologic Criteria of Malignancy

- Nuclear crowding and overlap (oval, polygonal, angular nuclei)
- Anisokaryosis
- Nuclear membrane contour irregularities
- Prominent nucleoli (large and irregular)
- Single cells or loss of cellular cohesion
- Mitotic figures, especially aberrant mitoses
- Increased nucleus-to-cytoplasm ratio

have resulted in a relatively high diagnostic sensitivity and specificity for the diagnosis of pancreatic adenocarcinoma ranging from 80% to 98% and 93% to 100%, respectively.[25] Similar standard criteria have not been developed in veterinary medicine. Given the increasing popularity of pancreatic FNA, objective cytologic criteria to diagnose pancreatic malignancy could be established for dogs and cats. Until that time, the criteria stated in human-based studies are compatible with the important criteria of malignancy noted by the author.

Criteria of malignancy defining pancreatic adenocarcinoma are listed in Box 19-3. In the initial study, major criteria of malignancy included nuclear crowding and overlap (nuclei became oval, angular, and polygonal, rather than round), nuclear membrane contour irregularities (grooving, notching), and irregular chromatin distribution (more applicable with alcohol-fixed specimens). Minor criteria included nuclear enlargement (or anisokaryosis, defined as a nucleus >2.5 times the size of a red blood cell), single epithelial cells, necrosis, and mitoses.[26] Later studies confirmed the utility of these initial criteria and suggested additional criteria, including increased cellularity, anisocytosis, prominent macronucleoli (large and irregular), cytoplasmic vacuolation, and coarsely clumped chromatin patterns. Mitoses, especially abnormal mitoses, favored malignancy.[27,28] Combined, the strongest indicators of malignancy that define human pancreatic adenocarcinomas include anisokaryosis, loss of cellular cohesion (single cells are common), irregular nuclear contours, nuclear crowding, prominent nucleoli, and aberrant mitoses (see Box 19-3).[25-28]

Aspirates of pancreatic carcinoma in small animals are characterized by high cellularity (Figure 19-3, Figure 19-8, and Figure 19-9). Individual cells have an increased nuclear-to-cytoplasmic (N:C) ratios, and anisokaryosis is frequently marked (Figure 19-8, Figure 19-9, and Figure 19-10). Irregular nuclear contours and nuclear molding may be noted along with polygonal and angular nuclei (Figure 19-8, Figure 19-9, and Figure 19-10). Although cytoplasmic vacuolization is frequently noted (Figure 19-8, Figure 19-9, and Figure 19-10), it also occurs with epithelial reactivity secondary to pancreatitis. Chromatin varies from reticulated to coarsely clumped, and prominent, irregular, and occasionally multiple nucleoli may be present (Figure 19-9 and Figure 19-10). The background may be necrotic, hemodilute, inflamed (macrophages and small lymphocytes) (Figure 19-9), or pink and cystic-appearing (Figure 19-10). Cytologic evaluations of well-differentiated pancreatic adenocarcinomas may result in false-negative

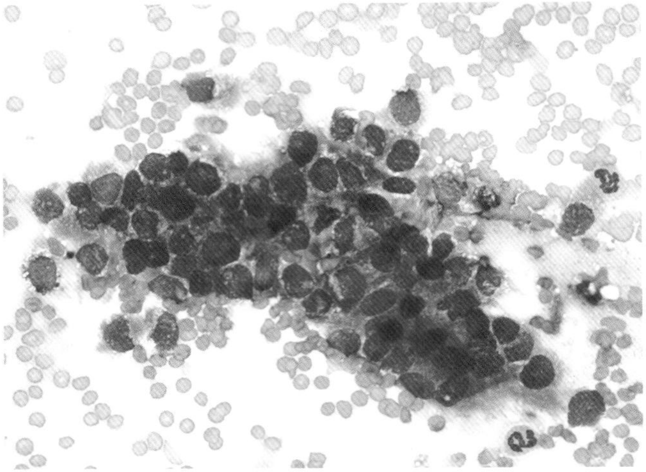

Figure 19-8 Fine-needle aspirate of pancreatic adenocarcinoma in a cat. These cells show a markedly increased nucleus-to-cytoplasm ratio and anisokaryosis. Additional criteria of malignancy include polygonal nuclei, nuclear overlap, irregular nuclear membranes, cytoplasmic vacuolization, and rare nucleoli. (Wright-Giemsa stain. Original magnification 500×.)

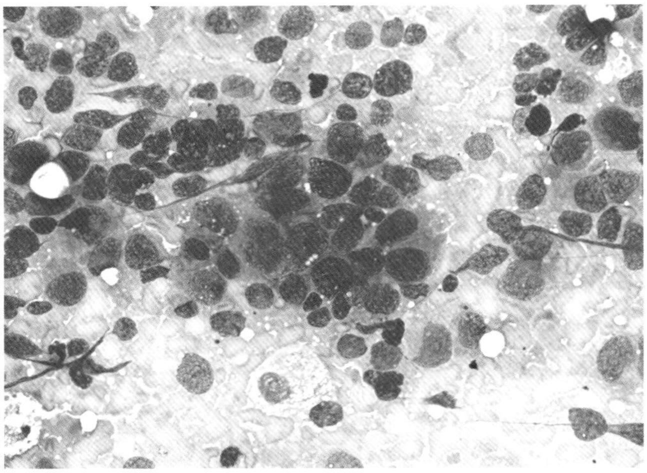

Figure 19-9 Fine-needle aspirate of pancreatic adenocarcinoma in a dog. Cells from this sample exfoliated in loosely cohesive sheets with many single cells present. Additional criteria of malignancy included marked anisokaryosis, increased nucleus-to-cytoplasmic ratios, nuclear crowding and molding, polygonal nuclei, punctate cytoplasmic vacuoles, and occasional nucleoli. (Wright-Giemsa stain. Original magnification 500×.)

cytologic interpretations. In one study, well-differentiated adenocarcinomas were differentiated from high-grade adenocarcinomas by the absence of necrosis, mitoses, and macronuclei.[25] Differential diagnoses for large sheets or clusters of fairly well-differentiated pancreatic epithelial cells should include normal pancreas, adenoma, nodular hyperplasia, or well-differentiated carcinoma (Figure 19-3).

Endocrine (Neuroendocrine) Tumors of the Pancreas: Neuroendocrine tumors of the pancreas (NETP) (i.e., tumors of pancreatic islet cells, islet cell adenomas, and

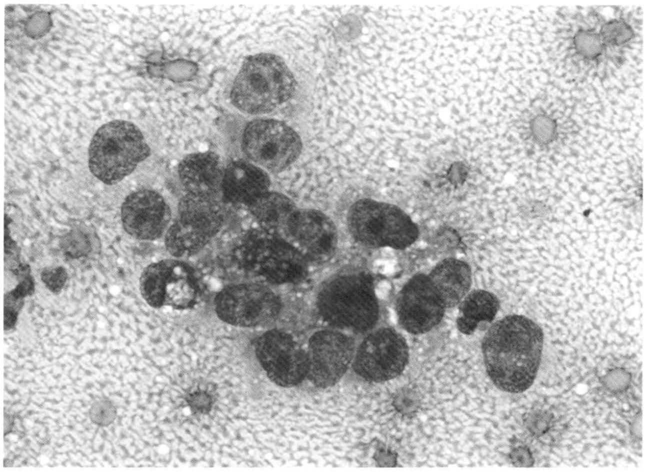

Figure 19-10 Fine-needle aspirate of pancreatic adenocarcinoma in a cat. This cluster of cells show marked nuclear and nucleolar criteria of malignancy. Note the markedly elevated nucleus-to-cytoplasm ratio, marked nuclear enlargement, irregular nuclear membrane contours, and prominent, deeply basophilic, single to multiple, occasionally irregular nucleoli. The dense, pink, stippled background of the slide may represent a cystic component to this neoplasm. (Wright-Giemsa stain. Original magnification 1000×.)

islet cell adenocarcinomas) include insulinomas (β-cell neoplasms), gastrinomas, somatostatinomas, glucagonomas, and carcinoid tumors.[19] In small animal patients, insulinomas are the most common NETP followed in frequency by gastrinoma. Somatostatinoma, glucagonoma, and carcinoid tumor are rarely or not yet reported in small animals. Most NETPs are multihormonal; as such, they may secrete or express one or more neuroendocrine markers, including pancreatic hormones (e.g., insulin, glucagon, pancreatic polypeptide, and somatostatin) and hormones not normally expressed in mammalian pancreas (e.g., gastrin, adrenocorticotropic hormone, and calcitonin). The majority of NETPs are immunohistochemically positive for insulin (89%), approximately 30% being positive for somatostatin, glucagon, and pancreatic polypeptide.[19,29] Amyloid deposits may be found in 17% to 32% of NETPs.[29]

Cytopathologists examining tissue from a pancreatic mass generally readily distinguish between tumors of the exocrine and endocrine (NETPs) pancreas (Figure 19-3). However, the biologic behavior of NETPs may be difficult to predict. Pancreatic NEPTs in human beings are classified as well-differentiated neuroendocrine tumors (benign, uncertain malignant potential, low-grade malignant) or poorly differentiated neuroendocrine carcinoma (high-grade malignant). Cytologic criteria are not used for distinguishing between these tumor types in humans. Rather, differentiation is based on tumor size, the presence of vascular invasion or metastases, the number of mitoses per high power field and the Ki67 proliferation index.[30] The degree of multihormonality and growth pattern show no correlation with biologic behavior.[29] In addition, cytologic features of the neoplastic cells are generally not helpful in differentiating between benign NETPs (islet cell adenomas) and their malignant counterparts (islet cell carcinomas) unless profound criteria of malignancy are met. The absence of anaplastic features cannot be used to rule out malignancy. Histologic evidence of invasion by the tumor cells through the capsule and into adjacent pancreatic parenchyma or lymphatics, or metastatic disease, are the most important criteria of malignancy for NETPs.[31,32] When the cytologic specimen is characterized by minimally pleomorphic neuroendocrine cells, in the absence of history or clinical findings, the cytologic diagnosis of neuroendocrine tumor or islet cell tumor is most appropriate.

Insulinomas are seen most frequently in dogs ages 5 to 12 years. Grossly, they appear as single, small nodules visible from the serosal surface of the pancreas; however, malignant tumors may be larger and multilobular and show extensive invasion into the adjacent parenchyma. Malignant insulinomas are more common than benign insulinomas in dogs.[31] In one study, 45% to 55% of insulin-producing NETPs were malignant in dogs (in contrast to 10% to 15% in human beings).[29] Metastasis to regional lymph nodes, liver, mesentery, and omentum is noted in about 50% of cases.[33] Many different breeds are affected; however, Boxers, Fox Terriers, Standard Poodles, and German Shepherds appear to be overrepresented. Both sexes appear to be affected equally.[31] Because most insulinomas are secretory, a tentative diagnosis may be made by demonstrating profound hypoglycemia and an abnormal insulin-to-glucose ratio. Surgical removal (partial pancreatectomy) may significantly increase median survival time.[33] In one study of dogs with insulinomas, it was reported that (1) dogs with higher preoperative serum insulin levels had shorter survival times, (2) dogs with tumors confined to the pancreas had longer disease-free intervals, and (3) younger dogs had significantly shorter survival time compared with older dogs.[33] Gastrinomas, although a rare tumor in veterinary medicine, frequently metastasize to regional lymph nodes and liver. Prognosis is considered grave.[32,34]

The cytologic and histologic appearance of NETPs is typical of other neuroendocrine tumors. They are generally highly cellular with prominent cellular dissociation, consisting of many single cells, small, poorly cohesive groups, or both (Figure 19-11; Figure 19-12). Aspirates frequently contain free (naked) nuclei embedded in a background of lightly basophilic cytoplasm (Figure 19-11 and Figure 19-12). Intact cells are of medium to large size with poorly defined cytoplasmic borders (Figure 19-11). The cytoplasm of intact cells is generally pale blue and may contain numerous small, punctate vacuoles (Figure 19-12). Anisokaryosis is usually mild to moderate, giving a monomorphic appearance to the cells (Figure 19-11 and Figure 19-12). Additional nuclear features may include nuclear molding, eccentrically placed nuclei (giving a plasmacytoid appearance), and binucleation. Chromatin is generally fine and granular with a single prominent nucleolus (Figure 19-11 and Figure 19-12).[12,33,35,36]

Nonepithelial Tumors: Nonepithelial pancreatic tumors in small animals are rare (Figure 19-3). Fibrosarcoma and multicentric system disease, including malignant histiocytosis, lymphoma (Figure 19-13), hemangiosarcoma, liposarcoma, malignant nerve sheath tumor, and malignant melanoma, have been described.[12,20,37] Bloodborne metastasis from thyroid and mammary gland carcinoma and direct extension from contiguous organs in alimentary

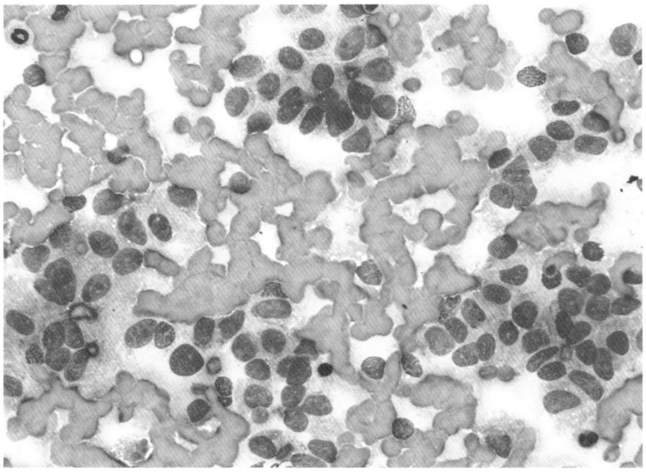

Figure 19-11 Fine-needle aspirate of a malignant insulinoma in a dog. The sample is highly cellular, with cells found in loosely cohesive groups. Cell-to-cell borders are indistinct, and free nuclei appear scattered in a mass of shared cytoplasm. Compared with adenocarcinomas, anisokaryosis is relatively mild, although rare large nuclei are noted. Overall, the cells have a monomorphic appearance. As with other neuroendocrine tumors, individual cells are generally nondescript. Definitive tumor classification can be made only in light of imaging findings, physical examination findings, and clinicopathologic data. This patient had a persistently low glucose of 23 milligrams per deciliter (mg/dL) (reference interval: 70-120 mg/dL) and a fasting insulin concentration of 138 international units per milliliter (IU/mL) (reference interval: 5-15 IU/mL). Necropsy confirmed metastases to mesenteric lymph nodes and liver. (Wright-Giemsa stain. Original magnification 500×.)

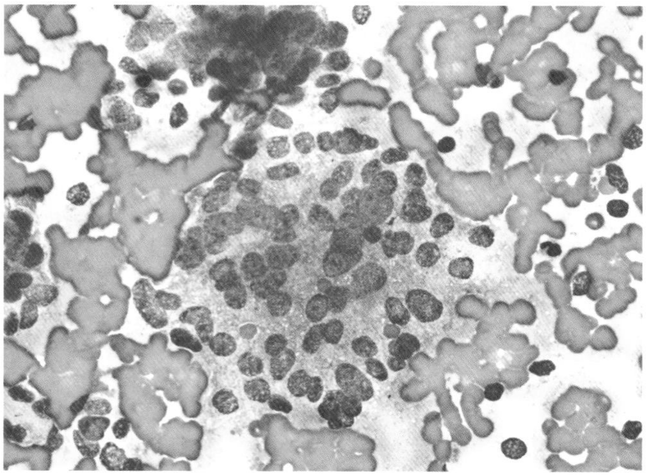

Figure 19-12 Fine-needle aspirate of a malignant insulinoma in a dog. A large cluster of cells is noted with free nuclei in a hemodiluted background. Individual cells have indistinct cytoplasmic borders, giving the appearance of naked nuclei in a sea of cytoplasm. In this case, anisokaryosis is moderate; nuclear crowding is evident; and single to multiple, small, deeply basophilic nucleoli are noted. Necropsy confirmed multiple metastatic lesions and positive immunohistochemical staining for insulin. (Wright-Giemsa stain. Original magnification 500×.)

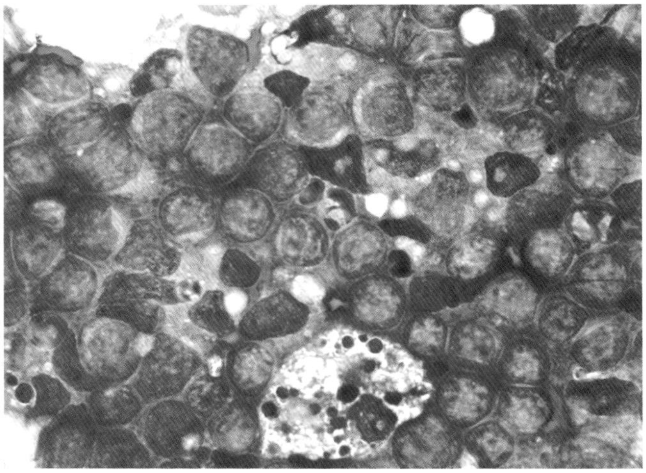

Figure 19-13 Fine-needle aspirate of pancreatic lymphoma in a dog. The sample is highly cellular; however, only rare pancreatic epithelial cells were noted in the aspirate (none are depicted in the image) as the pancreas was infiltrated with neoplastic lymphocytes. Individual lymphocytes are large and round with a small rim of basophilic cytoplasm. Chromatin is smooth, and single to multiple pale nucleoli are noted. A large macrophage or histiocyte is noted along with occasional dark, condensed, apoptotic cells. This patient had multisystemic lymphoma involving the liver, spleen, and pancreas at the time of presentation. (Wright-Giemsa stain. Original magnification 1000×.)

lymphoma and from carcinoma of gastric, duodenal or common bile duct origin have been noted.[18,38]

Nonneoplastic Lesions

Nonneoplastic lesions are common in the canine pancreas. Some initiative has been taken to develop a histopathologic grading classification scheme for exocrine pancreatic diseases in the dog.[3,39] In a published case series, the most common lesion was pancreatic hyperplastic nodules (80.2%), followed by lymphocytic inflammation (52.5%), fibrosis (49.5%), atrophy (46.5%), neutrophilic inflammation (31.7%), pancreatic fat necrosis (25.7%), pancreatic necrosis (16.8%), and edema (9.9%).[39]

Nodular Hyperplasia of Acinar Cells: Nodular hyperplasia of acinar cells (i.e., pancreatic exocrine nodular hyperplasia) is a common, often incidental, lesion in older dogs and cats (up to 80% of dogs may have nodular hyperplasia at necropsy).[40] In one study, the mean age of dogs with nodular hyperplasia was 9.5 years, whereas the mean age of dogs without nodular hyperplasia was 3.4 years.[40] Grossly, the lesion may be a solitary nodule or, more commonly, may appear as multiple, small, white to tan, well-circumscribed nodules. Ultrasonographically, nodular hyperplasia tends to manifest as multiple smaller lesions, compared with a single, large lesion for neoplasia; however, imaging findings for these entities overlap.[10] Histologically, nodular hyperplasia is distinguished from adenomas by their multiplicity, small size, lack of a capsule, and close resemblance to normal exocrine pancreatic tissue.[20,31] Fibrosis, atrophy, lymphocytic infiltration, or all of these may commonly accompany nodules.[39] These lesions are not preneoplastic, and patients are generally asymptomatic. Cytologically, nodular hyperplasia consists of sheets of well-differentiated exocrine pancreatic epithelial cells and, as such, is not distinguishable from an adenoma or well-differentiated carcinoma (Figure 19-3). In these cases, cytologic interpretation should be done in light of imaging findings.

Pancreatitis

Acute Pancreatitis: In human beings, a uniform classification system has been developed for pancreatitis.[41] *Acute pancreatitis* is defined as an acute inflammatory process (usually neutrophilic) of the pancreas, with variable involvement of other regional tissues or remote organ systems that does not lead to permanent changes. In dogs, neutrophilic inflammation may be associated with necrosis (pancreatic necrosis, pancreatic fat necrosis, or both).[39] *Chronic pancreatitis* is defined as a chronic inflammatory process (usually lymphocytic) of the pancreas, with variable involvement of other regional tissues or remote organ systems that leads to permanent changes, mainly fibrosis or atrophy and adhesions.[41] In addition, *acute necrotizing pancreatitis* is a severe form of acute pancreatitis, which is characterized by extensive pancreatic and peripancreatic necrosis, with severe forms progressing to dissolution of pancreatic parenchyma with accompanying hemorrhage, interstitial fluid accumulation, and deposition of fibrin and leukocytes.[41,42] This classification scheme may be loosely applied to both cats and dogs that manifest acute, uncomplicated pancreatitis; acute necrotizing pancreatitis; and chronic (fibrosing) pancreatitis.[12]

Pancreatitis is the most frequent disease process of the exocrine pancreas in dogs. For many canine patients, physical examination, biochemical testing, and imaging studies are adequate to support the diagnosis of acute pancreatitis in the absence of pancreatic cytologic evaluation.[2,3,11,39] However, increasingly, FNA of the pancreas is recommended to confirm the diagnosis, rule out secondary disease processes such as underlying neoplasia, or both.

Acute pancreatitis appears to be both less common and more difficult to diagnose in the cat.[5,6,8] Ultrasonography is of only moderate utility in the diagnosis of pancreatitis in cats. In one study, results of ultrasonography were consistent with a diagnosis of pancreatitis in only 7 of 20 cats with acute pancreatic necrosis.[6] In addition, in cats with clinical signs of pancreatitis, serum concentration of feline trypsin-like immunoreactivity was poorly associated with histopathologic diagnosis.[7] Together, findings suggest that feline acute necrotizing pancreatitis and chronic nonsuppurative pancreatitis cannot be reliably distinguished from each other or from other primary pancreatic diseases on the basis of history, physical examination findings, clinicopathologic testing, radiographic abnormalities, or ultrasonographic abnormalities.[5] As such, cytology may play a larger role in distinguishing between pancreatic inflammation and other pancreatic disorders (especially neoplasia) in feline patients. In cats, pancreatitis, pancreatic necrosis, pancreatic degeneration, or all of these may also occur in association with other diseases, including toxoplasmosis, hepatic lipidosis, feline infectious peritonitis, Easter lily toxicosis, and virulent systemic feline calicivirus infection.[43,44] Therefore, concurrent cytologic evaluation of the pancreas and other organs, notably the liver, the GI system, or both may prove useful for evaluating pancreatic manifestations of systemic disease. Histologically, acute pancreatitis consists of neutrophilic inflammation associated with interstitial edema, steatitis, and necrosis of mesenteric fat (Figure 19-14; Figure 19-15).[4] However, as with dogs, some degree of pancreatic inflammation, necrosis, fibrosis, or all of these is a very common histopathologic finding at necropsy, even with no clinical evidence of pancreatic disease. As such, the cytologic diagnosis of pancreatic inflammation should not be based solely on the number of inflammatory cells present but also on concurrent abnormalities, including necrosis, hemorrhage, epithelial reactivity, or all.

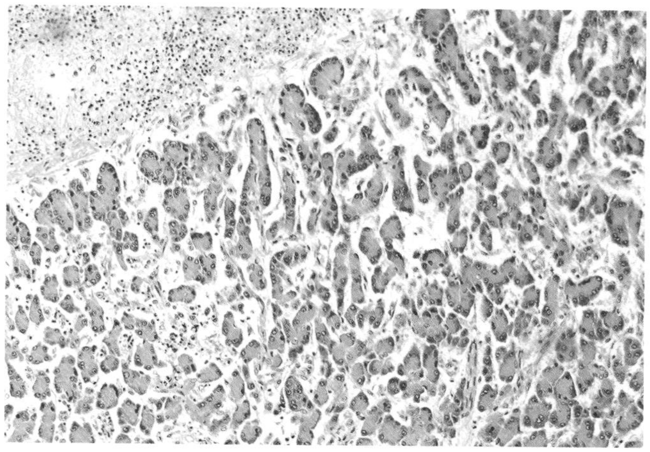

Figure 19-14 Histopathologic section of necrotizing pancreatitis in a dog. The section consists of relatively uniform tubulacinar secretory units separated by pale-pink material consistent with edema. Infiltrating neutrophils are focally abundant (*upper left area of section*) and dissect through pancreatic acinar cells. Multifocal clusters of acinar cells are degenerate and necrotic. (Hematoxylin and Eosin stain. Original magnification 100×.)

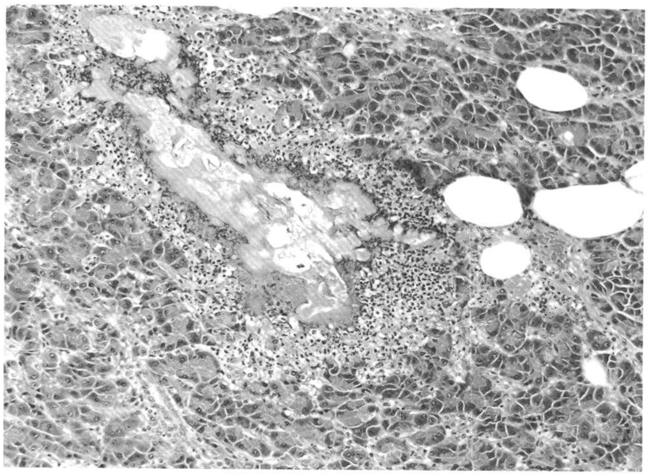

Figure 19-15 Histopathologic section of suppurative pancreatitis in a dog. The section consists of mildly atypical tubulacinar secretory units with a large focus of suppurative inflammation surrounding an area of eosinophilic material lacking histologic detail (fat necrosis, *center*). Areas of dissecting fibrosis (*upper right*) are also noted along with small areas of hemorrhage and mineralization. (Hematoxylin and Eosin stain. Original magnification 100×.)

Aspirates are generally highly cellular and characterized by abundant exocrine epithelial cells and a population of inflammatory cells (Figure 19-3; Figure 19-16). Neutrophils predominate in acute or acute necrotizing pancreatitis. The neutrophils are classically nondegenerate; however, they may appear ragged and mild to moderately degenerate, likely secondary to concurrent necrosis (Figure 19-16; Figure 19-17). Neutrophils are frequently noted in large aggregates, occasionally embedded in necrotic or cystic-appearing debris (see Figure 19-14, Figure 19-15, Figure 19-16, Figure 19-17, and Figure 19-19). The background may contain amorphous blue to pink material consistent with necrosis (see Figure 19-19) or aggregates of crystalline, clear material consistent with calcific debris (Figure 19-18). Necrosis may be accompanied by hemorrhage, as evidenced by activated, vacuolated, and hemosiderin-laden macrophages. Golden heme breakdown products may also be noted (Figure 19-19). Epithelial cells often appear atypical and reactive. They may have deeply

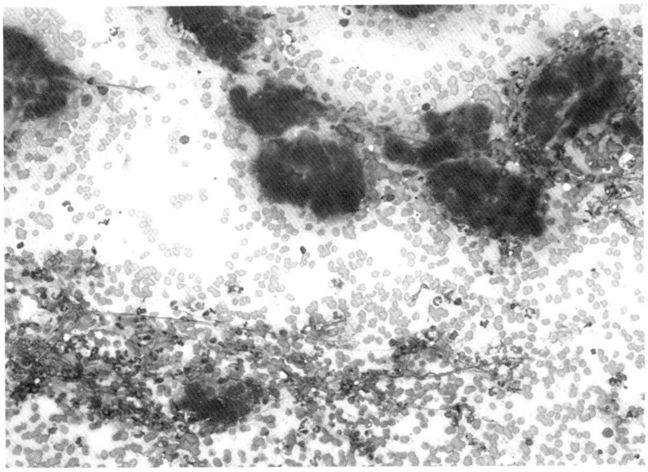

Figure 19-16 Fine-needle aspirate of acute pancreatitis in a dog. The sample consists of multiple cell populations, including exocrine pancreatic epithelial cells and mixed, primarily neutrophilic, inflammatory cells. Epithelial cells are highly cohesive. They have abundant pink or blue cytoplasm and a low nucleus-to-cytoplasm ratio. Inflammatory cells are present in large aggregates surrounding and adjacent to epithelial cells. (Wright-Giemsa stain. Original magnification 200×.)

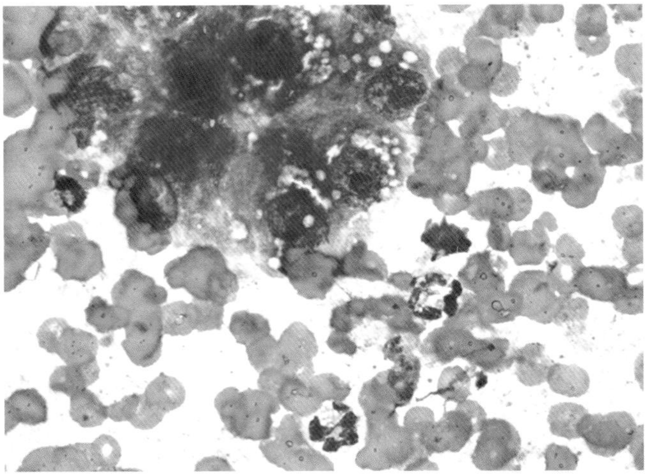

Figure 19-17 Fine-needle aspirate of acute pancreatitis in a dog. The sample consists of multiple cell populations. Note that the neutrophils appear ragged and one neutrophil contains clear, punctate cytoplasmic vacuoles. Epithelial cells are atypical and reactive (deeply basophilic) with some criteria of malignancy, including prominent nucleoli. In the absence of inflammation, these cellular changes could be mistaken as indicative of malignancy. (Wright-Giemsa stain. Original magnification 1000×.)

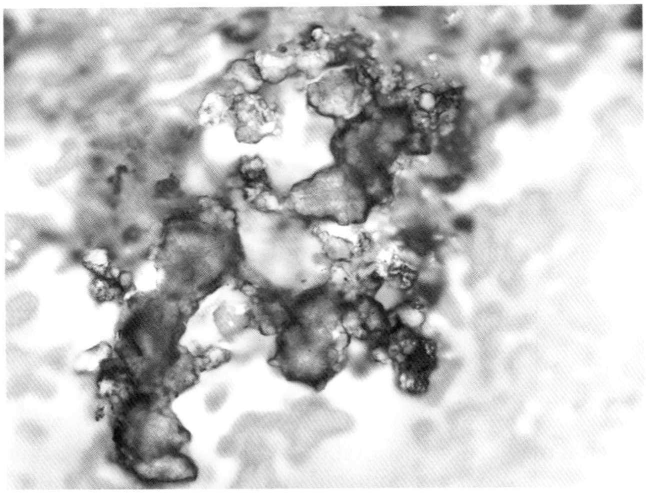

Figure 19-18 Calcific or mineralized debris obtained from fine-needle aspirate of canine pancreas. This debris is often multidimensional and refractile. It may be noted in large chunks, as depicted, or scattered throughout the background as crystalline material. It appears to be primarily associated with necrosis; however, it is not indicative of any specific pancreatic disorder. In this case, it was associated with necrotizing pancreatitis; however, it may also be noted if the necrotic center of a pancreatic adenocarcinoma is aspirated. (Wright-Giemsa stain. Original magnification 500×.)

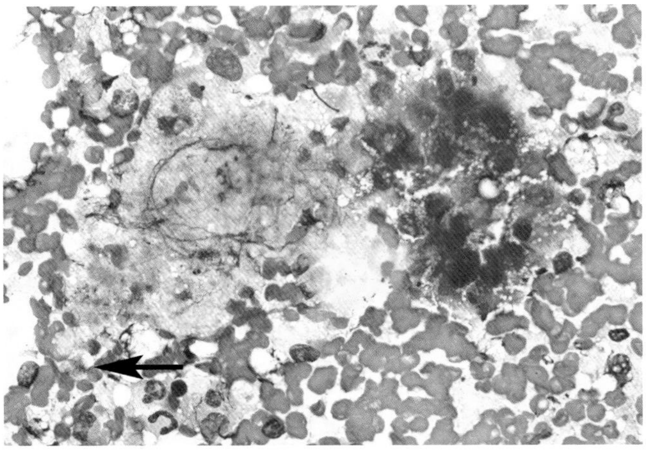

Figure 19-19 Fine-needle aspirate of acute pancreatitis in a dog. This aspirate was characterized by reactive, deeply basophilic, and atypical epithelial cells admixed with mixed inflammatory cells in a background of amorphous pink and blue material consistent with necrotic and cystic debris. Golden heme breakdown products were also noted consistent with hemorrhage (*arrow*). (Wright-Giemsa stain. Original magnification 500×.)

basophilic cytoplasm (with fewer distinct pink granules), cytoplasmic vacuolation, increased N:C ratios, and even prominent or small multiple nucleoli (see Figure 19-17). Although generally mild, the epithelial atypia can be fairly marked and may result in a false-positive diagnosis of pancreatic carcinoma if the presence of inflammatory cells or other evidence of pancreatitis is lacking (e.g., necrosis, hemorrhage, or fibrosis). Thus, distinguishing between pancreatitis with marked epithelial reactivity and pancreatic carcinoma with secondary inflammation and necrosis may present a challenge and should be recognized as a potential pitfall in the cytologic diagnosis of pancreatic disease. Finally, pancreatitis may be accompanied by ascites. This effusion is generally a modified transudate or a nonseptic, purulent exudate with neutrophils that have punctate clear, cytoplasmic vacuoles. The effusion may have a proteinaceous background that is basophilic or "dirty" and may indicate saponified fat.

Chronic Pancreatitis or Lymphocytic Inflammation: Histopathologically, chronic pancreatitis is characterized by focal aggregation of ducts and endocrine cells set in fibrous tissue infiltrated by chronic inflammatory cells.[18] Cavalier King Charles Spaniels, Collies, and Boxers may be predisposed to chronic pancreatitis, and Cocker Spaniels appear to have an increased relative risk of combined acute and chronic pancreatitis.[45] In addition, a chronic pancreatitis in English Cocker Spaniels that displays a periductular distribution of fibrosis and inflammation (primarily CD3+ T-lymphocytes) with duct destruction has been described. This duct destruction is evidently typical of autoimmune pancreatitis in humans.[46] The histopathologic lesions of chronic pancreatitis in cats are similar to chronic pancreatitis in humans with cystic degeneration and fibrosis being more prominent than inflammatory changes.[4] On imaging, the pancreas may appear fibrotic, nodular, or atrophied. As such, FNA of the lesions associated with chronic pancreatitis is rarely performed. Described morphologic features of chronic pancreatitis include low numbers of mixed acinar and ductal epithelial cells; mild epithelial reactivity or atypia (demonstrated by slight nuclear enlargement and slight nuclear contour irregularities); mixed inflammatory cells, especially small lymphocytes; calcified debris; and, possibly, wispy pink fibrous material (Figure 19-1).[47] Unfortunately, underlying carcinoma may be associated with, or surrounded by, lesions compatible with acute and chronic pancreatitis, which leads to a potential sample bias.

Occasionally, lymphocytic inflammation of the pancreas that is not associated with chronic pancreatitis may be noted. Considerations for increased numbers of small, well-differentiated lymphocytes in a pancreatic aspirate include lymphocytic inflammation of pancreatic islets associated with diabetes, underlying viral disease, or small cell lymphoma (see Figure 19-3).[48] In a cat with diabetes, it was hypothesized that immune-mediated islet cell destruction could have contributed to β-cell depletion.[48] However, inflammatory destruction of insulin-producing cells has not been proven to be involved in development of diabetes in cats.

Pancreatic Cysts: Pancreatic cysts are subcategorized into congenital cysts, acquired retention cysts, and pseudocysts. Congenital cysts have been rarely described in small animals.[49] Similarly, acquired retention cysts are rare. Pseudocysts are also rare but are the most common pancreatic cystic lesion seen in small animals.[49,50] In human beings, pseudocysts are a common sequela to acute and chronic pancreatitis. Pseudocysts are lined by granulation tissue and contain pancreatic enzymes and debris. They are suspected to result from the release of pancreatic secretions into the periductular connective tissue during an episode of acute pancreatitis. This may also hold true for dogs and cats; in one retrospective study, all 6 animals had a clinical diagnosis of pancreatitis.[50] Pseudocysts can be safely aspirated.[50,51] In addition, preferential localization of pseudocysts to the left pancreatic limb may occur.[50,51] Their fluid contents may be measured for amylase and lipase activities, and cytology may be performed to rule out an abscess. In one retrospective study, 6 animals had high lipase activity in the pseudocyst fluid, and in 2 dogs and 1 cat, the lipase activity in the fluid was greater than in serum.[50] Low pancreatic enzyme activity suggests a cystic neoplasm, whereas high levels of pancreatic enzyme activity suggest a pseudocyst. In human beings, many pseudocysts resolve spontaneously; however, they may also hemorrhage, rupture, or become secondarily infected.

Regardless of ontogeny, the cytologic appearance of cyst fluid derived from the pancreas is similar to that of cysts from any organ or structure. Aspirated samples are generally of low cellularity with a light-pink to deep-blue background that may contain abundant amorphous or crystalline debris (Figure 19-3; Figure 19-20 and Figure 19-21). Nucleated cells consist of rare nondegenerate neutrophils and occasional macrophages (Figure 19-20). Macrophages may be cytophagic, including erythrophagocytic or hemosiderin-laden, if hemorrhage is present (Figure 19-21). Pseudocyst fluid is aseptic and may have elevated total protein concentration. Cytologic evaluation of cystic

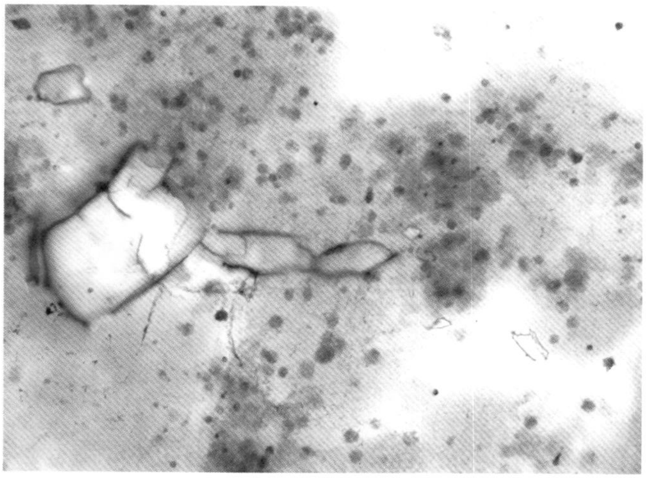

Figure 19-20 Fine-needle aspirate of a pancreatic cyst in a dog. The sample is of low cellularity with amorphous cellular and crystalline debris in a dense pink background. Epithelial cells are generally absent. Differential diagnoses should include a primary cyst (the type of cyst cannot be determined on cytologic examination alone) or cystic neoplasm. (Wright-Giemsa stain. Original magnification 500×.)

fluid from the pancreas is most useful in ruling out other significant differential diagnoses for fluid-filled masses of the pancreas, including abscesses and cystic neoplasms.

Pancreatic Abscesses: Primary pancreatic abscesses in small animals are rare. Sources of infection for abscesses include the biliary tract, the transverse colon, or the bloodstream. Aspirates of abscesses are highly cellular and dominated by degenerate neutrophils (Figure 19-3; Figure 19-22). Because of cell fragility, the slide background is frequently characterized by lysed nuclear and cellular debris. Neutrophil nuclei are swollen (degenerate) and intracellular bacteria may be seen (Figure 19-3; Figure 19-22 [*arrow*]). The absence of bacteria does not rule out an abscess; as such, if an abscess is suspected based on clinical or imaging findings, culture and sensitivity are warranted. The cytologic distinction between an abscess and acute pancreatitis is not always straightforward. Occasionally, an abscess may be characterized by nondegenerate neutrophils and scattered reactive epithelial cells in the absence of bacteria. This is most likely if the patient has been, or is currently being, treated with antibiotics. As such, differential diagnoses for purulent inflammation should include an abscess or acute pancreatitis in the absence of additional cytologic clues.

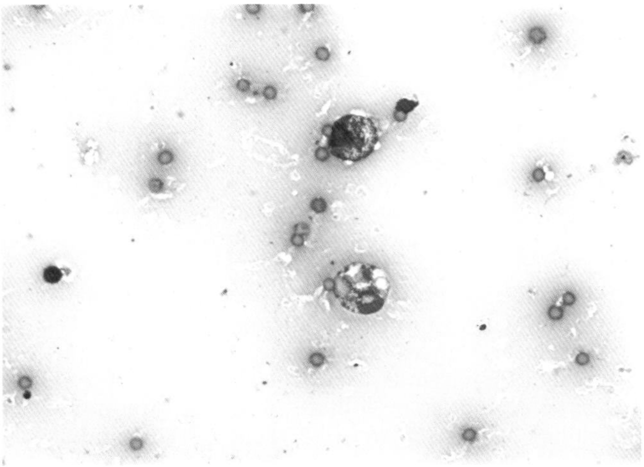

Figure 19-21 Fine-needle aspirate of a pancreatic cyst with mild hemorrhage in a cat. Samples are characterized by low cellularity and primarily activated erythrophagocytic macrophages. The background contains rare red blood cells and pink stippling consistent with increased protein. (Wright-Giemsa stain. Original magnification 500×.)

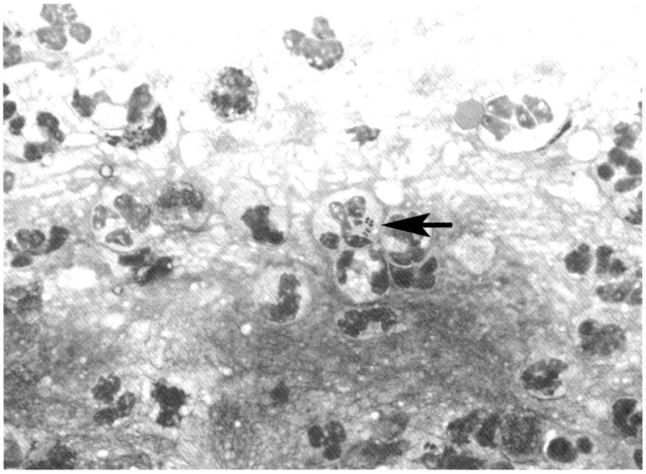

Figure 19-22 Fine-needle aspirate of a pancreatic abscess in a dog. The sample is highly cellular and dominated by degenerate neutrophils with swollen nuclei. Intracellular coccoid bacteria are present (*arrow*). As a result of cell fragility, the background contains abundant lysed nuclear and cellular material. This dog had a history of chronic pancreatic cyst. (Wright-Giemsa stain. Original magnification 1000×.)

ACKNOWLEDGEMENT

The author would like to thank Dr. Eric Johnson for the helpful review of the sampling technique section and Dr. Brian Murphy for review of histopathology images and figure legends.

References

1. Cordner AP, Armstrong PJ, Newman SJ, et al: Effect of pancreatic tissue sampling on serum pancreatic enzyme levels in clinically healthy dogs, J Vet Diagn Invest 22:702.
2. Steiner JM, Newman S, Xenoulis P, et al: Sensitivity of serum markers for pancreatitis in dogs with macroscopic evidence of pancreatitis, *Vet Ther* 9:263, 2008.
3. Trivedi S, Marks SL, Kass PH, et al: Sensitivity and specificity of canine pancreas-specific lipase (cPL) and other markers for pancreatitis in 70 dogs with and without histopathologic evidence of pancreatitis, *J Vet Intern Med* 25:1241.
4. De Cock HE, Forman MA, Farver TB, et al: Prevalence and histopathologic characteristics of pancreatitis in cats, *Vet Pathol* 44:39, 2007.
5. Ferreri JA, Hardam E, Kimmel SE, et al: Clinical differentiation of acute necrotizing from chronic nonsuppurative pancreatitis in cats: 63 cases (1996-2001), *J Am Vet Med Assoc* 223:469, 2003.
6. Saunders HM, VanWinkle TJ, Drobatz K, et al: Ultrasonographic findings in cats with clinical, gross pathologic, and histologic evidence of acute pancreatic necrosis: 20 cases (1994-2001), *J Am Vet Med Assoc* 221:1724, 2002.
7. Swift NC, Marks SL, MacLachlan NJ, et al: Evaluation of serum feline trypsin-like immunoreactivity for the diagnosis of pancreatitis in cats, *J Am Vet Med Assoc* 217:37, 2000.
8. Xenoulis PG, Steiner JM: Current concepts in feline pancreatitis, *Top Companion Anim Med* 23:185, 2008.
9. Hecht S, Henry G: Sonographic evaluation of the normal and abnormal pancreas, *Clin Tech Small Anim Pract* 22:115, 2007.
10. Hecht S, Penninck DG, Keating JH: Imaging findings in pancreatic neoplasia and nodular hyperplasia in 19 cats, *Vet Radiol Ultrasound* 48:45, 2007.
11. Hess RS, Saunders HM, Van Winkle TJ, et al: Clinical, clinicopathologic, radiographic, and ultrasonographic abnormalities in dogs with fatal acute pancreatitis: 70 cases (1986-1995), *J Am Vet Med Assoc* 213:665, 1998.
12. Jones TC, Hunt RD, King NW: *Veterinary pathology*, ed 6, Baltimore, MD, 1997, Williams & Wilkins.
13. Bacha WJ, Bacha LM: *Color atlas of veterinary histology*, ed 2, Baltimore, MD, 2000, Lippincott Williams & Wilkins.
14. Bjorneby JM, Kari S: Cytology of the pancreas, *Vet Clin North Am Small Anim Pract* 32(6):1293–1312, 2002.

15. Iseri T, Yamada K, Chijiwa K, et al: Dynamic computed tomography of the pancreas in normal dogs and in a dog with pancreatic insulinoma, *Vet Radiol Ultrasound* 48:328, 2007.
16. Bennett PF, Hahn KA, Toal RL, et al: Ultrasonographic and cytopathological diagnosis of exocrine pancreatic carcinoma in the dog and cat, *J Am Anim Hosp Assoc* 37:466, 2001.
17. O'Toole D, Palazzo L, Arotcarena R, et al: Assessment of complications of EUS-guided fine-needle aspiration, *Gastrointest Endosc* 53:470, 2001.
18. Head KW, Cullen J, Dubielzig RR, et al: *WHO histological classification of tumors of the alimentary system of domestic animals*, Washington DC, 2003, Armed Forces Institute of Pathology.
19. Kiupel M, Capen CC, Miller M, et al: *Histological classification of tumors of the endocrine system of domestic animals, World Health Organization international histological classification of tumors of domestic animals*, vol 12, Washington, D.C., 2008, Armed Forces Institute of Pathology.
20. Head KW, Else RW, Dubielzig RR: Tumors of the alimentary tract. In Meuten DJ, editor: *Tumors in domestic animals*, Ames, IA, 2002, Iowa State Press.
21. Priester WA: Data from eleven United States and Canadian colleges of veterinary medicine on pancreatic carcinoma in domestic animals, *Cancer Res* 34:1372, 1974.
22. Tasker S, Griffon DJ, Nuttall TJ, et al: Resolution of paraneoplastic alopecia following surgical removal of a pancreatic carcinoma in a cat, *J Small Anim Pract* 40:16, 1999.
23. Bright JM: Pancreatic adenocarcinoma in a dog with a maldigestion syndrome, *J Am Vet Med Assoc* 187:420, 1985.
24. Fabbrini F, Anfray P, Viacava P, et al: Feline cutaneous and visceral necrotizing panniculitis and steatitis associated with a pancreatic tumour, *Vet Dermatol* 16:413, 2005.
25. Lin F, Staerkel G: Cytologic criteria for well differentiated adenocarcinoma of the pancreas in fine-needle aspiration biopsy specimens, *Cancer* 99:44, 2003.
26. Robins DB, Katz RL, Evans DB, et al: Fine needle aspiration of the pancreas: in quest of accuracy, *Acta Cytol* 39:1, 1995.
27. Eloubeidi MA, Jhala D, Chhieng DC, et al: Yield of endoscopic ultrasound-guided fine-needle aspiration biopsy in patients with suspected pancreatic carcinoma, *Cancer* 99:285, 2003.
28. Ylagan LR, Edmundowicz S, Kasal K, et al: Endoscopic ultrasound guided fine-needle aspiration cytology of pancreatic carcinoma: a 3-year experience and review of the literature, *Cancer* 96:362, 2002.
29. Minkus G, Jutting U, Aubele M, et al: Canine neuroendocrine tumors of the pancreas: a study using image analysis techniques for the discrimination of metastatic versus nonmetastatic tumors, *Vet Pathol* 34:138, 1997.
30. Verbeke CS: Endocrine tumours of the pancreas, *Histopathology* 56:669.
31. Capen CC: Tumors of the endocrine gland. In Meuten DJ, editor: *Tumors in domestic animals*, Ames, IA, 2002, Iowa State Press.
32. Tobin RL, Nelson RW, Lucroy MD, et al: Outcome of surgical versus medical treatment of dogs with beta cell neoplasia: 39 cases (1990-1997), *J Am Vet Med Assoc* 215:226, 1999.
33. Caywood D, Klausner J, O'Leary T, et al: Pancreatic insulin-secreting neoplasms: clinical, diagnostic, and prognostic features in 73 dogs, *J Am Anim Hosp Assoc* 24:577, 1988.
34. Green RA, Gartrell CL: Gastrinoma: a retrospective study of four cases (1985-1995), *J Am Anim Hosp Assoc* 33:524, 1997.
35. Ardengh JC, de Paulo GA, Ferrari AP: EUS-guided FNA in the diagnosis of pancreatic neuroendocrine tumors before surgery, *Gastrointest Endosc* 60:378, 2004.
36. Jimenez-Heffernan JA, Vicandi B, Lopez-Ferrer P, et al: Fine needle aspiration cytology of endocrine neoplasms of the pancreas. Morphologic and immunocytochemical findings in 20 cases, *Acta Cytol* 48:295, 2004.
37. Hayden DW, Waters DJ, Burke BA, et al: Disseminated malignant histiocytosis in a golden retriever: clinicopathologic, ultrastructural, and immunohistochemical findings, *Vet Pathol* 30:256, 1993.
38. Swann HM, Holt DE: Canine gastric adenocarcinoma and leiomyosarcoma: a retrospective study of 21 cases (1986-1999) and literature review, *J Am Anim Hosp Assoc* 38:157, 2002.
39. Newman SJ, Steiner JM, Woosley K, et al: Histologic assessment and grading of the exocrine pancreas in the dog, *J Vet Diagn Invest* 18:115, 2006.
40. Newman SJ, Steiner JM, Woosley K, et al: Correlation of age and incidence of pancreatic exocrine nodular hyperplasia in the dog, *Vet Pathol* 42:510, 2005.
41. Bradley EL 3rd: A clinically based classification system for acute pancreatitis. Summary of the International Symposium on Acute Pancreatitis, Atlanta, GA, September 11 through 13, 1992, *Arch Surg* 128:586, 1993.
42. Newman S, Steiner J, Woosley K, et al: Localization of pancreatic inflammation and necrosis in dogs, *J Vet Intern Med* 18:488, 2004.
43. Rumbeiha WK, Francis JA, Fitzgerald SD, et al: A comprehensive study of Easter lily poisoning in cats, *J Vet Diagn Invest* 16:527, 2004.
44. Pesavento PA, MacLachlan NJ, Dillard-Telm L, et al: Pathologic, immunohistochemical, and electron microscopic findings in naturally occurring virulent systemic feline calicivirus infection in cats, *Vet Pathol* 41:257, 2004.
45. Watson PJ, Roulois AJ, Scase T, et al: Prevalence and breed distribution of chronic pancreatitis at post-mortem examination in first-opinion dogs, *J Small Anim Pract* 48:609, 2007.
46. Watson PJ, Roulois A, Scase T, et al: Characterization of chronic pancreatitis in English Cocker Spaniels, *J Vet Intern Med* 25:797, 2011.
47. Afify AM, al-Khafaji BM, Kim B, et al: Endoscopic ultrasound-guided fine needle aspiration of the pancreas: diagnostic utility and accuracy, *Acta Cytol* 47:341, 2003.
48. Hall DG, Kelley LC, Gray ML, et al: Lymphocytic inflammation of pancreatic islets in a diabetic cat, *J Vet Diagn Invest* 9:98, 1997.
49. Coleman MG, Robson MC, Harvey C: Pancreatic cyst in a cat, *N Z Vet J* 53:157, 2005.
50. VanEnkevort BA, O'Brien RT, Young KM: Pancreatic pseudocysts in 4 dogs and 2 cats: ultrasonographic and clinicopathologic findings, *J Vet Intern Med* 13:309, 1999.
51. Hines BL, Salisbury SK, Jakovljevic S, et al: Pancreatic pseudocyst associated with chronic-active necrotizing pancreatitis in a cat, *J Am Anim Hosp Assoc* 32:147, 1996.

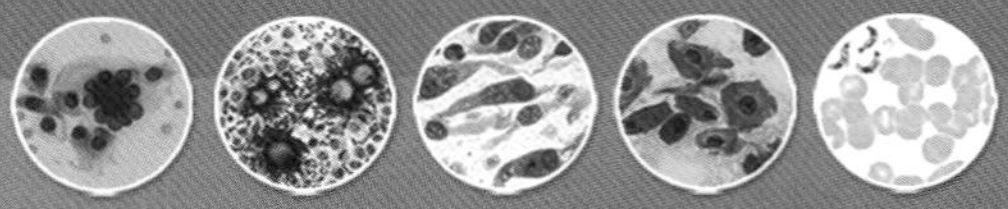

CHAPTER 20

The Liver

Tara P. Arndt and Sonjia M. Shelly

The liver is one of the most important organs and is involved in almost all functions of the living body, and as such, liver disease is commonly encountered in small animal veterinary medicine. Liver disease may be nonspecific and have many effects on other body systems, resulting in systemic alterations with various manifestations. Liver disease is often identified using a combination of data obtained from clinical signs (such as icterus, ascites, abnormal fecal or urine characteristics, gastrointestinal [GI] signs, weight loss, bleeding dyscrasias), blood work (e.g., elevated liver enzymes, altered hepatic function tests), imaging study abnormalities (e.g., radiography, ultrasonography, or computed tomography [CT]). These results may indicate liver disease in generic terms and, once identified, often requires additional diagnostics to arrive at a definitive diagnosis.

Cytologic examination of samples from the hepatobiliary system complements other diagnostic procedures and, in some cases, provides the specific, definitive diagnosis. Specimens for cytologic examination may be collected by percutaneous fine-needle aspiration (FNA), percutaneous needle core biopsy, or surgical biopsy. Cytologic examination of material collected by FNA or fine-needle biopsy (FNB), which are relatively inexpensive and safe procedures, determine whether additional sampling or exploratory surgery is warranted. Collection and examination of cytologic samples are most commonly performed on patients with nodular lesions, abnormal echogenicity, or generalized or lobar liver enlargement. It may also be used prior to therapy in patients with persistently increased liver enzymes or to stage certain neoplastic conditions such as lymphoma and mast cell neoplasia. The increasing availability of imaging procedures such as ultrasonography and CT, to direct specimen collection via FNA and FNB has increased the accuracy of sampling nodular lesions, thereby increasing the diagnostic acuity of liver cytology. Studies reported in the literature have shown that the accuracy of cytologic interpretations is greatest for diffuse hepatic disease and neoplasia, and least sensitive for subtle inflammatory conditions.[1,2]

Evaluation of hepatobiliary tissue by cytology should be preceded by assessment for abnormal liver size or function via physical examination, hematologic and clinical chemistry enzyme and function tests, and radiographic or ultrasound examinations. Cytologic examination is the logical next step when working through the differential diagnoses of suspected parenchymal, inflammatory, or neoplastic liver disease.

SAMPLING TECHNIQUES

Various techniques for percutaneous sampling of the hepatobiliary system have been described.[3-6] Complications following these procedures are rare and include hemorrhage and potential seeding of needle tracts with neoplastic cells. As compromised hemostasis is a life-threatening concern in animals with liver disease, the risk for prolonged or excessive bleeding should be assessed, particularly in cats with prolonged anorexia and in severely ill patients.[4,7] A thorough history taking should include querying the owner about any prior bleeding episodes or current treatment with prescribed or over-the-counter drugs such as aspirin or ibuprofen, which may alter normal coagulation. This is followed by a complete physical examination and laboratory testing to evaluate platelet number (platelet count or estimate from a peripheral blood smear), buccal mucosal bleeding time (BMBT), and coagulation assays (prothrombin time [PT], activated partial thromboplastin time [APTT], and protein-induced vitamin K absence). It must be kept in mind that normal coagulation testing profiles do not exclude potential bleeding episodes.[8] It is pragmatic to avoid aspirating the highly vascular liver if severe coagulation abnormalities, clinical signs of hemorrhage elsewhere in the body, or both exist. If a liver aspirate is deemed an acceptable risk in a patient with mildly prolonged coagulation tests, it is prudent to perform it early in the day so that the hematocrit can be followed and interventional treatments performed if excess bleeding is detected.

FNA and FNB are often performed using ultrasound guidance, especially when nodular lesions are detected. Sensitive imaging procedures such as ultrasonography facilitate accurate sampling of the liver, including sites with normal and abnormal echogenecity.[3,4] Blind sampling may be done with the patient in dorsal or right lateral recumbency but also in the standing position; chemical restraint may be unnecessary for some patients. With the patient in dorsal recumbency, a blind biopsy is performed by inserting (at a 30- to 45-degree angle to the skin in dogs, and almost vertically in cats) midway between the left costal arch and the end of the xiphoid process.[2] If the animal is standing or lying on the right side, the collection site is found by percussing the intercostal spaces to locate the liver beneath the rib cage. The next intercostal space caudal to the space where the sound of percussion changes from resonant to dull is usually a satisfactory site for aspiration. The collection site may be determined by palpation if an enlarged liver extends beyond the rib cage in which case the site would be just caudal to the costal arch.[5] In some cases, the clinician may sample on the right side at the tenth intercostal space at the level of the rib-cartilage junction.[5]

Cells from the hepatobiliary system may be aspirated using a 21- to 22-gauge, 1 to 2½-inch hypodermic needle and a 6- or 12-milliliter (mL) syringe. Alternatively, a 22-gauge spinal needle with a stylet may be used. The stylet prevents obstruction of the needle as it penetrates the body wall. With the needle in the liver, samples are aspirated by rapidly withdrawing the plunger of the syringe to the 5- or 6-mL mark. The suction is gently released before the needle is withdrawn. The specimen will consist of small pieces of parenchymal tissue mixed with fresh blood. Once the needle is withdrawn, the syringe should be detached and filled with 1 to 2 mL of air. After reattaching the syringe to the needle, a small drop of sample (6 to 8 millimeter [mm] diameter) is expelled onto each of several glass slides. The drops are placed near the center of the slide and spread gently into a smear by the squash method (see Chapter 1).

The liver may also be sampled by a nonaspiration technique, using a 26-gauge needle only, as described in Chapter 1. This method may reduce the amount of blood contamination but may result in exfoliation of fewer hepatobiliary cells.[5]

Smears of liver biopsies are prepared by imprinting the tissue on clean glass slides or by gently rolling a core of tissue along a slide. The surface of the tissue to be imprinted should be lightly blotted with absorbent, lint-free paper before the smears are made. Small fragments of tissue may be manipulated with fine forceps or skewered on a clean 25-gauge hypodermic needle, which provides a convenient handle for touching the cut surface of the specimen to the slides. Two to three impressions should be made on each of several slides, taking care to use minimal pressure to avoid crush artifact.

Smears should be dried thoroughly prior to placing in a protective slide case. Slides should be protected from exposure to formalin fumes or excess moisture, which may be detrimental to sample quality. Typically, if several smears are available, one or two may be stained in-house with a routine quick Romanowsky-type stain and then examined for cellularity. Additional unstained smears should be retained so that special stains can be performed later, if indicated. It is also possible to destain slides and re-apply special stains such as Fites, GMS (Gomori methenamine silver), rubeanic acid, or rhodamine, as indicated, after examination with Romanowsky-type stain.

MAJOR CYTOLOGIC CLASSIFICATIONS OF LIVER PROCESSES

Hepatocellular changes may be classified into many categories, and the major classifications will be described and illustrated in the following chapter.

Normal Liver

To accurately interpret hepatic aspirates, normal hepatocytes and biliary epithelium as well as normal parenchymal features should be recognized. Aspirates and impressions from normal livers consist largely of hepatocytes and variable amounts of peripheral blood. Hepatocytes exfoliate readily and are distributed in the smear as single cells, as sheets, and in cords and clusters. Normal hepatocytes are fairly uniform, large, round, or slightly oval to polyhedral cells that have round, centrally placed nuclei, with stippled coarse chromatin and a single large prominent nucleolus (Figure 20-1). Their abundant cytoplasm

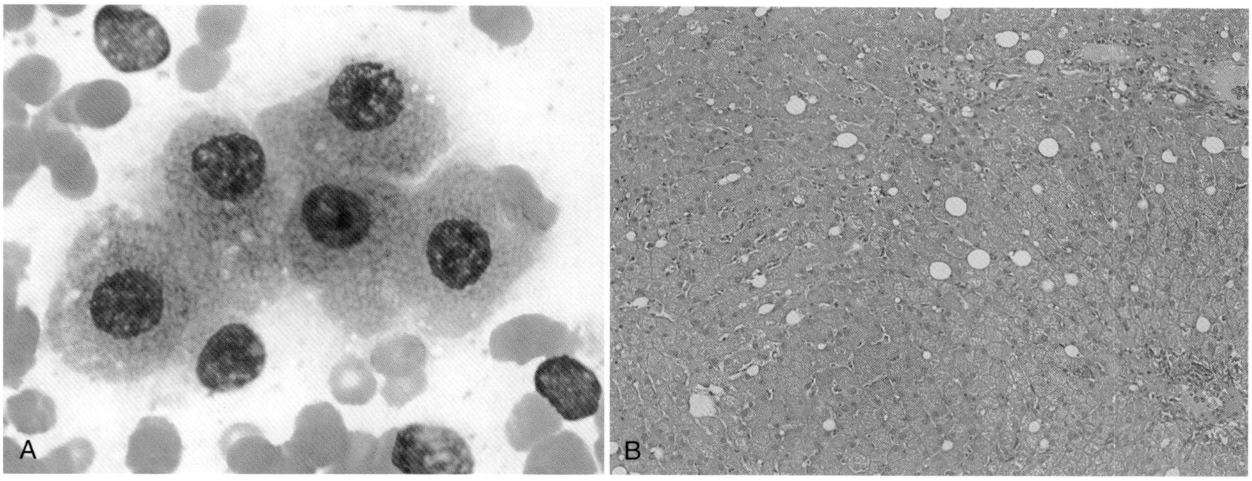

Figure 20-1 A, Cytologically normal hepatocytes from a dog. These cells may be from a normal liver, or an unaffected area of a diseased liver. Normal-appearing hepatocytes may be seen in areas of hyperplastic nodules, hepatic adenoma, or well-differentiated hepatic carcinoma. (Wright stain. Original magnification 400×.) B, Normal canine liver histology. (H&E stain. Original magnification 200×.)

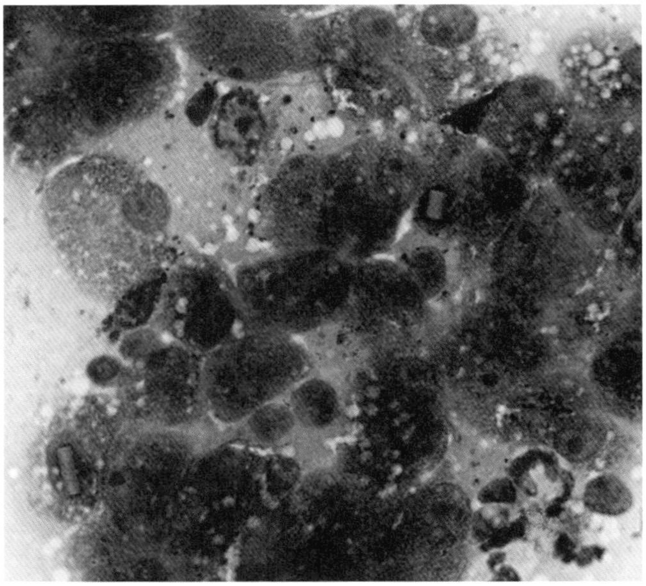

Figure 20-2 Liver aspirate from a 12-year-old Labrador Retriever presented for vomiting. Hyperplastic hepatocytes with occasional resident well-granulated mast cells are present (also note the intranuclear crystalline inclusions). (Wright stain. Original magnification 1000×.)

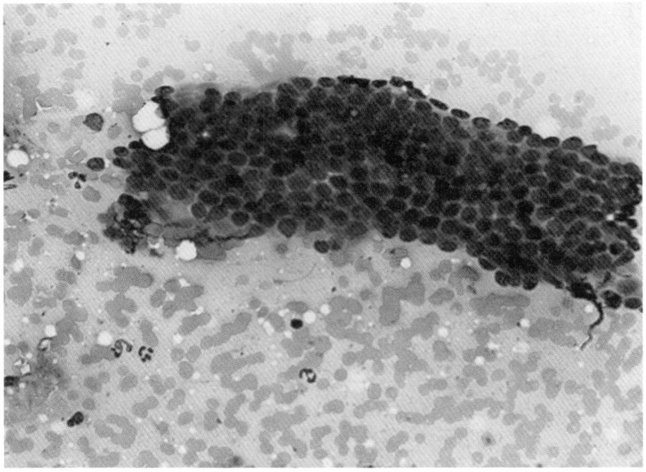

Figure 20-3 Normal biliary tract epithelial cells. Note the flat sheet of cuboidal to low columnar cells in a tubular structure and low numbers of neutrophils. (Wright stain. Original magnification 500×.)

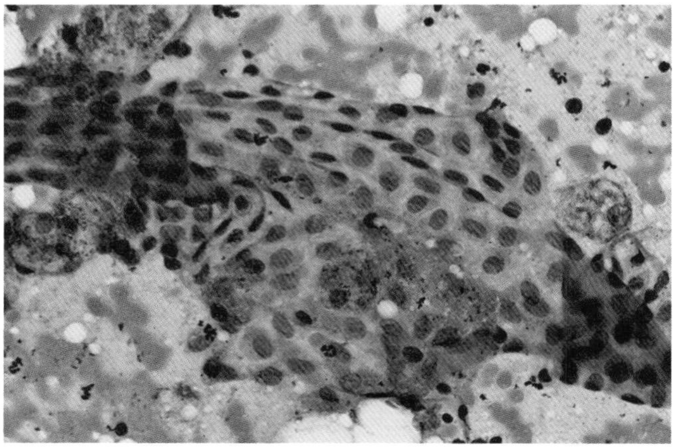

Figure 20-4 Liver aspirate from a dog. Note the regular angular cellular characteristics of exfoliated mesothelium and few normal hepatocytes. (Wright stain. Original magnification 500×.)

contains many ribosomes, which stain blue and other organelles that are unstained or slightly pink, giving the overall color of the cytoplasm in most normal hepatocytes a grainy light blue or lavender, with faint pink cytoplasmic granules. Hepatocytes in large clusters, which resist flattening, have a deeper blue cytoplasm compared with single cells or cells in flattened sheets. In older animals, pigment granules may be seen in the cytoplasm of the hepatocytes (see the section titled "Pigments" below). Nuclei typically are centrally located, uniform in size, and have coarsely reticular chromatin. A single nucleolus is often visible; however, in some intact cells, this may be obscured by heterochromatin. The nucleoli are more easily seen in the nuclei of ruptured or understained cells. Low numbers of binucleate hepatocytes are commonly present in liver aspirates from older dogs, and few rectangular crystalline intranuclear inclusions may also be noted (Figure 20-2). The pathologic significance of these inclusions is not clear; however, they are felt to be increased in cases of chronic liver insult or disease.[9] In some cases of canine herpes virus -1 or adenovirus (infectious canine hepatitis), viral intranuclear inclusions are identified and must be differentiated from cytoplasmic invaginations into the nucleus.[9]

Several other cell types are commonly encountered in normal liver aspirates. Biliary tract epithelial cells appear as uniform cuboidal to short columnar cells in small clusters or flat sheets (Figure 20-3). Rarely, distinct tubular arrangements may be seen. Biliary cells have a high nucleus-to-cytoplasm (N:C) ratio; have round, central nuclei with dense smooth chromatin; and scant pale blue cytoplasm, which distinguishes them from noticeably larger hepatocytes. Mesothelial cells may be difficult to distinguish from biliary epithelial cells but are generally larger, polygonal to spindloid, and found in flat sheets with a mosaic pattern (Figure 20-4). Occasional samples may include extrahepatic tissue such as adipocytes, lipid, or both when mesenteric fat is inadvertently aspirated. Most cytologic preparations of liver aspirates will contain some peripheral blood, and normal blood leukocytes are expected in numbers consistent with the complete blood count (CBC). Mast cells are normal resident perivascular cells, and therefore, with the highly vascular nature of the liver, few are anticipated in normal dog and cat liver aspirates (see Figure 20-2).

Resident hepatic macrophages (Kupffer cells) may be aspirated from normal liver, and rare lipid-laden Ito cells may be identified in some aspirates. In cats, low numbers of lymphocytes may also be seen and are of equivocal significance because a few lymphocytes may be found in the portal triads in healthy animals.[10]

A common and significant artifact of ultrasound-guided liver biopsies is the inadvertent contamination

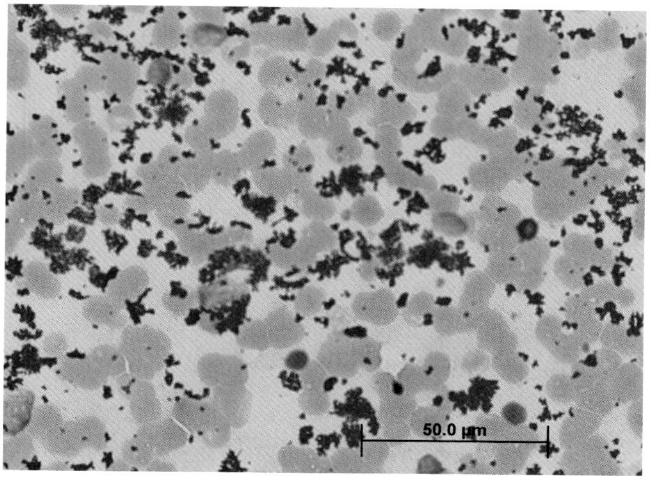

Figure 20-5 Ultrasound gel may be a common artifact obscuring sample detail and must be correctly identified. Canine liver. (Wright stain. Original magnification 1000×.)

with ultrasound gel. After staining with Romanowsky-type stains, this material often appears globular and dark magenta to metachromatic and may be mistaken for mast cell granules or large granules in lymphocytes. The presence of this material in samples may vary from slight interference of staining and appreciation of cellular detail to completely obscuring the sample (Figure 20-5). Ultrasound gel has been reported to cause cellular disruption in human cytology samples.[11] In the experience of the chapter authors, this also occurs in veterinary cytology specimens; however, this has not been documented in domestic animal cytology preparations.

Pigments

Several different pigments may be seen within hepatocytes in cytologic preparations and may be a normal finding or associated with extrahepatic or intrahepatic disease. The most common pigments include bile pigment, hemosiderin, lipofuscin, and copper. Specific staining is often required for differentiation, as in a recent study, it was determined that the blue-green pigment often interpreted as bile is, in fact, lipofuscin.[12] Differentiating the pigments solely on the basis of routine staining with Romanowsky stains such as Wright-Giemsa or modified Wright-Giemsa (Diff-Quik, Leukostat, or Quik-Dip) may be difficult, and special stains may be employed for specific identification, when required.

Bile Pigment: Bile accumulation within hepatocytes is recognized as variably sized, dark-green to black granules in cytologic preparations and yellow to green-brown on standard hematoxylin and eosin (H&E) histologic sections (Figure 20-6). Abundant intracytoplasmic bile pigment is suggestive of cholestasis and may precede hyperbilirubinemia and clinical icterus. More significant accumulations of bile result in bile-filled cannalicular plugs, which are easily recognized on cytologic preparations (Figure 20-7). In some cases, the cause of cholestasis may be determined by an accompanying inflammatory or neoplastic infiltrate; in other cases, the cause is not readily identified.

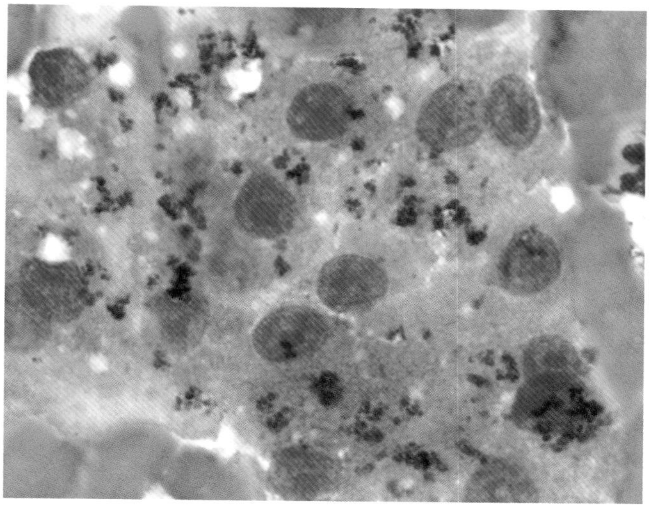

Figure 20-6 Liver aspirate from a dog with elevated γ-glutamyl transferase (GGT). Dark-green to black granular pigment suggests bile pigment, which is readily observed in cholestasis. (Wright stain. Original magnification 400×.)

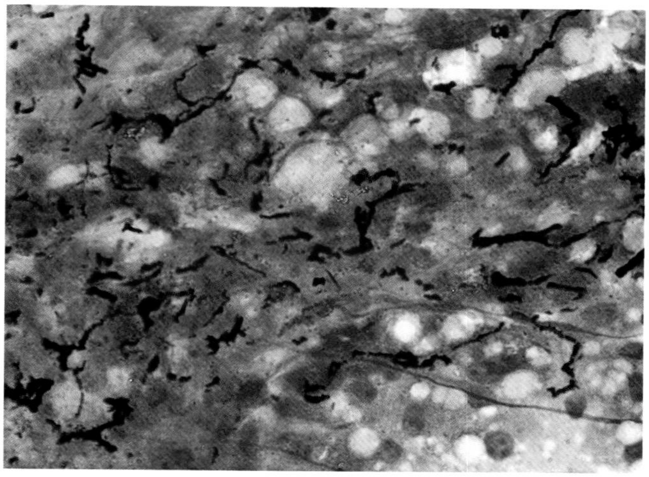

Figure 20-7 Liver aspirate from a 10-year-old dog on chemotherapy for high-grade lymphoma. Cholestasis and prominent bile cannalicular plugs are identified as intact and fragmented tubular accumulations of dark blue-green pigment. (Wright stain. Original magnification 1000×.)

Lipofuscin: Lipofuscin is a "wear and tear" pigment, composed of accumulated indigestible cellular residue within autophagolysosomes. Large amounts may be seen in hepatocytes from older cats and dogs. This is a normal feature of aging and does not represent a pathologic process. Granules of lipofuscin are similar in size to bile pigment and hemosiderin and range from brownish to blue-green (Figure 20-8). Lipofuscin is yellow-brown on standard H&E staining of histologic sections and often centrilobular in location. On the basis of one study, lipofuscin is the pigment most commonly observed within canine hepatocytes and correlates with a lack of supportive evidence of cholestasis such as hyperbilirubinemia, bile cannalicular plugs, or casts.[12] Lipofuscin granules specifically stain red with a modified Ziehl-Neelsen stain or Luxol fast blue.

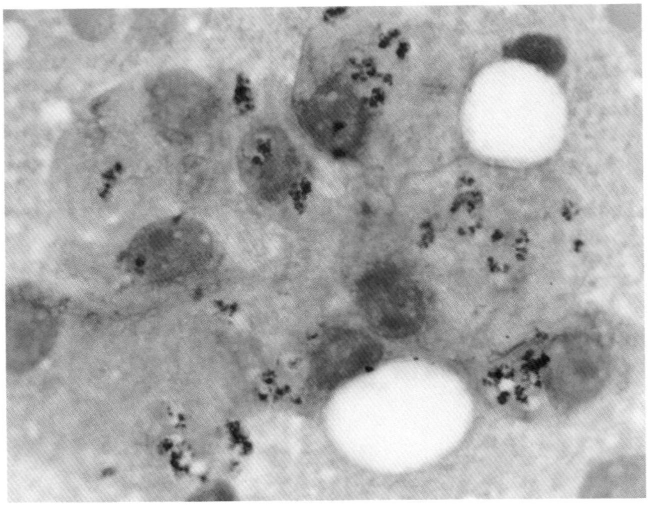

Figure 20-8 Liver aspirate from a 12-year-old dog with a hyperplastic hepatic nodule. The dark blue-green pigment in these canine hepatocytes is lipofuscin. (Wright stain. Original magnification 1000×.)

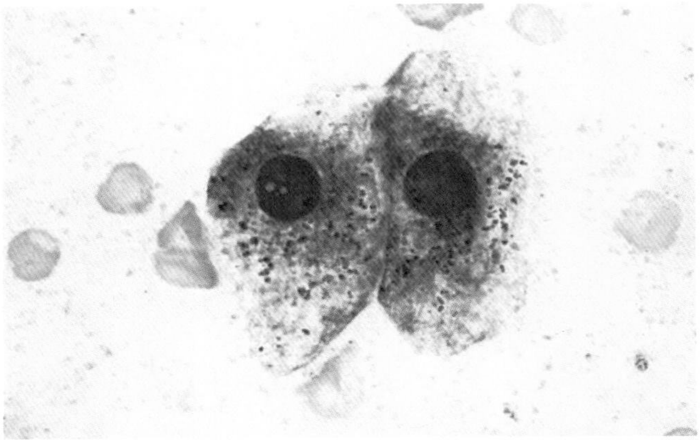

Figure 20-9 Hemosiderin may be recognized as golden-brown globular in hepatocytes. (Wright stain. Original magnification 400×.)

Hemosiderin: Hemosiderin is a globular, insoluble, iron-containing material, which appears golden-brown in hepatocytes (Figure 20-9) with Romanowsky-type stains and dark-blue with Prussian Blue stain. Histologically, with H&E staining, iron appears golden brown and refractile. In many cases, increased hemosiderin in hepatocytes is associated with increased iron turnover caused by hemolytic anemia or ineffective erythropoiesis (such as immune-mediated nonregenerative anemia). Iron also may accumulate because of decreased iron utilization associated with severely decreased erythropoiesis (pure red blood cell [RBC] aplasia, aplastic anemia). Repeated blood transfusions or administration of iron-containing compounds (especially by injection) also may increase hepatic iron content. In macrophages, hemosiderin may vary from gold to brown-black, depending on the amount within the cell. Macrophages containing phagocytized RBCs, hemosiderin, or both are concomitant findings in many patients with hemolytic or hemophagocytic disease.

Copper: When present in large amounts, copper may be visible in hepatocytes as coarsely clumped, refractile, pale blue-green cytoplasmic granules (Figure 20-10, *A*). Liver smears may be stained with rubeanic acid to confirm the presence of copper (see Figure 20-10, *B*). Large amounts of copper are often associated with a primary copper-accumulation hepatopathy.[9] Small amounts of stainable copper may be seen secondary to prolonged cholestatic liver disease and in cases of chronic hepatitis. Primary copper hepatopathy has been reported as a familial condition in Bedlington Terriers because of a genetic mutation in the *COMM-D* gene. This gene produces a defective protein involved in copper transport; thus, excessive copper accumulation occurs in the liver. Copper accumulation also seems to be familial in West Highland White Terriers, Skye Terriers, Doberman Pinschers, Labrador Retrievers, and Dalmations.[5,9,13-15] Copper-associated hepatopathy in a young Siamese cat has also been reported.[16] Excess copper in hepatocytes leads to injury or necrosis with inflammation.

NONNEOPLASTIC DISORDERS AND CONDITIONS

Degenerative Conditions

Hepatocellular vacuolar degeneration is a common yet nonspecific cytologic finding, and it results from the intracellular deposition of glycogen, lipid, or water and is recognized as either discrete, round vacuoles or poorly circumscribed, pale, feathery areas within the cytoplasm (Figure 20-11 and Figure 20-12). Hepatocellular steatosis may be seen as macrovesicular (vacuoles larger than the nucleus) or microvesicular (vacuoles smaller than the nucleus) inclusions. Microvesicular lipidosis is seen with more severe hepatocellular dysfunction and is correlated with lipid accumulation in mitochondria.[5] Discrete round vacuoles indicate lipid, whereas the less defined areas of feathery change or rarefaction often represent increased glycogen or water (hydropic degeneration) resulting from hypoxemia, cholestasis, or toxin exposure. If needed, lipid may be confirmed by staining an unfixed cytology smear with Sudan III; and glycogen may be confirmed by periodic acid-Schiff (PAS) staining. The most common vacuolar change recognized cytologically is hepatic lipidosis in feline samples and glucocorticoid-induced hepatopathy in canine liver aspirates.

In cats, hepatomegaly caused by the accumulation of fat in the liver is recognized as the syndrome of feline hepatic lipidosis (steatosis). In this condition, often a combination of macrovesicular and microvesicular vacuole accumulation occurs. Development of this disorder generally is triggered by a period of anorexia causing a catabolic state.[17] Primary lipidosis may be a result of inadequate food from owner-directed rapid weight loss, unacceptable food change, unintended food withdrawal, or stress. Secondary hepatic lipidosis may be affiliated with underlying systemic disease (lymphoma, pancreatitis, cholangiohepatitis, etc.).[5] Affected cats are often icteric and have enlarged livers caused by extensive, diffuse accumulation of lipid within hepatocytes. Most cats with hepatic lipidosis have increased serum alkaline phosphatase activity and hyperbilirubinemia with no or only a slight increase

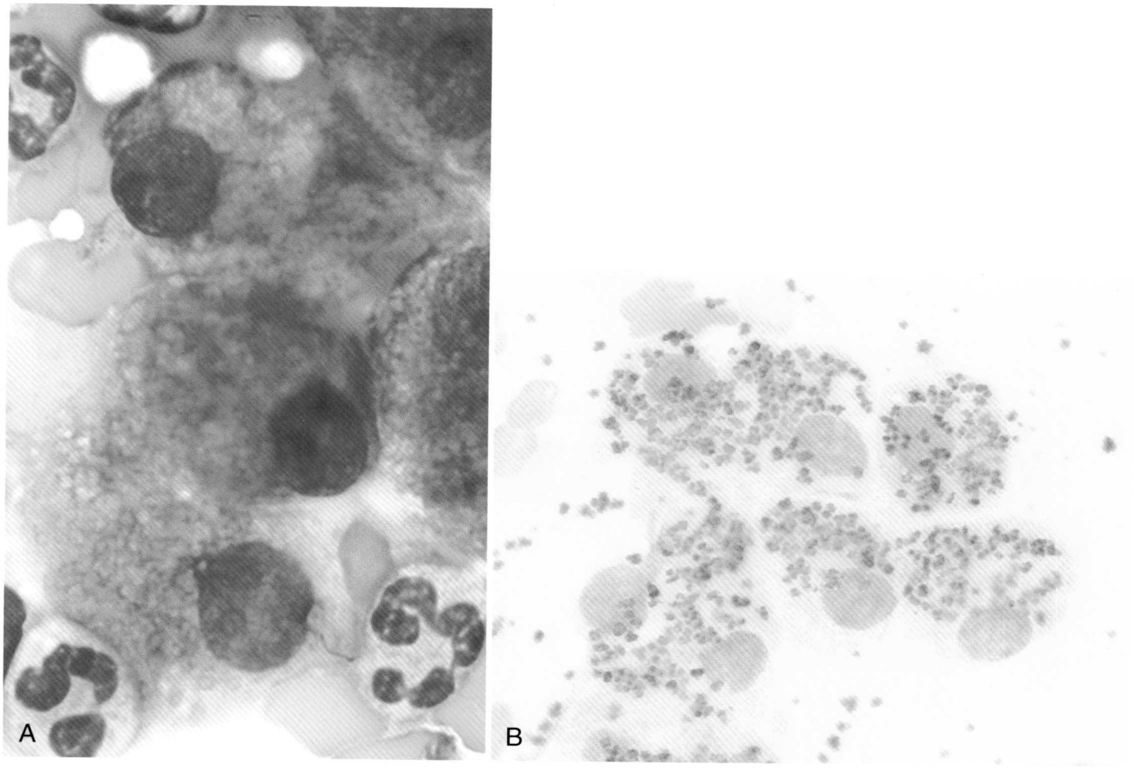

Figure 20-10 A, Liver aspirate from a 3-year-old Bedlington Terrier with copper-associated hepatopathy. Copper in hepatocytes appears as coarsely clumped, refractile, pale blue-green cytoplasmic granules. (Wright stain. Original magnification 400×.) **B,** Rubeanic acid highlights excess cytoplasmic copper in canine hepatocytes.(Rubeanic stain. Original magnification 400×.) (A, Case material from Dr. Michael Scott, 1991, ASVCP slide review session.)

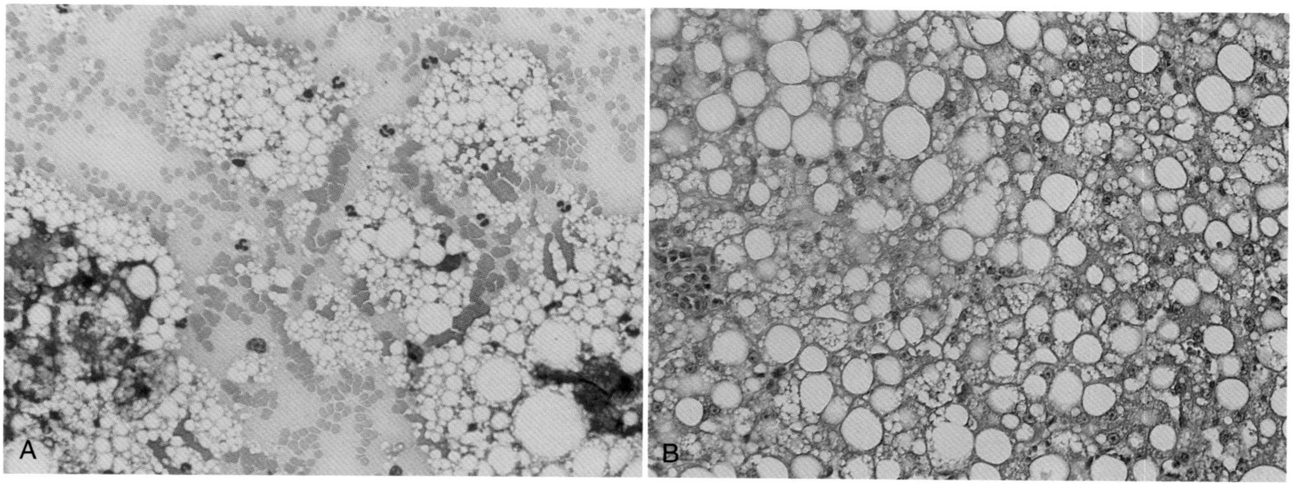

Figure 20-11 A, Hepatocytes from a 4-year-old cat with pancreatitis and hepatomegaly. Note the cytoplasmic hepatocellular vacuolar changes (demarcated, large and small discrete clear lipid - filled vacuoles) and increased neutrophils. Similar clear vacuoles are seen in the background released from ruptured hepatocytes. The cytologic diagnosis is lipidosis with suppurative inflammation (secondary lipidosis). (Wright stain. Original magnification 1000×.) **B,** Follow-up histologic section (liver biopsy taken two weeks after cytology due to persistently elevated alanine persistently elevated alanine aminotransferase) from the same patient with the histologic diagnosis of feline hepatic lipidosis (H&E stain. Original magnification 400×.)

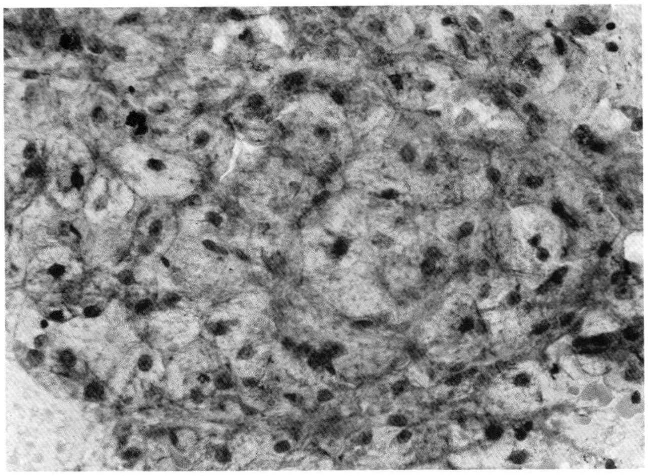

Figure 20-12 Hepatocytes from a 12-year-old dog with increased liver enzyme activity treated for 8 months with corticosteroids for a persistent cough. Note the feathery rarefaction of the cytoplasm (nondiscrete vacuolization), which suggests glycogen accumulation associated with glucocorticoid effects, ischemic damage, or hepatoxin exposure. The diagnosis, in this case, was hyperadrenocortism and hypothyroidism. (Wright stain. Original magnification 500×.)

in γ-glutamyltransferase activity. Hepatocytes from cats with hepatic lipidosis will contain round, sharply delineated empty vacuoles with a background punctuated with similar vacuolation. Most hepatocytes are distended by multiple vacuoles of various sizes that often peripheralize the nucleus and other organelles, leaving only a thin rim of visible cytoplasm. It is of utmost importance that the cytologist recognizes that feline hepatic steatosis may be primary or secondary and is therefore obligated to perform a thorough search for inflammation, infection, or neoplasia. Inherited lysosomal storage disease may produce similar vacuolar changes, but these conditions are very rare and more likely to cause recognizable changes in younger animals.

Hepatomegaly caused by lipid accumulation in hepatocytes is uncommon in dogs. Mild to moderate lipid vacuolization may develop secondary to various metabolic disorders in dogs and cats, especially diabetes mellitus. Severe hepatic lipidosis (microvesicular) with hypoglycemia may occur subsequent to anorexia in puppies of toy dog breeds.[18] Dogs with aflatoxicosis develop severe hepatic lipidosis, in which liver aspirates resemble those from cats with feline hepatic lipidosis.[19]

In dogs, high plasma concentrations of glucocorticoid hormones (endogenous or exogenous) produce recognizable biochemical changes (increased serum alkaline phosphatase activity without hyperbilirubinemia) and cytomorphologic changes (several-fold enlargement of hepatocytes with vacuolar changes). Canine vacuolar hepatopathy of this type may be attributed to hyperadrenocorticism (HAC) or exogenous corticosteroid therapy, or "steroid hepatopathy" (see Figure 20-12). These patients generally have characteristic accompanying clinical signs (polyuria, polydipsia, polyphagia) with hepatomegaly. Excess glycogen and water cause the cytoplasm of these hepatocytes to swell, displacing the blue-staining, ribonucleic acid (RNA)–containing organelles. Aspirates will contain a mixture of swollen affected hepatocytes and intact normal hepatocytes.

Similar, nonspecific vacuolar changes and increased alkaline phosphatase activity, secondary to a variety of conditions (e.g., neoplasia, congenital or acquired hepatobiliary disease, nodular hyperplasia, GI disease, stress), are common findings in dogs.[20]

Irreversible cellular injury leading to death and necrosis of hepatocytes may occur from a variety of toxins (e.g., aflatoxins, cycad toxicity, wild mushrooms), drugs (e.g., tetracycline and diazepam in cats, rimadyl and xylitol in dogs), immune-mediated disease, metabolic disturbances, ischemia, neoplasia, and infectious agents. Cell death may occur via two pathways: *apoptosis* and *necrosis*. The two are largely distinct pathways, with apoptosis being "programmed cell death" and necrosis reflecting a pathologic condition. Apoptosis is important in the development and homeostasis of renewable cell populations. Apoptotic cells have pyknotic or karyorrhectic nuclei but intact cell membranes and cytoplasmic features. Hepatocellular necrosis involves altered cell membrane permeability and cellular swelling and is recognized as pink cytoplasm because of loss of RNA and denaturation of cytoplasmic proteins (Figure 20-13). Nuclei are condensed or disrupted or not discernible.

Inflammatory Disorders

Reports in the literature vary with regard to the relative sensitivity of cytology compared with histologic evaluation in the diagnosis of various inflammatory diseases of the liver.[1,21,22] Cytology is less sensitive for conditions with minimal cellular infiltrates (such as low-grade chronic hepatitis or small multifocal lesions). The same effect of sample size applies when comparing histologic evaluation of needle and wedge biopsy specimens.[22] The absence of significant numbers of inflammatory cells does not exclude an inflammatory process. Blood contamination may also impair the ability to detect inflammation in liver aspirates and blurs the significance of leukocytes in light of a peripheral blood leukocytosis. Supportive evidence of inflammation includes finding cells not generally found in peripheral blood (e.g., macrophages and plasma cells), observing neutrophils intercalated between hepatocytes in clusters, and recognizing degenerate neutrophils and necrotic cellular debris.

Suppurative Inflammation: Suppurative inflammation is almost entirely composed of neutrophils, with macrophages and lymphocytes comprising usually less than 10% of the inflammatory cell population. Suppurative inflammation often represents bacterial infection (the most commonly reported bacterial pathogens in the liver of canines and felines are *E. coli*, *Streptococcus* spp., *Staphylococcus* spp., *Enterococcus* spp., and *Clostridium* spp.).[23] Organisms may reach the liver by ascending the biliary tree or, less commonly, by spreading hematogenously and producing focal or multifocal hepatic abscesses. Aspirates from livers with suppurative cholangiohepatitis typically include hepatocytes in addition to inflammatory cells. Intracellular bile pigment and bile casts are often present because of concomitant cholestasis (see Figure 20-6 and Figure 20-7).

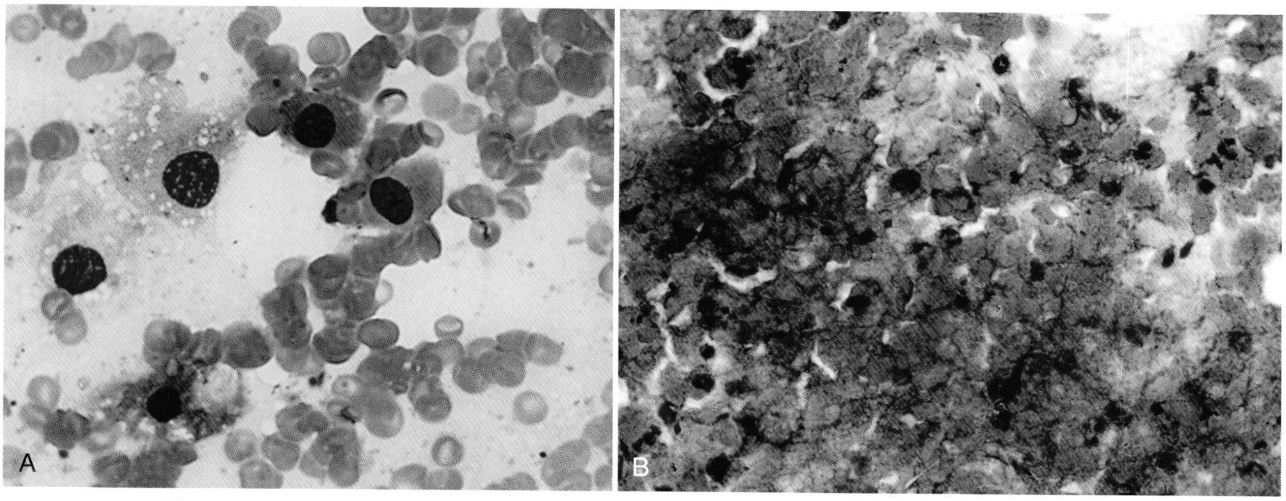

Figure 20-13 Hepatic necrosis in a liver aspirate from a young dog after eating wild mushrooms. A, Early stage typified by single cell eosinophilic cytoplasm and a pyknotic nucleus. (Wright stain. Original magnification 1000×.) **B,** Later stage necrosis with large amounts of amorphous basophilic material resembling blurred cytoplasmic membranes and nuclei. (Wright stain. Original magnification 1000×.)

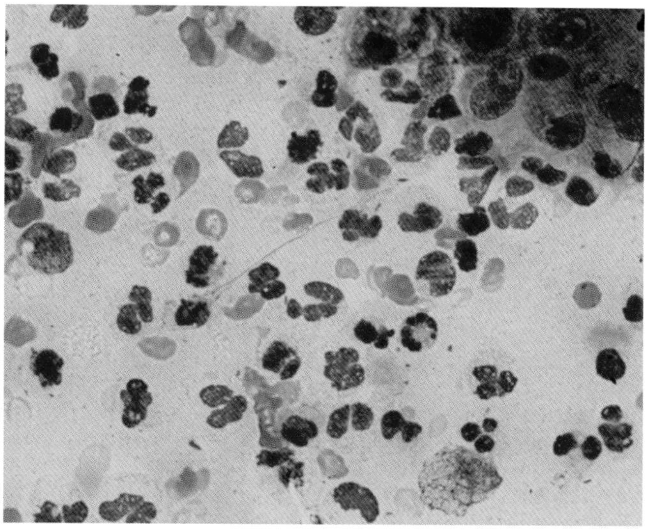

Figure 20-14 Aspirate from an 11-year-old Boston Terrier with increased liver enzymes and a hypoechoic mass. Diagnosis is septic suppurative hepatitis or abscess or bacterial cholangiohepatitis. Note the lipid-laden macrophages and numerous neutrophils, one containing bacteria, and several bacterial rods in the background. (Wright stain. Original magnification 1000×.)

In most cases, aspiration of suppurative inflammation with few or no hepatocytes from a focal lesion indicates a hepatic abscess. Phagocytized and extracellular bacteria may occasionally be found in some aspirates and are rewarding when identified (Figure 20-14).

Mixed or Chronic Inflammation: Mixed inflammatory cell infiltrates include a variety of cells such as neutrophils, eosinophils, macrophages, lymphocytes, plasma cells, and, in some cases, multinucleate giant macrophages (Langhans cells). The proportion of specific inflammatory cells is variable and depends on the cause. Chronic inflammation often has predominantly macrophages and is termed *granulomatous* or *pyogranulomatous* if a significant neutrophil component is present. Causes of chronic mixed cell inflammation include feline infectious peritonitis (FIP), mycotic infection (coccidioidomycosis, histoplasmosis, or aspergillosis), mycobacterial infection, bartonellosis, protozoal infection (hepatozoonosis, leishmaniasis, cytauxzoonosis, and toxoplasmosis), drug and toxic injury, and systemic immune-mediated disorders. In some cases, the specific cause of mixed inflammation remains undetermined even after histologic assessment of liver biopsies.

Lymphocytic (Nonsuppurative) Inflammation: Hepatic infiltrates composed of numerous small lymphocytes and a few plasma cells are commonly recognized in cats with nonsuppurative periportal hepatitis (Figure 20-15). Lymphocytes and a few plasma cells are typical of lymphocytic cholangiohepatitis in cats but are also consistent with certain forms of lymphoid neoplasia (i.e., chronic lymphocytic leukemia [CLL] and small cell lymphoma). The lymphocytes in CLL and small cell lymphoma are morphologically indistinguishable from nonneoplastic small lymphocytes and additional clinical data and diagnostics are often required to come to a firm diagnosis. CLL occurs in middle-aged to elderly cats and dogs and is characterized by persistent lymphocytosis and splenomegaly. Small cell lymphoma usually is differentiated from lymphocytic cholangiohepatitis by examining a liver biopsy histologically and by immunophenotyping. If an infiltrate consists mostly of a single lymphoid lineage (e.g., CD3+ T-cells), lymphoma is likely, whereas a mixed lymphoid infiltrate (T-cells and B-cells) is more characteristic of inflammatory diseases. It is becoming increasingly common to perform polymerase chain reaction (PCR) testing for clonal receptor gene rearrangements on lymphoid cells to determine if the infiltrate is neoplastic or reactive. This may be done on slides that have been stained (to confirm adequate

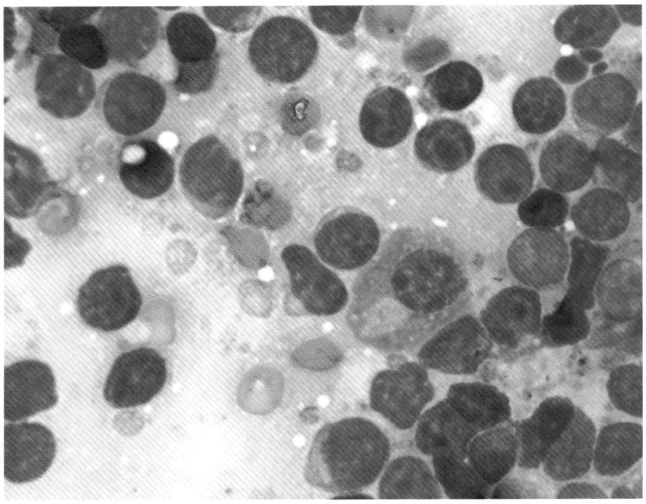

Figure 20-15 Nonsuppurative periportal hepatitis in an icteric cat. Note the many small mature lymphocytes and few plasma cells among the hepatocytes. Differentials include infiltrating well-differentiated lymphoma or chronic lymphocytic lymphoma. The histologic diagnosis was lymphocytic plasmacytic cholangiohepatitis. (Wright stain. Original magnification 500×.)

cellularity), since deoxyribonucleic acid (DNA) is not altered by staining. The cells may be scraped from the slides and the genes amplified to determine if the cells are derived from a single clone. Lymphocytic cholangiohepatitis is more prevalent than small cell lymphoma or CLL; and in most cases of hepatic lymphoma, the cells are large and immature.

Eosinophilic Inflammation: Eosinophils are often a nonspecific infiltrate in hepatopathies. Few conditions other than liver fluke infestation, seen in cats in Florida and Hawaii, elicit a purely eosinophil rich cell response.[24] Generalized or periportal infiltrates of eosinophils, lymphocytes, and plasma cells are found in some dogs and cats with eosinophilic enteritis, hypereosinophilic syndromes, eosinophilic leukemia, or mast cell tumors and occasionally in idiosyncratic drug reactions.[5]

Amyloidosis

The liver is a major site of amyloid deposition in dogs with reactive, or secondary, amyloidosis. Amyloid accumulation in the space of Disse in liver and other tissues such as kidney, spleen, lymph node, and skin may develop secondary to prolonged, intense systemic inflammation. In some animals, the primary disease is infectious (such as systemic mycosis or leishmaniasis). A familial inflammatory disorder culminating in severe amyloidosis is recognized in Chinese Shar Pei dogs, some of which have severe liver dysfunction.[25] Hepatic hemorrhage and rupture are major causes of morbidity and death in Oriental Shorthair and Siamese cats with systemic amyloidosis.[26] In smears of affected liver or other tissue, amyloid appears as amorphous, pink, extracellular material found between hepatocytes and may resemble necrotic cellular debris (Figure 20-16).

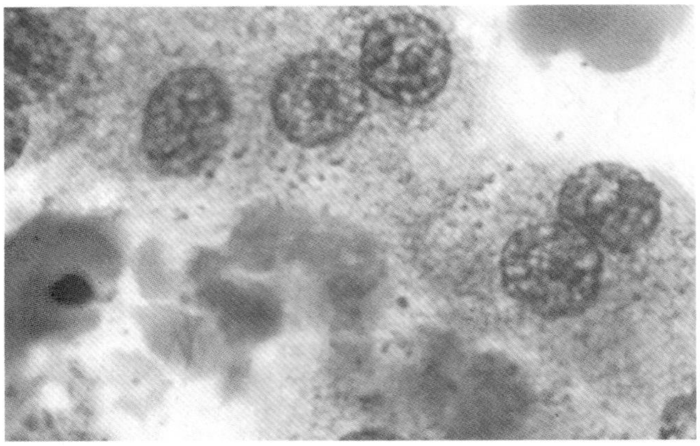

Figure 20-16 Chronic inflammatory disease of osteomyelitis in a dog. Note the pale eosinophilic amorphous slightly fibrillar extracellular material consistent with hepatic amyloid deposition. (Wright stain. Original magnification 1000×.)

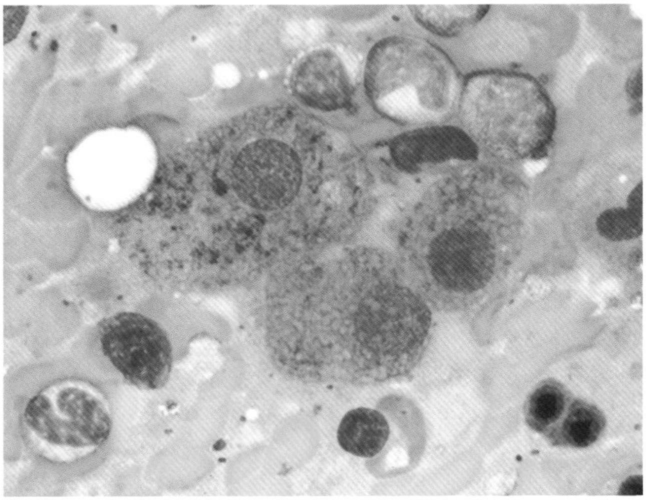

Figure 20-17 Liver aspirate from an anemic dog. Note the extramedullary hematopoiesis, including metarubricytes and metamyelocytes and intracellular hemosiderin pigment. (Wright stain. Original magnification 1000×.)

Extramedullary Hematopoiesis

Hematopoietic foci in the livers of dogs and cats may develop concurrently with accelerated hematopoiesis in marrow, usually in response to anemia or systemic inflammatory diseases. Occasionally, evidence of hepatic hematopoiesis is found in nonanemic dogs with chronic hepatitis or nodular hyperplasia. It may also be a normal finding in some older animals and other species (rodents and fish). Extramedullary hematopoiesis is defined by the presence of hematopoietic cells at all stages of maturation (Figure 20-17). The erythroid line is usually the predominant cell line and, in most cases, is accompanied by immature stages of the neutrophilic series. The hematopoietic cells are normal in appearance, and intermediate to late stages of maturation should be more numerous than earlier stages (synchronous expansion and maturation). Myelolipomas, which are tumorlike nodular masses composed of lipid-containing stromal cells and

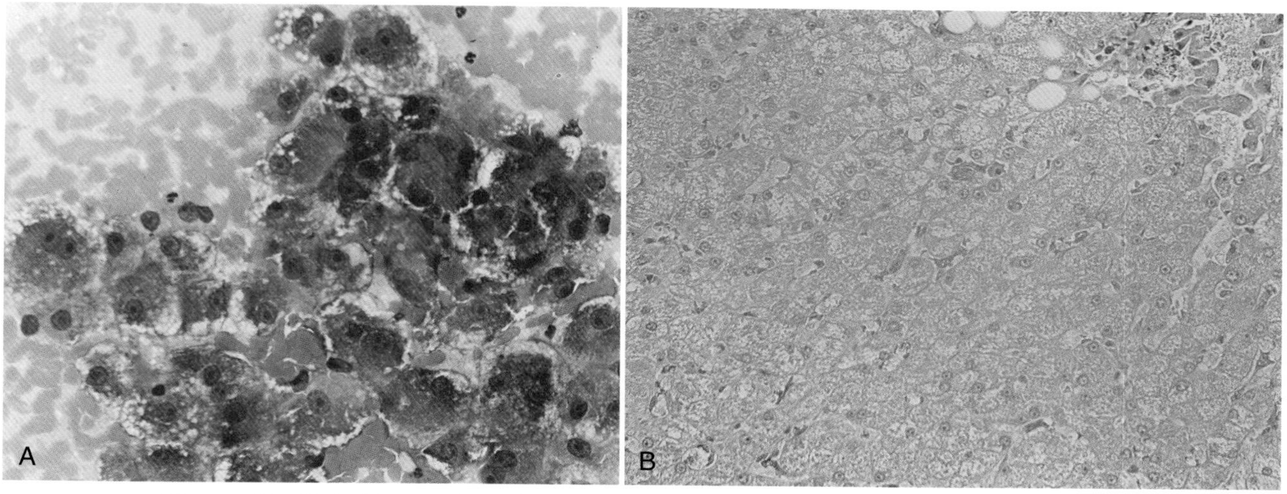

Figure 20-18 **A,** Liver aspirate from a 10-year-old Labrador Retriever with chronic liver disease and recent development of hepatic nodules. Cytologic interpretation is regenerative hepatic nodule. Note the mild anisocytosis, binucleate cells with normal nuclear morphology, and increased cytoplasmic basophilia and variable vacuole accumulation. (Wright stain. Original magnification 500×,) **B,** Histologic correlate from a hyperplastic nodule with variably vacuolated hepatocytes admixed with normal hepatocytes. (H&E. Original magnification 400×,)

hematopoietic cells, are rarely encountered in dogs and cats. Material aspirated from a myelolipoma is cytologically indistinguishable from normal marrow; however, often, accompanying adipocytes are seen.

Nodular Hepatic Hyperplasia (Hyperplastic Nodules)

Single or multiple distinct masses composed of normal-appearing hepatic parenchyma are commonly found in old dogs but are uncommon in cats. In livers of otherwise normal size and contour, randomly distributed masses are called hyperplastic nodules. In many dogs, these are incidental findings, often detected during abdominal ultrasonography. A concomitant mild to moderate increase in liver enzyme activity, especially alkaline phosphatase, is often seen. Hyperplastic nodules consist of hepatocyte proliferation or expansion with normal lobular architecture and may compress adjacent normal tissue. In contrast, regenerative nodules (regenerative hyperplasia) are believed to be outgrowths of residual hepatocytes as a sequela to chronic inflammation, necrosis, or both. In these nodules, often, abnormal lobular architecture, for example, often a single portal tract, is present.[5] In liver samples collected from hyperplastic nodules or areas of regenerative hyperplasia, the hepatocytes may be indistinguishable from normal hepatocytes, may display vacuolar degeneration, or may have only subtle cytologic features characteristic of hyperplastic tissue, including slightly increased cellular and nuclear size, increased N:C ratios, mild anisocytosis and anisokaryosis, and increased basophilia of the cytoplasm. Binucleate hepatocytes may be more numerous than in normal liver tissue and focal accumulations of lipid- or lipofuscin-laden macrophages (lipogranulomas) may also be appreciated (Figure 20-18). Hyperplastic masses may closely resemble primary or metastatic tumors based on radiographic and ultrasound findings. Furthermore, the cytologic features of such masses may be indistinguishable from those of hepatocellular adenoma and well-differentiated carcinoma (see the discussion on epithelial tumors later in this chapter). In some cases, hyperplastic nodules may be differentiated from hepatocellular tumors if cytologic findings are considered in addition to clinical history and findings of other diagnostic procedures. In other cases, histologic examination of liver biopsies to determine the architecture of the mass is needed for definitive diagnosis.

Gall Bladder Disorders

Gallbladder disease may be affiliated with obstructive processes (choleliths), mucoceles, or bacterial infection or in combination with some hepatic diseases. Biliary stasis may increase susceptibility to bacterial infection. Ultrasound examination may reveal abnormal gall bladder contents, obstruction, mucoceles, masses, or choleliths. Gallbladders are lined by tall simple columnar epithelium. In gallbladder disease, degrees of hemorrhage, inflammation, mucosal hyperplasia, and necrosis may exist. Cytologic evaluation via FNA may reveal inflammatory cells, bacteria, mucinous bile, hemorrhage, or neoplastic cells similar to material from cystadenomas recognized in feline livers (Figure 20-19).

Neoplastic Disorders

Differentiating primary and metastatic hepatobiliary tumors from nonneoplastic disease may often pose a diagnostic challenge. Primary hepatobiliary tumors are more common than metastatic disease in the cat, and these are more often benign; in dogs, metastatic neoplasia occurs 2.5 times more often than primary liver neoplasia.[27] The following serves to describe the cytologic features of hepatobiliary neoplasia, and further extensive descriptions

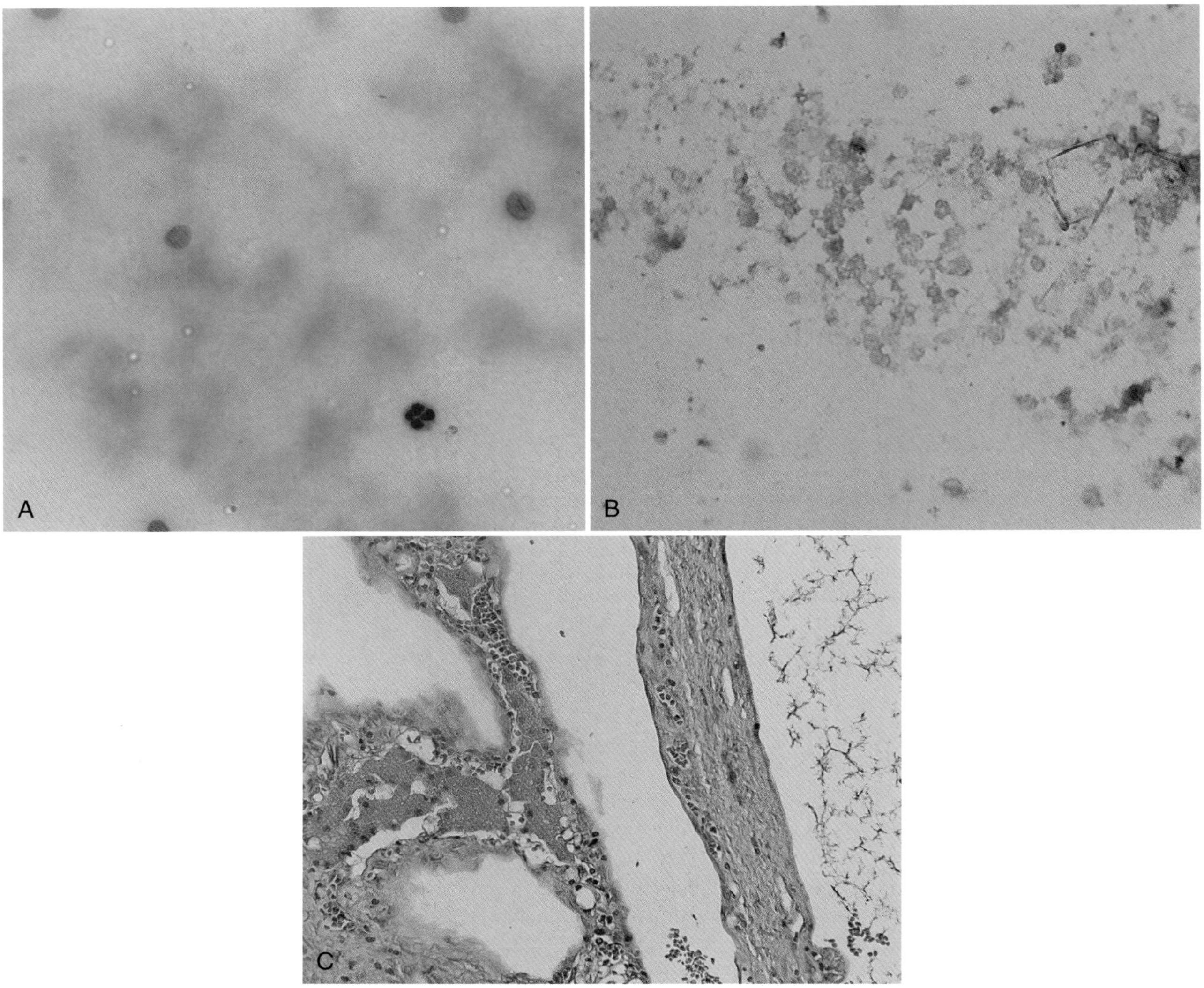

Figure 20-19 **A,** Aspirates from 10-year-old cat with ultrasonic evidence of a cystic hepatic mass. Lakes of mucin, and inflammatory cells. (Wright stain. Original magnification 1000×.) **B,** Coarse amorphous mucinous material and bilirubin crystals. (Wright stain. Original magnification 1000×.) **C,** Histologic section of a biliary cyst adenoma with variably dense mucin-filled cysts and adjacent islands of normal hepatocytes. (H&E stain. Original magnification 400×.)

are found in other sources that provide the clinical and histologic characteristics.[27-30]

Epithelial Tumors: Primary epithelial tumors of the hepatobiliary system in dogs and cats are hepatocellular adenomas and carcinomas and bile duct (cholangiocellular) adenomas and carcinomas. Hepatocellular and intrahepatic cholangiocellular carcinomas are classified on the basis of gross appearance (massive, nodular, or diffuse).[9,31,32] Massive carcinomas produce a single markedly enlarged liver lobe, often the left lobe. Nodular carcinomas form multiple, discrete masses of different sizes that are distributed through several lobes and may resemble the multiple, regenerative nodules of cirrhotic livers. Diffuse carcinomas infiltrate large areas of the liver and are nonencapsulated. Bile duct carcinomas may be intrahepatic or extrahepatic in bile ducts and in the gallbladder. Both benign and malignant cholangiocellular tumors may have a cystic component containing watery to mucinous material (see Figure 20-19).

Animals with diffuse and nodular carcinomas may have extrahepatic metastases at the time of diagnosis, with the lungs, peritoneum, and lymph nodes common sites of early metastases. The liver also acquires carcinomas from metastases of neoplasms arising in other tissues. In some cases, cytologic examination of aspirates or imprints from hepatic masses may distinguish between hepatocyte and biliary origins, but often the cytologist is limited in differentiating primary from metastatic processes. Features evident on imaging with radiography or ultrasonography may be similarly constrained, and in these cases, histologic assessment of architectural features offers the best chances of a definitive diagnosis.

Smears of aspirates and imprints of epithelial tumors typically are cellular and contain variably sized multicellular clusters. Cells from hepatocellular adenomas and

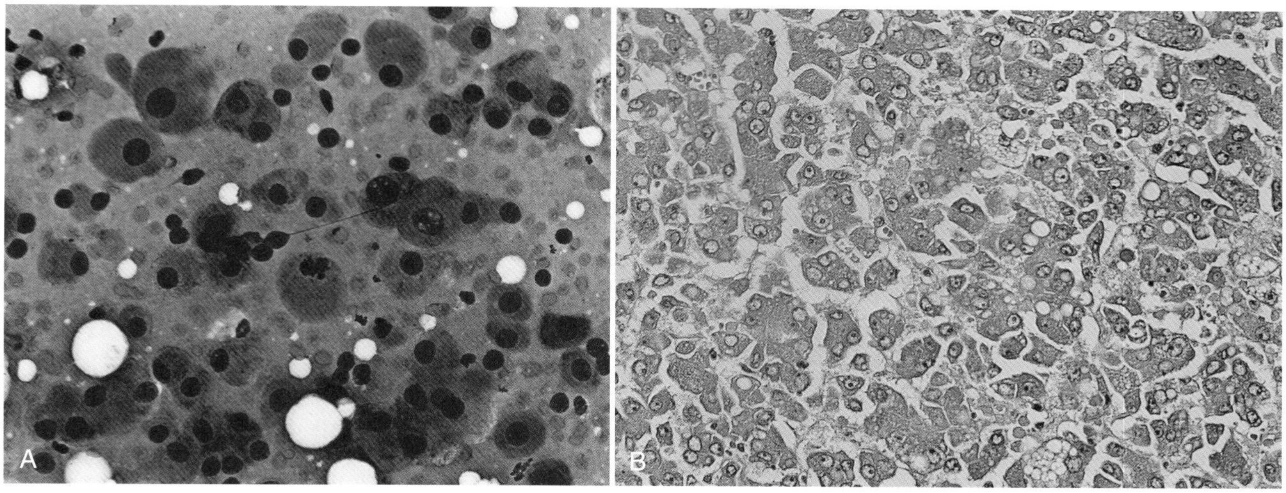

Figure 20-20 **A,** Liver aspirate from an 11-year-old cat with a large mass in the central liver lobe. Cytologic diagnosis of hepatocellular carcinoma based on the marked pleomorphism including anisocytosis and anisokaryosis, variable nuclear to cytoplasmic ratios, and prominent meganucleoli. (Wright stain. Original magnification 500×.) **B,** Histologic section from same mass. (H&E. Original magnification 400×.)

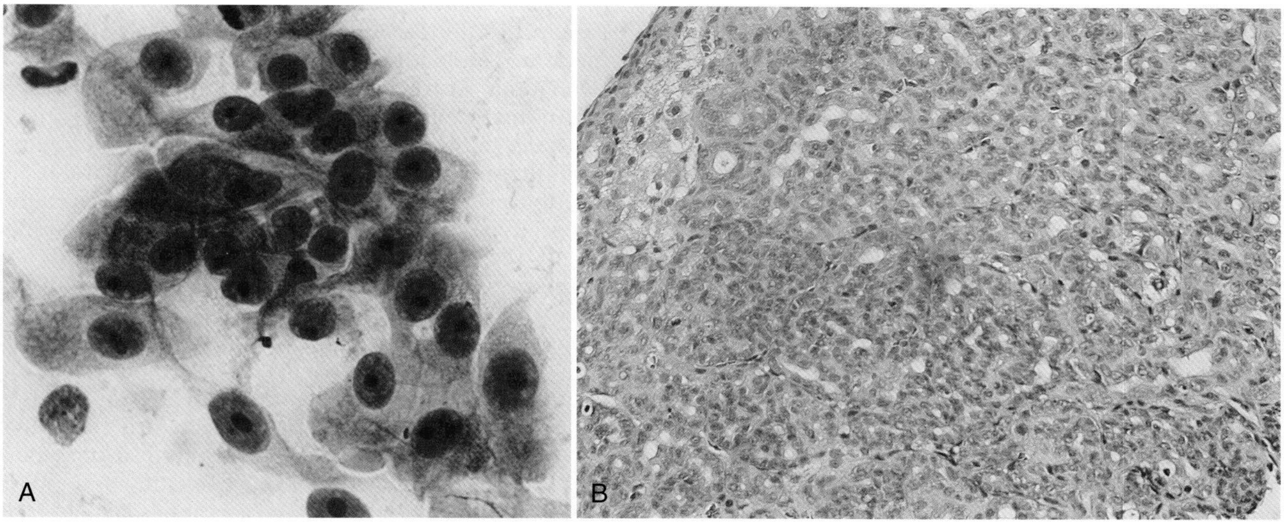

Figure 20-21 **A,** Liver aspirate from a 14-year-old cat with significant weight loss and a mass in the right liver lobe. Note the pleomorphism and resemblance to normal, but densely packed, biliary epithelial cells. The cytologic diagnosis is cholangiocellular neoplasia and the histologic diagnosis was bile duct carcinoma. (Wright stain. Original magnification 1000×.) **B,** Histologic section from the same patient. (H&E. Original magnification 400×.)

some well-differentiated hepatocellular carcinomas may be cytologically indistinguishable from normal hepatocytes or those from hyperplastic and regenerative nodules (see Figure 20-18, *A*). The presence of hepatocytes with marked cytologic atypical features (nuclear pleomorphism, high N:C ratios, large nucleoli, deeply basophilic cytoplasm, and marked anisocytosis and anisokaryosis) provides a reasonable basis for a cytologic diagnosis of hepatocellular carcinoma. In the chapter author's experience, hepatocellular carcinomas are typically cellular on aspiration, but cells often occur singly, rather than in cellular clusters (Figure 20-20). These tumors are not typically inflamed or necrotic, which helps distinguish them from hepatocellular regeneration in response to necrosis. If hepatocytes from a liver mass are not markedly atypical, the cytologic interpretation should acknowledge the possibility of nodular hyperplasia, hepatocellular adenoma, or well-differentiated carcinoma.

Cells exfoliated from well-differentiated cholangiocellular (bile duct) tumors (benign or malignant) are cuboidal to low columnar, arranged in sheets and clusters, some with tubular and acinar arrangements and are smaller than hepatocytes (Figure 20-21). Cells from these lesions may closely resemble normal biliary epithelium but tend to be tightly bound in irregular clusters (see Figure 20-3). Nuclei are round to oval and have smooth, finely reticular chromatin with faint to absent nucleoli. Poorly differentiated biliary carcinomas cannot be clearly distinguished

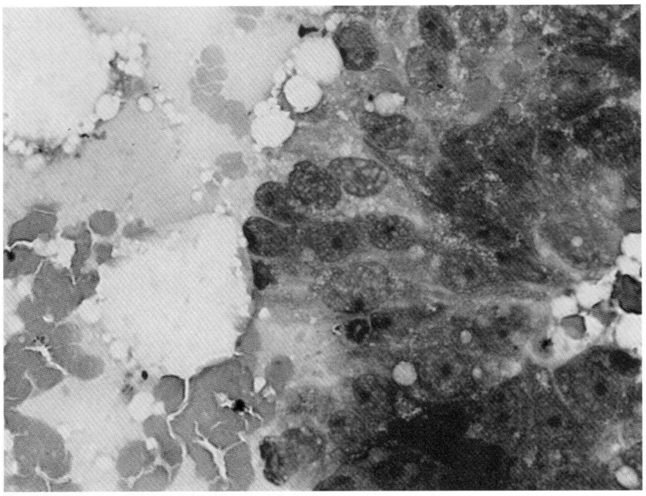

Figure 20-22 Liver aspirate from a cat. Cytologic diagnosis of mucinous carcinoma. Note the lakes of pale-blue mucin, with clusters of anaplastic carcinoma cells. (Wright stain. Original magnification 1000×.) Histologic diagnosis was metastatic intestinal mucinous carcinoma.

from other carcinomas by cytology alone (see the following discussion).

Aspirates from biliary cystadenomas and cystadenocarcinomas often consist primarily of fluid that may be mucinous, hemorrhagic, or clear. Cytologic examination of aspirates from cystadenomas or cystadenocarcinomas may consist of acellular coarse cloudy fluid, which stains gray-blue, or lakes of mucinous secretion, sometimes with inflammatory cells. It is not unusual to find scattered biliary cells or islands of hepatocytes on slides from aspirates. Similar fluid may be aspirated from nonneoplastic hepatobiliary cysts, gall bladder mucoceles, and some cholangiocellular tumors.

The cells of many metastatic carcinomas in liver aspirates are clearly identifiable as malignant but lack sufficient cellular differentiation for determination of specific tissue of origin. In some cases of metastatic pancreatic carcinoma, acinar structures may be seen and minute pink zymogen granules may be seen in the cytoplasm of highly basophilic epithelial cells consistent with pancreatic tissue. In mucin-secreting neoplasms from the bowel, pools of mucin may be seen (Figure 20-22).

Smears of anaplastic carcinomas consist of cells that are too poorly differentiated to allow specific identification. They usually contain large, dense clusters of adherent cells, indicating a possible epithelial origin (Figure 20-23). Further characterization often is achieved with immunophenotyping; however, some anaplastic neoplasms are too primitive to display developed antigens, which are needed for identification even with advanced diagnostics.

Neuroendocrine and Endocrine Tumors: Neuroendocrine tumors, or carcinoids, are derived from amine precursor uptake and decarboxylation (APUD) cells of the biliary system and occur in both dogs and cats.[31-33] In most cases, these tumors are found as multiple nodular masses dispersed throughout the liver, but they may also form masses in the extrahepatic bile ducts and gallbladder.[34]

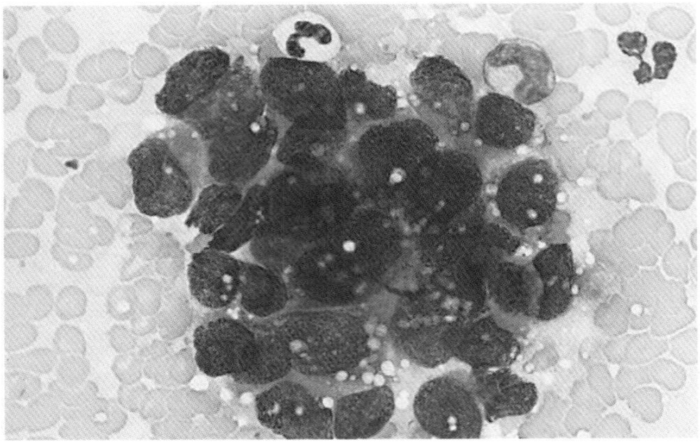

Figure 20-23 Liver aspirate from a dog with multiple masses in the liver and abdomen noted on ultrasonography. The cells display no characteristic features to indicate tissue of origin and the cytologic diagnosis is anaplastic undifferentiated carcinoma. (Wright stain. Original magnification 400×.)

Metastatic disease is present at diagnosis in nearly all animals with hepatobiliary carcinoids, and metastases may be present as widely dispersed nodules in the liver. Pancreatic islet cell tumor is the most common type of metastatic endocrine tumor, but others include pheochromocytoma, gastrinoma, intestinal carcinoid, and thyroid carcinoma. Cells in aspirates from these types of lesions generally may be identified as originating from neuroendocrine or endocrine tumors but cytologic features alone are not specific enough to reliably differentiate among the subtypes (Figure 20-24). The use of immunohistochemical stains to demonstrate the presence of different hormones such as gastrin, insulin, or thyroglobulin may also be helpful in identifying specific tumors.[32-35]

Smears of aspirates and imprints of neuroendocrine and endocrine tumors readily exfoliate and are usually very cellular, but the cells are quite fragile and easily disrupted. Typically, a high percentage of the cells are partly or completely disrupted during smear preparation, and bare nuclei outnumber intact cells in some preparations. Cells in imprints tend to form a mosaic pattern that occurs in small flat sheets or packets.

Mesenchymal Neoplasia: Malignant tumors of connective tissue origin (mesenchymal neoplasia, sarcoma) may arise in the liver, but metastatic sarcomas are much more common. Hemangiosarcoma, a neoplasm of endothelial origin, is the most common sarcoma involving the liver, where it may be either a primary or metastatic tumor. Aspirates or imprints of hepatic sarcomas may contain rare to many neoplastic cells, depending on the density of cells in the sampled location and the amount of collagen surrounding the area. Neoplastic mesenchymal cells are spindle to stellate shaped, with tapering tails of basophilic cytoplasmic that is often vacuolated and extends away from the nucleus (Figure 20-25). Cell borders are indistinct, and nuclei are typically oval and may be found near the center of the cell. Chromatin may be moderately condensed to finely reticular. Nucleoli may be faint or absent or prominent and large. Some sarcomas are quite uniform in their cellular and nuclear sizes, whereas others display

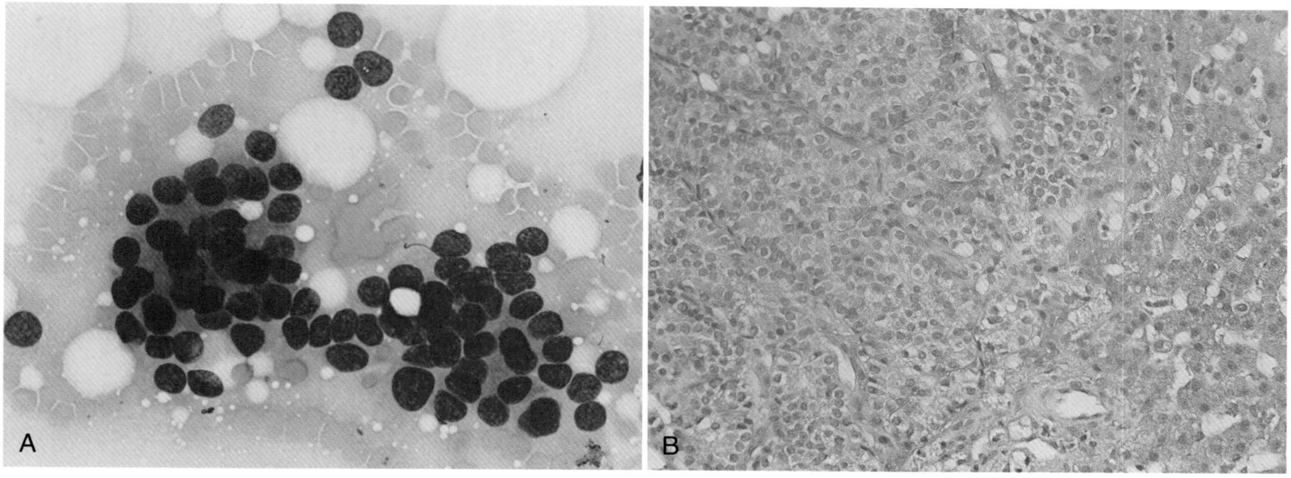

Figure 20-24 A, Liver aspirate from a 7-year-old French Bulldog with multifocal discrete hepatic nodules. Cytologic diagnosis of carcinoid with cell packeting and moderate anisokaryosis. Cells are fragile, and the background contains material consistent with cytoplasm released from disrupted cells. (Wright stain. Original magnification 1000×.) **B,** Biopsy of same nodule with diagnosis of hepatic carcinoid. (H&E stain. Original magnification 400×.)

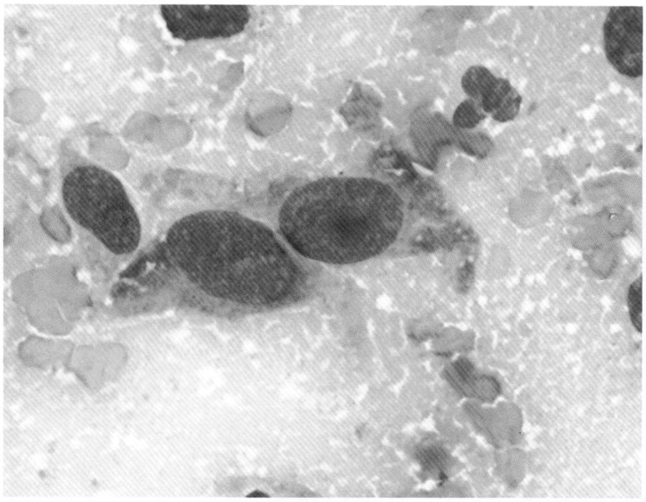

Figure 20-25 Liver mass aspirate from a cat. Note the wispy tails with vacuolated cytoplasm, anisocytosis and anisokaryosis and other anaplastic features. Cytologic diagnosis is sarcoma, and the histologic diagnosis is hemangiosarcoma. (Wright stain. Original magnification 250×.)

marked anisocytosis and anisokaryosis (Figure 20-26). Streaming bands of pink fibrillar extracellular matrix may be intimately associated with mesenchymal neoplastic populations. Although hemangiosarcoma is the most common mesenchymal neoplasm (primary from liver or metastatic from the spleen), often, a paucity of cells is seen in aspirates because of the poorly exfoliative nature of the tumor and large vascular spaces. Frequently, aspirates consist largely of blood and erythrophagocytic macrophages from cavernous sinuses within the tumor mass. Finding few to no identifiable tumor cells causes a diagnostic quandary, which is not uncommon for cytopathologists.

Histiocytic sarcoma, which is a tumor recognized with increased frequency in Bernese Mountain Dogs, Golden Retrievers, Labrador Retrievers, and Rottweilers, arises from interstitial dendritic cells (DC).[36] The tumor occurs in cats as well, but more commonly in dogs.[37,38] Hepatic involvement has been reported with the disseminated form of this disease in both species. Cytologically, the tumor cells are generally large, round to oval cells with eccentric, oval to indented nuclei with lacey chromatin. The cytoplasm is abundant, light to medium blue, and often contains discrete vacuoles. In some cases, the tumor cells are hemophagocytic, resulting in a clinical presentation that must be distinguished from benign hemophagocytic and immune-mediated syndromes.[38,39] In many cases, neoplastic histiocytes (DC origin)have markedly abnormal features such as giant, multiple nuclei; prominent nucleoli; and marked anisocytosis and anisokaryosis (see Figure 20-26). In other patients, the neoplastic cells are of macrophage lineage (CD11d+) and arise from splenic red pulp or bone marrow macrophages. These tumor cells do not appear remarkably different from inflammatory macrophages, and the diagnosis of neoplasia is more difficult to make. Demonstration of similar cells in other sites such as the spleen or bone marrow lends support to the diagnosis. In dogs or cats, immunophenotyping on air-dried cytologic specimens or on formalin-fixed histologic sections may be used to confirm histiocytic (or macrophage) origin.[36]

Hemolymphatic Neoplasia: Lymphoma (lymphosarcoma) is the most common neoplastic disease involving the liver in dogs and cats. In a small percentage of cases, the neoplastic lymphocytes are small, mature cells that are indistinguishable from normal lymphocytes. The differentiation of chronic lymphocytic leukemia from well-differentiated small cell lymphoma and lymphocytic cholangiohepatitis is discussed in the section on nonsuppurative inflammation. In the experience of one of the chapter authors, lymphocytes (of small cell lymphoma) are often slightly larger than normal small lymphocytes, have a cap of cytoplasm on one pole of the nucleus and slightly open chromatin. When many cells with this morphology are encountered in a liver sample, additional testing is suggested to characterize

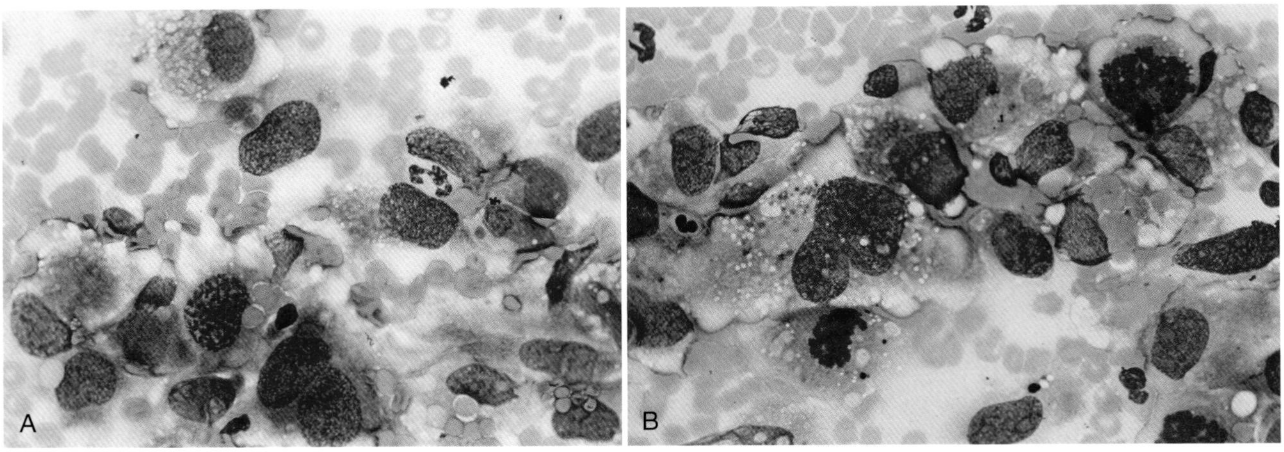

Figure 20-26 **A,** Liver aspirate from a Bernese Mountain Dog. Note the pleomorphic erythrophagocytic round to spindloid population admixed with neutrophils and small lymphocytes. Cytologic diagnosis is histiocytic sarcoma. Histiocytic lineage confirmed by CD18 +, CD31- immunocytochemisty. (Wright stain. Original magnification 1000×.) **B,** Liver aspirate from same dog. Note the marked nuclear pleomorphism and mitoses of the neoplastic population. (Wright stain. Original magnification 1000×.)

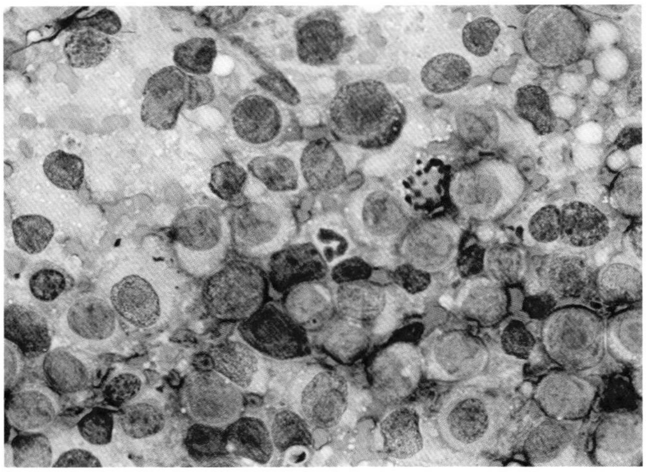

Figure 20-27 **Hepatic lymphoma in a liver aspirate from an 8-year-old cat with anorexia and neurologic signs and liver mass on ultrasonography.** Note the high numbers of large immature round cells interpreted as neoplastic lymphoblasts. (Wright stain. Original magnification 1000×.)

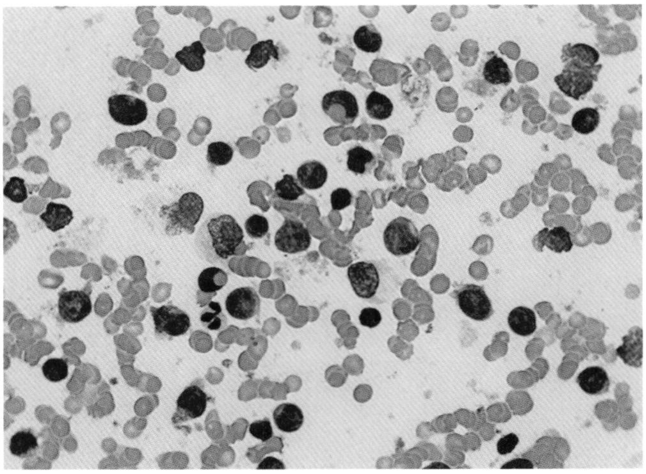

Figure 20-28 **Liver aspirate from a 12-year-old cat with weight loss and marked hepatosplenomegaly.** Cytologic diagnosis is hepatosplenic lymphoma. Note the highly cellular aspirate with immature lymphoid cells and erythrophagocytic neoplastic cells. (Wright stain. Original magnification 1000×.)

the phenotype (e.g., clonality or histopathology to evaluate architecture). In most cases of hepatic lymphoma, the infiltrating lymphocytes have the cytologic features of immature blast cells (Figure 20-27), are larger than normal lymphocytes, have finely or coarsely reticular chromatin and variable amounts of deep-blue cytoplasm, and may have indented nuclei. Immunophenotyping may be useful to differentiate T-cell and B-cell lymphomas. In these cases, immunocytochemical stains for lymphoid markers (e.g., CD3, CD79a, CD20) and, in some cases, additional stains (CD18) could be used to identify the cell lineage.

A recent report describes hepatosplenic lymphoma of γδ-T-cell origin in a dog.[40] This neoplasm is characterized by infiltration of the liver and spleen with large immature neoplastic lymphocytes. The nuclei are large and have irregular nuclear indentations. The chromatin is densely stained and uniformly dispersed. The cytoplasmic volume varies. That these neoplastic lymphoid cells can be erythrophagic is quite remarkable (Figure 20-28).[40] This condition is infrequently reported in both humans and dogs but is also seen in cats. Cells from lymphoma of granular lymphocytes contain distinctive pink to red granules that vary in size and number but are often found in a small area of cytoplasmic clearing adjacent to an indentation of the nucleus (Figure 20-29). Lymphoma of granular lymphocytes is a common neoplasm in cats and is less frequently seen in dogs. In cats, the tumor usually arises in the intestinal tract (jejunum, ileum, duodenum) and metastasizes readily to the mesenteric lymph nodes, liver, and other sites. Most granular lymphomas in cats appear to be CD8+ cytotoxic T-cells, originating from an intraepithelial lymphocyte.[41,42] Some cells from these lymphomas may have granules that are quite large, red to magenta, and found within a distinct cytoplasmic vacuole. The presence of low numbers of small granular lymphocytes does not always indicate neoplasia; these cells may also be seen as part of an inflammatory response (such as secondary to hepatic necrosis).

The liver is a common site of infiltration in dogs and cats with acute leukemia (either acute myeloid leukemia [AML] or acute lymphoblastic leukemia [ALL]). In smears stained with routine Romanowsky-type stains, monoblasts, and agranular myeloblasts may be indistinguishable from lymphoblasts; therefore, additional diagnostics (cytochemical staining, immunophenotyping, flow cytometry, or PCR) are needed to differentiate lymphoma from AML or ALL. Additionally, evaluating bone marrow and blood provides helpful information in many cases. Variable numbers of blast cells circulate in the blood in all three diseases (lymphoma, ALL, and AML), but patients with acute leukemia are more likely than patients with lymphoma to have a concurrent nonregenerative anemia, neutropenia, and thrombocytopenia. Cats with AML are commonly noted to have macrocytosis. Bone marrow aspirates are definitive; marrows aspirated from most patients with AML or ALL are hypercellular with blast cells greater than 20% of all nucleated cells and often lack cells of normal differentiation. Marrow from many patients with lymphoma contains a detectable, but highly variable, number of abnormal cells along with normal hematopoietic cells.

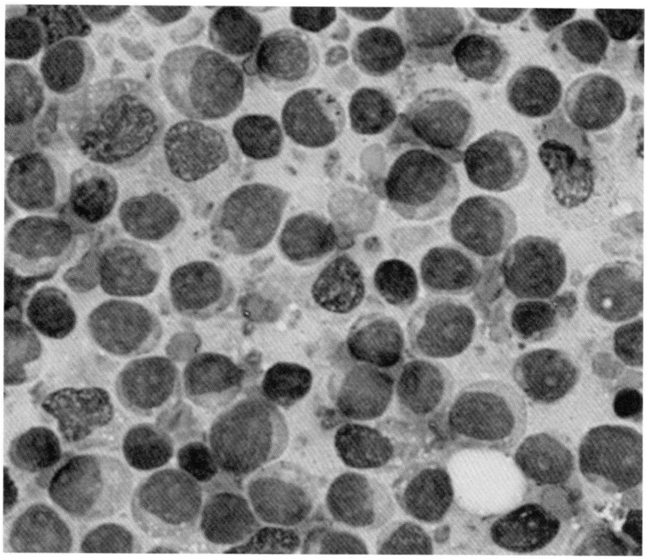

Figure 20-29 Liver aspirate from an 11-year-old Australian Shepherd dog with weight loss, increased liver enzyme activity, and an enlarged generally hypoechoic liver. Cytologic diagnosis of lymphoma of large granular lymphocytes (LGL). Note the distinctive pink to magenta cytoplastic granules in many of the neoplastic CD8+ cytotoxic T cells. (Wright stain. Original magnification 1000×.)

Hepatic involvement in disseminated mast cell neoplasia is often readily recognized by large numbers of mast cells, often pleomorphic, in liver aspirates. Neoplastic mast cells may infiltrate the liver secondary to cutaneous or systemic mast cell disease or as part of the syndrome of visceral mastocytosis, which typically arises in the spleen and is not associated with a primary skin tumor. Resident liver mast cells are typically lightly granulated and have small round nuclei (see the section titled "Normal Findings") and may be numerous in certain inflammatory diseases or secondary to nonspecific hepatocellular injury. Larger cells with more abundant cytoplasm and variable number and size of cytoplasmic granules are more likely to be neoplastic, particularly when seen in high numbers (Figure 20-30, *A*). Basophilic cytoplasm, binucleation, variably sized nuclei, and the presence of nucleoli are additional cytologic

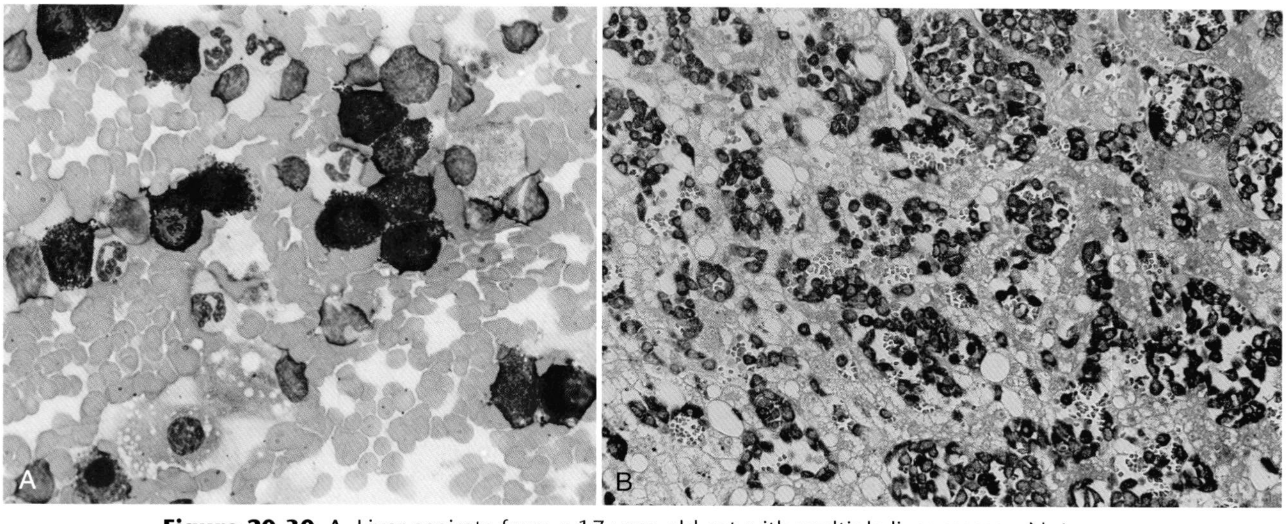

Figure 20-30 A, Liver aspirate from a 17-year-old cat with multiple liver masses. Note aggregates of well-differentiated, highly granulated mast cells. Cytologic diagnosis of hepatic mast cell tumor. (Wright stain. Original magnification 1000×.) **B,** Histologic section from the liver of the same patient highlighting the infiltrative nature of the neoplastic mast cell population. (Giemsa stain. Original magnification 400×.)

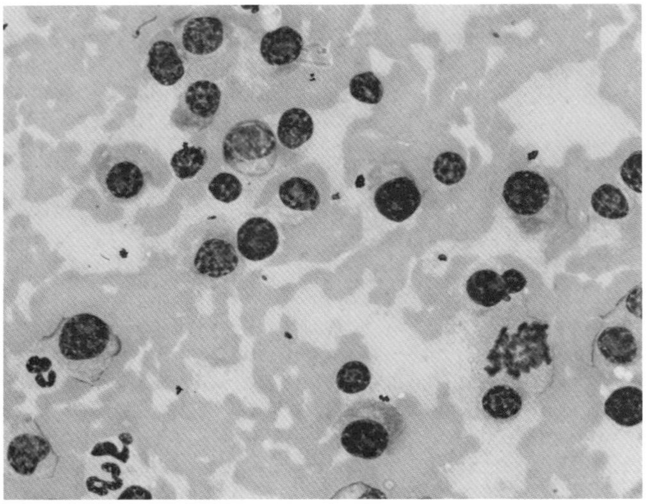

Figure 20-31 Liver aspirate from a 10-year-old cat with weight loss and multiple mixed echogenic hepatic masses. Note the pleomorphic, intermediately differentiated plasma cells with characteristic cytomorphology. Diagnosis of multiple myeloma with concomitant monoclonal gammopathy. (Wright stain. Original magnification 1000×.)

features that are indicative of malignancy in mast cell populations.

Plasma cell tumors are neoplasms of terminally differentiated B-cells, which may infiltrate the liver. Historically, extramedullary plasmacytomas were generally considered benign, and they rarely metastasized; however, recent reports in cats have shown that both cutaneous and noncutaneous extramedullary plasmacytomas commonly exhibit malignant and systemic behavior, and a visceral form with a more aggressive nature has been reported in both dogs and cats.[43] Multiple myeloma is a disseminated plasma cell neoplasm, which predominantly involves the bone marrow in humans and dogs. It has been shown that myeloma-related disease in cats often has marked extramedullary involvement at initial presentation, even if cells appear well differentiated, which is in contrast to the behavior of this condition in humans. Plasma cells may be recognized by their characteristic morphologic features (eccentrically located round nuclei with coarsely clumped chromatin and a moderate amount of deep-blue cytoplasm with a distinct perinuclear clear zone representing the Golgi apparatus) and may be further characterized as well differentiated, intermediate grade, or poorly differentiated (Figure 20-31). Moreover, morphologic features may be correlated to prognosis.[43-44] The tumor cells in plasma cell neoplasms may secrete excess quantities of a specific class of immunoglobulin (Ig), either IgA or IgG, resulting in an accompanying monoclonal gammopathy.

References and Suggested Reading

1. Roth L: Comparison of liver cytology and biopsy diagnoses in dogs and cats: 56 cases, *Vet Clin Pathol* 30:35–38, 2001.
2. Kristensen AT, et al: Liver cytology in cases of canine and feline hepatic disease, *Compend Cont Ed Pract Vet* 12:797–808, 1990.
3. Nyland TG, Mattoon JS: *Small animal diagnostic ultrasound*, ed 2, Philadelphia, PA, 2002, Saunders. pp. 30–48.
4. Hager DA, Nyland TG, Fisher P: Ultrasound-guided biopsy of the canine liver, kidney, and prostate, *Vet Radiol* 26:82–88, 1985.
5. Armstrong JP, Rothuizen J: Veterinary Clinics of North America, Small Animal Practiceed 2, *Hepatology*, vol. 39-3, St. Louis, MO, 2009, Elsevier. (pp. 395–418, 469-480, 599-616).
6. Meyer D: In Raskin R, editor: *Liver: canine and feline cytology*, ed 2, Philadelphia, PA, 2010, Saunders, pp 226–248.
7. Léveillé R, et al: Complications after ultrasound-guided biopsy of abdominal structures in dogs and cats: 246 cases (1984-1991), *J Am Vet Med Assoc* 203:413–415, 1993.
8. Bigge LA, Brown DJ, Penninck DG: Correlation between coagulation profile findings and bleeding complications after ultrasound-guided biopsies: 434 cases (1993-1996), *J Am Anim Hosp Assoc* 37:228–233, 2001.
9. Stalker M, Hayes A: Liver. In Maxie G, editor: *Jubb, Kennedy, and Palmer's pathology of domestic animals*, ed 5, Philadelphia, PA, 2007, Saunders, pp 297–388.
10. Weiss DJ, Gagne JM, Armstrong PJ: Characterization of portal lymphocytic infiltrates in feline liver, *Vet Clin Pathol* 24:91–95, 1995.
11. Lalzad A, Ristitsch D, Downey W, et al: Effect of ultrasound transmission gel on ultrasound-guided fine needle aspiration cytological specimens of thyroid, *Cytopathology* 23(5):330–333, 2012.
12. Scott M, Buriko K: Characterization of the pigmented cytoplasmic granules common in canine hepatocytes, *Vet Clin Pathol* 34(suppl):281–282, 2005.
13. Rolfe DS, Twedt DC: Copper-associated hepatopathies in dogs, *Vet Clin North Am Small Anim Pract* 25:399–417, 1995.
14. Haywood S, Rutgers HC, Christian MK: Hepatitis and copper accumulation in Skye terriers, *Vet Pathol* 25:408–414, 1988.
15. Webb CB, Twedt DC, Meyer DJ: Copper-associated liver disease in Dalmatians: a review of 10 dogs (1998-2001), *J Vet Intern Med* 16:665–668, 2002.
16. Haynes JS, Wade PR: Hepatopathy associated with excessive hepatic copper in a Siamese cat, *Vet Pathol* 32:427–429, 1995.
17. Center SA: Feline hepatic lipidosis, *Vet Clin North Am Small Anim Pract* 35:225–269, 2005.
18. van der Linde-Sipman JS, van den Ingh I, van Toor AJ: Fatty liver syndrome in puppies, *J Am Anim Hosp Assoc* 26:9–12, 1990.
19. Newman SJ, Joanne R, Smith JR, et al: Aflatoxicosis in nine dogs after exposure to contaminated commercial dog food, *J Vet Diagn Invest* 19:168–175, 2007.
20. Sepesy LM, et al: Vacuolar hepatopathy in dogs: 336 cases (1993-2005), *J Am Vet Med Assoc* 229:246–252, 2006.
21. Wang KY, et al: Accuracy of ultrasound-guided fine-needle aspiration of the liver and cytologic findings in dogs and cats: 97 cases (1990-2000), *J Am Vet Med Assoc* 224:75–78, 2004.
22. Weiss DJ, Blauvelt M, Aird B: Cytologic evaluation of inflammation in canine liver aspirates, *Vet Clin Pathol* 30:193–196, 2001.
23. Centre S: Hepatobiliary infections. In Greene CE, editor: *Infectious diseases of the dog and cat*, ed 3, Philadelphia, PA, 1990, Saunders, pp 915–918.
24. Crews LJ, Feeney DA, Jessen CR, et al: Clinical, ultrasonographic, and laboratory findings associated with gall bladder disease and rupture in dogs: 45 cases (1997-2007), *J am Vet Med Assoc* 234:359–366, 2009.
25. Watson TG, Croll NA: Clinical changes caused by the liver fluke metorchis conjunctus in cats, *Vet Pathol* 18:778–785, 1981.
26. Loeven KO: Hepatic amyloidosis in two Chinese Shar Pei dogs, *J Am Vet Med Assoc* 204:1212–1216, 1994.

27. Hammer AS, Sikkema DA: Hepatic neoplasia in the dog and cat, *Vet Clin North Am Small Anim Pract* 25:419–435, 1995.
28. Zuber RM: Systemic amyloidosis in Oriental and Siamese cats, *Aust Vet Pract* 23:66–70, 1993.
29. Liptak JM: Hepatobiliary tumors. In Withrow SJ, Vail DM, Page R, editors: *Withrow and MacEwen's small animal clinical oncology*, ed 4, Philadelphia, PA, 2007, Saunders, pp 483–491.
30. Cullen JM, Popp JA: Tumors of the liver and gallbladder. In Meuton DJ, editor: *Tumors in domestic animals*, ed 4, Ames, Iowa, 2002, Iowa State Press / Blackwell Publishing, pp 483–508.
31. Patnaik AK: A morphologic and immunocytochemical study of hepatic neoplasms in cats, *Vet Pathol* 29:405–415, 1992.
32. Patnaik AK, et al: Canine hepatic carcinoids, *Vet Pathol* 18:445–453, 1981.
33. Patnaik AK, et al: Hepatobiliary neuroendocrine carcinoma in cats: a clinicopathologic, immunohistochemical, and ultrastructural study of 17 cats, *Vet Pathol* 42:331–337, 2005.
34. Patnaik AK, et al: Canine hepatic neuroendocrine carcinoma: an immunohistochemical and electron microscopic study, *Vet Pathol* 42:140–146, 2005.
35. Morrell CN, Volk MV, Mankowski JL: A carcinoid tumor in the gallbladder of a dog, *Vet Pathol* 39:756–758, 2002.
36. Affolter VK, Moore PF: Localized and disseminated histiocytic sarcoma of dendritic cell origin in dogs, *Vet Pathol* 39:74–83, 2002.
37. Kraje AC, Patton C, Edwards D: Malignant histiocytosis in 3 cats, *J Vet Intern Med* 15:252–256, 2001.
38. Moore PF, Affolter VK, Vernau W: Canine hemophagocytic histiocytic sarcoma: a proliferative disorder of CD11d+ macrophages, *Vet Pathol* 43:632–645, 2006.
39. Weiss DJ: Flow cytometric evaluation of hemophagocytic disorders in canine bone marrow, *Vet Clin Pathol* 31:36–41, 2002.
40. Fry MM, et al: Hepatosplenic lymphoma in a dog, *Vet Pathol* 40:556–562, 2003.
41. Valli VE: T cell and NK cell Neoplasms. In Valli VE, editor: *Veterinary comparative hematopathology*, Ames Iowa, 2007, Blackwell publishing, pp 316–318.
42. Roccabianca P, et al: Feline large granular lymphocyte (LGL) lymphoma with secondary leukemia: primary intestinal origin with predominance of a CD3/CD8αα phenotype, *Vet Pathol* 43:15–28, 2006.
43. Mellor PJ, et al: Histopathologic, immunohistochemical, and cytologic analysis of feline myeloma-related disorders: further evidence for primary extramedullary development in the cat, *Vet Pathol 45* 2:159–173, 2008.
44. Patel RT, et al: Multiple myeloma in 16 cats: a retrospective study, *Vet Clin Pathol* 34:341–352, 2005.

CHAPTER 21

The Spleen

Peter S. MacWilliams and Patricia M. McManus

The spleen is the second largest lymphoid organ.[1] Splenic functions include initiation of immune-response to bloodborne antigens; storage of platelets and mature red blood cells (RBCs); maturation of reticulocytes; phagocytosis and destruction of senescent and damaged RBCs, platelets, and white blood cells (WBCs); phagocytosis of foreign particles and microorganisms; and extramedullary hematopoiesis.[1,2] Because of these highly varied and often independent functions, different systemic inflammatory and noninflammatory diseases and hematologic disorders will impact the gross and microscopic appearance of the spleen in vastly different ways. As with other organs, the spleen is subject to cell growth disturbances (e.g., hyperplasia, hypoplasia), circulatory abnormalities (e.g., hemorrhage, congestion, thrombosis, and infarction), inflammation, and neoplasia (primary and metastatic).[2] These processes, either alone or in combination, may result in splenic enlargement or changes in shape and echotexture.

Splenomegaly is usually detected by palpation or diagnostic imaging. Depending on the cause, splenomegaly may be accompanied by hematologic abnormalities such as anemia, thrombocytopenia, neutropenia, and leukemia. A complete blood count (CBC) and careful examination of morphologies of RBCs, WBCs, and platelets in a peripheral blood film may be very revealing regarding causative factors. Causes of splenomegaly in dogs and cats are listed in (Table 21-1).[2-7] Careful palpation and radiographic imaging should reveal the severity of splenomegaly and whether enlargement is diffuse or localized. Ultrasonographic examination provides a more detailed assessment of architectural abnormalities. By visualizing small nodules, target lesions, or changes in echogenicity in the spleen, ultrasonographic examination can reveal suspect areas of neoplasia, hyperplasia, inflammation, or extramedullary hematopoiesis and enables precise localization for fine-needle aspiration (FNA) or fine-needle biopsy (FNB).[8-10]

Indications for sampling of spleen are summarized in Box 21-1, but invasive collection of splenic tissue is not always needed if the cause is revealed by other means.[11,12] For example, splenomegaly is likely linked to immune-mediated disease if a patient tests positive for erythrocytic antiglobulins (Coombs test), antinuclear antibodies, or rheumatoid factor. Serologic tests may suggest fungal or protozoal infections. Detection of hemoparasites such as *Mycoplasma, Cytauxzoon*, or *Babesia* spp. in a peripheral blood film also supports an infectious cause for splenomegaly. Cytologic examination of bone marrow or peripheral lymph nodes may enable diagnosis of hematopoietic and lymphocytic neoplasia or systemic infections. When splenomegaly is accompanied by peritoneal effusion collection and cytologic evaluation of abdominal fluid is indicated prior to direct sampling of the spleen.

SAMPLING METHODS

Needle collections of splenic tissue are indicated when the cause of splenomegaly cannot be determined by other means. Specimens for cytologic assessment of the spleen may be collected by needle and syringe, by using material collected at the time of a surgical biopsy, and at necropsy.

Needle Methods

Collection of splenic samples by needle puncture should be carefully considered. An enlarged spleen may be turgid, friable, and engorged with blood. Profuse intraabdominal hemorrhage and tumor metastasis within the abdominal cavity are possible complications; however, several studies in dogs and humans concluded that thrombocytopenia, number of needle passes during collection, repeat collections, and core biopsies were not associated with an increase in the number or severity of complications.[13-15]

Fine-needle collections of the spleen can usually be done without general anesthesia. The size and location of the spleen within the abdominal cavity determine the actual site for penetration, which should be at the site where the spleen is most easily apposed to the abdominal wall. The site is prepared as if for surgery by clipping, washing, and applying an antiseptic. If the collection is aided by ultrasonographic imaging, care must be taken to not contaminate the skin, the slides, and the needles with lubricant, as this material stains a rich purple to magenta on slides and will interfere with microscopic evaluation (Figure 21-1). Infiltration of the abdominal wall with local anesthetic is usually unnecessary. A 22-gauge needle may be either directly attached to a 12-mL (milliliter) syringe for aspiration (FNA) or attached via an intravenous extension set

TABLE 21-1

CAUSES AND CHARACTERISTICS OF SPLENOMEGALY IN DOGS AND CATS

Cause	Type of Enlargement	Severity of Enlargement
Hyperplasia	Symmetric or nodular	Mild to moderate
Infection		
Immunologic disease		
Extramedullary hematopoiesis	Symmetric or nodular	Mild to moderate
Hemolymphatic neoplasia	Symmetric	Moderate to severe
Lymphoma or lymphocytic leukemia		
Myeloid neoplasms		
Systemic mastocytosis		
Plasma cell tumor or multiple myeloma		
Other neoplasia	Symmetric or nodular	Mild to severe
Hemangioma or hemangiosarcoma	Nodular	
Fibrosarcoma or undifferentiated sarcoma	Nodular	
Histiocytic sarcoma	Nodular	
Hemophagocytic histiocytic sarcoma	Symmetric	
Leiomyoma or leiomyosarcoma	Nodular	
Metastatic neoplasms	Asymmetric or nodular	
Other	Symmetric or nodular	Highly variable
Systemic histiocytosis		
Hemophagocytic syndrome		
Fibrohistiocytic nodules		
Hypereosinophilic syndrome		
Inflammation		
Circulatory disturbances		
Hematoma	Asymmetric	Mild to moderate
Thrombosis with infarction	Symmetric	May not be enlarged
Portal hypertension with splenic congestion	Symmetric	Mild to moderate
Torsion	Symmetric	Severe

Spangler WL, Culbertson MR: Prevalence and type of splenic diseases in cats: 455 cases (1985-1991), *J Am Vet Med Assoc* 201:773-776, 1992.

BOX 21-1

Indications for Cytologic Examination of the Spleen

- Diffuse or symmetric enlargement
- Splenic nodules or asymmetric enlargement
- Radiographic evidence of abnormal splenic architecture
- Abnormal ultrasonographic image of the spleen
  - Hyperechoic or hypoechoic areas
  - Abnormal variation in echogenicity
  - Nodular or focal lesions
- Diagnosis of neoplasia
- Tumor staging

From Spangler WL, Kass PH: Pathologic and prognostic characteristics of splenomegaly in dogs due to fibrohistiocytic nodules: 98 cases, *Vet Pathol* 35:488-498, 1998.

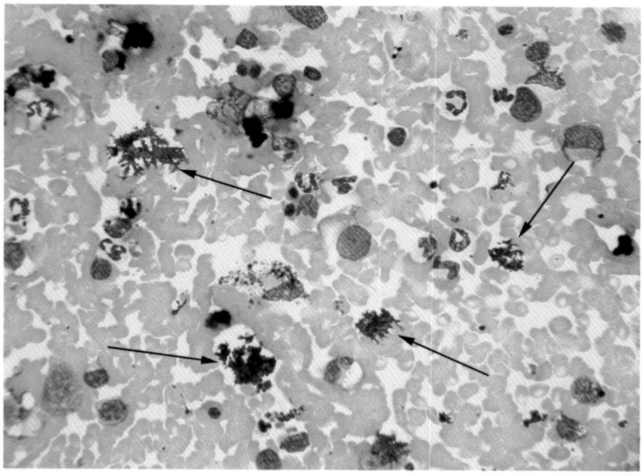

Figure 21-1 Canine spleen. The arrows indicate deposits of magenta-stained material, typical for aqueous lubricant used for ultrasound-guided fine needle methods. Heavy contamination can prevent evaluation of a slide. (Wright-Giemsa. Original magnification 50× oil objective.)

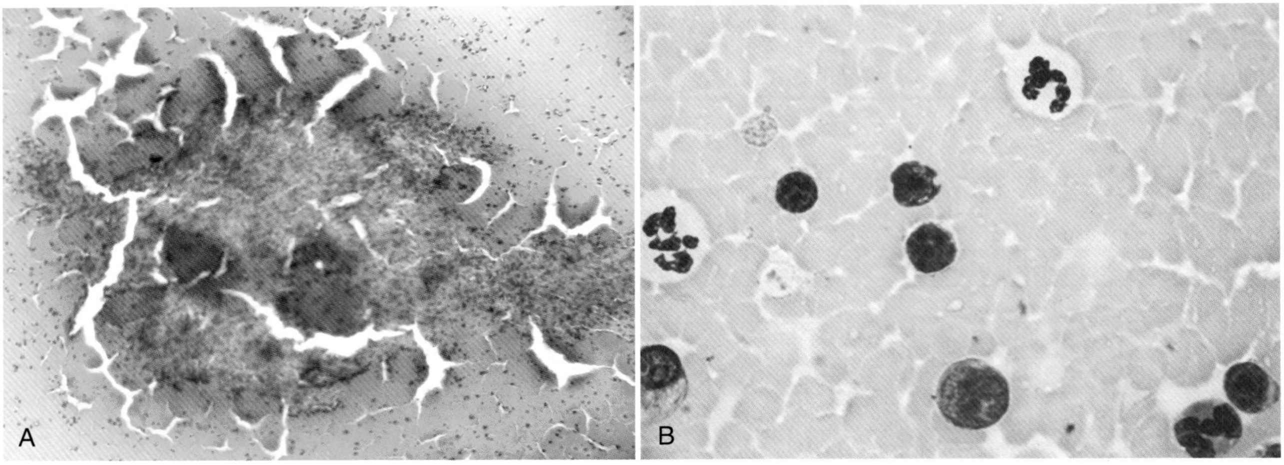

Figure 21-2 Canine spleen. A, This preparation is very thick and cracked due to slow drying of the thick areas. The splenic tissue fragment cannot be evaluated and most of the dispersed nucleated cells are difficult to identify. In this type of preparation, it is difficult to distinguish small lymphocytes from larger potentially neoplastic cells. However, detection of these fragments confirms successful aspiration of spleen. (Wright-Giemsa. Original magnification 10× objective.) **B,** In some cases, the smear cannot be evaluated at all, but, as this image demonstrates, patient examination of thinner areas between fragments will be rewarded by finding cells spread thin enough to identify and evaluate. (Wright-Giemsa. Original magnification 100× oil.)

for the nonaspiration method (FNB), which may reduce hemodilution of the sample, yield more highly cellular tissue fragments, and produce superior preparations.[16-17] Needle length is determined by the size of the animal, but usually a 1- or 1½-inch needle is adequate.

The spleen is gently pressed against the abdominal wall at the prepared site. The needle is inserted through the skin and muscle layer into the spleen. For the FNA method, the syringe plunger produces negative pressure while the needle is moved within the spleen along several axes. Maintaining suction while redirecting the needle in the parenchyma collects cells and tissue fragments from several areas. To minimize hemorrhage and dilution of the sample, negative pressure on the plunger should be released immediately if bloody fluid appears in the syringe tip. It is very important to release the syringe plunger before the needle is withdrawn from the spleen. Immediately after withdrawing the needle from the animal, small drops of the aspirate are applied to glass slides and prepared as described below.

For the FNB method, the needle is attached to an intravenous extension set, which is attached to the syringe.[16] The syringe is filled with air prior to penetration of the skin and does not need to be handled during the actual collection of specimen, unlike the FNA method. After the spleen is penetrated, the needle tip is rapidly moved in and out 8 to 10 times without changing its path and without allowing the tip of the needle to leave the spleen. This will dislodge a small sample that will be retained within the bore of the needle. The needle is then withdrawn, and the specimen contained within the needle is immediately expelled onto a glass slide using the air-filled syringe. Prepare the smear as described below. This method usually results in only a single slide per penetration; therefore, three to five collections are suggested, each time targeting different areas of the spleen or splenic nodule.

The consistency of the specimen determines the method of smear preparation. Most specimens collected by the aspiration method have the consistency of blood and slides are prepared in the same manner as blood films. Specimens that are thick or contain tissue fragments, for example, specimens collected by FNB, are prepared by the squash technique, with the material gently compressed between two slides. Too much material on the slide can result in slides that are too thick to evaluate (Figure 21-2). Chapter 1 contains a detailed description of slide preparation techniques.

Impression, Scraping, and Squash Preparations

Impression, scraping, and squash preparations of splenic tissue may be prepared from biopsies taken during surgical exploration and often complement histologic assessment. In some situations, an immediate diagnosis may be obtained. For example, a homogeneous population of large lymphoblasts (Figure 21-3) or a pure population of mast cells (Figure 21-4) confirms a diagnosis of lymphoma and mast cell neoplasia, respectively. Cytologic preparations of splenic tissue reveal nuclear and cytoplasmic details not visible in tissue sections. The different tinctorial characteristics of hematologic stains allow more accurate identification of erythroid precursors versus lymphocytes, basophils versus histiocytes, and mast cells versus other round cells. Although tissue architecture is lost in collection, recognition of individual cell types, fungi, protozoa, RBC parasites, and neoplastic cells is sometimes easier on Wright-stained slides. Cytologic preparations are particularly valuable in identifying subtle dysplastic morphologies. However, changes attributable to circulatory disturbances as causes of splenomegaly, for example, congestion, hemorrhage, torsion, or infarction, are better assessed by histologic evaluation.

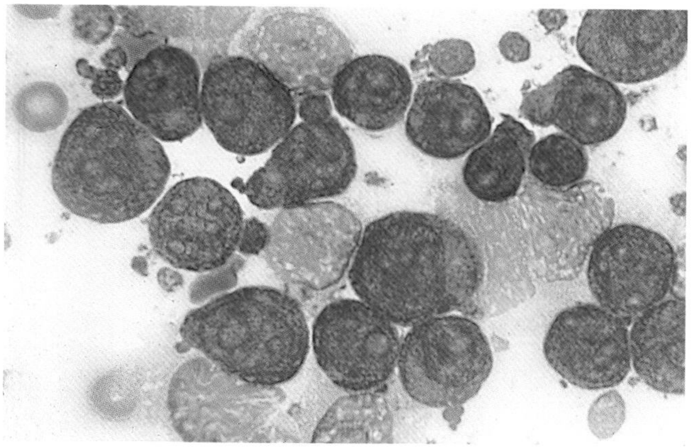

Figure 21-3 Canine spleen. Impression smear prepared from a splenic biopsy from a dog with lymphoma contains a homogeneous population of large lymphocytes characterized by multiple prominent nucleoli. (Wright stain. Original magnification 100× oil objective.)

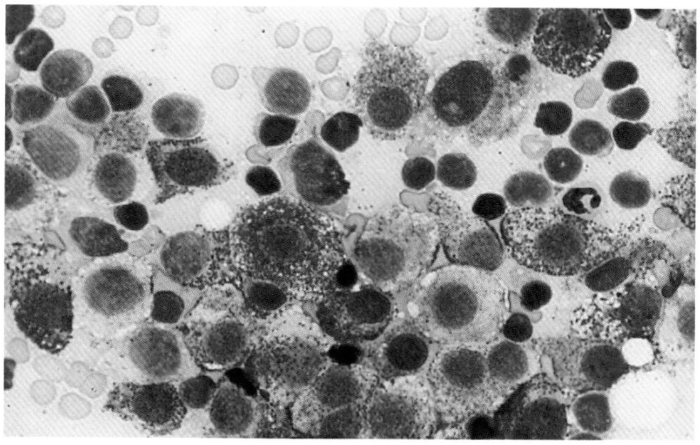

Figure 21-4 Feline spleen. Impression smear prepared from a splenic biopsy from a cat with systemic mastocytosis and marked symmetric splenomegaly. The spleen is diffusely infiltrated with neoplastic mast cells that have round nuclei and numerous intracytoplasmic purple granules. Numerous small lymphocytes, plus a single neutrophil in the upper right corner, are also present. (Wright stain. Original magnification 100× oil objective.)

Preliminary to making impression and scraping smears from whole tissue specimens, blot the tissue on a paper towel to remove excess blood and fluid. If feasible, trim the tissue with a scalpel blade to expose a fresh-cut surface. Then make tissue imprints on the slides or scrape the surface with the scalpel blade and spread the scrapings on the slide. Also making squash preparations from tissue fragments should be considered. Using a variety of techniques increases the likelihood of getting smears that contain adequate specimen with good preservation of cell morphology. Further details are provided in Chapter 1.

Staining

Wright-Giemsa stain or a similar Romanowsky stain is the ideal stain for splenic cytology because it provides excellent definition of cytoplasmic features, facilitates identification of cytoplasmic granulation, and allows evaluation

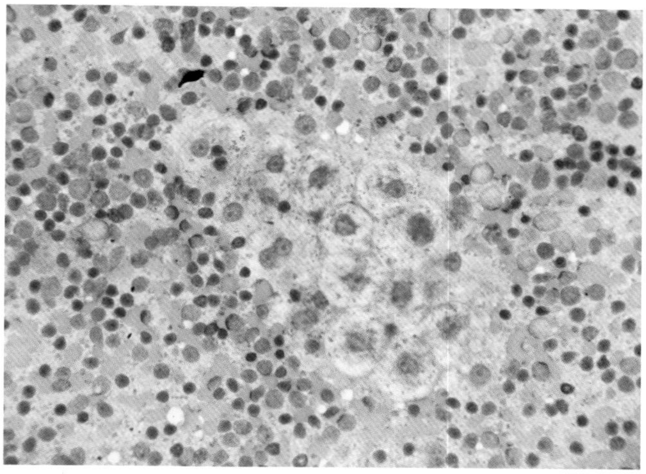

Figure 21-5 Canine spleen. Occasionally, hepatic tissue may be inadvertently included in an aspirate and should not be mistaken for metastatic carcinoma. (Wright stain. Original magnification 50× objective.)

of hematopoietic cells. If using "quick" or "rapid" modified Wright stains, fixation and staining times will need to be increased for preparations that are thicker than blood films. Cytoplasmic granulation (e.g., granular lymphocytes, mast cells, myeloid precursors) may not be preserved with quick stains, although longer fixation times may ameliorate that problem to some extent. Chapter 1 contains specific information on staining techniques.

MICROSCOPIC EXAMINATION

Low-power objectives (4× and 10×) are used to assess cellularity and stain quality, locate cellular clusters and tissue fragments, and select slides and microscopic fields for further examination under higher magnification. Occasionally, miscellaneous structures that have no clinical significance, for example, fragments of mechanically exfoliated mesothelial tissue or hepatic tissue that was inadvertently included will be found (Figure 21-5). The 40× (or 50× oil to allow examination without a coverslip) and 100× oil objectives are used to assess the general composition of the cell population and study the nuclear and cytoplasmic details of individual cells. At these magnifications, it is helpful to find a small lymphocyte or segmented neutrophil for size and color comparisons (see Figure 21-2; Figure 21-6). Small lymphocytes are smaller than segmented neutrophils and have round, slightly indented, or narrowly cleaved nuclei, dark condensed chromatin, no visible nucleoli, and scant light-blue cytoplasm.

Table 21-1 lists five general causes of splenic enlargement, but more than one mechanism may be operative in a given animal. For example, a dog with immune-mediated hemolytic anemia may have splenomegaly caused by both lymphoid hyperplasia and extramedullary hematopoiesis. Animals with infections such as *Histoplasma, Cytauxzoon,* and *Babesia* spp. infections (Figure 21-7 and Figure 21-8) may have splenomegaly from both lymphoid hyperplasia and granulomatous inflammation. Figure 21-9 presents an algorithm for classification of splenic cytologic findings.

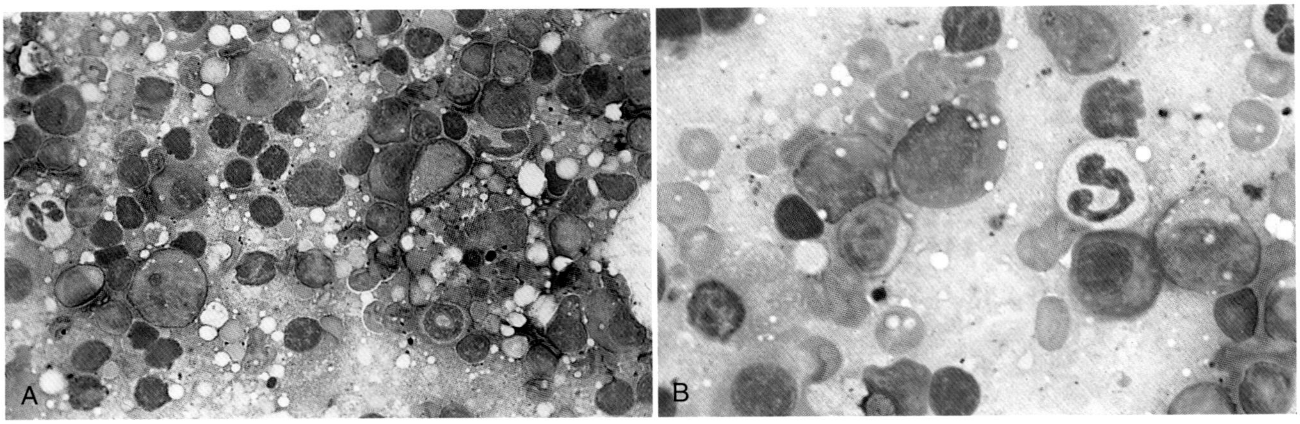

Figure 21-6 Canine spleen. Fine-needle aspirate of hyperplastic splenic tissue from a dog with immune-mediated hemolytic anemia. **A,** Small lymphocytes predominate, but increased numbers of large lymphocytes (*lower left*) and plasma cells (*upper left*) indicate hyperplasia. A large macrophage (*lower right*) contains many phagocytized erythrocytes. (Wright stain. Original magnification 48x objective.) **B,** Higher magnification reveals two lymphoblasts (*left*) adjacent to a small lymphocyte. A neutrophil, plasma cell, and lymphoblast are located to the right of center. The plasma cell is recognized by its round, eccentric nucleus; smooth blue cytoplasm; and prominent Golgi zone. Compare the sizes of the neutrophil, plasma cell, lymphoblast, and lymphocyte. (Wright stain. Original magnification 100× oil objective.)

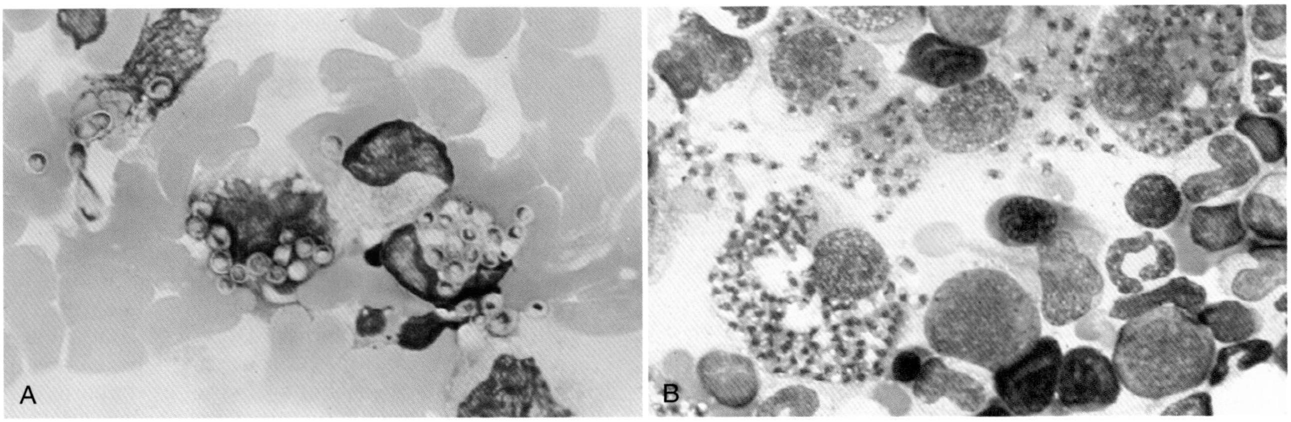

Figure 21-7 Canine spleen. Recognition of infectious agents in splenic aspirates. **A,** Fine-needle aspirate of spleen from a dog infected with the fungus *Histoplasma capsulatum*. Macrophages contain phagocytized *Histoplasma* organisms. One organism in the upper left appears to be budding. (Wright stain. Original magnification 100× oil objective.) **B,** Impression smear of spleen from a dog infected with the protozoan parasite of the genus *Leishmania*, most likely of the *L. donovani* complex, the cause of visceral leishmaniasis. Numerous *Leishmania* amastigotes are present in macrophages and in the background. The image also contains several plasma cells, neutrophils, and immature granulocytes. (Wright stain. Original magnification 100× oil objective.)

Normal Cytologic Features

Smears of normal splenic tissue have microscopic features similar to those of normal lymph nodes. A good preparation should be very cellular and contain a mixed population of many small lymphocytes, few to moderate numbers of larger lymphocytes, few macrophages, few plasma cells, few mast cells, and occasional hematopoietic cells (trilineage).[1,2,12] A good sample contains variably sized fragments of splenic tissue, which consist of reticular fibers, stroma cells (also called *myofibroblasts* and *fibrohistiocytes*), endothelial cells, macrophages, and plasma cells (Figure 21-10). Small lymphocytes predominate in most fields; however, because the spleen contains numerous lymphoid follicles with germinal centers, large lymphocytes may predominate in some areas (Figure 21-11). The larger lymphocytes may display loosely clumped to vesicular chromatin, and nucleoli may be visible, similar to neoplastic lymphocytes. Often, context is needed to rule out a neoplastic proliferation. Finding areas of the smears that contain a heterogeneous collection of lymphocytes and plasma cells precludes designation of these cells as neoplastic (Figure 21-12).

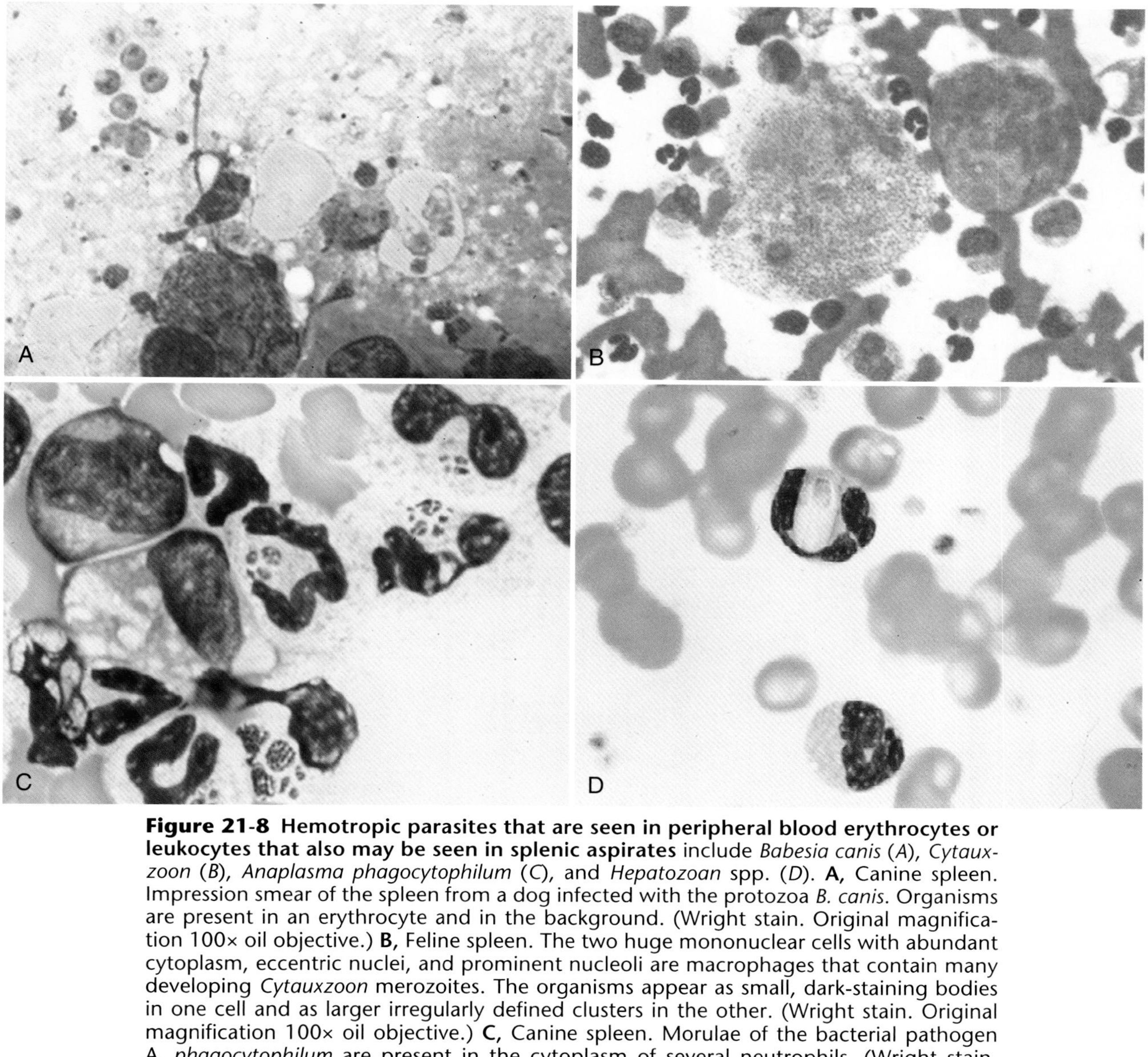

Figure 21-8 Hemotropic parasites that are seen in peripheral blood erythrocytes or leukocytes that also may be seen in splenic aspirates include *Babesia canis* (*A*), *Cytauxzoon* (*B*), *Anaplasma phagocytophilum* (*C*), and *Hepatozoan* spp. (*D*). **A,** Canine spleen. Impression smear of the spleen from a dog infected with the protozoa *B. canis*. Organisms are present in an erythrocyte and in the background. (Wright stain. Original magnification 100× oil objective.) **B,** Feline spleen. The two huge mononuclear cells with abundant cytoplasm, eccentric nuclei, and prominent nucleoli are macrophages that contain many developing *Cytauxzoon* merozoites. The organisms appear as small, dark-staining bodies in one cell and as larger irregularly defined clusters in the other. (Wright stain. Original magnification 100× oil objective.) **C,** Canine spleen. Morulae of the bacterial pathogen A. *phagocytophilum* are present in the cytoplasm of several neutrophils. (Wright stain. Original magnification 100× oil objective.) **D,** Canine spleen. A protozoal *Hepatozoon* organism is present in the cytoplasm of a neutrophil. Infected leukocytes may be seen in peripheral blood and may become entrapped in splenic sinusoids. Fine-needle aspirates of spleen are often diluted with peripheral blood. Red blood cells and platelets are present, indicating that some hemodilution has occurred. (Wright stain. Original magnification 100× oil objective.)

Macrophages may contain small to moderate amounts of cytoplasmic hemosiderin.

The microscopic appearance of fine-needle aspirates of splenic tissue is affected by the amount of hemodilution in the specimen. Depending on the amount of blood contamination and the peripheral leukocyte count, the background contains varying numbers of RBCs, WBCs, and platelets. A severe peripheral neutrophilia could potentially lead to misinterpretation as splenitis, when the actual inflammation causing the neutrophilia may be elsewhere.

Hyperplasia

Splenomegaly secondary to lymphocytic hyperplasia results from a variety of inflammatory diseases, both septic and nonseptic. Mild to moderate degrees of splenomegaly are found in immune-mediated disorders and in systemic infectious diseases caused by bacteria, rickettsiae, protozoa, and fungi. Cytologic findings in hyperplastic splenomegaly depend on the causative agent, mechanism of disease, and the host's immune response. In general, splenic hyperplasia is characterized by increased numbers of macrophages, plasma cells, and

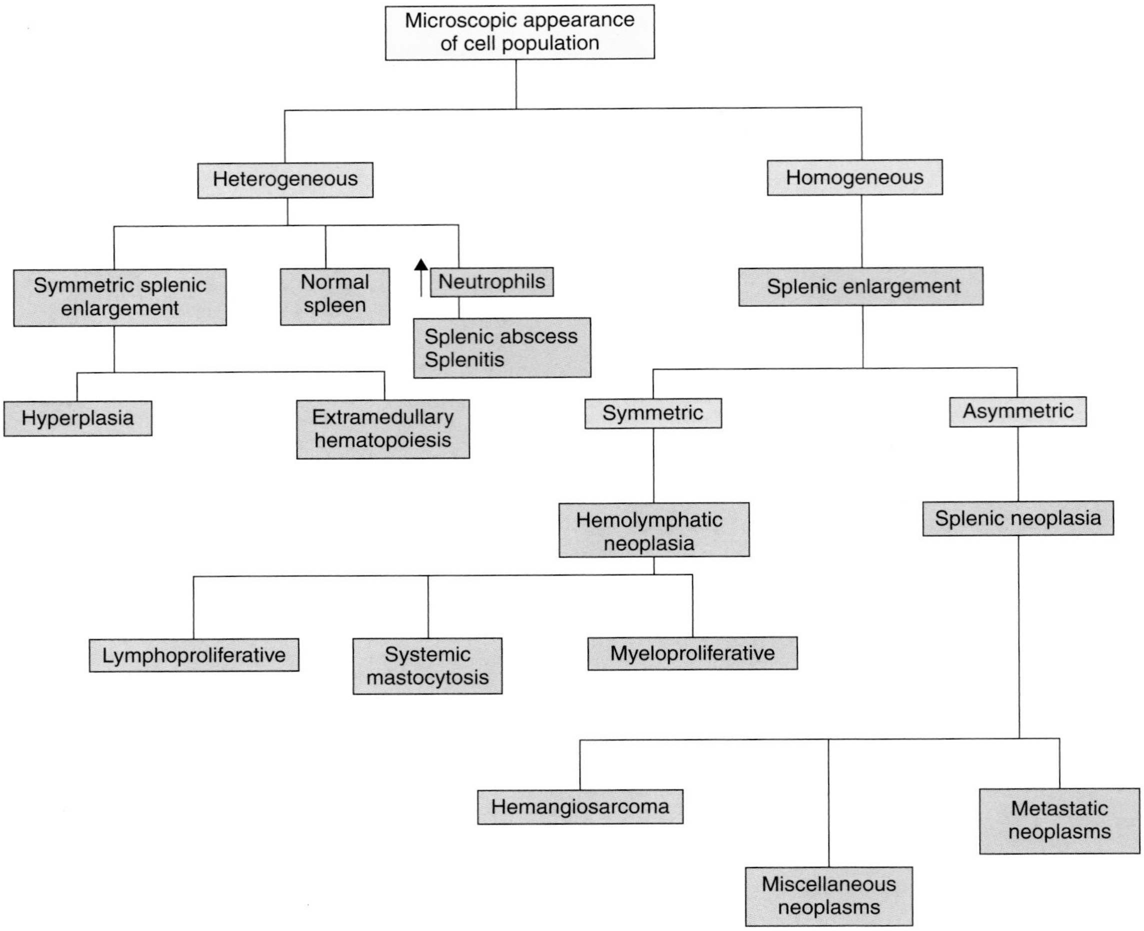

Figure 21-9 Cytologic classification of fine-needle aspirates and impression smears from the spleens of dogs and cats.

larger lymphocytes (see Figure 21-6). A relative decrease in numbers of small lymphocytes occurs; however, these cells remain the predominant cell type. A slight to occasionally moderate increase in neutrophil numbers is expected, but a marked predominance of neutrophils is uncommon and suggests splenitis, necrosis, abscessation, extramedullary granulopoiesis, or inflammation secondary to a neoplastic cell infiltrate. A marked increase in eosinophils may correlate with enteric parasites, severe allergies, some neoplasms, or idiopathic eosinophilic infiltrative disease. With some infections and immune responses, increases in macrophages and plasma cells are pronounced. When macrophages are increased, it is important to examine their cytoplasm for cellular debris, pigment, phagocytized erythrocytes (see Figure 21-6), bacteria, and organisms such as *Histoplasma* (see Figure 21-7, *A*) and *Leishmania* spp. (see Figure 21-7, *B*). Erythrocytes in background blood should be examined for *Babesia* (see Figure 21-8, *A*), *Cytauxzoon*, *Mycoplasma haemofelis,* and Heinz bodies and eccentrocytes.[11] Phagocytosis of erythrocytes (see Figure 21-6) is also increased with immune-mediated hemolytic anemia, but the thickness of the smear may prevent identification of spherocytes. Leukocytes should be scrutinized for morulae of *Anaplasma phagocytophilum* (see Figure 21-8, *C*) and *Hepatozoon* organisms (see Figure 21-8, *D*). Mast cells can also increase in a stimulated spleen; therefore, few to moderate numbers (and occasionally many mast cells, depending on other changes) are not sufficient to diagnose neoplastic systemic mastocytosis or mast cell tumor metastasis (Figure 21-13 and Figure 21-14). A marked increase in hemosiderin deposits within macrophages is often best assessed by examination of tissue fragments (see Figure 21-13). The change may be incidental as quantity will increase with age, but increases may also correlate with chronic congestion (e.g., with chronic liver or heart disease), hemorrhage, or hemolysis.

Extramedullary Hematopoiesis

Extramedullary hematopoiesis is the development of sites of hematopoiesis outside of bone marrow. Hematopoietic cells are often detected at a low frequency in splenic tissue from healthy cats and dogs, but disorders that markedly increase their numbers are numerous and diverse, for example, inflammatory disease, recovery from chemotherapy and other causes of cytotoxicity, bone marrow disorders, disseminated histiocytic sarcoma, hemangiosarcoma, myelolipomas, immune-mediated thrombocytopenia, and hemolytic anemia and hemorrhage. Responses are similar to bone marrow, with increases reflective of the current

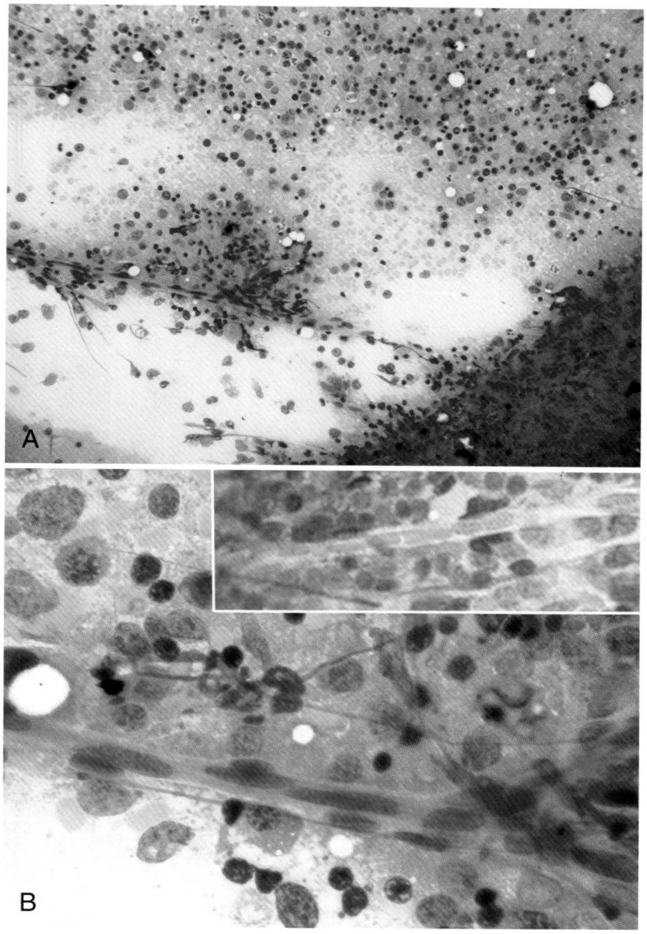

Figure 21-10 Canine spleen. **A,** Note the capillary fragment emerging from the thick splenic tissue fragment. A smaller fragment of splenic tissue is still adherent to it. The large fragment is too thick to evaluate, but the thinner areas between fragments contain nicely spread cells, amenable to evaluation (Wright-Giemsa. Original magnification 20× objective.) **B,** This is a higher magnification of that same blood vessel. Note the small, narrow oval nuclei. Cytoplasm of endothelial cells is often almost invisible as it stains a very light grey. (Wright-Giemsa. Original magnification 100× objective.) *Inset,* Note the capillary that still has erythrocytes within it. (Wright-Giemsa. Original magnification 100× objective.)

need, that is, predominantly a single lineage (myeloid, erythroid, megakaryocytic), bilineage, or trilineage. Splenomegaly and hypoechoic splenic foci are common manifestations in animals with extramedullary hematopoiesis, which may be encountered as the primary change or in combination with lymphocytic hyperplasia and neoplasia.

In hemolytic anemia caused by immunologic disease or infectious agents, the cytologic appearance is dominated by erythroid precursors, which frequently exfoliate as clusters around central macrophages (Figure 21-15). These clusters are referred to as *erythroblastic islets.* The central macrophages are considered intrinsic to the regulation of erythropoiesis and also phagocytize the nuclei from the maturing cells. Macrophages containing hemosiderin and phagocytized RBCs are also easily found (Figure 21-16). Late-stage erythroid precursors are numerous and recognized easily, but the more immature erythroid cells could be confused with lymphocytes (Figure 21-17). Features of immature RBCs that differentiate them from lymphocytes include an evenly round nucleus with irregularly clumped chromatin imparting a "wheel-spoke" or "checkerboard" appearance (see Figure 21-17). The cytoplasm is dark blue progressing to blue-gray to "polychromatophilic," with maturation as ribosomes decrease and hemoglobin increases. The less mature forms often display a small clear spot adjacent to the nucleus (see Figure 21-17). When these cells are found in conjunction with myeloproliferative disease or lymphoid neoplasia in the spleen, erythroid precursors are mixed with the neoplastic cells. Asynchronous nuclear and cytoplasmic development is often present, especially in cats (see Figure 21-17).

Myelolipomas are benign nodular lesions that are observed incidentally in the spleen of dogs and occasionally in cats. Their cytologic appearance is characterized by marked extramedullary hematopoiesis with small groups of normal adipocytes. The key difference between myelolipomas and extramedullary hematopoiesis as described above is the presence of embedded fat tissue in the former.

Lymphoid and Myeloid Neoplasms

The cells obtained from normal spleen are heterogeneous in terms of morphologies and lineage, whereas with a lymphocytic or myeloid neoplasm, the slides contain a homogeneous population of neoplastic cells. Replacement of parenchyma with these cells is nearly complete, leaving few normal lymphocytes, plasma cells, and macrophages.

In most dogs and cats with high-grade lymphoma and acute lymphocytic leukemia, normal cells are replaced by a homogeneous population of large to very large lymphocytes characterized by dark blue cytoplasm, round or indented nuclei, and multiple distinct nucleoli (see Figure 21-3). If only small fields are examined and the smears are thick, lymphoid hyperplasia may be mistaken for lymphoma (see Figure 21-11). Chronic lymphocytic leukemia and small cell lymphomas are more difficult to identify cytologically because the neoplastic cells are small, and difficult to differentiate from nonneoplastic lymphocytes. Surgical biopsy or other diagnostic methods, for example, immunocytochemistry (see Chapter 29), flow cytometric immunophenotyping (see Chapter 30), may be required. However, clues that the cells are neoplastic may include a lack of a plasmacytosis, extreme cellularity of the specimen, detection of consistently granulated cytoplasm (if a granular lymphocyte lymphoma), and clinical history, for example, severe splenomegaly, peripheral blood lymphocytosis, or hypercalcemia.

Splenic impression smears from cats with erythroid leukemia have a cellular profile that is similar to their marrow; that is, numerous large round cells with round nuclei, fine granular chromatin, single nucleoli, and dark blue cytoplasm are present. In some cells, the cytoplasm contains a small, localized clear zone (Figure 21-18). The relatively few late-stage erythroid precursors often display nucleus–cytoplasm asynchronous maturation.

Round cell tumors seen in spleen may be derived from granulocytes, monocytes, plasma cells (Figure 21-19),

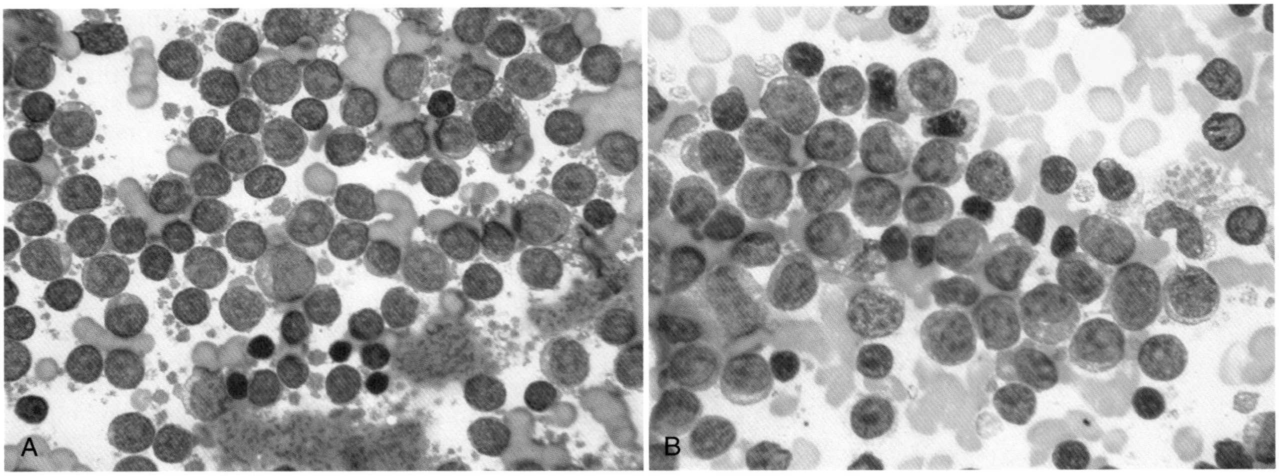

Figure 21-11 **A,** Feline spleen. Ultrasonographic evaluation of this 14-year-old cat showed liver and spleen enlargement and diffusely thickened intestines. Lymphoma was diagnosed based on detection of a diffuse and homogeneous infiltrate of these moderately large lymphocytes within the splenic fine-needle biopsy. No evidence of a plasmacytosis in any area of the aspirates was present, and very few small lymphocytes were seen. (Wright-Giemsa. Original magnification 100× objective.) **B,** Canine spleen. This is an area of a splenic aspirate from a dog with lymphocytic hyperplasia. It also contains a homogeneous collection of moderately large lymphocytes; however, a broader evaluation of several areas of the spleen revealed a heterogeneous population of smaller lymphocytes, plasma cells, and extramedullary hematopoiesis (see Figure 21-12). (Wright-Giemsa. Original magnification 100× objective.)

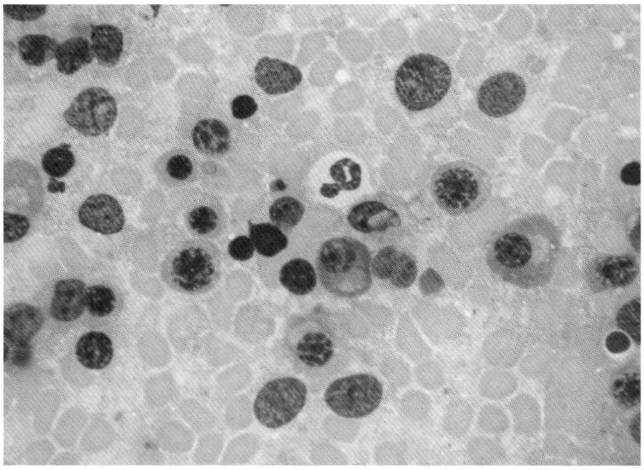

Figure 21-12 **Canine spleen.** This image was taken from the same aspirate as seen in Figure 21-11, *B*. Detection of significant numbers of plasma cells precludes designating the cells seen in Figure 21-11, *B*, as neoplastic. This image also contains numerous mid to late stage erythroid precursors. (Wright-Giemsa. Original magnification 100× objective.)

mast cells (see Figure 21-4), cells of uncertain lineage (Figure 21-20), or primitive, undifferentiated cells (Figure 21-21). A monotonous population of the involved cell type usually replaces normal lymphocytes and hematopoietic cells, although inflammatory cell infiltrates may be seen, for example, neutrophils, macrophages, and mast cells. Some of these neoplasms are described in more detail in Chapter 27.

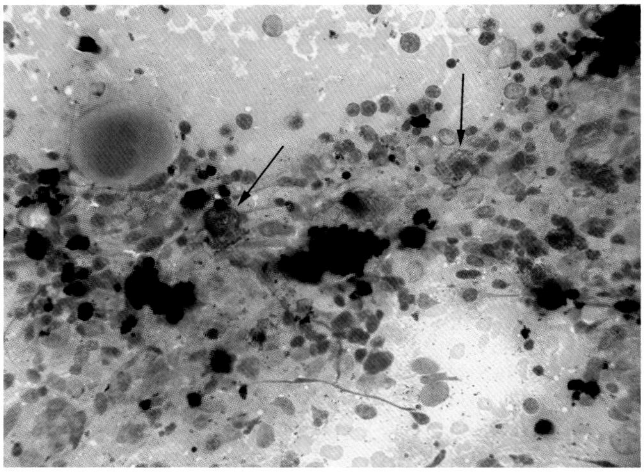

Figure 21-13 **Canine spleen.** This 13-year-old Labrador Retriever has splenic lymphocytic hyperplasia. The fragment of splenic tissue demonstrates increased hemosiderin deposits that may be seen not only in older animals but also in animals with hemolytic anemia, hemorrhage, and chronic congestion. Note that this dog also had a high frequency of mast cells (*arrows*) throughout its spleen, but frequency was not diagnostic for systemic mastocytosis or mast cell tumor metastasis. Note the megakaryocyte in the upper left. The area is too thick to clearly see its nucleus. (Wright-Giemsa. Original magnification 50× objective.)

Mesenchymal Neoplasms

Primary malignant mesenchymal neoplasms of the spleen include disseminated histiocytic sarcoma, hemophagocytic

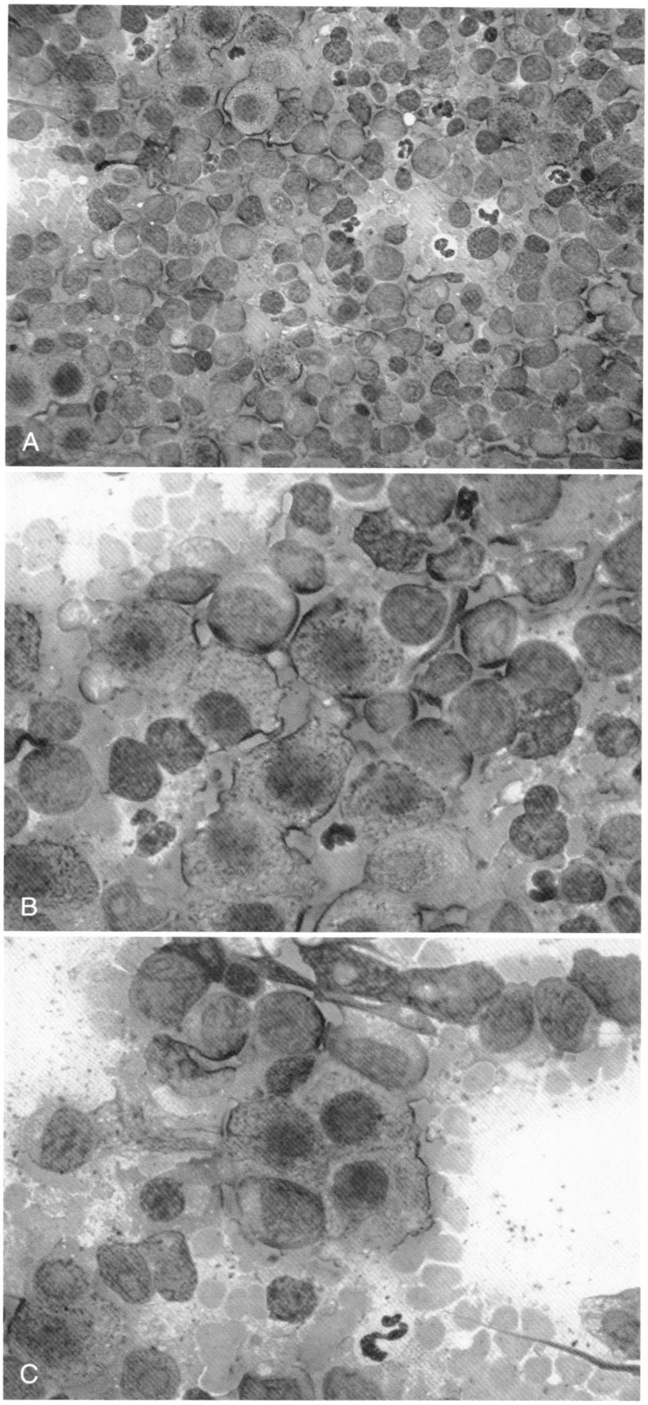

Figure 21-14 Canine spleen. This 11-year-old mixed breed dog had a confusing smear that included both large immature round cells and approximately equivalent numbers of mast cells. No morphologic progression connected the two cell types. The neoplastic round cells are most likely of lymphocytic lineage, although immunophenotyping is needed for confirmation. The mastocytosis may indicate concurrent mast cell neoplasia or the mastocytosis may be a reactive infiltrate secondary to lymphoma (considered more likely). The opinion was that regardless of whether or not the mast cells were neoplastic, they are likely of lesser importance in terms of long-term prognosis for this dog compared to high-grade lymphoma. (*All images,* Wright-Giemsa stained. **A,** Original magnification 50× objective; **B** and **C,** Original magnification 100× objective.)

histiocytic sarcoma, hemangiosarcoma, leiomyosarcoma, fibrosarcoma, and undifferentiated sarcoma.

Hemangiosarcomas may be recognized on impression smears and aspirates, but slides made from scrapings of fresh-cut surfaces of tissue are frequently superior. The microscopic appearance of hemangiosarcomas in a cytologic preparation (Figure 21-22) may be typical of other high-grade sarcomas, but in histologic sections, the cells characteristically line blood-filled sinuses (see Figure 21-22). Cells exfoliate individually or may be associated with vascular structures to appear almost epithelioid. Tumor cells are highly pleomorphic, with marked anisokaryosis and marked anisocytoosis. Giant forms are not unusual. Some cells are fusiform, with indistinct borders, and others are irregularly shaped, with angular margins. Nuclei are round to oval, with variable chromatin patterns and many large, pleomorphic nucleoli. Cytoplasm is light blue stained and variably abundant (see Figure 21-22). Erythroid precursors are often present, indicating extramedullary hematopoiesis. Because of associated hemorrhage, macrophages may contain abundant hemosiderin and numerous phagocytized erythrocytes.

Histiocytic sarcomas are more often diagnosed by FNA and FNB because the cells usually exfoliate readily, unlike hemangiosarcoma, and the cells may be embedded within highly cellular splenic tissue rather than associated with cavernous areas of hemorrhage. Splenic disseminated histiocytic sarcoma may contain many neoplastic cells and few lymphoid and hematopoietic elements (Figure 21-23), but this may also be reversed; that is, the neoplastic cells may be noted at a low frequency within highly cellular aspirates containing lymphocytes, plasma cells, nonneoplastic macrophages, neutrophils, and hematopoietic cells. When giant in size, they may be as large or larger than megakaryocytes (Figure 21-24).

Fibrosarcoma and leiomyosarcoma occur less frequently compared with hemangiosarcoma and histiocytic sarcoma and have the cytologic appearance of low- to intermediate-grade spindle cell tumors. The diagnostic criteria discussed in Chapter 2 may be used to identify these tumors. Fibrosarcoma is further discussed in Chapter 5.

CONCLUSION

Cytologic evaluation of splenic tissue may be key to achieving an accurate, clinically relevant diagnosis, but success hinges on the experience of the pathologist, the skill of the person collecting the specimen, and the quality of the slides.

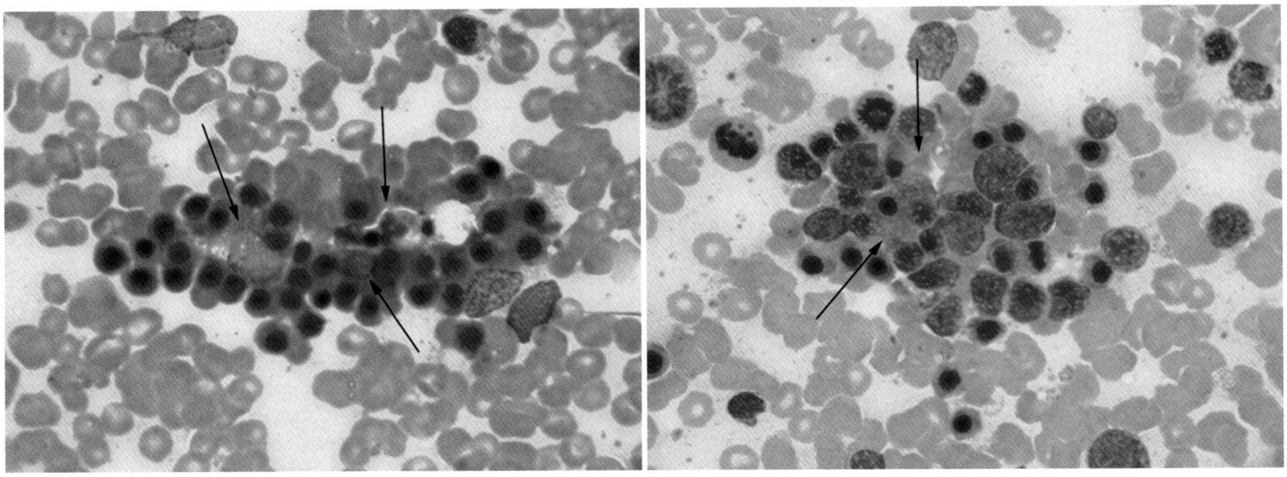

Figure 21-15 Canine spleen. These images were from the spleen of an 8-year-old Rottweiler with hemophagocytic histiocytic sarcoma (also see Figure 21-24). This dog has marked erythropoiesis. These images demonstrate the small islands of maturing erythroid precursors (erythroblastic islets) that are seen adherent to central macrophages (*arrows*). (*Both images,* Wright-Giemsa. Original magnification 100× objective.)

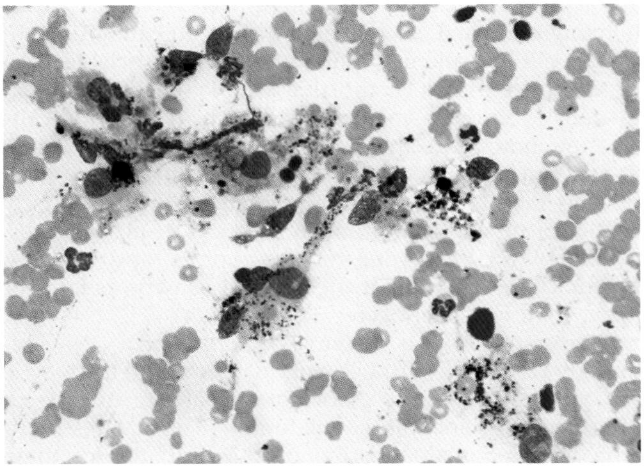

Figure 21-16 Canine spleen. This was an 8-year-old Cain Terrier with severe nonregenerative anemia and ineffective erythroid hyperplasia in the marrow. Destruction of red blood cells and their precursors was thought to be immune mediated. The spleen contained many macrophages that demonstrated phagocytosis of erythrocytes, their precursors, and apoptotic nuclear debris. Similar cells were seen in marrow. (Wright-Giemsa. Original magnification 50× objective.)

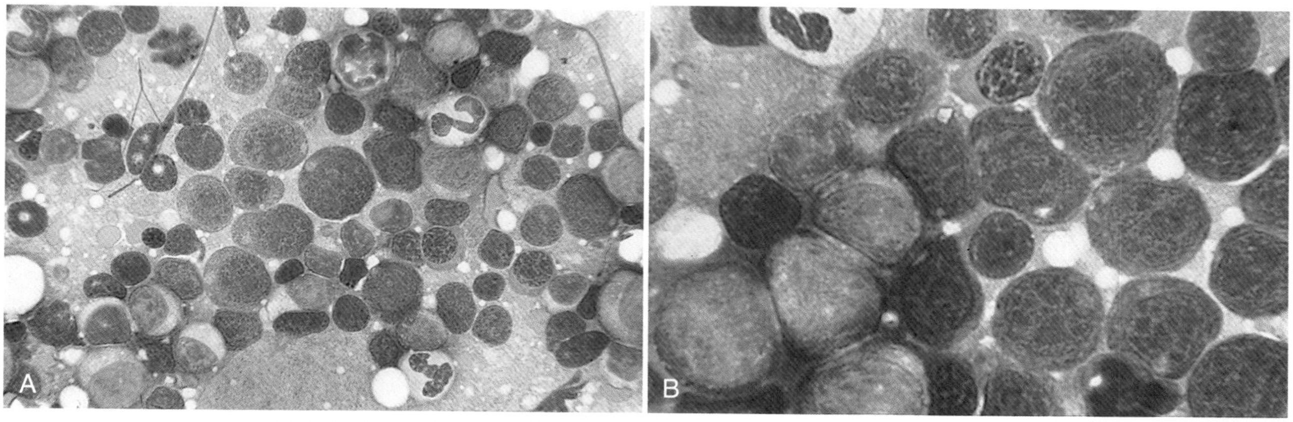

Figure 21-17 Feline spleen, with extramedullary hematopoiesis. A, Most of the cells are erythroid precursors at various stages of development, with a few neutrophils and several lymphocytes (*lower right*). The large round cells in the center are early to intermediate stage erythroid precursors. (Wright stain. Original magnification 48× objective.) **B,** Large lymphocytes are in the lower left, whereas erythroid precursors are on the right. These may be difficult to distinguish. Immunophenotypic analysis that demonstrates a lack of lymphocytic markers may be needed when the lineage of a round cell population is uncertain. Immature erythroid precursors at the rubriblast and prorubricyte stage have round nuclei, dark basophilic cytoplasm, coarse granular or loosely clumped chromatin, and, when visible, singular nucleoli. The metarubricyte at the top of the field has an immature nucleus but well-differentiated cytoplasm (nucleus–cytoplasm asynchrony). (Wright stain. Original magnification 100× objective.)

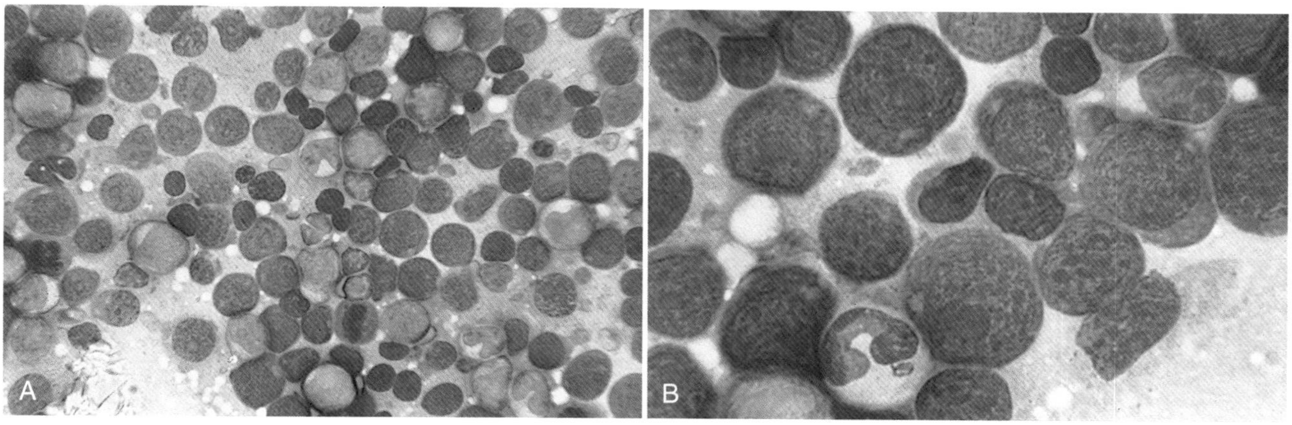

Figure 21-18 Feline spleen. Impression smear of splenic tissue from a cat with erythroid leukemia. **A,** Many large round cells have replaced the normal cell population. No differentiation toward more mature forms in the erythroid series is evident. (Wright stain. Original magnification 48× objective.) **B,** The neoplastic cells are similar to very early erythroid precursors. Morphologic features include a round nucleus, coarse granular chromatin, a single large nucleolus, and a small clear zone within dark blue cytoplasm. (Wright stain. Original magnification 100× oil objective.)

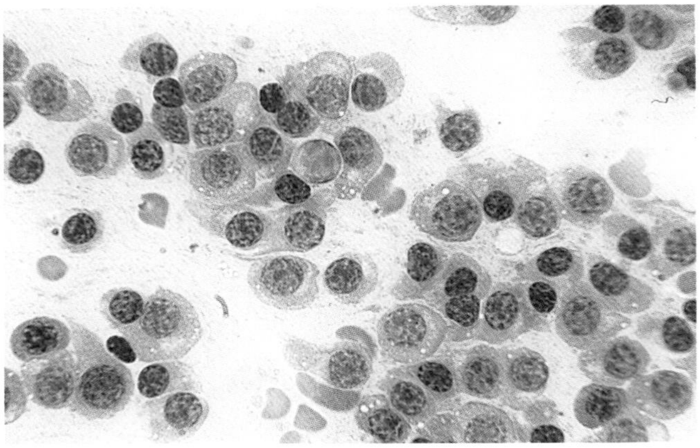

Figure 21-19 Canine spleen. Impression smear of splenic tissue from a dog with multiple myeloma. The spleen is effaced by a homogeneous population of neoplastic plasma cells. (Wright stain. Original magnification 48× objective.)

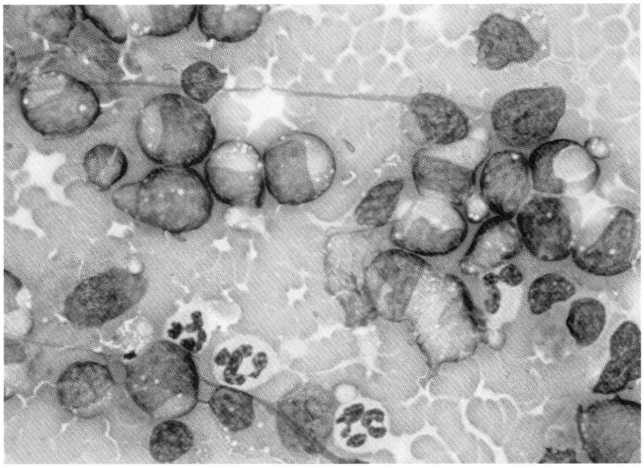

Figure 21-20 Canine spleen. Round cell tumor of uncertain lineage. This dog had hepatosplenomegaly and 10,900 per microliter (µL) unclassifiable cells in peripheral blood. The spleen contains many large, vacuolated cells of uncertain lineage. One cell in the upper left contains a phagocytized erythrocyte. Note the irregular shape of the nuclei and size relative to neutrophils and small lymphocytes. The chief differentials are high-grade lymphoma and acute monocytic leukemia. (Wright-Giemsa. Original magnification 100×.)

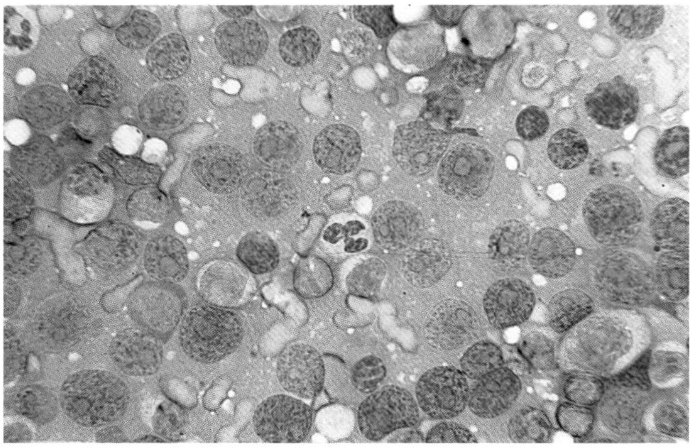

Figure 21-21 Feline spleen. Impression smear of splenic tissue from a cat with an undifferentiated round cell neoplasm. A neutrophil and several small lymphocytes in the center are surrounded by primitive cells with indistinct cell margins, round nuclei, vesicular chromatin, and singular prominent nucleoli. (Wright stain. Original magnification 48× objective.)

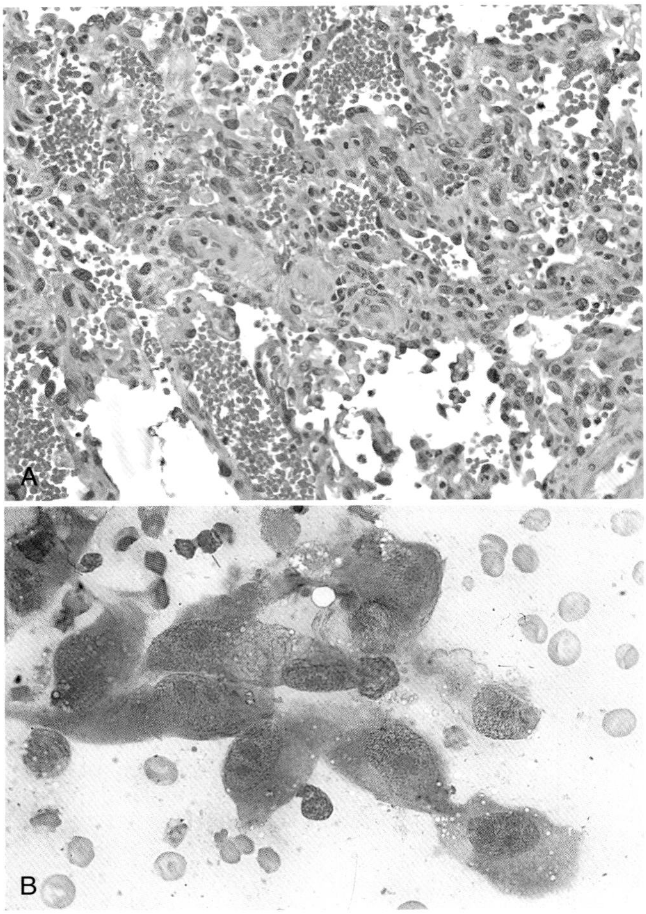

Figure 21-22 Canine spleen. A, Surgical biopsy of hemangiosarcoma in the spleen of a dog. Note the large blood filled sinuses lined by neoplastic cells. (H&E. Original magnification 20× objective.) (Contributed by Dr. Michael Goldschmidt, University of Pennsylvania, School of Veterinary Medicine, Department of Pathobiology, Philadelphia).**B,** Impression smear of splenic tissue from a dog with hemangiosarcoma. The neoplastic cells have features of a mesenchymal malignancy such as marked anisocytosis, indistinct cell margins, marked anisokaryosis, and variable nucleolar size, shape, and number. (Wright stain. Original magnification 100× oil objective.)

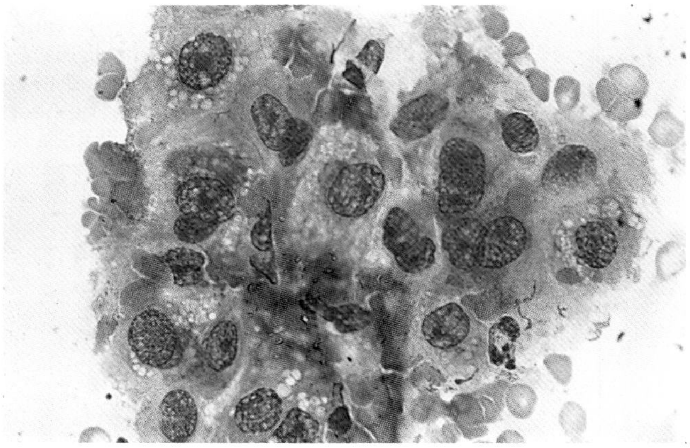

Figure 21-23 Canine spleen. Fine-needle aspirate of spleen from a dog with histiocytic sarcoma. Lymphoid cells normally present in the spleen have been replaced by pleomorphic cells characterized by marked anisocytosis, indistinct cell margins, cytoplasmic vacuolation, marked anisokaryosis, and irregular chromatin clumping. (Wright stain. Original magnification 100× oil objective.)

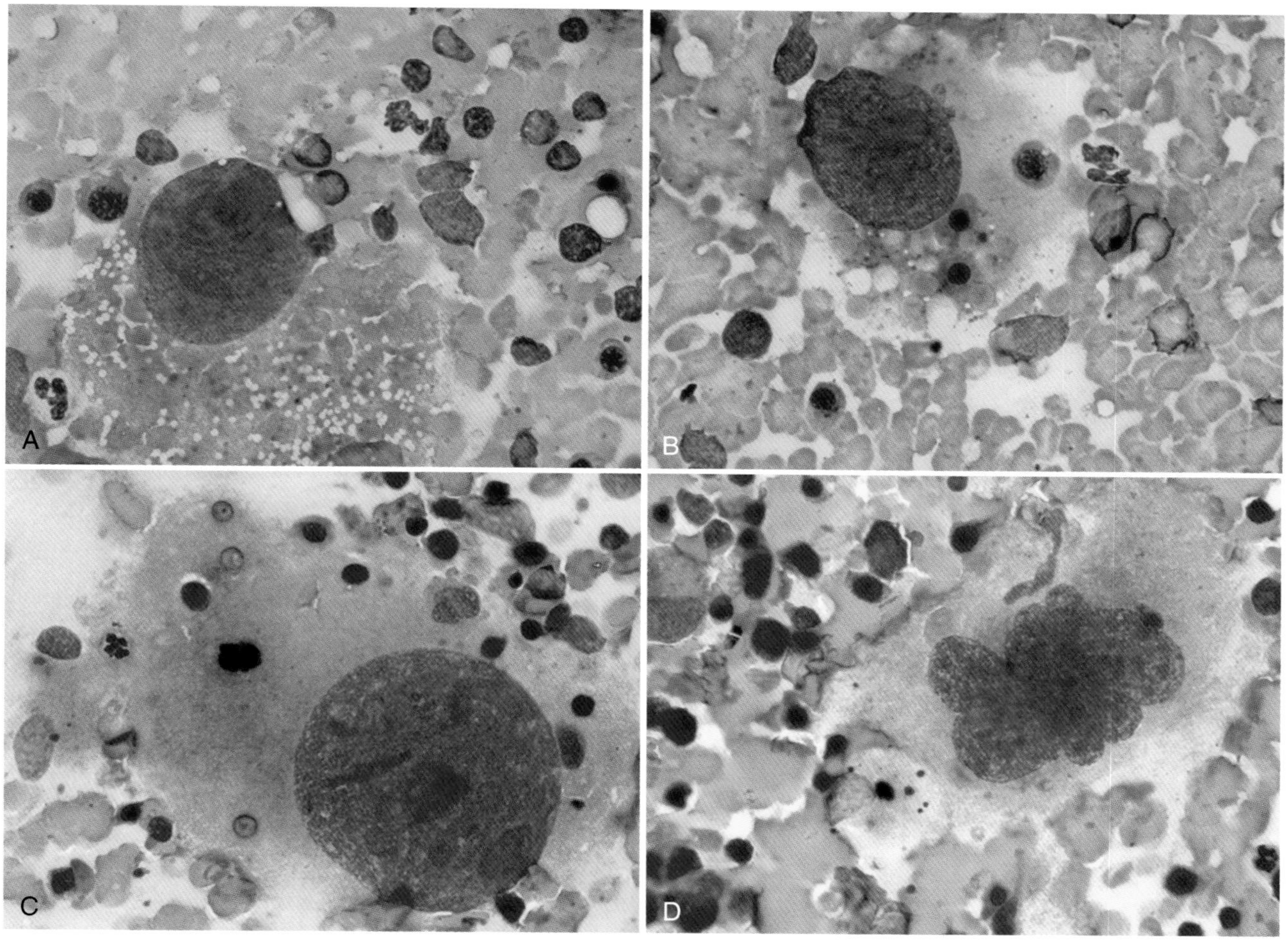

Figure 21-24 Canine spleen. Hemophagocytic histiocytic sarcoma. This was an 8-year-old female spayed Rottweiler with lethargy, decreased appetite, pale mucous membranes, splenomegaly, severe regenerative anemia (packed cell volume [PCV] 18%), and leukopenia. The splenic aspirate indicated marked extramedullary hematopoiesis (predominantly erythroid precursors) as well as lymphocytic hyperplasia. A low frequency of giant hemophagocytic cells, characterized by giant round nuclei, macronucleoli, and fine granular to lacey chromatin, was seen. **A,** This neoplastic macrophage (phagocytic histiocyte) displays a macronuclolus and phagocytosis of erythrocytes. (Wright-Giemsa stain. Original magnification 100× oil objective.) **B,** The neoplastic cell has phagocytized both erythrocytes and late-stage erythrocytic precursors. The nucleolus is giant and misshapen. Compare the size of the cell and its nucleus to the neutrophil next to it. (Wright-Giemsa stain. 100× oil objective.) **C,** The neoplastic cell displays multiple misshapen nucleoli and a particle of hemosiderin in its cytoplasm. (Wright-Giemsa stain. Original magnification 100× oil objective.) **D,** Compare the neoplastic cells in *A, B,* and *C* to this normal megakaryocyte found in the same aspirate and to a more typical macrophage to the left of the megakaryocyte. The megakaryocyte has a lobulated nucleus, moderately coarse chromatin, indistinct small nucleoli, and finely granular light purple stained cytoplasm. It is possible to occasionally detect cells within the cytoplasm of megakaryocytes (emperipolesis), but only a few should be present, and they are usually mature neutrophils rather than erythrocytes. (Wright-Giemsa stain. Original magnification 100× oil objective.)

References

1. Cesta MF: Normal structure, function, and histology of the spleen, *Toxicol Pathol* 34:455–465, 2006.
2. Valli VE: *Veterinary comparative hematopathology*, Ames, IA, 2007, Blackwell Publishing, pp 47–77.
3. Spangler WL, Culbertson MR: Prevalence, type, and importance of splenic diseases in dogs: 1,480 cases (1985-1989), *J Am Vet Med Assoc* 200:829–834, 1992.
4. Spangler WL, Culbertson MR: Prevalence and type of splenic diseases in cats: 455 cases (1985-1991), *J Am Vet Med Assoc* 201:773–776, 1992.
5. Spangler WL, Kass PH: Pathologic and prognostic characteristics of splenomegaly in dogs due to fibrohistiocytic nodules: 98 cases, *Vet Pathol* 35:488–498, 1998.
6. Spangler WL, Kass PH: Splenic myeloid metaplasia, histiocytosis, and hypersplenism in the dog (65 cases), *Vet Pathol* 36:583–593, 1999.
7. Sykes JE, et al: Idiopathic hypereosinophilic syndrome in 3 Rottweilers, *J Vet Int Med* 15:162–166, 2001.
8. Hanson JA, Papageorges M, Girard E, et al: Ultrasonographic appearance of splenic disease in 101 cats, *Vet Radiol Ultrasound* 42:441–445, 2001.
9. Ballegeer EA, Forrest LJ, Dickinson RM, et al: Correlation of ultrasonographic appearance of lesions and cytologic and histologic diagnoses in splenic aspirates from dogs and cats: 32 cases (2002-2005), *J Am Vet Med Assoc* 230:690–696, 2007.
10. Crabtree AC, et al: Diagnostic accuracy of gray-scale ultrasonography for the detection of hepatic and splenic lymphoma in dogs, *Vet Radiol Ultrasound* 51:661–664, 2010.
11. O'Keefe DA, Couto CG: Fine-needle aspiration of the spleen as an aid in the diagnosis of splenomegaly, *J Vet Int Med* 1:102–109, 1987.
12. Christopher MM: Cytology of the spleen, *Vet Clin North Am Small Anim Pract* 33:135–152, 2003.
13. Lal A, et al: Splenic fine needle aspiration and core biopsy: a review of 49 cases, *Acta Cytol* 47:951–959, 2003.
14. Watson AT, Penninck D, Knoll JS, et al: Safety and correlation of test results of combined ultrasound-guided fine-needle aspiration and needle core biopsy of the canine spleen, *Vet Radiol Ultrasound* 52:317–322, 2011.
15. McInnes MD, Kielar AZ, Macdonald DB: Percutaneous image-guided biopsy of the spleen: systematic review and meta-analysis of the complication rate and diagnostic accuracy, *Radiology* 260:699–708, 2011.
16. Papageorges M, et al: Ultrasound-guided fine-needle aspiration: an inexpensive modification of the technique, *Vet Radiol* 29:269–271, 1988.
17. Leblanc CJ, Head LL, Fry MM: Comparison of aspiration and nonaspiration techniques for obtaining cytologic samples from the canine and feline spleen, *Vet Clin Pathol* 38:242–246, 2009.

CHAPTER 22

The Kidneys

Patty J. Ewing, James H. Meinkoth, Rick L. Cowell, and Ronald D. Tyler

Cytologic examination (e.g., fine-needle aspiration [FNA]) is a useful tool in diagnosing certain renal lesions, especially neoplasms, in dogs and cats. The advantages and disadvantages of FNA (cytology) compared with incisional biopsy (histopathology) of the kidney are presented in Table 22-1. Although the examination of cytologic specimens does not provide the cellular architecture necessary to characterize many lesions in which structural relationships are important, it may sometimes provide sufficient diagnostic information to aid in the clinical management of cases and is less invasive and associated with fewer complications compared with full tissue biopsy. Major complications resulting from FNA of the kidney are relatively uncommon if appropriate procedures are followed.[1]

Disease conditions that are most likely and least likely to yield diagnostic cytologic results are presented in Box 22-1 and Box 22-2. The primary indication for FNA is abnormally sized or abnormally shaped kidneys. Cytologic specimens from patients with unilateral or bilateral renomegaly are most likely to yield diagnostic information; small or shrunken kidneys rarely yield positive diagnostic findings. Either fluid or solid tissue lesions may be encountered, and the results of cytologic analysis may help characterize the process as cystic, inflammatory, or neoplastic. Renal cytology is especially useful for the rapid confirmation of renal lymphoma in cats. Although positive cytologic findings are useful in establishing a diagnosis, tentative diagnoses cannot always be excluded on the basis of negative findings because representative material may not have been recovered during collection attempts.

Collecting adequately cellular specimens for evaluation is a limiting factor of renal cytology. FNA of the kidney is easier in cats because their kidneys are more easily palpated and immobilized against the body wall. Using ultrasonography to detect optimal sites for specimen collection and to provide additional information about the nature and extent of lesions may significantly increase diagnostic yield. Because of the highly vascular nature of the kidneys, blood contamination is a significant problem during sample collection. Use of a nonaspiration (i.e., capillary action) technique (see Chapter 1) facilitates the collection of cellular specimens that are not heavily contaminated with blood. Highly cellular, solid lesions (e.g., neoplasms) are also more likely to provide cellular samples than many degenerative or inflammatory diseases.

SAMPLING TECHNIQUE

FNA is associated with less tissue trauma compared with punch biopsies, and contraindications for collecting cytologic specimens from the kidneys are only a few. Contraindications for renal FNA are listed in Box 22-3. As with other renal biopsy procedures, the main complication is excessive hemorrhage.[1] Patients should be evaluated for the presence of coagulation defects prior to the procedure; adequate restraint is necessary to prevent unexpected movement during the procedure, and the kidney must be adequately immobilized against the body wall. Seeding of the needle tract with neoplastic cells during fine-needle sampling of malignant lesions has been suggested as a complication; however, clinical experience and results of retrospective studies in humans show such seeding to be uncommon.[2,3]

A blind, percutaneous technique may be used if the lesion appears diffuse (i.e., generalized renomegaly), and the kidney can be immobilized against the wall of the abdomen. The concurrent use of ultrasonography to facilitate sample collection is preferred, and tranquilization, sedation, or anesthesia is used, as necessary, to adequately restrain the patient, preventing unexpected movement during the procedure.

The skin at the site is clipped and prepared as for surgery. The patient is usually restrained in lateral recumbency, and the kidney is manually immobilized against the body wall. As mentioned previously, a nonaspiration technique is preferred to limit the amount of blood contamination.[4] A 22- or 23-gauge needle attached to a 10- to 12-milliliter (mL) syringe that has been prefilled with air is held at the base of the needle with the thumb and forefinger. Depending on the type of lesion, the needle is directed either into the lesion (focal lesions) or tangentially into the cortex of the kidney (diffuse lesions). Care should be taken to avoid the renal hilus, which contains large vascular structures. The needle is passed through approximately two thirds the thickness of the lesion about five to seven times with a stabbing motion. The repeated needle punctures should be along a single plane

TABLE 22-1

Advantages and Disadvantages of Renal Cytology Compared with Incisional Biopsy

Advantages	Disadvantages
Less invasive, fewer complications	Does not allow for assessment of tissue architecture
Less expensive	Does not allow for evaluation of glomeruli
Rapid diagnosis of some conditions such as feline lymphoma	Blood contamination and low cell yield often limit usefulness

BOX 22-1

Conditions *Most* Likely to Yield Diagnostic Renal Aspirates

- Unilateral renomegaly
- Bilateral renomegaly
- Solid mass lesions:
  - Neoplasms (especially lymphoma)
  - Abscesses
  - Fungal granulomas

BOX 22-2

Conditions *Least* Likely to Yield Diagnostic Renal Aspirates

- Small or shrunken fibrotic kidneys (end-stage kidneys)
- Renal tubular degeneration or necrosis
- Interstitial nephritis
- Glomerulonephritis

BOX 22-3

Contraindications for Renal Aspiration Cytology

- Marked thrombocytopenia (platelet count <50,000/μL)
- Platelet function disorder (increased buccal mucosal bleeding time)
- Coagulopathy (one-stage prothrombin time or activated partial thromboplastin time prolonged >20%)
- Patients at high risk for anesthesia or sedation
- Obstructive uropathy (severe hydronephrosis or septic pyonephrosis) if risk of abdominal cavity contamination is high

(similar to the action of a sewing machine) to minimize blood vessel rupture. Samples may be collected from different portions of the lesion using multiple (two or three) collection attempts. Collection of several slides (at least five) from different areas of the lesion helps increase the chances of obtaining a diagnostic specimen. Whenever blood is visible in the hub of the needle or syringe, collection should be stopped and the material spread onto a glass slide because continued collection attempts usually result in gross blood contamination, rendering the sample worthless.

After collection, the material in the needle (none is usually visible in the syringe) should be carefully dispersed on one end of a glass slide and gently spread out using a slide-over-slide technique (see Chapter 1). If fluid is obtained, direct and line smears should be made, and the remainder of the fluid put into an ethylenetetraacetic acid (EDTA) tube. If the fluid is clear (suggesting low cellularity) and sufficient sample has been obtained, concentrated sediment smears, which are similar to urine sediments, are prepared and air-dried.

Impression smears may be made from renal biopsy specimens or kidneys removed at surgery or necropsy before the specimen is fixed in formalin for histologic analysis. Before the impression smears are made, excess blood should be gently blotted from the tissue to increase the number of cells that transfer to the glass slides. Whenever sufficient tissue has been obtained for histologic analysis, it should be submitted in case the cytologic preparations are nondiagnostic. Samples for histologic and cytologic examinations must be mailed in separate packages because formalin fumes (even from sealed containers) will partially fix the cells on unstained smears, making evaluation impossible.

CYTOLOGIC EVALUATION

Normal and Abnormal Cell Types Encountered

The normal histologic anatomies of the canine and feline renal cortices are shown in Figure 22-1. The renal parenchyma consists of glomeruli, tubules, interstitium, and blood vessels. Renal tubules make up the bulk of the parenchyma. Findings in normal renal aspirates are listed in Table 22-2. Renal tubular epithelial cells are the predominant cell type seen in fine-needle aspirates from normal kidneys. They are rather large, round to polygonal cells that occur singly and in clusters (Figure 22-2, *A*). They have a round, centrally placed nucleus and abundant light blue cytoplasm, which, in cats, often contains several distinct, clear vacuoles from the presence of lipid droplets (see Figure 22-2, *B*). Clear cytoplasmic vacuoles may also occur in dogs with diabetes mellitus, long-term exposure to corticosteroids, or lysosomal storage disease (Box 22-4). Cells of the distal convoluted tubules and ascending limb of the loop of Henle may contain dark intracytoplasmic granules (see Figure 22-2, *C*).[3]

Differentiation of the various epithelial cell types is not practical or of diagnostic importance. The cells and their nuclei should be relatively uniform in size and shape; however, the different types of epithelial cells differ slightly in size. The nucleus-to-cytoplasm (N:C) ratio of normal tubular cells is low, except for feline lipid-laden proximal tubular epithelial cells, and tubular cells that are well spread out often have a single, visible nucleolus (see Figure 22-2). When present, nucleoli should be small and round. Renal tubular cells often remain together as recognizable tubule fragments of various sizes (Figure 22-3). Tubular casts may also be seen in renal aspirates from some animals (Figure 22-4). Their significance

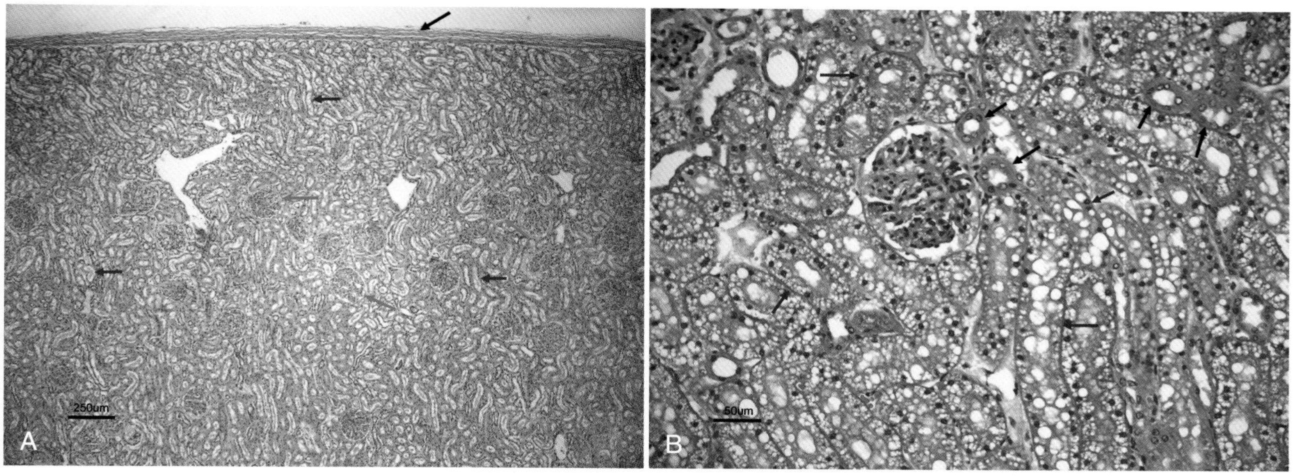

Figure 22-1 A, Histologic section of normal canine kidney. Renal tubules comprise the majority of the normal renal parenchyma. Note absence of vacuoles in the proximal tubular epithelial cells (*blue arrows*) in contrast to the cat kidney shown in *B*. Glomeruli (*green arrows*) are prominent structures in the renal cortex and consist of a tuft of interconnected capillaries enclosed in a capsule named after Bowman. Orange arrows identify dilated intralobular veins. The black arrow identifies the thick fibrous capsule through which the needle penetrates during the fine-needle aspiration procedure. (H&E stain.) **B,** Histologic section of normal feline kidney. Note prominent lipid vacuolation of proximal tubular epithelial cells (*blue arrows*). The lipid vacuolation is what accounts for the grossly pale tan-yellow appearance of a normal feline kidney. Note cuboidal cells without vacuoles that line the distal tubules (*black arrows*) and low cuboidal, nonvacuolated epithelial cells of the collecting duct (*orange arrows*). The green arrow identifies a glomerulus. (H&E stain.) (**A,** Courtesy of Dr. Pam Mouser. **B,** Courtesy of Dr. Pam Mouser)

TABLE 22-2

Findings in Normal Renal Aspirates

Cell Types or Structures	Appearance	Comments
Renal tubular epithelial cell (see Figure 22-2)	Medium to large, round to polygonal cells that occur singly and in clusters; central round nucleus with single visible nucleolus, light blue cytoplasm, which may have clear vacuoles (in cats)	Predominant cell type seen
Intact renal tubules (see Figures 22-3 and 22-4)	Densely packed cells as described above arranged in tubular arrays	Variably present
Glomeruli (see Figure 22-5)	Lobulated clusters of slender, oval to spindle-shaped cells	Infrequently seen
Collagen matrix	Strands of homogeneous, acellular pink material	Absent or present in only small amounts; collagen obtained from renal capsule or interstitium
Peripheral blood	Many erythrocytes with platelet aggregates and leukocytes (neutrophils, lymphocytes, and monocytes)	Marked blood contamination is common; subjective assessment of types and number of leukocytes present is only way to differentiate blood contamination versus inflammation

depends on the amount and type of cast present, similar to those in urine sediments. Glomeruli may be seen in cellular samples and appear as somewhat lobulated clusters of slender, spindloid cells (Figure 22-5).[5] Individual cells are difficult to see because they are tightly clustered. Abnormalities of the glomeruli (e.g., glomerulonephritis) are not readily discernible cytologically and require histologic analysis. A few homogeneous strands of acellular pink matrix (collagen) may be seen in normal renal aspirates. The matrix is typically obtained as the needle passes through the fibrous capsule of the kidney (Figure 22-1, *A*).

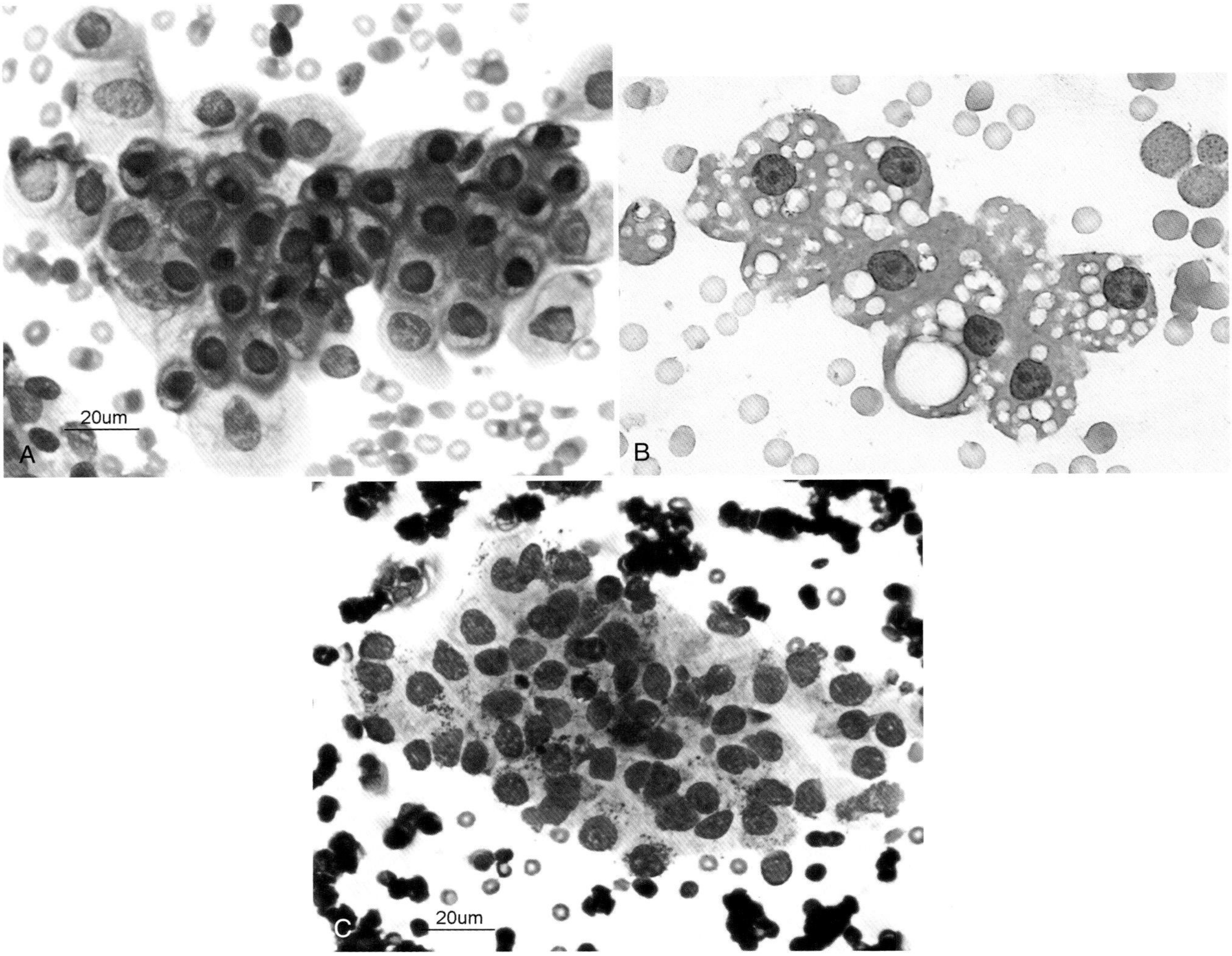

Figure 22-2 **A,** Renal fine-needle aspiration (FNA) from a dog. Numerous renal tubular cells showing mature, uniform nuclei with dark, mature chromatin. (Wright-Giemsa stain.) **B,** Renal FNA sample from a cat. Note the cluster of renal tubular epithelial cells with some blood contamination; feline renal tubular cells are often vacuolated. Nucleoli are visible but are small and round. (Wright stain. Original magnification 330×.) **C,** Cluster of renal tubular cells from a renal FNA sample from a cat. The cells are mature and uniform and show cytoplasmic granules. (Wright-Giemsa stain.)

BOX 22-4

Causes of Clear Vacuoles in Renal Tubular Epithelial Cells

- Normal cat renal proximal tubular cells (lipid)
- Diabetes mellitus in dogs (lipid)
- Long-term exposure to corticosteroids in dogs (glycogen)
- Lysosomal storage disorders—congenital or drug-induced (lipid or glycogen)

Some degree (often marked) of peripheral blood contamination is always present in renal aspirates. Various peripheral blood leukocytes (i.e., neutrophils, small mature lymphocytes, monocytes, and possibly eosinophils) and platelets, often in aggregates, will be present as a result of peripheral blood contamination. A subjective assessment of the number and type of leukocytes present compared with the amount of peripheral blood on the slide is the only way to assess whether the leukocytes most likely represent blood contamination or renal inflammation. Inflammation is suggested by a disproportionate number of leukocytes relative to red blood cells (RBCs) or the presence of cells not associated with peripheral blood (e.g., overt plasma cells, vacuolated or phagocytically active macrophages). Plasma cells are lymphoid cells with eccentric nuclei, increased amounts of deeply basophilic cytoplasm (compared with small lymphocytes), and a perinuclear clear area (Figure 22-6). Macrophages, which must be differentiated from peripheral blood monocytes, have more abundant cytoplasm that may have phagocytized cellular debris or many small vacuoles (see Figure 22-18 and Figure 22-25). Macrophage nuclei are usually round, unlike irregular, pleomorphic

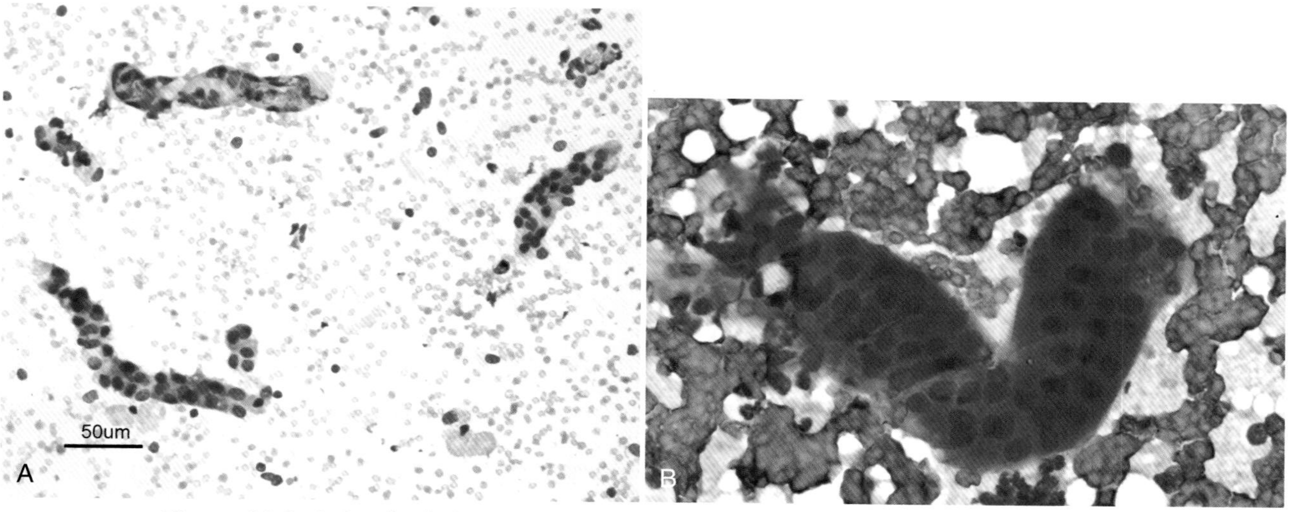

Figure 22-3 **A,** Small tubular fragments in a renal fine-needle aspiration (FNA) from a dog. (Wright stain. Original magnification 50×.) **B,** Higher magnification of tubular fragment in a renal FNA from a cat. Dark nuclei of individual tubular cells are visible, but cell margins are difficult to discern. (Wright stain. Original magnification 500×.)

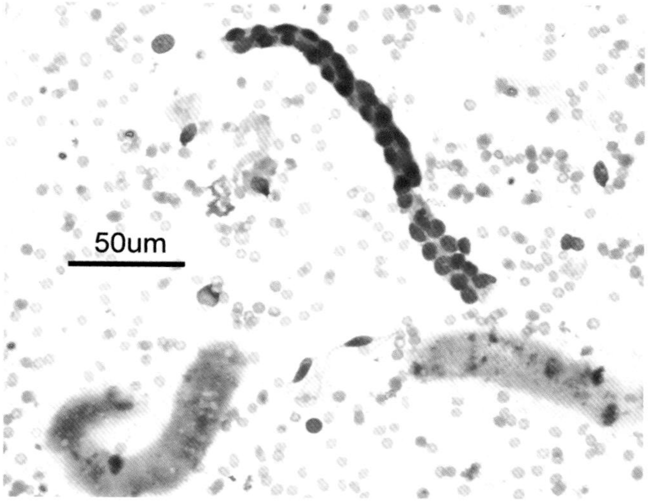

Figure 22-4 A renal tubular fragment and two casts in a renal fine-needle aspiration from a dog. (Wright stain. Original magnification 50×.)

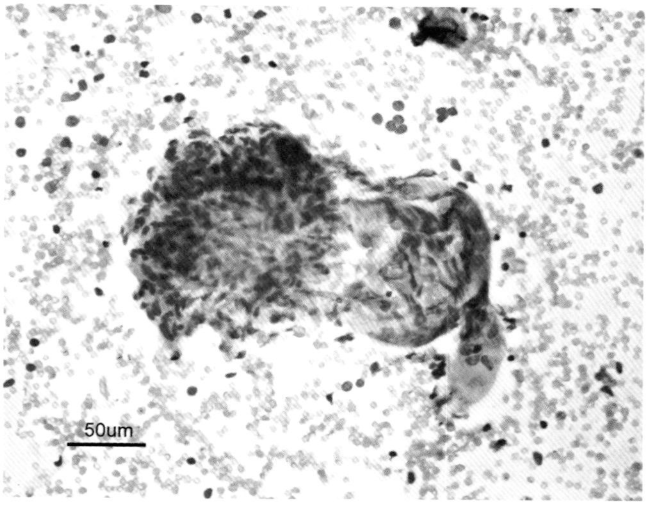

Figure 22-5 A glomerulus present in a renal fine-needle aspiration sample from a dog. (Wright stain. Original magnification 50×.)

monocyte nuclei. Additionally, finding neutrophils with degenerate changes (e.g., swelling of the nuclear lobes) and phagocytized bacteria (see Figure 22-18) is abnormal and indicates septic inflammation.

Small mature lymphocytes, which are approximately 10 micrometers (μm) in diameter (slightly smaller than neutrophils) and have only scant amounts of basophilic cytoplasm, are often present as the result of blood contamination. Their deep purple nuclei are round and slightly indented (see Figure 22-6). The presence of reactive lymphocytes (Figure 22-7) or prolymphocytes, which are slightly larger than small mature lymphocytes, suggests inflammatory infiltrates. Their nuclei are larger, stain a less dense color, and do not have prominent nucleoli. These cells also have moderately increased amounts of blue cytoplasm. Lymphoblasts are usually seen in cases of renal lymphoma. These cells are distinctly larger than the other lymphoid cells (larger than neutrophils) and have prominent nucleoli and less dense nuclear chromatin. Their cytoplasm is more abundant, is deeply basophilic, and often completely encircles the nucleus (Figure 22-8).

Cytologic Characteristics of Solid Lesions

Cytologic preparations from enlarged or abnormally shaped kidneys or discrete, solid kidney masses are evaluated for the presence of neoplasia or inflammatory responses (Figure 22-9).

Neoplasia: Confirming neoplasia from a patient with renomegaly or a renal mass is a situation in which renal cytology is most likely to be diagnostically rewarding.[1] Renal lymphoma is the most common neoplastic disease

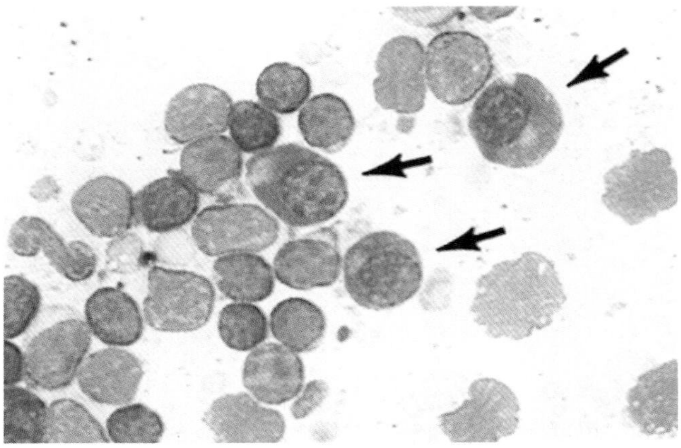

Figure 22-6 Plasma cells (*arrows*) characterized by an eccentric round nucleus with abundant, deep-blue cytoplasm and a prominent, clear Golgi apparatus, and small lymphocytes. (Wright stain. Original magnification 250×.)

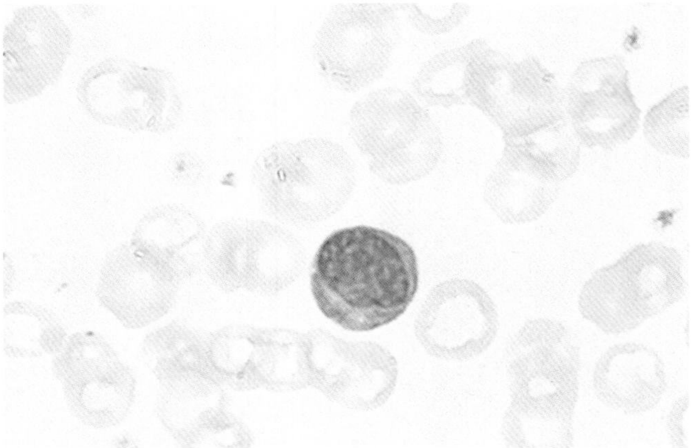

Figure 22-7 A reactive lymphocyte. (Wright stain. Original magnification 250×.)

affecting feline kidneys and may occur as a single, discrete nodule but more often causes diffuse renal enlargement (typically bilateral).[6] It is not usually limited to the kidneys. Aspirates are of high cellularity and consist almost entirely of lymphoid cells. In most cases, the majority of these cells (>80%) are large lymphoid cells (i.e., lymphoblastic lymphoma) (see Figure 22-8). Lymphoid cells are fragile, and slides may contain many ruptured cells. Nearly all cells may be ruptured if downward pressure is applied to the spreader slide during slide preparation. Depending on the degree to which the tumor has replaced normal tissue in the area sampled, renal tubular cells may be present. Slides made from animals with lymphoma are often very thick, and in many areas, the cells are not well spread out. In such areas, it is difficult to accurately classify the lymphoid cells. Lymphoblasts that are not well spread out appear smaller; their nucleoli are indistinct, and it is difficult to determine the amount of cytoplasm present. Thus, it is imperative to find thin areas of the smear where the cells have assumed their normal morphology. Forms of lymphoma in which the neoplastic cell populations cytologically appear as prolymphocytes or small lymphocytes occur, but these forms are much less common. In such cases, it may be difficult to differentiate these lesions from severe lymphocytic infiltrates resulting from chronic inflammatory conditions. Inflammatory lesions typically result in lower numbers of lymphoid cells admixed with normal renal tubular cells. A mixture of small lymphocytes, prolymphocytes, and some plasma cells may be present. Lymphoma is suggested if a dense, monotonous population of lymphoid cells exist in an extremely cellular smear from an enlarged kidney, but histologic confirmation or immunophenotyping (flow cytometry, polymerase chain reaction [PCR] for B-cell and T-cell receptor clonality on FNA specimens, or both) is often warranted.

In retrospective studies of primary renal neoplasia, excluding lymphoma, 94% or more of primary canine and feline renal tumors were malignant.[7,8] Carcinomas

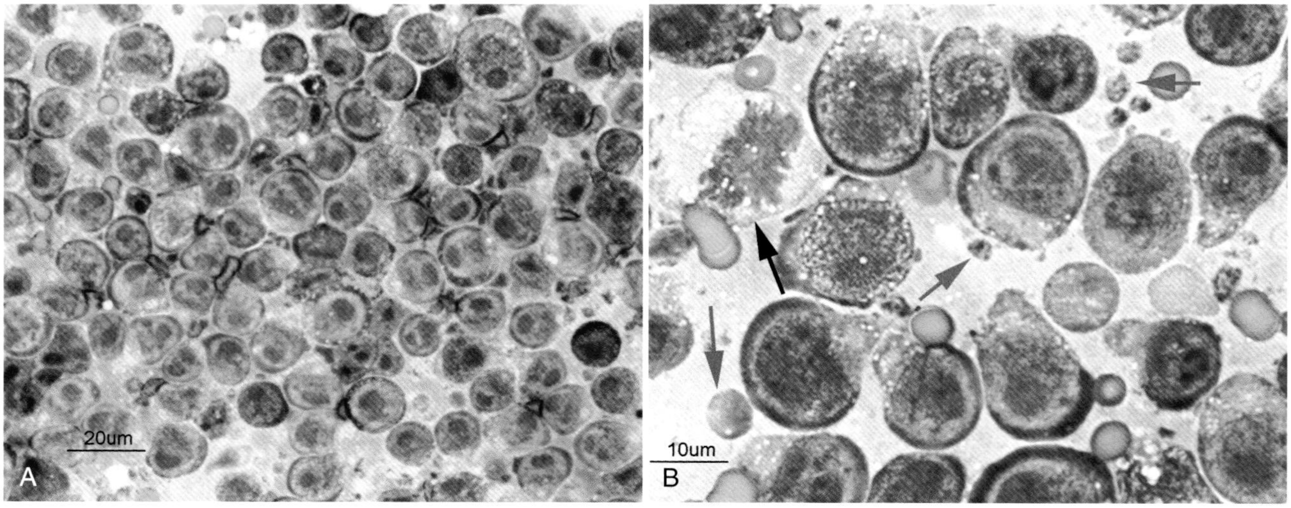

Figure 22-8 Fine-needle aspiration samples from a cat with renal lymphoma presenting as bilateral renomegaly. A, The specimen is densely cellular with a population of discrete cells. (Wright-Giemsa stain.) **B,** More than 90% of the cells present are lymphoblasts. Numerous lymphoglandular bodies are present (*red arrows*). One mitotic figure is seen (*black arrow*). (Wright-Giemsa stain.)

(e.g., tubular adenocarcinomas or renal cell carcinomas, transitional cell carcinomas, and squamous cell carcinomas of the renal pelvis) are the most common primary renal neoplasms of dogs and cats, but the overall incidence of renal cancer is fairly low (approximately 1% of all canine neoplasms and 1.5% to 2.5% of all feline neoplasms).[6] A diagnosis of carcinoma is made from smears containing a population of epithelial cells that demonstrate adequate criteria of malignancy (see Chapter 2). Aspirates from renal carcinomas are often of much higher cellularity than aspirates from normal kidneys or renal inflammatory diseases and yield a dense population of renal epithelial cells (Figure 22-10, *A*). Well-differentiated renal cell carcinomas may yield a majority of cells that are somewhat uniform, and cells demonstrating criteria of malignancy must be found among uniform cells (see Figure 22-10, *B*). The high cellularity of the aspirates correlates with the histologic finding of densely packed epithelial cells arranged in lobules (Figure 22-11). Poorly differentiated renal cell carcinomas as well as transitional cell carcinomas and squamous cell carcinomas typically show moderate to marked cytologic atypia (Figure 22-12 and Figure 22-13). Adrenal carcinomas may be encountered in animals with masses in the kidney area. If a blind aspirate is performed, these carcinomas are difficult or impossible to differentiate from renal carcinomas. Adrenal cortical cells are larger and have more abundant cytoplasm that often contains many fine vacuoles (Figure 22-14).[5,9] Adrenal carcinomas should be considered if the patient shows clinical evidence of hyperadrenocorticism; diagnostic imaging studies may help identify the location of the tumor in such cases.

Nephroblastoma is an uncommon embryonal tumor that occurs primarily in the kidney and thoracolumbar region of young dogs but has also been reported to occur as a primary renal tumor of cats.[7,8,10,11] Nephroblastomas typically present as a solitary unilateral mass at one pole

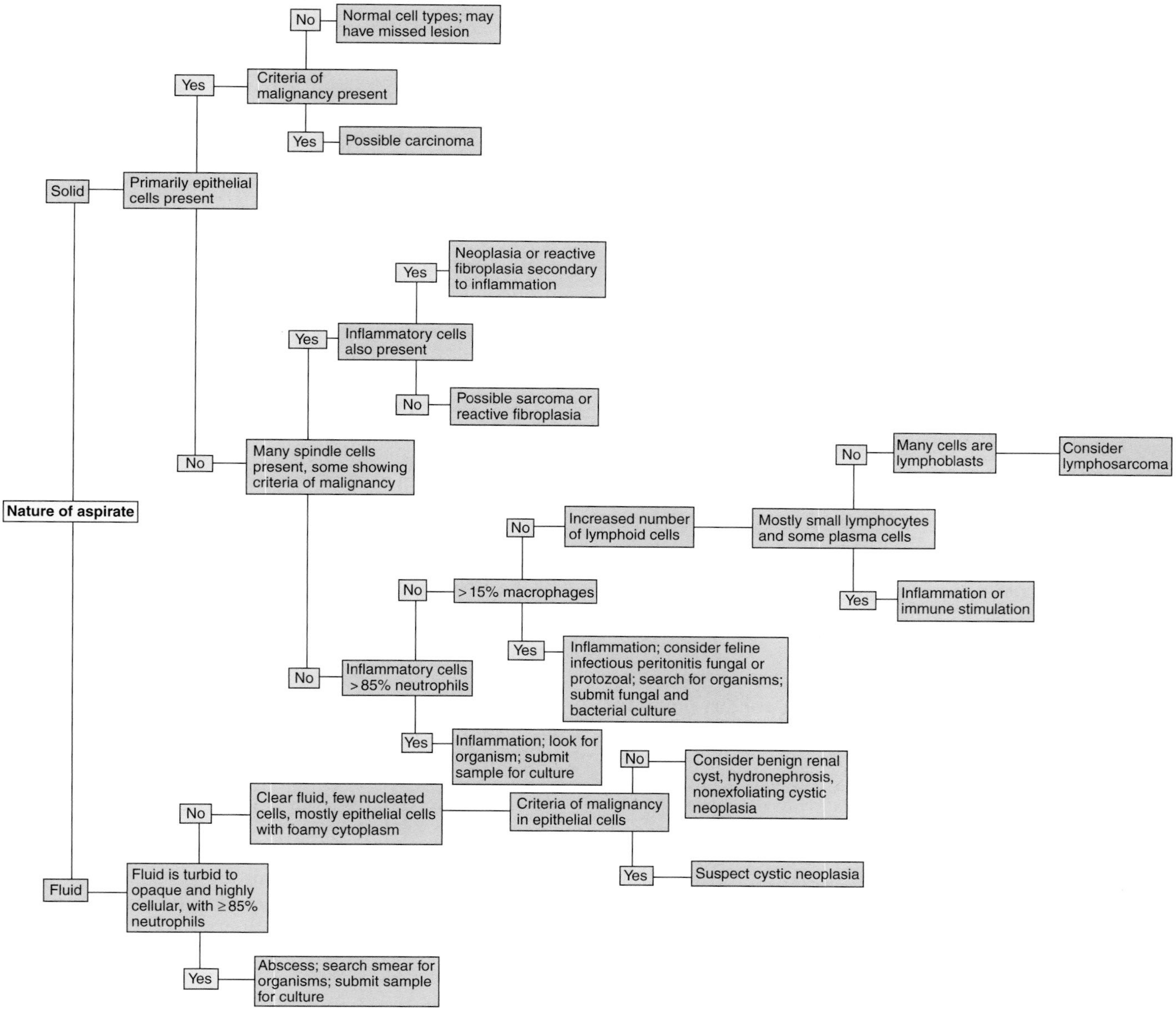

Figure 22-9 An algorithm to aid cytologic evaluation of renal aspirates and impression smears.

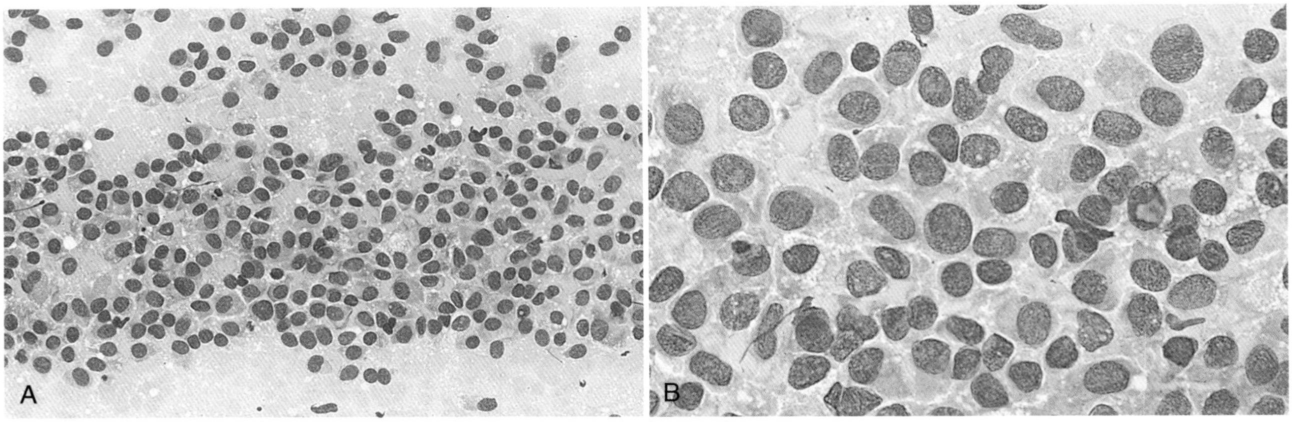

Figure 22-10 **Fine-needle aspirates from a mass involving the right kidney of a dog.** **A,** The samples are highly cellular, consisting of a single population of epithelial cells. (Wright stain. Original magnification 100×.) **B,** The epithelial cells present show criteria of malignancy, allowing a diagnosis of carcinoma. Histopathologic examination confirmed a diagnosis of renal cell carcinoma. (Wright stain. Original magnification 250×.)

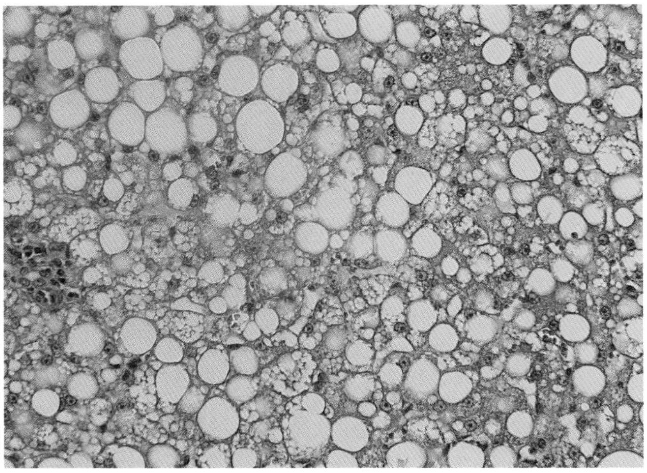

Figure 22-11 Histologic section of renal cell carcinoma from a dog. Note densely packed large polygonal epithelial cells divided into distinct lobules by fibrous connective tissue septa. Individual cells have abundant clear to granular eosinophilic cytoplasm and a centrally located round nucleus with vesicular chromatin and a single prominent nucleolus. (H&E stain. Original magnification 200×.)

of kidney located primarily in the cortex with possible extension through the capsule or as a solitary mass in the spinal cord (T3-L3). Aspirates or impression smears of nephroblastomas are highly cellular and composed of numerous large (12 to 30 µm in diameter) epithelioid mononuclear, round to oval cells arranged individually and in clusters often in combination with a mesenchymal cell population (Figure 22-15, *A*). They exhibit mild to moderate anisocytosis and anisokaryosis and a variable but high N:C ratio. The cells have eccentrically located round, oval, or pleomorphic nuclei with a finely granular to smudged chromatin, single to multiple small nucleoli, and a scant rim of basophilic and occasionally vacuolated cytoplasm. They may be mistaken for lymphoma cells given their high N:C ratio and finely granular chromatin. Nuclear molding and pseudorosette formation may be evident. Small spindloid cells with dark nuclei are frequently admixed with the round to oval mononuclear cells.[10,11] Confirmation of diagnosis via histologic evaluation is warranted (see Figure 22-15, *B*). The mesenchymal component exhibits immunopositivity for vimentin, and the epithelial component exhibits immunopositivity for cytokeratin. Immunohistochemical expression for marker WT-1 may also be useful in confirming a diagnosis of nephroblastoma.[12]

Mesenchymal tumors are less common than epithelial tumors, accounting for approximately 5% of feline and 34% of canine renal neoplasms.[7,8] Types of mesenchymal tumors that may be found in the canine or feline kidney include malignant fibrous histiocytoma (Figure 22-16), histiocytic sarcoma (Figure 22-17), neurofibroma, fibroleiomyosarcoma, leiomyosarcoma, hemangiosarcoma, hemangioma, angiomyolipoma, cortical fibroma, congenital mesoblastic nephroma, oncocytoma, chondrosarcoma, and extramedullary osteosarcoma.[6,7,8,13,14] Mesenchymal tumors of the kidney may be primary, disseminated, or metastatic.[6,7,8,11,12] An example of a disseminated round cell mesenchymal neoplasm that may occur in the kidney, especially in dogs, is histiocytic sarcoma. Histiocytic sarcoma is a tumor of neoplastic dendritic cells.[15] More common sites of involvement include periarticular regions, lung, spleen, liver, and lymph nodes. The neoplastic cells are large round cells occurring singly and in noncohesive aggregates. The round cells contain abundant basophilic cytoplasm, which may exhibit vacuolation or phagocytosis. Nuclei are large, round to indented, and eccentrically located with vesicular to coarse chromatin and one or more prominent nucleoli. Neoplastic cells frequently exhibit moderate to marked anisocytosis and anisokaryosis (see Figure 22-17). Neoplastic cells typically exhibit immunopositivity for the following markers: CD45, CD18, CD1, CD11c, and MHCII.

Inflammation: Most inflammatory diseases affecting the kidney (e.g., chronic interstitial nephritis, pyelonephritis,

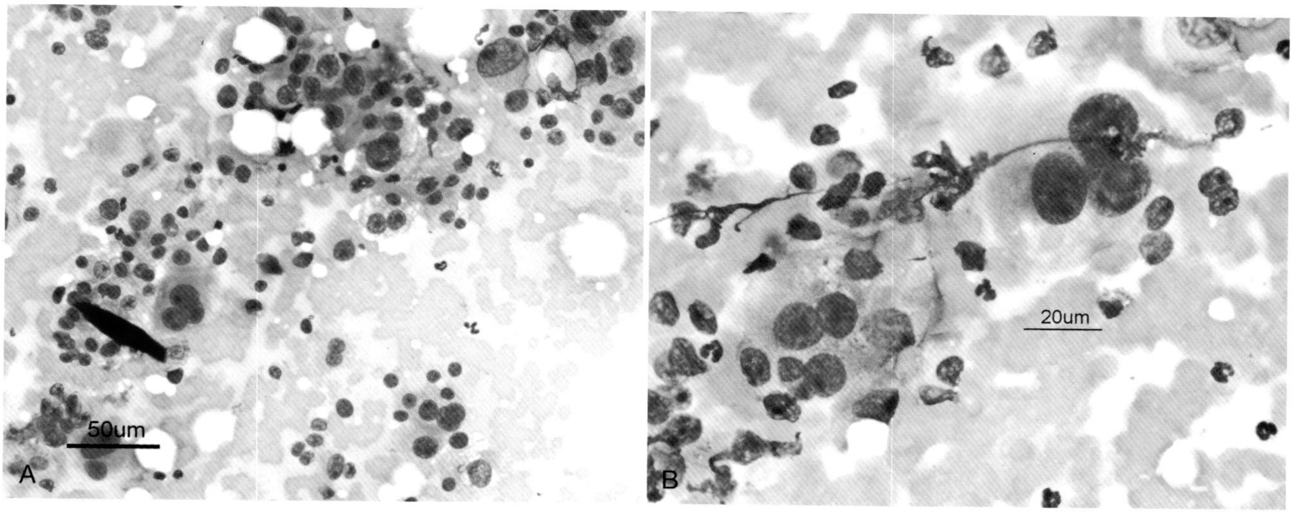

Figure 22-12 Fine-needle aspirates from a German Shepherd with renal cystadenocarcinoma. A, Slides are highly cellular and display marked atypia, including marked anisocytosis, marked anisokaryosis, multinucleation, and large prominent nuclei. (Wright-Giemsa stain.) **B,** Higher magnification shows multiple large, irregularly shaped nucleoli. (Wright-Giemsa stain.)

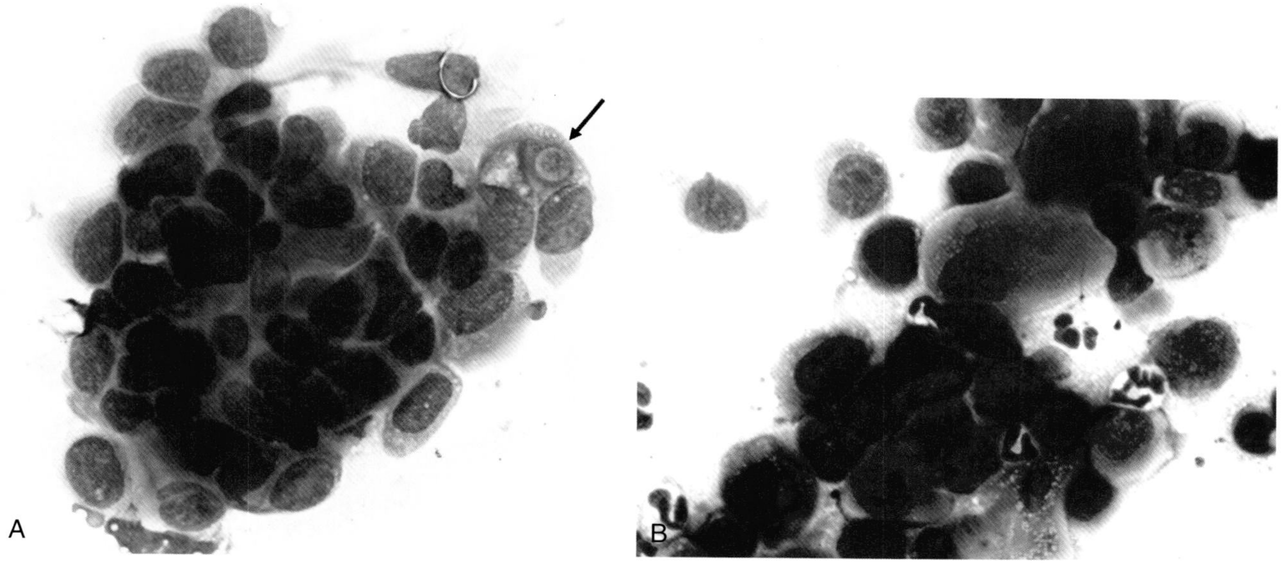

Figure 22-13 A, Fine-needle aspiration (FNA) of a renal transitional cell carcinoma from an English Springer Spaniel. Note cohesive aggregate of medium polygonal cells typical of an epithelial neoplasm. Cells exhibit increased N:C ratio, moderate anisocytosis and anisokaryosis, and a distinctive intracytoplasmic eosinophilic inclusion (*black arrow*). Histopathologic examination confirmed a diagnosis of transitional cell carcinoma arising from the renal pelvis. (Wright-Giemsa stain. Original magnification 500×.) **B,** FNA of a renal squamous cell carcinoma from a dog. Note large polygonal, angular and oval cells that exhibit marked anisocytosis, anisokaryosis, vesicular cytoplasm, and large oval to irregular multiple nucleoli. (Diff-Quik stain. Original magnification1000×.)

glomerulonephritis) are diagnosed on the basis of history, physical examination findings, and ancillary diagnostic procedure results. Cytologic examination is not usually indicated in such conditions; however, inflammatory responses are occasionally encountered in aspirates from clinical cases or impression smears taken at necropsy. Because kidneys are highly vascular, nearly all renal aspirates contain some inflammatory cells secondary to peripheral blood contamination. A diagnosis of inflammation depends on the presence of cells not typically found in blood (e.g., plasma cells, macrophages) or greater numbers of inflammatory cells than expected from the degree of blood contamination.

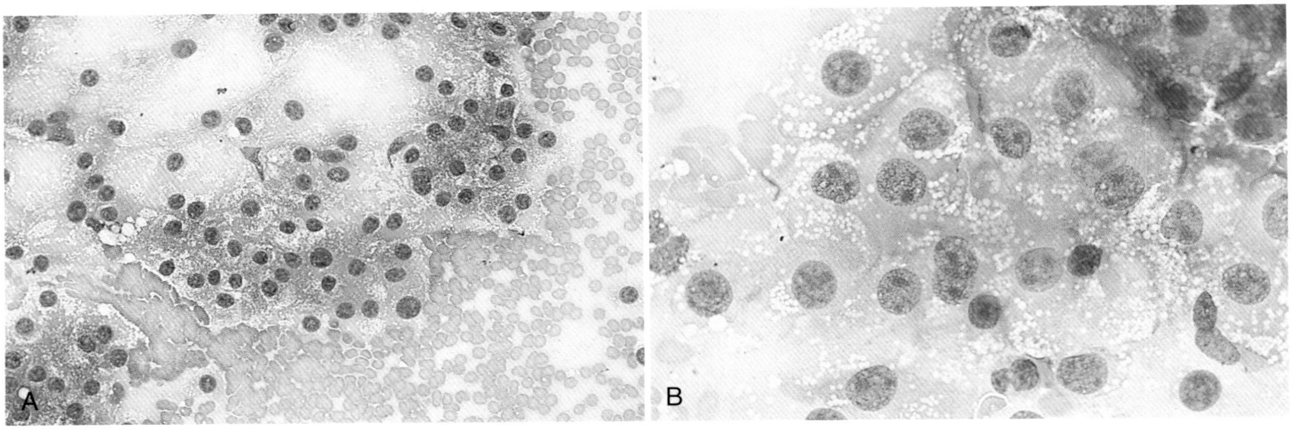

Figure 22-14 Fine-needle aspirates from an abdominal mass of a dog displaying signs of Cushing syndrome. Ultrasonography revealed an extremely large right adrenal gland mass. The left adrenal gland could not be seen. **A,** Samples are highly cellular and consist of finely vacuolated epithelial cells. (DipStat. Original magnification 100×.) **B,** Cells show moderate variability and prominent nucleoli. Some extremely large cells displaying macronuclei were present in other fields. (DipStat. Original magnification 250×.)

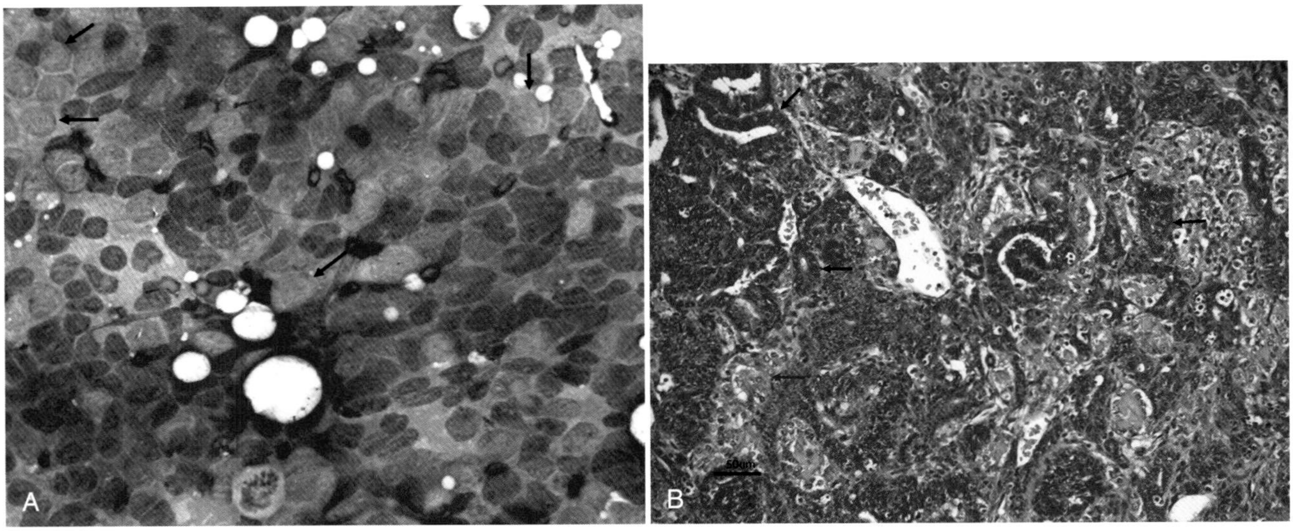

Figure 22-15 A, Fine-needle aspiration of canine nephroblastoma. Note predominance of round to oval epithelial cells in dense aggregates. The cells have a high N:C ratio, dispersed chromatin, and inapparent to indistinct nucleoli (*black arrows*). Fewer spindle (mesenchymal) cells with oblong nuclei are observed (*red arrows*). A bizarre mitotic figure is present (*green arrow*). (Wright-Giemsa stain. Original magnification 500×.) **B,** Histologic section of canine nephroblastoma. Densely packed epithelial cells form aggregates, primitive tubules (*black arrows*) and tuft-like invaginations (green arrow). Paler eosinophilic areas (*blue arrows*) represent stroma containing mesenchymal cells. (H&E stain.) (Courtesy of Dr. Pam Mouser.)

Purulent inflammation is denoted by a marked predominance of neutrophils (usually >90%) with only scattered macrophages and suggests inflammation produced by pyogenic bacteria (Figure 22-18) but may also result from noninfectious causes. Many species of pyogenic bacteria, which are usually the result of ascending infection from the lower urinary tract but may also be of hematogenous origin, have been cultured from dogs with acute pyelonephritis. Increased percentages of macrophages (>15%) are seen in cases of pyogranulomatous and granulomatous inflammation. Feline infectious peritonitis is one cause of such lesions that should be considered in cats with appropriate clinical features (Figure 22-19 and Figure 22-20). Slides should also be searched for the presence of atypical bacteria (e.g., *Mycobacterium* spp.), protozoal (e.g., *Leishmania* spp.), amoebic (e.g., *Balamuthia* spp.), systemic algae (e.g., *Prototheca zopfii*; refer to Chapter 3), and fungal organisms. Yeast phases of *Blastomyces dermatitidis*, *Cryptococcus neoformans*, *Coccidioides immitis*, *Histoplasma capsulatum*, and pseudohyphal forms of *Candida* spp. (Figure 22-21) have all been found in the kidneys of animals with disseminated disease, although such organisms are more commonly encountered in other

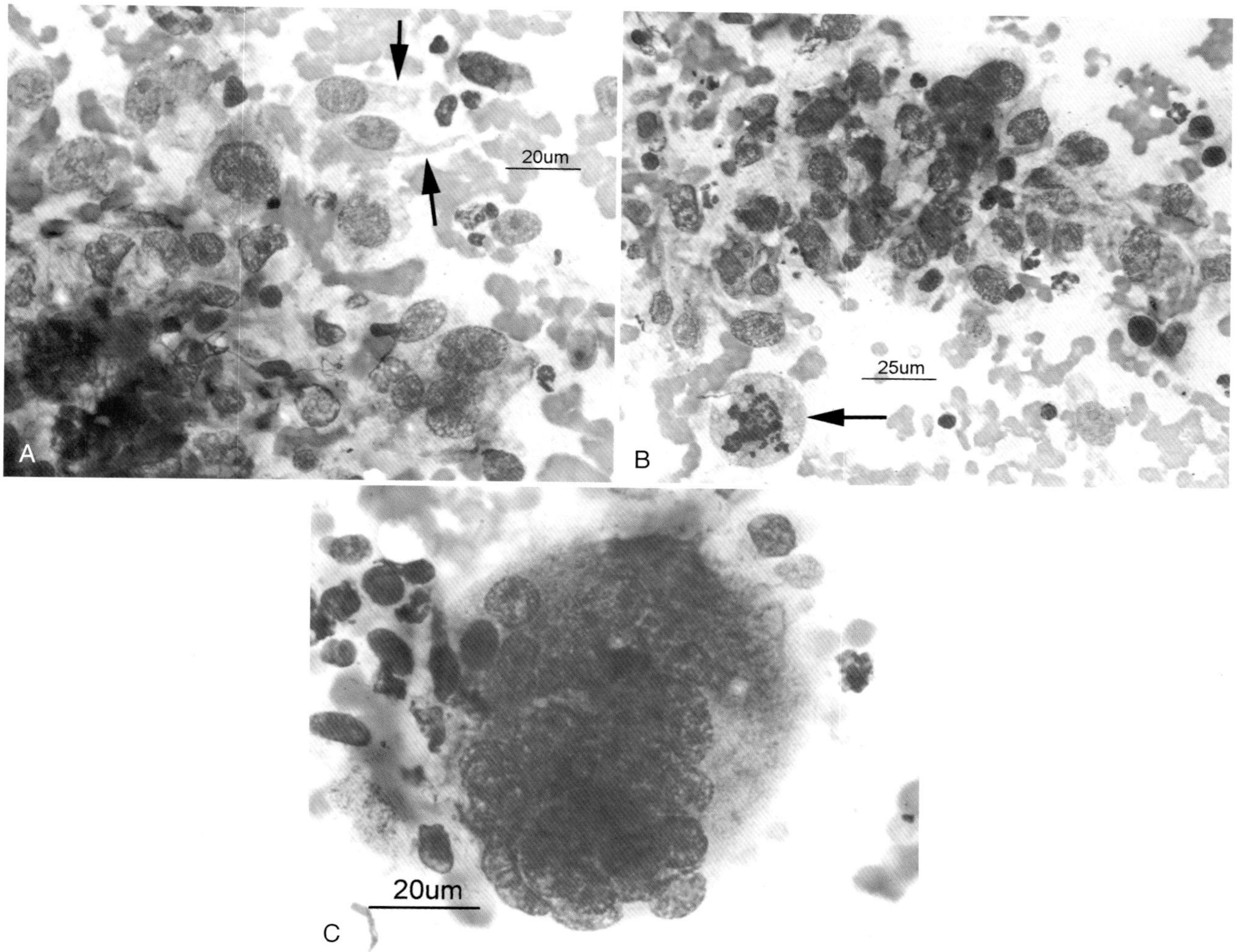

Figure 22-16 Fine-needle aspirates from a feline renal sarcoma (suspected malignant fibrous histiocytoma). A, Aspirates are highly cellular and show a pleomorphic population of mesenchymal cells. Tapered cytoplasm is evident in some cells (*arrows*). Most cells have large, prominent nucleoli. (Wright-Giemsa stain.) **B,** Image showing pleomorphic mesenchymal cells and a bizarre mitotic figure (*arrow*). (Wright-Giemsa stain.) **C,** Large multinucleated giant cells containing >20 nuclei are common, suggesting malignant fibrous histiocytoma. Further diagnostics were not performed. (Courtesy of Dr. Robin Allison.)

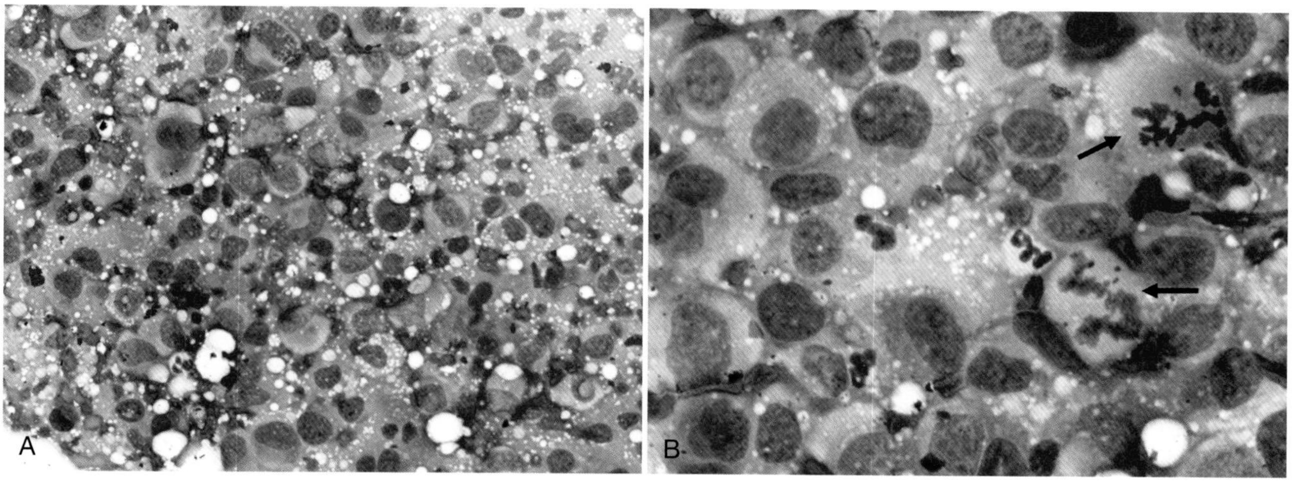

Figure 22-17 Fine-needle aspirates from a dog with disseminated histiocytic sarcoma involving the kidney. A, Aspirates are highly cellular and consist of singly occurring round cells of variable size. Some are binucleate or have vacuolated cytoplasm. (Wright-Giemsa stain. Original magnification 500×.) **B,** Higher magnification view showing neoplastic round cells with variable amounts (often abundant) of pale blue-grey cytoplasm and an eccentric large oval to irregularly round nucleus with smudged chromatin and multiple irregular nucleoli. Cells exhibit moderate anisocytosis and anisokaryosis. Two bizarre mitotic figures are present (*black arrows*). (Wright-Giemsa stain. Original magnification 1000×.)

tissues. The yeast phase of *Cryptococcus* spp. is typically characterized by a thick nonstaining capsule; however, nonencapsulated or poorly encapsulated forms of *Cryptococcus* spp. have been observed in the feline kidney (Figure 22-22). Nonencapsulated forms of *Cryptococcus* spp. may be difficult to differentiate morphologically from other fungal yeast and protozoal organisms. Fungal hyphae (Figure 22-23) may occasionally be found in imprints or aspirates, but culture is necessary to further identify the fungus. Special stains such as GMS (Gomori-Grocott methenamine silver) and PAS (periodic acid-Schiff) are often required to highlight the presence of fungal organisms in tissue specimens (Figure 22- 24), whereas routinely used Romanowsky-type stains such as Diff-Quik are typically sufficient to identify fungal organisms in cytologic specimens.

Inflammatory infiltrates characterized by a predominance of small, mature lymphocytes and plasma cells are typical of chronic inflammatory lesions and must be differentiated from cases of renal lymphoma, as previously discussed.

Cytologic Characteristics of Fluid Lesions

FNA may be performed to collect samples for cytologic examination and bacterial culture from animals with fluid lesions (e.g., hydronephrosis or abscesses).

Cysts: In humans, renal cysts are a commonly reported cause of space-occupying kidney lesions and have also been reported in domestic animals. Renal cysts may be single or multiple, congenital or acquired, and they frequently do not cause symptomatic disease. They may enlarge and induce local tissue hypoxia, however, resulting

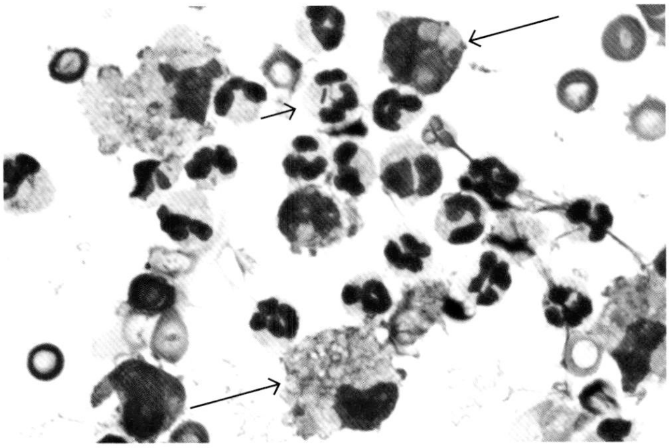

Figure 22-18 Fine-needle aspirates from the kidney of a dog with septic pyelonephritis. The smears are highly cellular and contain degenerate neutrophils, some of which contain phagocytized bacterial rods (*short arrow*). Macrophages containing cytoplasmic vacuoles or phagocytized cellular debris are present in lesser numbers (*long arrows*). (Diff-Quik. Original magnification 1000×.)

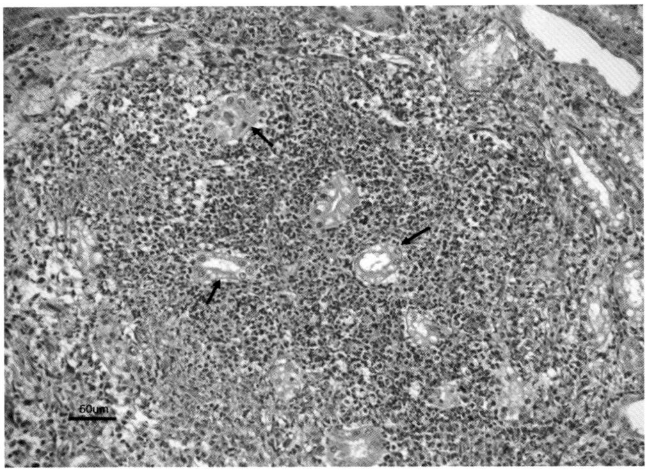

Figure 22-20 Histologic section of kidney from cat with feline infectious peritonitis. Renal parenchyma is largely replaced by sheets of inflammatory cells including lysed neutrophils and fewer macrophages, lymphocytes, and plasma cells. Renal tubules (*black arrows*) are widely separated by the interstitial inflammatory cell infiltrate (H&E.) (Courtesy of Dr. Pam Mouser.)

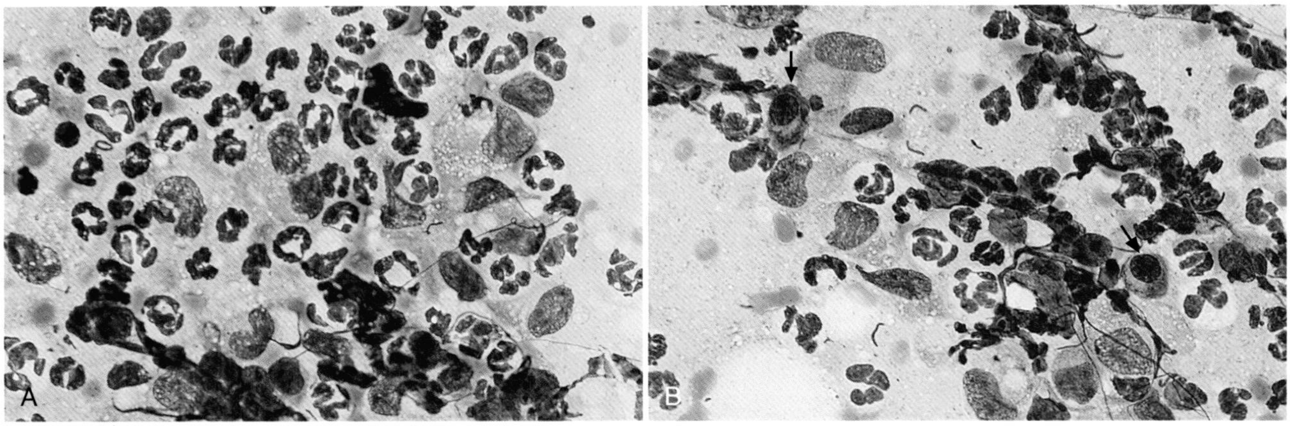

Figure 22-19 Fine-needle aspirates from the kidney of a cat with feline infectious peritonitis. The smears are highly cellular and contain a pyogranulomatous inflammatory response. **A,** Nondegenerate neutrophils and numerous macrophages are shown. In other areas of the smear, macrophages predominate. (Diff-Quik. Original magnification 250×.) **B,** Same slide as *A* and similar cell population as *A*. Note the presence of two mature plasma cells (*arrows*). (Diff-Quik. Original magnification 250×.)

in overproduction of erythropoietin with resultant polycythemia or causing sufficient loss of parenchyma from pressure atrophy that renal failure eventually develops. Aspiration of renal cysts may be performed to rule out other causes of renal enlargement and evaluate for secondary bacterial infection. Benign cysts contain a clear, straw-colored fluid that is of low cellularity but may contain a few cuboidal, epithelial lining cells. These cells occur singly and generally have foamy cytoplasm and a low N:C ratio with absent or small nucleoli. A few neutrophils and macrophages, including hemosiderophages or debris-laden macrophages, may also be present (Figure 22-25).

Some renal carcinomas are cystic and must be differentiated from benign cysts. Exfoliated cells should be evaluated for malignant changes (see Chapter 2), but not all cystic neoplasms exfoliate recognizably malignant cells into the fluid.

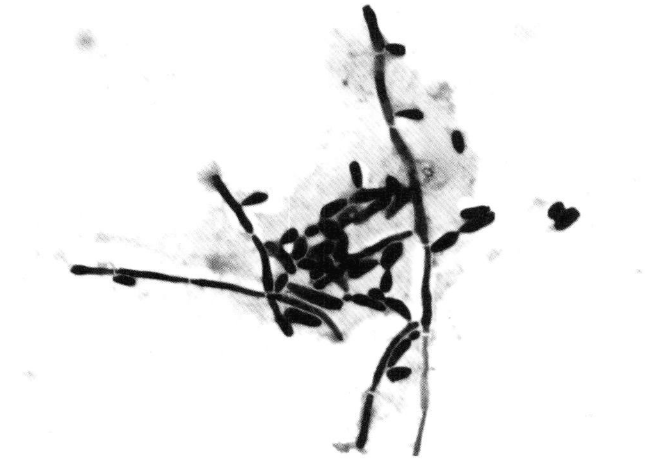

Figure 22-21 Urine sediment from dog with renal candidiasis. Basophilic pseudohyphae and blastospores of *Candida* spp. (Diff-Quik stain. Original magnification 1000×.)

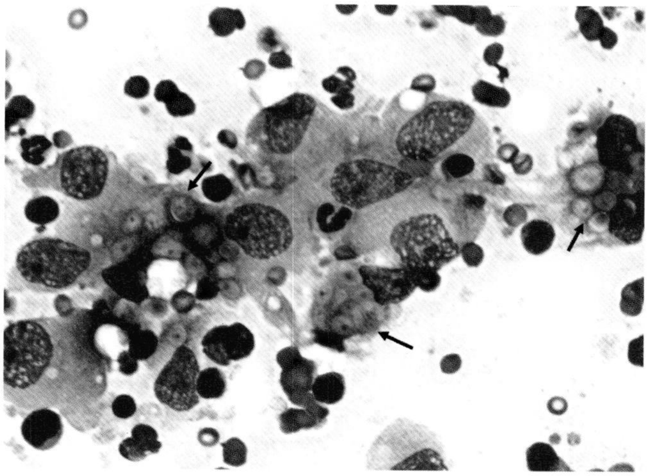

Figure 22-22 Fine-needle aspirates from the kidney of a cat with cryptococcosis. The very cellular smears contain macrophages, neutrophils, and lymphocytes consistent with pyogranulomatous inflammation. Macrophages contain several phagocytized *Cryptococcus* spp. organisms (*black arrows*) that lack a thick nonstaining capsule that this organism typically displays. Poorly encapsulated forms of *Cryptococcus* spp. must be differentiated from other fungal yeast and protozoal organisms. (Diff-Quik stain. Original magnification 1000×.)

Hydronephrosis: Hydronephrosis is the dilation of the renal pelvis and the associated parenchymal atrophy and cystic enlargement of the kidney that results from an obstruction of urine flow. The obstruction may be complete or partial, arise suddenly or progressively, and occur at any level of the urinary tract. A variable amount of clear fluid is recovered from aspiration, and smears of this fluid contain few cells; a few inflammatory cells and epithelial lining cells may be present. High numbers of inflammatory cells are seen with secondary infections. The causes of hydronephrosis, which may be radiographically distinguished from renal cysts, include ectopic ureters, calculi, neoplasia, benign prostatic hyperplasia, pregnancy, and inadvertent surgical ligation of the ureter.

Abscesses: Renal abscesses occur infrequently in dogs and cats but may occur secondary to a septic process such as pyelonephritis. The physical appearance of the aspirated material is like that of any other purulent exudate. Cytologically, the smears are highly cellular and typically consist of greater than 85% neutrophils with varying numbers of macrophages (see Figure 22-18). A search should be made for infectious agents, and material should be submitted for culture and sensitivity. Identifying bacterial rods or cocci helps in choosing antibiotic therapy while awaiting culture and sensitivity results. With Romanowsky-type stains, bacteria (both gram-positive and gram-negative) stain blue-black (see Figure 22-18). If bacterial rods (especially bipolar rods) are seen cytologically, an antimicrobial effective against gram-negative bacteria should be used while culture and sensitivity results are awaited. The pathologic bacterial cocci are generally *Staphylococcus* and *Streptococcus* spp.; therefore, when bacterial cocci are seen cytologically, an antimicrobial effective against gram-positive bacteria should be used while culture and sensitivity results are awaited.

Cytologic Characteristics of Crystals

Crystals are rarely encountered in FNA of normal or diseased kidneys but, when present, may provide important diagnostic clues in nephrotoxicosis cases. Calcium oxalate monohydrate crystals may be seen in FNA or impression smears of kidneys from dogs or cats with oxalate nephrosis, which occurs most commonly in ethylene glycol–poisoning cases. The calcium oxalate monohydrate crystals may appear as flat, elongated structures with pointed ends that resemble a picket fence or as groupings of crystals that resemble sheaves of wheat (Figure 22-26). The crystals exhibit birefringence when viewed under polarized light (see Figure 22-26, *B*). It is important to differentiate oxalate crystals from another important crystal type found in dogs and cats with nephrotoxicosis because of ingestion of contaminated pet food. Such crystals are thought to result from precipitation of melamine and cyanuric acid. They are pale yellow to golden, round to oval, polarizable crystals with distinctive radiating striations or globular dense green aggregates found in distal tubules and collecting ducts (Figure 22-27).[16]

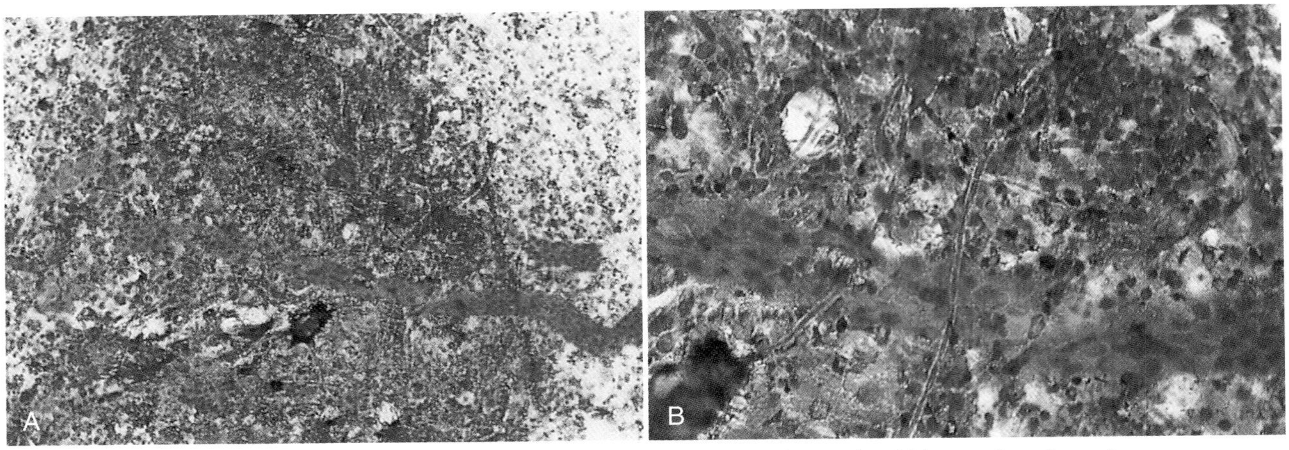

Figure 22-23 **Impression smears taken at necropsy from the kidney of a dog. A,** Highly cellular smear with recognizable tubules and fungal hyphae. (Wright stain. Original magnification 33×.) **B,** Higher magnification of the same area. (Wright stain. Original magnification 200×.)

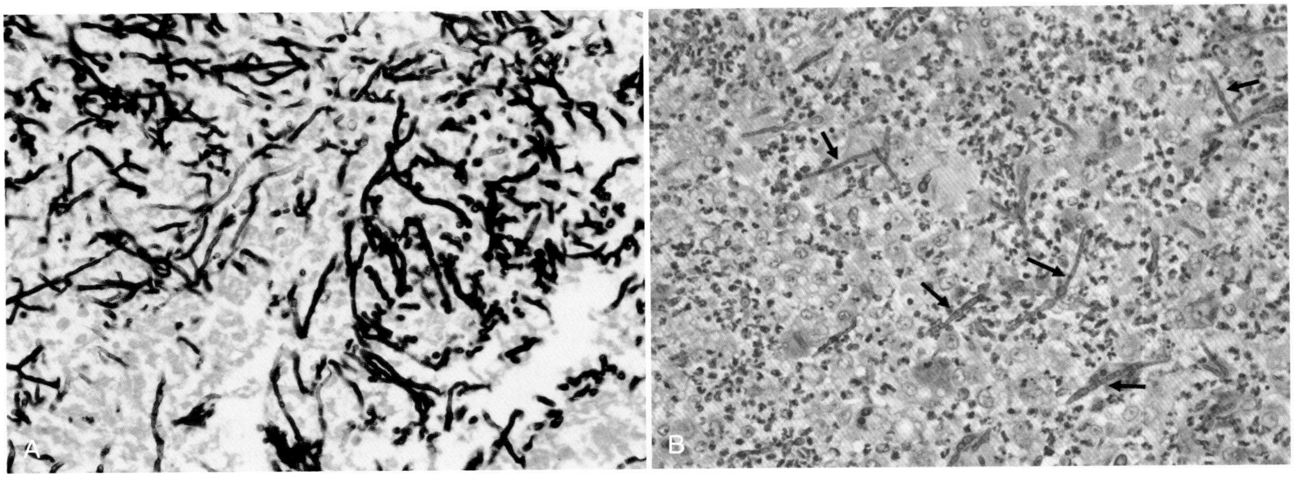

Figure 22-24 A, Histologic section of fungal nephritis in a Newfoundland dog. GMS stain highlights fungal hyphae in tissue as black branching structures against a pale green background. *Aspergillus terreus* was cultured from the patient (GMS stain. Original magnification 400×.) **B,** Histologic section of fungal nephritis in a cat. Periodic acid-Schiff (PAS) stain highlights fungal hyphae in tissue as pink branching structures (*black arrows*) in a background of pyogranulomatous inflammation. *Phialophora verrucosa* was cultured from the patient. (PAS stain. Original magnification 400×.) (Courtesy of Dr. Pam Mouser.)

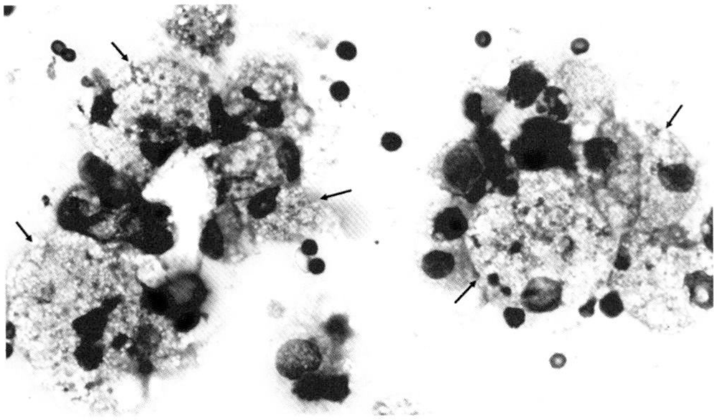

Figure 22-25 **Cytocentrifuge preparation of fluid collected from a renal cyst in a cat.** Several foamy macrophages, some containing phagocytized amorphous blue debris (*black arrows*), are found in the fluid. The findings in cystic fluid are relatively nonspecific. Histologic evaluation of the cyst wall is required for accurate classification of these types of lesions. (Diff-Quik stain. Original magnification 1000×.)

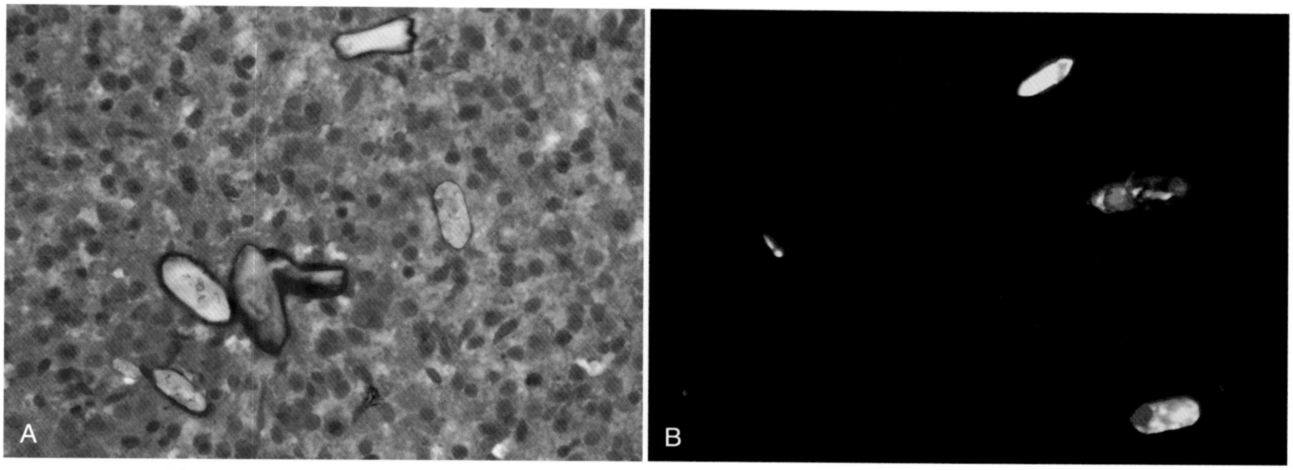

Figure 22-26 Impression smears taken at necropsy from the kidney of a dog. A, Highly cellular smear with degenerate tubular epithelial cells and calcium oxalate monohydrate crystals. Crystals resemble a picket fence with pointed ends. (Wright stain. Original magnification 500×.) **B,** Lower magnification of crystals as viewed under polarized light demonstrating birefringence. (Wright stain. Original magnification 250×.)

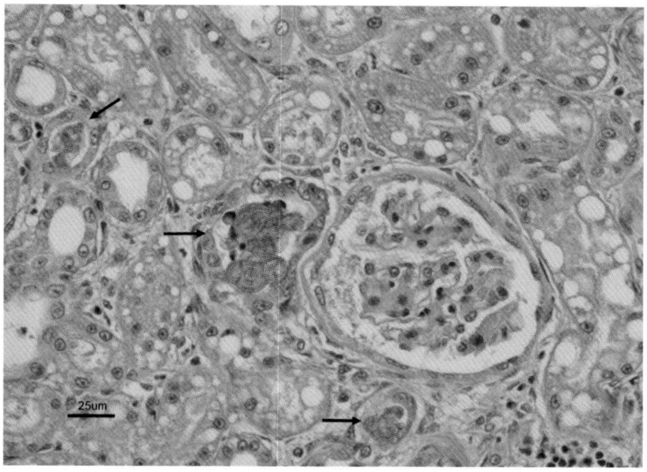

Figure 22-27 Histologic section of kidney from a cat that ingested pet food contaminated with melamine and cyanuric acid. Pale tan to golden, round to oval crystals with distinctive radiating striations or globular dense aggregates are found in lumens of distal tubules and collecting ducts. (H&E stain.) (Courtesy of Dr. Pam Mouser.)

References

1. Borjesson DL: Renal cytology, *Vet Clin North Am Small Anim Pract* 33:119–134, 2003.
2. Leiman G: Audit of fine needle aspiration cytology of 120 renal lesions, *Cytopathology* 1:65–72, 1990.
3. Nguyen GK: Percutaneous fine-needle aspiration biopsy cytology of the kidney and adrenal, *Pathol Annu* 1:163–197, 1987.
4. Menard M, Papageorges M: Technique for ultrasound-guided fine needle biopsies, *Vet Radiol Ultrasound* 36:137–138, 1995.
5. DeMay RM: *The art and science of cytopathology*, Chicago, IL, 1996, ASCP Press, pp 1083–1134.
6. Maxie MG, Newman SJ: Urinary System. In Maxie MG, editor: *Jubb, Kennedy, and Palmer's pathology of domestic animals*, vol 2, Philadelphia, PA, 2007, Saunders, pp 498–503.
7. Henry CJ, et al: Primary renal tumors in cats: 19 cases (1992-1998), *J Feline Med Surg* 1(3):165–170, 1999.
8. Bryan JN, et al: Primary renal neoplasia of dogs, *J Vet Intern Med* 20:1155–1160, 2006.
9. Barton: Cytology of the endocrine and neuroendocrine tumors, *Vet Can Soc Newslett* 17:5–9, 1993.
10. Gasser AM, et al: Extradural spinal, bone marrow, and renal nephroblastoma, *J Am Anim Hosp Assoc* 39(1):80–85, 2003.
11. Neel J, et al: A mass in the spinal column of a dog, *Vet Clin Pathol* 29(3):87–89, 2000.
12. Brewer DM, et al: Spinal cord nephroblastoma in dogs: 11 cases (1985-2007), *J Am Vet Med Assoc* 238(5):618–624, 2011.
13. Munday JS, et al: Renal osteosarcoma in a dog, *J Small Anim Pract* 45(12):618–622, 2004.
14. Hahn KA, et al: Bilateral renal metastases of nasal chondrosarcoma in a dog, *Vet Pathol* 34(4):326–352, 1997.
15. Affolter VK, Moore PF: Localized and disseminated histiocytic sarcoma of dendritic cell origin in the dog, *Vet Pathol* 39:74–83, 2002.
16. Brown CA, et al: Outbreaks of renal failure associated with melamine and cyanuric acid in dogs and cats in 2004 and 2007, *J Vet Diagn Invest* 19:525–531, 2007.

CHAPTER 23

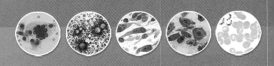

Examination of the Urinary Sediment

Heather L. Wamsley

SPECIMEN COLLECTION

In addition to the biologic variability of patients, urinalysis results are influenced by the urine collection method, the timing of urine collection, administration of therapeutic or diagnostic agents prior to collection, and how the sample is handled prior to analysis.[1] Ideally, at least 6 milliliters (mL) of urine should be collected prior to the administration of therapeutic or diagnostic agents to establish baseline information; however, in patients with cystitis and urge incontinence, this ideal may be challenging to attain. In urinalysis, 5 mL of urine may be used; 1 mL may be used for urine culture, if necessary. When choosing the urine collection method and the timing of urine collection, it is useful to consider the patient's clinical status, the logistics of the collection method, and the intended use of the sample (Table 23-1 and Table 23-2).

First morning, preprandial urine samples, which are inherently collected after a period of nil per os (NPO, nothing by mouth), will be the most concentrated with highest urine specific gravity and concentration of sediment; however, the cytomorphology of sediment contents and viability of fastidious microorganisms may be reduced because of the relatively prolonged retention of the urine within the bladder. If sediment examination and urine culture are primary goals, cystocentesis of a randomly timed urine sample may be preferred in patients lacking contraindications for cystocentesis (e.g., thrombocytopenia, urethral obstruction). Cystocentesis samples are also useful to localize urinalysis findings (e.g., sediment abnormalities, proteinuria) to the bladder or proximal urinary tract, since samples obtained via cystocentesis will lack modifications by the lower genitourinary tract.

Samples collected during natural, midstream micturition or by transurethral catheterization are also suitable for sediment examination and a specialized type of culture—quantitative urine culture—which should be interpreted using guidelines based on collection method and colony-forming units per milliliter (CFU/mL) (Table 23-3). Manual compression of the bladder to induce micturition should be avoided, since doing so may cause reflux of potentially infectious urine, traumatic hematuria, or rarely uroabdomen. Voided urine samples rescued from the examination room tabletop have limited utility; but, if the sediment is examined without delay, some components may still be assessed, specifically cells that might come from the patient (e.g., leukocytes, erythrocytes, atypical cells). Such a sample should not be used for biochemical analysis or to screen for bacteriuria.

In addition to routine urine sediment evaluation, urine samples may be converted to a dry-mount cytology;[2,3] this permits more sensitive detection of bacteria and more accurate assessment of bacterial morphology and greatly facilitates evaluation of atypical cells in-house or by a reference laboratory. The method is described in Box 23-1. If available, cytocentrifugation of urine sediment is equally useful. When applicable, obtaining cells directly from a mass (i.e., traumatic catheterization, ultrasound-assisted fine-needle biopsy [FNB], or surgical biopsy imprint) usually produces a sample with the best morphology for cytologic examination.

SPECIMEN HANDLING PRIOR TO URINALYSIS

With proper sample handling and testing, complete urinalysis may rapidly provide information about the genitourinary tract and screen for diseases of other body systems (e.g., endocrine, hepatic). Urine should be collected into a sterile, single-use vessel to avoid potential contamination by cleanser residues and microorganisms. The body of the container (not just the lid) should be labeled, and the container should be sealed to avoid sample leakage and evaporation of volatile compounds (e.g., ketones). To minimize postcollection artifacts and obtain results that are most representative of urine in vivo, urine samples should be evaluated within 30 minutes of collection.[4] If urinalysis will be delayed, the sample should be refrigerated and protected from light to prevent overgrowth of microorganisms and photodegradation of bilirubin, respectively. If necessary, samples may be stored for approximately 12 to 24 hours (i.e., overnight); however, depending on the initial sample composition (e.g., pH, concentration of crystallogenic substances), the sediment content may be modified from what was initially present immediately ex vivo—crystals may form with refrigerated storage (i.e., struvite, calcium oxalate dihydrate), renal tubular casts may degrade, cytomorphology may be detrimentally altered.[5] Freezing or routine use of chemical

TABLE 23-1

Methods of Urine Collection with Their Advantages and Disadvantages or Precautions

Collection Method	Advantages	Disadvantages / Precautions
Midstream, naturally voided	Noninvasive, relatively easy technique in dogs May be performed by clients and is useful to collect first morning, maximally concentrated urine samples from outpatients Unlike cystocentesis or catheterization, is not associated with iatrogenic hematuria Though not ideal, a freshly voided sample may be used for urine culture, as long as a quantitative urine culture is performed	Likely contaminated by a variable amount of material from the lower genitourinary tract (e.g., bacteria, epithelial cells, blood, sperm, debris), perineum, or environment (e.g., pollen), which may be observed in the urine sediment. Cleanser residues or microorganisms within the collection vessel may affect results. Urine should be collected into a sterile, single-use urine collection cup, rather than into a reusable container. Avoid manual bladder compression to induce micturition, which may cause reflux of urine into other organs (e.g., kidneys, prostate) or iatrogenic hematuria.
Transurethral catheterization	Useful collection method when an indwelling urinary catheter is already present for another reason Though not ideal, sample may be used for urine culture, as long as a quantitative urine culture is performed	Risk of traumatic catheterization, which may injure the patient and contaminate the sample with blood. Risk of iatrogenic infection, especially in patients predisposed to urinary tract infection (e.g., lower urinary tract disease, renal failure, diabetes mellitus, hyperadrenocorticism). Should be performed aseptically and atraumatically by a trained, experienced individual. Urine sample may be contaminated by variable numbers of epithelial cells, bacteria, and debris from the lower genitourinary tract, which may be observed in the urine sediment. Catheters that are chemically sterilized may contain residue of the antiseptic solution, which may irritate mucosal linings and affect results of urinalysis and urine culture. Catheterization may be technically challenging in female patients. May require use of a vaginal endoscope.
Antepubic cystocentesis	Avoids lower genitourinary tract contamination of urine sample Ideal sample for urine culture Less risk of iatrogenic infection compared with transurethral catheterization Easier than collection of a voided sample from cats Better tolerated than catheterization	Contraindicated in patients with urethral obstruction or bleeding diathesis (e.g., thrombocytopenia), may be performed with caution after cystotomy. An adequate volume of urine within the bladder is required. Blind cystocentesis without at least manual localization and immobilization of the bladder is not recommended. Ultrasound-guided needle placement is helpful, though not mandatory. Misdirection of the needle may lead to a nondiagnostic or contaminated sample (e.g., enterocentesis). A variable degree of iatrogenic microscopic hematuria, which cannot be readily distinguished from pathologic, disease-induced hematuria, may be caused by this collection method. This type of contamination may be particularly pronounced when the bladder wall is inflamed or congested. Iatrogenic hematuria may limit the utility of this collection method when monitoring the progression of disease in a patient that has pathologic hematuria.

TABLE 23-2

Timing of Urine Sample Collection, Indications, and Potential Effects on Urinalysis Results

Collection Time	Advantages	Disadvantages
First morning urine – Urine is formed after a several hour period of nil per os	Represents the patient's maximally concentrated urine and is, therefore, ideal for assessing renal tubular ability to concentrate urine Microscopic sediment will be more concentrated Postprandial alterations unlikely Urine more likely to be acidic, so casts may be better preserved (proteinaceous structures dissolve in alkaline urine)	Urine present within bladder for a relatively prolonged period May alter cellular morphology observed during microscopic examination May decrease viability of fastidious microorganisms, causing false-negative culture results
Postprandially	Useful to assess the effect of diets intended to modulate urinary pH when collected 3 to 6 hours postprandially More likely to detect hyperglycemic glucosuria when collected 3 to 4 hours postprandially	pH may be elevated by postprandial alkaline tide when collected within 1 hour postprandially
Randomly timed urine sample – Represents urine that has accumulated within the bladder for minutes to hours or urine that has been diluted by recent ingestion of water	Cytomorphology and viability of fastidious microorganisms may be better preserved since urine is stored within the bladder for relatively less time	If the urine is isosthenuric or minimally concentrated, no conclusion can be drawn about renal tubular concentrating ability

TABLE 23-3

Guidelines for Interpretation of Quantitative Urine Cultures

	Significant (CFU/mL)		Questionable (CFU/mL)		Contamination (CFU/mL)	
Collection Method	Dog	Cat	Dog	Cat	Dog	Cat
Cystocentesis	>1000	>1000	100–1000	>1000	<100	>1000
Catheterization	>10,000	>1000	1000–10,000	100–1000	<1000	<100
Voided	>100,000	>10,000	10,000–100,000	1000–10,000	<10,000	<1000

CFU/mL, colony-forming units per milliliter.

preservatives should be avoided. Refrigeration is the preferred means to preserve urine samples; however, since cold urine may influence urinalysis results (e.g., falsely increase specific gravity, inhibit enzymatic urine dipstick reactions, promote crystal formation), a sample that has been refrigerated should be permitted to warm to room temperature prior to urinalysis. If crystalluria is a medically important problem that is being evaluated, then the finding should be confirmed in a freshly obtained sample collected into a single-use container and analyzed within 30 to 60 minutes without intervening refrigeration.[4,5]

PREPARATION OF URINE SEDIMENT WET-MOUNT

Evaluation of urine sediment for the presence of increased concentrations of cells, casts, microorganisms, or crystals is useful to detect underlying urinary tract disease or disease of other organs (e.g., ammonium biurate crystalluria). Gross clarity of the urine sample should not be used as the sole means to detect potential sediment findings (i.e., cells, crystals, casts, microorganisms, lipid, mucus, or sperm), since even nonturbid samples may be microscopically abnormal. However, some advocate forgoing urine sediment evaluation when the sample is grossly normal (i.e., yellow and clear) and all of the urine dipstick tests are normal, keeping in mind that the small percentage of animals with concurrent microscopic abnormalities may go undetected.

The urine sample should be mixed well prior to removing an aliquot for centrifugation to avoid loss of formed elements by spontaneous sedimentation that may have occurred prior to urinalysis. Most urine sediment findings are reported semiquantitatively, though the coefficient of variation is high for microsopy.[6] To aid result interpretation and intersample result comparisons, laboratories should use a standardized technique for urine sediment preparation

BOX 23-1

Method to Prepare Urine Sediment Dry-Mount for Routine Cytologic Examination

- Centrifuge the urine at 400× to 500× g (~1000 – 1500 revolutions per minute [rpm]) in a conical centrifuge tube for 5 minutes.
- Remove the supernatant fluid by either gently decanting or using a transfer pipette to aspirate it.
- Use a transfer pipette to aspirate the sediment pellet from the bottom of the centrifuge tube.
- Place a small drop of the aspirated material onto a clean, glass microscope slide.
- Use a second clean, glass microscope slide to spread the material in a monolayer as is done for tissue aspirate cytology.
- Allow the slide to air-dry. Heat fixation is not necessary and will alter cell morphology.
- Stain as a routine cytology using quick Romanowsky-type stain. Alternatively, the slide may be stored in a covered container at room temperature and sent to a reference diagnostic laboratory for evaluation.

and evaluation (Box 23-2). The starting volume of urine used to prepare the sediment, the speed and duration of centrifugation, and the volume in which the sediment pellet is resuspended after centrifugation affect the concentration of the urine sediment. Ideally, both a standard starting volume of urine and a standard volume to resuspend the sediment pellet should be used. When possible, 5 mL of well-mixed urine should be centrifuged at 400 to 500 times gravity (g) (approximately 1000–1500 revolutions per minute [rpm]) in a conical centrifuge tube for 5 minutes; 4.5 mL of supernatant should be removed and either discarded or saved for subsequent biochemical testing (e.g., urine specific gravity, sulfosalicylic acid precipitation of protein). The sediment pellet should be gently resuspended in 0.5 mL of supernatant, which represents 10% of the original starting volume. When restricted by lesser urine sample volume, the volume of supernatant used to resuspend the pellet for wet-mounting should accordingly be reduced to 10% of the initial volume of urine centrifuged (see Box 23-2). Commercial systems for urine sediment preparation (e.g., Stat-Spin®, Kova®, IRIS International, Inc., Chatsworth, CA; HYCOR Biomedical, Indianapolis, IN, respectively) are available. Adherence to the manufacturer's guidelines will ensure standardized results. The urine sediment pellet may be gently resuspended by using a disposable transfer pipet to gently aspirate and expel the contents of the centrifuge tube to form a suspension or by holding the conical centrifuge tube between an index finger and thumb to form a fulcrum and gently flicking the tube with the contralateral index finger to create a weak vortex. Aggressive mixing may degrade fragile structures such as casts.

To prepare an unstained wet-mount, a single drop of the well-mixed pellet suspension should be transferred to a clean glass microscope slide and a coverslip applied. A stained wet-mount prepared using a drop of 0.5% new methylene blue or Sternheimer-Malbin stain (Sedi-Stain™, Becton Dickinson, Rutherford, NJ) added to the pellet suspension is helpful in identifying nucleated cells. Addition of stain will dilute the concentration of the sediment or may contaminate the sample with crystals or microorganisms. Semiquantitative results should be determined using an unstained wet-mount, and any crystals or microorganisms that are identified in a stained wet-mount should be confirmed in an unstained wet-mount. It may be useful to mount a stained wet-mount and an unstained wet-mount side by side on a single slide. In general, wet-mounts should be examined without delay. However, a humidified chamber prepared from a Petri dish, a thin layer of dampened absorbent material, and a halved cotton-tip applicator stick (Figure 23-1) may be used to temporarily preserve a wet-mount in instances when consultation with an in-house colleague is desired.

BOX 23-2

Guidelines for Urine Sediment Preparation and Evaluation

- Since cells, crystals, casts, and so on will spontaneously sediment because of gravity, mix the whole urine sample well before removing an aliquot for centrifugation to ensure that the urine sediment wet mount is representative of the whole sample.
- Use a standard volume aliquot of urine for centrifugation (e.g., 5 milliliters [mL]).
- Use a standard volume of urine supernatant to gently resuspend the sediment pellet (i.e., 10% of the original aliquot volume).
  - If 5 mL of urine are centrifuged, remove 4.5 mL of supernatant and resuspend the pellet in the remaining 0.5 mL.
  - If 4 mL of urine are centrifuged, remove 3.6 mL of supernatant and resuspend the pellet in the remaining 0.4 mL.
  - If 3 mL of urine are centrifuged, remove 2.7 mL of supernatant and resuspend the pellet in the remaining 0.3 mL.
  - If 2 mL of urine are centrifuged, remove 1.8 mL of supernatant and resuspend the pellet in the remaining 0.2 mL.
- Examine the whole coverslip and a standard number of microscopic fields (i.e., 10 fields) using both the 10× and 40× objectives and reduced illumination.
- Use the unstained wet-mount to determine the concentration of materials within the sediment, since the addition of stain dilutes the sediment.
- Staining (e.g., with new methylene blue) is helpful for identification of nucleated structures but may form crystals or may be contaminated with microorganisms. If crystals or microorganisms are observed in a stained sediment wet-mount, confirm their presence in an unstained wet-mount of the sediment.

MICROSCOPIC EXAMINATION OF URINE SEDIMENT

To enhance visualization of materials in wet-mounts, samples are observed with modified illumination to increase

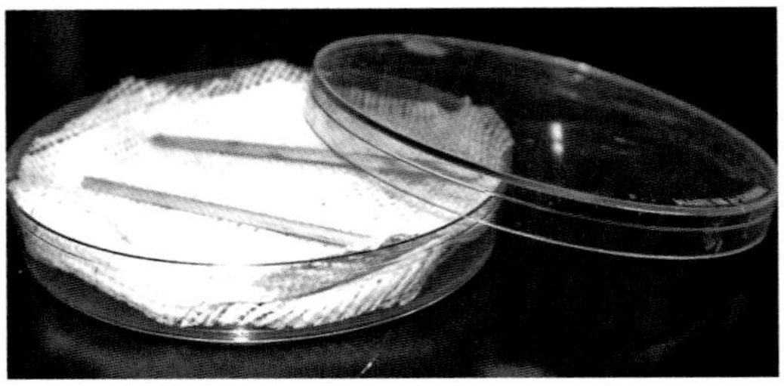

Figure 23-1 Wet-mounts may be temporarily preserved in a humidified Petri dish created by placing dampened material in the bottom of the dish with struts formed from the broken wooden handle of a cotton-tipped applicator.

the refraction of formed elements relative to the surrounding liquid. Proper illumination using a light microscope is achieved by either lowering the substage condenser a couple of centimeters or by partial closure of the iris diaphragm of the condenser; the latter is considered optically superior. In addition to scanning the entire coverslip, a standardized number of 10× and 40× microscopic fields, that is, 10 fields at each magnification, should be examined to determine the concentration of formed elements. Box 23-3 details steps for systematic microscopic urine sediment evaluation and reporting.

BOX 23-3

Detailed Steps for Microscopic Urine Sediment Evaluation

- Reduce the illumination of the microscope slide by either lowering the microscope's condenser to a couple centimeters below the stage or by partially closing the aperture of the iris diaphragm within the condenser.
- Scan the entire area of the wet-mount using the 10× objective to find the plane of focus in which material has settled and to detect larger structures, for example, casts, which tend to flow to the edges of the coverslip.
- Examine 10 microscopic fields of the slide from low power using the 10× objective for the presence of the following things and provide an assessment of their amounts in the unstained wet mount.
    - Crystals
        - Record type(s) present.
        - Record qualitative impression of the amount of each type of crystal (i.e., none, few, moderate, or many).
    - Casts
        - May be better visualized at the margins of the coverslip.
        - Record type(s) present (e.g., hyaline, cellular, granular, waxy).
        - Record the number of each cast type per 10× low power field (LPF) as a range (e.g., 0–2/LPF).
    - Epithelial cells
        - Record type(s) present.
        - Record the number of each type of epithelial cell per 10× LPF as a range (e.g., 0–4/LPF).
        - Observe cytomorphology for the presence of dysplastic or neoplastic changes.
    - Mucous threads
        - Record qualitative impression of the number of mucous threads (none, few, moderate, or many).
    - Helminth ova, larva, adult worms, or other parasites
        - Record qualitative impression of the number of parasite structures (none, few, moderate, or many).
- Examine 10 microscopic fields of the slide from higher power using the 40× objective.
    - Scrutinize the morphology of structures observed at low power.
        - Confirm the identification of the structures observed at low power.
        - Again, inspect epithelial cells for dysplastic or neoplastic cytomorphology.
    - Inspect the slide for the presence of the following things and provide an assessment of their amounts in the unstained wet mount:
        - Erythrocytes
            - Record the number of erythrocytes per 40× high power field (HPF) as a range (e.g., 2–4/HPF).
        - Leukocytes
            - Record the number of leukocytes per 40× HPF as a range (e.g., 0–3/HPF).
        - Microorganisms (e.g., bacteria, yeast, fungi, algae)
            - Record morphology of bacteria (e.g., cocci, bacilli, filamentous, spore-forming).
            - Record qualitative impression of the number of each type of microorganism (none, few, moderate, or many).
        - Lipid droplets
            - Lipid droplets need to be distinguished from erythrocytes.
            - Lipid droplets are variably sized, refractile, and often float above the focal plane.
            - Record qualitative impression of the number of lipid droplets (none, few, moderate, or many).
        - Sperm
            - Record qualitative impression of the number of sperm (none, few, moderate, or many).
        - Other structures or unidentified structures
            - Identify the structures or describe their morphology.
            - Record qualitative impression of the number of these structures (none, few, moderate, or many).

URINARY SEDIMENT FINDINGS

Cells (Table 23-4), microorganisms (see Table 23-4), casts (Table 23-5), crystals (Table 23-6 and Table 23-7), lipid, and contaminating substances may be found in urinary sediment. Urine obtained from healthy dogs and cats forms little sediment. Small numbers of epithelial cells, mucous threads, erythrocytes, leukocytes, hyaline casts, and various types of crystals may be found in the urine of most healthy animals. Bacteria and squamous epithelial

TABLE 23-4

Routine Microscopic Urine Examination: Cells, Cell-like Structures, Microorganisms, Parasites, and Confusing Artifacts

Finding	Normal	Interpretation If Increased	Follow-Up
Erythrocytes	<5/HPF	Bleeding: If voided, urethra, prepuce, and vagina (e.g., proestrus, estrus, postpartum) must be considered as well as bladder	Imaging, ultrasonography Culture if white blood cells (WBCs) are present
Leukocytes	<3/HPF, by cystocentesis <8/HPF, by catheterization or micturition	Inflammation: If voided, urethra, prepuce, and vagina (e.g., proestrus, estrus, postpartum) must be considered as well as proximal urinary tract	Culture, imaging, ultrasonography
Epithelial cells: Squamous	Rare in samples collected by cystocentesis	Presence of squamous epithelial cells in cystocentesis urine samples suggests squamous metaplasia of urinary bladder transitional cells; consider chronic irritation and/or neoplasia	Imaging, ultrasonography
	Variable by catheterization or micturition	None unless cellular abnormalities are noted	None, unless neoplasia is suspected, then cytology, imaging, and ultrasonography should be considered
Transitional	<5/LPF	Catheterization, inflammation (WBC should also be present), chronic irritation, neoplasia, chemotherapy	Cytology, imaging, and ultrasonography
Spermatozoa	Occasional in males	None in males; post-coitus in females	None
Microorganisms	Depends on collection method	Strongly suggestive of infection if sample collected by cystocentesis or catheterization (usually accompanied by WBCs). Voided samples may be contaminated with organisms from the prepuce, vagina, or vulva	Culture, look for WBCs in urine, check urine protein and glucose, consider possibility of diabetes mellitus, dry-mount cytology
Parasites	None	Fecal contamination, blood contamination, or *Capillaria plica* (bladder worm of dogs and cats) or *Dioctophyma renale* (kidney worm of dogs)	Imaging or ultrasonography if bladder or kidney worm suspected
Fat droplets	Cats: Frequent Dogs: Occasional	Increased numbers of fat droplets may be seen with lubricants used for catheterization, obesity, diabetes mellitus, and hypothyroidism	Physical examination for evidence of hypothyroidism and obesity, urine and serum glucose for diabetes mellitus
Artifacts: Air bubbles, glass chips, oil droplets, starch granules, pollen, fungal conidia, feces, yeast, bacteria, parasitic ova	Variable, depending on method of collection	Associated with contamination or slide preparation	Beware of contamination

HPF, high-power field (40× objective); *LPF*, low-power field (10× objective).

TABLE 23-5

Routine Microscopic Urine Examination: Casts and Confusing Artifacts

Cast Type	Normal	Interpretation If Increased	Follow-Up
Hyaline	≤2/LPF in moderately concentrated urine	Diuresis of dehydrated animals or proteinuria of preglomerular (e.g., fever, strenuous exercise, seizures) or renal etiology	Urine and serum protein concentration, physical examination, history
Granular	≤2/LPF in moderately concentrated urine	Acute to subacute renal tubular injury	Physical examination, history, CBC, serum chemistries
Cellular	None	Acute renal tubular injury	Physical examination, history, CBC, serum chemistries
Waxy	None	Chronic renal tubular injury	Physical examination, history, CBC, serum chemistries
Fatty	≤1/LPF	Excessive numbers suggest renal tubule necrosis or degeneration; more commonly seen in cats than dogs; occasionally seen in dogs with diabetes mellitus	Physical examination, history, CBC, serum chemistries (especially glucose)
Bilirubin	None	Indicate moderate to marked bilirubinuria	Check for hemolysis or hepatobiliary dysfunction
Hemoglobin or myoglobin (red-brown casts)	None	Hemoglobin casts and myoglobin casts both orange to red-brown and cannot be differentiated microscopically; hemoglobin casts occur with intravascular hemolysis, whereas myoglobin casts occur with severe myolysis	Check for intravascular hemolysis (CBC) and muscle injury (serum chemistries, especially LDH, CK, and AST)
Castlike artifacts (mucus threads, fibers)	Occasional	Urethral irritation or contamination with genital secretions	None
Other confusing artifacts: Hair, fecal material, fungal hyphae	None	Associated with contamination or slide preparation	Beware of contamination

AST, aspartate aminotransferase; CBC, complete blood count; CK, creatine kinase; LDH, lactate dehydrogenase; *LPF*, low-power field (10× objective).

cells derived from external genital surfaces may be present in voided and catheterized urine. When interpreting urine sediment, it is also necessary to keep in mind the biochemical findings that may influence the sediment content, for example, in dilute urine (specific gravity <1.008) erythrocytes will likely be lysed; highly alkaline urine may reduce the numbers of cells and casts; and urine pH influences crystal formation.

Epithelial Cells

Epithelial cells in urine vary markedly in size, depending on the origin. They are larger in the lower portions of the urinary tract than in the ureters, renal pelves, and renal tubules. It is routine to see fewer than 5 epithelial cells per 10× low-power field in normal urine samples. While using unstained wet-mount preparations, it may be challenging to distinguish the different types of epithelial cells, since transitional epithelial cells are highly pleomorphic, and all epithelial cells will become rounded within fluid and degrade when exposed to urine. When evaluation of cell morphology is critical, urine sediment dry-mount cytology is useful for examination in-house or by a reference laboratory. A greater number of epithelial cells are seen in urine samples collected by transurethral catheterization or in patients with inflamed, hyperplastic, or neoplastic mucosa. Methods to diagnose structural lesions within the urinary tract (e.g., ultrasonography, traumatic catheter biopsy, FNB, surgical biopsy imprint) are often more conclusive than urinalysis alone.

Squamous Epithelial Cells: Squamous epithelial cells line the distal third of the urethra, the vagina, and the prepuce and are usually not considered significant. They are the largest of the epithelial cells and the largest cell from the patient found in urine sediment. They are flat or rolled cells, which have at least one angular border and usually a single small, condensed nucleus, or they may be anucleate (Figure 23-2, Figure 23-3; Figure 23-16; Figure 23-17; Figure 23-18).

A variable number of squamous epithelial cells are most commonly observed with lower genitourinary tract contamination of voided or catheterized samples. Squamous epithelial cells are typically not present in samples collected by cystocentesis. A significant number of squamous epithelial cells are very rarely seen in cystocentesis samples because of squamous cell carcinoma of the bladder or squamous metaplasia of the bladder, which may occur with transitional cell carcinoma or chronic bladder

TABLE 23-6

Routine Microscopic Urine Examination: Crystals and Confusing Artifacts

Crystal	Causes
Struvite (magnesium ammonium phosphate)	• Refrigerated storage for more than 1 hour • Commonly seen in clinically normal animals • Urinary tract infection by urease-producing bacteria • Alkaline urine for reasons other than infection (e.g., diet, recent meal, renal tubular ammoniagenesis in cats, post-collection artifact) • Sterile or infection-associated uroliths of potentially mixed mineral composition
Calcium oxalate dihydrate	• Storage for more than 1 hour with or without refrigeration • Acidic urine (e.g., diet, postcollection artifact) • May be seen in clinically normal animals • Calcium oxalate urolithiasis • Hypercalciuria (e.g., from hypercalcemia or hypercortisolemia) • Hyperoxaluria (e.g., ingestion of oxalate-containing vegetables, ethylene glycol, or chocolate)
Calcium oxalate monohydrate	• Hyperoxaluria (e.g., ingestion of ethylene glycol or uncommonly chocolate)
Calcium carbonate	• Anecdotally reported rarely in dogs and cats • Sulfonamide crystals with similar morphology may be mistaken for calcium carbonate
Bilirubin	• A low number commonly found in concentrated canine urine, especially males • Altered bilirubin metabolism (e.g., hemolytic or hepatobiliary diseases)
Amorphous phosphates	• Insignificant finding in clinically normal animals
Amorphous urates Uric acid Ammonium biurate	• Portovascular malformation • Severe hepatic disease • Ammonium biurate urolithiasis • Breed-associated: Dalmatians, English Bulldogs, Weimaraners, others; may represent risk factor for urolithiasis, especially in males
Cystine	• Defect in proximal renal tubular transport of amino acids; represents risk factor for urolithiasis
Iatrogenic	• Antibiotic administration (e.g., sulfonamides, ciprofloxacin) • Other drugs: anticonvulsants (particularly with polytherapy, alkaline urine, and certain drugs), xanthine crystals with allopurinol administration • Radiocontrast medium crystals
Artifacts from contamination or slide preparation	• Starch granules • Glass chips • Fecal material and microorganisms • Pollen • Fungal micro- or macroconidia

TABLE 23-7

pH Influence on Crystalluria

Crystal	Acidic Urine	Neutral Urine	Alkaline Urine
Ammonium biurate	✓	✓	
Amorphous phosphates			✓
Amorphous urates	✓		
Bilirubin	✓		
Calcium carbonate			✓
Calcium oxalate dihydrate	✓	✓	✓ (in stored samples)
Calcium oxalate monohydrate	✓	✓	
Cystine	✓	✓	
Drug metabolites	✓	✓	✓
Struvite		✓	✓
Uric acid	✓		

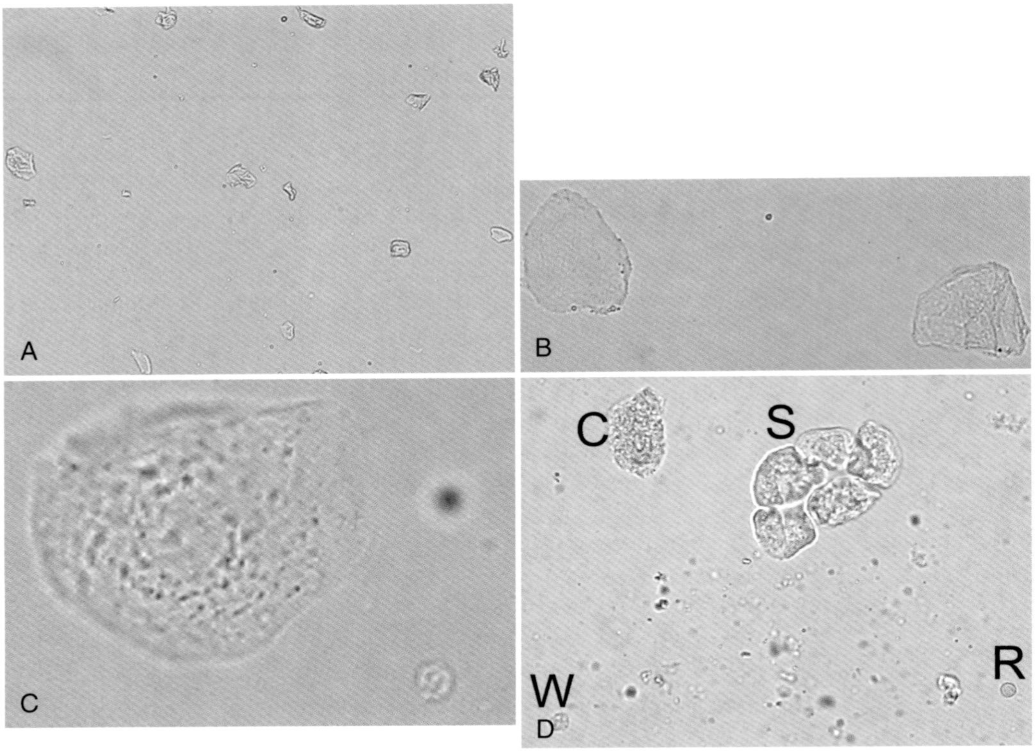

Figure 23-2 **A,** Voided urine sediment with squamous epithelial cells, which are lying flat or partially twisted. (Unstained. Original magnification 100×.) **B,** Two anucleate squamous epithelial cells with one of more angular borders. A small lipid droplet is in the center. (Unstained. Original magnification 400×.) **C,** Nucleated squamous epithelial cell with granular cytoplasm with a crenated erythrocyte (*lower right*). Note the relative size of these cells. (Unstained. Original magnification 400×.) **D,** A sheet of squamous epithelial cells (*S*), a leukocyte (*W*), an erythrocyte (*R*), and a granular cast fragment (*C*) (same dog as in Figure 23-40). The erythrocyte is biconcave and more translucent than the epithelial cells and the leukocyte. Small, refractile amorphous crystals are scattered in the background. (Unstained. Original magnification 400×.)

irritation. With transitional cell carcinoma, many other features suggestive of epithelial neoplasia, including an extreme number of epithelial cells with marked pleomorphism, are typically found. Squamous epithelial cells may also be found if the uterine body of an intact female is unintentionally penetrated during cystocentesis. Cells with squamous features may be found in the urine sediment of male dogs with conditions that cause squamous metaplasia of the prostate.

Transitional Epithelial Cells: Transitional epithelial cells line the proximal two thirds of the urethra, bladder, ureters, and renal pelves. They are highly pleomorphic, variably sized cells that are smaller than squamous epithelial cells and two to four times larger than leukocytes; those originating in the proximal urethra and bladder are the largest. They may be round, oval, pear-shaped, polygonal, or caudate and often have granular cytoplasm with a single nucleus that is larger than that of squamous epithelial cells (see Figure 23-3; Figure 23-22; Figure 23-39; Figure 23-51.

There should be less than 5 transitional epithelial cells per 10× low-power field in normal urine sediments. A greater number of transitional epithelial cells are seen in urine samples collected by catheterization or in patients with inflamed, hyperplastic, or neoplastic mucosa. Urine from animals with inflammation-induced epithelial hyperplasia also contains increased numbers of leukocytes (Figure 23-4). Urolithiasis and some chemotherapeutic agents (e.g., cyclophosphamide) may induce epithelial hyperplasia with mild to moderate atypia (Figure 23-5). Many epithelial cells are found in sediment from animals with transitional cell carcinomas, and a variable number of leukocytes are also often present because of secondary inflammation or infection. Neoplastic epithelial cells are found individually or in large cohesive sheets, tend to be larger than normal epithelial cells, usually vary markedly in size, and have a high nuclear to cytoplasm ratio along with other malignant features (Figure 23-6). Knowledge of the clinical context is important when determining the significance of atypical epithelial cells in urine sediment, for example, presence of uroliths, presence and location of urinary tract mass, or medication administration.

If a large number of atypical epithelial cells are found, dry-mount sediment cytology should be prepared and evaluated (see Box 23-1). Dry-mount cytology (Figure 23-7) affords the best opportunity for conclusive cytologic evaluation and is the best means to preserve atypical cells for evaluation by a pathologist at a reference laboratory. Cells degrade during transport in fluid; this is particularly true

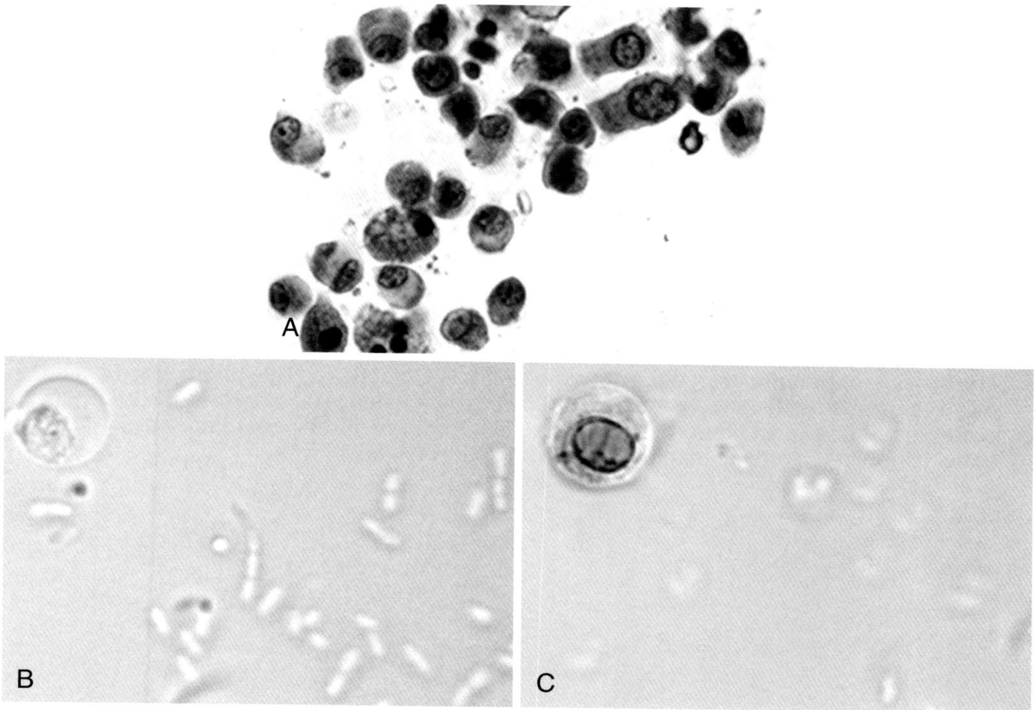

Figure 23-11 Urine sediment wet-mounts with renal tubular epithelial cells. A, Several individualized cells that can be confidently identified as renal tubular epithelial cells based on their cuboidal or oval shape with eccentric nuclei. (New methylene blue stain. Original magnification 400×.) **B,** Renal tubular epithelial cells (*upper left*) tend to become rounded once sloughed, which makes distinction from small transitional epithelial cells challenging. Several bacilli are also in the background. (Unstained. Original magnification 1000×.) **C,** Same specimen as shown in *B*. (New methylene blue stain. Original magnification 1000×.)

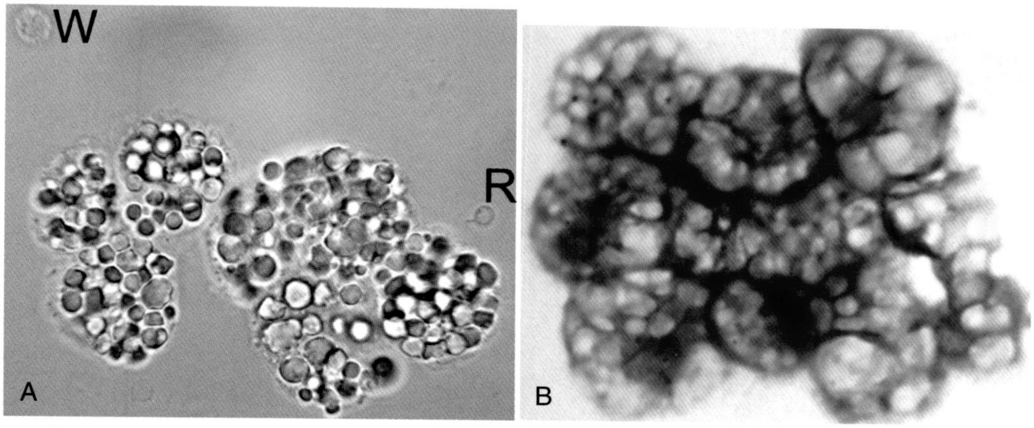

Figure 23-12 Urine sediment wet-mount and dry-mount cytology from a cat with sloughed lipid-laden renal tubular epithelial cells, sometimes referred to as *oval fat bodies*. **A,** A small group of round cells contain several refractile lipid vacuoles that project three-dimensionally from the focal plane. A leukocyte (*W*) and an erythrocyte ghost (*R*) are also present. (Unstained. Original magnification 500×.) **B,** Dry-mount sediment cytology of the same specimen shown in *A* shows an aggregate of partially degraded, lipid-laden renal tubular epithelial cells. (Wright-Giemsa stain. Original magnification 500×.)

a cytologic stain for confirmation (Figure 23-26). In the urine wet-mount, bacterial morphology is characterized, and their numbers are reported as none, few, moderate, or many. A large number of bacteria accompanied by a large number of leukocytes indicates infection with inflammation of the urinary tract, genital tract, or both, depending on how the sample was obtained (i.e., cystocentesis versus midstream micturition) (see Figures 23-23 and 23-26). Usually, when bacteria are found without accompanying increase in leukocytes, the sample has been contaminated (e.g., by external genitalia or nonsterile collection materials) (Figure 23-27), bacteria in the sample have overgrown

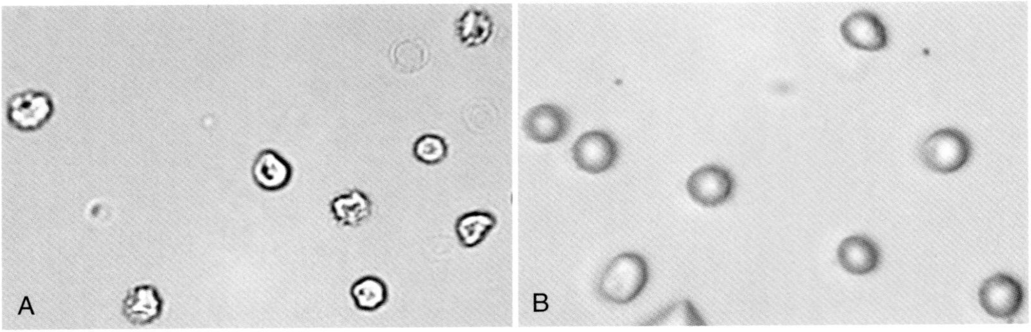

Figure 23-13 Urine sediment wet-mounts showing the effects of urine tonicity on erythrocyte appearance. Erythrocytes usually are pale orange-red due to hemoglobin and may maintain their biconcave shape. **A,** Shriveled, crenated, and ghost erythrocytes are present in highly concentrated urine. **B,** Swollen, round erythrocytes are present in dilute urine. (Unstained. Original magnification both images 500×.)

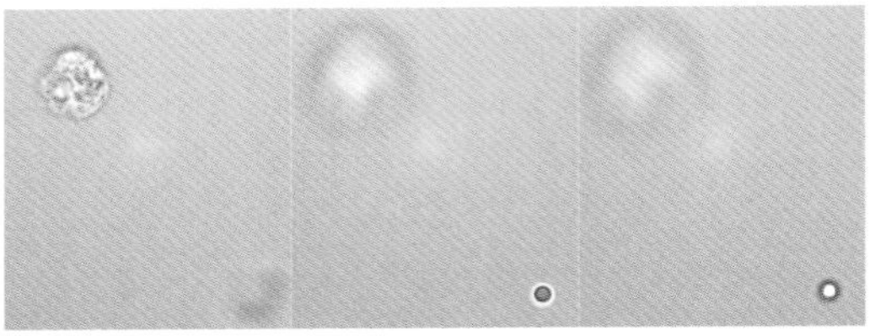

Figure 23-14 Three images of the same urine sediment wet-mount field showing a flat, round, refractile lipid droplet (*lower right*) that is floating above the focal plane of a leukocyte (*upper left*) with granular cytoplasm and visible nuclear lobule. (Unstained. Original magnification all images 1000×.)

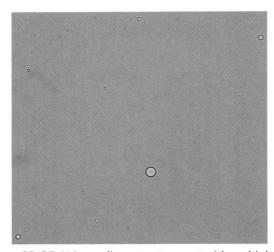

Figure 23-15 Urine sediment wet-mount with multiple variably sized, flat, round, refractile lipid droplets. (Unstained. Original magnification 400×.)

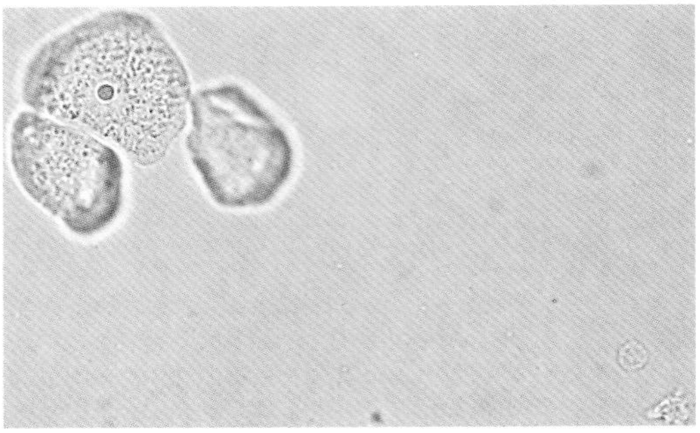

Figure 23-16 Urine sediment wet-mount with three large angular squamous epithelial cells (*upper left*) and a crenated erythrocyte (*lower right*). The squamous epithelial cell in the center has a small, round, condensed nucleus. Note the relative size of the cells. (Unstained. Original magnification 400×.)

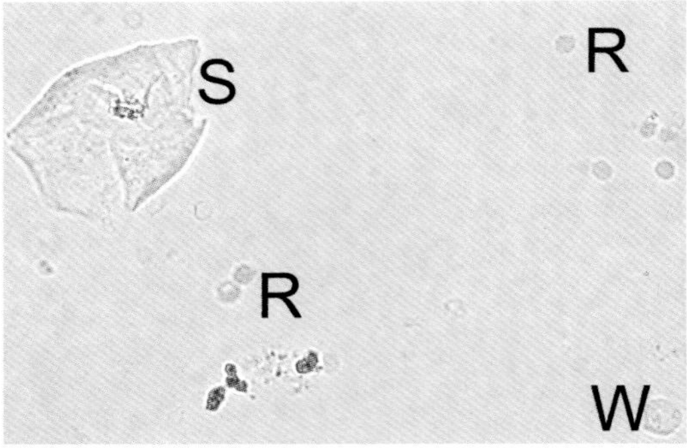

Figure 23-17 Relative sizes of a squamous epithelial cell (*S*), a leukocyte (*W*), and several erythrocytes that are often crenated (*R*) and a few erythrocytes ghosts in a urine sediment wet-mount. A few amorphous crystals are also in the background. (Unstained. Original magnification 400×.)

because of delayed urinalysis and lack of refrigeration, the observer is mistaking amorphous mineral precipitates for bacteria, or, less commonly, there is silent urinary tract infection. (see Figure 23-22). When bacteria or other microorganisms are observed in a stained wet-mount, it is useful to distinguish them from stain-contaminants by confirming their presence in an unstained wet-mount or by sediment dry-mount cytology.

Though bacteria may be confidently identified during urinalysis, occasionally urine cultures may be negative. Reasons for this disparity, for example, antimicrobial administration prior to sample collection, are listed in (Box 23-4). Uncommon infections by viruses or highly fastidious microorganisms (e.g., *Mycoplasma, Ureaplasma*) may yield negative urine culture results, even when infection is truly present.

Dependent on geographic distribution, other infectious agents such as fungi (e.g., *Candida* [Figure 23-28],

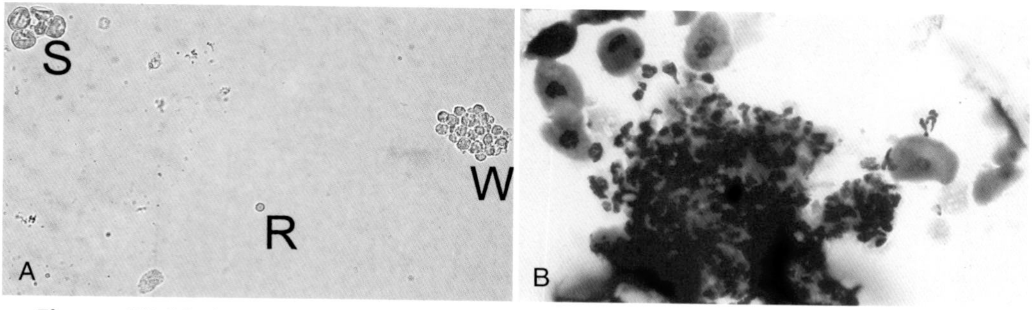

Figure 23-18 **A,** Aggregates of squamous epithelial cells (*S*) and leukocytes (*W*) with an erythrocyte (*R*). Note the relative sizes of the cells. (Unstained. Original magnification 400×.) **B,** Urine sediment dry-mount cytology of the same case with epithelial cells and a large clump of neutrophils. (Wright-Giemsa stain. Original magnification 500×.)

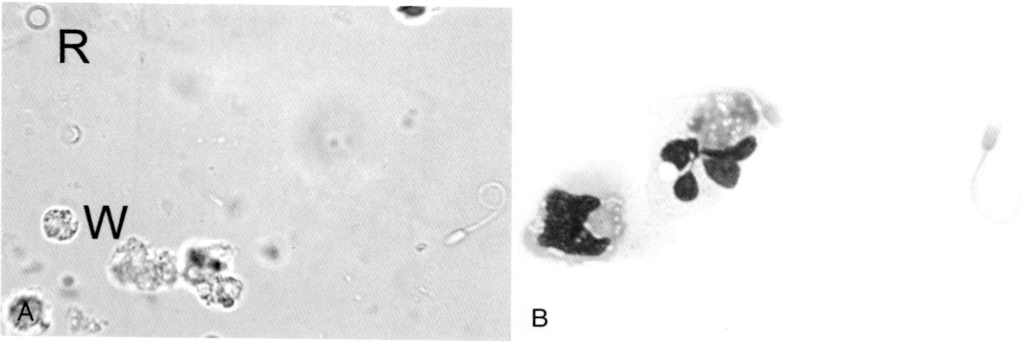

Figure 23-19 **A,** The leukocytes (*W*) are stippled and do not transmit as much light as the smaller erythrocyte (*R*). A sperm is present on the right. (Unstained. Original magnification 1000×.) **B,** Urine sediment dry-mount cytology of the same case with two leukocytes and two sperm. (Wright-Giemsa stain. Original magnification 1000×.)

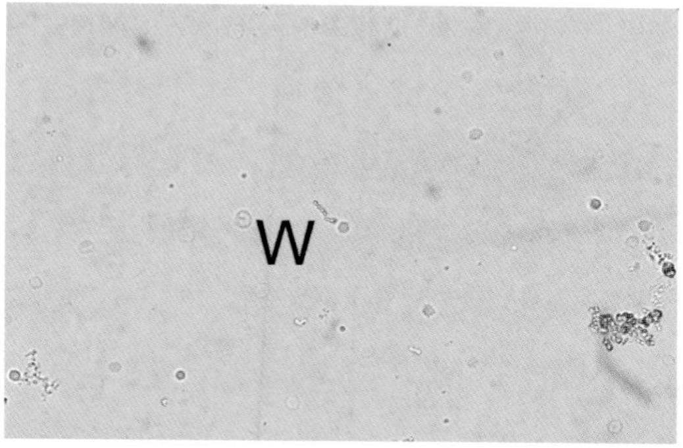

Figure 23-20 One leukocyte (*W*) with a U-shaped nucleus is present along with several erythrocytes and variably sized aggregates of amorphous crystals (Unstained. Original magnification 400×.)

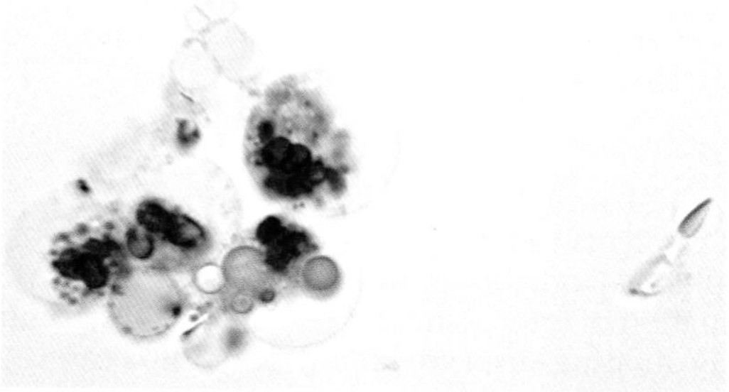

Figure 23-21 **A group of neutrophils in which the granules are visible and refractile.** In the wet-mount, the neutrophil granules may exhibit Brownian movement; these cells may be referred to as *glitter cells* by some. Lipid droplets overlay and surround the leukocytes, and a sperm is present (*right*). (New methylene blue stain. Original magnification 1000×.)

Aspergillus [Figure 23-29, Figure 23-30, Figure 23-31], *Blastomyces dermatitidis*, *Cryptococcus*); algae (e.g., *Prototheca* [Figure 23-32 and Figure 23-33]); and nematode ova, larvae, or adults (e.g., *Capillaria* [Figure 23-34], *Dirofilaria immitis* [Figure 23-35], *Dioctophyma renale*) are occasionally identified in urine sediment.

Yeast organisms may be confused with red blood cells or lipid droplets, but yeast organisms usually display characteristic budding, often have double refractile walls, and do not dissolve in acetic acid (see Figure 23-28). When found in low number, they usually are contaminants, and yeast infections of the external genitalia may cause them to be present in voided samples (e.g., snow shoe–shaped *Malassezia pachydermatis*). Long-term antimicrobial treatment is occasionally associated with secondary yeast infection (i.e., candidiasis).

Fungal hyphae (see Figure 23-29) are larger than bacteria, long, branched structures with parallel walls and perpendicular septa. Primary fungal infections of the urinary tract are uncommon. Systemic mycosis in German Shepherds or immunosuppressed patients may affect the kidneys (see

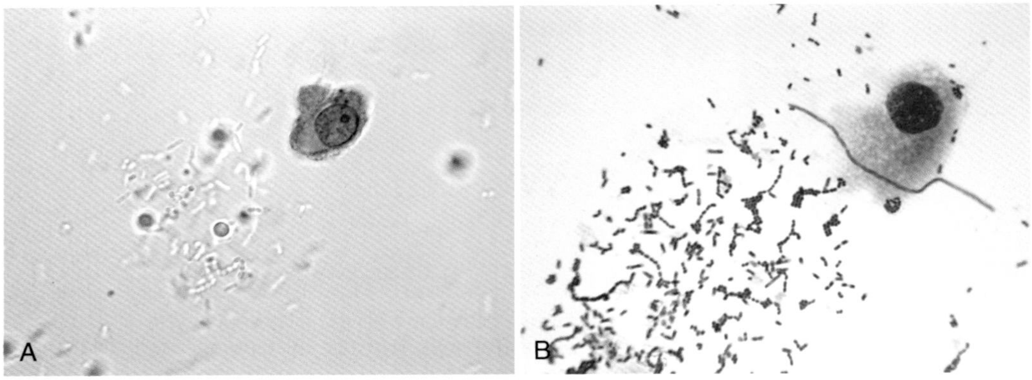

Figure 23-22 Diabetic canine cystocentesis urine sediment. A, Many bacilli and chains of cocci are present with a transitional epithelial cell. Note the lack of inflammatory response. (New methylene blue stain. Original magnification 1000×.) **B,** Urine sediment dry-mount cytology of the same case permits reliable identification of bacterial morphology. A lysed transitional epithelial cell is also present. (Wright-Giemsa stain. Original magnification 1000×.)

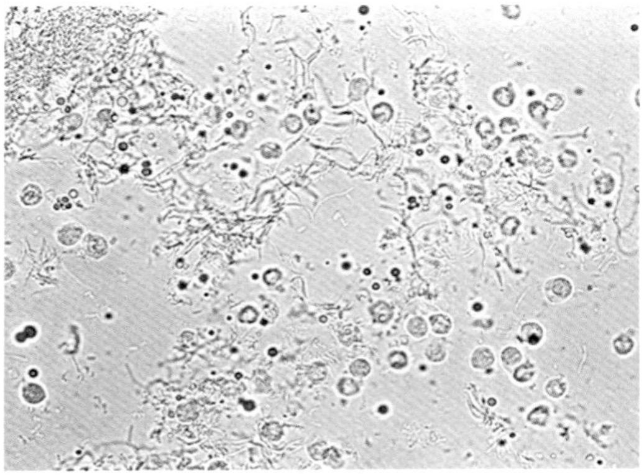

Figure 23-23 Evidence of a urinary tract infection with marked pyuria and numerous bacilli in mats and long chains. Small, refractile lipid droplets are dispersed throughout the field. (Unstained. Original magnification 400×.)

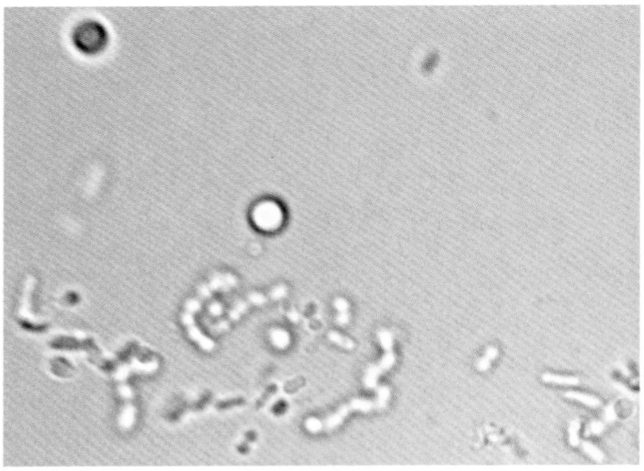

Figure 23-24 Urine sediment with bacilli and chains of cocci with two refractile lipid droplets. (Unstained. Original magnification 1000×.)

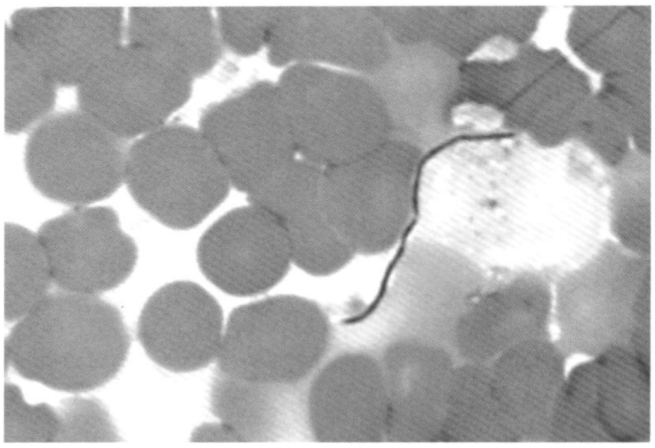

Figure 23-25 Urine sediment dry-mount cytology with a filamentous bacterium and hematuria. (Wright-Giemsa stain. Original magnification 1000×.)

Figure 23-30 and 23-31) and lower urinary tract, causing fungal elements to potentially be observed with leukocytes and epithelial cells in urine sediment (see Figure 23-29). Examination of urine sediment is also a useful screening test when evaluating suspected discospondylitis cases.

Trichuris (whipworm) ova may be present in samples contaminated by feces or enteric contents. These ova are similar to *Capillaria plica* ova (see Figure 23-34) but have important distinguishing features involving the positioning of their bipolar opercula and the texture of their outer shells. The bipolar opercula of *Capillaria* ova are slightly askew, rather than being perfectly bipolar as they are in *Trichuris* ova. The shells of *Capillaria* ova are knobby (i.e., mammillated), rather than perfectly smooth as they are in *Trichuris* ova. *Capillaria* may be an incidental finding in the urine of asymptomatic cats. However, *Capillaria* ova are rarely identified in cats with lower urinary tract signs, which resolve after appropriate treatment.

When evaluating the importance of potentially infectious agents in urine, it is important to consider whether clinical and microscopic evidence of urinary tract irritation or inflammation exists or if the animal has a condition that might inhibit such an inflammatory reaction (e.g., diabetes mellitus, hypercortisolemia). Consideration should also be given to the method of collection and the subsequent handling of the urine sample to assess the likelihood of contamination.

Casts and Castlike Artifacts

Casts (see Table 23-5) are formed in the lumen of the distal nephron (i.e., Henle's loop, distal tubule, collecting

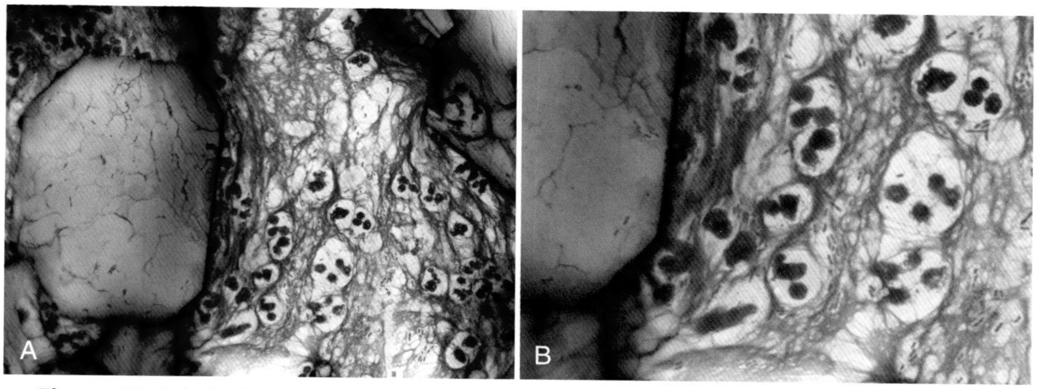

Figure 23-26 Canine urinary tract infection with struvite crystalluria. A, Urine sediment dry-mount cytology with struvite crystalluria, many degenerate neutrophils, abundant bacteria, and streaming, purple nucleoprotein. (Wright-Giemsa stain. Original magnification 500×.) **B,** Close examination facilitates accurate characterization of bacterial morphology, in this case bacilli. (Wright-Giemsa stain. Original magnification 1000×.)

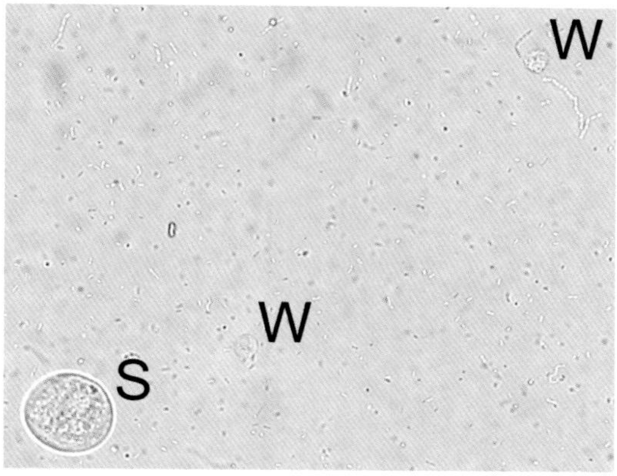

Figure 23-27 Voided urine sediment with abundant bacteria that are present individually and in chains. Although two leukocytes (*W*) are present in the field, their overall concentration is not increased. A squamous epithelial cell (*S*) is also present; this is the same case as Figure 23-39. (Unstained. Original magnification 400×.)

duct). The increased concentration and acidity of urine in the tubules promotes precipitation of protein present in the tubules. Because casts are formed in renal tubules, they are cylindrical with parallel sides. When cells in the tubules die and exfoliate, they are often incorporated into the precipitated meshlike mucoprotein matrix (i.e., Tamm-Horsfall mucoprotein). During microscopic sediment evaluation, cellular casts are further classified as epithelial, leukocyte, or erythrocyte casts, if the constituent cells are discerned. Once locked within the proteinaceous matrix, cells continue to degrade, progressing from intact cells, to granular cellular remnants, and finally to a waxy, cholesterol-rich end product. A cast may dislodge from a given renal tubular lumen at any time during this degenerative process and may be observed in the urine sediment. Other material such as lipid from degenerated renal tubular epithelial cells, hemoglobin during hemolytic disease, and bilirubin may be trapped within the proteinaceous matrix. Casts are fragile and prone to degeneration, particularly in alkaline urine; therefore, fresh urine and proper technique should be used when

BOX 23-4

Causes of a Negative Urine Culture Despite Identification of Bacteria in the Urine Sediment

- Observed bacteria represent contaminants of the urine sample incurred during collection or processing.
- Observed bacteria may actually be nonbacterial structures in the sediment that were mistakenly identified as bacteria during urinalysis.
- Observed bacteria may not be viable for the following reasons:
  - Prior antimicrobial administration
  - Prolonged urine storage
  - Fastidious nutritional and culture requirements
- Observed bacteria may not grow because of improper culture technique.

preparing specimens for evaluation. In most instances, cylindruria (i.e., casts in the urine sediment) is an insensitive, but specific indicator of renal tubular disease.

Very low numbers (i.e., 0 to 2 per 10× low-power field) of hyaline or granular casts may be seen in normal urine, but higher numbers of casts suggest a renal tubular lesion. The number of casts observed in the sediment does not correlate with the severity of renal disease or its reversibility; and the absence of casts from urine sediment cannot be used to exclude the possibility of renal disease. When hyaline or granular casts are present in increased numbers or when other cast types are observed, the only conclusion is that the renal tubules are diseased, but the severity and reversibility are indeterminate. The type of cast observed may provide additional information. Leukocyte casts indicate active renal tubulointerstitial inflammation. Waxy casts reflect a chronic tubular lesion. To recognize the onset of nephrotoxicity in patients receiving aminoglycoside antibiotic therapy, it is useful to monitor urine sediment for the appearance of tubular casts, which should prompt withdrawal of the antibiotic. Other abnormalities seen with aminoglycoside-induced nephrotoxicity include isosthenuria,

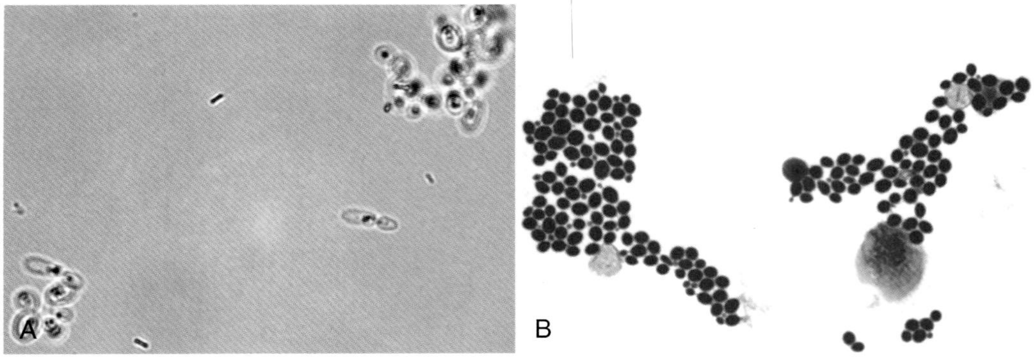

Figure 23-28 Yeast in feline cystocentesis urine sediment after chronic antibiotic administration. A, Small, budding yeast are present individually and in two aggregates with scant amorphous crystals. (Unstained. Original magnification 1000×.) **B,** Urine sediment dry-mount cytology of the same case with numerous small, budding yeast, consistent with *Candida*. A few erythrocytes and a degraded epithelial cell are also present. (Wright-Giemsa stain. Original magnification 1000×.)

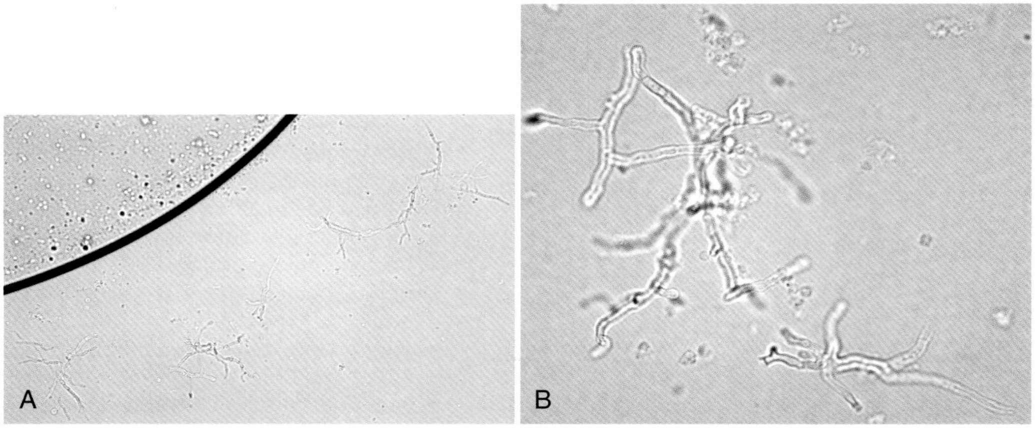

Figure 23-29 Canine systemic fungal infection after chronic immunosuppressant administration. A, Urine sediment with three mats of fungal hyphae, pyuria, hematuria, and an air bubble artifact (*top left*). (Unstained. Original magnification 200×.) **B,** Perpendicular septa are visible in the branching fungal hyphae; pyuria is also present. Compare with bacilli growing in chains in Figure 23-23. (Unstained. Original magnification 500×.) Figure 23-30 shows renal fine-needle biopsy specimen of the same case.

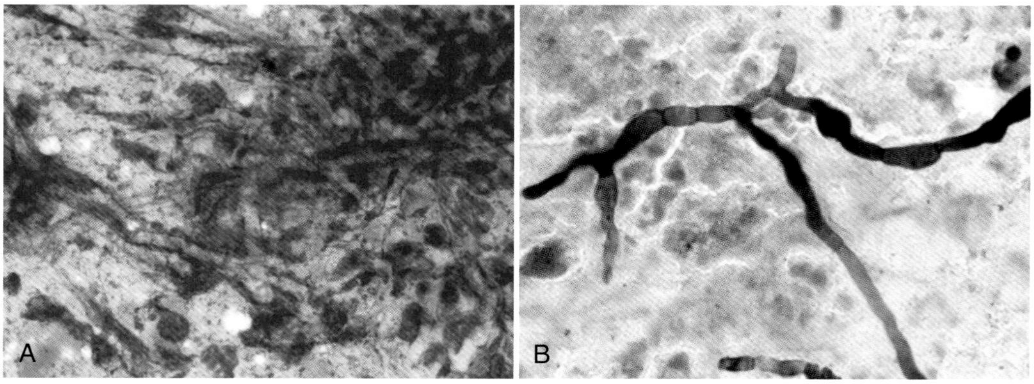

Figure 23-30 Canine systemic fungal infection after chronic immunosuppressant administration. A, Renal fine-needle biopsy (FNB) specimen with a dense mat of negatively stained, branched fungal hyphae, which is outlined by purple nucleoproteinaceous material and highly karyolytic cells. A single golden hematoidin crystal (*top middle*) indicates chronic hemorrhage. (Wright-Giemsa stain. Original magnification 1000×.) **B,** Renal FNB with branching, septate fungal hyphae stained black by silver stain. (Gomori methenamine silver stain. Original magnification 1000×.) Figure 23-29 shows urine sediment of the same case.

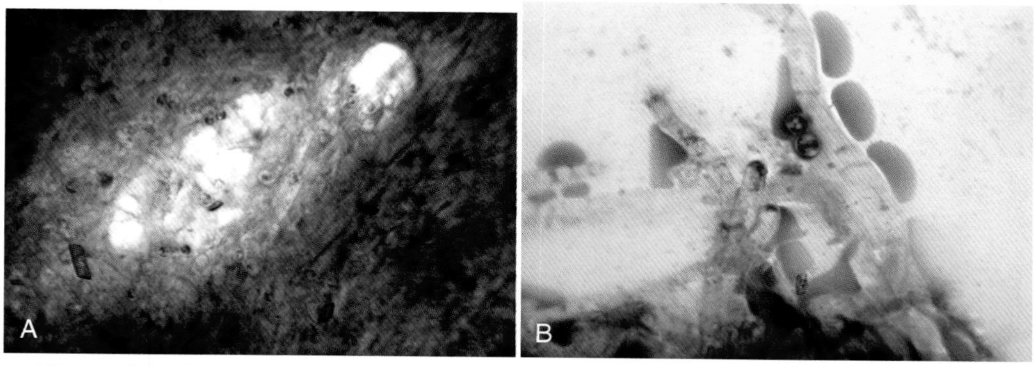

Figure 23-31 Renal pelvis fine-needle biopsy specimen. A, A three-dimensional mat of partially stained fungal hyphae is present with several partially stained microconidia and golden, rhomboid hematoidin crystals. (Wright-Giemsa stain. Original magnification 500×.) **B,** Closer view with two thinly encapsulated microconidia, partially stained hyphal termini, and hematoidin. (Wright-Giemsa stain. Original magnification 1000×.)

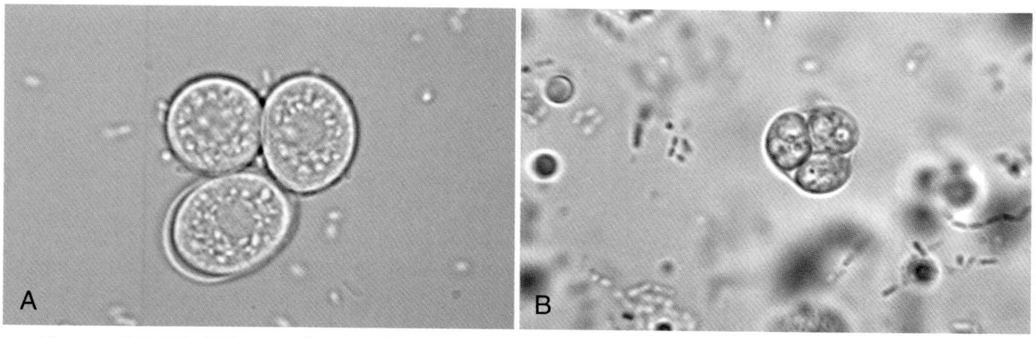

Figure 23-32 Urine sediment from a dog with cystic lesions in the kidneys and brain. A, Three algal sporangiospores and bacteria in a different focal plane. (Unstained. Original magnification 1000×.) **B,** An endosporulated sporangiospore with bacteria and lipid droplets. (New methylene blue stain. Original magnification 1000×.) Figure 23-33 shows fine-needle biopsy specimen of a cystic renal mass from same case.

proteinuria, glucosuria, and aminoaciduria, all of which may precede the onset of azotemia.

Mucous threads or fibers, which are much more common than cylindruria, should not be mistaken for casts during sediment evaluation. Mucous threads are distinguished by their variable width, curvilinear shape, and tapered ends (Figure 23-36). Mucous threads are an expected finding in horses and may also be seen with urethral irritation or contamination by genital secretions. Fibers are typically larger than the surrounding cells and may contain a repetitive internal geometric structure (Figure 23-37 and Figure 23-38; Figure 23-57, *A*).

Hyaline Casts: A few (i.e., 0 to 2 per 10× low-power field) hyaline casts, which are clear, colorless, and refractile, may be seen in moderately concentrated urine from animals without renal disease (Figure 23-39). Similar to all casts, hyaline casts are cylindrical, with parallel sides and rounded termini. Diuresis of dehydrated animals or proteinuria of preglomerular (e.g., fever, strenuous exercise, seizures) or renal etiology may cause an increased number of hyaline casts in urine. Hyaline casts may also be increased with renal tubular disease, which should typically be accompanied by an inappropriately low urine specific gravity.

Granular Casts: Granular casts are commonly seen in urine sediment (Figure 23-38; Figure 23-40 and Figure 23-41). A few (i.e., 0 to 2 per 10× low-power field) granular casts may be seen in moderately concentrated urine from animals without renal disease. Granular casts may be increased with renal tubular injury and are more specific than hyaline casts.

Cellular Casts: Cellular casts may contain epithelial cells, leukocytes, or erythrocytes (Figure 23-42). Epithelial cell casts are formed when dead epithelial cells are sloughed intact from the renal tubules and the cast is passed into the urine before the cells degenerate to granular material. Leukocyte casts are uncommon but indicate active tubulointerstitial inflammation. Erythrocyte casts are also uncommon but may form with renal hemorrhage. Granular casts usually accompany cellular casts, and mixed cellular and granular casts may occur (Figure 23-43).

Waxy Casts: Waxy casts, which indicate chronic tubular injury, look somewhat like hyaline casts but usually are wider, have blunt, square ends instead of round, and are dull, homogenous, and waxy (Figure 23-44; Figure 23-46). They are more opaque than hyaline casts and may appear to have fissures.

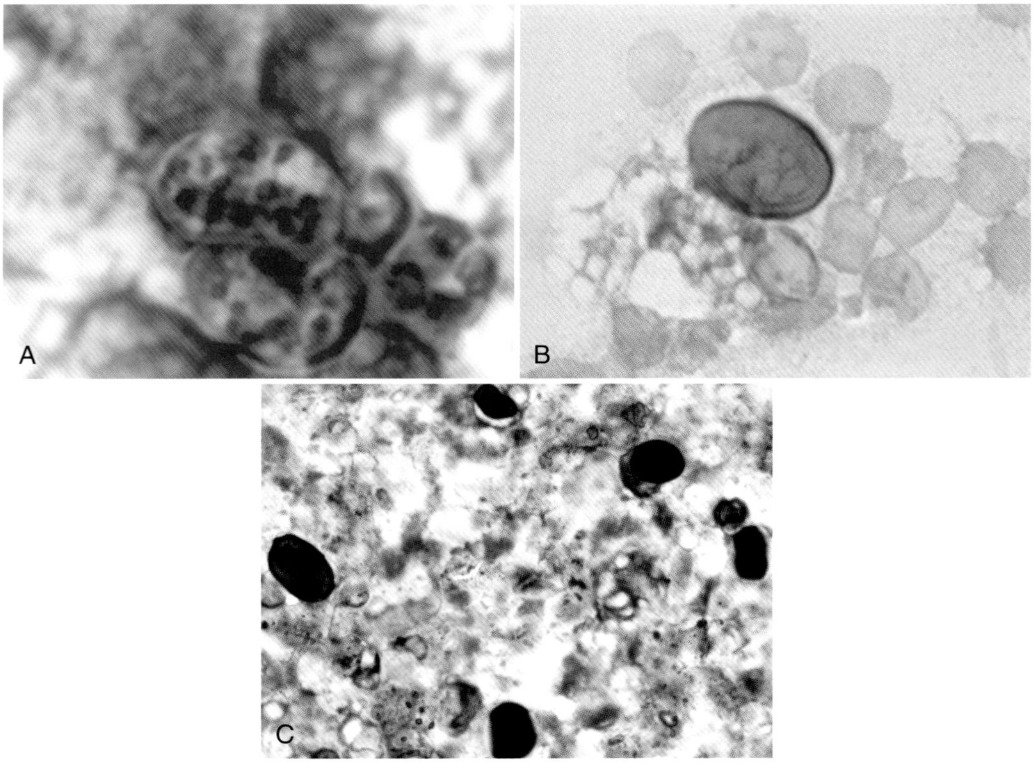

Figure 23-33 Fine-needle biopsy specimen of a cystic renal lesion; Figure 23-32 shows urine sediment from the same case. A, Two sporangiospores are adjacent to a neutrophil with free purple nucleoproteins in the background. (Wright-Giemsa stain. Original magnification 1000×.) **B,** A sporangiospore and an empty theca within a degraded macrophage. The staining pattern distinguishes *Prototheca* from *Chlorella*; in the former, only the wall is PAS-positive, the latter contains starch granules that are strongly PAS-positive. (Periodic acid-Schiff stain. Original magnification 1000×.) **C,** Several GMS-positive sporangiospores (Gomori methenamine silver stain. Original magnification 1000×.)

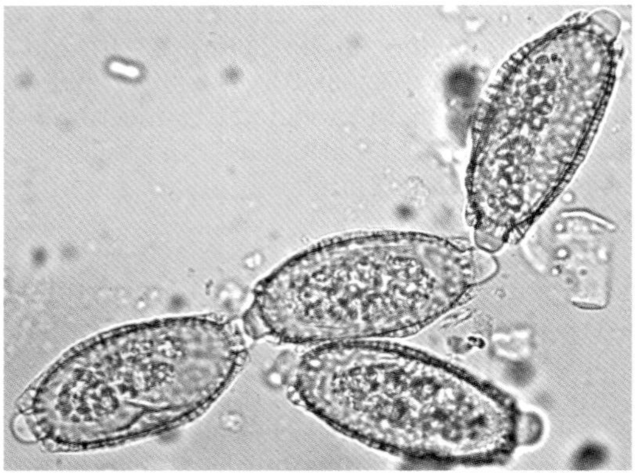

Figure 23-34 Four ***Capillaria plica*** **ova in feline urine sediment.** Note the mammillated shell and askew polar opercula. (Unstained. Original magnification 500×.)

Fatty Casts: Fatty casts contain many small fat droplets, which are round, highly refractile bodies (Figure 23-45). They are frequently seen in cats, as cats have fat in their renal tubular epithelial cells, and are occasionally seen in dogs with diabetes mellitus. Numerous fatty casts suggest renal tubule degeneration.

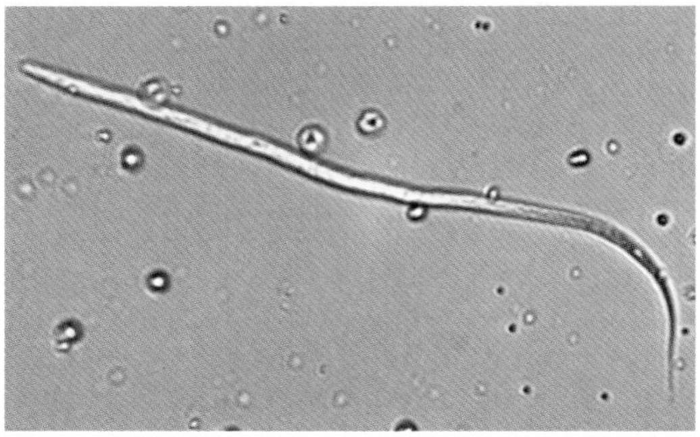

Figure 23-35 *Dirofilaria immitis* microfilaria in canine urine sediment with hematuria. (Unstained. Original magnification 200×.)

Other Casts: The matrix of casts is occasionally admixed with other materials such as bilirubin, hemoglobin, myoglobin, or crystalline precipitates (i.e., calcium oxalate monohydrate).[7] Bilirubin-stained casts indicate the presence of moderate to marked bilirubinuria (Figure 23-46). Hemoglobin and myoglobin both impart a red to red-brown tint. The presence of hemoglobin casts suggests intravascular hemolysis (Figure 23-47). Myoglobin-stained casts may be seen with widespread myolysis.

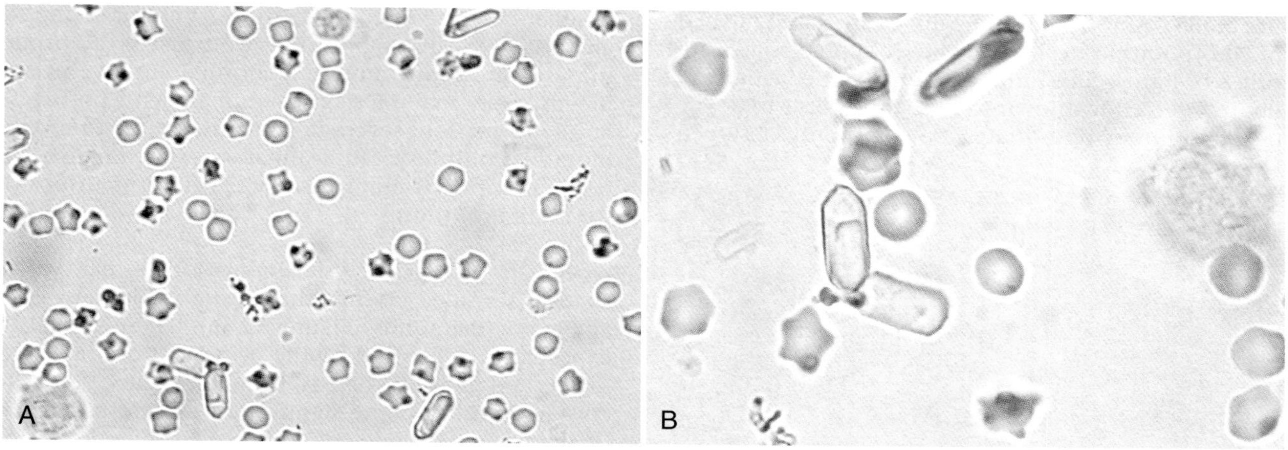

Figure 23-51 **A,** Calcium oxalate monohydrate as flat picket fence board–like crystals in a cat with ethylene glycol intoxication and hematuria, a leukocyte (*top center*), and a transitional epithelial cell (*lower left*). (Unstained. Original magnification 500×.) **B,** Same cat with calcium oxalate monohydrate crystalluria, hematuria, and a transitional epithelial cell (*right*). (Unstained. Original magnification 1000×.)

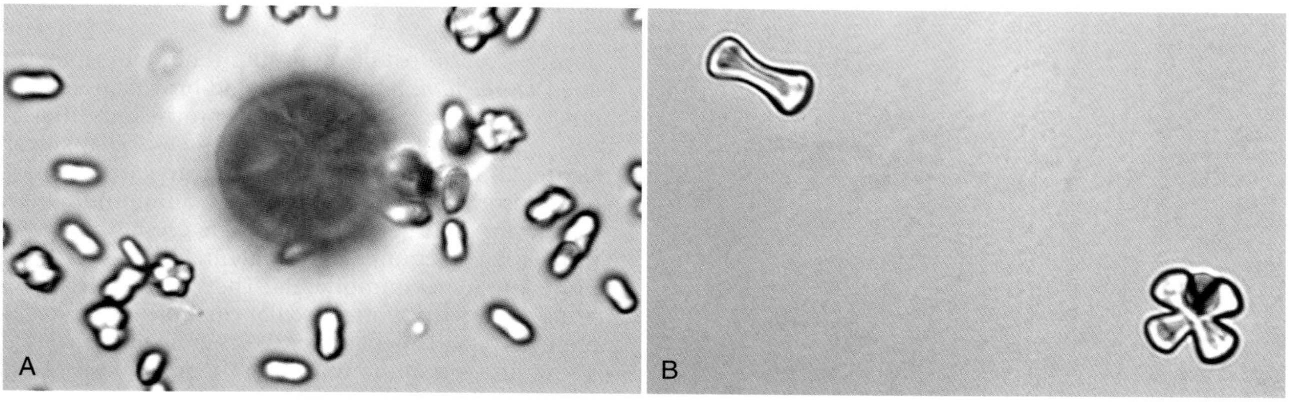

Figure 23-52 **Pleomorphic calcium carbonate crystals in elephant urine.** **A,** A spherical calcium carbonate crystal with radiating striations is present with smaller elongated oval forms. (Unstained. Original magnification 500×.) **B,** Dumbbell-shaped and cloverleaf-like calcium carbonate crystals. (Unstained. Original magnification 500×.)

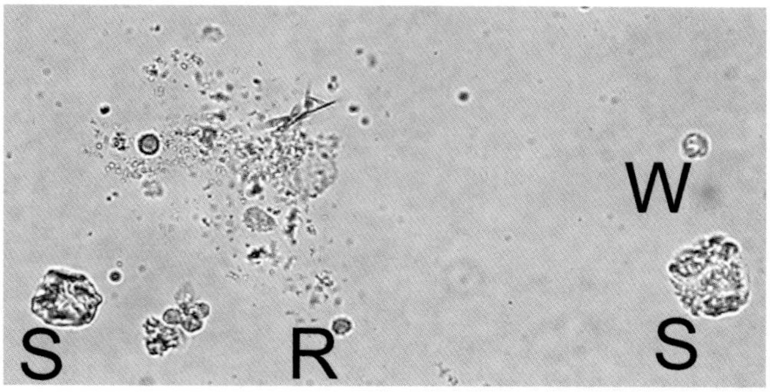

Figure 23-53 Bilirubin as small bundle of copper, acicular crystals in canine urine with squamous epithelial cells (*S*), a leukocyte (*W*), and an erythrocyte (*R*). (Unstained. Original magnification 400×.)

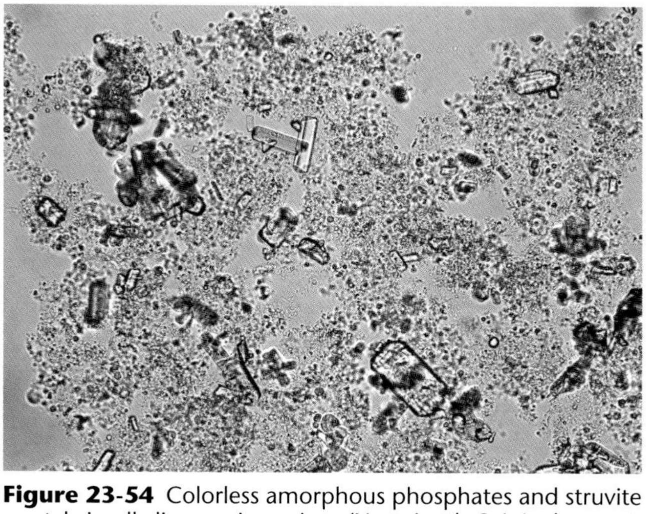

Figure 23-54 Colorless amorphous phosphates and struvite crystals in alkaline canine urine. (Unstained. Original magnification 200×.)

Figure 23-55). Amorphous phosphates are distinguished from amorphous urates in two ways: (1) phosphates are colorless or light yellow and form in alkaline urine; and (2) urates are yellow-brown to black and form in acidic urine. Amorphous phosphates are commonly observed in alkaline urine of clinically normal animals, and they are not clinically significant. Conversely, amorphous urates are an uncommon abnormal finding in most breeds. They may be seen in animals with portovascular malformation, severe hepatic disease, or ammonium biurate urolithiasis. In Dalmatians and English Bulldogs, amorphous urates may represent a predisposition for urate urolithiasis.

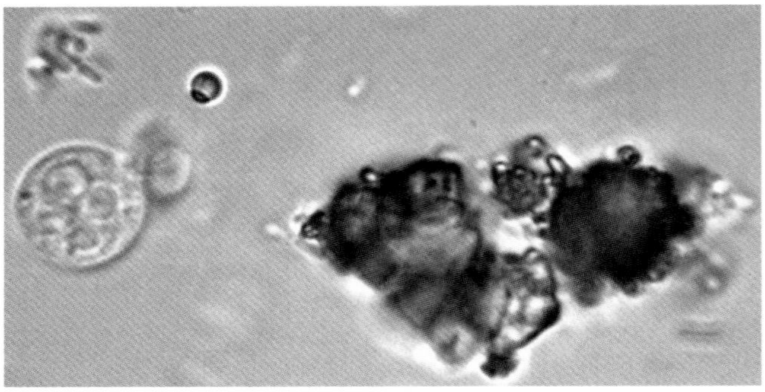

Figure 23-55 Yellow-brown amorphous urates in acidic Dalmatian urine with a neutrophil (*left*) and bacilli (*top left*) that are less refractile than the crystals. (Unstained. Original magnification 1000×.)

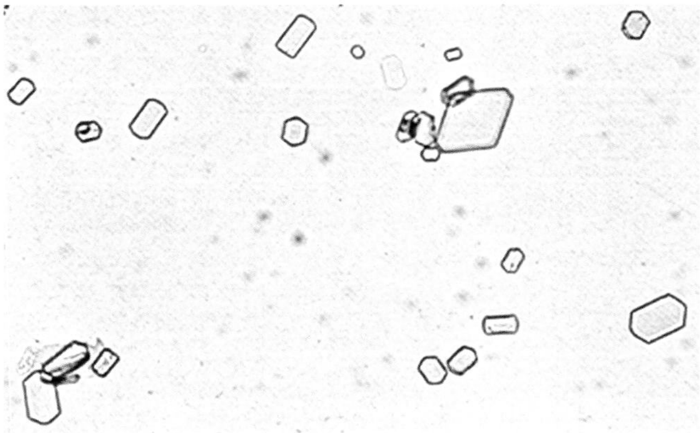

Figure 23-56 Colorless, flat, pleomorphic, six-sided uric acid crystals forming blunt ovals and a diamond. (Unstained. Original magnification 400×.)

Uric Acid: Uric acid crystals are colorless, flat, variably shaped, six-sided crystals that occur as blunt ovals, triangles, or diamonds (Figure 23-56). These crystals are expected in avian and reptile urine, but are rarely seen in cats and most dog breeds. In cats and most dogs, these crystals have the same significance as amorphous urate or ammonium biurate crystals. Some canine breeds (e.g., Dalmatian, English Bulldog, Black Russian Terrier, Weimaraner, and others) have an autosomal-recessive trait that causes hyperuricosuria, which is a risk factor for urate urolithiasis.[8] Males are more likely than females to develop urate urolithiasis, which may be an important consideration when selecting chronic preventive therapy.[9]

Ammonium Biurate: Ammonium biurate (sometimes called *ammonium urate*) are golden-brown in color and spherical shaped, with irregular protrusions that render a thorn-apple or sarcoptic mange-like appearance (Figure 23-57). They may occur as aggregates of smooth spheroids in cats. In most instances, ammonium biurate crystals are considered a pathologic crystal observed in animals with acquired or congenital causes of hepatic failure and hyperammonemia. They are commonly seen in animals with portovascular malformation or, less commonly, with hepatoxicity, other acquired causes of liver failure, or ammonium biurate urolithiasis. Ammonium biurate crystals may uncommonly be found in low numbers in the urine of Dalmatians and English Bulldogs and may represent a predisposition for urate urolithiasis.

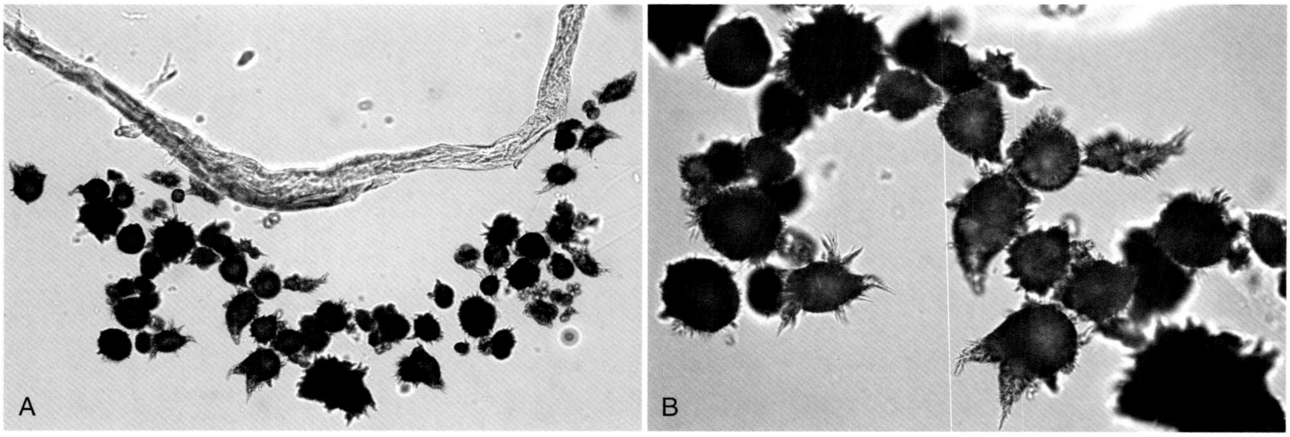

Figure 23-57 **A,** Ammonium biurate crystalluria in a dog with acquired hepatic failure caused by intoxication with the glycoside, cycasin, after sago palm ingestion. A large contaminating fiber is also present (*top*). (Unstained. Original magnification 200×.) **B,** Dark amber to brown ammonium biurate crystals with thorn apple–like or sarcoptic mange-like appearance. (Unstained. Original magnification 500×.)

Cystine: Cystine crystals are pathologic and occur as colorless, flat hexagonal plates that may have unequal sides. Daughter crystals form as hexagons that bud vertically from the seed crystal (Figure 23-58). Crystals occur in cystinuric patients that have concentrated, acidic urine. Cystinuria is a predisposition for the development of cystine urolithiasis, which often lodge at the base of the os penis and may be missed on survey radiographs, since they are relatively radiolucent. Cystinuria may be caused by acquired proximal renal tubular disease or a congenital defect of proximal renal tubular transport of several amino acids (i.e., arginine, cystine, lysine, ornithine). Among dogs, male Dachshunds, Basset Hounds, English Bulldogs, Yorkshire Terriers, Irish Terriers, Chihuahuas, Mastiffs, Rottweilers, and Newfoundlands are affected with increased frequency. Female dogs and other breeds also may be affected. In cats, this disease has been recognized in male and female Siamese and American Domestic Shorthairs.

Iatrogenic: Crystals may be seen with administration of some antibiotics (e.g., sulfonamides, ciprofloxacin); anticonvulsants (e.g., zonisamide, acetazolamide, polytherapy);[10,11] xanthine crystals with allopurinol administration, particularly when dietary protein and purine are not concurrently restricted; and radiocontrast medium administration. Sulfonamide crystals (Figure 23-59) are more likely to be observed in acidic urine as pale yellow crystals that may form haystack-like bundles or round globules with radiant striations. The latter morphology may be mistaken for calcium carbonate crystals. Zonisamide is a sulfonamide antiepileptic that has been reported to cause crystalluria and urolithiasis in children on ketogenic diets;[11] antiepileptic polytherapy is also a risk factor for crystalluria in children.[10] Veterinary publications are currently lacking; however, the crystals in Figure 23-60 were observed in the urine sediment of a dog receiving polytherapy that included zonisamide.

Uncommon Crystals of Unknown Significance: Cholesterol crystals are large, flat rectangles with a notched border (Figure 23-61). These crystals are uncommon, and their significance is unknown, but they may be found in

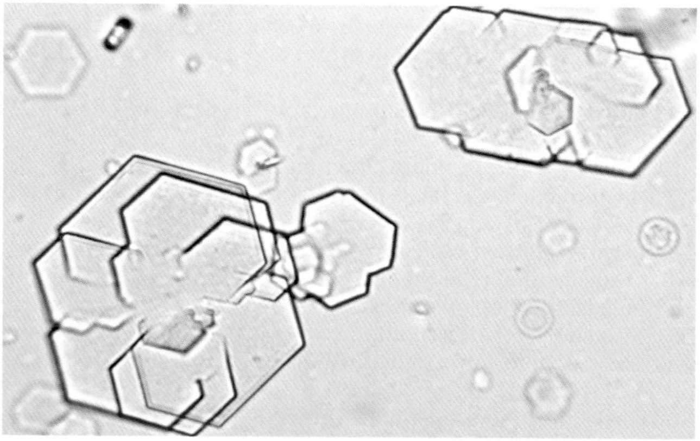

Figure 23-58 Cystine crystalluria in a dog with hematuria. Cystine crystals form colorless, flat hexagonal plates that bud in three-dimensions. (Unstained. Original magnification 500×.)

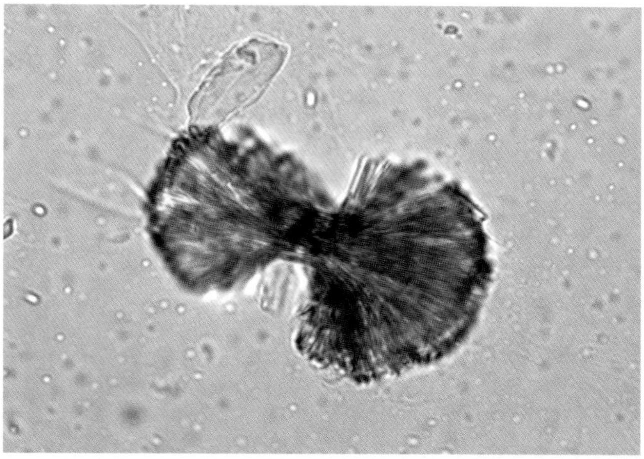

Figure 23-59 Iatrogenic crystalluria in a dog treated with trimethoprim sulfamethoxazole. This sulfa crystal exhibits the sheaf-of-wheat-like appearance. (Unstained. Original magnification 500×.)

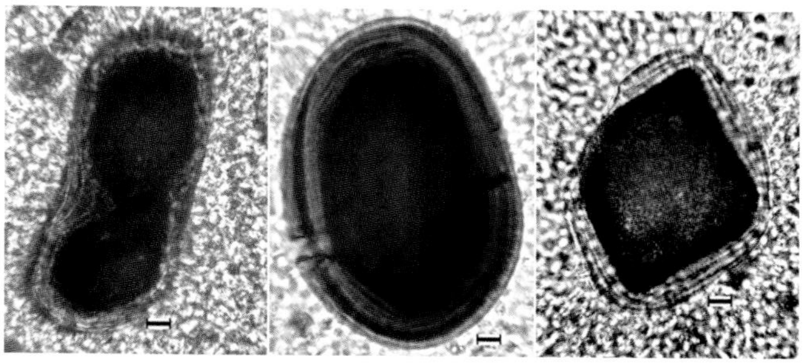

Figure 23-60 Iatrogenic crystalluria in acidic urine from a dog receiving polytherapy that included zonisamide (a sulfonamide), levetiracetam, dexamethasone, acetylcysteine, furosemide, mannitol, and other medications. Erythrocytes and amorphous debris are abundant in a different, background focal plane. (Unstained, bar = 10 μm. Original magnification 500×.)

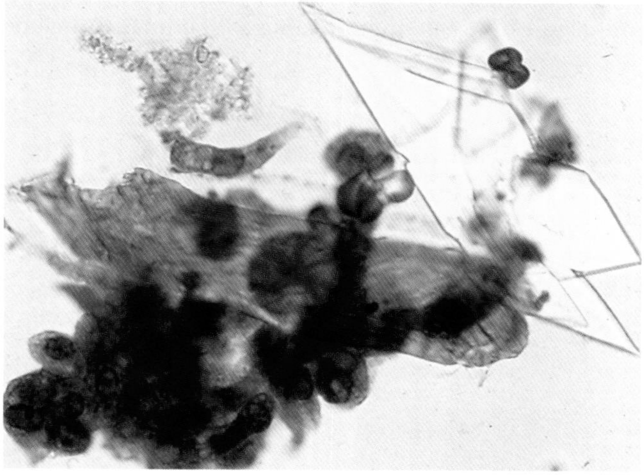

Figure 23-61 A flat, notched cholesterol crystal (*right*) with a dense aggregate of nucleated cells (*bottom*), a fiber (*center*), and amorphous crystals (*top left*). (New methylene blue stain. Original magnification 500×.)

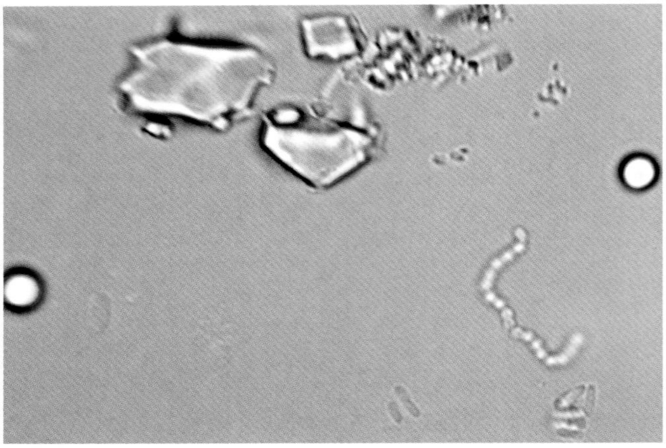

Figure 23-62 Fragments of coverslip glass (*top*) with a chain of cocci, two small groups of bacilli, and two refractile lipid droplets. (Unstained. Original magnification 1000×.)

the urine of animals with previous urinary tract hemorrhage or diseases with cellular degeneration. Leucine and tyrosine crystals are rarely observed in humans with certain hereditary diseases or severe hepatic failure, and their significance in animal urine is poorly defined. Tyrosine crystals are dark, fine acicular crystals found individually or in small clusters. Leucine crystals appear as large spheroids with concentric striations.

Common Contaminants

Urine sample contaminants are common and may arise from the environment or from the patient, depending on sample collection method (e.g., epithelial cells or sperm from the distal genitourinary tract [see Figure 23-47]). Care should be taken to distinguish common contaminants from other relevant sediment findings. Starch granules from powdered gloves or coverslip glass chips (Figure 23-62) may be mistaken for crystalluria; plant pollen could be mistaken for transitional epithelial cells or ova; and hair or synthetic fibers could be misconstrued as casts (see Figures 23-37, 23-38, 23-57A, and Figure 23-61). Other possible contaminants include air bubbles (see Figure 23-29, *A*), personal lubricant from catheters, bacteria, yeast, fungal macroconidia, or feces. Abundant pleomorphic bacilli and possibly intestinal parasite ova without accompanying pyuria may be found with fecal contamination of the urine sample.

References

1. Osborne CA, Stevens JB: In Osborne CA, Stevens JB, editors: *Urinalysis: a clinical guide to compassionate patient care*, ed 1, Shawnee Mission, Kansas, 1999, Veterinary Learning Systems, Bayer Corporation.
2. Swenson CL, et al: Evaluation of modified Wright-staining of urine sediment as a method for accurate detection of bacteriuria in dogs, *J Am Vet Med Assoc* 224:1282–1289, 2004.
3. Swenson CL, et al: Evaluation of modified Wright-staining of dried urinary sediment as a method for accurate detection of bacteriuria in cats, *Vet Clin Pathol* 40:256–264, 2011.
4. Gunn-Christie RG, Flatland B, Friedrichs KR, et al: American Society for Veterinary Clinical Pathology (ASVCP): ASVCP quality assurance guidelines: control of preanalytical, analytical, and postanalytical factors for urinalysis, cytology, and clinical chemistry in veterinary laboratories, *Vet Clin Pathol* 41:18–26, 2012.
5. Albasan H, Lulich JP, Osborne CA, et al: Effects of storage time and temperature on pH, specific gravity, and crystal formation in urine samples from dogs and cats, *J Am Vet Med Assoc* 222:176–179, 2003.
6. Block DR, Lieske JC: Automated urinalysis in the clinical lab, *MLO Med Lab Obs* 44:8–10, 2012. 12.
7. Morfin J, Chin A: Images in clinical medicine. Urinary calcium oxalate crystals in ethylene glycol intoxication, *N Engl J Med* 353:e21, 2005.
8. Karmi N, Brown EA, Hughes SS, et al: Estimated frequency of the canine hyperuricosuria mutation in different dog breeds, *J Vet Intern Med* 24:1337–1342, 2010.
9. Albasan H, et al: Evaluation of the association between sex and risk of forming urate uroliths in Dalmatians, *J Am Vet Med Assoc* 227:565–569, 2005.
10. Go T: Effect of antiepileptic drug polytherapy on crystalluria, *Pediatr Neurol* 32:113–115, 2005.
11. Paul E, Conant KD, Dunne IE, et al: Urolithiasis on the ketogenic diet with concurrent topiramate or zonisamide therapy, *Epilepsy Res* 90:151–156, 2010.
12. From Quigley RR, Knowles KE, Johnson GC: Disseminated chlorellosis in a dog, *Vet Pathol* 46:439-443, 2009.

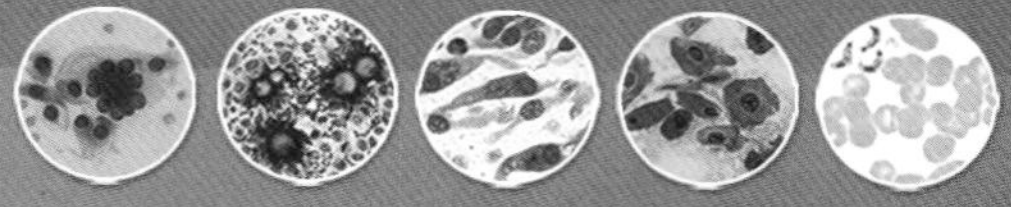

CHAPTER 24

Male Reproductive Tract: Prostate, Testes, Penis, and Semen

*Sabrina Vobornik and Mary B. Nabity**

The most commonly evaluated organs of the male reproductive system are the prostate and the testes. Enlargement of either the prostate gland or testicle(s) and testicular tumors are the primary reasons for evaluation of these organs. Testicular fine-needle aspiration (FNA) may also be used to evaluate for male infertility concerns. While prostatic disease is frequently encountered in dogs, especially intact, older dogs, it is extremely rare in cats.[1,2] Clinical signs that suggest enlargement of the prostate include difficulty with defecation or micturition, although difficulty with the latter occurs less frequently. Sometimes, urine is tinged red by blood, or blood or pus may drip from the penis. Males may also have decreased fertility or loss of libido. When any of these signs occurs, rectal palpation of the prostate may reveal symmetric or unilateral enlargement, focal bumpiness, or softness.[3,4] Such prostate abnormalities detected by palpation or, occasionally, radiographic examination are the primary indications for obtaining material from the gland for cytologic evaluation. Testicular tumors rarely cause clinical signs, and enlargement of the testes or palpation of a mass on physical examination is the most common means for identifying testicular tumors. Aspiration of the testicle does not appear to have immediate or long-term adverse effects on male sexual performance or fertility.[5,6] Penile and preputial cytology may also be helpful if a lesion is present, although limited published information is available.

PROSTATE GLAND

Collecting and Preparing Samples

Material from the prostate may be obtained directly through the urethra or by FNA of the gland. To collect via the urethra, digitally massage the prostate while aspirating through a urinary catheter passed to the level of the gland.[7,8] More prostatic material may be obtained by washing the part of the urethra near the prostate with a small amount of saline through gentle injection and aspiration while gently massaging the prostate. Material may also be obtained from the prostate through ejaculation.[4,8] The prostate is gently massaged during the process to increase the amount of material of prostatic origin because this method may contain contaminants from other parts of the reproductive tract. The first part of the ejaculate contains material primarily derived from the prostate gland.[4,8] The sample size is usually large and has a moderate concentration of cells. In addition to prostatic epithelial cells, ejaculated samples may contain numerous spermatozoa and other cells of reproductive tract and urethral origin. Simultaneously collecting and evaluating urethral wash specimens and urine samples (by antepubic cystocentesis) may alleviate some of the problems of interpreting the cytologic and microbiologic findings of the material collected by ejaculation.

The prostate may also be sampled by direct aspiration with a small-gauge needle. It should be noted that aspiration of the prostate is contraindicated when a prostatic abscess is suspected, as it is possible to seed the needle tract with organisms.[1] Ultrasound-guided aspiration is superior to all other methods for obtaining specimens, especially from focal lesions such as cysts. The inguinal area is anesthetized, and the area is prepared as for surgery. Sterile petroleum jelly is applied to the skin to provide an acoustic coupler between the skin and the scanhead, and a small stab incision may be made in the skin to facilitate needle passage. While the ultrasound scanhead is held stationary and needle advancement is monitored on the screen, the needle is directed to the prostate or a specific location within the prostate. When the needle has reached the proper site, a small amount of specimen is aspirated into a sterile syringe.[8]

The prostate may be sampled by digital guidance of a needle as well, which may be passed through the posterior abdominal wall or the perineal region, although the latter method has not been widely used in veterinary medicine. At either site, local anesthesia is necessary to prevent discomfort and facilitate needle guidance. When the prostate is so enlarged that it can be palpated through the abdominal wall, the needle may be guided to the prostate while the dog is in either lateral or dorsal recumbency and the prostate is immobilized with one hand. This method is usually effective only when the prostate is markedly enlarged.[8] From the perineal area, a finger is placed in

*The authors wish to acknowledge the contribution of Dr. Joseph G. Zinkl, DVM, PhD, DACVP, who authored this chapter for the previous editions of the book. His contribution served as the foundation for the material appearing in this edition.

the rectum, and the needle is passed through the skin in the perineal area and guided into the prostate along the finger. With both methods, the gland is gently aspirated while the needle is moved within it.[8] Occasionally, only a small amount of material is obtained by aspiration, but it is usually adequate for making one or two direct smears.

Preparation and staining of the slides of prostate material are similar to that of other samples. When samples of low cellularity are obtained (e.g., from cysts), they should be concentrated by centrifugation or with a cytofuge to obtain slides with sufficient material for proper evaluation.

Cytologic Evaluation of Normal Prostate

The cytologic features of the normal prostate vary, depending on the method of obtaining materials. Samples obtained by direct aspiration contain fewer contaminating cells and are usually more cellular than samples obtained from ejaculation, massage, or urethral washes. Glandular cells of the normal prostate are found in small to medium clusters, are uniform in size, cuboidal to columnar in shape and have a centrally to eccentrically located nucleus, which displays a finely stippled or reticular pattern. The cytoplasm has a fine, granular appearance and may be vacuolated (Figure 24-1, Figure 24-2, and Figure 24-3). If a prostatic wash was performed, a few contaminant bacteria may be present in association with squamous epithelial cells; however, in general, bacteria are not normally present in samples from the canine prostate gland. Cells and contaminating material from other locations in the urogenital tract may be found (Figure 24-4).

Spermatozoa: Sperm heads characteristically stain aqua with the Wright method. Spermatozoa, which often adhere to other cells, possibly with many attached to a single epithelial cell, are most frequently found in ejaculated material but may also be found in massage or wash samples (see Figure 24-4; Figure 24-5).

Squamous Cells: Squamous epithelial cells are large cells with a flattened, floppy appearance. More differentiated squamous cells have a pyknotic or karyorrhectic nucleus, and immature squamous cells are difficult to differentiate from urothelial cells and possibly even prostatic epithelial cells. Because they originate from the distal urethra or the external genitalia, squamous cells are found not only in ejaculate, massage, and wash samples but also in prostatic squamous metaplasia (Figure 24-6 and Figure 24-7). Large, flat, and angular or rolled squamous particles may be obtained from the external skin surface as well; these particles do not usually contain even a remnant of a nucleus. Contamination by such particles may be nearly eliminated by cleaning the skin before obtaining a sample.

Urothelial Cells: Urothelial cells (i.e., transitional epithelial cells) usually appear individually but may also be present in small clusters. They are larger than prostatic epithelial cells and have homogeneous, lightly basophilic cytoplasm and a lower nucleus-to-cytoplasm (N:C) ratio

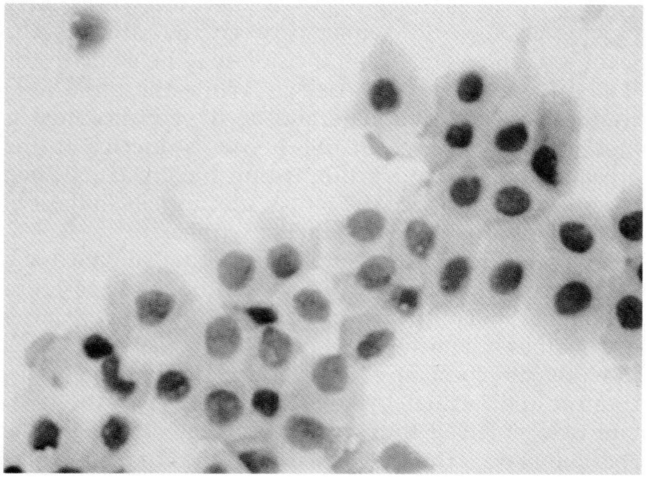

Figure 24-1 Epithelial cells from a normal prostate. The cells are in large clusters and have mildly acidophilic cytoplasm and relatively large nuclei. Prostatic massage slightly concentrated by centrifugation. (Wright-Giemsa stain.)

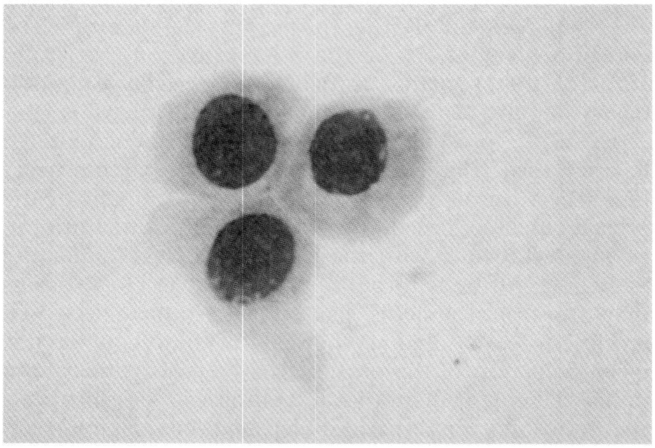

Figure 24-2 Epithelial cells from a normal prostate. The cytoplasm is grainy and acidophilic, and the nuclei are centrally located and have a moderately reticular chromatin network. Prostatic massage slightly concentrated by centrifugation. (Wright-Giemsa stain.)

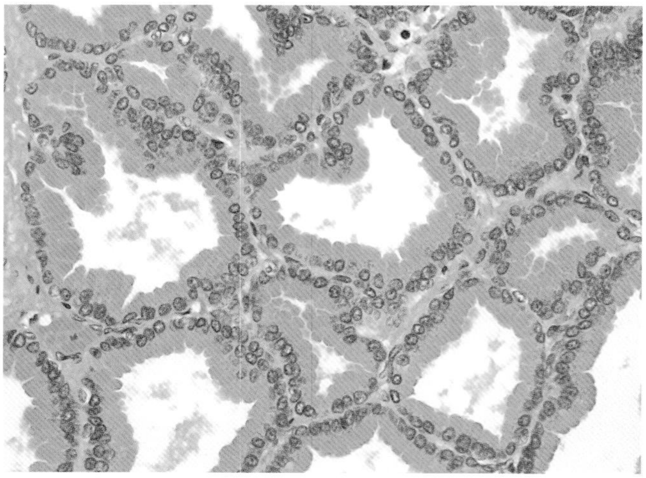

Figure 24-3 Histology of normal prostate. Uniform cuboidal to columnar epithelial cells with apical eosinophilic cytoplasm are forming single-layered tubular structures. (H&E stain. Original magnification 400×.) (Courtesy of Dr. John Edwards.)

than prostatic cells (see Figure 23-1). Urothelial cells originate from the bladder and the tubular structures of the urinary and genital tracts and are most frequently found in samples obtained by ejaculation, massage, and washing.

Other Epithelial Cells: Cells of the ductus deferens and the epididymis are difficult to distinguish from prostatic cells.

Ultrasound Contact Gel: The gel used to ensure adequate acoustic coupling of the ultrasound scanhead to the body wall may contaminate the material obtained with ultrasound assistance. This typically appears as magenta granular material, found individually or in large aggregates. When a large amount of material is present, the cells may be obscured or not be stained sufficiently for evaluation. The amount of contamination may be minimized by wiping excess gel from the skin before introducing the needle. Enough gel usually remains on the skin and scanhead to ensure sufficient contact for visualization of the prostate and accurate guidance of the needle.

Prostatic Cysts

Prostatic cysts may be present as incidental findings but are often present in dogs with concurrent benign prostatic

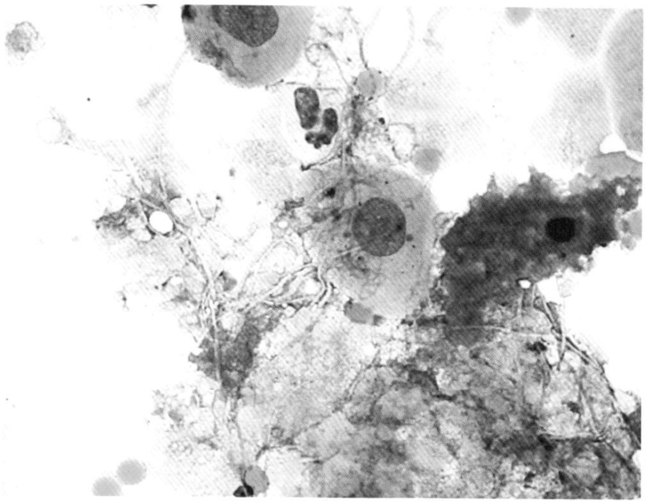

Figure 24-4 Prostatic wash from a normal dog. Many spermatozoa, few epithelial cells, and a small amount of blood (few red blood cells and rare neutrophils) are present. (Wright-Giemsa stain. Original magnification 1000×.) (Courtesy of Dr. Rick Cowell.)

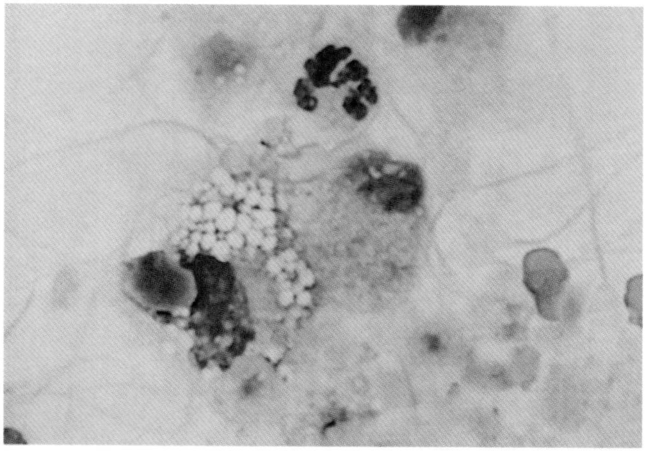

Figure 24-5 A prostatic epithelial cell, neutrophil, macrophage, and many spermatozoa from a dog with mild prostatitis. The background contains proteinaceous material, which is probably the product of prostatic epithelial cells. Spermatozoa characteristically stain aqua with Wright stain. Prostatic ejaculate slightly concentrated by centrifugation. (Wright-Giemsa stain.)

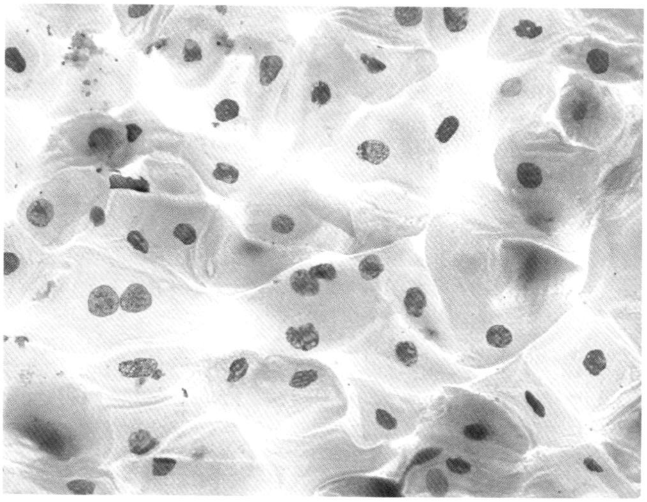

Figure 24-6 Squamous metaplasia of the prostatic epithelium in a dog with a Sertoli-cell tumor. The cells are large and pale-staining, and some contain karyorrhectic nuclei. Prostatic massage concentrated by centrifugation. (Wright-Giemsa stain. Original magnification 500×.) (Courtesy of Dr. Rick Cowell.)

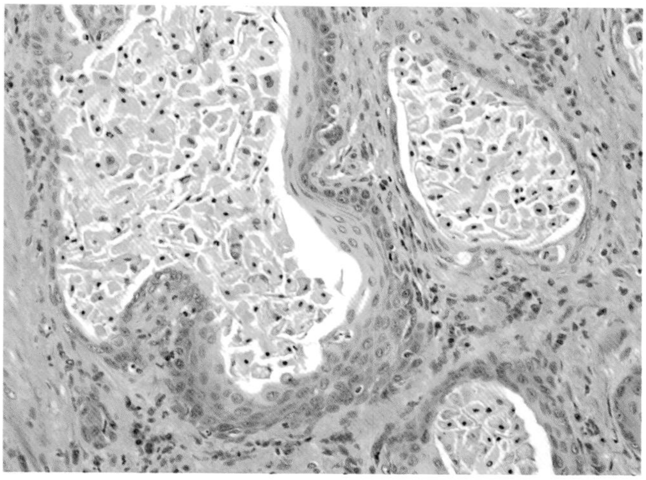

Figure 24-7 Histology of the prostate of a dog with squamous metaplasia caused by a Sertoli cell tumor. Glandular epithelium has been replaced by a stratified squamous epithelium, and numerous sloughed squamous cells are present within the lumens. Note increased connective tissue between acini. (H&E stain. Original magnification 200×.) (Courtesy of Dr. John Edwards.)

hyperplasia or other prostatic diseases.[1,9] A paraprostatic cyst has been reported in a cat.[2] Prostatic cysts are quite variable cytologically. Some contain poorly cellular serosanguinous to brown fluid, which, even when concentrated, contains only a few epithelial cells, rare neutrophils, and some debris. Sometimes, moderate numbers of normal or slightly hyperplastic (e.g., basophilic) epithelial cells are found. Squamous cells are rarely obtained. The protein concentration of prostatic cysts is usually similar to transudate fluid.

Prostatitis

Bacterial prostatitis is the most common prostatic disease diagnosed in intact dogs.[2,10] It occurs as either an acute infection or a chronic infection. Cytologic evaluation reveals predominantly suppurative inflammation. In septic prostatitis, the neutrophils typically have features that indicate degenerative change, including karyolysis and foamy cytoplasm (Figure 24-8). Usually, variable numbers of macrophages exist, especially in chronic prostatitis, which typically have abundant, foamy cytoplasm. Bacteria may be found both intracellularly and extracellularly, and when they are found, it is necessary to determine whether they are actually the cause of the inflammation or are contaminants from other locations in the genital or urinary tract.[7] If the sample was obtained by an aspiration technique, the bacteria should be considered the cause, but if the sample was obtained through the urogenital ductal system, it is necessary to determine if the bacteria are contaminants from the external genitalia or from an inflammatory lesion elsewhere in the urinary or genital system. Intracellular bacteria are certainly a strong indication that the inflammatory process is septic. Organisms frequently isolated include *Escherichia coli* (most common), *Proteus* spp., *Staphylococcus* spp., *Brucella canis*, *Mycoplasma* spp., and *Streptococcus* spp. Fungal causes of prostatitis are infrequent but have been reported.[1,11] In addition to inflammatory cells, clusters of variably-sized epithelial cells may be obtained. In aspirates obtained from an inflamed prostate, prostatic cells appear to have loose cohesion. Additionally, their cytoplasm usually shows increased basophilia, indicating that the prostatic epithelium is hyperplastic secondary to the inflammation (Figure 24-9).

Prostatic abscesses are focal areas of severe inflammation within the prostate, and they are a sequela to chronic prostatitis or prostatic cysts.[1] Abscesses may be single, large accumulations of pus or multiple, small accumulations. Degenerated neutrophils with karyolysis and foamy cytoplasm present in a background of cellular debris are found. Features of prostatic hyperplasia may accompany prostatic abscesses. In addition to hyperplasia, the prostatic epithelium may also develop squamous metaplasia secondary to inflammation (see the discussion on squamous metaplasia later).

Benign Prostatic Hyperplasia

Benign prostatic hyperplasia (BPH) is a distinct entity that usually occurs in older, intact male dogs, and although the pathogenesis is not completely understood, it is apparently caused by a sex hormone imbalance.[1,12] It includes both increases in cell number and cell size.[1] Additionally, prostatic hyperplasia usually accompanies inflammatory lesions of the prostate, and the epithelium that lines prostatic cysts is often hyperplastic. Clinical signs associated with BPH are typically absent. However, enlargement of the gland may result in constipation, tenesmus, and stranguria. Mild hemorrhagic urethral discharge may also be seen. Prostatic palpation often reveals a symmetrically enlarged, nonpainful gland; however, an irregular surface or prostatic cysts may also be palpated. The cytologic features of the epithelial cells are similar regardless of the cause of the hyperplasia. Moderate cell numbers are usually found, often in variably sized clusters, although many individual cells are also found. In cell clusters, acinar-like arrangements may be seen, and cytoplasmic borders are usually indistinct. The cells are typically uniform and similar in appearance to normal prostatic epithelium. The cytoplasm is often abundant, basophilic, and slightly granular with or without small punctate vacuoles. Nuclei

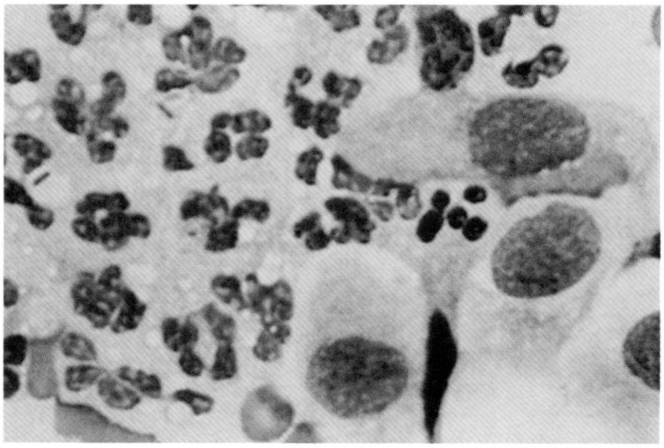

Figure 24-8 Neutrophils and prostatic epithelial cells from a dog with acute prostatitis. Bacilli are in some of the neutrophils, which are mildly degenerative with acidophilic, foamy cytoplasm and minimal nuclear degeneration. Prostatic massage slightly concentrated by centrifugation. (Wright-Giemsa stain.)

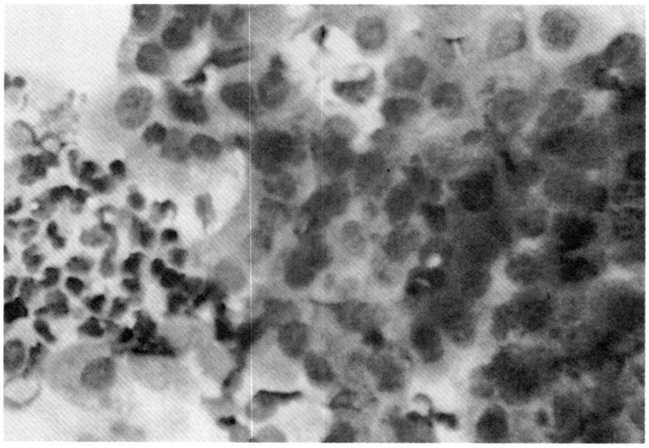

Figure 24-9 Hyperplasia of the prostatic epithelium from a dog with prostatitis. The cells are basophilic and have an increased nucleus-to-cytoplasm ratio. Pleomorphism is minimal, and differentiation is suggested along the edges of the cell clusters. Prostate massage slightly concentrated by centrifugation. (Wright-Giemsa stain.)

are round to oval and somewhat large, with finely reticulated or stippled chromatin patterns. Nucleoli are not usually observed. The N:C ratio is increased compared with that of normal prostatic cells (Figure 24-10 and Figure 24-11). When hyperplasia is not accompanied by inflammation, it should be considered a preneoplastic change.[13]

Squamous Metaplasia

Under the influence of the estrogen-like hormone activity that occurs with Sertoli cell tumors and rarely interstitial cell tumors, the epithelium of the prostate may undergo metaplasia to become a squamous-like epithelium (see Figures 24-6 and 24-7). Squamous metaplasia may also occur as a sequela to chronic irritation or inflammation, but the most prominent squamous metaplastic changes occur in dogs with Sertoli cell tumors or treated with exogenous estrogens.[7,14] One case report in a cat described squamous metaplasia associated with interstitial cell neoplasia in a retained testicle, although hormone assays were not obtained.[15] Aspirates are moderately cellular, and large cells (many individual, some in clusters) with slightly basophilic to slightly acidophilic cytoplasm are found. The cells are very large and appear flattened and floppy (see Figure 24-6). Cells occasionally contain a pyknotic or karyorrhectic nucleus. Inflammatory and hyperplastic prostatic epithelial cells are occasionally found.

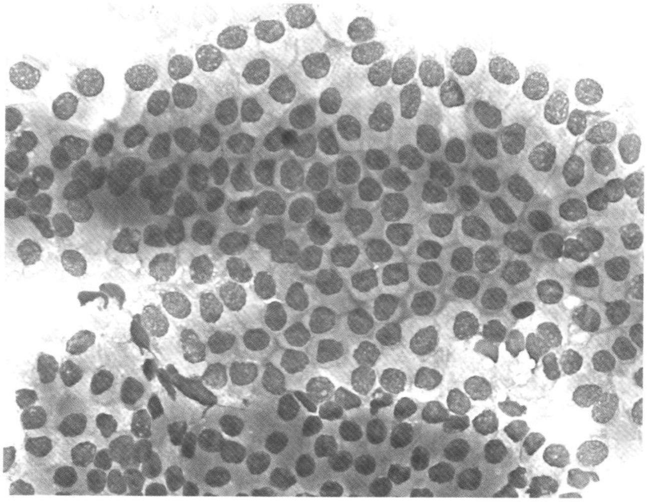

Figure 24-10 A large cluster of uniform prostatic epithelial cells from an older dog with benign prostatic hyperplasia. The cells have moderate amounts of purple granular cytoplasm that often contains vacuoles (fine-needle aspiration and biopsy). (Wright-Giemsa stain. Original magnification 500×.) (Courtesy of Dr. Rick Cowell.)

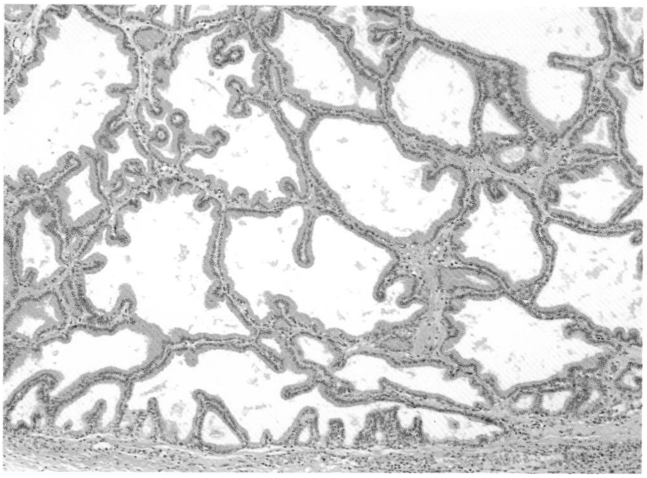

Figure 24-11 Histology of the prostate of a dog with benign prostatic hyperplasia. Glandular lumens are dilated, and papillary projections extend into the lumen. (H&E stain. Original magnification 100×.) (Courtesy of Dr. John Edwards.)

Prostatic Neoplasia

Although less frequent, prostatic neoplasia does occur in both dogs and cats. In dogs, carcinomas or adenocarcinomas of the prostate are most commonly diagnosed.[1,16] Although no breed predilection exists, most affected dogs tend to be medium- to large-breed, and tumors may develop in both intact and neutered animals.[1,16] Prostatic carcinomas or adenocarcinomas have rarely been reported in cats.[2,17,18] Prostatomegaly and its accompanying signs occur in dogs with prostatic carcinomas. Most prostatic carcinomas arise from the urothelium or transitional epithelial cells instead of the glandular prostate.[14] On rectal palpation, the prostate may be very large, irregular, and asymmetrical, and in some cases, it is very painful.[1,3,13,16] Cats with prostatic neoplasia may present with clinical signs associated with lower urinary tract disease, obstruction, or both. Cellularity of a cytologic sample is moderate to marked, and criteria of malignancy may be prominent and include anisocytosis, anisokaryosis, nuclear enlargement and irregularity, and marked increases in the N:C ratio (Figure 24-12, Figure 24-13, and Figure 24-14). However, some carcinomas may demonstrate only mild cellular atypia (Figure 24-15). Nucleoli are often present and are

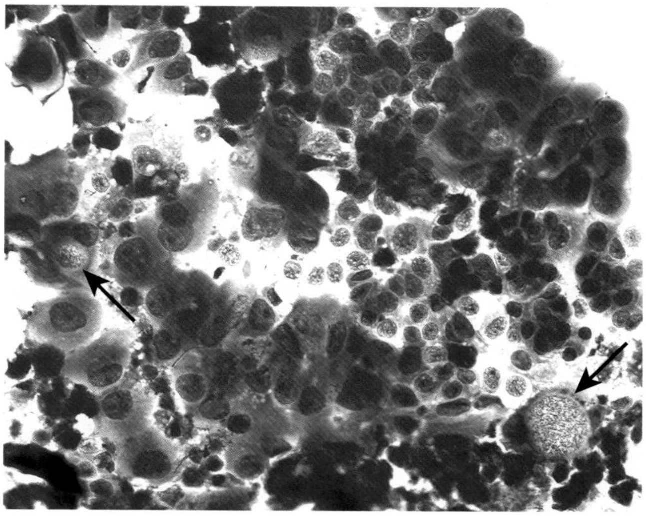

Figure 24-12 Clusters of neoplastic epithelial cells demonstrating marked criteria of malignancy. Note the occasional intracellular vacuoles containing pink granular material, typical of prostatic and transitional cell carcinomas (*arrows*) (fine-needle aspiration and biopsy). (Wright-Giemsa stain. Original magnification 500×.) (Courtesy of Dr. Amy Valenciano.)

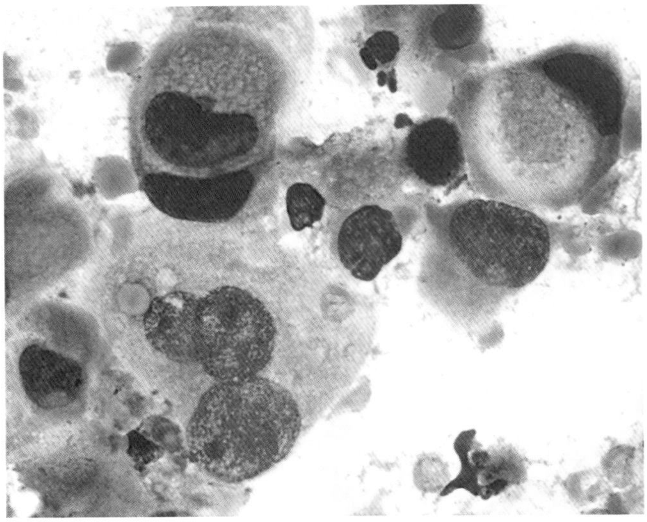

Figure 24-13 A group of neoplastic epithelial cells from a prostatic carcinoma, demonstrating multinucleation, prominent nucleoli, and moderate to marked anisocytosis and anisokaryosis. One cell contains intracellular magenta material (fine-needle aspiration and biopsy). (Wright-Giemsa stain. Original magnification 1000×.)

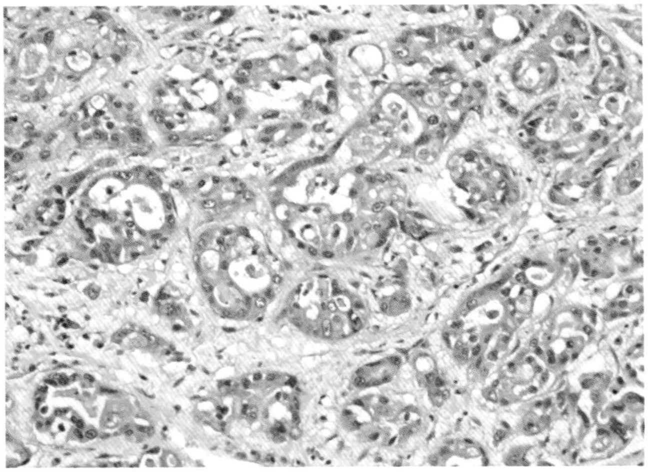

Figure 24-14 Histology of the prostate of a dog with prostatic carcinoma. Cells display marked atypia and form nests and occasionally tubelike structures separated by a fibroblastic response. (H&E stain. Original magnification 200×.) (Courtesy of Dr. John Edwards.)

usually small, single, and uniform, but sometimes large, irregular nucleoli are found. Cell membranes may be distinct in well-differentiated neoplasms but are indistinct in poorly differentiated tumors. Cell cohesion is often apparent, and acinar-like formation is rarely present within some of the cell clusters. It is difficult to distinguish prostatic carcinomas that arise from the transitional cells from those that arise from the glandular area of the prostate by cytologic examination. Both may contain occasional cytoplasmic aggregates of eosinophilic granular material characteristic of these tumors (see Figures 24-12 and 24-13). However, when acinar-like structures are found, adenocarcinomas are more likely than transitional cell carcinomas.

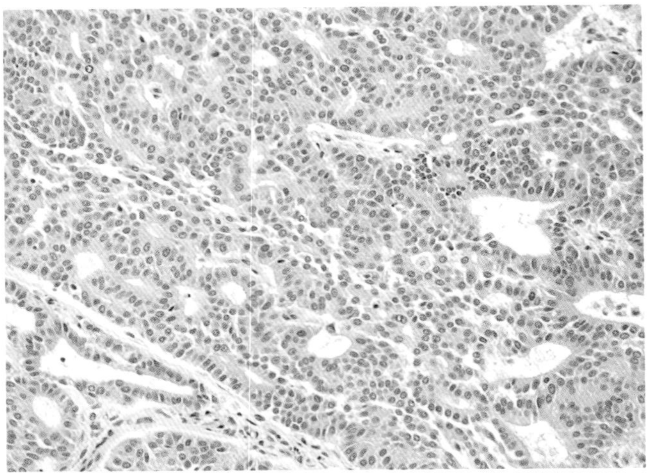

Figure 24-15 Histology of the prostate of a dog with a prostatic carcinoma. Cellular atypia is mild but glandular structures are disorganized, and apical eosinophilic cytoplasm is lost. The neoplasm metastasized widely. (H&E stain. Original magnification 200×.) (Courtesy of Dr. John Edwards.)

Prostatic carcinomas frequently metastasize to the iliac and sublumbar lymph nodes; thus, nodular palpation and evaluation are indicated in suspected cases of prostatic neoplasia.[3,13] In addition, mineralization of the prostate and metastatic bone lesions, especially in the pelvis and lumbar vertebrae, may also occur.[1,16] In fact, neutered dogs with prostatic mineralization are extremely likely to have prostatic neoplasia. Although mineralization is also associated with neoplasia in intact dogs, other prostatic diseases should be considered.[19]

TESTES

Obtaining Testicular Samples

Enlargement, either unilateral or bilateral, is the major indication for FNA and cytologic evaluation of the testes and may help differentiate inflammatory from neoplastic causes.[14,20] The epididymis may be enlarged and may be sampled via FNA. Decreased testicular size with increased firmness suggests atrophy. FNA of atrophic testicles does not usually yield a sample that is adequate for cytologic evaluation, and biopsy with histopathologic evaluation may be required for an informed diagnosis (Figure 24-16).[20] Semen evaluation may also provide information on testicular lesions, although it is mainly valued for determining sperm quality.

Cytologic Evaluation of Normal Testes

The cellularity of a sample obtained from an aspirate or core of a normal testicle may be quite variable, depending on the aggressiveness of sampling. A pleomorphic population of cells is typically seen, including spermatozoa and their precursors (spermatogonia, spermatocytes, and spermatids), Sertoli cells, and occasionally interstitial cells. The material obtained from normal testicles is often contaminated with blood, and many bare nuclei and cytoplasmic fragments may be observed in the background.[21] Spermatogonia are difficult to identify but appear as medium-sized

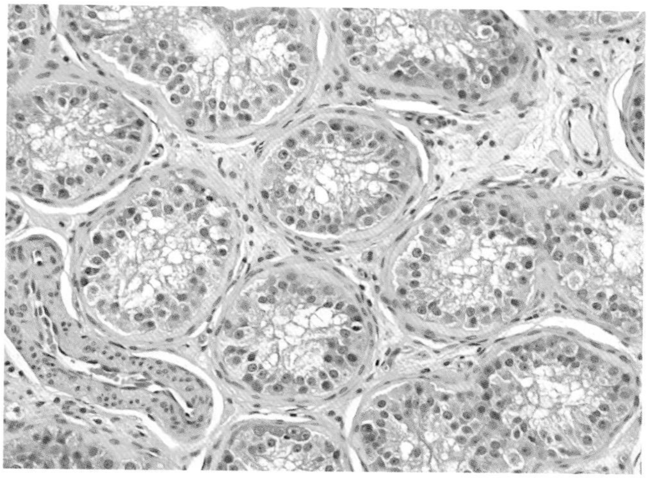

Figure 24-16 Histology of testicular degeneration in a dog secondary to an intrascrotal Sertoli cell tumor. Tubules are atrophied with a thick basement membrane and no maturing spermatids but are lined by Sertoli cells and some spermatogonia indicating this testis could return to function. (H&E stain. Original magnification 200×.) (Courtesy of Dr. John Edwards.)

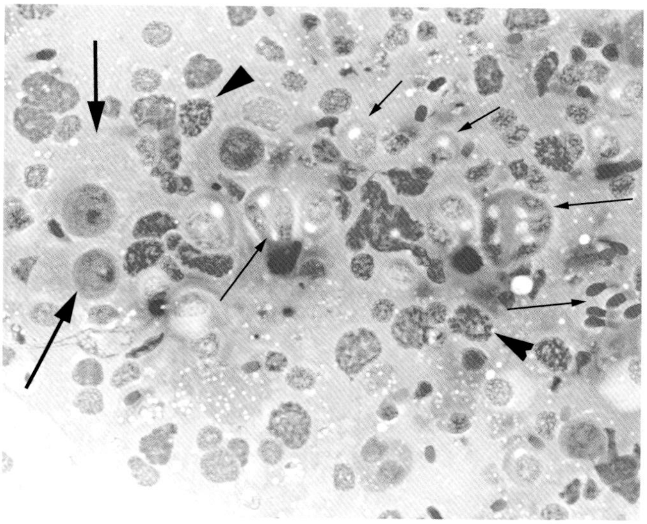

Figure 24-17 Aspirate of a normal testicle. Numerous lysed and intact cells are present, with many cytoplasmic fragments observed in the background. Few Sertoli cells (*thick arrows*), few spermatocytes (*arrow heads*), and many early and late spermatids (*thin arrows*) are present. (Diff-Quik stain. Original magnification 500×.)

round cells with an oval-shaped nucleus that may display a distinct parachromatin condensation with a semilunar shape.[21] Spermatocytes are the largest of the spermatozoa precursor cells and appear as round, occasionally multinucleate cells with a round nucleus and cordlike chromatin.[21] Spermatids are the most common precursors observed. Early spermatids are slightly smaller than spermatocytes and contain a small to moderate amount of basophilic cytoplasm, often with a single perinuclear vacuole or several small, dispersed vacuoles. They have a round to oval nucleus with an indistinct nucleolus, and they often appear multinucleate (Figure 24-17 and Figure 24-18). Late

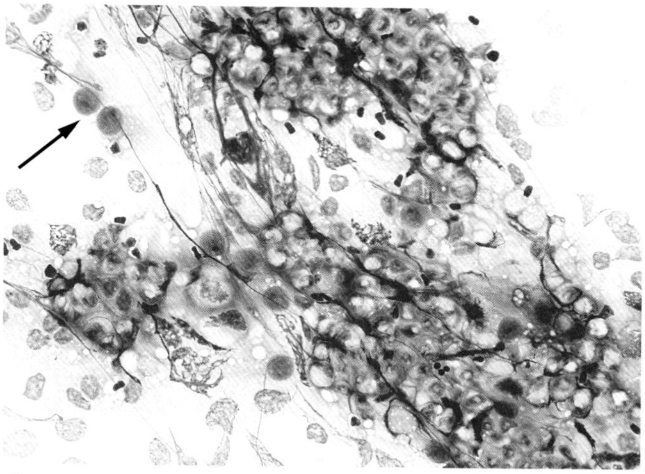

Figure 24-18 Impression smear from a normal testicle. Nuclear streaming is present, and the majority of cells appear to be spermatids in various stages of maturation, with the earlier stages resembling lymphocytes. Few Sertoli cells (*arrow*) and mitotic figures are observed. (Wright-Giemsa stain. Original magnification 500×.) (Courtesy of Dr. Amy Valenciano.)

stage spermatids are differentiated by their more elongated and dark nucleus as the chromatin becomes more clumped with maturation. Sertoli cells may be identified as round to slightly oval cells, with poorly defined cell borders and abundant amounts of pale cytoplasm surrounding a large round nucleus with finely stippled to reticular chromatin and a single, prominent, round nucleolus (see Figures 24-17 and 24-18). Although rare, Leydig (interstitial) cells may be seen in small sheets and are round in shape with abundant basophilic cytoplasm that contains multiple, variably sized punctuate vacuoles. The nucleus is eccentrically located, round in shape, and displays a coarsely clumped chromatin pattern with one to two small nucleoli. Because multinucleate cells and large cells with prominent nucleoli may be apparent, care should be taken not to diagnose malignant neoplasia. In addition, some of the spermatogenic precursors may appear similar to large lymphocytes, and a misdiagnosis of lymphoma is possible (see Figure 24-18). It is helpful to remember that normal testes will contain a variety of spermatozoa precursors (see Figure 24-17; Figure 24-19).

Testicular Inflammation (Orchitis and Epididymitis)

The cytologic findings of orchitis and epididymitis are similar to the cytologic findings of other tissue inflammation. Neutrophils with variable degenerative changes are the predominant cells, but other inflammatory cells (especially macrophages) may be found. The cause of inflammation may occasionally be determined by cytologic or microbiologic methods. In some cases of blastomycosis, *Blastomyces dermatitidis* organisms may be observed in testicular aspirates, but in cases of brucellosis orchitis and epididymitis, *Brucella canis* is rarely seen.[11,20,22,23] In both blastomycosis and brucellosis of the testes, macrophages, including multinucleated phagocytes (i.e., giant cells), may be present. Intranuclear or intracytoplasmic inclusions may be seen in dogs that develop orchitis due to distemper infection. Although rare, other etiologies involved in testicular inflammation in dogs include *Mycoplasma canis* as a cause of chronic epididymitis and Rocky Mountain Spotted Fever as a cause of orchitis.[24]

Testicular Neoplasia

The three major tumors of canine testes are Sertoli cell tumors, seminomas, and interstitial cell tumors.[16,25,26] Testicular tumors may occur in both intact and neutered animals.[27] In neutered animals, tumors may be located in the scrotum or at the prescrotal incision site and are thought to arise from embryologic testicular remnants, ectopic testis-like tissue (including polyorchidism), or transplanted testicular tissue from trauma to the testes during castration.[27] Testicular tumors may be difficult to differentiate cytologically, despite a reported 100% specificity in one study.[25] However, when evaluated with clinical signs and history, a diagnosis is usually possible. The differentiation of testicular neoplasia from inflammation, the other major cause of testicular enlargement, is relatively simple. Testicular tumors are rare in cats and only a few isolated case reports exist.[16,28,29] It is not uncommon for an animal to have more than one type of testicular tumor.[25]

Sertoli Cell Tumors: Sertoli cell tumors are a type of sex cord stromal tumor. They commonly occur in the testicles of older dogs or the undescended testicles of cryptorchid dogs. Many dogs have feminization syndrome, which, along with many other signs, results in atrophy of the contralateral testicle (see Figure 24-16). Feminization has not been reported in cats with Sertoli cell tumors.[28] Although rare, extratesticular Sertoli cell tumors have been reported.[27] It is possible to obtain material from intra-abdominal Sertoli cell tumors with ultrasound assistance, and inguinal cryptorchid testicles are easily aspirated.

Cytologically, Sertoli cell tumors are variably cellular consisting of round to columnar shaped cells present individually or in distinct palisading arrangements (Figure 24-20).[25] Cells may vary in size and amount of cytoplasm. The most unique feature is the abundant light-staining cytoplasm, often containing few irregularly sized, distinct, clear vacuoles (see Figures 24-20, Figure 24-21, and Figure 24-22). Nuclei are predominantly round and display a finely reticulated chromatin pattern with one to three prominent, round nucleoli. Mitotic figures may be identified. Call-Exner bodies have been reported in two dogs.[30] These structures are more typically seen in ovarian granulosa cell tumors, but in Sertoli cell tumors, they are characterized by rows of neoplastic Sertoli cells arranged in pseudorosettes surrounding deeply eosinophilic hyaline material.

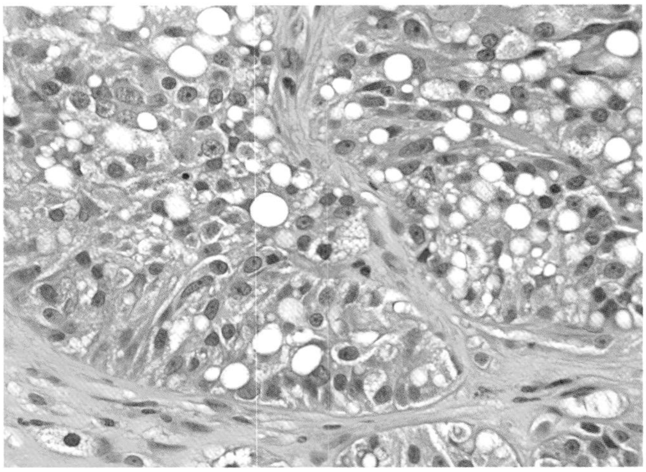

Figure 24-20 Histology of a Sertoli cell neoplasm in a dog, demonstrating the palisading arrangement seen in this tumor. Cells have variably sized, intracytoplasmic vacuoles. (H&E stain. Original magnification 400×.) (Courtesy of Dr. John Edwards.)

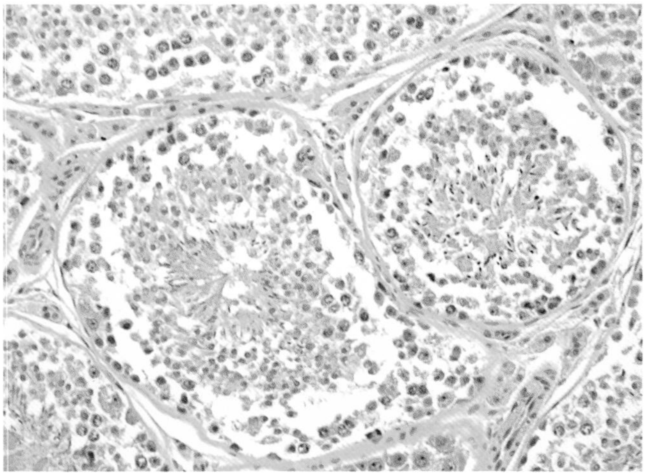

Figure 24-19 Histology of a normal testicle from an 8-year-old dog. Cells display orderly progression through maturation within each tubule, with immature cells present along the periphery and mature spermatids and spermatozoa within the lumen. (H&E stain. Original magnification 200×.) (Courtesy of Dr. John Edwards.)

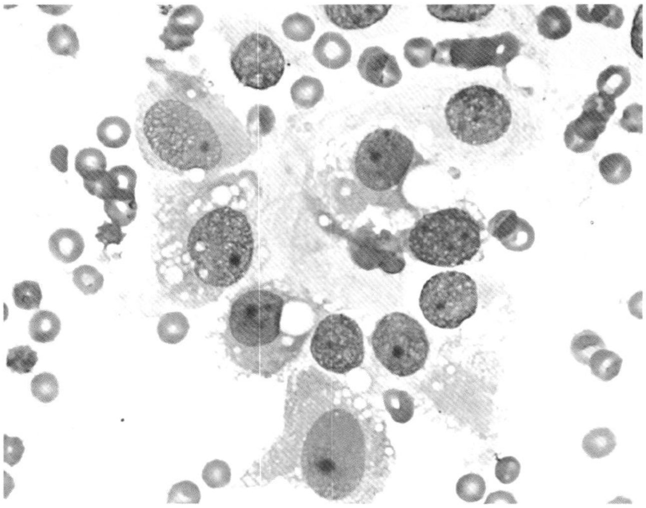

Figure 24-21 A group of lightly vacuolated cells aspirated from a Sertoli cell tumor. The cells have abundant cytoplasm with variably sized, clear vacuoles and coarse nuclear chromatin. (Wright-Giemsa stain. Original magnification 1000×.) (Courtesy of Dr. Rick Cowell.)

Seminomas: Seminomas are derived from the germ cells in the testes. Few clinical signs are seen in dogs that have seminomas, except when a Sertoli cell tumor coexists, which is a moderately common occurrence. Seminomas are frequently associated with cryptorchidism and undescended testicles have an increased risk of seminoma development.[31] An increased incidence of seminoma development within the right testicle in dogs has also been reported.[31] Some dogs may have feminization syndrome (if a concurrent Sertoli cell tumor is present), and prostatitis, prostatic hyperplasia, and perianal adenomas may occur. The major feature of seminomas is testicular enlargement, which is usually unilateral but occasionally may be bilateral. Seminomas may cause multiple enlargements in one or both testicles. Although relatively uncommon, of the major testicular tumors, metastasis is most likely with seminomas.[16]

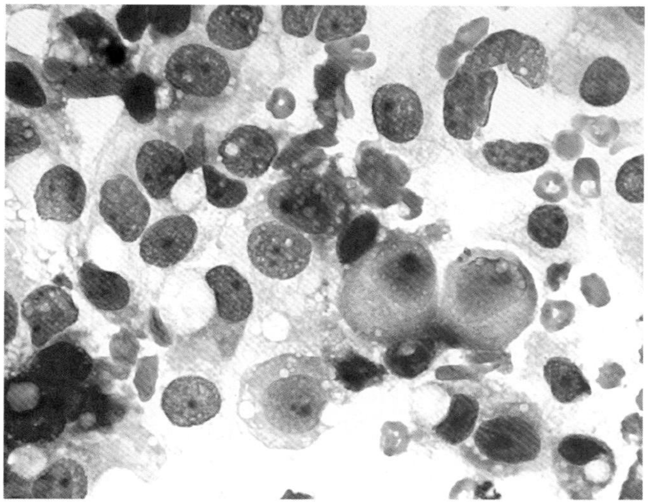

Figure 24-22 A group of cells aspirated from a Sertoli cell tumor. The cells have a moderate amount of wispy, vacuolated cytoplasm. The two large cells on the right have prominent large nucleoli often seen with these tumors. (Wright-Giemsa stain. Original magnification 1000×.) (Courtesy of Dr. Rick Cowell.)

Aspiration usually yields moderate to large numbers of discrete round cells that contain a sparse to moderate amount of cytoplasm, which is typically lightly basophilic and homogeneous (Figure 24-23). Nuclei contain characteristic coarsely reticular to irregularly clumped chromatin. Multinucleation is common (see Figure 24-23, Figure 24-24, and Figure 24-25). Relatively large nucleoli are found, and mitotic figures are frequent (see Figure 24-23). The presence of a granular, lacey eosinophilic background (tigroid background), lymphocytic infiltrate (Figure 24-26 and Figure 24-27), and atypical mitoses (see Figure 24-23) are diagnostic features commonly observed with seminomas.[25]

Interstitial Cell Tumors: Interstitial cell tumors are a type of sex cord stromal tumor that arise from the Leydig cells. Clinical signs are unusual in dogs with interstitial cell tumors, although they may rarely produce estrogen resulting in feminization.[32] Aspirates of interstitial cell tumors may be variably cellular. Cell clusters frequently surround an endothelial-lined capillary (perivascular pattern), which is a distinguishing hallmark in the diagnosis (Figure 24-28 and Figure 24-29).[27] Cells vary in size but frequently are round to spindle in shape, and they usually have abundant cytoplasm that stains basophilic.[25] As opposed to Sertoli cell tumors, interstitial cell tumors comprise cells containing numerous fine, punctate, clear vacuoles (microvacuoles), which are also often present in the background due to cell rupture (see Figure 24-29, Figure 24-30).[25] Fine, blue to black granules are occasionally seen in a few cells (Figure 24-31), and the N:C ratio is usually low. Nuclei are small to medium, have a finely stippled to reticular chromatin pattern, and may contain visible nucleoli. Nuclear pseudoinclusions, appearing as small vacuoles embedded within the nucleus, may also be identified as a distinguishing cytologic characteristic.[25]

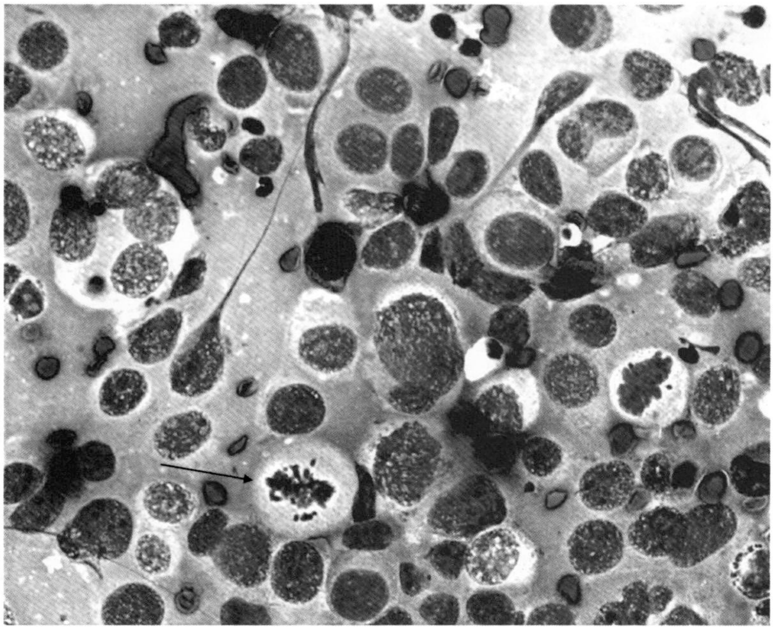

Figure 24-23 An aspirate from a seminoma containing many intact and lysed cells. Cells have a high nucleus-to-cytoplasm ratio and a finely reticular chromatin pattern. Multinucleation and frequent mitotic figures, including an atypical mitotic figure (arrow), are seen. (Diff-quik stain. Original magnification 500×.)

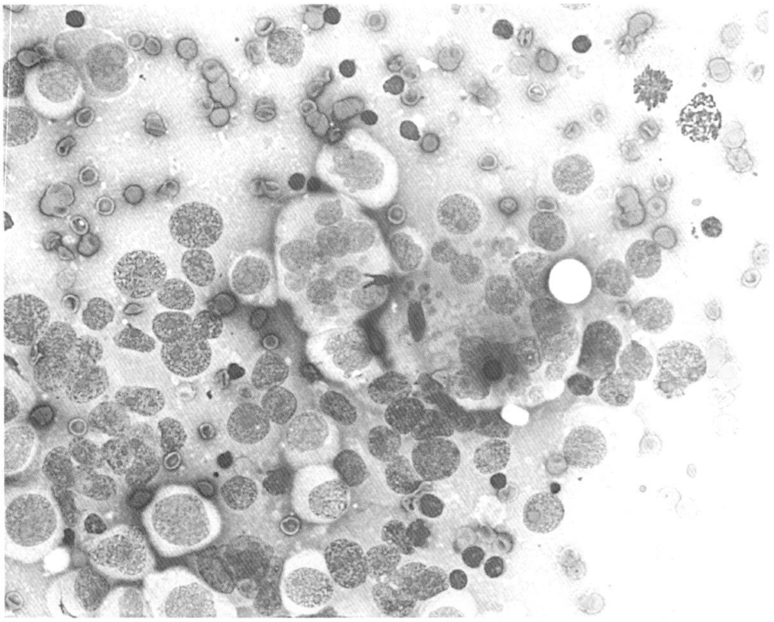

Figure 24-24 Impression smear from a seminoma. Large multinucleated cells containing numerous nuclei and satellite nuclei are seen, along with several other intact and lysed neoplastic cells and few small lymphocytes. Mitotic figures are present. (Diff-Quik stain. Original magnification 400×.)

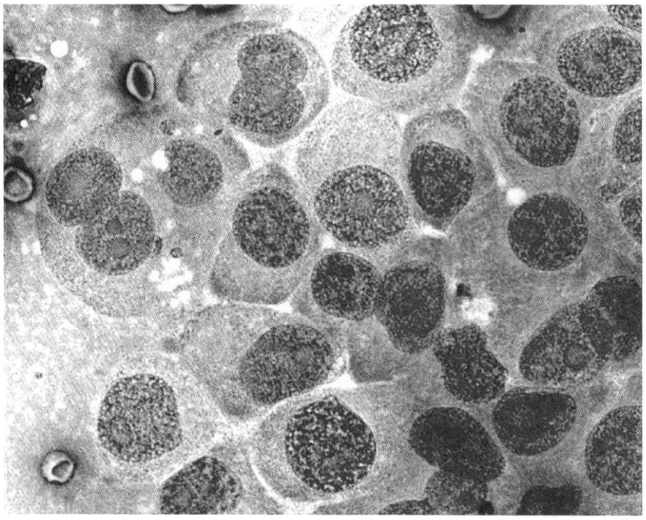

Figure 24-25 Impression smear from a seminoma. Characteristic round cells with a high nucleus-to-cytoplasm ratio, a reticular chromatin pattern, and prominent, variably sized nucleoli are present, including a trinucleate cell with satellite nuclei. (Diff-Quik stain. Original magnification 1000×.)

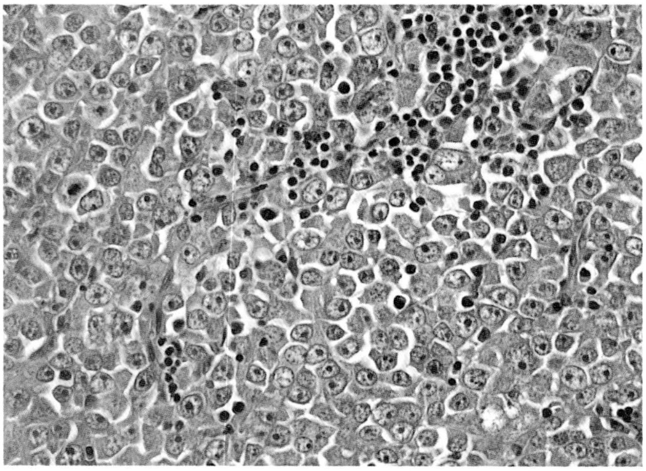

Figure 24-26 Histology of a seminoma from a dog, solid variant. Cells are arranged in a solid sheet with a mild infiltrate of lymphocytes. Neoplastic cells have a large, round nucleus with vesicular chromatin and typically a single prominent nucleolus. (H&E stain. Original magnification 400×.) (Courtesy of Dr. John Edwards.)

Other Testicular Neoplasms

In addition to the tumors listed above, other testicular tumors may occur, although they are rare. Metastases to the testes are also rare but have been reported.

Mixed Germ Cell-sex Cord-stromal Tumors: These testicular neoplasms are characterized by a mixture of atypical germ cells and sex cord stromal derivatives (Sertoli cells or Leydig cells). Grossly, these tumors are difficult to distinguish from other testicular tumors, appearing as firm, gray-white to tan, single to multilobed masses.[33] Mixed germ cell stromal tumors should be suspected when two populations of neoplastic cells are observed cytologically, most commonly a mixture of neoplastic germ cells, as in seminomas, and Sertoli cells. Mixed gonadal tumors are differentiated histologically from collision tumors (two individual tumors that have grown into one another) based on the degree of intermingling of the two cell populations.

Teratomas: A teratoma is a type of germ cell tumor that is composed of multiple germ layers in various stages of maturation. It is extremely rare in small animals with only one published case reported in a cryptorchid testicle

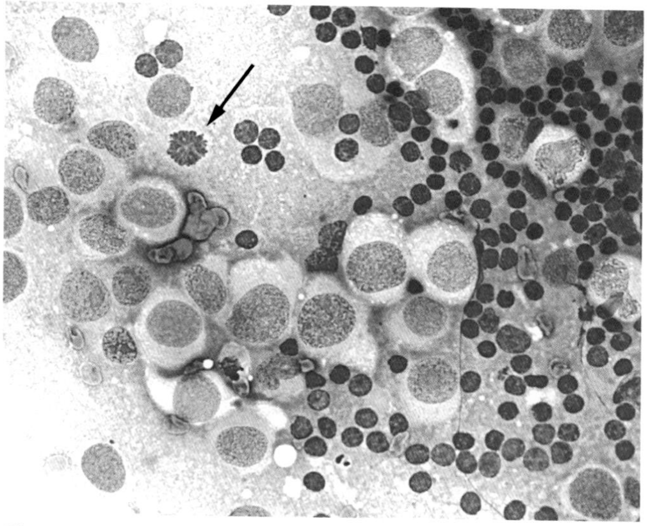

Figure 24-27 Impression smear from a seminoma. Characteristic round cells with a high nucleus-to-cytoplasm ratio, a reticular chromatin pattern, and prominent nucleoli are present, in addition to a large number of small lymphocytes. A mitotic figure is also observed (*arrow*). (Diff-Quik stain. Original magnification 500×.)

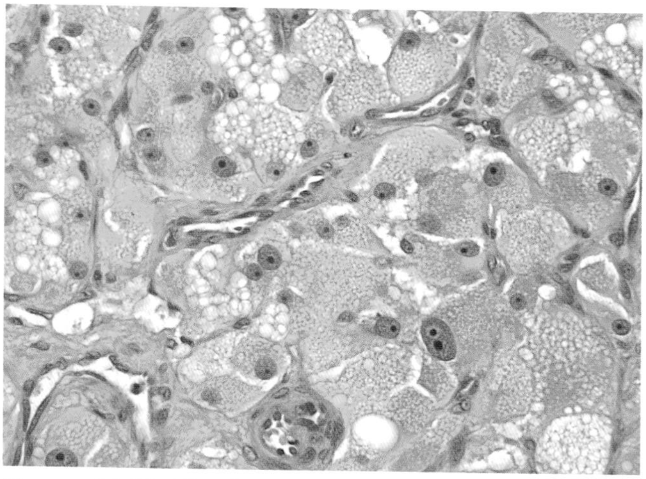

Figure 24-29 Histology of an interstitial cell neoplasm from a dog. Cells display numerous fine to moderately sized vacuoles and moderate anisocytosis and anisokaryosis. Frequent capillaries are observed throughout the neoplasm. (H&E stain. Original magnification 400×.) (Courtesy of Dr. John Edwards.)

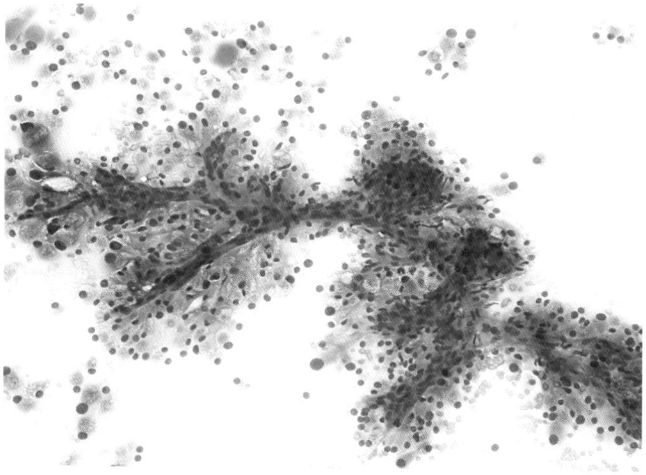

Figure 24-28 An aspirate from an interstitial cell tumor composed of round to polygonal cells surrounding a capillary. Cells typically contain many fine, clear vacuoles and cell borders are indistinct. Few macronuclei are present. (Wright-Giemsa stain. Original magnification 200×.) (Courtesy of Dr. Amy Valenciano.)

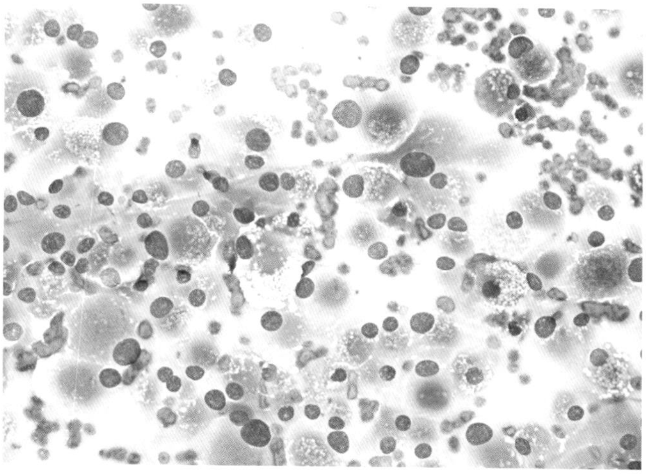

Figure 24-30 Cells from an aspirate of an interstitial cell tumor demonstrate moderate to marked anisocytosis and anisokaryosis. Note the often numerous, relatively uniformly sized vacuoles. (Wright-Giemsa stain. Original magnification 500×.) (Courtesy of Dr. Amy Valenciano.)

of a cat.[34] However, various textbooks have discussed teratomas occurring in canine testes. These tumors tend to be benign, although malignant teratomas may occur.

Sperm Granulomas

Sperm granulomas develop because of a chronic inflammatory response elicited by extravasation of spermatozoa from the reproductive tract. Granuloma development has been associated with congenital alterations of the epididymal duct and following trauma, infection, or surgical procedures.[35,36] Grossly, granulomas are visualized as variably sized, white to gray, firm nodules.[35,37] Cytologically, inflammation (mostly macrophages and lymphocytes) may be observed.[36]

PENIS AND PREPUCE

Cytologic Evaluation of the Normal Penis

Cytologic evaluation of the penis using the impression smear or aspiration technique may be helpful in assessing for inflammatory conditions and neoplasia of the penis. The most prevalent cell of normal penile cytology is the nucleated squamous epithelial cell. In addition, variable numbers of nondegenerate to slightly degenerate neutrophils

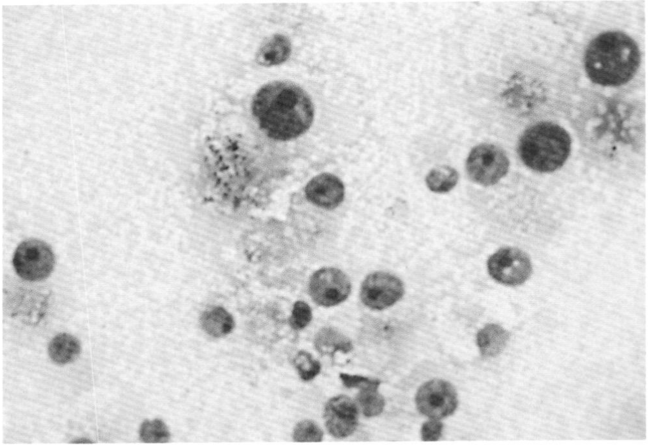

Figure 24-31 Fine-needle aspirate of an interstitial cell tumor. The cells and their nuclei vary in size and show prominent vacuolization. Some cells contain blue-black cytoplasmic granules. (Diff-Quik stain.)

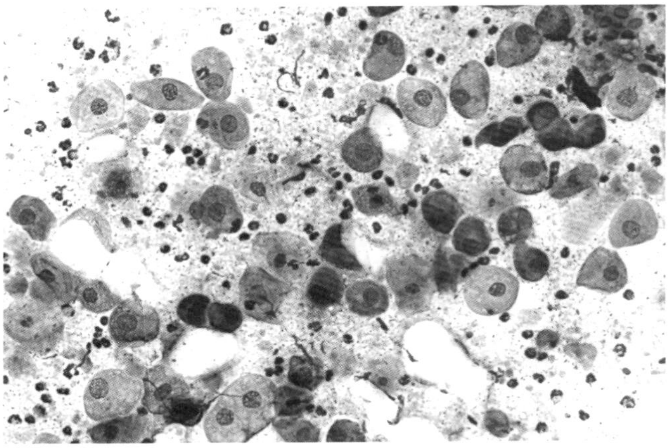

Figure 24-32 Impression smear from the tip of the penis of an intact dog. Many nucleated squamous epithelial cells, neutrophils, and bacteria are present. Mild variation in cell appearance is evident among the epithelial cells. (Diff-Quik stain. Original magnification 200×.)

are present, and bacteria may be found both extracellularly and intracellularly (Figure 24-32). *Simonsiella* spp. from oral contamination may also be observed. Because the preputial covering is an extension of the skin, criteria used for cytologic evaluation of the skin may be applied.

Posthitis

It is not uncommon for male dogs to have a small amount of greenish-yellow, purulent discharge (smegma) extruding at the tip of the penis and prepuce. Copious amounts of this material, however, may be an indication of an underlying infection. The penis should be extruded from the preputial sheath and examined closely for a foreign body, discoloration, masses, or all of these signs. Excessive licking from a number of causes may lead to hyperemia. Cytologic evaluation of the purulent material may reveal a nonspecific inflammatory response, including macrophages, variably degenerate neutrophils, intracellular and extracellular bacteria, or all of these. Bacterial culture is

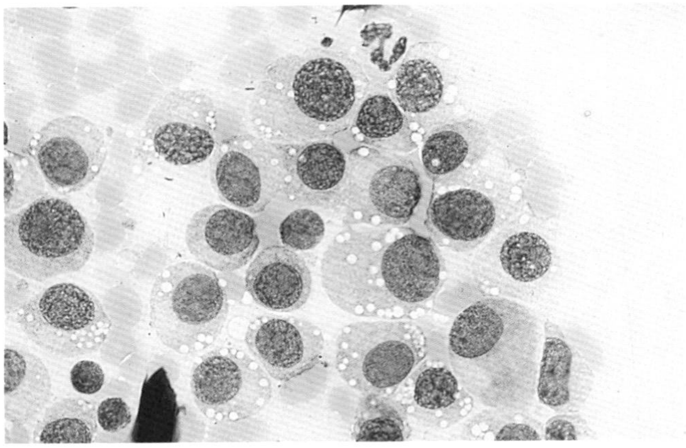

Figure 24-33 Numerous transmissible venereal tumor cells with coarse chromatin and smoky gray vacuolated cytoplasm are shown. (Wright stain.)

typically not helpful unless a true bacterial infection that does not resolve with antibiotic therapy is suspected.

Penile Squamous Papilloma

Dogs with penile squamous papillomas may present for preputial swelling and intermittent hematuria.[38] Evaluation of the penis reveals a variably sized, single, pedunculated, soft, pinkish red, cauliflower-like mass. Cytologic evaluation may reveal a homogeneous population of squamous epithelial cells, with minimal atypia in conjunction with a variable inflammatory response, predominantly neutrophilic. Papillomas may be associated with infection of a papilloma virus but may also be related to trauma or may be idiopathic.[38]

Penile and Preputial Neoplasia

Although not common, neoplasia of the penis has been reported in dogs. Not having knowledge of normal canine anatomy, some owners may mistake the swelling of the bulbus glandus of the penis for an abnormal "mass." Cytologic evaluation may be done by using an impression smear technique or FNA.

Canine Transmissible Venereal Tumors: Transmissible venereal tumors (TVTs) usually occur on the external genitalia of dogs, but they may also be found in the nasal cavity, mouth, and pharynx (especially near the tonsils) and on nongenital skin; a TVT may occasionally metastasize to other locations. Impression smears or smears of aspirated material are usually quite cellular, and the tumor cells have distinct characteristics. Cells are medium-sized, with an N:C ratio that is moderately increased because the nuclei are large and they have a moderate amount of cytoplasm. Nuclei are immature with a finely reticulated chromatin pattern. Large, round nucleoli may be found in a few cells. The cytoplasm variably stains from light to dark blue. Most cells contain distinct, small (1 to 2 micrometers [μm] in diameter), punctate vacuoles (Figure 24-33). Mitotic cells are frequently found. Reports in the recent literature have suggested that it may be beneficial to classify the different morphologies of TVT into the subtypes plasmacytoid, lymphocytoid, and mixed, as it may influence biologic behavior of the tumor.[39]

Other cells may be seen in cytologic preparations of TVTs. During the regressive stage, many lymphocytes are present, along with a few neutrophils and macrophages. Impression smears made from the surface of ulcerated tumors may contain bacteria, neutrophils, and epithelial cells.

Other Neoplasms: Penile squamous cell carcinoma has been reported in dogs.[40] Additional penile neoplastic diseases that have been reported in dogs include, but are not limited to, penile lymphosarcoma, osteosarcoma of the os penis, chondrosarcoma in the penile urethra, ossifying fibroma, hemangiosarcoma, and lipoma.[41-43]

As mentioned previously, because the prepuce is a continuation of the skin, any cutaneous neoplasms may be encountered, such as mast cell tumors.[44] The skin of the prepuce does contain few perianal gland cells (modified sebaceous glands), and thus, perianal gland tumors may also occur here.

SEMEN

Semen is usually evaluated as part of a routine breeding-soundness examination or to determine its quality in infertile or subfertile males.[5,45] Because semen contains material derived from the testes and from the remainder of the reproductive tract, including the prostate gland, semen examination may also provide information on lesions in the genital tract of male dogs, such as some inflammatory or neoplastic lesions of the reproductive tract.

Semen Collection

Semen is often collected into an artificial vagina while the penis is manually manipulated in the presence of a teaser female. The male's interest is enhanced by applying a solution of a 1:100 dilution of p-hydroxybenzoate methyl ester to the perineum of the teaser female. The technique is more fully described elsewhere.[45,46] Semen may be collected from cats with the use of an artificial vagina or electroejaculation.[46] Dogs produce from 1 to 40 milliliters (mL) of semen ejaculate, and cats produce up to 0.5 mL.[45,47] FNA of the testicle may also be used as a tool for semen evaluation to provide information on procession of spermatogenesis.[5] Identification of cells is described in the discussion on normal testicle cytology above.

Semen Evaluation

The gross characteristics of the fluid, including color and consistency, should be determined immediately after collection. Normal semen is milky and moderately viscous. A red or pink color indicates that blood is present in the sample, and yellow discoloration suggests the presence of urine. Serous, greenish, or grayish semen indicates inflammation, especially when small flecks of material are present.

The number of spermatozoa per ejaculate is the most important piece of information when evaluating the breeding potential of a male dog.[45] Sperm concentration is determined using a hemocytometer after appropriate dilution. A portion of semen is diluted 1:100 with saline or a red cell Unopette (Becton Dickinson), and the total number of sperm in the central primary square is counted. This number is then multiplied by 106 and the volume of the ejaculate (in milliliters) to determine the total sperm count. In samples with low numbers of sperm, either the sample is diluted less or a greater area of the hemocytometer is used for counting. Appropriate adjustments of the multiplication factor are made for calculating the total sperm count.

Sperm motility should be evaluated immediately after collection. The sample should be maintained at body temperature or warmed to body temperature in an incubator. A drop is placed on a warm slide, which is immediately covered with a coverslip. Samples with a high concentration of spermatozoa may be diluted 1:1 with warm physiologic saline or 2.9% sodium citrate.

Progressive, forward motility of individual sperm is estimated at high-dry magnification. Such movement is thought to reflect viability and ability to fertilize the ovum. Spermatozoa may have side-to-side motion without forward progression, move in small circles, or be nonmotile or hypomotile. A normal semen sample should have greater than 70% motility. Decreased motility may be found in semen contaminated with urine or exposed to inflammation. Overall sperm motility of the first ejaculate after a long period of sexual inactivity is decreased because of the increased percentage of old and dead sperm.[45]

Sperm morphology is assessed by bright field microscopy of a new methylene blue–stained smear or phase-contrast microscopy of an unstained smear. For bright field microscopy, an air-dried smear is mounted in a drop of 0.5% new methylene blue (NMB) stain. A total of at least 200 sperm should be evaluated and classified as *normal sperm, abnormal head, abnormal midpiece, coiled tail, head only, protoplasmic droplet,* and *abnormal head attachment* (Figure 24-34).

In semen of high quality, nearly all sperm should be morphologically normal. Increased percentages of abnormalities indicate poor quality and breeding potential; however, correlations between percentages of sperm abnormalities and conception rate have not been determined in dogs.[45] Although not sensitive for identifying subtle infertility problems, FNA of the testicle has been shown to correlate well with clinical findings in dogs with infertility, especially in those with suspected obstructive azoospermia.[5]

Wright-Giemsa–stained semen should be examined after Wright staining when inflammation or neoplasia is suspected. Neutrophils indicate inflammation in the reproductive tract; however, when abnormal cells are found, contamination from the external surface of the penis and inflammation of the urethra or bladder must be ruled out. Ejaculates, especially the first portion of the ejaculate, occasionally contain cells from the prostate gland, so the diagnosis of prostate gland inflammation or neoplasia may be suggested from such observations. Evaluation of the prostate is indicated with these findings.

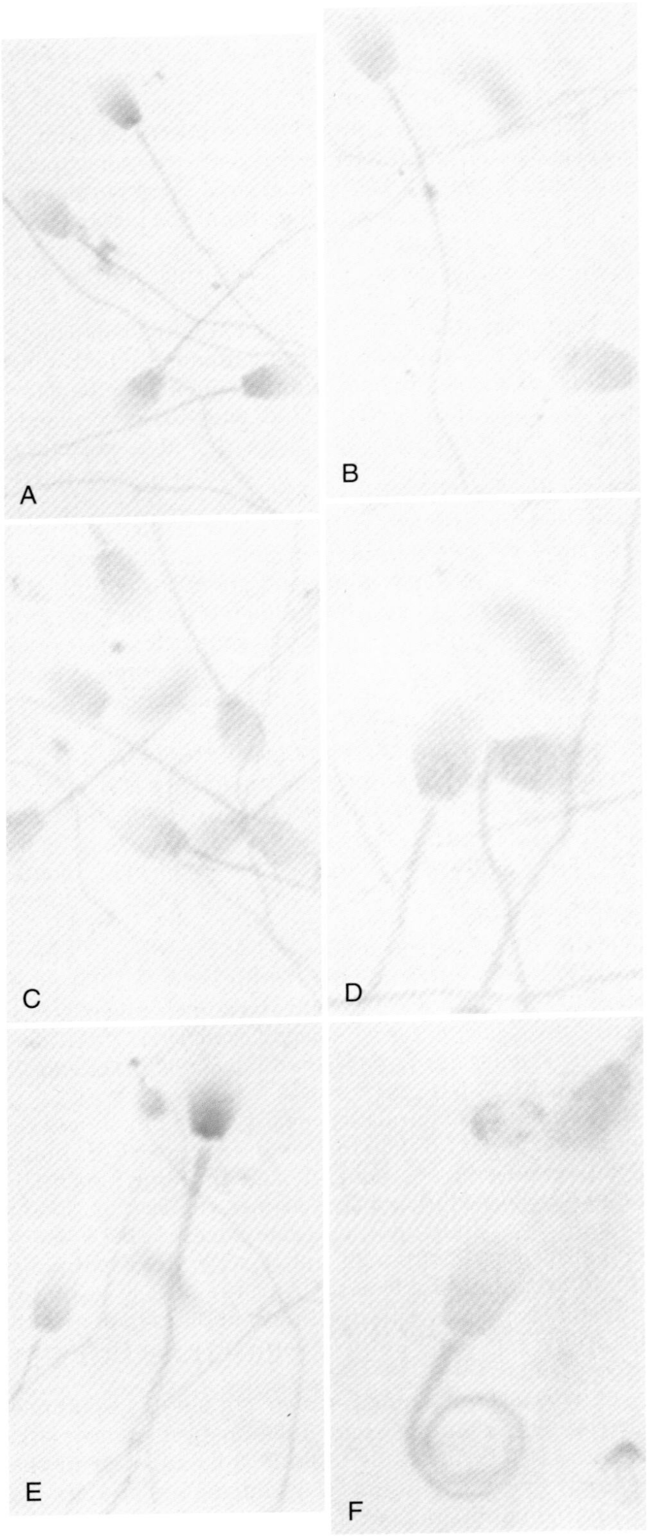

Figure 24-34 **A,** Normal spermatozoa. **B,** Spermatozoa with a protoplasmic droplet. **C,** Detached sperm head. **D,** Spermatozoa with an abnormally attached head. **E,** Spermatozoa with a double tail. **F,** Spermatozoa with a coiled tail. (New methylene blue stain.)

References

1. Smith J: Canine prostatic disease: a review of anatomy, pathology, diagnosis, and treatment, *Theriogenology* 70: 375–383, 2008.
2. Mordecai A, Liptak JM, Hofstede T, et al: Prostatic abscess in a neutered cat, *J Am Anim Hosp Assoc* 44:90–94, 2008.
3. Ling GV, et al: Canine prostatic fluid: Techniques of collection, quantitative bacterial culture, and interpretation of results, *J Am Vet Med Assoc* 183:201–206, 1983.
4. Ling GV: In Ling GV, editor: *Lower urinary tract diseases of dogs and cats*, St. Louis, MO, 1995, Mosby, pp 129–141.
5. Dahlbom M, Makinen A, Suominen J: Testicular fine needle aspiration cytology as a diagnostic tool in dog infertility, *J Small Anim Pract* 38:506–512, 1997.
6. Gouletsou PG, Galatos AD, Sideri AI: Impact of fine- or large-needle aspiration on canine testes: clinical, in vivo ultrasonographic and seminological assessment, *Reprod Domest Anim* 46:712–719, 2011.
7. Thrall DE, Olson ON, Freemyer FG: Cytologic diagnosis of canine prostatic disease, *J Am Anim Hosp Assoc* 21:95–102, 1985.
8. Ling GV: In Ling GV, editor: *Lower urinary tract diseases of dogs and cats*, St. Louis, MO, 1995, Mosby, pp 49–59.
9. Black GM, et al: Prevalence of prostatic cyst in adult, large-breed dogs, *J Am Anim Hosp Assoc* 34:177–180, 1998.
10. Krawiec DR, Heflin D: Study of prostatic disease in dogs: 177 cases (1981-1986), *J Am Vet Med Assoc* 200:1119–1122, 1992.
11. Totten AK, Ridgway MD, Sauberli DS: *Blastomyces dermatitidis* prostatic and testicular infection in eight dogs (1992-2005), *J Am Anim Hosp Assoc* 47:413–418, 2011.
12. Rogers KS, Wantschek L, Lees GE: Diagnostic evaluation of the canine prostate, *Compend Contin Educ* 8:799–811, 1986.
13. Madewell BR, Theilen GH: *Veterinary cancer medicine*, ed 2, Philadelphia, PA, 1987, Lea & Febiger, pp 583–600.
14. DeNicola DB, Rebar AH, Boon GD: *Cytology of the canine male urogenital tract*, St. Louis, 1980, MO, Ralston-Purina.
15. Tucker AR, Smith JR: Prostatic squamous metaplasia in a cat with interstitial cell neoplasia in a retained testis, *Vet Pathol* 45:905–909, 2008.
16. McEntee MC: Reproductive oncology, *Clin Tech Small Anim Pract* 17(3):133–149, 2002.
17. Tursi M, et al: Adenocarcinoma of the disseminated prostate in a cat, *J Feline Med Surg* 10:600–602, 2008.
18. Caney SMA, Holt PE, Day MJ, et al: Prostatic carcinoma in two cats, *J Small Anim Pract* 39:140–143, 1998.
19. Bradbury CA, Westropp JL, Pollard RE: Relationship between prostatomegaly, prostatic mineralization, and cytologic diagnosis, *Vet Radiol Ultrasound* 50(2):167–171, 2009.
20. Larsen RE: Testicular biopsy in the dog, *Vet Clin North Am* 7:747–755, 1977.
21. Santos M, Marcos R, Caniatti M: Cytologic study of normal canine testis, *Theriogenology* 73:208–214, 2010.
22. Legendre AM: *Infectious diseases of the dog and cat*, ed 4, St. Louis, MO, 2012, Saunders. 606–614.
23. Greene CE, Carmichael LE: *Infectious diseases of the dog and cat*, ed 4, St. Louis, MO, 2012, Saunders, pp 398–411.
24. Ober CP, Spaulding K, Breitscherdt EB, et al: Orchitis in two dogs with Rocky Mountain Spotted Fever, *Vet Radiol Ultrasound* 45:458–465, 2004.
25. Masserdotti C, Bonfanti U, De Loenzi D, et al: Cytologic features of testicular tumors in dog, *J Vet Med* 52:339–346, 2005.
26. Grieco V, Riccardi E, Greppi GF, et al: Canine testicular tumours: a study on 232 dogs, *J Comp Path* 138:86–89, 2008.

27. Doxsee AL, et al: Extratesticular interstitial and sertoli cell tumors in previously neutered dogs and cats: a report of 17 cases, *Can Vet J* 47:763–766, 2006.
28. Miller MA, Hartnett SE, Ramos-Vara JA: Interstitial cell tumor and sertoli cell tumor in the testis of a cat, *Vet Pathol* 44:394–397, 2007.
29. Miyoshi N, Yasuda N, Kamimura Y, et al: Teratoma in a feline unilateral cryptorchid testis, *Vet Pathol* 38:729–730, 2001.
30. Masserdotti C, De Lorenzi D, Gasparotto L: Cytologic detection of Call-Exner bodies in Sertoli cell tumors from 2 dogs, *Vet Clin Pathol* 37:112–114, 2008.
31. Bush JM, Gardiner DW, Palmer JS, et al: Testicular germ cell tumours in dogs are predominantly of spermatocytic seminoma type and are frequently associated with somatic cell tumours, *Int J Androl* 34:288–295, 2011.
32. Suess RP Jr, et al: Bone marrow hypoplasia in a feminized dog with an interstitial cell tumor, *J Am Vet Med Assoc* 200(9):1346–1348, 1992.
33. Patnaik AK, Mostofi FK: A clinicopathologic, histologic, and immunohistochemical study of mixed germ cell-stromal tumors of the testis in 16 dogs, *Vet Pathol* 30:287–295, 1993.
34. Miyoshi N, Yasuda N, Kamimura Y, et al: Teratoma in a feline unilateral cryptorchid testis, *Vet Pathol* 38:729–730, 2001.
35. Batista-Arteaga M, Santana M, Lozano O, et al: Bilateral epididymal sperm granulomas following urethrostomy in a German Shepherd dog, *Reprod Dom Anim* 46:731–733, 2011.
36. Pérez-Marín CC, et al: Clinical and pathological findings in testis, epididymis, deferens duct and prostate following vasectomy in a dog, *Reprod Dom Anim* 41:169–174, 2006.
37. Kawakami E, et al: Sperm granuloma and sperm agglutination in a dog with asthenozoopermia, *J Vet Med Sci* 65(3):409–412, 2003.
38. Cornegliani L, Vercelli A, Abramo F: Idiopathic mucosal penile squamous papillomas in dogs, *Vet Dermatol* 18: 439–443, 2007.
39. Flórez MM, et al: Cytologic subtypes of canine transmissible venereal tumor, *Vet Clin Path* 41(1):4–5, 2012.
40. Wakui S, Furusato M, Nomura Y, et al: Testicular epidermoid cyst and penile squamous cell carcinoma in a dog, *Vet Pathol* 29:543–545, 1992.
41. Michels GM, Knapp DW, David M, et al: Penile prolapse and urethral obstruction secondary to lymphoma of the penis in a dog, *J Am Anim Hosp Assoc* 37:474–477, 2001.
42. Peppler C, Weissert D, Kappe E, et al: Osteosarcoma of the penile bone (os penis) in a dog, *Aust Vet J* 87:52–55, 2009.
43. Davis GJ, Holt D: Two chondrosarcomas in the urethra of a German shepherd dog, *J Small Anim Pract* 44:169–171, 2003.
44. Vandis M, Knoll JS: Cytologic examination of a cutaneous mast cell tumor in a boxer, *Vet Med* 102(3):165–168, 2007.
45. Feldman EC, Nelson RW: *Canine and feline endocrinology and reproduction*, ed 3, St. Louis, MO, 2004, Saunders, pp 930–952.
46. Threlfall WR: *Textbook of veterinary internal medicine*, ed 7, St. Louis, MO, 2010, Elsevier, pp 1934–1939.
47. Seager SWJ: In Kirk R, editor: *Current veterinary therapy VI: small animal practice*, Philadelphia, PA, 1977, Saunders, pp 1252–1254.

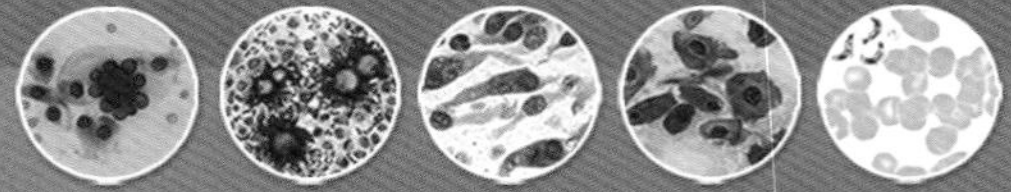

CHAPTER 25

Vaginal Cytology

Robin W. Allison

Examination of exfoliated cells from the vagina is a simple technique that is useful to monitor the progression of proestrus and estrus in dogs and cats.[1-3] The vaginal epithelium undergoes a predictable hyperplastic response to increasing plasma estrogen concentrations during proestrus. Starting as only a few cell layers, the epithelium becomes 20 to 30 cell layers thick, eventually exfoliating large numbers of superficial epithelial cells during estrus. Vaginal cytology, often in tandem with hormone analysis, may provide valuable information about the stage of the ovarian cycle.[4] In addition, vaginal cytology has proven useful to detect inflammatory and neoplastic conditions in the female reproductive tract.[5]

VAGINA

Collecting Vaginal Samples

Cells are obtained by passing a cotton-tipped swab into the caudal vagina (Figure 25-1 and Figure 25-2). A narrow spreading speculum may be used to allow unimpeded swab passage. If no vaginal discharge is present, the swab may be moistened with sterile saline to avoid discomfort. The swab should be directed craniodorsad when entering the vaginal vault to avoid the clitoral fossa; keratinized epithelium normally present in the fossa could lead to an inappropriate cytologic interpretation (Figure 25-3).[3] Once cranial to the urethral orifice, the vaginal wall is gently swabbed. The cells are then transferred to a glass slide by gently rolling the swab with minimal pressure to avoid rupturing cells. The smear is allowed to air-dry thoroughly before staining. Romanowsky-type stains typically used for blood films (Wright or modified Wright-Giemsa stains, including quick-type stains) provide good morphologic detail.

Classifying Vaginal Cells

Vaginal epithelial cells are described beginning with the deepest, most immature layer near the basement membrane and progressing superficially to the most mature layer nearest the vaginal lumen (Figure 25-4).

Basal Cells: Basal cells give rise to all epithelial cell types observed in a vaginal smear. They are small cells with round nuclei and a high nucleus-to-cytoplasm (N:C) ratio and are rarely observed in vaginal smears.

Parabasal Cells: Parabasal cells are small round cells with round vesiculated nuclei and a small amount of cytoplasm and are usually quite uniform in size and shape (see Figure 25-4, *A*). Large numbers of parabasal cells may exfoliate when the vagina of a prepubertal animal is swabbed.

Intermediate Cells: Intermediate cells vary in size, depending on the amount of cytoplasm present. Although the nuclei of both small and large intermediate cells are similar in size to parabasal cell nuclei, intermediate cells are about twice the size of parabasal cells (see Figure 25-4, *B* and *C*). Intermediate cells still have vesiculated nuclei, but as they increase in size, their cytoplasm becomes irregular, folded, and angular, similar to the cytoplasm of superficial cells. Large intermediate cells are sometimes called *superficial intermediate cells* or *transitional intermediate cells*.

Superficial Cells: Superficial cells are the largest epithelial cells seen in vaginal smears (see Figure 25-4, *D*). These are dead cells, whose nuclei become pyknotic and then faded, often progressing to anucleate forms (see Figure 25-4, *E*). Their cytoplasm is abundant, angular, and folded. As cells degenerate, their cytoplasm may develop small vacuoles (Figure 25-5). The degeneration process of stratified squamous epithelial cells into large, flat, dead cells is called *cornification*; superficial epithelial cells are commonly called *cornified cells*. Superficial cells with small pyknotic nuclei and anuclear superficial epithelial cells have the same significance.

Other Normal Cytologic Findings: Metestrum cells have been described as vaginal epithelial cells containing neutrophils in their cytoplasm (Figure 25-6).[3,6] They are not specific for any stage of the cycle and may be seen whenever neutrophils are present.

The vagina of dogs and cats contains normal bacterial flora, and bacteria are frequently observed on vaginal cytology slides.[7,8] Unless the bacteria are accompanied by large numbers of neutrophils, they are generally considered normal flora.

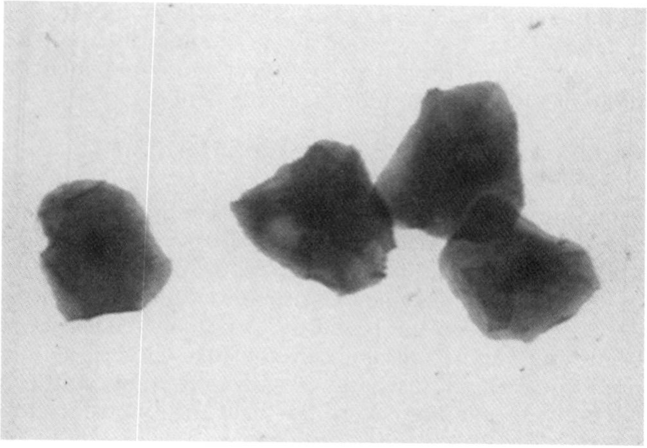

Figure 25-12 Vaginal smear from a dog in estrus. Note superficial epithelial cells with pyknotic nuclei. (Wright stain. Original magnification 100×.)

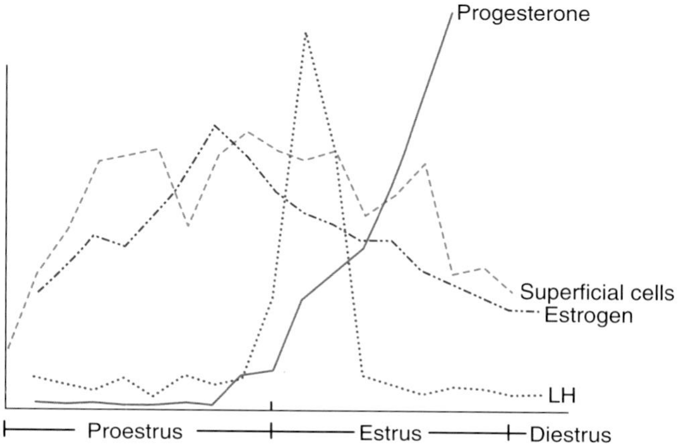

Figure 25-13 Illustration of hormone fluctuations and vaginal cytology during the average canine estrous cycle. (Adapted from Feldman EC, Nelson RW: Ovarian cycle and vaginal cytology. In: Feldman EC, Nelson RW, editors: *Canine and feline endocrinology and reproduction*, ed 3, Philadelphia, PA, 2004, Saunders, p. 755.)

increase.[6] Neutrophils appear in variable numbers and usually coincide with increased numbers of parabasal and intermediate cells (Figure 25-15). Some bitches have few or no neutrophils in cytologic preparations made during diestrus (Figure 25-16). Erythrocytes and bacteria may or may not be present. Bacteria engulfed by neutrophils are occasionally seen during diestrus in normal bitches.[5] Behavioral diestrus is defined by the bitch's refusal of the male and usually lags behind cytologic diestrus by several days.[3]

Individual cytologic preparations made during the transition period from late estrus to early diestrus, without benefit of prior preparations, may appear very similar to smears made in early or mid-proestrus. At both times, a similar mixture of superficial and nonsuperficial cells may be present, as well as both erythrocytes and neutrophils. Vaginoscopy, vulvar examination, and the animal's behavior are usually helpful in making differentiations. When in doubt, repeating vaginal cytology in 3 or 4 days should clarify the situation.

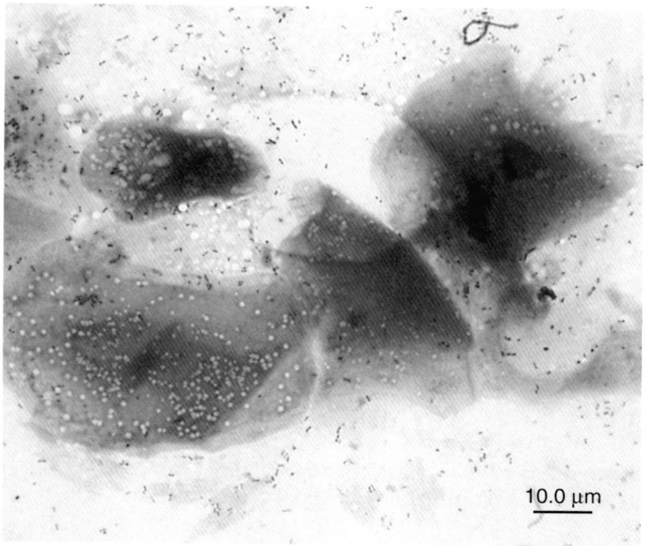

Figure 25-14 Vaginal smear from a dog in estrus. Superficial cells predominate, and many bacteria are present in the background and adhered to the epithelial cells. (Wright stain. Original magnification 1000×.)

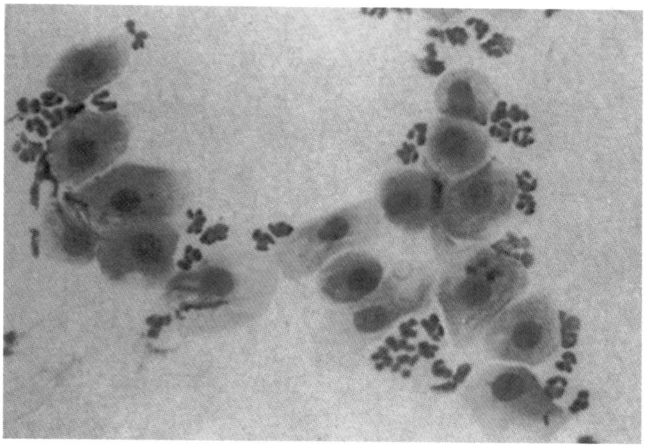

Figure 25-15 Vaginal smear from a dog in diestrus. Note the numerous neutrophils and intermediate cells. (Wright stain. Original magnification 100×.)

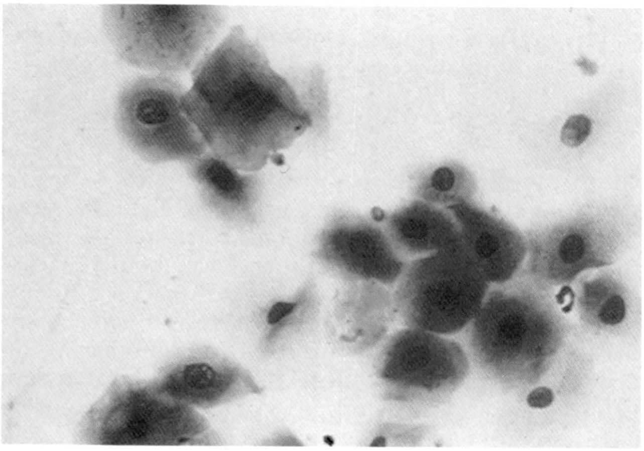

Figure 25-16 Vaginal smear from a dog in diestrus that contains very few neutrophils. (Wright stain. Original magnification 100×.)

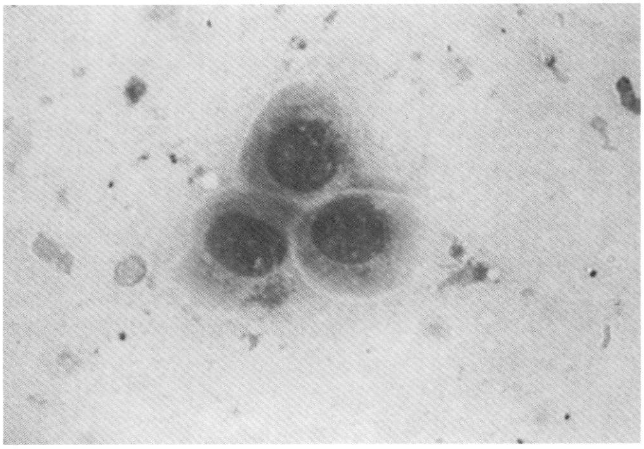

Figure 25-17 Parabasal cells in a vaginal smear from a dog in anestrus. (Wright stain. Original magnification 400×.)

Anestrus

Parabasal and intermediate cells predominate during anestrus (Figure 25-17). If present, neutrophils and bacteria are few in number.

MANAGEMENT OF BREEDING

Considerable variation exists in the duration of proestrus and estrus in normal bitches. Although the average length of time from the onset of proestrus to standing heat (when the bitch will accept a male) is 9 days, it may be as short as 2 or as long as 25 days in normal animals.[6] Some bitches have no discernible behavioral proestrus or estrus, yet they ovulate normally. These variations may cause confusion about the best time to attempt breeding. Vaginal cytology is useful to suggest appropriate breeding times, but cytology alone cannot reliably distinguish between late proestrus and estrus and does not give specific information about the date of ovulation.

Normal, healthy bitches should be bred every 3 to 4 days throughout the period when greater than 90% of vaginal epithelial cells are superficial.[3,9] Because canine spermatozoa can survive for at least 4 to 6 days in the uterus of bitches in estrus, mating may be successful from shortly before the time of ovulation to about 4 days after ovulation. Once diestrus occurs, fertility rapidly declines. Breedings are unlikely to be successful if delayed more than 24 hours after the onset of cytologic diestrus.

Hormone Analysis

Ovulation has been shown to occur about 48 hours (range 24 to 72 hours) after the LH surge.[9,10] Serum LH concentrations may be measured but stay elevated only 12 to 24 hours, making them inconvenient as a marker of ovulation for routine breedings; however, measuring LH levels may be justified in animals experiencing reproductive difficulties or when frozen semen is used for artificial insemination. By contrast, serum progesterone levels rise from basal levels of less than 0.5 nanogram per milliliter (ng/mL) to greater than 1 ng/mL shortly before the LH surge, 2 to 4 ng/mL during the LH surge, and typically reach greater than 4 ng/mL by the time ovulation occurs.[4,9,11] Commercial laboratories now offer 24-hour turnaround time on serum progesterone assays, making them a convenient adjunct to vaginal cytology, with the benefit of more precise estimation of the fertile period.

Combining Vaginal Cytology and Hormone Analysis

Determining serial progesterone levels and vaginal cytology during proestrus and estrus will provide the most information about the fertile period and have proven useful in the management of animals with variable estrus cycles.[4] A protocol proposed by Goodman recommends beginning vaginal cytology at the first clinical sign of proestrus (vaginal discharge or vulvar swelling) and following with cytology every few days until cornification reaches 70%.[9] A baseline progesterone level should be performed at the time of the first vaginal cytology. When cornification reaches 70%, serial progesterone assays should be performed every other day until the progesterone level is greater than 2 ng/mL, at which point breeding should begin and continue every other day for at least two or three breedings. Vaginal cytology should be evaluated concurrently with the progesterone assays to ensure that cornification progresses to 80% to 100%. Following vaginal cytology throughout the breeding period is suggested to identify the onset of diestrus, and at least one additional progesterone assay is suggested to be sure that concentrations continue to rise.

STAGING THE FELINE ESTROUS CYCLE

Female cats (queens) are seasonally polyestrous. Coitus is necessary for ovulation, and successive estrous periods occur in the absence of ovulation. The mean duration of estrus is about 8 days (range 3 to 16 days). The average interval between estrous periods is 9 days (range 4 to 22 days) if ovulation does not occur. Ovulation and the subsequent pseudopregnancy delay the return to estrus for about 45 days. Vaginal smears may be examined to accurately detect estrus in cats.[12-16] Ovulation may be induced while obtaining cells for vaginal cytologic preparations.

Vaginal cytologic characteristics of the queen are similar to those of the bitch; the differences are outlined below.

Proestrus

Proestrus is usually difficult to detect because queens do not typically have a vaginal discharge as observed in the bitch.[2] Duration of proestrus is short (0.5 to 2 days).[17] Erythrocytes and leukocytes are not usually present on cytologic samples, but clearing of the background mucus is seen on vaginal smears because of increasing estrogen levels prior to the onset of estrus. Epithelial cells consist of a mixture of intermediate and nucleated superficial cells, with low numbers of parabasal cells and anuclear superficial cells.[16]

Estrus

Epithelial cells become progressively cornified as serum estrogen levels rise above 20 picogram per milliliter (pg/mL) during estrus.[16] The proportion of anuclear superficial cells increases to greater than10% on the first day of

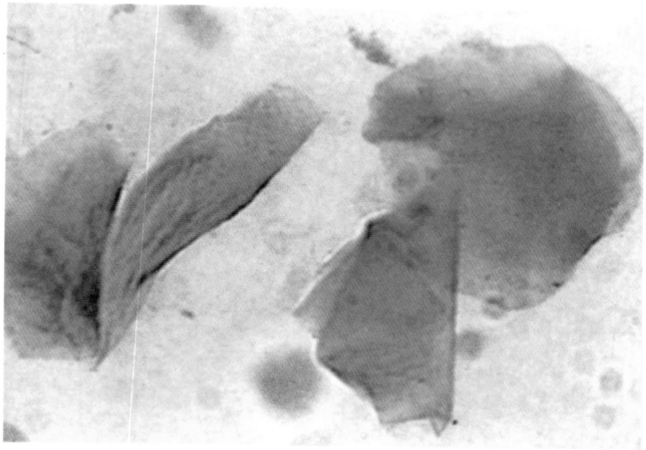

Figure 25-18 **Vaginal smear from a cat in estrus.** Note the anuclear superficial epithelial cells with folded angular cytoplasm. (Wright stain. Original magnification 400×.)

estrus. By the fourth day of estrus, about 40% of the cells are anuclear superficial cells, whereas intermediate cell numbers decrease to less than 10% (Figure 25-18).[16] Numbers of anuclear superficial cells remain relatively constant during the remainder of estrus, ranging from 40% to 60% of the total. Neutrophils and parabasal cells are absent during estrus. It has been suggested that the pronounced clearing of the background mucus and debris on vaginal smears obtained during estrus may be the most sensitive indicator of estrogen activity in cats.[16]

Interestrous Period and Diestrus

Estrus is followed by the interestrous period (if no ovulation occurs) or diestrus (if ovulation occurs). As estrus ends, background debris and parabasal cells reappear on vaginal smears. Anuclear superficial cell numbers decrease, and the majority of cells are a mixture of intermediate and nucleated superficial cells. Low numbers of neutrophils are occasionally present.[16]

Anestrus

Vaginal cytology during anestrus is similar to that of the interestrous period. Epithelial cells are predominantly intermediate, with up to 40% nucleated superficial cells and about 10% parabasal cells.[17,18]

CYTOLOGIC CHARACTERISTICS OF VAGINITIS AND METRITIS

Cytologic samples obtained from animals with inflammation of the vagina or uterus are characterized by large numbers of neutrophils (Figure 25-19). If a bacterial infection is the cause, neutrophils often show degenerative changes (swollen, pale nuclei with loss of segmentation) and may contain phagocytized bacteria. Cytologic samples from bitches in early diestrus also contain many neutrophils and may contain bacteria that may occasionally be phagocytized by neutrophils.[5] Thus, vaginal smears from early diestrus may resemble those from bitches with vaginal or uterine inflammation; however, the number of neutrophils in smears from normal bitches in diestrus markedly decreases by 1 week postestrus. Mucus and a few macrophages and lymphocytes may be seen in cases of chronic vaginitis (Figure 25-20).[5]

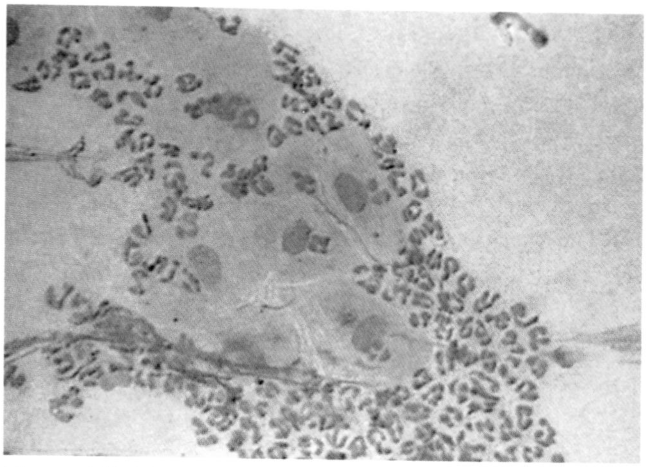

Figure 25-19 Large numbers of neutrophils and intermediate epithelial cells from a puppy with vaginitis. (Wright stain. Original magnification 100×.)

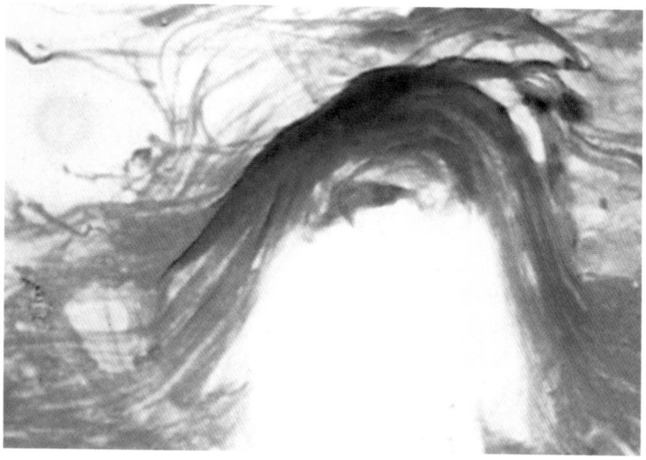

Figure 25-20 Mucus in a vaginal smear from a bitch with a chronic vulvar discharge. (Wright stain. Original magnification 400×.)

Vaginitis is often caused by noninfectious factors (e.g., vaginal anomalies, clitoral hypertrophy, foreign bodies, or vaginal immaturity), in which case nondegenerate neutrophils will be present. Epithelial intracytoplasmic inclusions that are morphologically similar to *Chlamydia* or *Mycoplasma* spp. have been observed in bitches with vaginitis, but their significance is not known (Figure 25-21). Vaginal smears from animals with pyometra or metritis usually contain large numbers of degenerate neutrophils, and bacteria are frequently observed (Figure 25-22). Muscle fibers from decomposing fetuses may rarely be seen in bitches with metritis secondary to dystocia (Figure 25-23).

CYTOLOGIC CHARACTERISTICS OF NEOPLASIA

Neoplasia of the urinary and reproductive tracts may occasionally be diagnosed by cytologic examination of vaginal smears, although direct aspiration of the mass is

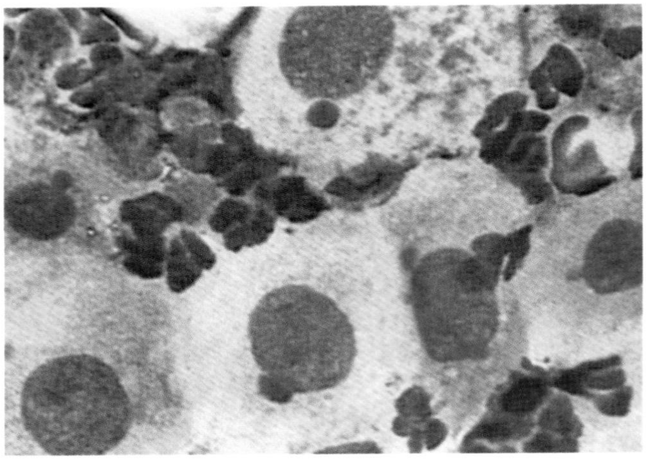

Figure 25-21 Basophilic intracytoplasmic inclusions in epithelial cells in a vaginal smear from a bitch with vaginitis. (Wright stain. Original magnification 400×.)

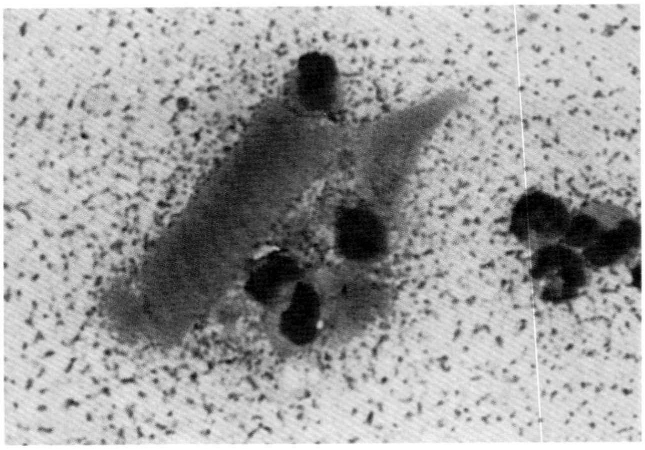

Figure 25-23 Neutrophils and muscle fibers from decomposing puppies in a vaginal smear from a bitch with a herniated uterus and metritis. (Wright stain. Original magnification 400×.)

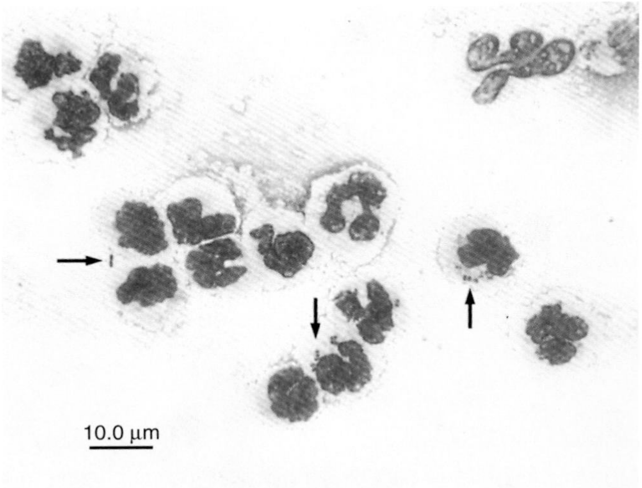

Figure 25-22 Degenerate neutrophils and bacteria *(arrows)* in a vaginal smear from a bitch with metritis. (Wright stain. Original magnification 1000×.)

often more useful. The most common vaginal tumors in dogs are of smooth muscle or fibrous tissue origin (leiomyoma, fibroma, and leiomyosarcoma), which do not exfoliate cells readily and so are not generally recognized with routine vaginal cytology.[19,20] If directly aspirated, cytologic samples from benign tumors will contain fairly uniform cells with round to oval nuclei and relatively abundant spindled cytoplasm, present individually or in aggregates. Aspirates from sarcomas will contain similar cells, but with prominent pleomorphism and other criteria of malignancy (Figure 25-24).

Canine transmissible venereal tumors (TVTs) may be diagnosed by vaginal cytology or direct mass aspiration. These contagious tumors are sexually transmitted and occur not only on genitalia but also in other locations (oral and nasal cavity, rectum, skin, subcutaneous tissue).[21] The malignant cells are discrete round cells containing round nuclei with stippled to coarse chromatin and often prominent nucleoli. They have a moderate amount of pale basophilic cytoplasm, which usually contains multiple clear, punctate vacuoles (Figure 25-25). Because these tumors are frequently ulcerated and inflamed, variable numbers of neutrophils, macrophages, and lymphocytes may also be present on cytologic samples.[21]

Vaginal carcinomas are less common, but sometimes result from extension of urinary tract carcinomas into the vagina or vestibule (Figure 25-26 and Figure 25-27). These carcinomas may be of transitional cell or squamous cell origin because the distal portion of the canine urethra is lined by modified squamous epithelium.[22] In one report of seven dogs with urinary tract carcinomas involving the vagina or vestibule, six dogs had vaginal smears performed and neoplastic epithelial cells were identified in all six samples.[23]

Cytologic features of vaginal carcinomas are the same as those occurring in other locations; see discussion of cell types and criteria of malignancy in Chapter 2 and cutaneous carcinomas in Chapter 5.

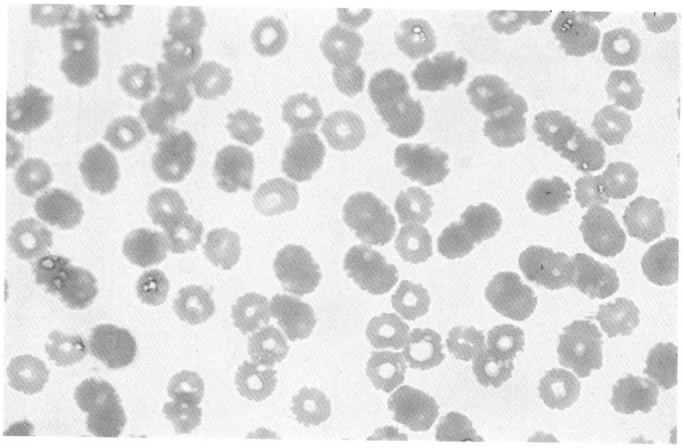

Figure 26-3 This blood film was inadequately dried before staining. The punched out, unstained regions in the red blood cells are a result of moisture interfering with the contact between cells and stain. (Diff-Quik stain. Original magnification 250×.)

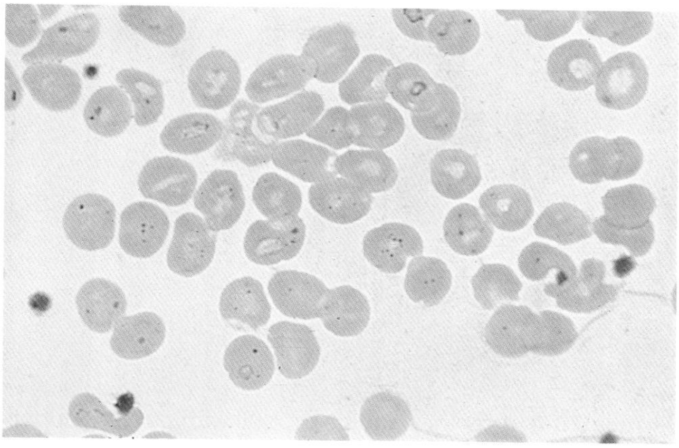

Figure 26-4 Drying artifact. The eosin component of the Diff-Quik stain has precipitated around red blood cell areas that were inadequately dried. This artifact could be mistaken for erythroparasites, cytoplasmic inclusions, or basophilic stippling. (Diff-Quik stain. Original magnification 330×.)

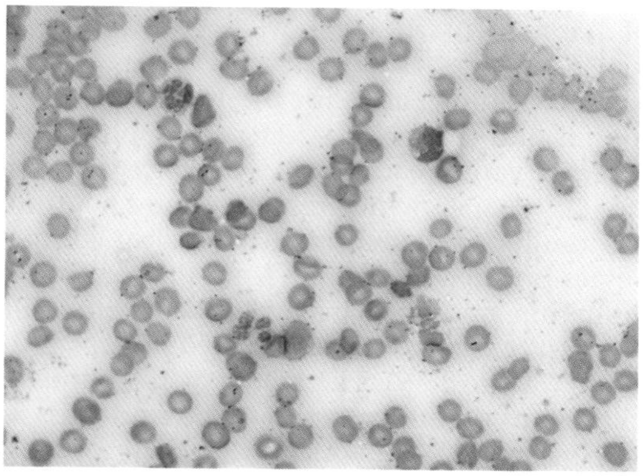

Figure 26-5 Erythrocytes showing a pale, hazy, and basophilic appearance characteristic of formalin fume exposure. (Wright stain, original magnification 100×.) (Photo courtesy of Dr. Amy Valenciano.)

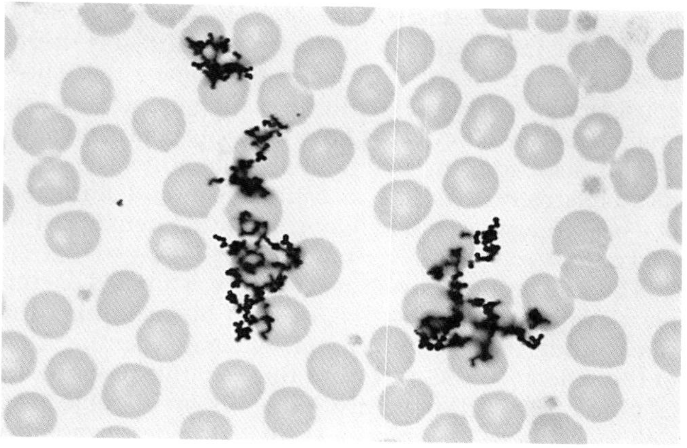

Figure 26-6 The granular stain precipitate appears in and out of the plane of focus for the smear. The precipitate formed as a result of insufficient washing of Wright stain after buffer application. The granular precipitate that forms in the stain during storage may also be deposited on blood smears. The latter may be prevented by filtering the stain before use. (Wright stain. Original magnification 330×.)

Stain Precipitate: Stain precipitate is more often a problem with Wright stains than with quick stains. Wright stain will precipitate in storage, if incubated on a slide too long, or if insufficiently washed from a slide after incubation. Precipitate formed during storage and from insufficient washing occurs as random aggregates of spherical and dumbbell-shaped granules that appear both in and out of the smear's plane of focus (Figure 26-6). With prolonged incubation time, stain precipitate appears throughout the smear as uniformly dispersed, irregular globules of stain. Precipitate formed during storage may be removed by filtering the stain through Whatman filter paper into clean vials.

BLOOD SMEAR EVALUATION

Smears should be initially examined from the thickest region to the feathered edge using the 10× or 20× objective. At this low magnification, blood films may be checked for staining, overall thickness, smooth transitions in thickness, cell distribution, and adequacy of the monolayer area. The monolayer is generally found within the distal half of the smear adjacent to the feathered edge and is luminescent when the unstained slide is held under indirect light. The monolayer represents the limited region where cell morphology is most reliably evaluated. WBCs should be fairly uniformly distributed within this region and only mildly clustered along the feathered edge. Examination of the borders, especially the feathered edge of the smear under low magnification, may demonstrate the presence of platelet aggregates, microfilaria, large atypical cells, or cells with phagocytized organisms.

A rough approximation of the patient's hematocrit may be obtained by examining a blood smear at low magnification. Blood films from nonanemic animals generally have RBCs that are closely apposed in the monolayer as well as several RBC layers at the thick end of the smear that obstruct penetrance of most condenser light. In contrast, smears from animals that are moderately to markedly anemic usually have RBCs that are widely separated from one another in the monolayer and only one or two RBC layers in the thick end of the smear that allow considerable condenser light to penetrate. Unless the angle between slides was adjusted during smear preparation of hemoconcentrated samples, the monolayer occupies a relatively reduced area. Estimates should ultimately be checked against the patient's measured hematocrit or packed-cell volume.

The WBC count may also be roughly estimated or simply classified as low, normal, or high by examining the smear under low magnification. Accurate identification of the different WBC types and their relative proportions is more easily performed using the 40× or 50× objective. Cell morphology is typically evaluated under magnifications of 40× to 100×; platelet number and morphology are assessed at the highest of these magnification levels.

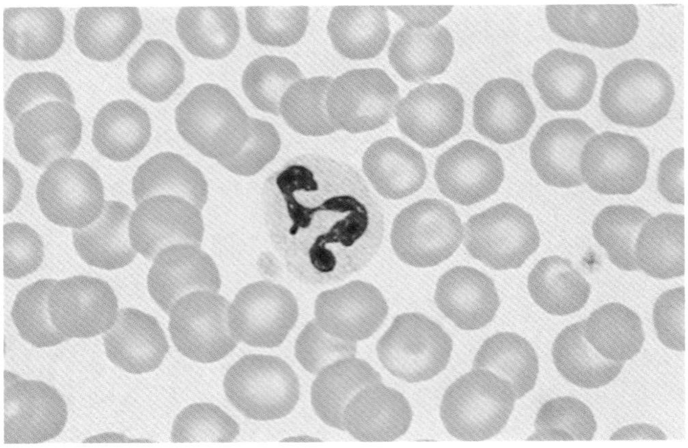

Figure 26-7 A canine neutrophil with pale, eosinophilic cytoplasm and a lobulated nucleus containing mostly dense heterochromatin. (Wright stain. Original magnification 330×.)

NORMAL CELL COMPONENTS OF BLOOD

Red Blood Cells

RBC morphology is primarily evaluated within the monolayer where artifactual distortion induced during preparation and differences in smear thickness are less apt to influence cell appearance. Nearly all significant morphologic abnormalities of RBCs may be detected at 40× or 50× magnification, although some alterations may require additional examination at higher magnification. Initial examination of RBC morphology with the 100× objective, however, often results in overdiagnosis of aberrations.

Mature RBCs in healthy adult dogs are about 7 micrometers (μm) in diameter (slightly larger than the 5.5- to 6.0-μm diameter of feline RBCs). As is apparent in the monolayer of blood smears, canine RBCs are biconcave with an area of central pallor occupying about one third of the cell's diameter. Feline RBCs do not consistently have discernible central pallor and tend to vary slightly more in shape than canine RBCs. Both species have mild RBC anisocytosis and may show an occasional immature polychromatophilic cell on peripheral blood smears.

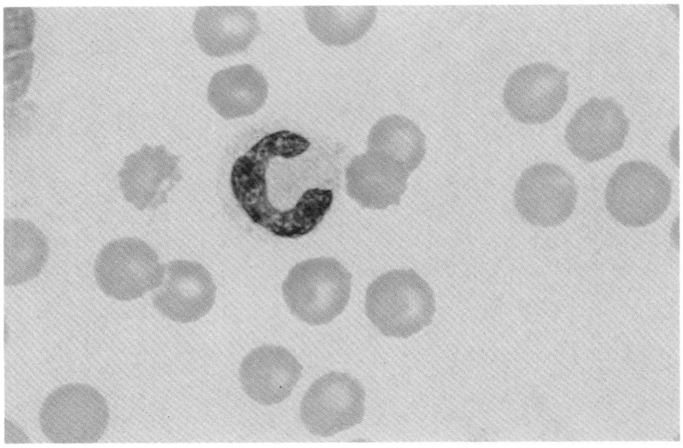

Figure 26-8 A canine band neutrophil with pale eosinophilic cytoplasm that is similar to a mature cell and a U-shaped nucleus lacking distinct segmentation. (Wright stain. Original magnification 330×.)

White Blood Cells

Neutrophils: Canine and feline neutrophils have similar appearance on blood films (Figure 26-7). The neutrophil nucleus is elongate and separated into multiple lobules by invaginations of the nuclear border. Demarcations between lobules are seldom distinct enough to be considered filamentous. Chromatin is organized into dense clumps of dark purple to black staining heterochromatin separated by narrow areas of less condensed euchromatin. Cytoplasm is clear, pale eosinophilic to faintly basophilic with a fine grainy texture and, rarely, contains one or two small vacuoles. Neutrophil granules range from indiscernible to faintly eosinophilic but are pale and much smaller than the prominent granules of mature eosinophils.

Band Neutrophils: Band neutrophils, low numbers of which occur in the peripheral blood of healthy dogs and cats, have an elongate, U- or J-shaped to slightly twisted nucleus with less chromatin condensation compared with mature neutrophils (Figure 26-8). Nuclear lobulation is absent or poorly defined. Constrictions of canine band neutrophil nuclei are less than half the width of the remainder (nonconstricted sections) of the nucleus; feline band neutrophils lack nuclear constrictions entirely. Cytoplasm is similar in granule content and staining to that of mature neutrophils.

Monocytes: Canine and feline monocytes are larger than neutrophils and similar in size to eosinophils and basophils. Nuclei vary greatly in morphology, ranging from elongate "U" shapes, which resemble band neutrophils to irregular multilobulated forms. The nuclear chromatin of monocytes is generally distinct from that of both mature and immature granulocytes and is characteristically lacy to ropy with only a few small isolated clumps of heterochromatin (Figure 26-9). The moderate to abundant gray-blue cytoplasm of monocytes has a ground-glass texture, is often sparsely dusted with minute eosinophilic granules, and occasionally contains vacuoles. Cytoplasmic borders are usually irregular, sometimes with fine, filamentous, pseudopodia-like extensions. Because of their relatively large size, monocytes may be concentrated

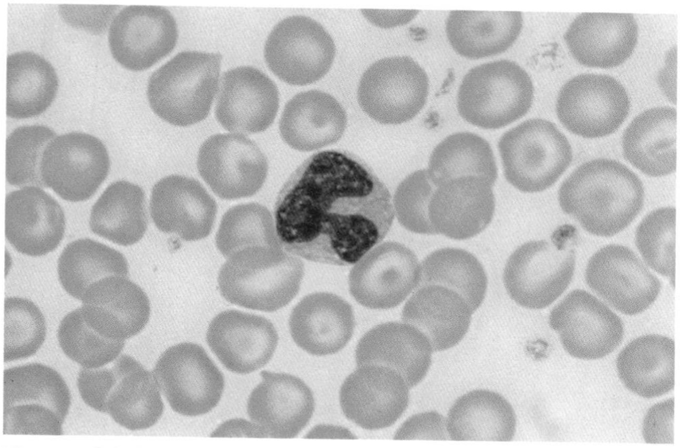

Figure 26-9 This canine monocyte has an irregular nucleus with a ropey chromatin pattern and grainy basophilic cytoplasm. (Wright stain. Original magnification 330×.)

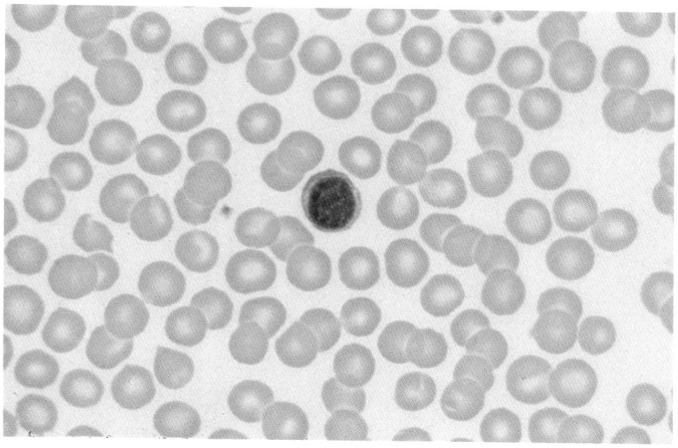

Figure 26-10 A canine lymphocyte with densely clumped nuclear chromatin and scant basophilic cytoplasm. (Wright stain. Original magnification 330×.)

along the feathered edge, and their proportion underestimated in blood smear differential WBC counts.

Lymphocytes: Lymphocytes vary in size in the peripheral blood of dogs and cats, with small cells predominating. Small lymphocytes have densely staining, round to oval nuclei that are sometimes slightly indented and usually have large, well-defined chromatin clumps (Figure 26-10). Alternatively, nuclear chromatin may appear smudged, especially when stained with a quick stain. The moderately blue cytoplasm of small lymphocytes is scant, and cytoplasmic borders are partially obscured by the nuclei, particularly with feline lymphocytes. Larger lymphocytes in peripheral blood have less densely staining, but still clearly clumped, nuclear chromatin. Cytoplasm of the larger cells is more abundant and ranges from light to moderately basophilic. Some lymphocytes have a few variably sized eosinophilic cytoplasmic granules that are usually concentrated within a single perinuclear cell area (Figure 26-11).

Eosinophils: Eosinophils, which are slightly larger than neutrophils, may usually be found in very low numbers

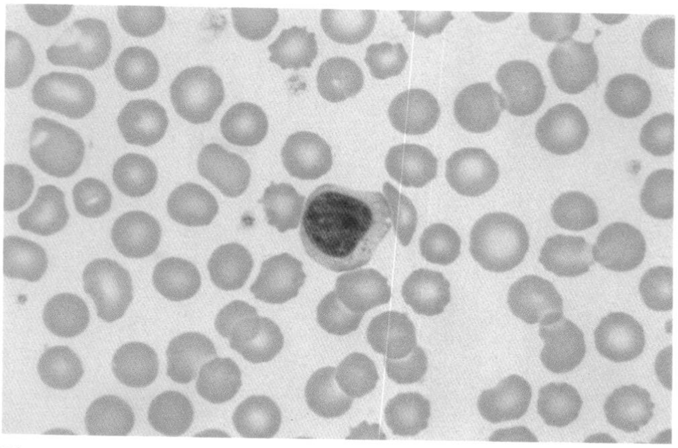

Figure 26-11 **A large granular lymphocyte in a healthy dog.** Both canine and feline lymphocytes occasionally contain a few eosinophilic granules in a moderate amount of homogeneous basophilic cytoplasm. (Wright stain. Original magnification 330×.)

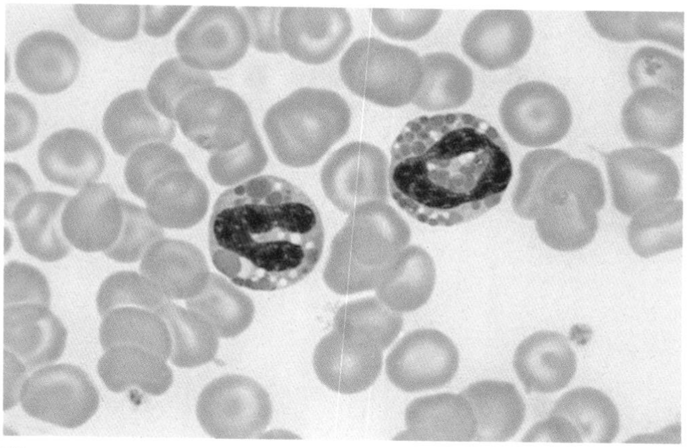

Figure 26-12 Two canine eosinophils, one of which has partially degranulated cytoplasm. Eosinophil nuclei are less condensed and lobulated than those of neutrophils. (Wright stain. Original magnification 330×.)

on blood smears of healthy dogs and cats. Nuclei are less lobulated (often being divided into only two distinct lobules) with less condensed chromatin (Figure 26-12) than those of mature neutrophils. Cytoplasm is clear to faintly basophilic and contains prominent pink granules, which are abundant, small, and rod-shaped in cats (Figure 26-13) but vary widely in number and size in dogs. Canine eosinophils occasionally contain a single, large granule that may be mistaken for an inclusion body or unusual organism (Figure 26-14). Eosinophils of Greyhounds are peculiar in that they may appear vacuolated on smears—a breed difference that has been attributed to differential staining properties of the specific granules (Figure 26-15).[10] Eosinophil granules that are ruptured in vitro are also sometimes freely scattered in the background of canine and feline blood smears.

Basophils: Basophils are the largest of the mature granulocytic cell types and rare in peripheral blood of healthy dogs and cats. Nuclei are less densely staining and have fewer lobulations and a more elongated, ribbon-like

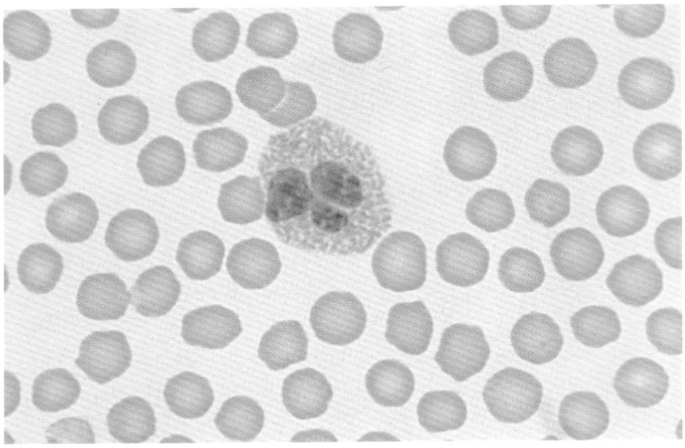

Figure 26-13 A feline eosinophil with small, rod-shaped, eosinophilic granules filling the cytoplasm and partially obscuring the nucleus. (Wright stain. Original magnification 330×.)

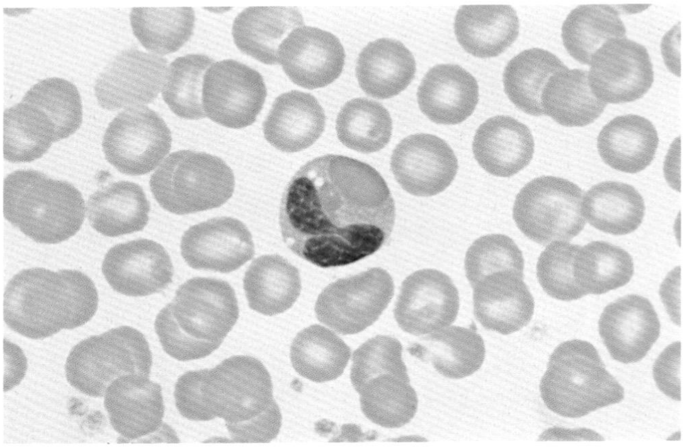

Figure 26-14 A canine eosinophil with only two large cytoplasmic granules. (Wright stain. Original magnification 330×.)

appearance than the nuclei of other granulocytic cell types (Figure 26-16). Cytoplasm is moderately blue-gray to slightly purple and usually contains granules. In dogs, basophil granules are usually low in number and stain dark blue to metachromatic. Canine basophils also occasionally lack obvious granules but are recognizable by their size, nuclear morphology, and cytoplasmic staining (Figure 26-17). In cats, basophils contain abundant oval, pale lavender to gray specific granules (Figure 26-18), although immature basophils may also contain a few primary, dark purple granules.

Platelets

Canine and feline platelets appear oval, round, or rod shaped on peripheral blood smears. Their clear to pale gray cytoplasm usually contains a central cluster of eosinophilic to metachromatic granules. Platelets normally vary in size from about one fourth to two thirds of the diameter of RBCs in canine blood, and occasionally are even larger than the RBCs in feline blood. These larger platelets may be noted as macroplatelets in hematology reports. Partially activated platelets have a spider-like

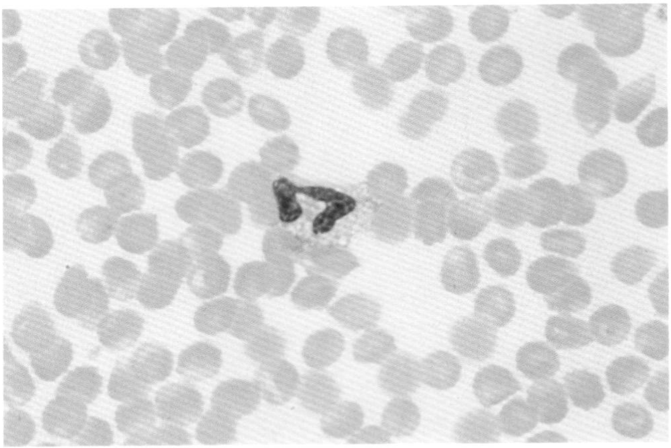

Figure 26-15 Vacuolated appearing "grey" eosinophil from a Greyhound. (Wright stain. Original magnification 100×.) (From *Hematology atlas of the dog and cat*; slide courtesy of Dr. Theresa Rizzi at Oklahoma state; image courtesy of Dr. Amy Valenciano.)

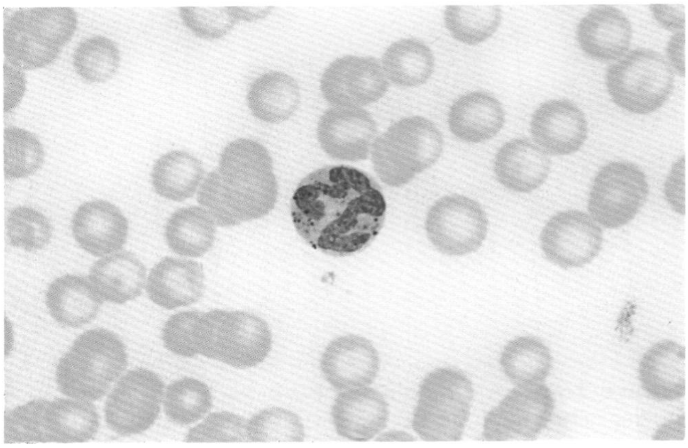

Figure 26-16 A canine basophil with metachromatic granules scattered in the cytoplasm. (Wright stain. Original magnification 250×.)

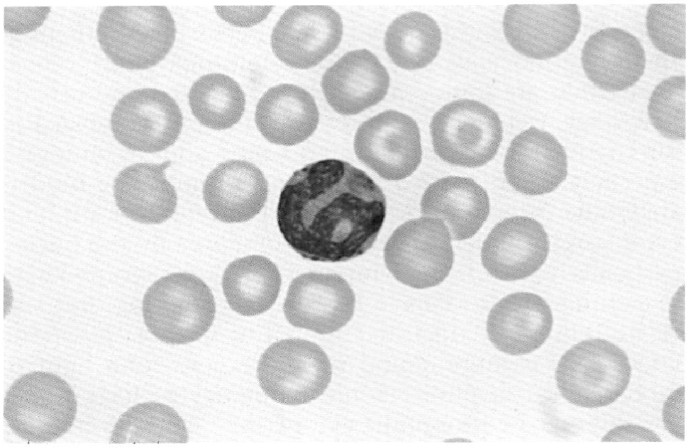

Figure 26-17 A poorly granulated canine basophil, which may be identified as such by its size, ribbonlike nuclear shape, and cytoplasmic staining, despite the near absence of cytoplasmic granules. (Wright stain. Original magnification 330×.)

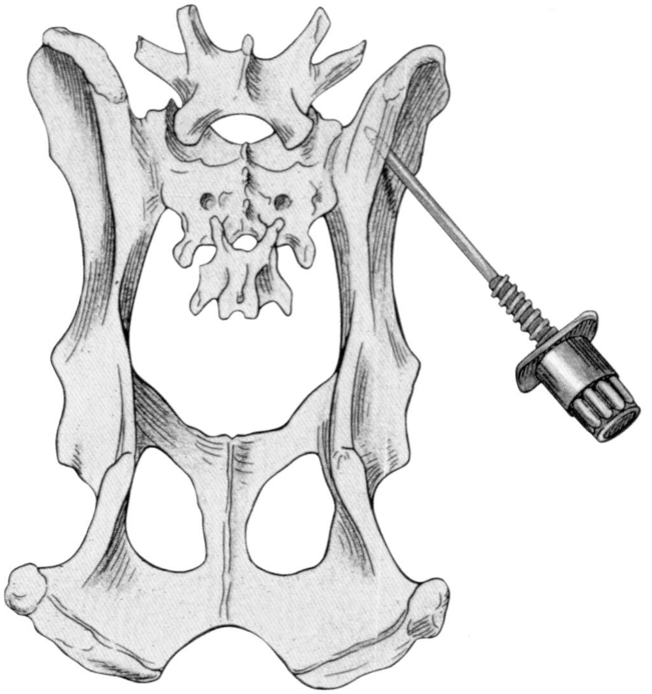

Figure 27-4 Bone marrow biopsy site for the wing of the ilium. For small dogs and cats the lateral approach to the wing of the ilium is a good location for core biopsies. (Reprinted with permission from Grindem CB: Bone marrow biopsy and evaluation, *Vet Clin Small Anim* 19[4]:673-4, 1989).

Smear Preparation with EDTA: If EDTA or isotonic saline is used, once the marrow sample is collected, the plunger is released to relieve the negative pressure, and the needle is detached from the syringe. The stylet is replaced in the needle, and the needle remains embedded in the bone. The contents of the syringe are thoroughly mixed, and the anticoagulated marrow sample is expelled into a watch glass or clear Petri dish. If the sample does not contain marrow flecks, the needle is repositioned by slight advancement and rotation. The stylet is removed, another syringe containing EDTA or saline solution is attached, and the aspiration procedure is repeated. After two or three aspiration attempts, or when marrow flecks are recovered, the needle is removed.

Marrow samples collected in EDTA or isotonic saline solution and expelled into a Petri dish are prepared as follows. The Petri dish is tilted, rotated, or both under a soft light so that the marrow flecks are seen and distinguished from fat droplets. Marrow flecks are clear to slightly opaque and light gray; fat droplets are clear and glisten. Marrow flecks may be slightly irregular in shape; fat droplets are spherical. Generally, marrow flecks are easily located if an adequate sample has been collected.

Flecks are transferred from the sample in the Petri dish to glass microscope slides by tilting the Petri dish, causing the sample to drain to one side of the dish. Some flecks cling to the bottom of the Petri dish, and the fluid portion of the sample drains away from them. These flecks are harvested with a microhematocrit capillary tube, one end of which is touched to the side of the fleck. Often the fleck is partially aspirated into the capillary tube and is transferred to the glass microscope slide. If the fleck does not partially aspirate into the capillary tube, the tube is

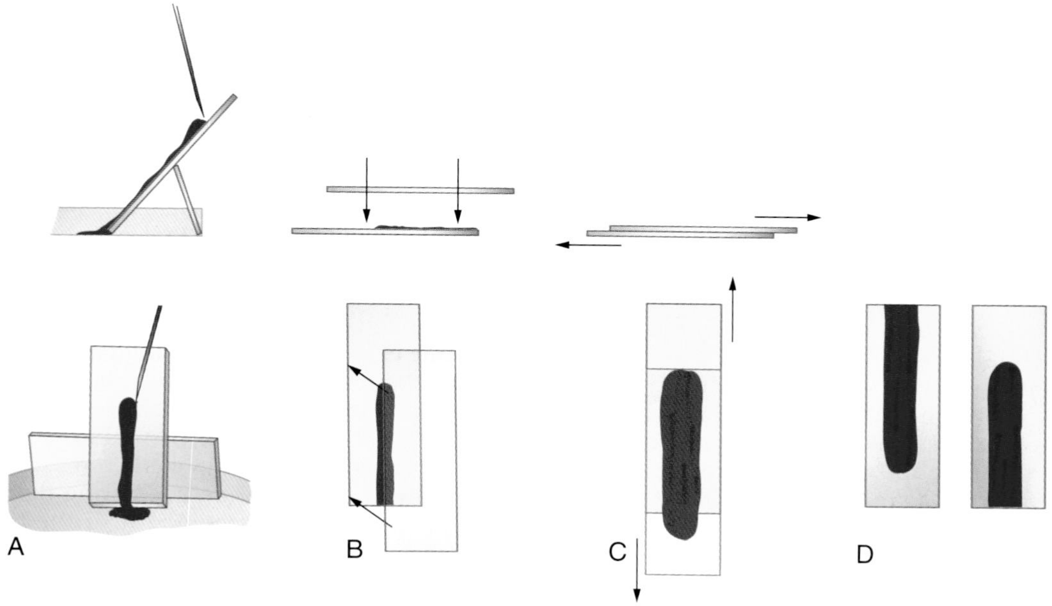

Figure 27-5 Smear preparation for bone marrow aspirates not collected in ethylenediaminetetraacetic acid (EDTA) or isotonic saline solution. **A,** Some of the aspirate is expelled onto a tilted glass microscope slide. The slide is propped up with another glass slide braced against the side of a Petri dish. Marrow flecks tend to adhere to the slide as the marrow runs down it. **B,** Another glass slide is placed over the slide containing the aspirate, which spreads the aspirate. **C,** The two slides are slid apart. **D,** This produces two preparations.

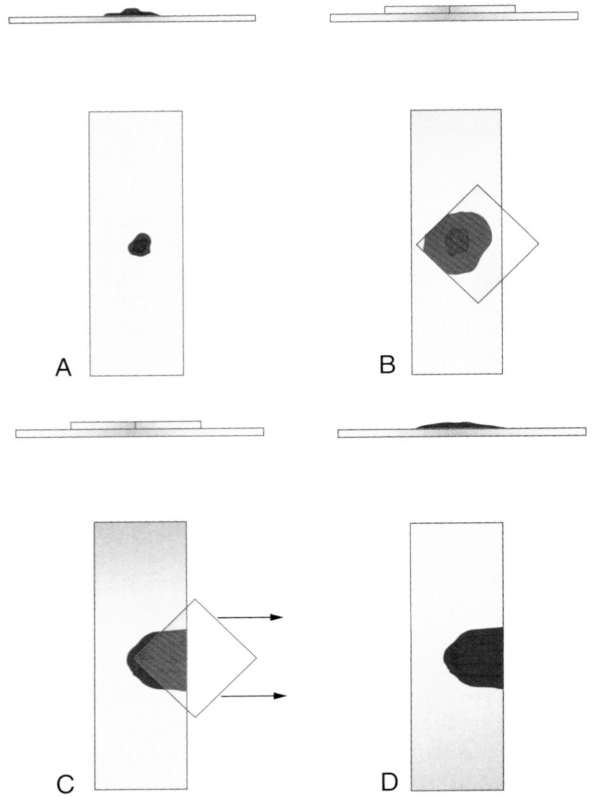

Figure 27-6 Smear preparation for bone marrow aspirates collected in ethylenediaminetetraacetic acid (EDTA) or isotonic saline solution. A, A fleck, collected from the Petri dish containing the sample, is placed on a glass microscope slide. **B,** A microscope slide coverslip is placed over the fleck at a 45-degree angle to the slide. This spreads the fleck and accompanying fluid. **C,** The coverslip is slid horizontally and smoothly off the glass slide. **D,** Both the glass microscope slide preparation and coverslip preparation are used. However, the coverslip preparation is usually hard to handle during staining and is often discarded. Multiple preparations are made on a glass slide, and multiple slides are prepared.

gently advanced, forcing the fleck into it. The marrow fleck is then transferred onto the glass microscope slide by tapping the capillary tube end containing the fleck on the slide. Any excessive fluid transferred is removed by touching the fluid with a piece of absorbent paper or cloth.

After the fleck is transferred to the glass microscope slide, a 22- × 22-millimeter (mm) coverslip is placed over the fleck at a 45-degree angle to the glass microscope slide, allowing one corner of the coverslip to hang over the edge of the microscope slide (Figure 27-6). When the coverslip is placed over the fleck, the fleck spreads to about twice its previous size. Some smears should be made without any pressure other than that caused by the coverslip, and others should be made with gentle thumb pressure sufficient to cause the smears to spread to about twice the diameter caused by coverslip pressure alone. This ensures that some of the flecks are spread optimally.

Excessive pressure, which causes cell rupture, is the most common error when preparing cytologic smears of marrow flecks. When making smears from marrow samples in EDTA or isotonic saline solution, using another glass microscope slide instead of a coverslip to spread the fleck may cause excessive pressure and result in rupture of nucleated cells.

If the smears do not have adequate cellularity, the EDTA specimen is placed into a Wintrobe or small tube and centrifuged, the buffy coat harvested, and additional squash preps made.

Core Biopsy

Core biopsies are collected with a Jamshidi infant (cats and small dogs) or pediatric (large dogs) marrow biopsy needle. The same procedure, as described for collecting marrow aspirate biopsies, is used for collecting core biopsies; however, in this case, after the point of the needle has penetrated the cortex of the bone and entered the marrow cavity, the stylet is removed from the needle and the needle is advanced about 3 mm with a rotating motion.[7,8,10,11,14-16] This cuts and collects a core of bone marrow. The needle is removed from the animal, and the core of marrow is forced onto a glass microscope slide by passing the stylet through the barrel of the needle from the hub end or retrograde from the needle end if the biopsy needle is tapered.

Using the point of the needle, the core of marrow is gently rolled the length of the microscope slide. After making one or two slide preparations in this manner, the core of marrow is placed in a container filled with 10% neutral buffered formalin.[17] If the cytologic preparations are to be sent to an outside laboratory, they should not be mailed with the formalin-filled container because formalin vapors alter the cells' staining qualities.

COLLECTING MARROW SAMPLES FROM DEAD ANIMALS

Bone marrow samples are occasionally collected from dead animals. If a complete evaluation of the marrow is expected, the samples must be collected and the cytologic preparations made immediately (within 30 minutes) after the animal's death. When collection, preparation, or both are delayed, the preparations are evaluated for cellularity, organisms, mast cell infiltration, plasmacytosis, erythrophagocytosis, and iron-containing pigments, but they should not be evaluated for myeloid or lymphoid neoplasia. Delay in sample preparation may result in rupture of all of the cells.

Although samples are collected from most flat bones and the extremities of most long bones of dead animals, it is advisable to collect marrow samples from the same location(s) used in live animals (see Figures 27-2, 27-3, and 27-4). It should be kept in mind that in adults, the central areas of long bones contain mostly fat. Access to the marrow may be gained by sawing the bone, cutting it with rongeurs, or fracturing it. If the bone is sawed, heat generated at the saw line may damage adjacent cells; therefore, samples from sawed bones should be collected well away from the saw line. Marrow is dug from between bony trabeculae, trying to avoid collecting bone spicules. The marrow is placed on one end of a glass microscope slide and gently rolled (by lifting upward with a needle or other instrument at the back of the sample) the length of the slide. Several slides are prepared from samples

TABLE 27-1

Nucleated Erythroid Cell Developmental Stages and Their Relative Percentage, Description, and Schematic Morphology

Developmental Stage	APPROXIMATE PERCENTAGE OF CLASSIFIABLE NUCLEATED ERYTHROID CELLS OF MARROW*		Description	Morphology
	Dogs	Cats		
Rubriblast	0.5	0.5	*Cell:* large; small to moderate amount of dark blue cytoplasm *Nucleus:* large; 1–2 nucleoli; dense granular chromatin	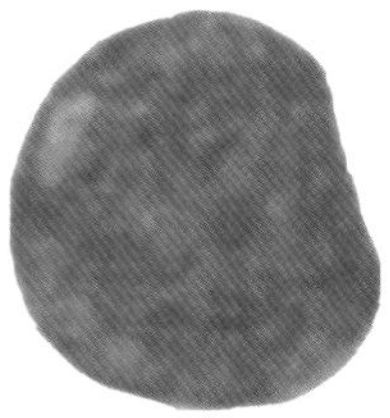
Prorubricyte	2.0	3.5	*Cell:* medium to large; moderate amount of medium to dark-blue cytoplasm *Nucleus:* medium to large; nucleoli usually not visible; coarse chromatin pattern	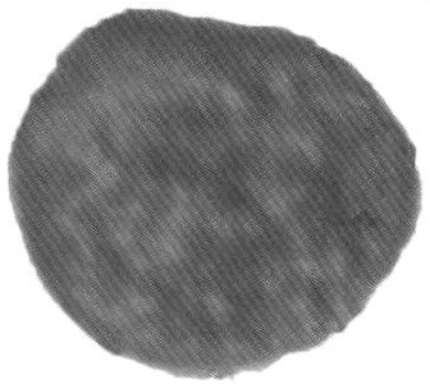
Rubricyte	65	75	*Cell:* medium to small; small to moderate amount of medium blue (basophilic) to blue-pink (polychromatophilic) to orange (orthochromic) cytoplasm *Nucleus:* medium to small; no visible nucleoli; coarse, clumped chromatin pattern with clear spaces	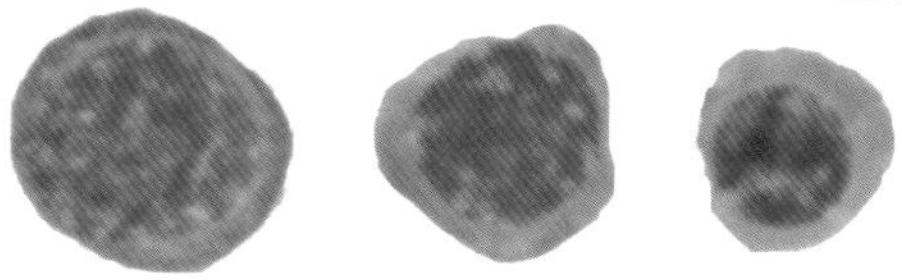
Metarubruicyte	32.5	21	*Cell:* small, small amount of blue-pink (polychromatophilic) to orange (orthochromic) cytoplasm *Nucleus:* small and pyknotic; no nucleoli visible; chromatin is densely clumped with few or no clear spaces	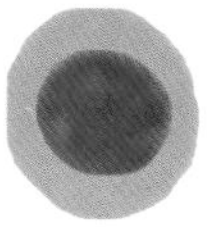

*Broad variations may occur in normal animals because of the influence of things such as the subjectivity of cell classification and normal variation among individuals.

collected from several different areas of the bone marrow. The slides are air-dried and stained as described later.

STAINING MARROW PREPARATIONS

After fleck smears or core biopsy or necropsy imprints are made, they are air-dried. The general Romanowsky-type staining procedures for staining blood smears are followed, except the stains and buffers are left in contact with the cells for a longer time. The extent to which the times must be lengthened depends on the thickness and cell density of the smears, but staining times must usually be increased two times or more. Macroscopically, the marrow fleck streaks in the smear appear blue-purple to purple when the smear is properly stained.

CELLS IN MARROW

To evaluate bone marrow preparations, one must be able to recognize the normal cells that occur in bone marrow, the neoplastic cells that have a propensity for infiltrating bone marrow, the organisms that can infect the marrow, and the processes (e.g., erythrophagia) that occur in some pathologic conditions.[7-12, 16,18]

Erythroid Series

During proliferation and maturation, erythroid progenitor cells undergo four to five mitoses, producing 16 to 32 daughter cells. As they mature, erythroid cells decrease in size, their nuclei condense, and their cytoplasm changes from dark blue to red-orange. The general characteristics of the different cell stages of erythroid production

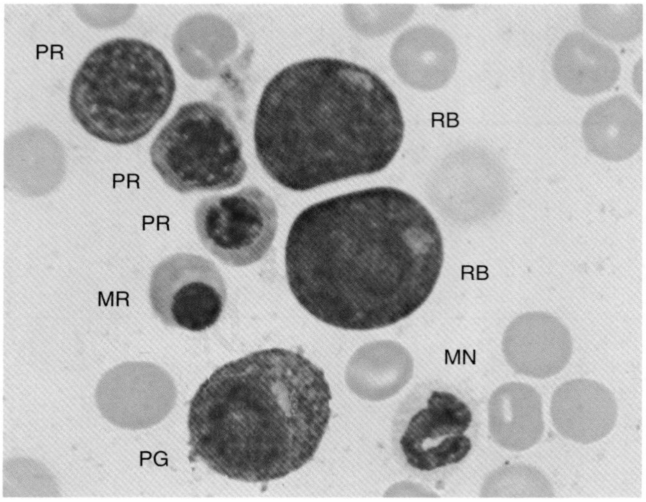

Figure 27-7 Bone marrow aspirate. Rubriblasts (*RB*), polychromatophilic rubricytes (*PR*), metarubricyte (*MR*), progranulocyte (*PG*), and mature neutrophil (*MN*) are indicated. (Wright-Giemsa stain. Original magnification 250×.)

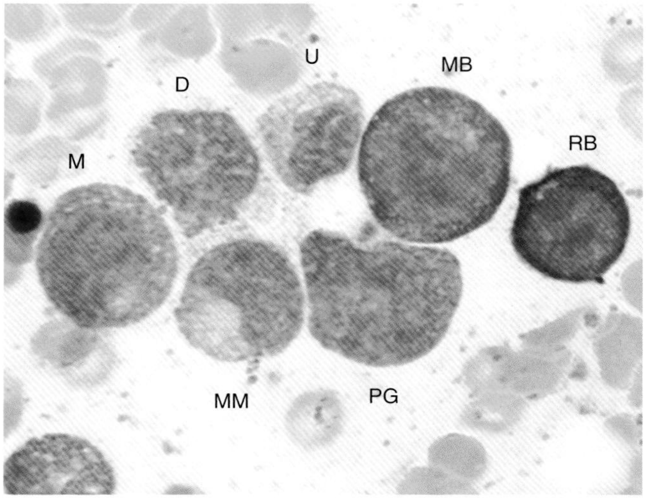

Figure 27-8 Bone marrow aspirate. Rubriblast (*RB*), myeloblast (*MB*), progranulocyte (*PG*), early myelocyte (*M*), metamyelocyte (*MM*), damaged cell nucleus (*D*), and an unidentified late stage granulocyte (*U*), most likely distorted band neutrophil, are indicated. (Wright-Giemsa stain. Original magnification 250×.)

are described later. Table 27-1 lists the different stages of erythroid development and provides an estimate of the relative proportions and a brief description and a generalized schematic of the classic morphology of each stage.

Rubriblasts: The rubriblast is the most immature identifiable erythroid cell. Its nucleus is round with a smooth nuclear border, a fine granular chromatin pattern, and one or two pale to medium blue nucleoli (Figure 27-7 and Figure 27-8). Its cytoplasm is intensely basophilic and forms a narrow rim around the nucleus. The rubriblast has the highest nucleus-to-cytoplasm (N:C) ratio of the erythroid series.

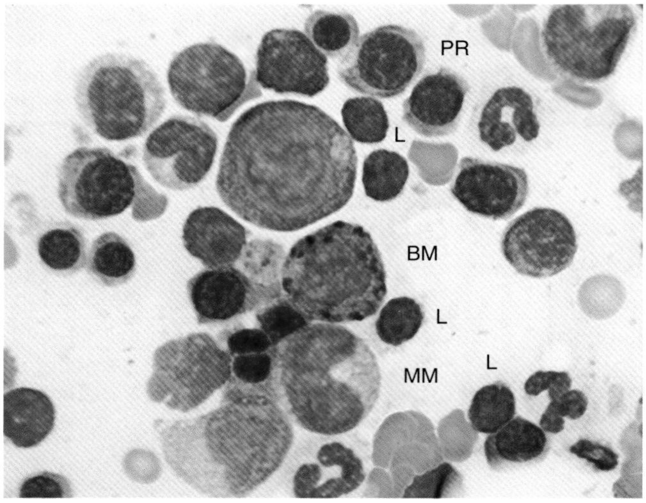

Figure 27-9 Bone marrow from a healthy cat. Small lymphocytes (*L*) are usually less than 10% of nucleated cells in the bone marrow of healthy cats. Basophilic myelocyte (*BM*), neutrophilic metamyelocyte (*MM*), polychromatophilic rubricytes (*PR*), and lymphocytes are indicated. Basophil precursors have prominent magenta to blue-black granules. Also, note that metamyelocytes may be difficult to impossible to distinguish from monocytes in the bone marrow. (Wright-Giemsa stain. Original magnification 250×.)

Prorubricytes: The next maturation stage of the erythroid series is the prorubricyte. Its nucleus is round with a smooth nuclear border and a nuclear chromatin pattern that is slightly coarser than that of the rubriblast. Nucleoli are usually not visible in the prorubricyte stage. Cytoplasm is slightly less intensely blue and forms a thicker rim around the nucleus. The N:C ratio is less than that of the rubriblast but greater than that of the rubricyte (the next stage of maturation).

Rubricytes: The next stage of erythroid maturation is the rubricyte. This stage is divided into basophilic and polychromatophilic rubricytes or sometimes divided into basophilic, polychromatophilic, and orthochromic rubricytes. The rubricyte and its nucleus are smaller than the prorubricyte and its nucleus. The rubricyte nucleus has an extremely coarse chromatin pattern that may resemble the spokes of a wheel. Cytoplasm is blue (basophilic) to bluish-red-orange (polychromic or polychromatophilic) to red-orange (orthochromic) (Figure 27-9 and Figure 27-10; see Figure 27-7). The N:C ratio is less than that of prorubricytes but greater than that of metarubricytes (the next stage of maturation). Mitosis occurs in the early rubricyte stage but ceases by the later rubricyte stages.

Metarubricytes: The next stage of erythroid development is the metarubricyte. Its nucleus is extremely pyknotic and appears black, without a distinguishable chromatin pattern (see Figure 27-7). Cytoplasm may be polychromatophilic or orthochromic.

Polychromatophilic Erythrocytes: The next stage of development is the polychromatophilic erythrocyte. In blood smears stained with Romanowsky-type stains,

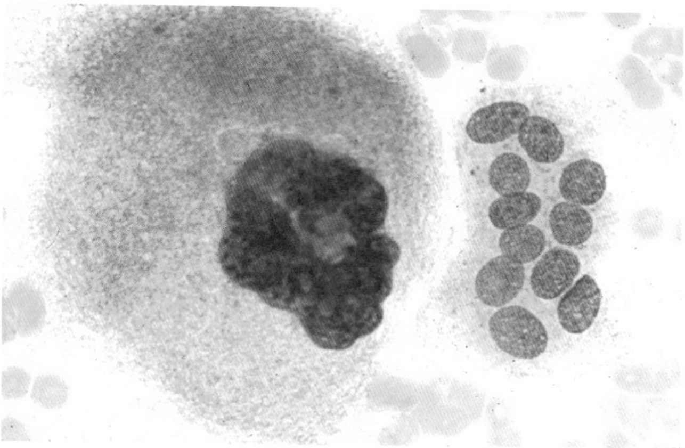

Figure 27-17 Bone marrow aspirate. Mature megakaryocyte with a condensed multilobulated nucleus and eosinophilic, granular cytoplasm on the left and a multinucleated osteoclast on the right. Osteoclasts are uncommonly seen in bone marrow aspirates and are associated with bone remodeling such as in young animals or animals with renal disease, metabolic bone disease, or neoplasia. (Wright-Giemsa stain. Original magnification 240×). (Reprinted with permission from Grindem CB: Bone marrow biopsy and evaluation, *Vet Clin Small Anim* 19[4],680, 1989.)

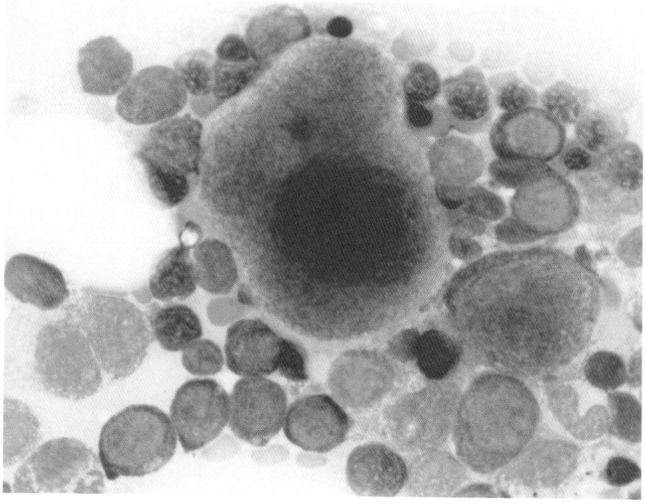

Figure 27-18 Bone marrow aspirate from a dog with megakaryocyte hyperplasia. A promegakaryocyte with two nuclei is in the lower left, an almost mature megakaryocyte with eosinophilic cytoplasm is in the center, and an immature basophilic megakaryocyte is on the right. Note the concurrent erythroid hyperplasia with left shifting (more immature precursors). (Wright-Giemsa stain. Original magnification 1000×.)

megakaryocytes that have shed their cytoplasm as platelets into the peripheral blood or megakaryocytes whose cytoplasm has been torn from their nuclei during smear preparation.

Histopathology of Megakaryocyte Series: Megakaryocytes are the largest cells encountered in the bone marrow (see Figure 27-12 and 27-13). Mature megakaryocytes have more condensed chromatin pattern and more abundant

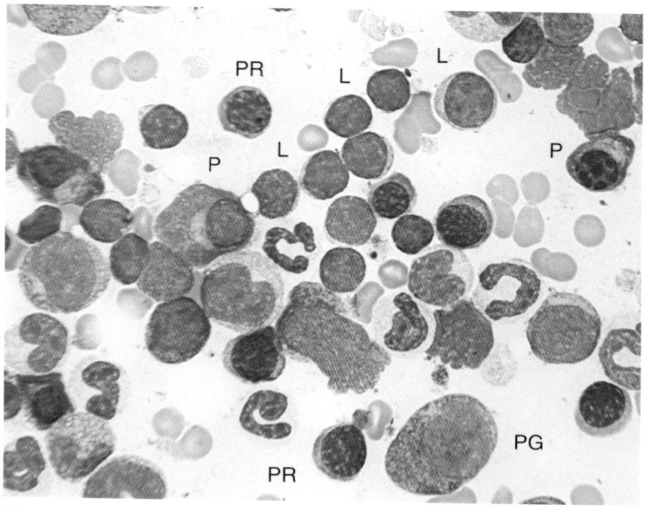

Figure 27-19 Bone marrow from a healthy cat. A focal area of numerous small lymphocytes is present. Small lymphocytes (*L*) may easily be confused with nucleated red blood cells, but small lymphocytes have scant to almost no visible cytoplasm and often a less coarsely clumped nuclear chromatin pattern. Small lymphocytes usually comprise less than 5% of nucleated bone marrow cells in healthy dogs and less than 10% in cats. Progranulocyte (*PG*), polychromatophilic rubricytes (*PR*), plasma cell (*P*), and lymphocytes are indicated. (Wright-Giemsa stain. Original magnification 250×.)

eosinophilic cytoplasm than immature megakaryocytes. Megakaryoblasts are difficult to distinguish from other blast cells. Megakaryocytes appear randomly distributed within the interstitium but, in fact, are adjacent to inconspicuous sinusoids. Generally two to four megakaryocytes per high-power magnification (40×) is regarded as adequate.[1] Since osteoclasts are another large cell identified in histologic sections, it is important to distinguish between these and megakaryocytes. Megakaryocytes will have a multilobulated nucleus, rather than the multiple small distinct nuclei in osteoclasts, and megakaryocytes will often be distributed in an interstitial or peri-sinusoidal location, rather than in the paratrabecular location of osteoclasts. Also, multinucleate inflammatory, or neoplastic giant cells may be differentiated from megakaryocytes by the "company they keep." These multinucleate cells will be associated with other inflammatory cells or neoplastic cells, rather than with hematopoietic cells.

Lymphocytes and Plasma Cells

Small lymphocytes (Figure 27-19; see Figure 27-9) are recognizably smaller than neutrophils and have a scant amount of light- to medium-blue cytoplasm and an indented but otherwise round nucleus with a dense smudged chromatin pattern without visible nucleoli. Intermediate-sized lymphocytes (often referred to as *prolymphocytes*) are about the same size as neutrophils and have a little more medium to light-blue cytoplasm compared with small lymphocytes. Their nuclei are round, other than an indentation in one area of the nucleus where the cytoplasm is most visible. The nuclear chromatin pattern appears smudged and nucleoli are rarely visible. Large lymphocytes, frequently called *lymphoblasts* when their nucleoli are prominent

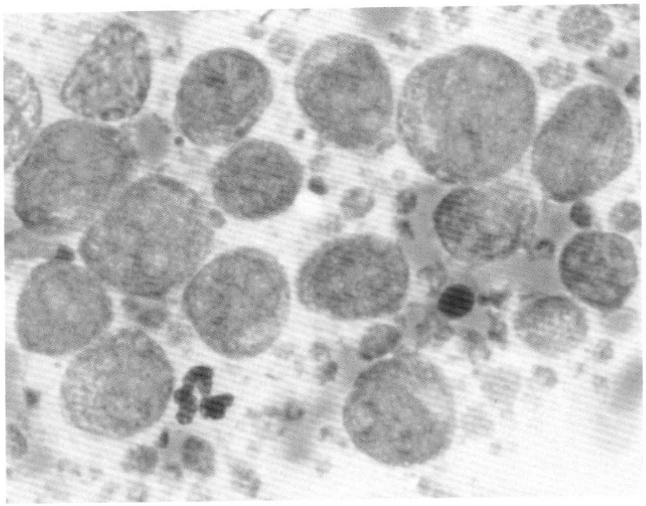

Figure 27-20 Bone marrow aspirate from a dog with lymphoma. Numerous lymphoblasts are on a pale basophilic background that contains lymphoglandular bodies. Although lymphoglandular bodies (cytoplasmic fragments) may be seen with any rapidly dividing cell population, they are most often associated with lymphoma. (Wright-Giemsa stain. Original magnification 1000×.)

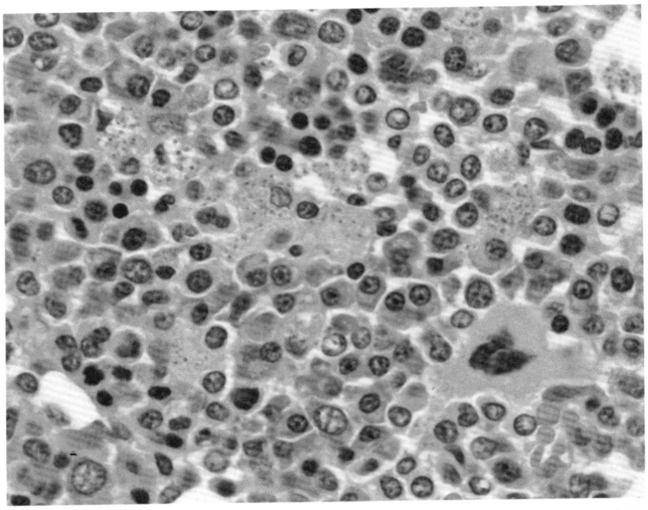

Figure 27-21 Bone marrow core biopsy from a dog with leishmaniasis. This is a hypercellular marrow with numerous macrophages containing multiple small amastigotes. Note the increased numbers of plasma cells. (H&E stain. Original magnification 1000×.)

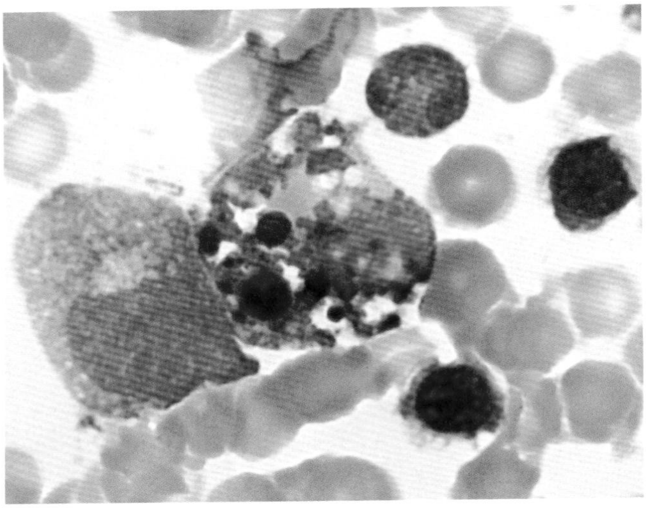

Figure 27-22 Bone marrow aspirate. The large macrophage in the center of the field contains pyknotic debris, red blood cell fragments, and golden-brown hemosiderin pigment. (Wright-Giemsa stain. Original magnification 250×.)

(Figure 27-20), are larger than neutrophils and have a small to moderate amount of light- to dark-blue cytoplasm. Their nuclei may be indented or irregular and have a fine reticular or lacy chromatin pattern. Multiple prominent nucleoli often are present.

Plasma cells are about the same size as or slightly larger than neutrophils (see Figures 27-10 and 27-19). They have round, eccentric nuclei and a moderate to abundant amount of deep blue cytoplasm. The Golgi apparatus is recognized as a clear area in the cytoplasm adjacent to the nucleus where the cytoplasm is most abundant. Sometimes, the cytoplasm contains round structures called *Russell bodies*, which are areas of rough endoplasmic reticulum that are markedly dilated by immunoglobulin. Plasma cells packed with Russell bodies are called *Mott cells*.

The bone marrow of normal dogs and cats usually contains less than 5% and less than 10% lymphocytes, respectively, and less than 2% plasma cells (both dogs and cats).[8-10,16,18,19] However, higher lymphocyte ranges have been reported (<15% in dogs and <20% in cats).[5,7,15] Lymphocytes and plasma cells are not uniformly distributed throughout the bone marrow; therefore, their proportions vary from area to area and fleck to fleck. On histopathology, small lymphocytes are normally dispersed in the interstitial areas of the bone marrow and are very difficult to distinguish from nucleated red cells or extruded red cell nuclei. Plasma cells, however, are recognized by their eccentric nuclei and deeply eosinophilic cytoplasm, which is more abundant than that of nucleated red cells. Plasma cells frequently occur in small perivascular clusters (Figure 27-21).

Macrophages

Usually less than 2% of the cells in normal canine and feline marrow are macrophages. Marrow macrophages are large but often not as large as early myeloid precursor cells (Figure 27-22). Their nuclei are usually eccentric, and their cytoplasm is abundant and stains light blue with indistinct boundaries. The cytoplasm is often vacuolated and may contain phagocytized material such as pyknotic nuclear debris, WBCs, RBCs, and their breakdown products, or organisms (e.g., *Histoplasma capsulatum* or *Leishmania spp.*).

Osteoclasts and Osteoblasts

Osteoclasts and osteoblasts are occasionally encountered in bone marrow aspirates. Osteoclasts are giant multinucleate cells that phagocytize bone and may be confused with megakaryocytes (see Figure 27-17). Osteoclast nuclei are discernibly separate, whereas megakaryocyte nuclei are fused. The cytoplasm of osteoclasts stains blue and

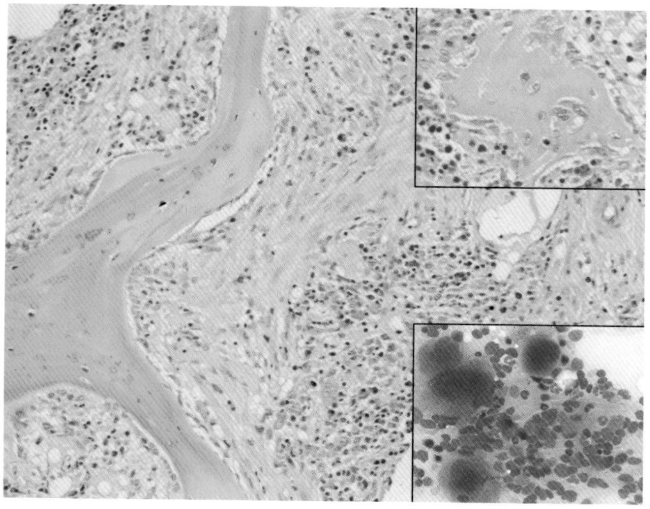

Figure 27-23 Bone marrow core biopsy from a dog with myelofibrosis. Marrow space has been replaced by pale eosinophilic stroma (myelofibrosis) with proliferating fibroblasts. Bony changes include endosteal bony proliferation (pale protrusions on the trabecular bone) and new bone formation (inset in upper right corner). Areas of cellular marrow and iron are located in the lower right and upper left corners. The lower inset is the cytologic sample illustrating megakaryocytic hyperplasia, a common finding with myelofibrosis, and an increased eosinophilic extracellular matrix. (H&E stain. Original magnification 200×) (Wright-Giemsa stain (cytology). Original magnification 500×.)

often contains azurophilic granular material. Osteoclasts are more common in aspirates from young animals than from old animals.

Osteoblasts are relatively large cells that cytologically somewhat resemble plasma cells. They have eccentric nuclei and basophilic, sometimes foamy, cytoplasm. The Golgi apparatus may be visible as a clear area adjacent to the nucleus. Osteoblasts are larger and have less condensed nuclear chromatin than plasma cells. Their nuclei are round to oval with a reticular chromatin pattern and one or two nucleoli. As with osteoclasts, they are more common in bone marrow aspirates from young, growing animals than from older animals.

On histopathology, osteocytes are small, flattened cells present within the lacunae of the trabecular or cortical bone, bone lining cells are flattened cells present along quiescent bone, and osteoblasts are plump stellate-shaped cells lining the bone in areas of bony remodeling or reactivity (see Figure 27-1; Figure 27-23). Osteoclasts are often also present in areas of bony remodeling or reactivity and may be identified in scalloped indentations within the bone surface known as *Howship lacunae*. A mild degree of bony remodeling may be seen at site of previous core biopsy samples; however, increased bone turnover is associated with inflammation, infection, neoplasia, or other processes (see Figure 27-23).

Miscellaneous Cells

Fat cells (adipocytes, lipocytes), endothelial cells (Figure 27-24), a few fibrocytes or fibroblasts, a few mast cells (see Figure 27-24), unidentifiable blast cells, and free nuclei

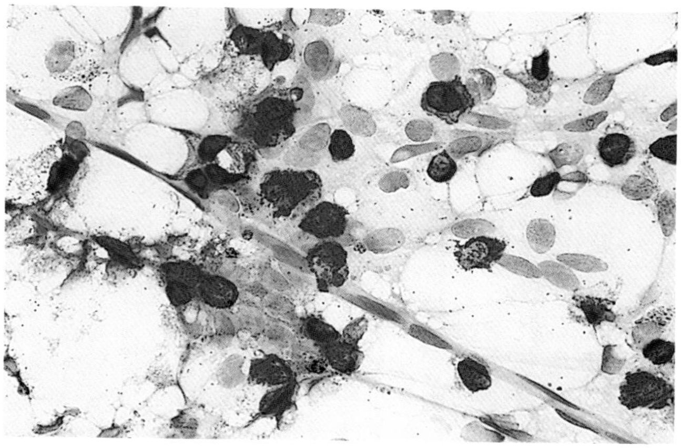

Figure 27-24 Hypocelluar bone marrow from a pancytopenic dog with chronic ehrlichiosis. Numerous well-differentiated mast cells are present along with capillaries and stromal cells. Prolonged treatment with doxycycline resulted in recovery of the marrow and resolution of the pancytopenia, although increased numbers of mast cells were still present in the marrow. (Wright stain. Original magnification 160×.)

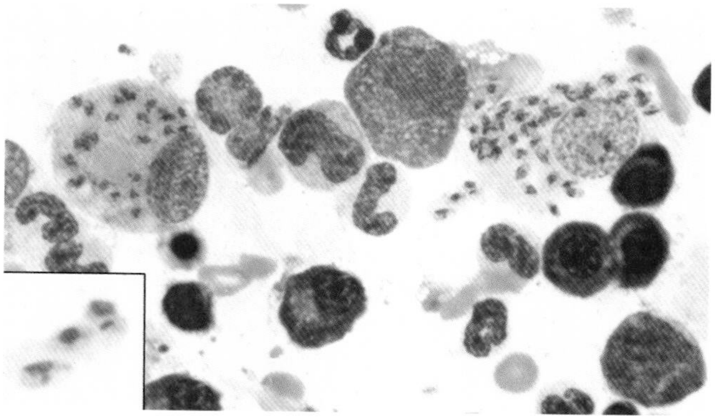

Figure 27-25 Bone marrow from a cat with disseminated histoplasmosis. Several large macrophages are present, each containing numerous *Histoplasma* organisms. Note the half-moon appearance of the organisms. (Wright stain. Original magnification 250×.)

may be found in aspirates from normal animals. The free nuclei may be small, round, condensed nuclei shed from metarubricytes or basket cells (large, free nuclei with dispersed lacelike chromatin from ruptured cells).

Adipose tissue is expected in bone marrow core biopsies and the relative amount of fat tissue and hematopoietic tissue identified is used to determine marrow cellularity. With age, adipose tissue increases and hematopoietic tissue decreases. The medullary cavity of long bones in adult animals is virtually all fat, so these areas should not be used to evaluate bone marrow.

ORGANISMS IN MARROW

Although bacterial infections may involve bone marrow, the organisms usually sought on bone marrow preparations are *H. capsulatum* (Figure 27-25), *L. infantum* or *L. donovani* (see Figure 27-21; Figure 27-26), *Mycobacterium*

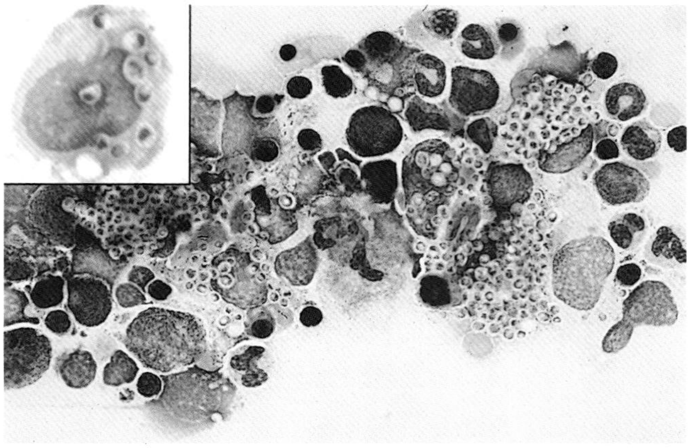

Figure 27-26 Bone marrow from a dog with disseminated leishmaniasis. Round to oval amastigotes of *Leishmania* with the "parachute men" appearance of small dark-staining rod-shaped kinetoplasts and paler round nuclei are seen within macrophages and in the background. Amastigotes are approximately 2.5 to 5 micrometers (μm) long and 1.5 to 2 μm wide. Plasma cells are increased. (Wright-Giemsa stain. Original magnification 1000×.)

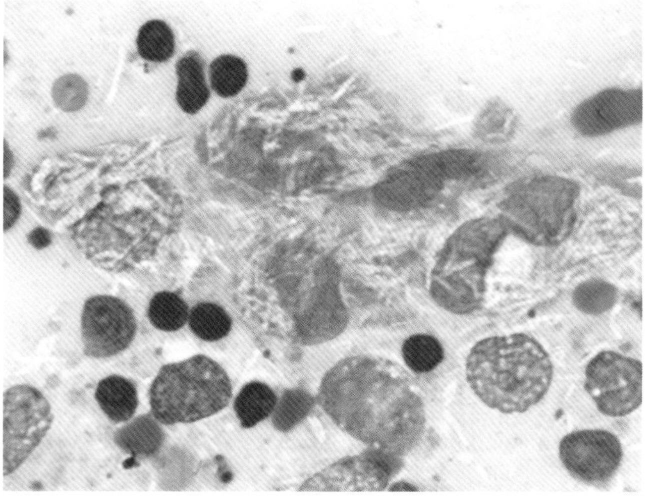

Figure 27-27 Bone marrow from an anemic feline immunodeficiency virus–positive cat with mycobacteriosis. Note the numerous intracellular and extracellular linear nonstaining rods (0.2 to 0.5 micrometer [μm] wide, 1 to 3 μm long). Organisms are most often observed in macrophages but only occasionally in granulocytes. Reexamination of the peripheral blood smear revealed rare mycobacterial organisms in neutrophils. Acid-fast staining for mycobacteriosis was positive. Culture and classification or polymerase chain reaction are necessary for determination of *Mycobacterium* species. (Wright-Giemsa stain. Original magnification 1000×.)

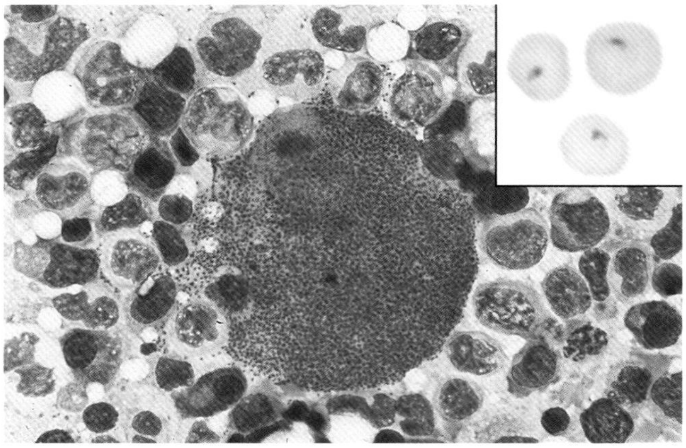

Figure 27-28 Necropsy bone marrow from a cat with cytauxzoonosis. A large macrophage containing a schizont of *Cytauxzoon felis* is surrounded by slightly degenerative-appearing myeloid cells and a few nucleated red blood cells, lymphocytes, and plasma cells. Cytauxzoon piroplasms were seen in the peripheral blood of this cat prior to death (*inset*). Scanning bone marrow smears at low power are helpful in identifying the large schizonts. (Wright-Giemsa stain. Original magnification 250×.) (Case courtesy of Dr. Jaime Tarigo.)

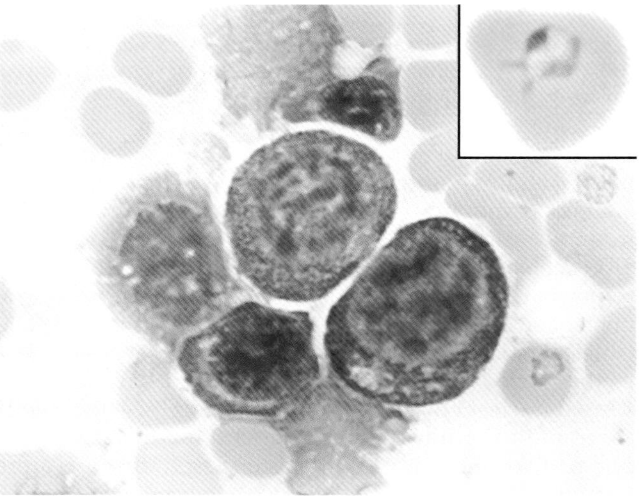

Figure 27-29 Bone marrow from a pancytopenic dog with babesiosis. Erythroid hyperplasia with pleomorphic large intracellular *Babesia* organisms in the red cells in the background. Organisms occurred singly or in doublets, but most organisms were irregular in shape; however, a few classic tear drop-shaped *Babesia* organisms were seen. The large size is consistent with *B. canis* (2.4 to 5 micrometers [μm]) in contrast to the smaller *B. gibsoni* (1 to 3.2 μm). (Wright-Giemsa stain. Original magnification 250×.)

spp. (Figure 27-27), *Cytauxzoon felis* (Figure 27-28), *Babesia spp.* (Figure 27-29), *Mycoplasma spp.* (Figure 27-30), *Toxoplasma gondii, Blastomyces dermatitidis* (Figure 27-31), and *Ehrlichia* or *Anaplasma* spp. *H. capsulatum* (see Figure 27-25) is one of the most common organisms identified in bone marrow preparations from dogs and cats.[20] Systemic histoplasmosis often causes nonregenerative anemia, thrombocytopenia, neutropenia, or all of these. In a very high proportion of systemic histoplasmosis cases, the organism is identified in bone marrow cytologic preparations. Macrophages containing amastigotes of leishmania are frequently observed in the bone marrow of dogs with visceral leishmaniasis. The small dark-staining kinetoplast and nucleus distinguish leishmania "parachute men" from histoplasma "half-moons" (see Figures 27-25 and 27-26). Megakaryocytic dysplasia, erythrophagocytosis, erythroid dysplasia, and emperipolesis

TABLE 27-5

Some Causes of Nonregenerative Anemia in Dogs and Cats

Disease	Prominent Marrow Features	Helpful Diagnostic Procedures
Anemia of chronic disease	Erythroid hypoplasia and granulocytic hyperplasia with increased marrow iron and plasma cells	History, physical examination, clinical signs, marrow iron, serum ferritin
Renal insufficiency	Erythroid hypoplasia	History, physical examination, clinical signs, BUN, serum creatinine concentration, or both; urinalysis
Nutritional iron deficiency or chronic blood loss	Erythroid hypoplasia; absent or decreased iron stores; small RBC precursors with scant, ragged cytoplasm	History, physical examination, clinical signs, marrow iron, serum ferritin
FeLV marrow suppression (in cats)	Erythroid hypoplasia with or without maturation arrest and/or abnormal morphology (e.g., megaloblastic erythroid cells); granulocytic hypoplasia may also be present.	Increased MCV on hemogram, the presence of megaloblastic erythrocytes in peripheral blood smears, or both; ELISA, IFA, PCR, or virus isolation testing for FeLV
Ehrlichiosis (in dogs)	*Early:* Variable findings often hypercellular	*Ehrlichia spp.* titer or PCR, response to therapy, or both
	Late: Erythroid hypoplasia, usually granulocytic and megakaryocytic hypoplasia, increased plasma cells, rarely cytoplasmic morulae	
Estrogen toxicity (in dogs)	Erythroid, granulocytic, and megakaryocytic hypoplasia/aplasia; increase in lymphocytes, mast cells, and plasma cells.	History and physical examination
Drug toxicity (e.g., trimethoprim or sulfadiazine, chemotherapy drugs)	Usually granulocytic and megakaryocytic hypoplasia but erythroid hypoplasia or aplasia may be observed	History
Marrow necrosis	Erythroid, granulocytic, and megakaryocytic hypoplasia with pink homogeneous strands of necrotic nuclear material; early changes include cytoplasmic and nuclear vacuolation	History, core biopsy
Myelofibrosis (sclerosis)	*Erythroid hypoplasia:* flecks are sparse, collected flecks may be normocellular or hypercellular	Core biopsy is necessary to confirm myelofibrosis
Histoplasmosis	*Organisms present:* variable findings, but most commonly erythroid hypoplasia and granulocytic hyperplasia	Refer slide for identification, culture, titers
Hypothyroidism	Erythroid hypoplasia, variable iron stores	Thyroid panel, physical examination, clinical signs, hypercholesterolemia
Nonerythroid neoplasia (e.g., granulocytic leukemia, lymphocytic leukemia, lymphoma)	Erythroid hypoplasia with marked increase in cells of the neoplastic cell line; blast cells make up >30% of the cell population	Cytochemistry, flow cytometry, or both; or immunohistochemistry (core biopsy) to specifically identify the type of neoplasia, PCR for lymphoma
Erythroid neoplasia (in cats, extremely rare in dogs)	Increased erythroid cells often with a maturation arrest and/or abnormal morphology; may need to repeat aspirate to separate from early regenerative response	Refer bone marrow cytologic sample and peripheral blood smear for interpretation; ELISA, IFA, PCR, or virus isolation testing for FeLV

BUN, blood urea nitrogen; *ELISA,* enzyme-linked immunosorbent assay; *FeLV,* feline leukemia virus; *IFA,* indirect fluorescent antibody; *MCV,* mean cell volume; *PCR,* polymerase chain reaction; *RBC,* red blood cell;.

deficiency), myelofibrosis, lymphoma, and marrow hypocellularity (especially chronic canine ehrlichiosis) has been reported.[24] In these cases, the low cellularity of the marrow accentuates the presence of the mast cells (see Figure 27-24). Bone marrow evaluation may not be indicated for routine staging of canine cutaneous mast cell neoplasia but should be considered when abnormal hematologic findings, tumor regrowth, and disease progression occur.[25] The overall marrow cellularity, plus the absolute number and morphology of mast cells, is used to differentiate mast cell hyperplasia from mast cell neoplasia (see Figure 27-49).

BOX 27-7

Interpretation of Bone Marrow Iron Stores

Increased Iron Stores
- Hemolytic anemia
- Anemia of chronic disease
- Multiple blood transfusions
- Old age
- Hemochromatosis or hemosiderosis
- Parenteral administration of iron

Decreased Iron Stores
- Newborn or young animal
- Nutritional iron deficiency
- Chronic blood loss
- Chronic phlebotomies

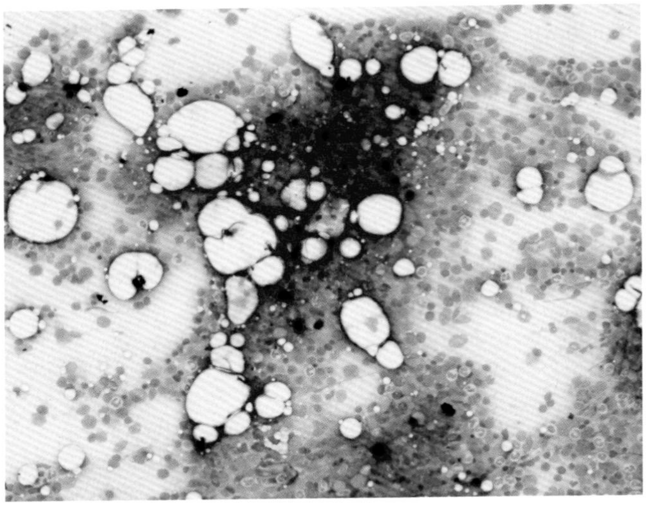

Figure 27-52 Bone marrow from a dog. Black aggregates of iron are associated with the dense unit particles. Increased iron stores may be seen with accelerated red cell turnover (hemolytic anemia), blood transfusions, parenteral iron injections, or old age. Bone marrow iron stores are not usually visible in cat bone marrow. (Wright-Giemsa stain. Original magnification 200×.)

Myelofibrosis is the displacement of normal marrow elements (myelophthisis) by fibrous tissue.[26] A few pockets of marrow usually persist within the fibrous tissue and undergo compensatory hyperplasia. Aspiration usually does not yield any marrow flecks, but occasionally a few small flecks may be recovered. These flecks usually contain very little fat and, therefore, appear hypercellular. Myelofibrosis may be primary as part of a myeloproliferative disorder, or may be secondary as a result of bone marrow necrosis, neoplasia, inflammation, or infection. Bone marrow core biopsy is necessary to definitively diagnose myelofibrosis. Histopathology reveals an increased amount of marrow stromal connective tissue, often with regions of decreased cellularity, and residual lymphocytes, plasma cells, and hemosiderin-laden macrophages may or may not be apparent (see Figure 27-23; Figure 27-55).

Examinations of Bone Marrow for Organisms

Bone marrow preparations may be examined for organisms such as *H. capsulatum* (see Figure 27-24), *Leishmania spp.* (see Figures 27-21 and 27-26), *Mycobacterium spp.* (see Figure 27-27), *C. felis* (see Figure 27-28), *Babesia spp.* (see Figure 27-29), *Mycoplasma* spp. (see Figure 27-30), *Blastomyces dermatitidis* (see Figure 27-31), *T. gondii*, *Ehrlichia* spp., and *Anaplasma spp.*, using the 40× or 50× and 100× (oil-immersion) objectives.[16] On cytology, the areas of the smear adjacent to the fleck and the edges of the fleck are usually the most rewarding because they tend to contain a greater concentration of marrow macrophages compared with other areas. When the presence of organisms is suspected, a short search should be performed. If they are not found quickly, the cytologic preparations should be sent to a consultant with more experience in identifying organisms and time to search for them. However, the examiner who has the time and enjoys bone marrow perusal should not be dissuaded from performing longer searches.

Diagnosis of Leukemia, Lymphoma, and Metastatic Neoplasia

The differentiation of neoplastic and myelodysplastic proliferative bone marrow disorders may be difficult (Box 27-8) (see Figure 27-44).[4-11,18-20, 23,24,26-28] Primary bone marrow neoplasia may be subdivided into myeloproliferative, meaning myeloid, erythroid, or megakaryocytic (see Figures 27-44 through 27-46, 27-51; Figure 27-56); lymphoid (Figure 27-57 and Figure 27-58; see Figure 27-20); histiocytic (see Figure 27-53); and undifferentiated or poorly differentiated (Figure 27-59). The diagnosis of neoplasia may be especially challenging when the marrow has not been totally effaced by tumor cells. Early bone marrow recovery (e.g., repopulation after parvovirus infection or after chemotherapy or radiotherapy) or an early regenerative response may look neoplastic with increased blast cells approaching 20% to 30%.[27,28] Therefore, it is imperative to scrutinize all available information, and if doubt persists, the CBC and, if necessary, the marrow should be reevaluated in 3 to 5 days. By that time, an early regenerative marrow will exhibit orderly maturation, whereas neoplasia will have the same or increased blast population. A useful guideline for diagnosing neoplasia is finding 20% to 30% blast cells (leukemia), 30% or more lymphoblasts or lymphocytes (lymphoma), 15% or more plasma cells (multiple myeloma), and sheets or large clusters of cells (metastatic mast cell tumor, histiocytic sarcoma, metastatic carcinoma, or sarcoma). In addition to numbers, cellular atypia may also suggest neoplasia, in spite of relatively few neoplastic-appearing cells (e.g., atypical plasma cells or mast cells) (see Figure 27-49). Suspected myelodysplastic syndromes, chronic leukemias, and specific classification of leukemia need to be referred to an experienced clinical pathologist.

Lymphoid neoplasia often infiltrates bone marrow (see Figures 27-20, 27-57, and 27-58). However, it is important to remember that although uncommon, normal dog and cat marrow can contain up to 15% and 20% lymphocytes, respectively.[4-11,13-16,18,19] Increased small lymphocytes may occasionally occur in reactive processes often associated with increased plasma cells. But, whenever

BOX 27-11

Some Causes of Bone Marrow Dysfunction

Bone Marrow Damage

Infections*
- Viral
  - FeLV
  - FIV
  - Parvovirus
  - Canine distemper
- Rickettsial
  - Ehrlichiosis
  - Anaplasmosis
- Bacterial
  - Mycobacteriosis
  - Any septicemia
- Mycoplasma-like
  - *M. haemofelis*
  - *M. haemominutum*
  - *M. haemocanis*
- Protozoal
  - Cytauxzoonosis
  - Babesiosis
  - Leishmaniasis
- Fungal or Yeast
  - Histoplasmosis
  - Any systemic fungi

Toxic Drugs
- Chemotherapy drugs
- Estrogen*
- Trimethoprim or sulfadiazine
- Phenylbutazone
- Medicated skin creams
- Thiacetarsamide
- Griseofulvin
- Meclofenamic acid
- Quinidine
- Fenbendazole

Radiation

Immunologic Mechanism
- Pure red blood cell aplasia
- Anti-rhEPO antibodies

Bone Marrow Replacement

Leukemia
Lymphoma
Myelofibrosis
Myelonecrosis
Osteosclerosis
Metastatic neoplasia
Infectious granulomas

Microenvironment or Hereditary Factors

Acquired Deficiencies or Defects
- Inflammation
  - Iron utilization defect
- Erythropoietin
  - Renal disease
  - Liver disease?
- Nutritional deficiencies
  - Iron deficiency
  - Starvation (protein)
  - Vitamin B_{12} or folic acid deficiency
- Toxins
  - Lead
  - Uremic toxins
- Hypothyroidism

Hereditary or Congenital
- Pyruvate kinase deficiency
- Canine cyclic hematopoiesis
- Leukocyte adhesion deficiency
- Chediak-Higashi syndrome
- Pelger-Huët syndrome†
- Poodle macrocytosis
- Vitamin B_{12} malabsorption – Giant Schnauzers
- Congenital dyserythropoiesis – English Springer Spaniels

*Cellularity varies with stage of disease.
†Hyposegmented granulocytes (neutrophils and eosinophils) without clinical disease effects.
FeLV, feline leukemia virus; *FIV,* feline immunodeficiency virus; *rhEPO*, recombinant human erythropoietin.

References

1. Fourcar K, Reichard K, Czuchlewski D: *Bone marrow pathology*, ed 3, Chicago, IL, 2010, ASCP Press.
2. Bain B, Clark D, Wilkins B: *Bone marrow pathology*, ed 4, Hoboken, NJ, 2010, Wiley-Blackwell.
3. Travlos GS: Normal structure, function, and histology of bone marrow, *Toxicol Pathol* 34:548–565, 2006.
4. Kearns SH, Ewing P: Causes of canine and feline pancytopenia, *Comp Cont Ed Pract Vet* 28:122–133, 2006.
5. Neel JA, Birkenheuer AJ, Grindem CB: Infectious and immune-mediated thrombocytopenia. In Bonagura JD, Twedt DC, editors: *Kirk's Current Veterinary Therapy XIV*, St Louis, MO, 2009, Saunders Elsevier, pp 281–287.
6. Weiss DJ: A retrospective study of the incidence and the classification of bone marrow disorders in the dog at a veterinary teaching hospital (1996-2004), *J Vet Intern Med* 20:955–961, 2006.
7. Grindem CB, Neel JA, Juopperi TA: Cytology of bone marrow, *Vet Clin Small Anim* 32:1313–1374, 2002.
8. Harvey JW: *Atlas of veterinary hematology*, Philadelphia, PA, 2001, Saunders.
9. Jain NC: Examination of the blood and bone marrow. In Jain NC, editor: *Essentials of veterinary hematology*, Philadelphia, PA, 1993, Lea & Febiger, pp 1–18.
10. Thrall MA, Weiser G, Jain N: Laboratory evaluation of bone marrow. In Thrall MA, editor: *Veterinary hematology and clinical chemistry*, Baltimore, MD, 2004, Lippincott Williams & Wilkins, pp 149–178.

11. Wellman ML, Radin MJ: *Bone marrow evaluation in dogs and cats*, Wilmington, DE, 1999, The Gloyd Group.
12. Harvey JW: Canine bone marrow: normal hematopoiesis, biopsy techniques and cell identification and evaluation, *Comp Cont Ed Pract Vet* 6:909–927, 1984.
13. Hoff B, Lumsden JH, Valli VEO: An appraisal of bone marrow biopsy in assessment of sick dogs, *Can J Comp Med* 49:34–42, 1985.
14. Friedrichs KR, Young KM: How to collect diagnostic bone marrow samples, *Vet Med* 100:578–588, 2005.
15. Relford RL: The steps in performing a bone marrow aspiration and core biopsy, *Vet Med* 86:670–688, 1991.
16. Grindem CB: Bone marrow biopsy and evaluation, *Vet Clin North Am Small Anim Pract* 19:669–696, 1989.
17. Weiss DJ: A review of the techniques for preparation of histopathologic sections for bone marrow, *Vet Clin Pathol* 16:90–94, 1987.
18. Mischke R, Busse L: Reference values for the bone marrow aspirates in adult dogs, *J Vet Med Assoc* 49:499–502, 2002.
19. Weiss DJ: Differentiating benign and malignant causes of lymphocytosis in feline bone marrow, *J Vet Intern Med* 19:855–859, 2005.
20. Greene CE: *Infectious diseases of the dog and cat*, ed 4, St. Louis, MO, 2011, Saunders.
21. Manzillo VF, Restucci B, Pagano A, et al: Pathological changes in the bone marrow of dogs with leishmaniosis, *Vet Rec* 158:690–694, 2006.
22. Mischke R, Busse L, Bartels D, et al: Quantification of thrombopoietic activity in bone marrow aspirates of dogs, *Vet J* 164:269–274, 2002.
23. DeHeer HL, Grindem CB: Histiocytic disorders. In Feldman BF, Zinkl JG, Jain NC, editors: *Schalm's veterinary hematology*, ed 5, Philadelphia, PA, 2000, Lippincott Williams & Wilkins, pp 696–705.
24. Plier ML, MacWilliams PS: Systemic mastocytosis and mast cell leukemia. In Feldman BF, Zinkl JG, Jain NC, editors: *Schalm's veterinary hematology*, ed 5, Philadelphia, PA, 2000, Lippincott Williams & Wilkins, pp 747–754.
25. Endicott MM, Charney SC, McKnight JA, et al: Clinicopathological findings and results of bone marrow aspiration in dogs with cutaneous mast cell tumours: 157 cases (1999-2002), *Vet Comp Oncol* 5:31–37, 2007.
26. Blue JT: Myelodysplastic syndromes and myelofibrosis. In Feldman BF, Zinkl JG, NC Jain, editors: *Schalm's veterinary hematology*, ed 5, Philadelphia, PA, 2000, Lippincott Williams & Wilkins, pp 682–688.
27. Juopperi TA, Bienzle D, Bernreuter DC, et al: Prognostic markers for myeloid neoplasms: a comparative review of the literature and goals for future investigation, *Vet Pathol* 48:182–197, 2011.
28. McManus PM: Classification of myeloid neoplasms: a comparative review, *Vet Clin Pathol* 34:189–212, 2005.
29. Raskin RE, Krehbiel JD: Histopathology of canine bone marrow in malignant lymphoproliferative disorders, *Vet Pathol* 25:83–88, 1988.
30. Weiss DJ: Histopathology of canine non-neoplastic bone marrow, *Vet Clin Pathol* 15:7–11, 1986.
31. Weiss DJ: Bone marrow pathology in dogs and cats with non-regenerative immune-mediated haemolytic anaemia and pure red cell aplasia, *J Com Path* 138:46–53, 2008.

CHAPTER 28

The Adrenal Gland

Tamara B. Wills and Gary J. Haldorson

The increased availability and use of modern imaging techniques such as ultrasonography, computed tomography (CT), and magnetic resonance imaging (MRI) have resulted in increased detection of adrenal masses and adrenomegaly. While some of these lesions may be incidental findings, some cases may require a definitive diagnosis, and cytology may be a valuable tool for initial evaluation. However, caution should be taken when considering adrenal fine-needle aspiration (FNA), especially in canine patients, as aspiration of pheochromocytomas may result in significant patient morbidity or possibly mortality from hypertensive or hypotensive emergencies and cardiac arrhythmias.[1]

NORMAL CELLULAR COMPONENTS

The adrenal glands are composed of two parts: (1) the cortex and (2) the medulla. The cortex is derived from the mesoderm and is divided into three zones functionally and histologically. Adjacent to the capsule is the *zona glomerulosa*, followed by the *zona fasciculata* and the *zona reticularis*, which is closest to the medulla. The cells in the zona glomerulosa (Figure 28-1) produce and secrete aldosterone and are arranged in irregular columns histologically.[2] The middle zone, the zona fasciculata (see Figure 28-1), is the thickest layer of the cortex and functions with the thinner inner layer, the zona reticularis, to produce cortisol and androgens respectively.[2] Histologically, these two layers may be difficult to differentiate.

In the human medical literature, the cells from the zona fasciculata and glomerulosa appear similar cytologically and are oval to polygonal with abundant, foamy to vacuolated cytoplasm because of intracytoplasmic lipids; cytologic descriptions in dogs and cats are similar.[3,4] Cells from the zona reticularis are lipid poor, containing eosinophilic granular cytoplasm with no vacuoles, but some cells from this zone may contain lipofuscin granules.[3,4] The medulla, derived from neuroectoderm, secretes catecholamines. Cytologically, these cells appear different from adrenocortical cells and are sometimes described as resembling small-sized hepatocytes, with centrally to eccentrically located nuclei and finely granular cytoplasm.[4]

ABNORMALITIES OF THE ADRENAL GLAND

Adrenal nodules, masses, or diffuse adrenomegaly are common reasons for cytologic evaluation of the adrenal gland in small animals. In addition to fine-needle aspirates, impression smears of surgically removed adrenal glands may also be encountered. Enlargement of the adrenal glands may occur with hyperplasia, primary or metastatic neoplasia, and less commonly with inflammation.

Nonneoplastic Conditions

Adrenalitis: Primary adrenalitis is uncommonly reported in the literature, but when observed, canine and feline adrenalitis is often seen with septicemia or disseminated disease. Adrenalitis may occur with bacterial septicemia; disseminated fungal infections such as *Coccidioides immitus, Histoplasma capsulatum,* and *Cryptococcus neoformans*; and some protozoal infections such as *Toxoplasma gondii* and *Babesia* spp.[4] Granulomatous inflammation may be seen with fungal organisms, whereas some protozoal infections elicit mild histiocytic infiltration and necrosis.[4,5] Depending on the inciting cause, edema and hemorrhage may also cause adrenomegaly with systemic infections.[5]

Adrenocortical Hyperplasia: Adrenocortical nodular hyperplasia is most common in older cats and dogs. Diffuse cortical hyperplasia may also result in adrenomegaly, typically caused by oversecretion of adrenocorticotrophic hormone (ACTH) by a pituitary neoplasm.[2] Histologically, hyperplasia of the adrenal cortex results in increased width of the cortex, often because of multiple nodules of hyperplasia, consisting primarily of the zona reticularis and the zona fasciculata (Figure 28-2).[2,5] Fine-needle aspirates of these areas contain cells resembling those described from the normal zona fasciculata. Cytologic preparations are often cellular, and cells may be more tightly arranged than typical adrenocortical cells. Binucleate cells are commonly reported in aspirates from human adrenocortical hyperplasia.[3] Differentiation of adrenocortical nodular hyperplasia from well-differentiated adrenal neoplasms may be challenging cytologically and will be further discussed in the next section.

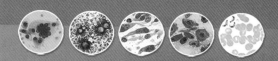

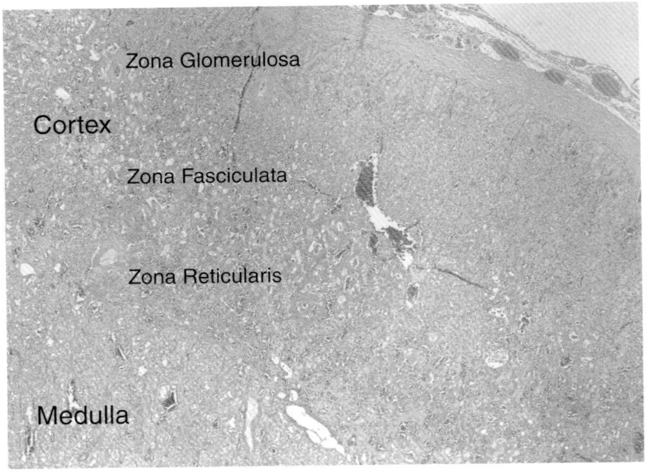

Figure 28-1 In this histologic section of normal canine adrenal gland, the cortex and medulla may be differentiated and the layers of the cortex may be observed. (H&E stain. Original magnification 100×.)

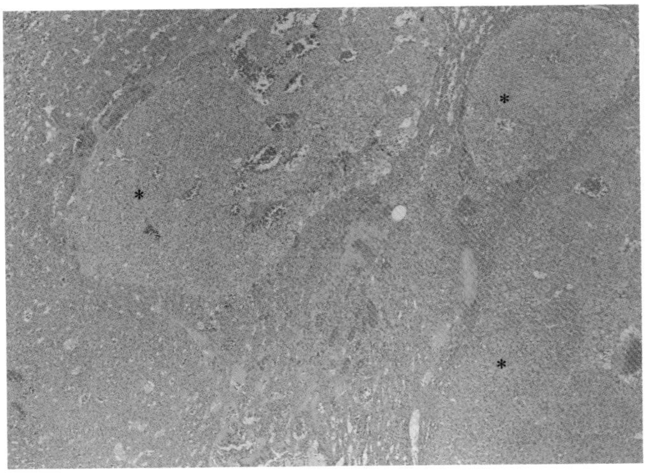

Figure 28-2 Histopathology of a canine nodular adrenal gland reveals three nonencapsulated, poorly demarcated nodules of cortical cells (*) that have slightly different staining characteristics relative to the adjacent normal cells (adrenocortical nodular hyperplasia). (H&E stain. Original magnification 100×.)

Primary Tumors of the Adrenal Cortex

Functional adrenal cortical neoplasms are reported to be the underlying cause of approximately 10% to 15% cases of canine hyperadrenocorticism.[4] Rare cases of feline hyperaldosteronism are associated with adrenal neoplasms.[6,7] Neither cytology nor histopathology can determine whether a tumor is functional and serum adrenal function tests are necessary.

FNA cytology of adrenal nodules cannot be used to assess encapsulation or invasiveness, which may make cytology a difficult tool for definitive classification of adrenocortical nodules.[3] Even histologic classification of adrenal lesions, including differentiation of normal from hyperplastic tissue, hyperplastic nodules from adenomas, and in some cases differentiation of adenomas from carcinomas, may be challenging. Distinguishing

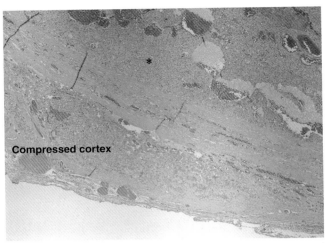

Figure 28-3 Histopathology of a canine adrenocortical adenoma reveals an expansile, densely cellular, encapsulated mass (*) compressing normal cortex (*labeled*). Cells are arranged in packets supported by thin wisps of fibrovascular stroma. On higher power, individual cells were large, polygonal, with prominently vacuolated eosinophilic cytoplasm and clearly defined cellular borders. (H&E stain. Original magnification 100×.)

adrenocortical carcinomas from pheochromocytomas may also be problematic in some cases.[2] In general, with increased malignancy of adrenocortical neoplasms, decreased lipid and increased nuclear atypia are encountered.[3] Necrosis is reportedly a common feature in human adrenal tumors.[3] Overlapping features of benign versus malignant adrenocortical nodules exist; however, cellular features at opposite ends of the spectrum, for example, benign adrenal cortical nodules may often be differentiated from a poorly differentiated adrenal cortical carcinoma.[3] Regardless, limitations of cytology should be recognized and cytologic findings should be used in conjunction with the patient history, clinical signs, blood work abnormalities, and imaging, if available.

Adrenocortical Adenomas and Carcinomas: Adrenal adenomas are common in older dogs and found only rarely in cats.[2] Histologically, adrenal adenomas are surrounded by a capsule and compress adjacent normal cortex (see Figure 28-3). Cells within adrenocortical adenomas resemble the zona fasciculata or reticularis.[4] Cytologically, adenomas are composed of cells similar to the normal zona fasciculata or reticularis and are round to polygonal, often containing several discrete vacuoles within moderate to abundant amounts of eosinophilic cytoplasm (Figure 28-4). Nuclei are typically round, and indistinct nucleoli are occasionally observed. Cells may exhibit mild anisocytosis and anisokaryosis.[5] In humans, adrenal adenomas may sometimes exhibit more cellular pleomorphism.[3] Some adenomas will also contain extramedullary hematopoiesis (Figure 28-5).[8]

Adrenocortical carcinomas occur less frequently compared with adenomas in dogs and rarely occur in cats.[8] These tumors are larger than adenomas and may invade into surrounding tissue, including the caudal vena cava.[8] Neoplastic cells in carcinomas are typically

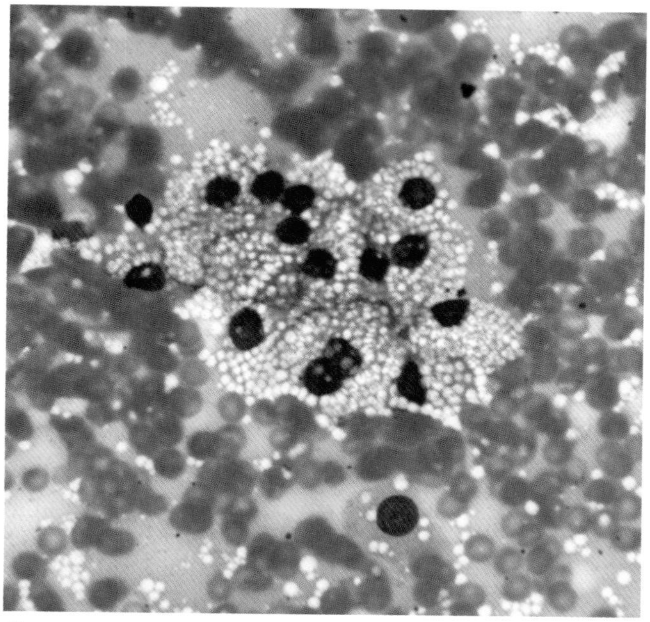

Figure 28-4 Aspirates from a canine cortical adenoma contain a cohesive cluster of polygonal cells with abundant, highly vacuolated cytoplasm. Mild anisocytosis and anisokaryosis are observed. (Wright stain. Original magnification 500×.)

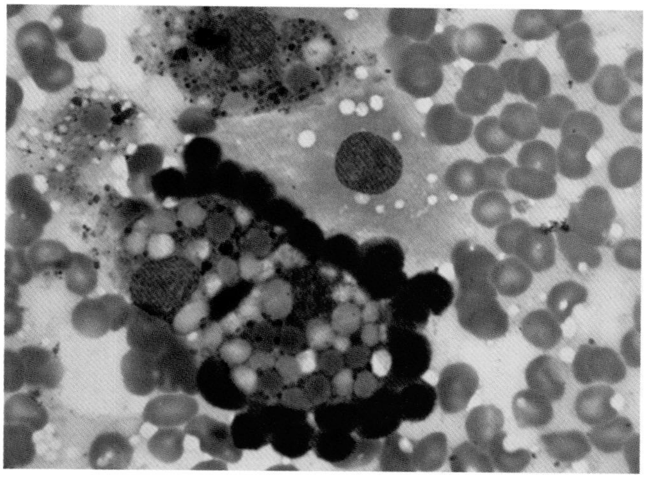

Figure 28-5 Aspirates from a canine cortical nodule, diagnosed histopathologically as an adrenal cortical adenoma, contain macrophages containing numerous erythrocytes and dark pigment (hemosiderin) surrounded by erythroid precursors. Adjacent is one polygonal cell with abundant eosinophilic cytoplasm with few discrete vacuoles, compatible with adrenocortical origin. (Wright stain. Original magnification 1000×.)

more pleomorphic compared with neoplastic cells from adenomas, although an overlap in cellular pleomorphism exists in these two entities. Tumor cells are often large, oval to polygonal, with basophilic cytoplasm containing several discrete vacuoles, although some may contain dense eosinophilic cytoplasm (Figure 28-6 and Figure 28-7).[7] Nucleoli are often prominent.[8]

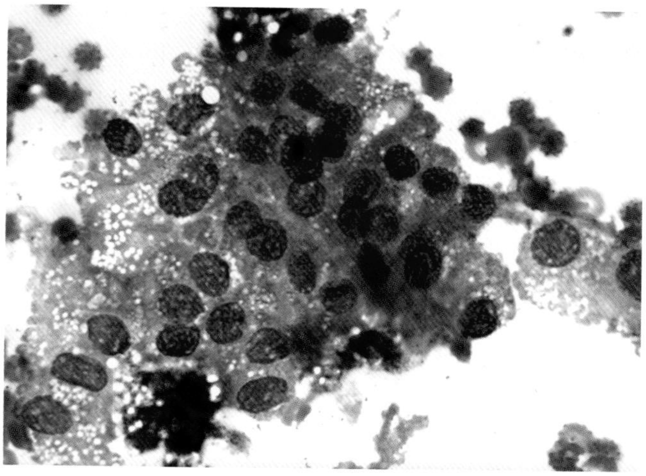

Figure 28-6 Aspirates from an adrenal mass diagnosed histopathologically as an adrenal cortical carcinoma contain disorganized clusters of oval to polygonal cells with moderate to abundant amounts of vacuolated basophilic cytoplasm. The neoplastic cells exhibit mild to moderate pleomorphism. (Wright stain. Original magnification 1000×.)

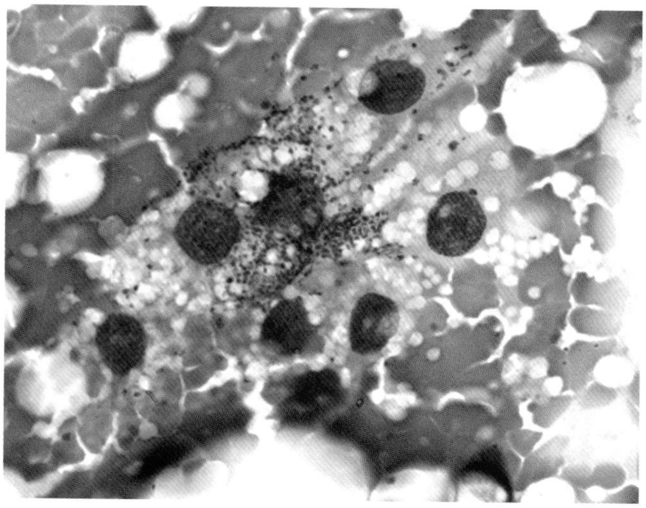

Figure 28-7 Aspirates of a histopathologically confirmed adrenal cortical carcinoma in a dog contain cells that appear more similar to those aspirated from the adrenal cortical adenoma in Figures 28-4 and 28-5. (Wright stain. Original magnification 1000×.) (Courtesy of Dr. Andrea Bohn, Fort Collins, CO.)

Myelolipoma: Myelolipomas are very uncommon in dogs but have been reported.[9] These tumors are benign and often originate in the cortex but may extend into the medulla. Expected cytologic findings would include lipid and mature adipocytes admixed with hematopoietic cells and macrophages containing hemosiderin.[9]

Primary Tumors of the Adrenal Medulla

Pheochromocytomas are the most common adrenal medulla tumors in dogs and cats; however, they are quite rare in cats.[8,10] Other tumors such as neuroblastomas and ganglioneuromas may develop from the neuroectodermal cells within the adrenal medulla.[8]

Pheochromocytoma: Pheochromocytomas are more common in dogs than in cats and are frequently found in middle-aged and older dogs.[8] Pheochromocytomas are often locally invasive and may metastasize to the lung, liver, kidney, spleen, and pancreas.[11] Serum and urine tests measuring the levels of catecholamines and metabolites may be used to diagnose pheochromocytomas, but these tests are not widely available for dogs and cats.[12] Cytology and histopathology are often necessary for diagnosis. Because manipulation of pheochromocytomas may result in cardiac and blood pressure instability greatly increasing risk of morbidity and mortality, FNA should be avoided. Histopathologically, the cells are arranged in nests, packets, and small lobules, separated by fine fibrovascular stroma (see Figure 28-8). Cytologic specimens are often highly cellular, with occasional papillary formations described;[13] and the cells may range from small and round, to polyhedral (Figures 28-9, Figure 28-10, Figure 28-11), to large, pleomorphic cells with eosinophilic to slightly basophilic, granular cytoplasm.[8,13] If a surgical specimen is obtained,

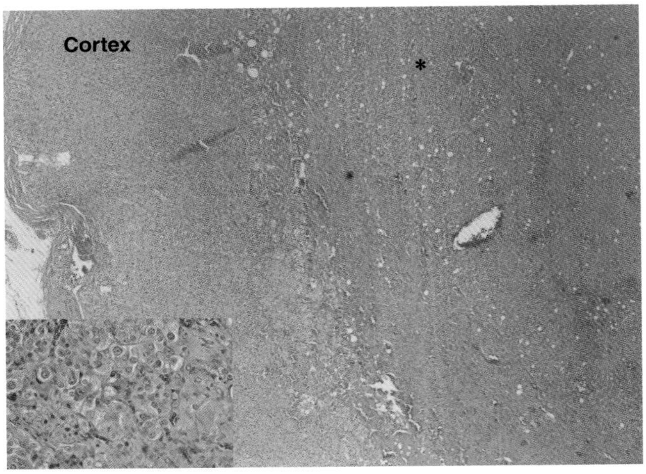

Figure 28-8 Histopathology of a canine pheochromocytoma reveals a poorly demarcated, unencapsulated, highly cellular, nodular mass expanding the medulla (*). Cells are arranged in sheets, nests, and packets separated by a delicate fibrovascular stroma. Morphologic features of the cells are better appreciated in the inset. Cells have indistinct margins with moderate to abundant, finely granular, and eosinophilic cytoplasm. Nuclei are round to oval, vesicular, and have a small nucleolus. (H&E stain. Original magnification 100×.) (*Inset*: H&E stain. Original magnification 400×.)

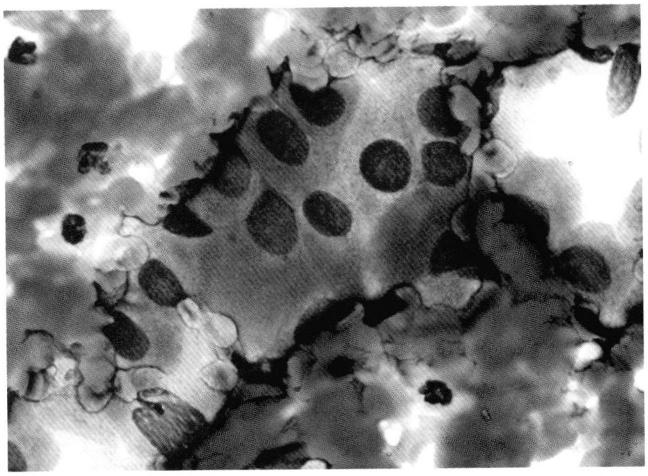

Figure 28-10 Cells from an aspirate of a dog with a pheochromocytoma contain individual and cohesive polygonal cells with moderate amounts of eosinophilic, granular cytoplasm. Mild to moderate pleomorphism is observed. (Wright stain. Original magnification 1000×.) (Courtesy of Dr. Andrea Bohn, Fort Collins, CO.)

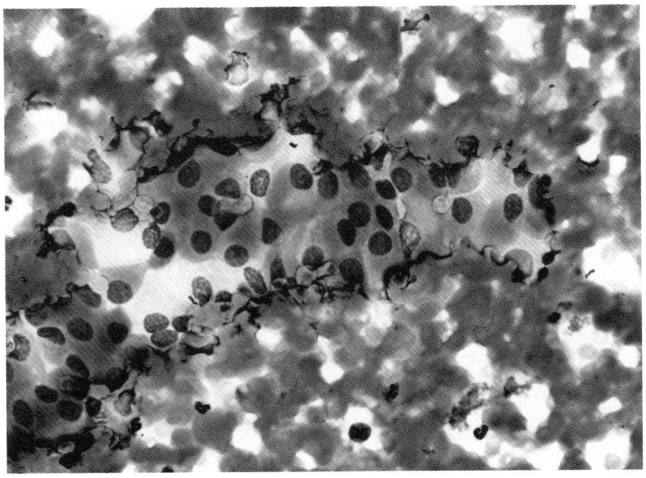

Figure 28-9 An aspirate from a canine pheochromocytoma contains sheets of polygonal cells containing moderate amounts of eosinophilic granular cytoplasm. The nuclei are round with a stippled chromatin pattern, occasionally containing a nucleolus. (Wright stain. Original magnification 500×.) (Courtesy of Dr. Andrea Bohn, Fort Collins, CO.)

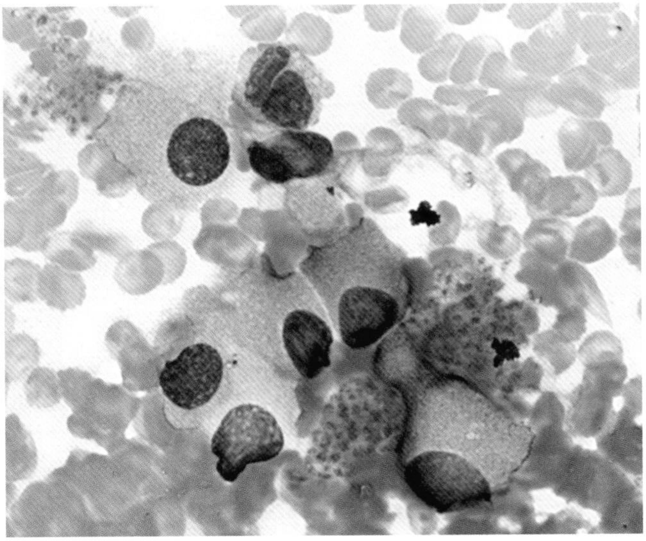

Figure 28-11 An aspirate of a canine pheochromocytoma contains individual polygonal cells with moderate amounts of eosinophilic, granular cytoplasm. Mild to moderate pleomorphism is observed. (Wright stain. Original magnification 1000×.) (Courtesy of Dr. Andrea Bohn, Fort Collins, CO.)

TABLE 29-1

Advantages and Disadvantages of Sample Type

	Advantages	Disadvantages
Direct smear	Slides from the original sample may be used, if multiple submitted	Increased background artifact Prior staining may affect results Variability of cellularity between slides Use of panels is limited because of limited numbers of slides
Cytospins	Useful with limited material Panels possible because multiple slides can be prepared May control cellularity May be used for fluids or transport media	Background artifact Extra sampling of patient may be required Added expense of transport media and cytospin preparation
Cell block	Histology laboratory can handle like routine material Materials, including controls, may be stored long term	Low cellular samples cannot be used Antigen retrieval necessary Added expense and time of cell block preparation

an effusion for ICC is the ability to make multiple slides from one sample, allowing for a panel of antibodies to be used rather than just one antibody. Using a combination of possible negative and positive antibodies will result in higher diagnostic yield than the use of one antibody.[6,15] Each of these methods of sample preparation has advantages and disadvantages (Table 29-1). When submitting a sample, the sample should be sent overnight, and if transport media are being used, the sample should be sent on ice.

CLINICAL APPLICATIONS OF IMMUNOHISTOCHEMISTRY

One of the advantages of cytology is the relatively low cost and rapid turnaround time. The use of ICC will increase the cost and likely the turnaround time of sample. Therefore, ICC is not necessary for every sample but should be reserved for very specific purposes. No one specific marker for neoplasia exists, so the diagnosis needs to be made on cytology or histopathology prior to ICC.[6] After a diagnosis of neoplasia is made from the Romanowsky-stained cytology specimen, ICC may be able to assist with the specificity of the diagnosis. Ideally, the slides used for ICC are obtained from the same aspirate or at least from the same location as the original cytology. In addition to increasing the specificity of a neoplasia diagnosis, ICC may allow for identification of small numbers of cells within a tissue (e.g., identification of epithelial cells in a thymoma or micrometastasis within a lymph node), or for immunophenotyping of neoplasms for prognostic information or assistance with therapeutic decisions.

Diagnosis

Cytology has limits in diagnoses, especially in identifying the tissue of origin in poorly differentiated tumors. Many antibodies have been validated for use in cytology to assist with the identification of tissue type. Some antibodies such as vimentin and cytokeratin are used to identify broader tissue types. Cytokeratin and vimentin are cytoplasmic intermediate filaments and are fairly specific for mesenchymal and epithelial tissues, respectively. Cells that express cytokeratin and do not express vimentin are considered epithelial in origin, so cytokeratin is fairly specific in identifying epithelial cells. Pancytokeratin antibodies, as well as more specific antibodies directed against single cytokeratins (such as cytokeratin 7), have been evaluated for cytology.[16] Vimentin is an intermediate filament found in mesenchymal cells. Antibodies to vimentin are used to identify tumors of connective tissue origin. Vimentin has been validated for use in cytology of imprints and fine-needle aspirates.[17,18] A tumor that expresses vimentin, not cytokeratin, is a mesenchymal tumor. A small group of neoplasms and benign tissues are known to express both cytokeratin and vimentin; these include synovial cell sarcoma, mesothelioma and benign mesothelium, papillary renal cell carcinoma, non–small cell lung carcinoma, carcinosarcoma, and melanoma, among others.[19-23] For this reason, panels of antibodies are much more useful than single antibodies. The sample should be evaluated for both cytokeratin and vimentin, in addition to more specific antibodies.

Additional antibodies such as Melan A for melanoma (Figure 29-6), CD31 and vWF for endothelial cells, and CD18 for histiocytic and granulocytic origin are available to allow for a more specific diagnosis. A more complete list of available antibodies is provided in Box 29-2. Many of these antibodies have been specifically evaluated for cytology.[8,17,24,25] This may be limiting in cytology because few slides may be available for evaluation.

Lymphoma, leukemia, and other round cell neoplasms may be phenotyped with immunocytochemistry.[26,27] Lymphomas are initially evaluated for expression of CD3 or CD79 (Figure 29-7) to determine T- or B-cell origin, respectively, but if they are of T-cell origin, they may then be further evaluated for expression of CD4 or CD8.[28] At this time, the specific CD subtype of T-cell lymphoma is not known to impact prognosis or therapy; however, over time and with subsequent studies, it may be found that such details do provide important prognostic and therapeutic information. Because of the similar morphology of many round cells of different

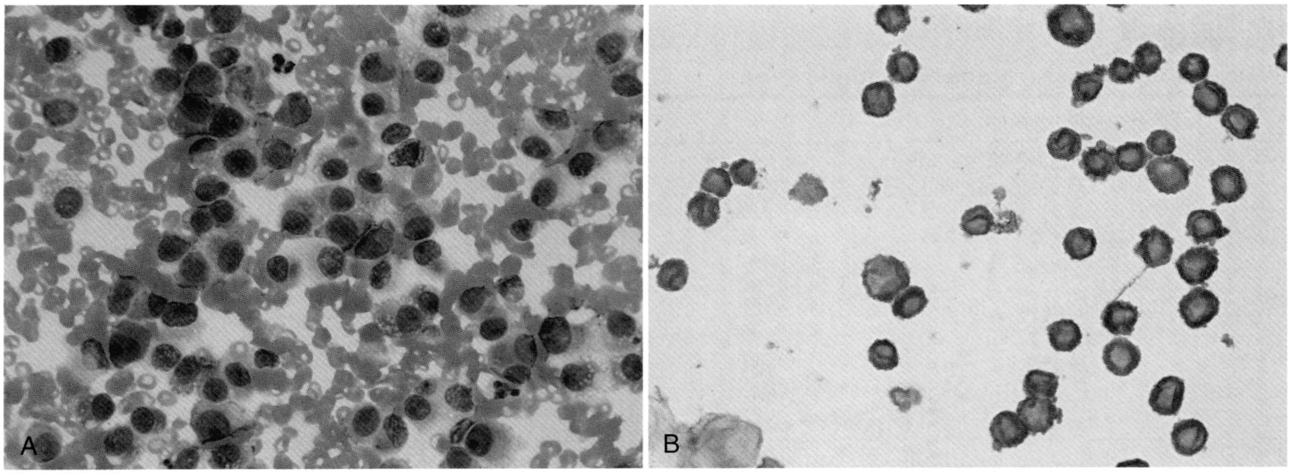

Figure 29-6 Fine-needle aspirate from a digital mass in a dog. A, The aspirate is cellular and consists of a population of round neoplastic cells with prominent nucleoli, amelanotic melanoma is likely. (Wright-Giemsa stain. Original magnification 500×.) **B,** Melan A performed on an unstained slide; cells are strongly positive. (Hematoxylin counter-stain. Original magnification 500×.)

BOX 29-2

Incomplete List of Antibodies Used in Immunohistochemistry

Antibody	Positive Tissue
CD3	T-lymphocytes
CD4	T-helper lymphocytes, neutrophils, macrophages
CD8	Cytotoxic T-lymphocytes
CD18	Macrophages, granulocytes
CD20	B-lymphocytes
CD31	Endothelial cells, platelets, monocytes
CD34	Stem cells
CD41	Platelets and megakaryocytes
CD79a	B-cells
CD 117 (cKit)	Mast cells, stem cells
-κ-light chains	B-cells
MUM1	Plasma cells
Cytokeratin	Epithelial cells
Vimentin	Mesenchymal cells
Melan-A	Melanocytes

lineages, a panel of antibodies is necessary to evaluate leukemias. Lymphoid markers such as CD3 and CD79 are valuable but myeloperoxidase, CD18, CD45, and Granzyme B should be included in the panel to identify tumors of myeloid, dendritic cell, and natural killer (NK) cell origin.[29]

Identification of Low Numbers of Cells

ICC may also be useful in identifying low numbers of cells in a tissue. In a study of dogs, the sensitivity of diagnosis of metastatic carcinoma was increased from 88% to 99% with the addition of cytokeratin ICC.[30] Identification of neoplastic cells within a draining lymph node may assist in prediction of behavior of the tumor and may also alter the therapeutic plan for the patient.

Prognostic Information

Different groups of antibodies have been evaluated to try to predict behavior or assist with grading of neoplasms. Most of these studies have been done with IHC and are often used in conjunction with other architectural changes used for tumor grading. Two such examples are antibodies directed against proliferating nuclear cell antigen (PCNA) and Ki67. PCNA is a highly conserved protein found in all eukaryotic cells. PCNA is an accessory protein to DNA polymerase δ and acts as a clamp to lock the enzyme on the leading strand.[31] PCNA has been evaluated in several different tumors, including mast cell tumors, testicular neoplasms, mammary tumors, and soft tissue sarcomas such as hemangiopericytomas.[32-36] Ki67 is a murine monoclonal antibody that recognizes a nuclear antigen expressed in the G1, S, G2, and M phases of the cell cycle and is used to evaluate the proliferative activity of neoplasms.[31] This antibody has been evaluated in mast cell tumors, melanomas, gastrointestinal stromal tumors, meningiomas, and lymphoma among others.[34,37-40] These proliferative markers are probably most useful with histopathology because they may be interpreted with the architecture and used as part of a grading scheme. A panel of proliferative markers, including Ki67, PCNA, and AgNOR, may be used in the evaluation of canine mast cell tumors. In addition to the proliferative markers, localization of the KIT receptor and identification of c-KIT mutations are also used to evaluate behavior of mast cell tumors.[33,41] The combination of Ki67, AgNOR, and KIT localization have been shown to be prognostic for mast cell tumor behavior and may potentially be used in cytology for prognostic information.[41]

ICC is a useful diagnostic tool, and its use is increasing in popularity. Currently, ICC is used primarily to

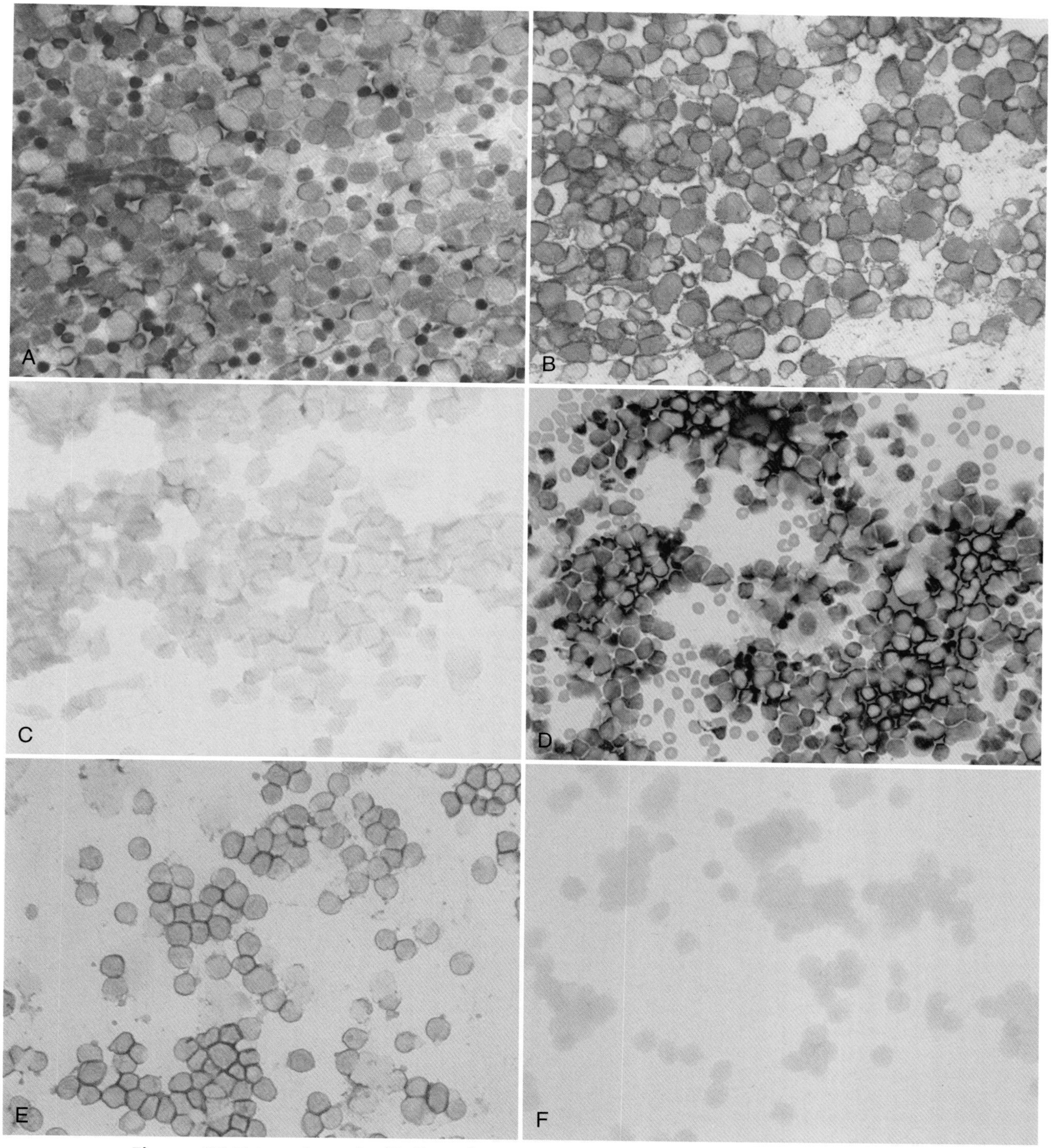

Figure 29-7 Lymph node (A-C) and Urinalysis (D-F) A, Mixed lymphoid population predominated by large lymphocytes. (Wright-Giemsa stain. Original magnification 500×.) **B,** Cells express CD79a. (Original magnification 500×.) **C,** Cells are negative for CD3. (Original magnification 500×.) **D** to **F,** Cytospin preparations from urine. **D,** A population of neoplastic round cells. (Wright-Giemsa stain. Original magnification 500×.) **E,** Cells express CD3. (Original magnification 500×.) **F,** Cells do not express CD79a. (Original magnification 500×.)

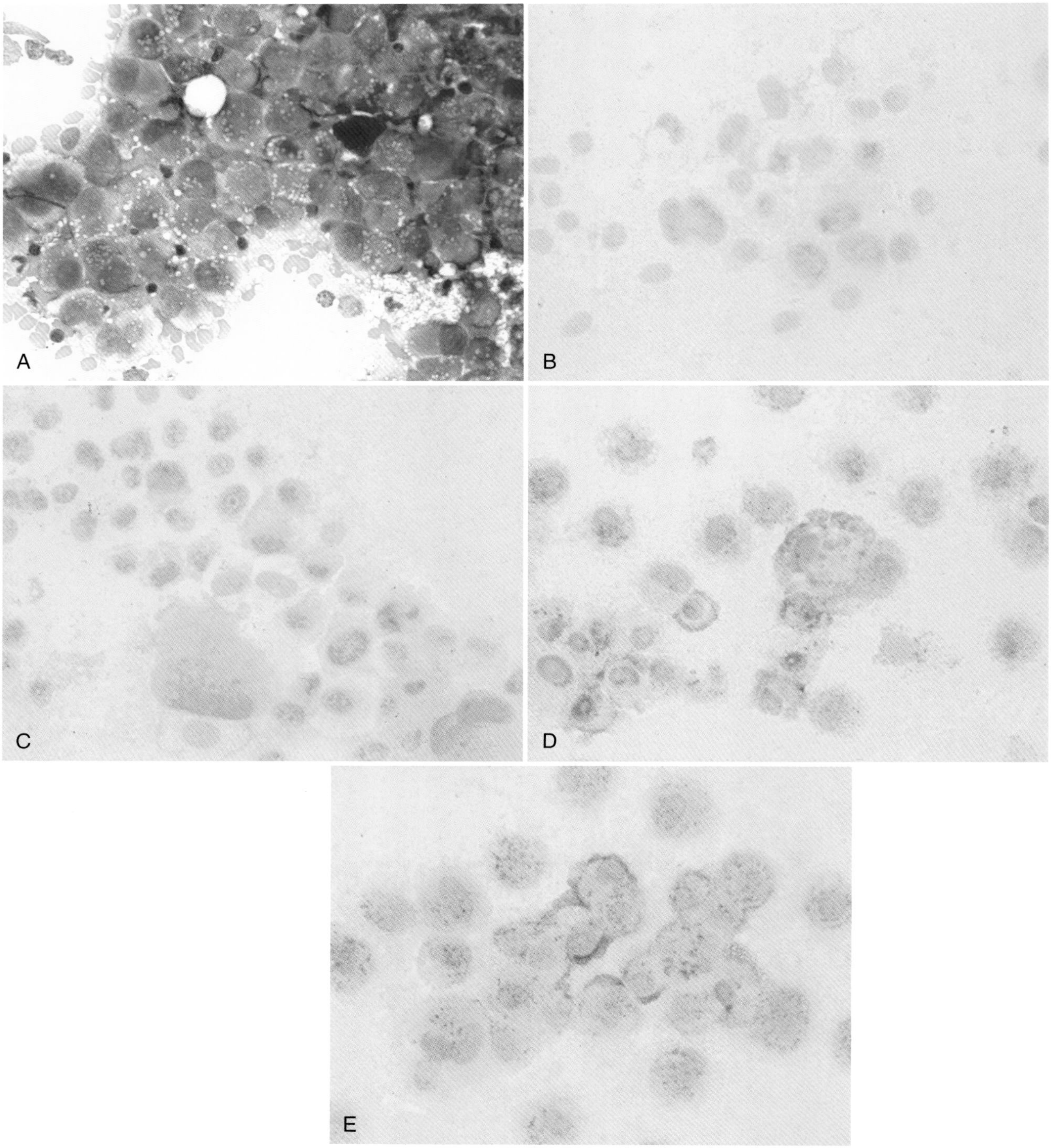

Figure 29-8 Lung mass from a dog, sample submitted in transport media, direct smears prepared. Population of neoplastic cells (*A*); cells vary from round to spindle with a moderate rim of cytoplasm. (Wright-Giemsa stain. Original magnification 500×.) Cells do not express CD3 (*B*) or CD79a (*C*) but do express CD18 (*D*) and vimentin (*E*). (Original magnification 500×.)

assist in tumor phenotyping. Cellularity of the sample and type of sample used greatly impact the quality of the results. Use of transport media allows for more standardization of the cellularity of the slides and the ability to produce multiple fairly uniform slides, which will allow for evaluation of a panel of antibodies rather than just one or two (Figure 29-8). Communication with the laboratory and pathologist providing and interpreting the ICC is critical for appropriate interpretation of the sample.

cases of B-cell lymphoma, and dogs with Burkitt-like B-cell lymphoma typically have a short survival time.[35,36] These types of lymphoma are relatively uncommon in dogs.[36-38] Evaluation of tissue architecture on a lymph node biopsy is necessary to diagnose these types of lymphoma. Breed predispositions to B-cell or T-cell lymphoid neoplasia have been identified, and examples include a predominance of T-cell disease in Boxers and B-cell disease in Cocker spaniels.[39,40]

Indications for Immunophenotyping in Lymphoma

Lymphoma in dogs is commonly diagnosed by FNA cytology when greater than 50% of the lymphocytes are immature and large.[41] FNA may also be performed to collect a sample for flow cytometry.[42] It is important to note that flow cytometry should be used as an adjunctive test after a cytologic or histologic diagnosis of lymphoma has been made to differentiate between T-cell and B-cell lymphoma.[43] Large cell multicentric lymphoma is the most common type of lymphoma in dogs, with small cell (low grade) lymphoma reported as 5% to 25% of cases in recent studies.[44] Small cell lymphoma is difficult to differentiate from lymphoid hyperplasia on the basis of cytology alone, and diagnosis and grading often requires histopathologic evaluation. Flow cytometry may be helpful in these cases to differentiate between a heterogeneous lymphoid population consistent with hyperplasia and a homogeneous lymphoid population with aberrant marker expression indicating lymphoid neoplasia.

Sample Information

Flow cytometry is most useful for homogeneous populations of lymphocytes.[43] Aspirates need to be placed in fluid (cell media or saline with added protein or patient serum) for transport, processing, and analysis by flow cytometry. Typically, two to three aspirates provide adequate numbers of cells for analysis.[45] Samples with low cellularity may not be diagnostic. It is also important to collect FNA cytology slides at the same time to ensure the neoplastic cell population is represented in the sample.[45] Occasionally, the neoplastic cells in the sample may be particularly fragile and lyse, leaving predominantly small lymphocytes from the residual normal lymphoid population of the node, and testing may be non-diagnostic. In patients with lymphoma, lymph nodes tend to exfoliate well for collection of samples for flow cytometry, but samples from the spleen, liver, intestinal masses, or cutaneous lesions may exfoliate poorly or be nondiagnostic because of cell disruption.[45]

Data Analysis

Differentiation between T-cell and B-cell lymphomas is based on gating of an intact cell population that corresponds to the neoplastic cells identified on cytology, and evaluation of the surface or cytoplasmic markers expressed by this population. A cutoff value of 60% T- or B-cells has been used to differentiate between T-cell or B-cell lymphoma, but in many reported cases, the percentage of cells expressing a single phenotype exceeds 80% of the population.[34] Figures 30-7, Figure 30-8, Figure 30-9, and Figure 30-10 provide examples of immunophenotyping results from canine lymphomas with corresponding cytology images.

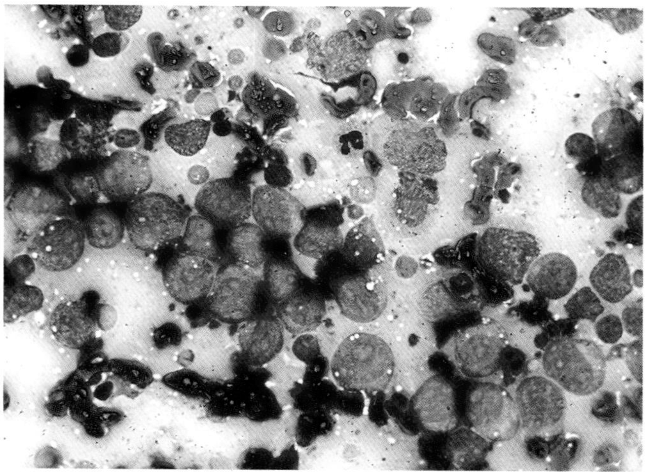

Figure 30-7 Lymph node aspirate (1000×) from an 8-year-old mixed breed dog. A homogeneous population of large lymphocytes is present, with finely stippled chromatin, multiple nucleoli, and deeply basophilic cytoplasm. Immunophenotyping findings are shown in Figure 30-8.

Aberrant Immunophenotypes in Lymphoma

Aberrant surface marker expression has been identified in cases of canine lymphomas and includes patterns not observed on normal or reactive lymphocytes or markers not commonly expressed by cells from the anatomic site that was sampled.[34,38] A few cases of canine B-cell lymphoma have been documented to express CD34 (which is typically expressed by stem cells associated with acute leukemia) in conjunction with CD21.[34,38] In a recent study, expression of CD34 in conjunction with CD21 did not affect prognosis.[46] However, decreased expression of class II major histocompatibility complex (MHC class II) in dogs with B-cell lymphoma was associated with a poorer prognosis.[46]

Implications for Therapy

In addition to providing prognostic information, immunophenotyping may help guide treatment decisions. A recent study reported that dogs with B-cell lymphoma have a significantly higher response rate to doxorubicin therapy compared with those with T-cell lymphoma.[47] Another study evaluating treatment of dogs with T-cell lymphoma found a greater response to L-asparaginase, mechloroethamine, vincristine, prednisone, and procarbazine (L-asp]/MOPP) than to cyclophosphamide, doxorubicin, vincristine, and prednisone (CHOP).[48] As immunophenotyping becomes more common in veterinary medicine, future studies will likely add to this body of knowledge, helping guide treatment for dogs with lymphoma.

IMMUNOPHENOTYPING OF LYMPHOMA IN CATS

In cats, immunophenotyping by flow cytometry is less commonly used than in dogs. The immunophenotype of lymphoma has not been strongly associated with prognosis as documented in dogs.[30,31] Lymphoma in cats often

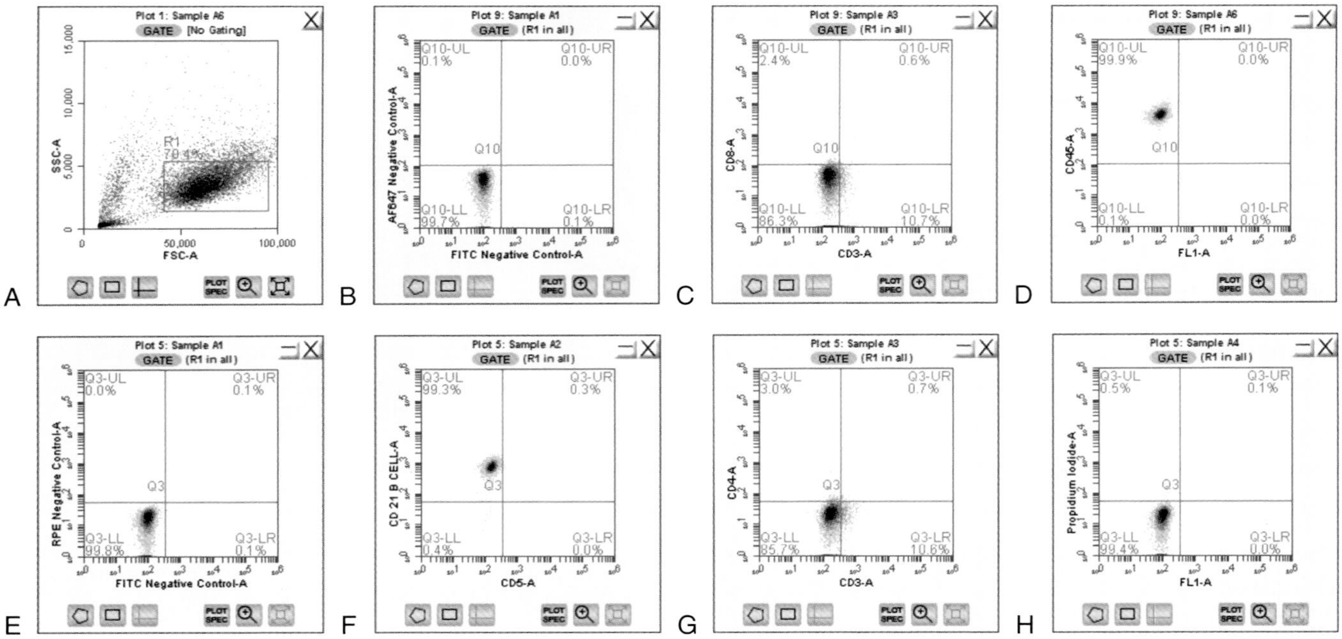

Figure 30-8 Immunophenotyping of lymph node aspirate with large cell B-cell lymphoma in a mixed breed dog (cytology shown in Figure 30-7). **A,** The cells of interest are gated on the forward versus side scatter plot. In this sample, most cells are large with similar light scatter properties. **B,** Negative isotype control for two fluorochromes, fluorescein isothiocyanate (FITC) and Alexa-Fluor 647 (AF647) to set a cutoff to eliminate nonspecific fluorescence. **C,** Expression of surface CD3 and CD8 is minimal. **D,** Positive expression of CD45 in 99.9% of the cells on the y-axis with no antibody added for the x-axis. **E,** Negative isotype control for two fluorochromes, FITC and *R-phycoerythrin* (RPE). **F,** Strong expression of CD21 in more than 99% of the cells indicating B-cell lineage, negative expression of CD5. **G,** Expression of surface CD3 and CD4 is minimal. **H,** Less than 1% of the cells in the gated population stain with propidium iodide and are not intact.

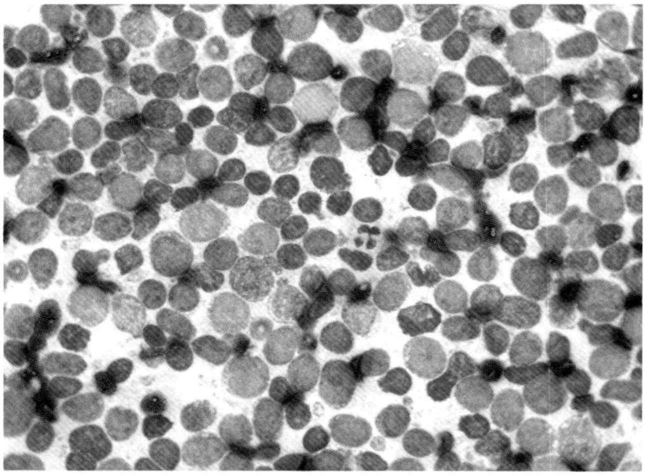

Figure 30-9 Lymph node aspirate (1000×) from a 6-year-old Boxer dog. Most of the lymphocytes are intermediate to large and have oval nuclei with fine to finely stippled chromatin and occasional indistinct nucleoli. See Figure 30-10 for immunophenotyping findings.

involves the alimentary tract or other internal organs that may be difficult to successfully sample for flow cytometry.[49] Lymphoma of large granular lymphocytes has been identified as a subtype of lymphoma with a poor prognosis in cats.[50] The immunophenotype of this disorder has been described, and these typically express CD3 and CD8, but neoplastic large granular lymphocytes are typically easily recognized on Wright-Giemsa–stained cytology slides and immunophenotyping is generally not necessary for diagnosis. The granules in these cells may dissolve with rapid aqueous stains such as Diff-Quik.

MEDIASTINAL MASS ASPIRATES

Immunophenotyping by flow cytometry may also be helpful in differentiating between lymphocyte rich thymomas and small cell thymic lymphoma. Thymic lymphocytes are T-cells that express both CD4 and CD8, whereas most T-cell lymphomas express only CD4, CD8, or neither marker. Identification of more than 10% small lymphocytes that coexpress CD4 and CD8 has been reported in dogs with thymoma.[51] As thymomas are typically treated with surgery or radiation and lymphoma is typically treated with chemotherapy, distinction between these two disorders may be useful. Correlation with the cytologic appearance on FNA is also important in these cases.

EVALUATION OF IMMUNE-MEDIATED HEMOLYTIC ANEMIA

The Coombs test is commonly used to support a diagnosis of immune-mediated hemolytic anemia (IMHA) in dogs.

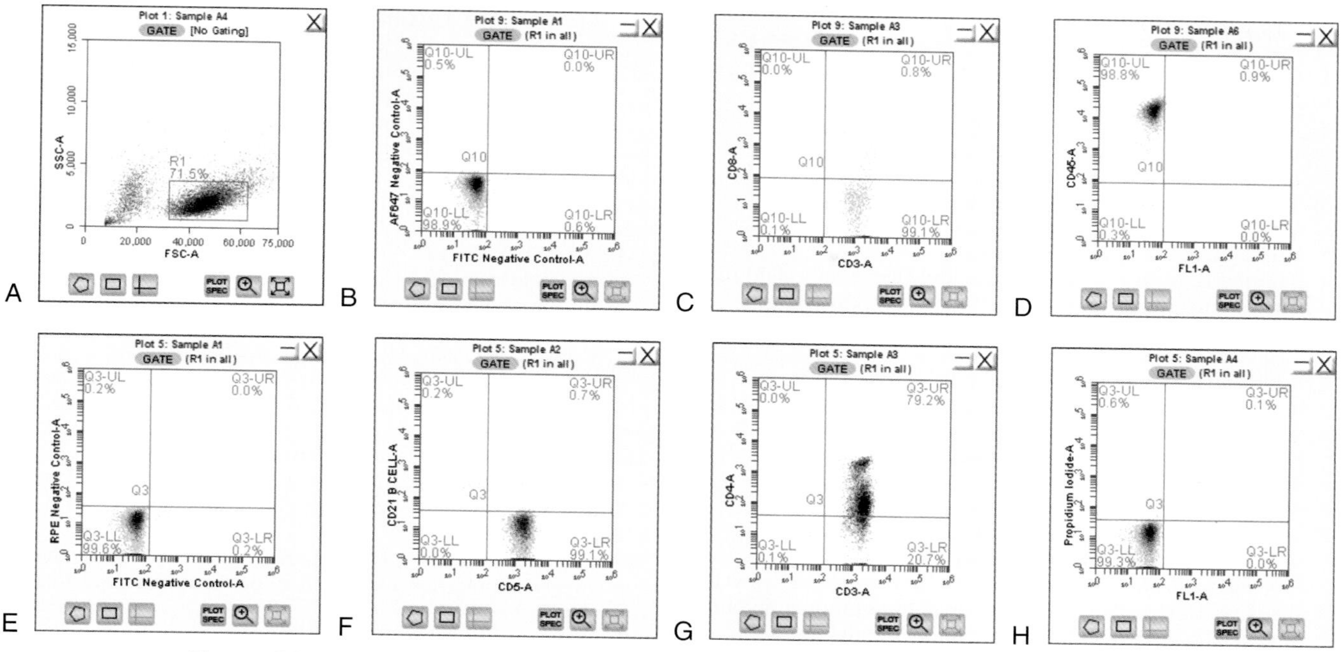

Figure 30-10 Immunophenotyping of a lymph node aspirate with helper T-cell lymphoma in a Boxer dog (same patient as Figure 30-9). **A,** The cells of interest are gated on the forward versus side scatter plot. In this sample, the cell population is homogeneous and most cells are intermediate to large in size (these have less forward scatter and are smaller than the B-cells in Figure 30-8). **B,** Negative isotype control for fluorescein isothiocyanate (FITC) and Alexa-Fluor 647 (AF647) to set cutoff to eliminate nonspecific fluorescence. **C,** More than 99% of the cells express CD3, but less than 1% express CD8. **D,** Positive expression of CD45 by more than 98% of the cells on the y-axis with no antibody added for the x-axis. **E,** Negative isotype control for two fluorochromes, FITC and *R-phycoerythrin* (RPE). **F,** More than 99% of the cells express CD5, but less than 1% are B-cells expressing CD21. **G,** The neoplastic cells co-express CD3 and CD4, indicating helper T-cell lineage. Many cells have dim CD4 expression and this is weaker than normal helper T-cells. **H,** Less than 1% of the cells in the gated population stain with propidium iodide and are not intact.

This test detects increased binding of immunoglobulin G (IgG), immunoglobulin M (IgM), complement, or all of these to RBCs in patients with IMHA, but the sensitivity of this test can be low.[52] Flow cytometry may be used to measure IgG, IgM, and complement (C3) bound to RBCs as well and has been shown to have greater sensitivity. In two studies, the sensitivity of the flow cytometric method was more than 90% compared with 53% to 58% for Coombs test, so this method may be helpful in patients with equivocal results on Coombs test.[53,54] Both Coombs test and flow cytometry assay are reportedly highly specific, but these studies did not evaluate anemic patients without IMHA to better determine the number of false positive results. Positive Coombs test results are occasionally seen in patients without evidence of hemolytic anemia, so correlation with the RBC parameters, morphology, and clinical findings is important.[52]

EVALUATION OF IMMUNE-MEDIATED THROMBOCYTOPENIA

A flow cytometric assay has been developed to measure IgG binding to platelets in dogs.[55] Increased platelet surface IgG is reported in approximately 70% to 80% of dogs with primary immune-mediated thrombocytopenia (IMT) but is also usually present in dogs with secondary IMT caused by infectious agents such as *Babesia gibsoni*, anaplasmosis, ehrlichiosis, leptospirosis, leishmaniasis; neoplasia (lymphoma and histiocytic sarcoma), drug-induced thrombocytopenia, and other inflammatory conditions.[56-58] Primary and secondary immune-mediated IMT are not differentiated by this assay. Nonspecific binding of IgG occurs over time, so blood samples should be analyzed within 24 hours of collection to prevent false positive results.[56,59]

CONCLUSION

Flow cytometry has been widely used in research in veterinary medicine for years, and assays with clinical utility to practicing veterinarians are becoming more widely available through university and private reference laboratories. In addition to its common application for obtaining reticulocyte counts and leukocyte differentials, flow cytometry may be used to immunophenotype lymphomas and leukemias, which provides important prognostic information and may help guide therapy. Flow cytometry may also be helpful to support a diagnosis of IMHA or ITP. Additional applications will likely develop from current research.

References

1. Craig FE, Foon KA: Flow cytometric immunophenotyping for hematologic neoplasms, *Blood* 111:3941, 2008.
2. Moritz A, Becker M: Automated hematology systems. In Weiss DJ, Waldrop KJ, editors: *Schalm's veterinary hematology*, ed 6, Ames, IA, 2010, Wiley-Blackwell.
3. Weiss DJ, Wilkerson MJ: Flow cytometry. In Weiss DJ, Waldrop KJ, editors: *Schalm's veterinary hematology*, ed 6, Ames, IA, 2010, Wiley-Blackwell.
4. Tvedten H, Moritz A: Reticulocyte and Heinz body staining and enumeration. In Weiss DJ, Waldrop KJ, editors: *Schalm's veterinary hematology*, ed 6, Ames, IA, 2010, Wiley-Blackwell.
5. Nguyen D, Diamond LW, Braylan RC: *Flow cytometry in hematopathology*, ed 2, Totowa, NJ, 2007, Humana Press.
6. Lana SE, Jackson TL, Burnett RC, et al: The utility of PCR for antigen receptor rearrangement (PARR) in staging and predicting prognosis in canine lymphoma, *Vet Comp Oncol* 3:40, 2005.
7. Avery A: Immunophenotyping and determination of clonality. In Weiss DJ, Waldrop KJ, editors: *Schalm's veterinary hematology*, ed 6, Ames, IA, 2010, Wiley-Blackwell.
8. Yagihara H, Uematsu Y, Koike A, et al: Immunophenotyping and gene rearrangement analysis in dogs with lymphoproliferative disorders characterized by small-cell lymphocytosis, *J Vet Diagn Invest* 21:197, 2009.
9. Avery A, Avery P: Determining the significance of persistent lymphocytosis, *Vet Clin North Am Small Anim Pract* 37:267, 2007.
10. Williams MJ, Avery AC, Lana SE, et al: Canine lymphoproliferative disease characterized by lymphocytosis: immunophenotypic markers of prognosis, *J Vet Intern Med* 22:596, 2008.
11. Comazzi S, Gelain ME, Martini F, et al: Immunophenotype predicts survival time in dogs with chronic lymphocytic leukemia, *J Vet Intern Med* 25:100, 2011.
12. Vernau W, Moore PF: An immunophenotypic study of canine leukemias and preliminary assessment of clonality by polymerase chain reaction, *Vet Immunol Immunopathol* 69:1454, 1999.
13. McDonough SP, Moore PF: Clinical, hematologic, and immunophenotypic characterization of canine large granular lymphocytosis, *Vet Pathol* 37:637, 2000.
14. Heeb HL, Wilkerson MJ, Chun R, et al: Large granular lymphocytosis, lymphocyte subset inversion, thrombocytopenia, dysproteinemia, and positive *Ehrlichia* serology in a dog, *J Am Anim Hosp Assoc* 39:379, 2003.
15. Gleich S, Hartmann K: Hematology and serum biochemistry of feline immunodeficiency virus-infected and feline leukemia virus-infected cats, *J Vet Intern Med* 23:552, 2009.
16. Reichard MV, Meinkoth JH, Edwards AC, et al: Transmission of *Cytauxzoon felis* to a domestic cat by *Amblyomma americanum*, *Vet Parasitol* 161:110, 2009.
17. Workman HC, Vernau W: Chronic lymphocytic leukemia in dogs and cats: the veterinary perspective, *Vet Clin North Am Small Anim Pract* 33:1379, 2003.
18. Campbell MW, Hess PR, Williams LE: Chronic lymphocytic leukaemia in the cat: 18 cases (2000-2010), *Vet Comp Oncol.* 2012 DOI:10.1111/j.1476-5829.2011.00315.x. Epub Feb 28.
19. Workman HC, Vernau W, Schmidt PS, et al: Chronic lymphocytic leukemia in cats is primarily a T helper cell disease. Abstract Presented at the 55th Annual Meeting of the American College of Veterinary Pathologists, Orlando, 2004.
20. Jain NC, Blue JT, Grindem CB, et al: Proposed criteria for classification of acute myeloid leukemia in dogs and cats, *Vet Clin Pathol* 20:63, 1991.
21. McManus PM: Classification of myeloid neoplasms: a comparative review, *Vet Clin Pathol* 34:189, 2005.
22. Tasca S, Carli E, Caldin M, et al: Hematologic abnormalities and flow cytometric immunophenotyping results in dogs with hematopoietic neoplasia: 210 cases (2002-2006), *Vet Clin Pathol* 38:2, 2009.
23. Usher SG, Radford AD, Villiers EJ, et al: RAS, FLT3, and C-KIT mutations in immunophenotyped canine leukemias, *Exp Hematol* 37:65, 2009.
24. Adam F, Villiers E, Watson S, et al: Clinical pathological and epidemiological assessment of morphologically and immunologically confirmed canine leukaemia, *Vet Comp Oncol* 7:181, 2009.
25. Comazzi S, Gelain ME, Bonfanti U, et al: Acute megakaryoblastic leukemia in dogs: a report of three cases and review of the literature, *J Am Anim Hosp Assoc* 46:327, 2010.
26. Willmann M, Müllauer L, Schwendenwein I, et al: Chemotherapy in canine acute megakaryoblastic leukemia: a case report and review of the literature, *In Vivo* 23:911, 2009.
27. Suter SE, Vernau W, Fry MM, et al: CD34+, CD41+ acute megakaryoblastic leukemia in a dog, *Vet Clin Pathol* 36:288, 2007.
28. Ameri M, Wilkerson MJ, Stockham SL, et al: Acute megakaryoblastic leukemia in a German Shepherd dog, *Vet Clin Pathol* 39:39, 2010.
29. Juopperi TA, Bienzle D, Bernreuter DC, et al: Prognostic markers for myeloid neoplasms: a comparative review of the literature and goals for future investigation, *Vet Pathol* 48:182, 2011.
30. Kisseberth WC, Helfand SC: General features of leukemia and lymphoma. In Weiss DJ, Waldrop KJ, editors: *Schalm's veterinary hematology*, ed 6, Ames, IA, 2010, Wiley-Blackwell.
31. Vail DM: Hematopoietic tumors. In Ettinger SJ, Feldman EC, editors: *Textbook of veterinary internal medicine*, ed 7, St. Louis, MO, 2010, Saunders.
32. Teske E, van Heerde P, Rutteman GR, et al: Prognostic factors for treatment of malignant lymphoma in dogs, *J Am Vet Med Assoc* 15:1722, 1994.
33. Kiupel M, Teske E, Bostock D: Prognostic factors for treated canine malignant lymphoma, *Vet Pathol* 36:292, 1999.
34. Wilkerson MJ, Dolce K, Koopman T, et al: Lineage differentiation of canine lymphoma/leukemias and aberrant expression of CD molecules, *Vet Immunol Immunopathol* 106:179, 2005.
35. Flood-Knapik KE, Durham AC, Gregor TP, et al: Clinical, histopathological and immunohistochemical characterization of canine indolent lymphoma, *Vet Comp Oncol.* 2012 DOI: 10.1111/j.1476-5829.2011.00317.x. Epub Feb 2.
36. Ponce F, Magnol JP, Ledieu D, et al: Prognostic significance of morphological subtypes in canine malignant lymphomas during chemotherapy, *Vet J* 167:158, 2004.
37. Sözmen M, Tasca S, Carli E, et al: Use of fine needle aspirates and flow cytometry for the diagnosis, classification, and immunophenotyping of canine lymphomas, *J Vet Diagn Invest* 17:323, 2005.
38. Gelain ME, Mazzilli M, Riondato F, et al: Aberrant phenotypes and quantitative antigen expression in different subtypes of canine lymphoma by flow cytometry, *Vet Immunol Immunopathol* 121:179, 2008.
39. Modiano JF, Breen M, Burnett RC, et al: Distinct B-cell and T-cell lymphoproliferative disease prevalence among dog breeds indicates heritable risk, *Cancer Res* 65:5654, 2005.
40. Lurie DM, Milner RJ, Suter SE, et al: Immunophenotypic and cytomorphologic subclassification of T-cell lymphoma in the boxer breed, *Vet Immunol Immunopathol* 125:102, 2008.

D

E

I

J

K